CHAPTER	TITLE*	PROCEDURE†	CASE STUDY‡
20	Toxoplasmosis	Rapid TORCH procedure	*CASE 20-1* A 24-year-old woman with a history of AIDS presented for evaluation of left-sided weakness. She had also been experiencing headaches and seizures, and others had observed an alteration in her mental status.
21	Cytomegalovirus	Passive latex agglutination for detection of antibodies to cytomegalovirus Quantitative determination of IgG antibodies to cytomegalovirus	*CASE 21-1* A 35-year-old man had recently been the recipient of a kidney transplant. He had been feeling well until 2 weeks ago, when he experienced a sore throat, fever, chills, profound malaise, and myalgia.
22	Infectious Mononucleosis	Paul-Bunnell screening test Davidsohn differential test MonoSlide test	*CASE 22-1* A female college freshman reported to the infirmary, complaining of extreme fatigue, frequent headaches, and a sore throat.
23	Viral Hepatitis	Rapid HCV test	*CASE 23-1* Several workers at a local fast food restaurant called in sick and reported to the local ambulatory clinic for treatment. They all complained of extreme fatigue. In addition, another 26-year-old food handler, who had returned from visiting his relatives in Costa Rica a month ago, was sick. *CASE 23-2* A 30-year-old phlebotomist presented with fever, persistent fatigue, and joint pain. She reported that a needle in a plastic garbage bag had nicked her finger about 2 months ago. *CASE 23-3* A 75-year-old white woman had an 18-month history of right-sided abdominal pain and progressive fatigue. Her other medical problems include insulin-dependent diabetes mellitus and hypertension. *CASE 23-4* A 45-year-old previously healthy medical technologist visited her primary care physician because of increasing fatigue and loss of appetite.
24	Rubella Infection	Passive latex agglutination test for rubella	*CASE 24-1* A 20-year-old college junior went to the student health office because she had been exposed to rubella during a recent outbreak at the college. She had been immunized as a child.
25	Acquired Immunodeficiency Syndrome	Rapid HIV antibody test	*CASE 25-1* A 40-year-old man with a history of IV drug use went to the emergency room because of a rash and fever. In addition, the patient complained of a several-day history of malaise, fatigue, fever, headache, and sore throat.
26	Hypersensitivity Reactions	Rapid test for food allergy Direct antiglobulin test	*CASE 26-1* A 60-year old man was stung by a bee while gardening. *CASE 26-2* A 35-year-old woman saw her gynecologist when she was 8 weeks pregnant. Her first pregnancy 4 years ago was unremarkable. The patient reported that her second and third pregnancies had resulted in a stillbirth at 36 weeks and a spontaneous abortion at 10 weeks of gestation. *CASE 26-3* A young man with a medical history including frequent sore throats as a child had been treated with antibiotics, particularly penicillin. Eventually, he developed a rash. He was told that he had developed an allergy to penicillin and should not have it again. *CASE 26-4* A 19-year-old college student went to the student health service because she had a slowly developing rash on both earlobes, hands and wrists, and around her neck. *CASE 26-5* A 35-year-old woman reported that she had experienced three bouts of urticaria of unknown origin about 10 years ago.
27	Immunoproliferative Disorders	Bence Jones protein screening procedure	*CASE 27-1* A 58-year-old nuclear power plant worker went to his physician because of increasing fatigue and weakness.
28	Autoimmune Disorders	Rapid slide test for antinucleoprotein Autoimmune enzyme immunoassay ANA screening test	*CASE 28-1* A 50-year-old white woman visited her primary care provider because of extreme fatigue. She also reported experiencing mild pain in her abdominal region. *CASE 28-2* A 25-year-old woman with no significant medical history came to the emergency department because of a sudden onset of slurred speech.
29	Systemic Lupus Erythematosus	Antinuclear antibody visible method Rapid slide test for antinucleoprotein Autoimmune enzyme immunoassay	*CASE 29-1* A 39-year-old African-American woman had been diagnosed with SLE 20 years ago. *CASE 29-2* A 27-year-old white woman sought medical attention because of persisting pain in her wrists and ankles and an unexplained skin irritation on her face.
30	Rheumatoid Arthritis	Rapid RA latex agglutination Quantitative determination of IgM rheumatoid factor in human serum	*CASE 30-1* A 62-year-old woman had been experiencing pain in her left knee unrelated to trauma. The pain occurred primarily with weight-bearing. She was currently being treated for hypertension, but was otherwise healthy. *CASE 30-2* A 31-year-old woman was referred to a rheumatologist with increasing pain and stiffness in her fingers and wrists. Before her last pregnancy 3 years earlier, she had experienced similar symptoms, but these had gone away. Since the birth of her last child, she had found it progressively more awkward to carry out a variety of tasks and hobbies, such as needlepoint.
31	Solid Organ Transplantation	MHC-HLA matching	*CASE 31-1* A 40-year-old woman had been seen by her family physician after several episodes of painless hematuria. On direct questioning, she complained of worsening malaise and swelling of her legs and hands over the previous 2 weeks. She also reported that despite a high fluid intake, she was urinating much less frequently than normal. She had no significant medical history.
32	Bone Marrow Transplantation	MHC-HLA matching	*CASE 32-1* An obese 46-year-old white woman with diabetes came to the emergency department with complaints of rectal bleeding and a feeling of significant fatigue.
33	Tumor Immunology	Rapid PSA screening	*CASE 33-1* A 59-year-old white man visited his primary care provider because of his need to urinate frequently and urgently. Over the last several years, his urine output had been in small volumes, with a decreasing flow rate. *CASE 33-2* A 65-year-old African-American woman visited her primary care provider for an annual examination, including a routine pelvic examination. Although she had gained some weight since her last examination, she reported that her general health was good, but that she had been experiencing some gastrointestinal problems over the last 6 weeks.

*Digital enrichment files for animated content, virtual labs, web-based videos, and additional chapter-specific online web resources are available on the Elsevier Evolve website for approved textbook adopters (instructors).

†The entire case study and associated questions are published in the respective chapters. A full discussion of the questions for each case study is posted on the Elsevier Evolve website for approved textbook adopters (instructors).

‡The principles and clinical applications of these procedures is explained in the textbook. Procedural protocols and other technical details are posted and explained on the Elsevier Evolve website for approved textbook adopters (instructors).

Immunology & Serology

in Laboratory Medicine

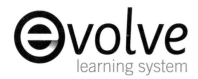
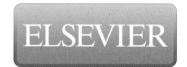
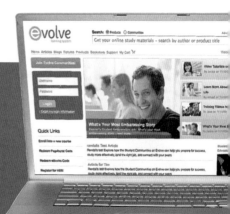

FIFTH EDITION

Immunology & Serology

in Laboratory Medicine

MARY LOUISE TURGEON, EdD, MLS(ASCP)CM

Clinical Laboratory Education Consultant
Mary L. Turgeon and Associates
Boston, Massachusetts; St. Petersburg, Florida

Adjunct Professor
Northeastern University
College of Professional Studies
Boston, Massachusetts

Adjunct Professor
South University
Physician Assistant Program
Tampa, Florida

Clinical Adjunct Assistant Professor
Tufts University
School of Medicine
Boston, Massachusetts

With 204 illustrations

ELSEVIER
MOSBY

3251 Riverport Lane
St. Louis, Missouri 63043

IMMUNOLOGY & SEROLOGY IN LABORATORY MEDICINE ISBN: 978-0-323-08518-2

Notices

Knowledge and best practice in this field are constantly changing. As new research and experience broaden our understanding, changes in research methods, professional practices, or medical treatment may become necessary.

Practitioners and researchers must always rely on their own experience and knowledge in evaluating and using any information, methods, compounds, or experiments described herein. In using such information or methods, they should be mindful of their own safety and the safety of others, including parties for whom they have a professional responsibility.

With respect to any drug or pharmaceutical products identified, readers are advised to check the most current information provided (i) on procedures featured or (ii) by the manufacturer of each product to be administered to verify the recommended dose or formula, the method and duration of administration, and contraindications. It is the responsibility of practitioners, relying on their own experience and knowledge of their patients, to make diagnoses, to determine dosages and the best treatment for each individual patient, and to take all appropriate safety precautions.

To the fullest extent of the law, neither the Publisher nor the authors, contributors, or editors assume any liability for any injury and/or damage to persons or property as a matter of products liability, negligence or otherwise, or from any use or operation of any methods, products, instructions, or ideas contained in the material herein.

Library of Congress Cataloging-in-Publication Data or Control Number
Turgeon, Mary Louise.
  Immunology & serology in laboratory medicine / Mary Louise Turgeon.–5th ed.
    p. ; cm.
  Immunology and serology in laboratory medicine
  Rev. ed. of: Immunology and serology in laboratory medicine / Mary Louise Turgeon. 4th ed. c2009.
  Includes bibliographical references and index.
  ISBN 978-0-323-08518-2 (hardcover : alk. paper)
  I. Turgeon, Mary Louise. Immunology and serology in laboratory medicine . II. Title. III. Title: Immunology and serology in laboratory medicine.
  [DNLM: 1. Immunologic Techniques–Laboratory Manuals. 2. Immune System Diseases–immunology–Laboratory Manuals. 3. Immune System Phenomena–Laboratory Manuals. 4. Serology–methods–Laboratory Manuals. QW 525]
  616.07′56–dc23
                                                                                                2012043280

Publishing Director: Andrew Allen
Content Manager: Ellen Wurm-Cutter
Publishing Services Manager: Catherine Jackson
Senior Project Manager: Rachel E. McMullen
Designer: Ashley Eberts

Printed in China

Last digit is the print number: 9 8 7 6 5 4 3 2 1

To the adventure of learning and exploring distant shores.

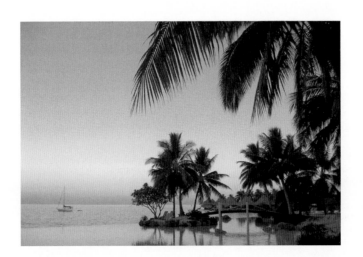

Cynthia R. Callahan, MEd, MT(ASCP)
Program Head
Medical Laboratory Technology
Stanly Community College
Locust, North Carolina

Jill Dennis, MEd, CLS
Chair of Math and Science
CLS Program Director
Thomas University
Thomasville, Georgia

Amy R. Kapanka, MS, MT(ASCP)SC
MLT Program Director
Hawkeye Community College
Waterloo, Iowa

Patricia Kelly, MT (AMT) (ASCP)BB
MLT Program Director
Mississippi Delta Community College
Moorhead, Mississippi

Marguerite E. Neita, PhD, MT(ASCP)
Chairperson and Program Director
Department of Clinical Laboratory Science
College of Nursing and Allied Health Sciences
Howard University
Washington, DC

Kyle Miller
Class of 2014
University of the South
Sewanee, Tennessee

The principles and practice of immunology and serology affect every aspect of the clinical laboratory. Immunology and serology have come to represent the bedrock of laboratory diagnostics by underlying principles or practical applications.

The intention of this fifth edition of *Immunology and Serology in Laboratory Medicine* is to continue to fulfill the needs of medical laboratory technician (MLT) and medical laboratory science (MLS) students and their instructors for an entry-level text that encompasses the most current theory, practice, and clinical applications in the fields of immunology and serology. This textbook is written specifically for students and practitioners in clinical laboratory science.

Content delivery is competency-based to provide the framework for theory and practice, with a strong emphasis on clinical applications. Critical thinking is essential and has a renewed emphasis in this edition, with many more clinical case studies. Every chapter has applicable cases with extensively developed presentations, case-related multiple-choice questions, and critical analysis group discussion questions. These cases not only promote critical thinking and stimulate an overall interest in medicine, but highlight the essential role of the laboratory in patient diagnosis and treatment.

The organization of the book allows for tremendous flexibility in instructional design and delivery. The book is well suited for traditional on-campus instruction, hybrid or blended modes of teaching, and online delivery of courses. A new category of content is the emphasis on Internet-delivered references to sites for virtual laboratories and for the enhancement of learning the content presented in the book.

Students in the digital age are becoming more visual learners. Extensive use is made of new and highly acclaimed illustrations originally published in the *New England Journal of Medicine,* as well as classic presentations from highly regarded immunology reference books. This adds a contemporary and exciting flair to a traditional college textbook. To accommodate student preference for visual presentation of information, the learning experience is enhanced with links to video animations and other digital resources in the textbook, on the Evolve website, and on the author's website. More tables and boxes have been added to chapters.

Each chapter has the principle and clinical application of at least one related procedure. In some cases, this provides the requisite information for a course. The procedural protocol, including specimen collection, the required materials, actual procedure, and expected reference results, are published on the Evolve websites for students and instructors who wish to select that laboratory exercise in their curriculum. Instructors can easily select procedures and create a customized laboratory manual that students can print, as needed. The benefits include reduction in the risk of soiling or contaminating their textbook in a wet laboratory. By reducing the number of pages devoted to laboratory procedures in the text, which may not be desired in a course, the planet gets a little greener with associated savings in the cost of production. Because the diversity in immunology and serology laboratory delivery ranges from a full semester of student laboratories to courses without any on-campus student laboratories, the new edition of this book is linked to a variety of virtual laboratories.

ORGANIZATION

The major topical areas are organized into four primary sections. The entire content of the book has been reviewed and updated with the newest technical and clinical information. Content of the book represents the basic knowledge required for certification examinations for MLT- and MLS-level graduates. Beyond basic knowledge and skills requirements, the text presents interdisciplinary topics and niche topics of transplantation and tumor immunology.

Parts I and II provide foundational knowledge and skills that progress from basic immunologic mechanisms and serologic concepts to the theory of laboratory procedures, including molecular techniques. Parts III and IV emphasize medical applications of importance to clinical laboratory science. In addition, they contain representative disorders of infectious and immunologic origin, as well as topics such as transplantation and tumor immunology. The sequence of the parts has been designed to accommodate the core needs of clinical laboratory students in basic concepts, the underlying theory of procedures, and immunologic manifestations of infectious diseases. Because the needs of some students are more advanced in immunopathology, these topics are presented later in the text to allow students to analyze, evaluate abnormalities, and exercise critical thinking skills based on their knowledge of the preceding parts. Students may study specific components of the text, depending on the level, length, and objectives of the course.

DISTINCTIVE FEATURES AND LEARNING AIDS

As an individually authored textbook, unlike edited books with multiple contributors, students gain the advantage of consistency in writing style and format from chapter to chapter. This fifth edition of *Immunology and Serology in Laboratory Medicine* capitalizes on the strengths of previous editions, beginning with the first edition in 1990.

To address the needs of new learners, key terms and expanded glossary are featured in this edition.
- Key words and a topical outline are presented at the beginning of each chapter. These outlines should be of value to students in the organization of the material and may be of convenience to instructors in preparing lectures.
- The latest illustrations, photographs, and summary tables are used to clarify various conceptual themes and information visually.
- Chapter highlights and review questions are provided at the conclusion of each chapter.
- Additional fully developed clinical case studies, with detailed answers to questions and more review questions, have been added to this edition.

To streamline this text, the principles and clinical applications of representative procedures appear in every chapter of the text. Complete procedural protocols, organized according to the format suggested by the Clinical Laboratory Standards Institute (CLSI), appear in the online Evolve website.

NEW TO THIS EDITION

What is significant that is new in this fifth edition? The knowledge base in the field of immunology and serology continues to expand logarithmically.

Every chapter has been reviewed and analyzed by clinical laboratory science students and instructors and has been updated, as needed. Each chapter has at least one relevant case study and reference to at least one related procedure. Suggestions for web-based videos and virtual laboratories have been compiled by chapter and presented on the Evolve site.

- In Part I, recent advances in medicine related to inflammation and T lymphocytes have been added, as well as representative procedures.
- Part II, "The Theory of Immunologic and Serologic Procedures," has been enhanced. Representative procedures have been added. The chapter on molecular diagnostics (see Chapter 14) continues to expand because of the increasing emphasis on this method of testing.
- In Part III, a unique chapter, Chapter 16, "A Primer on Vaccines," has been expanded as the importance of vaccines continues to become more evident. This chapter is unique and not available in competing textbooks. Representative case studies have been added to the chapters in this section.
- Part IV, "Immune Disorders," presents the latest information related to transplantation. In addition, information related to tumor immunology has been revised.

Although the content of immunology continues to expand, *Immunology and Serology in Laboratory Medicine* is written for clinical laboratory students in immunology who need an emphasis on the medical aspects of the discipline and the practical aspects of serology. The fifth edition should provide students with a basic foundation in the theory and practice of clinical immunology and practical serology in a one- or two-term course at MLT or MLS levels of instruction.

ANCILLARIES

For the Instructor

Evolve

The companion Evolve website offers several features to aid instructors:

- **Critical Analysis Group Discussion Questions:** Complete explanations are on the instructor's side of Evolve for the open-ended, case-related discussion questions.

- **Test Bank:** This is a test bank of more than 990 multiple choice questions that feature answers, explanations, and cognitive levels. The test bank can be used as review in class or for test development. More than 330 of the questions in the instructor test bank are available for student use.
- **PowerPoint Presentations:** One PowerPoint presentation is given per chapter; this feature can be used as is or as a template to prepare lectures.
- **Image Collection:** All the images from the book are available as *.jpg* files and can be downloaded into PowerPoint presentations. The figures can be used during lectures to illustrate important concepts.
- **Case Studies:** Case studies are provided for additional opportunities for student application of chapter content in real-life scenarios.
- **Procedures:** This feature presents the priniciples and application of procedures in every chapter.
- **Sample syllabi for MLT and MLS Students:** One- and two-semester courses are available.
- **Answers to Additional Review Questions:** Students have access to more than 330 questions that test their knowledge on the concepts presented in the text. The questions and answers are available to instructors.
- **Chapter-linked Digital Enrichment References:** References to videos, animations, and virtual laboratories are available.

For the Student

Evolve

The student resources on Evolve include the following:
- **Additional Review Questions:** A set of more than 330 multiple choice questions provides extra review and practice.

Mary L. Turgeon
Boston, Massachusetts
St. Petersburg, Florida
mary@mlturgeon.com

ACKNOWLEDGMENTS

Special thanks are given to the following student reviewers for their participation in the book review process:

Vicki Bickford
Class of 2012
Department of Medical Laboratory Science
University of North Dakota
Grand Forks, ND

Lucy Cole
Class of 2014
Medical Laboratory Technology Program
Diablo Valley College
Pleasant Hill, CA

Mariestell Dimalanta
Class of 2014
Medical Laboratory Technology Program
Diablo Valley College
Pleasant Hill, CA

Janel Flanary
Class of 2014
Medical Laboratory Technology Program
Diablo Valley College
Pleasant Hill, CA

Mark Gallardo
Class of 2014
Medical Laboratory Technology Program
Diablo Valley College
Pleasant Hill, CA

Andre Hall
Class of 2014
Medical Laboratory Technology Program
Diablo Valley College
Pleasant Hill, CA

Allison Harvey
Class of 2012
Department of Medical Laboratory Science
University of North Dakota
Grand Forks, ND

Boniphace Madoshi
Class of 2014
Medical Laboratory Technology Program
Diablo Valley College
Pleasant Hill, CA

Kim Nguyen
Department of Medical Laboratory Science
Wichita State University
Wichita, KS

Anthea Sabol
Class of 2013
Medical Laboratory Technology Program
Brevard Community College
Cocoa, FL

Meixin Tu
Class of 2014
Medical Laboratory Technology Program
Diablo Valley College
Pleasant Hill, CA

Thanks also to the following MLS faculty:

Jean Bricklee
Department of MLS
Wichita State University
Wichita, KS

Kathleen Faraday
Diablo Valley College
Pleasant Hill, CA

Karen Peterson
University of North Dakota
Grand Forks, ND

Mary Louise Turgeon, EdD, MLS(ASCP)^{CM} is an educator, author, and consultant in medical laboratory science education. Her career as an educator includes 15 years as a community college professor and program director and 14 years as an undergraduate and graduate university professor and administrator. She currently teaches online for the College of Professional Studies, Northeastern University, Boston, and is a graduate Physician Assistant Lecturer at South University, Tampa, Florida.

Dr. Turgeon is the author of medical laboratory science books (sold in more than 45 countries):

- *Immunology and Serology in Laboratory Medicine*, fifth edition (2014)
- *Linné & Ringsrud's Clinical Laboratory Science*, sixth edition (2012)
- *Clinical Hematology*, fifth edition (2012)
- *Fundamentals of Immunohematology*, second edition (1995)

Immunology and Serology in Laboratory Medicine has been translated into Italian and Chinese. *Clinical Hematology* has been translated into Spanish. Dr. Turgeon is the author of numerous professional journal articles.

The presentation of professional workshops and lectures complement the author's teaching and writing activities. Her consulting practice, Mary L. Turgeon and Associates (www.mlturgeon.com), focuses on new program development, curriculum revision, and increasing teaching effectiveness through the use of technology.

Dr. Turgeon's career in medical laboratory science has spanned the globe. Her professional involvement has offered her the opportunity to meet and collaborate with medical laboratory science colleagues in the United States and worldwide, including China, Italy, Japan, Qatar, Saudi Arabia, and the United Arab Emirates. Professional volunteer activities have taken her to Cambodia and Lesotho, Africa.

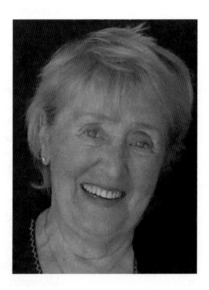

CONTENTS

Cell type	Principal function(s)
Lymphocytes: B lymphocytes; T lymphocytes; natural killer cells 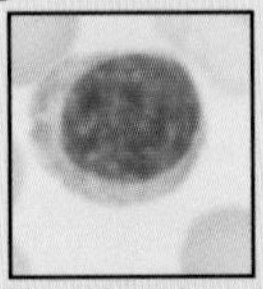 *Blood lymphocyte*	Specific recognition of antigens: B lymphocytes: mediators of humoral immunity T lymphocytes: mediators of cell-mediated immunity Natural killer cells: cells of innate immunity
Antigen-presenting cells: dendritic cells; macrophages; follicular dendritic cells 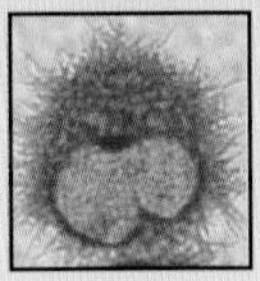 *Dendritic cell* 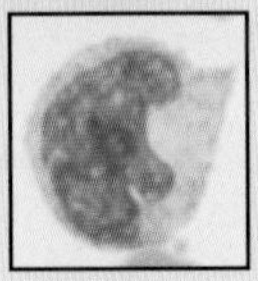 *Blood monocyte*	Capture of antigens for display to lymphocytes: Dendritic cells: initiation of T cell responses Macrophages: initiation and effector phase of cell-mediated immunity Follicular dendritic cells: display of antigens to B lymphocytes in humoral immune responses
Effector cells: T lymphocytes; macrophages; granulocytes 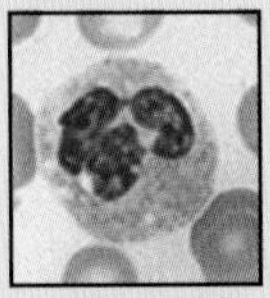 *Neutrophil*	Elimination of antigens: T lymphocytes: helper T cells and cytotoxic T lymphocytes Macrophages and monocytes: cells of the mononuclear-phagocyte system Granulocytes: neutrophils, eosinophils

Color Plate 1   **The Principal Cells of the Immune System.** The major cell types involved in immune responses, and their functions, are shown. Micrographs in the left panels illustrate the morphology of some of the cells of each type. Note that tissue macrophages are derived from blood monocytes. *(From Abbas AK, Lichtman AH: Basic immunology: functions and disorders of the immune system, updated edition, ed 3, Philadelphia, 2011, Saunders.)*

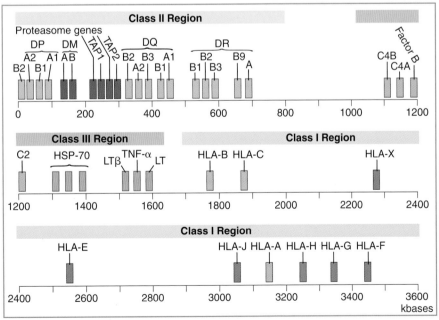

Color Plate 2   Human major histocompatibility complex. *(From Abbas AK et al: Cellular and molecular immunology, ed 7, Philadelphia, 2012, Saunders.)*

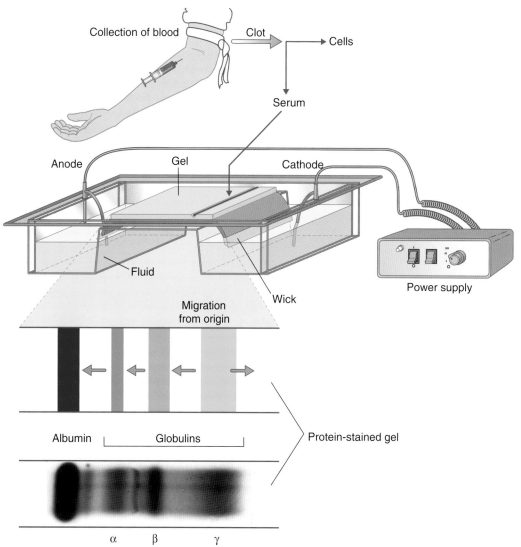

Color Plate 3 Separation of serum proteins by electrophoresis. *(Adapted from Peakman M, Vergani D: Basic and clinical immunology, St. Louis, 2009, Elsevier.)*

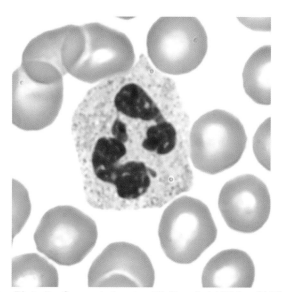

Color Plate 4 Segmented neutrophil. *(From Rodak BF, Carr JH: Clinical hematology atlas, ed 4, St Louis, 2013, Saunders.)*

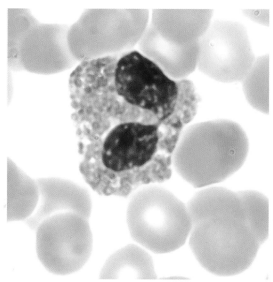

Color Plate 5 Eosinophil. *(From Rodak BF, Carr JH: Clinical hematology atlas, ed 4, St Louis, 2013, Saunders.)*

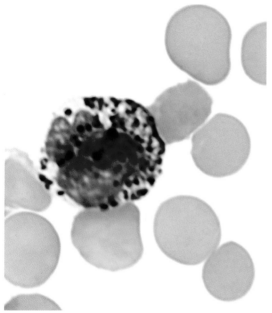

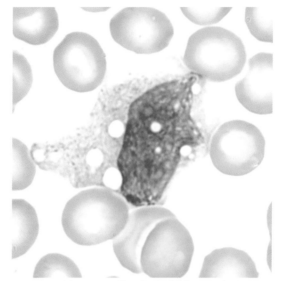

Color Plate 7 Monocyte. *(From Rodak BF, Carr JH: Clinical hematology atlas, ed 4, St Louis, 2013, Saunders.)*

Color Plate 6 Basophil. *(From Rodak BF, Carr JH: Clinical hematology atlas, ed 4, St Louis, 2013, Saunders.)*

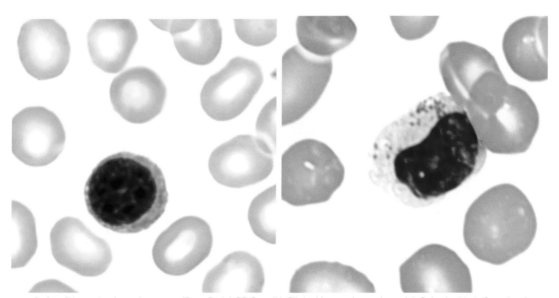

Color Plate 8 Lymphocytes. *(From Rodak BF, Carr JH: Clinical hematology atlas, ed 4, St Louis, 2013, Saunders.)*

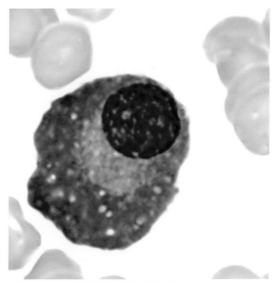

Color Plate 9 Plasma Cell. *(From Rodak BF, Carr JH: Clinical hematology atlas, ed 4, St Louis, 2013, Saunders.)*

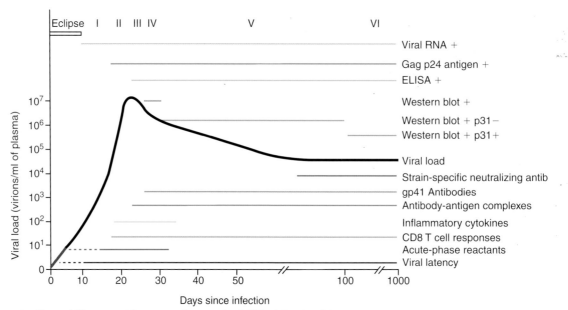

Color Plate 10   Natural History and Immunopathogenesis of HIV-1 Infection. The progression of HIV-1 infection can be depicted as six discrete stages (indicated by Roman numerals). These stages are defined according to the results of standard clinical laboratory tests (listed above the curve for viral load). The stages are based on the sequential appearance in plasma of HIV-1 viral RNA; the gag p24 protein antigen; antibodies specific for recombinant HIV-1 proteins, detected with the use of an enzyme-linked immunosorbent assay (ELISA); and antibodies that bind to fixed viral proteins, including p31, detected on Western immunoblot. A plus sign indicates a positive test result, a minus sign a negative result, and a plus–minus sign a borderline-positive result. The lines below the viral-load curve show the timing of key events and immune responses that cannot be measured with standard clinical laboratory assays, beginning with the establishment of viral latency. Acute-phase reactants include elevated levels of serum amyloid protein A. CD8 T-cell responses lead to the appearance of escape mutants concurrently with inflammatory cytokines in plasma. Immune complexes of antibodies with viral proteins, such as the HIV-1 envelope glycoprotein (gp41), precede the first appearance of free antibodies to gp41. Strain-specific antibodies to gp41 that neutralize the virus do not appear until sometime close to day 80. The portion of the line for viral latency that is dotted reflects uncertainty as to exactly when latency is first established; the dotted line for acute-phase reactants indicates that not all patients have elevated levels of reactants at this early point in the process of infection; the gray segment of the black line for viral load reflects the inability to measure very low viral loads. *(From Cohen MS, Shaw GM, McMichael AJ, et al: N Engl J Med 2011; 364:1943-1954, May 19, 2011.)*

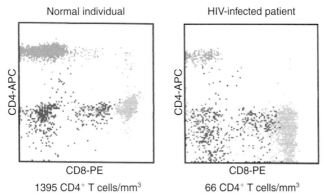

Color Plate 11   Flow Cytometry HIV Patient. *(From Abbas AK, Lichtman AH: Basic immunology: functions and disorders of the immune system, updated edition, ed 3, Philadelphia, 2011, Saunders.)*

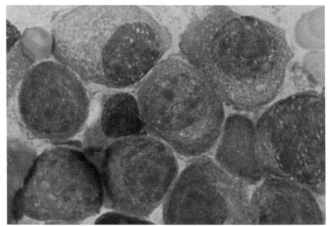

Color Plate 12   Bone Marrow Myeloma. *(From Nairn R, Helbert M: Immunology for medical students, ed 2, St Louis, 2007, Mosby.)*

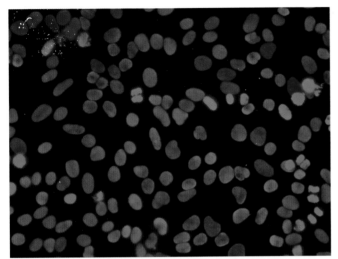

Color Plate 13 Antinuclear Antibody (ANA). *Homogeneous* or *Diffused:* A solid staining of the nucleus with or without apparent masking of the nucleoli. **Nuclear antigens present:** dsDNA, nDNA, DNP histone. **Disease association:** High titers are suggestive of systemic lupus erythematosus (SLE); lower titers are suggestive of SLE or other connective tissue diseases. *(Courtesy INOVA Diagnostics, Inc, San Diego, Calif.)*

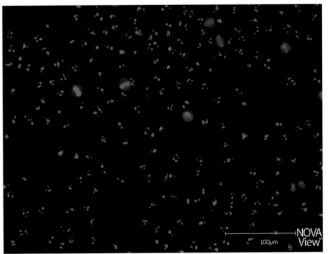

Color Plate 15 Antinuclear Antibody (ANA). *Nucleolar.* *(Courtesy INOVA Diagnostics, Inc, San Diego, Calif.)*

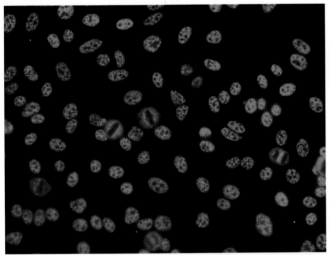

Color Plate 14 Antinuclear Antibody (ANA). *Coarse Speckled.* *(Courtesy INOVA Diagnostics, Inc, San Diego, Calif.)*

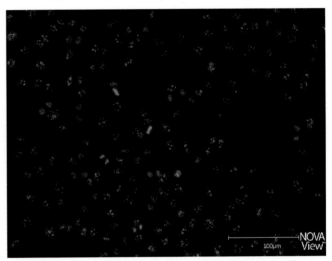

Color Plate 16 Antinuclear Antibody (ANA). *Centromere.* *(Courtesy INOVA Diagnostics, Inc, San Diego, Calif.)*

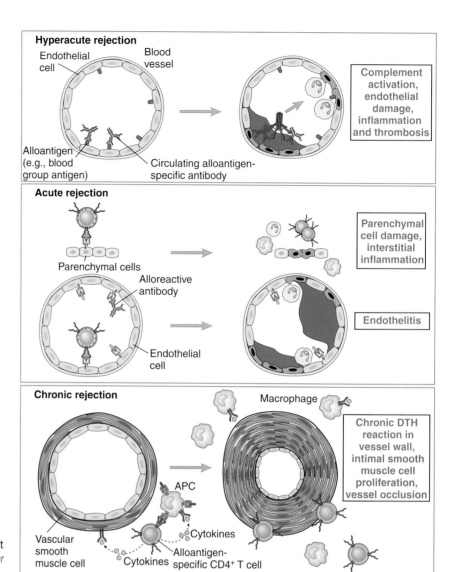

Color Plate 17 Immune mechanism of graft rejection. *(From Abbas AK et al: Cellular and molecular immunology, ed 7, Philadelphia, 2012, Saunders.)*

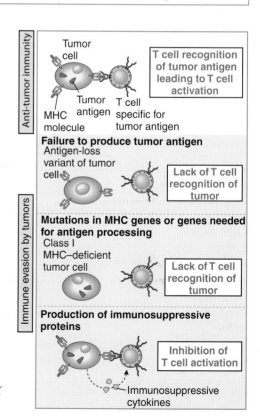

Color Plate 18 Mechanisms by which tumors escape immune defenses. *(From Abbas AK et al: Cellular and molecular immunology, ed 7, Philadelphia, 2012, Saunders.)*

PART I

Basic Immunologic Mechanisms

CHAPTER 1

An Overview of Immunology

Learning Objectives

At the conclusion of this chapter, the reader should be able to:

- Compare an immunogen and an antigen
- Define the term *immunology*.
- Explain the functions of the immune system.
- Describe the first, second, and third lines of body defense against microbial diseases.
- Compare innate and adaptive immunity.
- Analyze a case study related to immunity.

- Correctly answer case study related multiple choice questions.
- Be prepared to participate in a discussion of critical thinking questions.
- Describe the characteristics of five mature leukocytes and their immune function.
- Correctly answer end of chapter review questions.

Key Terms

acquired immunity
active immunity
adaptive immune system
allografts
antibodies
antigen
autoimmune disorder
cell-mediated immunity
complement
cytokines
endogenous

exogenous
genome
hematopoietic cells
humoral-mediated immunity
immunocompetent
immunoglobulins
immunology
inflammation
innate immune system
innate resistance
interleukins

major histocompatibility complex (MHC)
mononuclear phagocyte system
nonself
passive immunity
pathogen-associated molecular patterns (PAMPs)
pattern recognition receptors (PRRs)
phagocytosis
vaccination

HISTORY OF IMMUNOLOGY

The science of immunology arose from the knowledge that those who survived one of the common infectious diseases of the past rarely contracted the disease again. As early as 430 BC, during the plague in Athens, Thucydides recorded that individuals who had previously contracted the disease recovered and he recognized their "immune" status.

Beginning about 1000 AD, the Chinese practiced a form of immunization by inhaling dried powders derived from the crusts of smallpox lesions. In the 15th century, powdered smallpox "crusts" were inserted with a pin into the skin. When this practice became popular in England, it was discouraged at first, partly because the practice of inoculation occasionally killed or disfigured a patient.

Louis Pasteur is generally considered to be the Father of Immunology. Table 1-1 lists some historic benchmarks in immunology.

WHAT IS IMMUNOLOGY?

Immunology is defined as resistance to disease, specifically infectious disease. Immunology consists of the following: the study of the molecules, cells, organs, and systems responsible for the recognition and disposal of foreign **(nonself)** material; how body components respond and interact; the desirable and undesirable consequences of immune interactions; and the ways in which the immune system can be advantageously manipulated to protect against or treat disease (Box 1-1). Immunologists in the Western Hemisphere generally exclude from the study of immunology the relationship among cells during embryonic development.

The immune system is composed of a large complex set of widely distributed elements, with distinctive characteristics. Specificity and memory are characteristics of lymphocytes (see Chapter 4). Various specific and nonspecific elements of the immune system demonstrate mobility, including T and B lymphocytes, **immunoglobulins** (antibodies), complement, and **hematopoietic cells.**

CELLS OF THE IMMUNE SYSTEM

Cooperation is required for optimal functioning of the immune system. This cooperative interaction involves specific cellular elements, cell products, and nonlymphoid elements.

Cells of the immune system consist of lymphocytes, specialized cells that capture and display microbial antigen, and effector cells that eliminate microbes (see Color Plate 1). The principal functions of the major cell types involved in the immune response are as follows:

Box 1-1	Role of the Immune System
Defending the body against infections Recognizing and responding to foreign antigens Defending the body against the development of tumors	

Table 1-1	Significant Milestones in Immunology	
Date	**Scientist(s)**	**Discovery**
1798	Jenner	Smallpox vaccination
1862	Haeckel	Phagocytosis
1880-1881	Pasteur	Live, attenuated chicken cholera and anthrax vaccines
1883-1905	Metchnikoff	Cellular theory of immunity through phagocytosis
1885	Pasteur	Therapeutic vaccination First report of live "attenuated" vaccine for rabies
1890	Von Behring, Kitasata	Humoral theory of immunity proposed
1891	Koch	Demonstration of cutaneous (delayed-type) hypersensitivity
1900	Ehrlich	Antibody formation theory
1902	Portier, Richet	Immediate-hypersensitivity anaphylaxis
1903	Arthus	Arthus reaction of intermediate hypersensitivity
1938	Marrack	Hypothesis of antigen-antibody binding
1944		Hypothesis of allograft rejection
1949	Salk, Sabin	Development of polio vaccine
1951	Reed	Vaccine against yellow fever
1953		Graft-versus-host reaction
1957	Burnet	Clonal selection theory
1957		Interferon
1958-1962		Human leukocyte antigens (HLAs)
1964-1968		T-cell and B-cell cooperation in immune response
1972		Identification of antibody molecule
1975	Köhler	First monoclonal antibodies
1985-1987		Identification of genes for T cell receptor
1986		Monoclonal hepatitis B vaccine
1986	Mosmann	Th1 versus Th2 model of T helper cell function
1996-1998		Identification of toll-like receptors
2001		FOXP3, the gene directing regulatory T cell development
2005	Frazer	Development of human papillomavirus vaccine

- Specific recognition of antigens
- Capture of antigens for display to lymphocytes
- Elimination of antigens

FUNCTION OF IMMUNOLOGY

The function of the immune system is to recognize self from nonself and to defend the body against nonself. Such a system is necessary for survival. The distinction of self from nonself is made by an elaborate, specific recognition system. Specific cellular elements of the immune system include the lymphocytes. The immune system also has nonspecific effector mechanisms that usually amplify the specific functions. Nonspecific components of the immune system include mononuclear phagocytes, polymorphonuclear leukocytes, and soluble factors (e.g., complement).

Nonself substances range from life-threatening infectious microorganisms to a lifesaving organ transplantation. The desirable consequences of immunity include natural resistance, recovery, and acquired resistance to infectious diseases. A deficiency or dysfunction of the immune system can cause many disorders.

Undesirable consequences of immunity include allergy, rejection of a transplanted organ, or an **autoimmune disorder**, in which the body's own tissues are attacked as if they were foreign. Over the last decade, a new concept, the danger theory, has challenged the classic self-nonself viewpoint; although popular, it has not been widely accepted by immunologists (see Chapter 4).

BODY DEFENSES: RESISTANCE TO MICROBIAL DISEASE

First Line of Defense

Before a pathogen can invade the human body, it must overcome the resistance provided by the body's first line of defense (Fig. 1-1). The first barrier to infection is unbroken skin and mucosal membrane surfaces. These surfaces are essential in forming a physical barrier to many microorganisms because this is where foreign materials usually first contact the host. Keratinization of the upper layer of the skin and the constant renewal of the skin's epithelial cells, which repairs breaks in the skin, assist in the protective function of skin and mucosal membranes. In addition, the normal flora (microorganisms

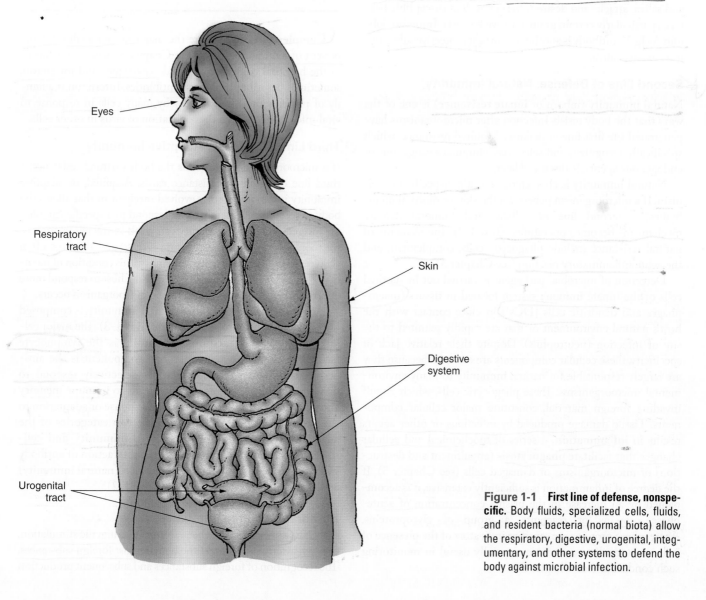

Figure 1-1 First line of defense, nonspecific. Body fluids, specialized cells, fluids, and resident bacteria (normal biota) allow the respiratory, digestive, urogenital, integumentary, and other systems to defend the body against microbial infection.

normally inhabiting the skin and membranes) deter penetration or facilitate elimination of foreign microorganisms from the body.

Secretions are also an important component in the first line of defense against microbial invasion. Mucus adhering to the membranes of the nose and nasopharynx traps microorganisms, which can be expelled by coughing or sneezing. Sebum (oil) produced by the sebaceous glands of the skin and lactic acid in sweat both possess antimicrobial properties. The production of earwax (cerumen) protects the auditory canals from infectious disease. Secretions produced in the elimination of liquid and solid wastes (e.g., urinary and gastrointestinal processes) are important in physically removing potential pathogens from the body. The acidity and alkalinity of the fluids of the stomach and intestinal tract, as well as the acidity of the vagina, can destroy many potentially infectious microorganisms. Additional protection is provided to the respiratory tract by the constant motion of the cilia of the tubules.

In addition to the physical ability to wash away potential pathogens, tears and saliva also have chemical properties that defend the body. The enzyme lysozyme, which is found in tears and saliva, attacks and destroys the cell wall of susceptible bacteria, particularly certain gram-positive bacteria. Immunoglobulin A (IgA) antibody is another important protective substance in tears and saliva.

Second Line of Defense: Natural Immunity

Natural immunity (inborn or **innate resistance**) is one of the ways that the body resists infection after microorganisms have penetrated the first line of defense. Acquired resistance, which specifically recognizes and selectively eliminates exogenous or endogenous agents, is discussed later.

Natural immunity is characterized as a nonspecific mechanism. If a microorganism penetrates the skin or mucosal membranes, a second line of cellular and humoral defense mechanisms becomes operational (Box 1-2). The elements of natural resistance include phagocytic cells, complement, and the acute inflammatory reaction (see Chapter 3).

Detection of microbial pathogens is carried out by sentinel cells of the innate immune system located in tissues (macrophages and dendritic cells [DCs]) in close contact with the host's natural environment or that are rapidly reunited to the site of infection (neutrophils). Despite their relative lack of specificity, these cellular components are essential because they are largely responsible for natural immunity to many environmental microorganisms. These phagocytic cells, which engulf invading foreign material, constitute major cellular components. Tissue damage produced by infectious or other agents results in **inflammation**, a series of biochemical and cellular changes that facilitate **phagocytosis** (engulfment and destruction) of microorganisms or damaged cells (see Chapter 3). If the degree of inflammation is sufficiently extensive, it is accompanied by an increase in the plasma concentration of acute-phase proteins or reactants, a group of glycoproteins. Acute-phase proteins are sensitive indicators of the presence of inflammatory disease and are especially useful in monitoring such conditions (see Chapter 5).

Box 1-2   Components of the Natural Immune System: The Second Line of Defense

Cellular
Mast cells
Neutrophils
Macrophages

Humoral
Complement
Lysozyme
Interferon

Box 1-3   Components of the Adaptive Immune System

Cellular
T lymphocytes
B lymphocytes
Plasma cells

Humoral
Antibodies
Cytokines

Complement proteins are the major humoral (fluid) component of natural immunity (see Chapter 5). Other substances of the humoral component include lysozymes and interferon, sometimes described as natural antibiotics. Interferon is a family of proteins produced rapidly by many cells in response to viral infection; it blocks the replication of virus in other cells.

Third Line of Defense: Adaptive Immunity

If a microorganism overwhelms the body's natural resistance, a third line of defensive resistance exists. Acquired, or adaptive, immunity is a more recently evolved mechanism that allows the body to recognize, remember, and respond to a specific stimulus, an antigen. Adaptive immunity can result in the elimination of microorganisms and recovery from disease and the host often acquires a specific immunologic memory. This condition of memory or recall (acquired resistance) allows the host to respond more effectively if reinfection with the same microorganism occurs.

Adaptive immunity, as with natural immunity, is composed of cellular and humoral components (Box 1-3). The major cellular component of **acquired immunity** is the lymphocyte (see Chapter 4); the major humoral component is the antibody (see Chapter 2). Lymphocytes selectively respond to nonself materials (antigens), which leads to immune memory and a permanently altered pattern of response or adaptation to the environment. Most actions in the two categories of the adaptive response, **humoral-mediated immunity** and **cell-mediated immunity**, are exerted by the interaction of antibody with complement and the phagocytic cells (natural immunity) and of T cells with macrophages (Table 1-2).

Humoral-Mediated Immunity

If specific antibodies have been formed to antigenic stimulation, they are available to protect the body against foreign substances. The recognition of foreign substances and subsequent production

Table 1-2	Characteristics of Two Types of Adaptive Immunity	
	Humoral-Mediated Immunity	**Cell-Mediated Immunity**
Mechanism	Antibody mediated	Cell mediated
Cell type	B lymphocytes	T lymphocytes
Mode of action	Antibodies in serum	Direct cell-to-cell contact or soluble products secreted by cells
Purpose	Primary defense against bacterial infection	Defense against viral and fungal infections, intracellular organisms, tumor antigens, and graft rejection

of antibodies to these substances define immunity. Antibody-mediated immunity to infection can be acquired if the antibodies are formed by the host or if they are received from another source; these two types of acquired immunity are called active immunity and passive immunity, respectively (Table 1-3).

Active immunity can be acquired by natural exposure in response to an infection or natural series of infections, or through intentional injection of an antigen. The latter, **vaccination** (see Chapter 16), is an effective method of stimulating antibody production and memory (acquired resistance) without contracting the disease. Suspensions of antigenic materials used for immunization may be of animal or plant origin. These products may consist of living suspensions of weak or attenuated cells or viruses, killed cells or viruses, or extracted bacterial products (e.g., altered and no longer poisonous toxoids used to immunize against diphtheria and tetanus). The selected agents should stimulate the production of antibodies without clinical signs and symptoms of disease in an **immunocompetent** host (host is able to recognize a foreign antigen and build specific antigen-directed antibodies) and result in permanent antigenic memory. Booster vaccinations may be needed in some cases to expand the pool of memory cells. The mechanisms of antigen recognition and antibody production are discussed in Chapter 2.

Artificial **passive immunity** is achieved by the infusion of serum or plasma containing high concentrations of antibody or lymphocytes from an actively immunized individual. Passive immunity via pre-formed antibodies in serum provides immediate, temporary antibody protection against microorganisms (e.g., hepatitis A) by administering preformed antibodies. The recipient will benefit only temporarily from passive immunity for as long as the antibodies persist in the circulation. Immune antibodies are usually of the IgG type (see Chapter 2, Antigens and Antibodies) with a half-life of 23 days.*

The main strategies for cancer immunotherapy aim to provide antitumor effectors (T lymphocytes and antibodies) to

patients. The purpose is to immunize patients actively against their own tumors and to stimulate the patient's own antitumor immune responses.

In addition, passive immunity can be acquired naturally by the fetus through the transfer of antibodies by the maternal placental circulation in utero during the last 3 months of pregnancy (Fig. 1-2). Maternal antibodies are also transferred to the newborn after birth. The amount and specificity of maternal antibodies depend on the mother's immune status to infectious diseases that she has experienced.

Passively acquired immunity in newborns is only temporary because it starts to decrease after the first several weeks or months after birth. Breast milk, especially the thick yellowish milk (colostrum) produced for a few days after the birth of a baby is very rich in antibodies. However, for a newborn to have lasting protection, active immunity must occur.

Cell-Mediated Immunity

Cell-mediated immunity consists of immune activities that differ from antibody-mediated immunity. Lymphocytes are the unique bearers of immunologic specificity, which depends on their antigen receptors. The full development and expression of immune responses, however, require that nonlymphoid cells and molecules primarily act as amplifiers and modifiers.

Cell-mediated immunity is moderated by the link between T lymphocytes and phagocytic cells (i.e., monocytes-macrophages). A B lymphocyte can probably respond to a native antigenic determinant of the appropriate fit. A T lymphocyte responds to antigens presented by other cells in the context of **major histocompatibility complex (MHC)** proteins (see Chapter 31). The T lymphocyte does not directly recognize the antigens of microorganisms or other living cells, such as **allografts** (tissue from a genetically different member of the same species, such as a human kidney), but recognizes when the antigen is present on the surface of an antigen-presenting cell (APC), the macrophage. APCs were at first thought to be limited to cells of the **mononuclear phagocyte system.** Recently, other types of cells (e.g., endothelial, glial) have been shown to possess the ability to present antigens.

Lymphocytes are immunologically active through various types of direct cell-to-cell contact and by the production of soluble factors (see Chapter 5). Nonspecific soluble factors are made by or act on various elements of the immune system. These molecules are collectively called **cytokines.** Some mediators that act between leukocytes are called **interleukins.**

Under some conditions, the activities of cell-mediated immunity may not be beneficial. Suppression of the normal adaptive immune response by drugs or other means is necessary in conditions or procedures such as organ transplantation, hypersensitivity, and autoimmune disorders.

COMPARISON OF INNATE AND ADAPTIVE IMMUNITY

Traditionally, the immune system has been divided into innate and adaptive components, each with a different function and role. The **innate immune system,** an ancient form of host

*Antibody half-life is a measure of the mean survival time of antibody molecules following their formation. It is usually expressed as the time required to eliminate 50% of a known quantity of immunoglobulin from the body. Half-life varies from one immunoglobulin class to another.

Table 1-3	Comparison of Types of Acquired Immunity			
	Type	Mode of Acquisition	Antibody Produced by Host	Duration of Immune Response
Active	Natural	Infection	Yes	Long[*],[†]
	Artificial	Vaccination	Yes	Long[*],[†]
Passive	Natural	Transfer in vivo or colostrum	No	Short
	Artificial	Infusion of serum/plasma	No	Short

[*]Immunocompetent host.
[†]IgG immune antibody half-life is 23 days. Memory cells (memory lymphocytes) lifespan is years.

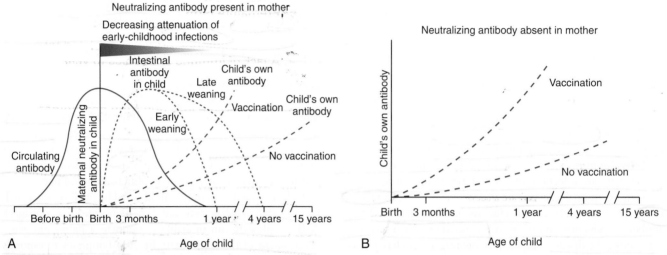

Figure 1-2   Protective effect of maternal antibodies in serum and milk. A, Maternal neutralizing antibodies cross the placenta to protect the offspring and attenuate systemic infections for 6 to 12 months after birth. The timing of weaning, early or late, influences the levels of intestinal antibodies derived from breast milk and the rate of attenuation of gastrointestinal infection. **B,** The absence of specific neutralizing antibodies in maternal serum leads to the absence of a protective effect. *(From Zinkernagel RM: Maternal antibodies, childhood infections, and autoimmune diseases, N Engl J Med 345:1331–1335, 2001.)*

defense, appeared before the adaptive immune system. Mechanisms of innate immunity (e.g., phagocytes) and the alternative complement pathways are activated immediately after infection and quickly begin to control multiplication of infecting microorganisms. By comparison, the **adaptive immune system** (Table 1-4) is organized around two classes of cells, T and B lymphocytes. When an individual lymphocyte encounters an antigen that binds to its unique antigen receptor site, activation and proliferation of that lymphocyte occur. This is called clonal selection and is responsible for the basic properties of the adaptive immune system.

Random generation of a highly diverse database of antigen receptors allows the adaptive immune system to recognize virtually any antigen. The downside to this recognition is the inability to distinguish foreign antigens from self antigens. Activation of the adaptive immune response can be harmful to the host when the antigens are self or environmental antigens. Environmental antigens are epitopes that can be found in infectious microorganisms or dietary sources. They can mimic other antigens and trigger an autoimmune condition.

Some form of innate immunity probably exists in all multicellular organisms. Innate immune recognition is mediated by germline-encoded receptors, which means that the specificity

of each receptor is genetically predetermined. Germline-encoded receptors evolved by natural selection to have defined specificities for infectious microorganisms. The problem is that every organism has a limit as to the number of genes it can encode in its genome.

Consequently, the innate immune response may not be able to recognize every possible antigen, but may focus on a few large groups of microorganisms, called **pathogen-associated molecular patterns (PAMPs).** The receptors of the innate immune system that recognize these PAMPs are called **pattern recognition receptors** (PRRs; e.g., Toll-like receptors).

Pathogen-Associated Molecular Patterns and Pattern Recognition Receptors

PAMPs are molecules associated with groups of pathogens that are recognized by cells of the innate immune system. PRRs are found in plants and animals.

Pattern Recognition Receptors

Three groups of PRRs exist:
1. Secreted PRRs are molecules that circulate in blood and lymph; circulating proteins bind to PAMPs on the surface of many pathogens. This interaction triggers the

Table 1-4	Comparison of Innate and Adaptive Immunity
Innate Immunity	**Adaptive Immunity**
Pathogen recognized by receptors encoded in the germline	Pathogen recognized by receptors generated randomly
Receptors have broad specificity, i.e., recognize many related molecular structures (PAMPs)	Receptors have very narrow specificity; i.e., recognize a specific epitope
Immediate response	Slow (3-5 days) response
Little or no memory of prior antigenic exposure	Memory of prior antigenic exposure

complement cascade, leading to the opsonization of the pathogen and its speedy phagocytosis (discussed in Chapter 3).

2. Phagocytosis receptors are cell surface receptors that bind the pathogen, initiating a signal leading to the release of effector molecules (e.g., cytokines). Macrophages have cell surface receptors that recognize PAMPs containing mannose.

3. Toll-like receptors (TLRs) are a set of transmembrane receptors that recognize different types of PAMPs. TLRs are found on macrophages, dendritic cells, and epithelial cells.

  • Mammals have multiple TLRs, with each exhibiting a specialized function, frequently with the aid of accessory molecules, in a subset of PAMPs. In this way, TLRs identify the nature of the pathogen and turn on an effector response appropriate for counteracting with it. These signaling cascades lead to the expression of various cytokine genes. Examples include TLR-1, which binds to the peptidoglycan of gram-positive bacteria and TLR-2, which binds lipoproteins of gram-negative bacteria.

In all these cases, binding of the pathogen to the TLR initiates a signaling pathway, leading to the activation of nuclear factor κB (NF-κB, light-chain enhancer of activated B cells). This transcription factor turns on many cytokine genes, such as tumor necrosis factor α (TNF-α), interleukin-1 (IL-1), and chemokines. All these effector molecules lead to the inflammation site (see Chapter 5).

CASE STUDY

A 1-month-old infant female neonate born 6 weeks premature was admitted for surgery to her foot. Several days after hospital discharge, her parents brought her back to the emergency department because she had a high fever and was crying all of the time. Physical examination revealed increased body temperature, increased respiration rate, and increased heart rate. She also had redness around the site of an inserted percutaneous central line related to her surgery.

Her blood count was normal except for a decreased concentration of blood platelets. A smear and a culture

were taken from the inflamed area. The direct smears revealed the presence of yeast. Pending results of the culture, the patient was started on antifungal therapeutics. She was admitted to the hospital, where her condition improved within the first 24 hours.

Subsequently, the culture demonstrated *Candida albicans.*

Questions

1. A risk factor for the development of a fungal infection in this child is:
   a. Gender
   b. Body weight
   c. Premature birth
   d. Decreased blood platelet count
2. The child's immune problem is related to:
   a. A lack of immune antibodies to yeast
   b. Defect in her cellular immune response
   c. Lack of sunshine and vitamins
   d. Acquiring the infection from her mother

See Appendix A for the answers to these questions.

Critical Thinking Group Discussion Questions

1. Why is the child at risk for developing an infection of this type?
2. Why did this child acquire an infection?

See Instructor site ⊖volve for a discussion of the answers to these questions.

Identification of Leukocytes Related to Immune Function

Principle

A whole blood smear is prepared and stained for microscopic examination. Five mature leukocytes with various immune functions can be identified.

See ⊖volve for a complete discussion of the method.

Results

The specific leukocytes and their related immune functions are as follows:

Band and segmented neutrophils = phagocytosis
Lymphocytes = recognition of foreign antigens and transformation to antibody producing cells
Monocytes = phagocytosis
Eosinophils = allergic reactions
Basophils = anaphylactic reactions

CHAPTER HIGHLIGHTS

• Immunology is defined as the study of the molecules, cells, organs, and systems responsible for the recognition and disposal of nonself material; how body components

respond and interact; desirable or undesirable conse=
quences of immune interactions; and how the immune
system can be manipulated to protect against or treat
disease.
- The function of the immune system is to recognize self
from nonself and to defend the body against nonself.
- The first line of defense against infection is unbroken skin,
mucosal membrane surfaces, and secretions.
- Natural immunity consisting of cellular and humoral
defense mechanisms forms the second line of body
defenses.   *INATE IMMUNITY* -
- If a microorganism overwhelms the body's natural
resistance, a third line of defensive resistance, acquired (or
adaptive) immunity, allows the body to recognize,
remember, and respond to a specific stimulus, an antigen.
Antibody-mediated immunity to infection can be acquired
if the antibodies are formed by the host (active immunity)
or received from another source (passive immunity).
- Cell-mediated immunity differs from antibody-mediated
immunity.   *Lymp*   *Humoral* .
- Lymphocytes are immunologically active through direct
cell to cell contact and production of cytokines for specific
immunologic functions, such as recruitment of phagocytic
cells to the site of inflammation.
- The main difference between the innate and adaptive
immune systems is the mechanisms and receptors used for
immune recognition.

REVIEW QUESTIONS

1-5. Match the following terms to their appropriate definitions or descriptions. (Use each answer only once.)

1. __E__ Immune system
2. __A__ Lymphocytes
3. __B__ Cooperative interaction
4. __C__ Nonspecific immune elements
5. __D__ Autoimmune disorder
  a.   T and B types
  b.   Specific cellular elements, cell products, and nonlym-
       phoid elements
  c.   Mononuclear phagocytes
  d.   Condition in which the body's own tissues are
       attacked as if they were foreign
  e.   Can protect against or be manipulated to treat
       disease

6. The first line of defense in protecting the body from
   infection includes all the following components except:
  a.   Unbroken skin
  b.   Normal microbial flora
  c.   Phagocytic leukocytes
  d.   Secretions such as mucus

7. Natural immunity is characterized as being:
  a.   Innate or inborn
  b.   Able to recognize exogenous or endogenous agents
       specifically
  c.   Able to eliminate exogenous or endogenous agents
       selectively
  d.   Part of the first line of body defenses against
       microbial organisms

8 and 9. Complete the chart below from the following list of
   choices:
  a.   Lymphocytes
  b.   Macrophages
  c.   Mucus
  d.   Interferons

Components of the Natural Immune System

Cellular	Mast cells
	Neutrophils
	8. __B__
Humoral	Complement
	Lysozyme
	9. __D__

10. Another term for adaptive immunity is:
  a.   Antigenic immunity
  b.   Acquired immunity
  c.   Lymphocyte reactive immunity
  d.   Phagocytosis

11. Humoral components of the adaptive immune system
    include:
  a.   T lymphocytes
  b.   B lymphocytes
  c.   Antibodies
  d.   Saliva

12-23. Complete the table below, choosing from the
    following answers:
Possible answers for questions 12-15:
  a.   Infusion of serum of plasma
  b.   Transfer in vivo or by colostrum
  c.   Vaccination
  d.   Infection

Comparison of the Types of Adaptive Immunity

Type	Mode of Acquisition
Active natural	D 12. __D__
Artificial active	C 13. __C__
Passive natural	14. __A__
Artificial passive	15. __A__

Comparison of the Types of Adaptive Immunity

Possible answers for questions 16-19:
  a.   Yes
  b.   No

Type	Antibody Produced by Host
Active natural	16. _____
Artificial active	17. _____
Passive natural	18. _____
Artificial passive	19. _____

Comparison of the Types of Adaptive Immunity

Possible answers for questions 20-23:

a. Short
b. Long

Type	Duration of Response
Active natural	20. _____
Artificial active	21. _____
Passive natural	22. _____
Artificial passive	23. _____

BIBLIOGRAPHY

Abbas AK, Lichtman AH: Basic immunology: functions and disorders of the immune system, updated edition, ed 3, Philadelphia, 2011, Saunders.

Bergsma J: Illness, the mind, and the body: cancer and immunology: an introduction, Theor Med 15:337–347, 1994.

Claman HN: The biology of the immune system, JAMA 268:2888–2892, 1992.

Lencer WI, von Andrian UH: Eliciting mucosal immunity, N Engl J Med 365:1151–1153, 2011.

Medzhitov R, Janeway C Jr: Innate immunity, N Engl J Med 343:338–344, 2000.

Peakman M, Vergani D: Basic and clinical immunology, ed 2, St Louis, 2009, Elsevier.

Antigens and Antibodies

Learning Objectives

At the conclusion of this chapter, the reader should be able to:
- Define the terms *antigen* and *antibody*.
- Compare the characteristics of major histocompatibility complex (MHC) classes I and II.
- Name and compare the characteristics of each of the five immunoglobulin classes.
- Draw and describe a typical immunoglobulin G (IgG) molecular structure.
- Name the four phases of an antibody response.
- Describe the characteristics of a primary and secondary (anamnestic) response.
- Compare the terms antibody *avidity* and antibody *affinity*.

- Describe the method of production of a monoclonal antibody.
- Analyze a case study related to antigens or antibodies.
- Correctly answer case study related multiple choice questions.
- Be prepared to participate in a discussion of critical thinking questions.
- Describe the principle and agglutination reactions in ABO blood grouping.
- Describe the principle, expected results, reference values, and clinical interpretation of the serum protein electrophoresis procedure.
- Correctly answer end of chapter review questions.

Key Terms

adjuvant
affinity
alloantibodies
anamnestic response
antibodies
antigens
autoantigen
avidity

clonal selection
epitope
haptens
human leukocyte antigen (HLA)
hybridoma
idiotypes
immune complex
immunogens

major histocompatibility complex
 (MHC)
monoclonal antibody (MAb)
precipitating
soluble
zeta potential

ANTIGEN CHARACTERISTICS

General Characteristics of Immunogens and Antigens

An immune response is triggered by **immunogens,** macromolecules capable of triggering an adaptive immune response by inducing the formation of **antibodies** or sensitized T cells in an immunocompetent host (a host capable of recognizing and responding to a foreign antigen). Immunogens can specifically react with corresponding antibodies or sensitized T lymphocytes. In contrast, an **antigen** is a substance that stimulates antibody formation and has the ability to bind to an antibody or a T lymphocyte antigen receptor but may not be able to evoke an immune response initially. For example, lower molecular weight particles, haptens, can bind to an antibody but must be attached to a macromolecule as a carrier to stimulate a specific immune response. In reality, all immunogens are antigens but not all antigens are immunogens. The two terms, *immunogens* and *antigens,* are frequently used interchangeably without making a distinction between the two terms.

Foreign substances can be immunogenic or antigenic (capable of provoking a humoral and/or cell-mediated immune response) if their membrane or molecular components contain(s) structures recognized as foreign by the immune system. These structures are called antigenic determinants, or epitopes. An **epitope,** as part of an antigen, reacts specifically with an antibody or T lymphocyte receptor.

Not all surfaces act as antigenic determinants. Only prominent determinants on the surface of a protein are normally recognized by the immune system and some of these are much more immunogenic than others. An immune response is directed against specific determinants and resultant antibodies will bind to them, with much of the remaining molecule being immunogenic.

The cellular membrane of mammalian cells consists chemically of proteins, phospholipids, cholesterol, and traces of polysaccharide. Polysaccharides (carbohydrates) in the form of glycoproteins or glycolipids can be found attached to the lipid and protein molecules of the membrane. When antigen-bearing cells, such as red blood cells (RBCs) from one person, a donor, are transfused into another person, a recipient, they can be immunogenic. Outer surfaces of bacteria, such as the capsule or the cell wall, as well as the surface structures of other microorganisms, can also be immunogenic.

Cellular antigens of importance to immunologists include histocompatibility antigens, autoantigens, and blood group antigens (see later, "ABO Blood Grouping Procedure"). The normal immune system responds to foreignness by producing antibodies. For this reason, microbial antigens are also important to immunologists in the study of the immunologic manifestations of infectious disease.

Histocompatibility Antigens

Nucleated cells such as leukocytes and tissues possess many cell surface–protein antigens that readily provoke an immune response if transferred into a genetically different (allogenic) individual of the same species. Some of these antigens, which constitute the **major histocompatibility complex (MHC)** (see Color Plate 2),

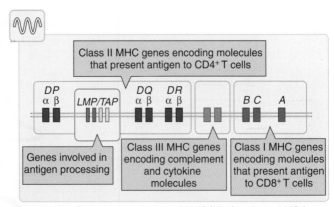

Figure 2-1 Genetic organization of MHC (HLA) antigen. *LMP,* Large multifunctional protease; *TAP,* transporter associated with antigen presentation. *(From Nairn R, Helbert M: Immunology for medical students, ed 2, St Louis, 2007, Mosby.)*

Table 2-1	Comparison of MHC Class I and Class II	
	Class I	**Class II**
Loci	HLA-A, -B, and -C	HLA-DN, -DO, -DP, -DQ, and -DR
Distribution	Most nucleated cells	B lymphocytes, macrophages, other antigen-presenting cells, activated T lymphocytes
Function	To present endogenous antigen to cytotoxic T lymphocytes	To present endogenous antigen to helper T lymphocytes

are more potent than others in provoking an immune response. The MHC is referred to as the **human leukocyte antigen (HLA)** system in humans because its gene products were originally identified on white blood cells (WBCs, leukocytes). These antigens are second only to the ABO antigens in influencing the survival or graft rejection of transplanted organs. HLAs are the subject of numerous scientific investigations because of the strong association between individual HLAs and immunologic disorders (see Chapter 31 for more discussion of the MHC).

Major Histocompatibility Complex Regions

The MHC is divided into four major regions (Fig. 2-1)—D, B, C, and A. The A, B, and C regions are the classic or class Ia genes that code for class I molecules. The D region codes for class II molecules. Class I includes HLA-A, HLA-B, and HLA-C. The three principal loci (A, B, and C) and their respective antigens are numbered, for example, as 1, 2, 3. The class II gene region antigens are encoded in the HLA-D region and can be subdivided into three families, HLA-DR, HLA-DC (DQ), and HLA-SB (DP).

Classes of HLA Molecules

Structurally, there are two classes of HLA molecules, class I and class II (Table 2-1). Both class I and class II antigens function as

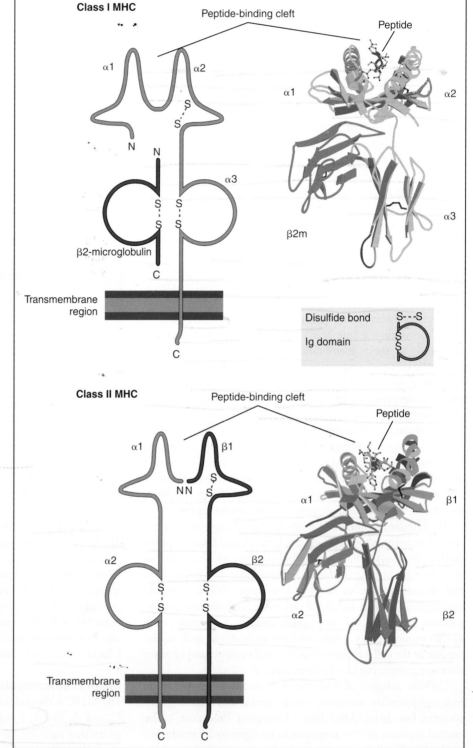

Figure 2-2 Structure of class I and class II MHC molecules. The schematic diagrams *(left)* and models *(right)* of the crystal structures of class I and class II MHC molecules illustrate the domains of the molecules and the fundamental similarities between them. Both types of MHC molecules contain peptide-binding clefts and invariant portions that bind CD8 (the α_3 domain of class I) or CD4 (the β_2 domain of class II). *$\beta_2 m$, β_2-Microglobulin.* *(From Abbas AK, Lichtman AH: Basic immunology: functions and disorders of the immune system, updated edition, ed 3, Philadelphia, 2011, Saunders; crystal structures courtesy Dr. P. Bjorkman, California Institute of Technology, Pasadena, Calif.)*

targets of T lymphocytes (see Chapter 4 for a further discussion of lymphocytes) that regulate the immune response (Fig. 2-2). Class I molecules regulate interaction between cytolytic T cells and target cells and class II molecules restrict the activity of regulatory T cells. Thus, class II molecules regulate the interaction between helper T cells and antigen-presenting cells (APCs). Cytotoxic T cells directed against class I antigens are inhibited by CD8 cells; cytotoxic T cells directed against class II antigens are inhibited by CD4 cells. Many genes in the class I and class II gene families have no known function.

Autoantigens

The evolution of a recognition system that can recognize and destroy nonself material must also have safeguards to prevent damage to self antigens. The body's immune system usually exercises tolerance to self antigens but, in some situations, antibodies may be produced in response to normal self antigens. This failure to recognize self antigens can result in autoantibodies directed at hormones, such as thyroglobulin (see Chapter 28).

Blood Group Antigens

Blood group substances are widely distributed throughout the tissues, blood cells, and body fluids. When foreign RBC antigens are introduced to a host, a transfusion reaction or hemolytic disease of the fetus and newborn can result (see Chapter 26). In addition, certain antigens, especially those of the Rh system, are integral structural components of the erythrocyte (RBC) membrane. If these antigens are missing, the erythrocyte membrane is defective and results in hemolytic anemia. When antigens do not form part of the essential membrane structure (e.g., A, B, and H antigens), the absence of antigen has no effect on membrane integrity.

CHEMICAL NATURE OF ANTIGENS

Antigens, or immunogens, are usually large organic molecules that are proteins or large polysaccharides and, rarely, if ever, lipids. Antigens, especially cell surface or membrane-bound antigens, can be composed of combinations of biochemical classes (e.g., glycoproteins, glycolipids). For example, histocompatibility HLAs are glycoprotein in nature and are found on the surface membranes of nucleated body cells composed of solid tissue and most circulating blood cells (e.g., granulocytes, monocytes, lymphocytes, thrombocytes).

Proteins are excellent antigens because of their high molecular weight and structural complexity. Lipids are considered inferior antigens because of their relative simplicity and lack of structural stability. However, when lipids are linked to proteins or polysaccharides, they may function as antigens. Nucleic acids are poor antigens because of relative simplicity, molecular flexibility, and rapid degradation. Anti–nucleic acid antibodies can be produced by artificially stabilizing them and linking them to an immunogenic carrier. Carbohydrates (polysaccharides) by themselves are considered too small to function as antigens. In the case of erythrocyte blood group antigens, protein or lipid carriers may contribute to the necessary size and the polysaccharides present in the form of side chains confer immunologic specificity.

Adjuvant

The response to immunization can be enhanced by a number of agents, collectively called adjuvants. One of the best-known emulsifying agents in vaccine studies is Freund's complete adjuvant. An **adjuvant** is a substance, distinct from antigen, that enhances T cell activation by promoting the accumulation of APCs at a site of antigen exposure and by enhancing the expression of costimulators and cytokines by the APCs.

PHYSICAL NATURE OF ANTIGENS

Important factors in the effective functioning of antigens include foreignness, degradability, molecular weight (MW), structural stability, and complexity.

Foreignness

Foreignness is the degree to which antigenic determinants are recognized as nonself by an individual's immune system. The immunogenicity of a molecule depends to a great extent on its degree of foreignness. For example, if a transplant recipient receives a donor organ with several major HLA differences, the organ is perceived as foreign and is subsequently rejected by the recipient. Normally, an individual's immune system does not respond to self antigens.

Degradability

For an antigen to be recognized as foreign by an individual's immune system, sufficient antigens to stimulate an immune response must be present. Foreign molecules are rapidly destroyed and thus cannot provide adequate antigenic exposure. In the case of vaccination, an adequate dose of vaccine at appropriate intervals must be administered for an immune response to be stimulated.

Molecular Weight

The higher the MW, the better the molecule will function as an antigen. The number of antigenic determinants on a molecule is directly related to its size. For example, proteins are effective antigens because of a large MW.

Although large foreign molecules (MW 10,000 daltons [Da]) are better antigens, haptens, which are tiny molecules, can bind to a larger carrier molecule and behave as antigens. If a hapten is chemically linked to a large molecule, a new surface structure is formed on the large molecule, which may function as an antigenic determinant.

Structural Stability

If a molecule is an effective antigen, structural stability is mandatory. If a structure is unstable (e.g., gelatin), the molecule will be a poor antigen. Similarly, totally inert molecules are poor antigens. Ther structural stability of an antigen is important in cases where the goal is to elicit a patient antibody response when adminstering a vaccine.

Complexity

The more complex an antigen, the greater is its effectiveness. Complex proteins are better antigens than large repeating polymers such as lipids, carbohydrates, and nucleic acids, which are relatively poor antigens.

GENERAL CHARACTERISTICS OF ANTIBODIES

Antibodies are specific proteins referred to as immunoglobulins. Many antibodies can be isolated in the gamma globulin fraction of protein by electrophoresis separation (Fig. 2-3). The term *immunoglobulin* (Ig) has replaced gamma globulin because not all antibodies have gamma electrophoretic mobility. Antibodies can be found in blood plasma and in many body fluids (e.g., tears, saliva, colostrum).

The primary function of an antibody in body defenses is to combine with antigen, which may be enough to neutralize bacterial toxins or some viruses. A secondary interaction of an

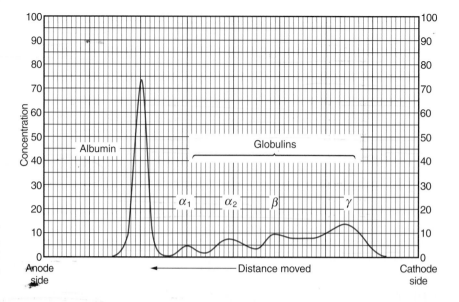

Figure 2-3 Tracing of the electrophoretic pattern of normal serum. *(Adapted from Kaplan LA, Pesce AJ, Kazmierczak SC, editors: Clinical chemistry: theory, analysis, correlation, ed 4, St Louis, 2003, Mosby.)*

Table 2-2	Characteristics of Immunoglobulin Classes				
	IgM	IgG	IgA	IgE	IgD
Molecular weight (daltons, Da)	900,000	160,000	360,000	200,000	160,000
Sedimentation coefficient (Σ)	19	7	11	8	7
Carbohydrate (%)	12	8	7	12	12
Subclasses	—	IgG1-4	α1, α2	—	—
Serum concentration, adults (mg/mL)	1.5	13.5	3.5	0.05	Trace
Serum half-life (days)*	5	23	6	2.5	3

*Half life (days) = the amount of time to reach ½ activity concentration. Serum values are average concentrations in normal, healthy individuals. Adapted from Peakman M, Vergani D: Basic and clinical immunology, St Louis, 2009, Elsevier, p 41.

antibody molecule with another effector agent (e.g., complement) is usually required to dispose of larger antigens (e.g., bacteria).

Determining Ig concentration can be of diagnostic significance in infectious and autoimmune diseases. Test methods to detect the presence and concentration of immunoglobulins are discussed in Part II and in chapters relating to specific diseases.

IMMUNOGLOBULIN (IG) CLASSES

Five distinct classes of immunoglobulin molecules are recognized in most higher mammals—IgM, IgG, IgA, IgD, and IgE. These Ig classes differ from each other in characteristics such as MW and sedimentation coefficients (Table 2-2).

Immunoglobulin M

Immunoglobulin M accounts for about 10% of the Ig pool and is largely confined to the intravascular pool because of its large size. This antibody is produced early in an immune response and is largely confined to the blood. IgM is effective in agglutination and cytolytic reactions. In humans, IgM is found in smaller concentrations than IgG or IgA. The molecule has five individual heavy chains, with an MW of 65,000 Da; the whole molecule has an MW of 900,000 Da and sedimentation coefficient, Σ, of 19.

Normal values of IgM are 60 to 250 mg/dL (70 to 290 IU/mL) for males and 70 to 280 mg/dL (80 to 320 IU/mL) for females. At 4 months of age, 50% of the adult level is present; adult levels are reached by 8 to 15 years. Cord blood contains greater than 20 mg/dL. IgM is usually undetectable in cerebrospinal fluid (CSF).

IgM is decreased in primary (genetically determined) Ig disorders as well as secondary Ig deficiencies (acquired disorders associated with certain diseases). IgM can be increased in the following conditions:

- Infectious diseases, such as subacute bacterial endocarditis, infectious mononucleosis, leprosy, trypanosomiasis, malaria, and actinomycosis
- Collagen disorders, such as scleroderma
- Hematologic disorders, such as polyclonal gammopathies, monocytic leukemia, and monoclonal gammopathies (e.g., Waldenström's macroglobulinemia)

Immunoglobulin G

The major immunoglobulin in normal serum is IgG. It diffuses more readily than other immunoglobulins into the extravascular spaces and neutralizes toxins or binds to microorganisms in extravascular spaces. IgG can cross the placenta. In addition, when IgG complexes are formed, complement can be activated. IgG accounts for 70% to 75% of the total Ig pool. It is a 7S molecule, with an MW of approximately 150,000 Da. One of the subclasses, IgG3, is slightly larger (170,000 Da) than the other subclasses.

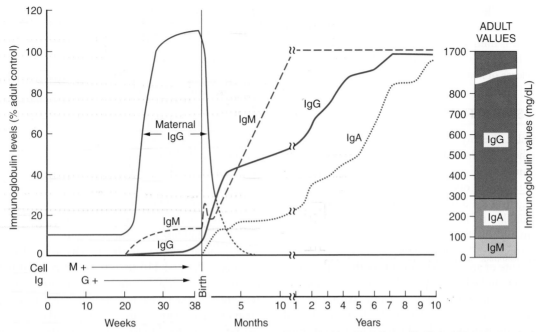

Figure 2-4 Immunoglobulin concentration in newborns, infants, and children. *(Adapted from Bauer JD: Clinical laboratory methods, ed 9, St Louis, 1982, Mosby.)*

Normal human adult serum values of IgG are 800 to 1800 mg/dL (90 to 210 IU/mL). In infants 3 to 4 months old, the IgG level is approximately 350 to 400 mg/dL (40 to 45 IU/mL), gradually increasing to 700 to 800 mg/dL (80 to 90 IU/mL) by the end of the first year of life (Fig. 2-4). The average adult level is achieved before age 16 years. Other body fluids containing IgG include cord blood (800 to 1800 mg/dL) and CSF (2 to 4 mg/dL).

Decreased levels of IgG can be manifested in primary (genetic) or secondary (acquired) Ig deficiencies. Significant increases of IgG are seen in the following conditions:

- Infectious diseases, such as hepatitis, rubella, and infectious mononucleosis
- Collagen disorders, such as rheumatoid arthritis and systemic lupus erythematosus
- Hematologic disorders, such as polyclonal gammopathies, monoclonal gammopathies, monocytic leukemia, and Hodgkin's disease

Immunoglobulin A

Immunoglobulin A represents 15% to 20% of the total circulatory Ig pool. It is the predominant immunoglobulin in secretions such as tears, saliva, colostrum, milk, and intestinal fluids. IgA is synthesized largely by plasma cells located on body surfaces. If produced by cells in the intestinal wall, IgA may pass directly into the intestinal lumen or diffuse into the blood circulation. As IgA is transported through intestinal epithelial cells or hepatocytes, it binds to a glycoprotein called the secretory component. The secretory piece protects IgA from digestion by gastrointestinal proteolytic enzymes. It forms a complex molecule termed *secretory IgA*, which is critical in protecting body surfaces against invading

microorganisms because of its presence in seromucous secretions (e.g., tears, saliva, nasal fluids, colostrum).

IgA monomer is present in relatively high concentrations in human serum; it has a concentration of 90 to 450 mg/dL (55 to 270 IU/mL) in normal adult humans. At the end of the first year of life, 25% of the adult IgA level is reached, and 50% at 3.5 years of age. The average adult level is attained by age 16 years. IgA concentration in cord blood is greater than 1 mg/dL; CSF contains 0.1 to 0.6 mg/dL of IgA.

IgA is decreased in primary or secondary Ig deficiencies. Significant increases in serum IgA concentration are associated with the following:

- Infectious diseases, such as tuberculosis and actinomycosis
- Collagen disorders, such as rheumatoid arthritis
- Hematologic disorders, such as polyclonal gammopathies, monocytic leukemia, and monoclonal gammopathy (e.g., IgA myeloma)
- Liver disease, such as Laennec's cirrhosis and chronic active hepatitis

Immunoglobulin D

Immunoglobulin D is found in very low concentrations in plasma, accounting for less than 1% of the total Ig pool. IgD is extremely susceptible to proteolysis and is primarily a cell membrane Ig found on the surface of B lymphocytes in association with IgM.

Immunoglobulin E

Immunoglobulin E is a trace plasma protein found in the blood plasma of unparasitized individuals (MW, 188,000 Da). IgE is crucial because it mediates some types of hypersensitivity (allergic) reactions, allergies, and anaphylaxis and is generally responsible for an individual's immunity to invading parasites. The IgE molecule is unique in that it binds strongly to a receptor on mast cells and basophils and, together with antigen, mediates the release of histamines and heparin from these cells.

ANTIBODY STRUCTURE

Antibodies exhibit diversity among the different classes, which suggests that they perform different functions in addition to their primary function of antigen binding. Essentially, each Ig molecule is bifunctional; one region of the molecule involves binding to antigen, and a different region mediates binding of the immunoglobulin to host tissues, including cells of the immune system and the first component (C1q) of the classic complement system.

The primary core of an antibody consists of the sequence of amino acid residues linked by the peptide bond. All antibodies have a common, basic polypeptide structure, with a three-dimensional configuration. The polypeptide chains are linked by covalent and noncovalent bonds, which produce a unit composed of a four-chain structure based on pairs of identical heavy and light chains. IgG, IgD, and IgE occur only as monomers of the four-chain unit, IgA occurs in both monomeric and polymeric forms, and IgM occurs as a pentamer with five four-chain subunits linked together.

Typical Immunoglobulin Molecule

The basic unit of an antibody structure is the homology unit, or domain. A typical molecule has 12 domains, arranged in two heavy (H) and two light (L) chains, linked through cysteine residues by disulfide bonds so that the domains lie in pairs (Fig. 2-5). The antigen-binding portion of the molecule (N-terminal end) shows such heterogeneity that it is known as the variable (V) region; the remainder is composed of relatively constant amino acid sequences, the constant (C) region. Short segments of about 10 amino acid residues within the variable regions of antibodies (or T cell receptor [TCR] proteins) form loop structures called complementary-determining

regions (CDRs). Three hypervariable loops, also called CDRs, are present in each antibody H chain and L chain. Most of the variability among different antibodies or TCRs is located within these loops.

The IgG molecule provides a classic model of antibody structure, appearing Y-shaped under electron microscopy (Fig. 2-6). If the molecule is studies by chemical treatment and the interchain disulfide bonds are broken, the molecule separates into four polypeptide chains. Light chains are small chains (25,000 Da) common to all Ig classes. The L chains are of two subtypes, kappa (κ) and lambda (λ), which have different amino acid sequences and are antigenically different. In humans, about 65% of Ig molecules have κ chains, whereas 35% have λ chains. The larger H chains (50,000 to 77,000 Da) extend the full length of the molecule.

A general feature of the Ig chains is their amino acid sequence. The first 110 to 120 amino acids of both L and H chains have a variable sequence and form the V region; the remainder of the L chains represents the C region, with a similar amino acid sequence for each type and subtype. The remaining portion of the H chain is also constant for each type and has a hinge region. The class and subclass of an Ig molecule are determined by its H-chain type.

Fab, Fc, and Hinge Molecular Components

A typical monomeric IgG molecule consists of three globular regions (two Fab regions and an Fc portion) linked by a flexible hinge region. If the molecule is digested with a proteolytic enzyme such as papain, it splits into three approximately equal-sized fragments (Fig. 2-7). Two of these fragments retain the ability to bind antigen and are called the antigen-binding fragments (Fab fragments). The third fragment, which is relatively homogeneous and is sometimes crystallizable, is called the Fc portion. If IgG is treated with another proteolytic enzyme,

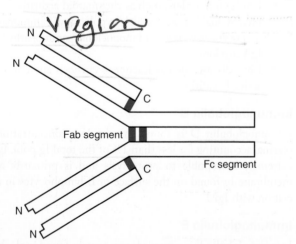

Figure 2-5 Basic immunoglobulin configuration. *(Adapted from Turgeon ML: Fundamentals of immunohematology, ed 2, Baltimore, 1995, Williams & Wilkins.)*

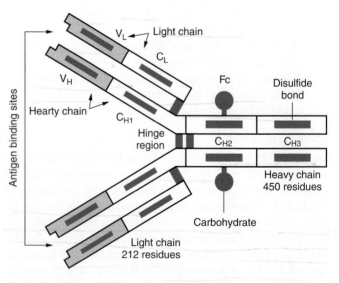

V_L and V_H = Variable regions
C_L and C_H = Constant regions

Figure 2-6 Basic structure of IgG. *(Adapted from Turgeon ML: Fundamentals of immunohematology, ed 2, Baltimore, 1995, Williams & Wilkins.)*

pepsin, the molecule separates somewhat differently. The Fc fragment is split into tiny peptides and thus is completely destroyed. The two Fab fragments remain joined to produce a fragment called F(ab)′2. This fragment possesses two antigen-binding sites. If F(ab)′2 is treated to reduce its disulfide bonds, it breaks into two Fab fragments, each of which has only one antigen-binding site. Further disruption of the interchain disulfide bonds in the Fab fragments shows that each contains a light chain and half of a heavy chain, which is called the Fd fragment.

Electron microscopy studies of IgG have revealed that the Fab regions of the molecule are mobile and can swing freely around the center of the molecule as if it were hinged. This hinge consists of a group of about 15 amino acids located between the C_{H1} and C_{H2} regions. The exact sequence of amino acids in the hinge is variable and unique for each Ig class and subclass. Because amino acids can rotate freely around peptide bonds, the effect of closely spaced proline amino acid residues is production of a so-called universal joint, around which the Ig chains can swing freely. A remarkable feature of the hinge region is the presence of a large number of hydrophilic and proline residues. The hydrophilic residues tend to open up this region and thus make it accessible to proteolytic cleavage with

enzymes such as pepsin and papain. This region also contains all the interchain disulfide bonds except for IgD, which has no interchain links.

Structures of Other Immunoglobulins

Immunoglobulin M

The IgM molecule is structurally composed of five basic subunits. Each subunit consists of two κ or two λ light chains and two mu (μ) heavy chains. The individual monomers of IgM are linked together by disulfide bonds in a circular fashion (Fig. 2-8). A small, cysteine-rich polypeptide, the J chain, must be considered an integral part of the molecule. IgM has carbohydrate residues attached to the C_{H3} and C_{H4} domains. The site for complement activation by IgM is located on this C_{H4} region. IgM is more efficient than IgG in activities such as complement cascade activation and agglutination.

Immunoglobulin A

In humans, more than 80% of IgA occurs as a typical four-chain structure consisting of paired κ or λ chains and two heavy chains (Fig. 2-9). The basic four-chain monomer has an MW of 160,000 Da; however, in most mammals, plasma IgA occurs mainly as a dimer. In dimeric IgA, the molecules are joined by a J chain linked to the Fc regions. Secretory IgA exists mainly in the 11S dimeric form and has an MW of 385,000 Da (Fig. 2-10). This form of IgA is present in fluids and is stabilized against proteolysis when combined with another protein, the secretory component. In humans, variations in the heavy chains account for the subclasses IgA1 and IgA2.

Immunoglobulin D

The IgD molecule has an MW of 184,000 Da and consists of two κ or α light chains and two delta (δ) heavy chains (Fig. 2-11). It has no interchain disulfide bonds between its heavy chains and an exposed hinge region.

Immunoglobulin E

The IgE molecule is composed of paired κ or α light chains and two epsilon (ε) heavy chains (Fig. 2-12). It is unique in that its Fc region binds strongly to a receptor on mast cells and basophils and, together with antigen, mediates the release of histamines and heparin from these cells.

IMMUNOGLOBULIN VARIANTS

An antigenic determinant is the specific chemical determinant group or molecular configuration against which the immune response is directed. Because they are proteins, immunoglobulins themselves can function as effective antigens when used to immunize mammals of a different species. When the resulting antiimmunoglobulins or antiglobulins are analyzed, three principal categories of antigenic determinants can be recognized—isotype, allotype, and idiotype (Fig. 2-13; Table 2-3).

Isotype Determinants

The isotypic class of antigenic determinants is the dominant type found on the immunoglobulins of all animals of a species.

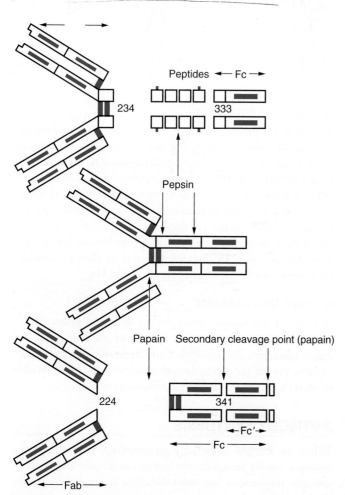

Figure 2-7   Enzymatic cleavage of human IgG1. *(Adapted from Turgeon ML: Fundamentals of immunohematology, ed 2, 1995, Williams & Wilkins.)*

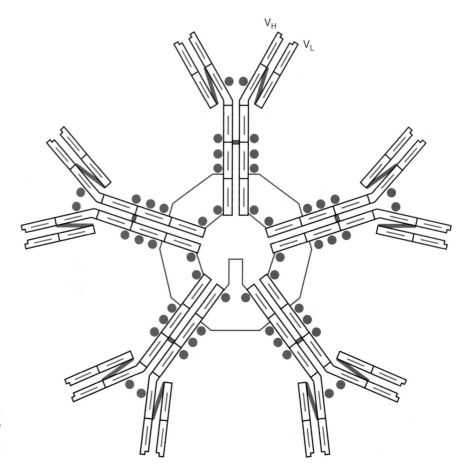

Figure 2-8 Pentameric polypeptide chain structure of human IgM. *(Adapted from Turgeon ML: Fundamentals of immunohematology, ed 2, Baltimore, 1995, Williams & Wilkins.)*

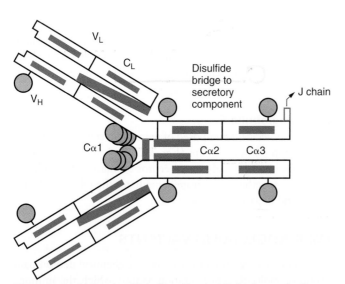

Figure 2-9 Molecule of IgA. *(From Turgeon ML: Fundamentals of Immunohematology, ed 2, Baltimore, 1995, Williams & Wilkins.)*

The heavy-chain, constant region structures associated with the different classes and subclasses are termed *isotypic variants.* Genes for isotypic variants are present in all healthy members of a species. Determinants in this category include those specific for each Ig class, such as gamma (γ) for IgG, mu (μ) for IgM, and alpha (α) for IgA, as well as the subclass-specific determinants κ and λ.

Allotype Determinants

The second principal group of determinants is found on the immunoglobulins of some, but not all, animals of a species. Antibodies to these allotypes (**alloantibodies**) may be produced by injecting the immunoglobulins of one animal into another member of the same species. The allotypic determinants are genetically determined variations representing the presence of allelic genes at a single locus within a species. Typical allotypes in humans are the Gm specificities on IgG (Gm is a marker on IgG). In humans, five sets of allotypic markers have been found—Gm, Km, Mm, Am, and Hv.

Idiotype Determinants

A result of the unique structures on light and heavy chains, individual determinants characteristic of each antibody are called **idiotypes.** The idiotypic determinants are located in the variable part of the antibody associated with the hypervariable regions that form the antigen-combining site.

ANTIBODY SYNTHESIS

When an antigen is initially encountered, the cells of the immune system recognize the antigen as nonself and elicit an immune response or become tolerant of it, depending on the circumstances. An immune reaction can take the form of cell-mediated immunity (immunity dependent on T cells and macrophages) or may involve the production of

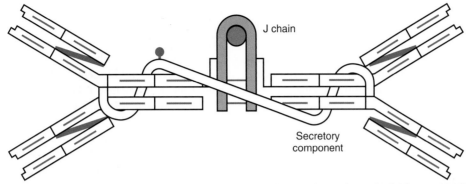

Figure 2-10 Molecule of secretory IgA. *(From Turgeon ML: Fundamentals of Immunohematology, ed 2, Baltimore, 1995, Williams & Wilkins.)*

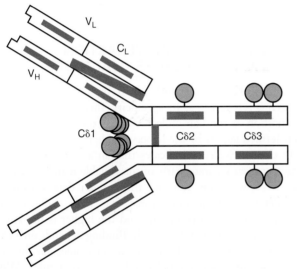

Figure 2-11 Molecule of IgD. *(From Turgeon ML: Fundamentals of Immunohematology, ed 2, Baltimore, 1995, Williams & Wilkins.)*

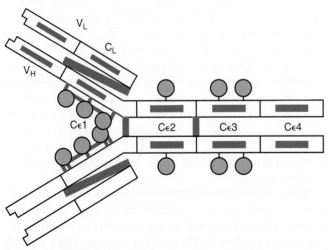

Figure 2-12 Molecule of IgE. *(From Turgeon ML: Fundamentals of Immunohematology, ed 2, Baltimore, 1995, Williams & Wilkins.)*

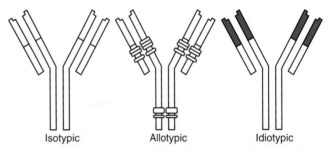

Figure 2-13 Variants of antibodies—antigenic determinants. *(Adapted from Turgeon ML: Fundamentals of immunohematology, ed 2, Baltimore, 1995, Williams & Wilkins.)*

Table 2-3	**Immunoglobulin Variants**		
Variant	**Distribution**	**Location**	**Examples**
Isotype	All variants in normal persons	C_H	IgM, IgE
		C_H	IgA1, IgA2
		C_L	Kappa subtype
		C_L	Lambda subtype
Allotype	Genetically controlled alternate forms; not present in all individuals	Mainly C_H/C_L Sometimes V_H/V_2	Gm groups in humans
Idiotype	Individually specific to each immunoglobulin molecule	Variable regions	Probably one or more hypervariable regions forming the antigen-combining site

C, Constant regent; *Gm,* marker on IgG; *H,* heavy chain; *L,* light chain; *V,* variable region.

antibodies (B lymphocytes and plasma cells) directed against the antigen.

Production of antibodies is induced when the host's lymphocytes come into contact with a foreign antigenic substance that binds to its receptor. This triggers activation and proliferation, or **clonal selection.** Clonal expansion of lymphocytes in response to infection is necessary for an effective immune response (Fig. 2-14). However, it requires 3 to 5 days for a sufficient number of clones to be produced and to differentiate into antibody-producing cells. This allows time for most pathogens to damage host tissues and cells.

Whether a cell-mediated response or an antibody response takes place depends on how the antigen is presented to the lymphocytes; many immune reactions display both types of responses. The antigenicity of a foreign substance is also related to the route of entry. Intravenous and intraperitoneal routes are stronger stimuli than subcutaneous and intramuscular routes.

Subsequent exposure to the same antigen produces a memory response, or **anamnestic response,** and reflects the outcome of the initial challenge. In the case of antibody production, the quantity of IgM-IgG varies.

Primary Antibody Response

Although the duration and levels of antibody (titer) depend on the characteristics of the antigen and the individual, an IgM antibody response proceeds in the following four phases after a foreign antigen challenge (see Fig. 2-14):
1. Lag phase—no antibody is detectable.
2. Log phase—the antibody titer increases logarithmically.
3. Plateau phase—the antibody titer stabilizes.
4. Decline phase—the antibody is catabolized.

Secondary (Anamnestic) Response

Subsequent exposure to the same antigenic stimulus produces an antibody response that exhibits the same four phases as the primary response (see Fig. 2-14). Repeated exposure to an antigen can occur many years after the initial exposure, but clones of memory cells will be stimulated to proliferate, with subsequent production of antibody by the individual. An anamnestic response differs from a primary response as follows:
1. Time. A secondary response has a shorter lag phase, longer plateau, and more gradual decline.
2. Type of antibody. IgM-type antibodies are the principal class formed in the primary response. Although some IgM antibody is formed in a secondary response, the IgG class is the predominant type formed.
3. Antibody titer. In a secondary response, antibody levels attain a higher titer. The plateau levels in a secondary response are typically 10-fold or greater than the plateau levels in the primary response.

An example of an anamnestic response can be observed in hemolytic disease, when an Rh-negative mother is pregnant with an Rh-positive baby (see Chapter 26). During the mother's first exposure, the Rh-positive RBCs of the fetus leak into the maternal circulation and elicit a primary response. Subsequent pregnancies with an Rh-positive fetus will elicit a secondary (anamnestic) response.

Vaccination is the application of primary and second responses. Humans can become immune to microbial antigens through artificial and natural exposure. A vaccine is designed to provide artificially acquired active immunity to a specific disease (e.g., hepatitis B). Booster vaccine (repeated antigen exposure) allows for an anamnestic response, with an increase in antibody titer and clones of memory cells (see Chapter 16).

FUNCTIONS OF ANTIBODIES

The principal function of an antibody is to bind antigen, but antibodies may also exhibit secondary effector functions and behave as antigens. The significant secondary effector functions of antibodies are complement fixation and placental transfer (Table 2-4). The activation of complement is one of most important effector mechanisms of IgG1 and IgG3 molecules (see Chapter 5). IgG2 seems to be less effective in activating complement; IgG4, IgA, IgD, and IgE are ineffective in terms of complement activation. IgG-4 related disease is a newly recognized inflammatory condition characterized by often but not always elevated serum IgG4 concentrations.

In humans, most IgG subclass molecules are capable of crossing the placental barrier; no consensus exists on whether IgG2 crosses the placenta. Passage of antibodies across the placental barrier is important in the etiology of hemolytic disease of the fetus and newborn and in conferring passive immunity to the newborn during the first few months of life.

ANTIGEN-ANTIBODY INTERACTION: SPECIFICITY AND CROSS-REACTIVITY

The ability of a particular antibody to combine with a particular antigen is referred to as its specificity. This property resides in the portion of the Fab molecule called the combining site, a cleft formed largely by the hypervariable regions of heavy and light chains. Evidence indicates that an antigen may bind to larger, or even separate, parts of the variable region. The closer the fit between this site and the antigen determinant, the stronger are the noncovalent forces (e.g., hydrophobic or electrostatic bonds) between them, and the higher is the affinity between the antigen and antibody. Binding depends on a close three-dimensional fit, allowing weak intermolecular forces to overcome the normal repulsion between molecules. When more than one combining site interacts with the same antigen, the bond has greatly increased strength.

Antigen-antibody reactions can show a high level of specificity. Specificity exists when the binding sites of antibodies directed against determinants of one antigen are not complementary to determinants of another dissimilar antigen. When some of the determinants of an antigen are shared by similar antigenic determinants on the surface of apparently unrelated molecules, a proportion of the antibodies directed against one type of antigen will also react with the other type of antigen; this is called cross-reactivity. Antibodies directed against a protein in one species may also react in a detectable manner with the homologous protein in another species.

Cross-reactivity occurs between bacteria that possess the same cell wall polysaccharides as mammalian erythrocytes. Intestinal bacteria, as well as other substances found in the environment, possess A-like or B-like antigens similar to the A and B erythrocyte antigens. If A or B antigens are foreign to an individual, production of anti-A or anti-B occurs, despite lack of previous exposure to these erythrocyte antigens. Cross-reacting antibodies of this type are termed *heterophile antibodies.*

Antibody Affinity

Affinity is the initial force of attraction that exists between a single Fab site on an antibody molecule and a single epitope or

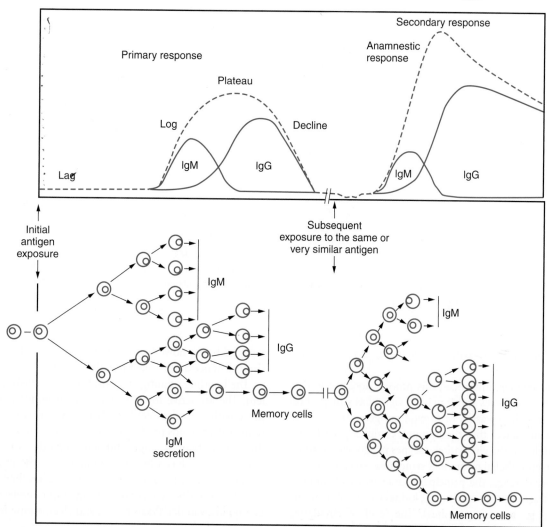

Figure 2-14 Primary and secondary antibody response. *(Adapted from Turgeon ML: Fundamentals of immunohematology, ed 2, Baltimore, 1995, Williams & Wilkins.)*

Table 2-4	**Comparison of Properties of Immunoglobulins**				
	IgM	**IgG**	**IgA**	**IgD**	**IgE**
Complement fixation	3+	0-2+	No	No	No
Placental transfer	No	Yes	No	No	No

determinant site on the corresponding antigen. The antigen is univalent and is usually a hapten. Several types of noncovalent bonds hold an epitope and binding site close together (see later, "Type of Bonding").

Antibody Avidity

Each four-polypeptide–chain antibody unit has two antigen-binding sites, which allows them to be potentially multivalent in their reaction with an antigen. The functional combining strength of an antibody with its antigen is called **avidity**, in contrast to affinity, the binding strength between an antigenic determinant (epitope) and an antibody-combining site

(Fig. 2-15). When a multivalent antigen combines with more than one of an antibody's combining sites, the strength of the bonding is significantly increased. For the antigen and antibody to dissociate, all the antigen-antibody bonds must be broken simultaneously.

Decreased avidity can result when an antigen (e.g., hapten) has only one antigenic determinant (monovalent).

Immune Complexes

The noncovalent combination of antigen with its respective specific antibody is called an **immune complex**. An immune complex may be of the small (**soluble**) or large (**precipitating**) type, depending on the nature and proportion of antigen and antibody. Under conditions of antigen or antibody excess, soluble complexes tend to predominate. If equivalent amounts of antigen and antibody are present, a precipitate may form. However, all antigen-antibody complexes will not precipitate, even at equivalence.

Antibody can react with antigen that is fixed or localized in tissues or that is released or present in the circulation. Once formed in the circulation, the immune complex is usually removed by phagocytic cells through the interaction of the Fc

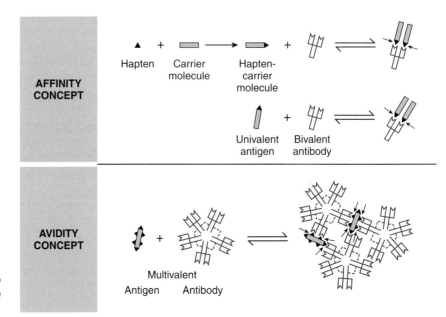

Figure 2-15 Affinity versus avidity. *(From Zane HD: Immunology: theoretical and practical concepts in laboratory medicine, Philadelphia, 2001, Saunders.)*

portion of the antibody with complement and cell surface receptors.

Under normal circumstances, this process does not lead to pathologic consequences and it may be viewed as a major host defense against the invasion of foreign antigens. It is only in unusual circumstances that the immune complex persists as a soluble complex in the circulation, escapes phagocytosis, and is deposited in endothelial or vascular structures—where it causes inflammatory damage, the principal characteristic of immune complex disease—or in organs (e.g., kidney), or inhibits useful immunity (e.g., tumors, parasites). The level of circulating immune complex is determined by the rate of formation, rate of clearance and, most importantly, nature of the complex formed. Detection of immune complexes and identification of the associated antigens are important to the clinical diagnosis of immune complex disorders.

MOLECULAR BASIS OF ANTIGEN-ANTIBODY REACTIONS

The basic Y-shaped Ig molecule is a bifunctional structure. The V regions are primarily concerned with antigen binding. When an antigenic determinant and its specific antibody combine, they interact through the chemical groups found on the surface of the antigenic determinant and on the surface of the hypervariable regions of the Ig molecule. Although the C regions do not form antigen-binding sites, the arrangement of the C regions and hinge region give the molecule segmental flexibility, which allows it to combine with separated antigenic determinants.

Types of Bonding

Bonding of an antigen to an antibody results from the formation of multiple, reversible, intermolecular attractions between an antigen and amino acids of the binding site. These forces require proximity of the interacting groups. The optimum distance separating the interacting groups varies for different

types of bond; however, all these bonds act only across a very short distance and weaken rapidly as that distance increases.

The bonding of antigen to antibody is exclusively noncovalent. The attractive force of noncovalent bonds is weak compared with that of covalent bonds, but the formation of multiple noncovalent bonds produces considerable total binding energy. The strength of a single antigen-antibody bond (antibody affinity) is produced by the summation of the attractive and repulsive forces. The four types of noncovalent bonds involved in antigen-antibody reactions are hydrophobic bonds, hydrogen bonds, van der Waals forces, and electrostatic forces.

Hydrophobic Bonds

The major bonds formed between antigens and antibodies are hydrophobic. Many of the nonpolar side chains of proteins are hydrophobic. When antigen and antibody molecules come together, these side chains interact and exclude water molecules from the area of the interaction. The exclusion of water frees some of the constraints imposed by the proteins, which results in a gain in energy and forms an energetically stable complex.

Hydrogen Bonds

Hydrogen bonding results from the formation of hydrogen bridges between appropriate atoms. Major hydrogen bonds in antigen-antibody interactions are O–H–O, N–H–N, and O–H–N.

Van der Waals Forces

Van der Waals forces are nonspecific attractive forces generated by the interaction between electron clouds and hydrophobic bonds. These bonds result from minor asymmetry in the charge of an atom caused by the position of its electrons. They rely on the association of nonpolar hydrophobic groups so that contact with water molecules is minimized. Although extremely weak, van der Waals forces may become collectively important in an antigen-antibody reaction.

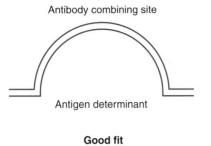

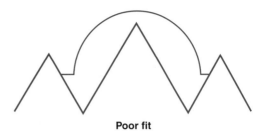

Figure 2-16 Goodness of fit.

Electrostatic Forces

Electrostatic forces result from the attraction of oppositely charged amino acids located on the side chains of two amino acid residues. The relative importance of electrostatic bonds is unclear.

Goodness of Fit

The strongest bonding develops when antigens and antibodies are close to each other and when the shapes of the antigenic determinants and the antigen-binding site conform to each other. This complementary matching of determinants and binding sites is referred to as goodness of fit (Fig. 2-16).

A good fit will create ample opportunities for the simultaneous formation of several noncovalent bonds and few opportunities for disruption of the bond. If a poor fit exists, repulsive forces can overpower any small forces of attraction. Variations from the ideal complementary shape will produce a decrease in the total binding energy because of increased repulsive forces and decreased attractive forces. Goodness of fit is important in determining the binding of an antibody molecule for a particular antigen.

Detection of Antigen-Antibody Reactions

In vitro tests detect the combination of antigens and antibodies. Agglutination is the process whereby particulate antigens (e.g., cells) aggregate to form larger complexes in the presence of a specific antibody. Agglutination tests are widely used in immunology to detect and measure the consequences of antigen-antibody interaction. Other tests include the following:

- Precipitation reactions combine soluble antigen with soluble antibody to produce insoluble complexes that are visible.
- Hemolysis testing involves the reaction of antigen and antibody with a cellular indicator (e.g., lysed RBCs).
- The enzyme-linked immunosorbent assay (ELISA) measures immune complexes formed in an in vitro system.

The principles of immunologic methods are discussed in Part II of this text. Detection and quantitation of immunoglobulins is important in the laboratory investigation of infectious diseases and immunologic disorders (Table 2-5).

Influence of Antibody Types on Agglutination

Immunoglobulins are relatively positively charged and, after sensitization or coating of particles, they reduce the **zeta potential,** which is the difference in electrostatic potential

Table 2-5	**Role of Specific Immunoglobulins in Diagnostic Tests**		
	IgG	**IgM**	**IgA**
Agglutination	1+	3+	Negative
Complement fixation	1+	3+	1+
Time of appearance after exposure to antigen (days)	3-7	2.5	3-7
Time to reach peak titer (days)	7-21	5-14	7-21

between the net charge at the cell membrane and the charge at the surface of shear (see Fig. 10-4). Antibodies can bridge charged particles by extending beyond the effective range of the zeta potential, which results in the erythrocytes closely approaching each other, binding, and agglutinating.

Antibodies differ in their ability to agglutinate. IgM-type antibodies, sometimes referred to as complete antibodies, are more efficient than IgG or IgA antibodies in exhibiting in vitro agglutination when the antigen-bearing erythrocytes are suspended in physiologic saline (0.9% sodium chloride solution). Antibodies that do not exhibit visible agglutination of saline-suspended erythrocytes, even when bound to the cell's surface membrane, are considered to be nonagglutinating antibodies and have been called incomplete antibodies. Incomplete antibodies may fail to exhibit agglutination because the antigenic determinants are located deep within the surface membrane or may show restricted movement in their hinge region, causing them to be functionally monovalent.

MONOCLONAL ANTIBODIES

Monoclonal antibodies are purified antibodies cloned from a single cell. These antibodies exhibit exceptional purity and specificity and are able to recognize and bind to a specific antigen.

Discovery of the Technique

In 1975, Köhler, Milstein, and Jerne discovered how to fuse lymphocytes to produce a cell line that was both immortal and a producer of specific antibodies. These scientists were awarded the Nobel Prize in Physiology and Medicine in 1984 for developing this **hybridoma** (cell hybrid) from different lines of cultured myeloma cells (plasma cells derived from malignant tumor strains). To induce the cells to fuse, they used Sendai

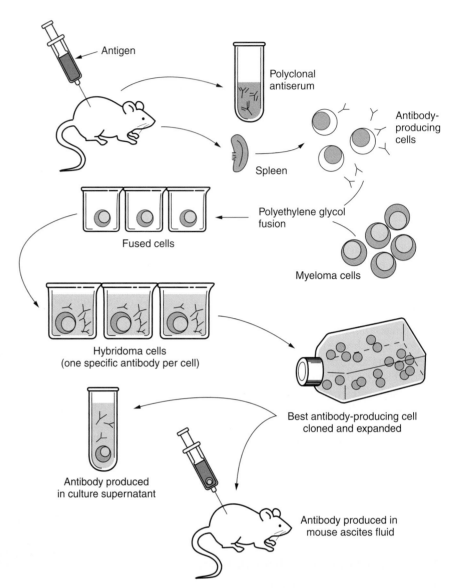

Figure 2-17 Production of monoclonal antibody (MAb). *(Adapted from Forbes BA, Sahm DF, Weissfeld AS: Bailey & Scott's diagnostic microbiology, ed 12, St Louis, 2007, Mosby.)*

virus, an influenza virus that characteristically causes cell fusion. Initially, the scientists immunized donors with sheep erythrocytes to provide a marker for the normal cells. The hybrids were tested to determine whether they still produced antibodies against the sheep erythrocytes. Köhler discovered that some of the hybrids were manufacturing large quantities of specific anti–sheep erythrocyte antibodies.

Hybrid cells secrete the antibody that is characteristic of the parent cell (e.g., anti–sheep erythrocyte antibodies). The multiplying hybrid cell culture is a hybridoma. Hybridoma cells can be cloned. The immunoglobulins derived from a single clone of cells are termed *monoclonal antibodies (MAbs)*.

Monoclonal Antibody Production

Modern methods for producing MAbs are refinements of the original technique. Basically, the hybridoma technique enables scientists to inoculate crude antigen mixtures into mice and then select clones producing specific antibodies against a single cell surface antigen (Fig. 2-17). The process of producing MAbs takes 3 to 6 months.

Mice are immunized with a specific antigen; several doses are given to ensure a vigorous immune response. After 2 to 4 days, spleen cells are mixed with cultured mouse myeloma cells. Myeloma parent cells that lack the enzyme, hypoxanthine phosphoribosyl transferase, are selected. Mouse myeloma cell lines usually do not secrete immunoglobulins, thus simplifying the purification process.

Polyethylene glycol (PEG) rather than Sendai virus is added to the cell mixture to promote cell membrane fusion. Only 1 in 200,000 spleen cells actually forms a viable hybrid with a myeloma cell. Normal spleen cells do not survive in culture. The fused cell mixture is placed in a medium containing hypoxanthine, aminopterin, and thymidine (HAT medium). Aminopterin is a drug that prevents myeloma cells from making their own purines and pyrimidines; they cannot use hypoxanthine from the medium, so they die.

Hybrids resulting from the fusion of spleen cells and myeloma cells contain transferase provided by the normal spleen cells. Consequently, the hybridoma cells are able to use the hypoxanthine and thymidine in the culture medium and survive. They divide rapidly in HAT medium, doubling in number every 24 to 48 hours. About 300 to 500 hybrids can be generated from the cells of a single mouse spleen, although not all will be making the desired antibodies. After the hybridomas have been growing for 2 to 4 weeks, the supernatant is tested for specific antibody using methods such as ELISA. Clones that produce the desired antibody are grown in mass culture and recloned to eliminate non–antibody-producing cells.

Antibody-producing clones lose their ability to synthesize or secrete antibody after being cultured for several months. Hybridoma cells usually are frozen and stored in small aliquots. The cells may then be grown in mass culture or injected intraperitoneally into mice. Because hybridomas are tumor cells, they grow rapidly and induce the effusion of large quantities of fluid into the peritoneal cavity. This ascites fluid is rich in MAbs and can be easily harvested.

Uses of Monoclonal Antibodies

The greatest impact of MAbs in immunology has been on the analysis of cell membrane antigens. Because they have a single specificity rather than the range of antibody molecules present in the serum, MAbs have multiple clinical applications, including the following:

- Identifying and quantifying hormones
- Typing tissue and blood
- Identifying infectious agents
- Identifying clusters of differentiation for the classification of leukemias and lymphomas and follow-up therapy
- Identifying tumor antigens and autoantibodies
- Delivering immunotherapy (see Chapter 33)

CASE STUDY

History and Physical Examination

A 38-year-old white woman presented to the emergency department of her local hospital with increasing difficulty in breathing. She also reported that she had experienced chronic diarrhea for the past 18 months.

Her physical examination revealed a cachectic woman with bilateral rales and splenomegaly. After a chest x-ray film confirmed the presence of pneumonia and bronchiectasis, the patient was admitted to the hospital.

The patient's condition worsened. Her respiratory insufficiency increased and she developed renal failure and disseminated intravascular coagulation (DIC). She was subsequently transferred to a tertiary care medical center.

Medical History

The patient had a childhood history of multiple episodes of bronchitis and middle ear infections (otitis media). In her late 20s, she developed sinusitis, frequent diarrhea, and a chronic productive cough. She had two bouts of pneumonia, one of which required hospitalization. One year before the current episode, the patient developed extreme difficulty in breathing when exercising. During the past year she lost almost 30 pounds and became so weak that she could no longer lead a normal life.

Family History

She had no family history of frequent infections, immunodeficiency, or autoimmune disorders.

Laboratory Data

On admission to the tertiary medical center, a blood count, serum protein, serum protein electrophoresis, immunoglobulin electrophoresis, stool culture, and ova and parasite examination were performed.

Assay	Patient's Results	Reference Range
Complete Blood Count		
Hemoglobin	9.8 g/dL	11.5-13.5 g/dL
Hematocrit	24%	34%-42%
Total leukocyte count	9.0×10^9/L	$4.5\text{-}9.0 \times 10^9$/L
Polymorphonuclear leukocytes	87%	40%-60%
Lymphocytes	13%	20%-40%
Absolute lymphocytes	1.17×10^9/L	$>1.1 \times 10^9$/L
Other Tests		
Stool culture	Normal biota (flora)	Normal biota (flora)
Ova and parasite examination	*Giardia lamblia*	Negative for all ova and parasites
Serum total protein	5.5 g/dL	
Immunoelectrophoresis		
IgM	0.7 g/L	0.6-2.5 g/L
IgG	2.2 g/L	6.8-15.5 g/L
IgA	Undetectable	0.7-3.0 g/L
Follow-Up		
CD4+	20%	35%-55%
CD8+	26%	18%-32%
Absolute CD4+ count	0.26×10^9/L	$>0.43 \times 10^9$/L

The patient was found to be anergic. Tetanus, rubella, and diphtheria titers were nonprotective, despite previous immunizations.

The patient was diagnosed with common variable immunodeficiency (CVID). She was treated with IV immunoglobulin monthly. She also received metronidazole for *Giardia lamblia* intestinal infection. After 1 year of Ig therapy, the patient gained weight and returned to a normal lifestyle.

Continued

ABO Blood Grouping (Forward Antigen Typing)

Principle

The ABO blood groups (A, B, AB, and O) represent the antigens expressed on the erythrocytes (red blood cells, RBCs) of each group.

Reagent typing sera contains specific antibodies to A antigen and B antigen. When an unknown patient's RBCs are mixed with known antibody A or antibody B, agglutination of the RBCs will occur if a specific antigen-antibody reaction occurs. This is called direct blood typing.

Agglutination Reactions		
Anti-A	Anti-B	Blood Group
Positive	Negative	A
Negative	Positive	B
Positive	Positive	AB
Negative	Negative	O

Refer to ⊖volve for the procedural protocol, sources of error, and clinical notes.

Serum Protein Electrophoresis

Principle

Serum protein electrophoresis is used to separate and quantitate serum proteins based on electrophoretic mobility on cellulose acetate (see Color Plate 3 and Fig. 11-2).

Proteins are large molecules composed of amino acids. Depending on electron distributions resulting from covalent or ionic bonding of structural subgroups, proteins have different electrical charges at a given pH. Based on electrical charge, serum proteins can be fractionated into five fractions: albumin, alpha-1 (α1), alpha-2 (α2), beta (β), and gamma (γ) proteins. For the following method, the pH is 8.8. After the proteins are separated, the plate is placed in a solution of sulfosalicylic acid and Ponceau S to stain the protein bands. The intensity of the stain for each band is related to protein concentration.

Results

The fastest moving band, and normally the most prominent, is the albumin band found closest to the anodic edge of the plate. The faint band next to this is alpha-1 globulin, followed by alpha-2, beta, and gamma globulins. Prealbumin is seldom visible with this system.

Reference Values

Each laboratory should establish its own range. The following reference values are for illustrative purposes only.

Protein Fraction	Concentration (g/dL)
Albumin	3.63-4.91
Alpha-1	0.11-0.35
Alpha-2	0.65-1.17
Beta	0.74-1.26
Gamma	0.58-1.74

Clinical Interpretation

Electrophoresis is used to identify the presence or absence of aberrant proteins and to determine when different groups of proteins are increased or decreased in serum or urine. It is frequently ordered to detect and identify monoclonal proteins—excessive production of one specific immunoglobulin. Protein and immunofixation electrophoresis are ordered to help detect, diagnose, and monitor the course and treatment of conditions associated with these abnormal proteins (e.g., multiple myeloma).

CHAPTER HIGHLIGHTS

- Foreign substances can be immunogenic if their membrane or molecular components contain structures (antigenic determinants or epitopes) recognized as foreign by the immune system. The normal immune system responds to foreignness by producing antibodies.
- Cellular antigens of importance to immunologists include MHC groups and HLAs, autoantigens, and blood group antigens. Some of these antigens (e.g., MHC) are more potent than others in provoking an immune response.
- Antigens are usually large organic molecules that are proteins or polysaccharides. Although large foreign molecules are better antigens, haptens can bind to larger carrier molecules and behave like antigens.
- Antibodies that are specific proteins are known as immunoglobulins. Many antibodies can be isolated in the

gamma globulin fraction of protein by electrophoretic separation. The primary function of an antibody in body defenses is to combine with antigen.

- Five distinct classes of immunoglobulin molecules are recognized—IgM, IgG, IgA, IgD, and IgE. Antibodies exhibit diversity among the different classes, suggesting different functions in addition to their primary function of antigen binding.
- A typical monomeric IgG molecule consists of three globular regions (two Fab regions and Fc portion) linked by a flexible hinge region.
- An antigenic determinant is the specific chemical determinant group or molecular configuration against which the immune response is directed. Because they are proteins, immunoglobulins can function as effective antigens when used to immunize mammals of a different species. When the resulting antiimmunoglobulins or antiglobulins are analyzed, three principal categories of antigenic determinants can be recognized—isotype, allotype, and idiotype.
- Production of antibodies is induced when the host's immune system comes into contact with a foreign antigenic substance and reacts to this antigenic stimulation. When an antigen is encountered initially, the cells of the immune system recognize the antigen as nonself and elicit an immune response or become tolerant of it. An immune reaction can be cell-mediated immunity (dependent on T cells and macrophages) or may involve the production of antibodies directed against the antigen.
- After a foreign antigen challenge, an IgM antibody response proceeds in four phases—lag, log, plateau, and decline. Subsequent exposure to the same antigenic stimulus produces an anamnestic (secondary) response, which exhibits the same four phases but differs from a primary response in time, type of antibody produced, and antibody titer.
- Specificity is the ability of a particular antibody to combine with one antigen instead of another.
- Affinity is the bonding strength between an antigenic determinant and antibody-combining site, whereas avidity is the strength with which a multivalent antibody binds a multivalent antigen.
- Agglutination and other tests (e.g., precipitation reactions, hemolysis testing, ELISA) are widely used in immunology to detect and measure the consequences of antigen-antibody interaction.
- Monoclonal antibodies (MAbs) are purified antibodies cloned from a single cell. MAbs bound to cell surface antigens now provide a method for classifying and identifying specific cellular membrane characteristics and leukocyte antigens.

REVIEW QUESTIONS

1. A synonym for an antigenic determinant is:
   a. Immunogen
   b. Epitope
   c. Binding site
   d. Polysaccharide

2. Genetically different individuals of the same species are referred to as:
   a. Allogenic
   b. Heterogenic
   c. Autogenic
   d. Isogenic

3. Antigenic substances can be composed of:
   a. Large polysaccharides
   b. Proteins
   c. Glycoproteins
   d. All of the above

4. Which of the following characteristics of an antigen is the least important?
   a. Foreignness
   b. Degradability
   c. Molecular weight
   d. Presence of large repeating polymers

5. The chemical composition of an antibody is:
   a. Protein
   b. Lipid
   c. Carbohydrate
   d. Any of the above

6-10. Match the following characteristics with the appropriate antibody class (use an answer only once).

6. __C__ IgM
7. __A__ IgG
8. __D__ IgA
9. __B__ IgE
10. __E__ IgD
   a. Highest in plasma or serum concentration in normal individuals
   b. Shortest half-life
   c. 19S
   d. Can exist as a dimer
   e. No known subclasses

11-15. Match the following characteristics with the appropriate antibody (use an answer only once).

11. __A__ IgG
12. __E__ IgM
13. __C__ IgA
14. __D__ IgD
15. __C__ IgE
   a. Predominant immunoglobulin in secretions
   b. Increased in infectious diseases, collagen disorders, and hematologic disorders
   c. Mediates some types of hypersensitivity reactions
   d. Primarily a cell membrane immunoglobulin
   e. Produced early in an immune response

16-18. Match each of the following antigenic determinant terms with its appropriate definition.

16. ___D___ Isotype
17. ___A___ Allotype
18. ___C___ Idiotype
    a. Found on the immunoglobulins of some, but not all, animals of a species
    b. Dominant type found on immunoglobulins of all animals of a species
    c. Individual determinants characteristic of each antibody

19-22. Arrange the sequence of events of a typical antibody response.

19. ___B___ C
20. ___C___ B
21. ___A___ A
22. ___D___ D
    a. Plateau
    b. Lag phase
    c. Log phase
    d. Decline

23. Which of the following statements is false about an anamnestic response versus a primary response?
    a. Has a shorter lag phase
    b. Has a longer plateau
    c. Antibodies decline more gradually.
    d. IgM antibodies predominate.

24. Which type of antibody is capable of placental transfer?
    a. IgM
    b. IgG
    c. IgA
    d. IgD

25-28. Match the following terms and their respective definitions.

25. ___C___ Specificity
26. ___A___ Affinity
27. ___D___ Avidity
28. ___B___ Immune complex
    a. Strength of a bond between a single antigenic determinant and an individual combining site
    b. Noncovalent combination of an antigen with its respective specific antibody
    c. Ability of an antibody to combine with one antigen instead of another
    d. Strength with which a multivalent antibody binds to a multivalent antigen

29. Which of the following type(s) of bonding is (are) involved in antigen-antibody reactions?
    a. Hydrophobic
    b. Hydrogen
    c. Van der Waals
    d. All of the above

30. Monovalent antibodies have also been referred to as:
    a. Complete antibodies
    b. Incomplete antibodies

31. Which of the following is an accurate statement about monoclonal antibodies (MAbs)?
    a. MAbs are antibodies engineered to bind to a single epitope.
    b. MAbs are purified antibodies cloned from a single cell.
    c. MAbs are used to classify and identify specific cellular membrane characteristics.
    d. All of the above are correct.

32. Antigens are characterized by all the following except that they:
    a. Are usually large organic molecules
    b. Are usually lipids
    c. Can be glycolipids or glycoproteins
    d. Are also called immunogens

33. The immunogenicity of an antigen depends greatly on:
    a. Its biochemical composition
    b. Being structurally unstable
    c. Its degree of foreignness
    d. Having a low molecular weight

34. Antibodies are also referred to as:
    a. Immunoglobulins
    b. Haptens
    c. Epitopes
    d. Gamma globulins

35-39. Match the following immunoglobulins with the appropriate description.

35. ___A___ IgM
36. ___E___ IgG
37. ___C___ IgA
38. ___B___ IgE
39. ___D___ IgD
    a. Accounts for 10% of Ig pool, largely confined to the intravascular space
    b. Mediates some types of hypersensitivity
    c. Found in tears, saliva, colostrum, milk, and intestinal secretions
    d. Makes up less than 1% of total immunoglobulins
    e. Diffuses more readily into extravascular spaces, neutralizes toxins, and binds to microorganisms

40 and 41. Label the components of the basic immunoglobulin (Ig) configuration in the following figure.

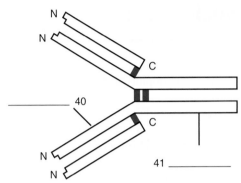

(Adapted from Turgeon ML: Fundamentals of immunohematology, ed 2, Baltimore, 1995, Williams & Wilkins.)

Possible answers for question 40:
a. Fc segment
b. Fab segment
c. Hinge region
d. Disulfide bond

Possible answers for question 41:
a. Fc segment
b. Fab segment
c. Hinge region
d. Disulfide bond

42. Which of the following statements about IgM is false?
a. Composed of five basic subunits
b. More efficient in the activation of the complement cascade and agglutination than IgG
c. Predominant in an initial antibody response
d. Predominant in a secondary (anamnestic) response

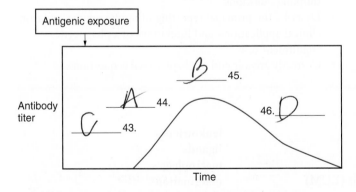

(Adapted from Turgeon ML: Fundamentals of immunohematology, ed 2, Baltimore, 1995, Williams & Wilkins.)

43-46. Label the four phases of an antibody response on the following figure, choosing from the following answers:
a. Log
b. Plateau
c. Lag
d. Decline

47. In a secondary (anamnestic) response, all the following characteristics are correct *except:*
a. IgG is the predominant antibody type
b. It has a shorter lag phase
c. The antibody titer is lower
d. It has a more gradual decline in antibody response

48. Bonding of antigen to antibody exists exclusively as:
a. Hydrogen bonding
b. Van der Waals forces
c. Electrostatic forces
d. Noncovalent bonding

49. The strongest bond of antigen and antibody chiefly results from the:
a. Type of bonding
b. Goodness of fit
c. Antibody type
d. Quantity of antibody

50. Monoclonal antibodies have all the following characteristics except:
a. Purified antibodies
b. Cloned from a single cell
c. Engineered to bind to a single specific antigen
d. Frequent occurrence in nature

BIBLIOGRAPHY

Abbas AK, Lichtman AH: Basic immunology: functions and disorders of the immune system, updated edition, ed 3, Philadelphia, 2011, Saunders.
Forbes BA, Sahm DF, Weissfeld AS: Bailey and Scott's diagnostic microbiology, ed 12, St Louis, 2007, Mosby.
McDougal JS, McDuffie FC: Immune complexes in man: detection and clinical significance, Adv Clin Chem 24:1–60, 1985.
Medzhitov R, Janeway C: Innate immunity, N Engl J Med 343:338–344, 2000.
Peakman M, Vergani D: Basic and clinical immunology, ed 2, London, 2009, Churchill Livingstone.
Ritzmann SE, editor: Physiology of immunoglobulins, New York, 1982, Alan R Liss.
Ritzmann SE, Daniels JC, editors: Serum protein abnormalities, Boston, 1985, Little, Brown.
Turgeon ML: Fundamentals of immunohematology, ed 2, Baltimore, 1995, Williams & Wilkins.

CHAPTER 3

Cells and Cellular Activities of the Immune System: Granulocytes and Mononuclear Cells

Learning Objectives

At the conclusion of this chapter, the reader should be able to:

- Describe the general functions of granulocytes, monocytes-macrophages, and lymphocytes and plasma cells as components of the immune system.
- Explain the process of phagocytosis.
- Describe the composition and function of neutrophil extracellular traps (NETs).
- Discuss the role of monocytes and macrophages in cellular immunity.
- Define and compare acute inflammation and sepsis.
- Briefly describe cell surface receptors.
- Name and compare the signs and symptoms of disorders of neutrophil function.

- Compare the signs and symptoms of two monocyte or macrophage disorders.
- Describe states involving the leukocyte integrins.
- Analyze case studies related to defects of neutrophils.
- Correctly answer case study related multiple choice questions.
- Be prepared to participate in a discussion of critical thinking questions.
- Describe the principal reporting of results, sources of error, clinical applications, and limitations of a phagocytic engulfment test.
- Correctly answer end of chapter review questions.

Key Terms

bacteremia
cell adhesion molecules (CAMs)
cell surface receptors
Chédiak-Higashi Syndrome
chemoattractant
chemokines
chemotaxis
chronic granulomatous disease (CGD)
complement receptor

diapedesis
endotoxin
exocytosis
extracellular matrix (ECM)
extravasation
exudate (pus)
Gaucher's disease
inflammation
interferon
leukocyte integrins

leukotrienes
ligands
macrophages
margination
neutrophil extracellular traps (NETs)
Niemann-Pick disease
opsonization
reactive oxygen species (ROS)
selectin
sepsis

Roxanne Serrano.

The entire leukocytic cell system is designed to defend the body against disease. Each cell type has a unique function and behaves independently and, in many cases, in cooperation with other cell types. Leukocytes can be functionally divided into the general categories of granulocyte, monocyte-macrophage, and lymphocyte–plasma cell. The primary phagocytic cells are the polymorphonuclear neutrophil (PMN) leukocytes and the mononuclear monocytes-macrophages. The response of the body to pathogens involves cross-talk among many immune cells, including **macrophages,** dendritic cells, and CD4 T cells (Fig. 3-1). The lymphocytes participate in body defenses primarily through the recognition of foreign antigens and production of antibody. Plasma cells are antibody-synthesizing cells.

ORIGIN AND DEVELOPMENT OF BLOOD CELLS

Embryonic blood cells, excluding the lymphocyte type of white blood cell (WBC), originate from the mesenchymal tissue that arises from the embryonic germ layer, the mesoderm. The sites of blood cell development, hematopoiesis, follow a definite sequence in the embryo and fetus:

1. The first blood cells are primitive red blood cells (RBCs; erythroblasts) formed in the islets of the yolk sac during the first 2 to 8 weeks of life.
2. Gradually, the liver and spleen replace the yolk sac as the sites of blood cell development. By the second month of gestation, the liver becomes the major site of hematopoiesis, and granular types of leukocytes have made their initial appearance. The liver and spleen predominate from about 2 to 5 months of fetal life.

3. In the fourth month of gestation, bone marrow begins to produce blood cells. After the fifth fetal month, bone marrow begins to assume its ultimate role as the primary site of hematopoiesis.

The cellular elements of the blood are produced from a common, multipotential, hematopoietic (blood-producing) cell, the stem cell. After stem cell differentiation, blast cells arise for each of the major categories of cell types—erythrocytes, megakaryocytes, granulocytes, monocytes-macrophages, lymphocytes, and plasma cells. Subsequent maturation of these cells will produce the major cellular elements of the circulating blood, the erythrocytes (RBCs), thrombocytes, and specific types of leukocytes (WBCs). In normal peripheral or circulating blood, the following types of leukocytes can be found, in order of frequency: neutrophils, lymphocytes, monocytes, eosinophils, and basophils.

GRANULOCYTIC CELLS ♡ *Eric Vela* ♡

Granulocytic leukocytes can be further subdivided on the basis of morphology into neutrophils, eosinophils, and basophils. Each of these begins as a multipotential stem cell in the bone marrow.

Neutrophils

Neutrophilic leukocytes, particularly the polymorphonuclear (PMN) type (see Color Plate 4), provide an effective host defense against bacterial and fungal infections. The antimicrobial function of PMNs is essential in the innate immune response. Although the monocytes-macrophages and other granulocytes are also phagocytic cells, the PMN is the principal leukocyte

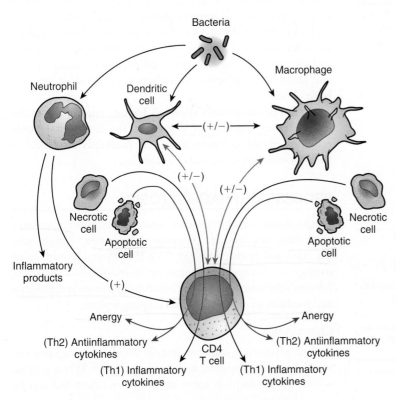

Figure 3-1 Response of pathogens, involving cross-talk among many immune cells, including macrophages, dendritic cells, and CD4 T cells. Macrophages and dendritic cells are activated by the ingestion of bacteria and by stimulation through cytokines (e.g., IFN-γ) secreted by CD4 T cells. Alternatively, CD4 T cells that have an antiinflammatory profile (type 2 helper T cell [Th2]) secrete IL-10, which suppresses macrophage activation. CD4 T cells become activated by stimulation through macrophages or dendritic cells. For example, macrophages and dendritic cells secrete IL-12, which activates CD4 T cells to secrete inflammatory (type 1 helper T cell [Th1]) cytokines. Depending on numerous factors (e.g., type of organism and site of infection), macrophages and dendritic cells respond by inducing inflammatory or antiinflammatory cytokines or causing a global reduction in cytokine production (anergy). Macrophages or dendritic cells that have previously ingested necrotic cells induce an inflammatory cytokine profile (Th1). Ingestion of apoptotic cells can induce an antiinflammatory cytokine profile or anergy. A plus sign indicates upregulation and a minus sign indicates downregulation; in cases in which both a plus sign and a minus sign appear, upregulation or downregulation may occur, depending on a variety of factors. *(Adapted from Hotchkiss RS, Karl IE: The pathophysiology and treatment of sepsis. N Engl J Med 348:138–150, 2003.)*

associated with phagocytosis and a localized inflammatory response. The formation of an inflammatory **exudate (pus)**, which develops rapidly in an inflammatory response, is composed primarily of neutrophils and monocytes.

PMNs can prolong **inflammation** by the release of soluble substances, such as cytokines and chemokines. The role of neutrophils in influencing the adaptive immune response is believed to include shuttling pathogens to draining lymph nodes, antigen presentation, and modulation of T helper types 1 and 2 responses. Functionality of neutrophils is no longer considered as limited as it once was because new research has discovered that PMNs have a 5.4 day lifespan.

Mature neutrophils are found in two evenly divided pools, the circulating and marginating pools. The marginating granulocytes adhere to the vascular endothelium. In the peripheral blood, these cells are only in transit to their potential sites of action in the tissues. Movement of granulocytes from the circulating pool to the peripheral tissues occurs by a process called **diapedesis** (movement through the vessel wall). Once in the peripheral tissues, the neutrophils are able to carry out their function of phagocytosis.

The granules of segmented neutrophils contain various antibacterial substances (Table 3-1). During the phagocytic process, the powerful antimicrobial enzymes that are released also disrupt the integrity of the cell itself. Neutrophils are also steadily lost to the respiratory, gastrointestinal (GI), and urinary systems, where they participate in generalized phagocytic activities. An alternate route for the removal of neutrophils from the circulation is phagocytosis by cells of the mononuclear phagocyte system.

Eosinophils and Basophils

Although capable of participating in phagocytosis, eosinophils and basophils possess less phagocytic activity. The ineffectiveness of these cells results from the small number of cells in the circulating blood and lack of powerful digestive enzymes. Both eosinophils and basophils, however, are functionally important in body defense.

Eosinophils

The eosinophil (see Color Plate 5) is considered to be a homeostatic regulator of inflammation. Functionally, this means that the eosinophil attempts to suppress an inflammatory reaction to prevent the excessive spread of the inflammation. The eosinophil may also play a role in the host defense mechanism because of its ability to kill certain parasites.

A functional property related to the membrane receptors of the eosinophil is the cell's ability to interact with the larval stages of some helminth parasites and damage them through oxidative mechanisms. Certain proteins released from eosinophilic granules damage antibody-coated *Schistosoma* parasites and may account for damage to endothelial cells in hypereosinophilic syndromes.

Basophils

Basophils (see Color Plate 6) have high concentrations of heparin and histamine in their granules, which play an important role in acute, systemic, hypersensitivity reactions (see Chapter 26). Degranulation occurs when an antigen such as pollen binds to two adjacent immunoglobulin E (IgE) antibody molecules located on the surface of mast cells. The events resulting from the release of the contents of these basophilic granules include increased vascular permeability, smooth muscle spasm, and vasodilation. If severe, this reaction can result in anaphylactic shock.

A class of compounds known as **leukotrienes** mediates the inflammatory functions of leukocytes. The observed systemic reactions related to leukotrienes were previously attributed to the slow-reacting substance of anaphylaxis.

PROCESS OF PHAGOCYTOSIS

Phagocytosis can be divided into six stages—chemotaxis, adherence, engulfment, phagosome formation, fusion, and digestion and destruction (Fig. 3-2). The physical occurrence of damage to tissues, by trauma or microbial multiplication, releases substances such as activated complement components and products of infection to initiate phagocytosis.

Chemotaxis

Various phagocytic cells continually circulate throughout the blood, lymph, GI system, and respiratory tract. When trauma occurs, the neutrophils arrive at the site of injury and can be

Table 3-1	**Function and Types of Granules in Neutrophils**	
Function	**Azurophilic (Primary) Granules**	**Specific (Secondary) Granules**
Microbicidal	Myeloperoxidase	Cytochrome b558 and other respiratory burst components
	Lysozyme	Lysozyme
	Elastase	Lactoferrin
	Defensins	
	Cathepsin G	
	Proteinase-3	
	Bacterial permeability-increasing protein (BPI)	
Cell migration		Collagenase
		CD11b–CD18 (CR-3)
		N-formulated peptides (e.g., *N*-formyl-methionyl-leucylphenylalanine receptor [FMLP-R])

Adapted from Peakman M, Vergani D: Basic and clinical immunology, ed 2, Edinburgh, 2009, Churchill Livingstone, p 24.

found in the initial exudate in less than 1 hour. Monocytes are slower in moving to the inflammatory site. Macrophages resident in the tissues of the body are already in place to deal with an intruding agent. Additional macrophages from the bone marrow and other tissues can be released in severe infections.

Recruitment of PMNs is an essential prerequisite in innate immune defense. Recruitment of PMNs consists of a cascade of events that allows for the capture, adhesion, and **extravasation** of the leukocyte. Activities such as rolling binding and diapedesis have been well characterized but receptor-mediated processes, mechanisms attenuating the electrostatic repulsion between the negatively charged glycocalyx of leukocytes and endothelium, are poorly understood. Research has demonstrated that myeloperoxidase (MPO), a PMN-derived heme protein, facilitates PMN recruitment becaue of its positive surface charge.

Neutrophils have been shown to activate complement when stimulated by cytokines or coagulation-derived factors. Neutrophils activate the alternative complement pathway and release C5 fragments, which further amplify neutrophil proinflammatory responses. This mechanism may be relevant to complement involvement in neutrophil-mediated diseases.

Segmented neutrophils are able to gather quickly at the site of injury because they are actively motile. The marginating pool of neutrophils, adhering to the endothelial lining of nearby blood vessels, migrates through the vessel wall to the interstitial tissues. Mediators produced by microorganisms and by cells participating in the inflammatory process include interleukin-1 (IL-1), which is released by macrophages in response to infection or tissue injury. Another is histamine, released by circulating basophils, tissue mast cells, and blood platelets. Mediators cause capillary and venular dilation.

Cells are guided to the site of injury by **chemoattractant** substances. This event is termed *chemotaxis.* A chemotactic response is defined as a change in the direction of movement of a motile cell in response to a concentration gradient of a specific chemical, chemotaxin. Chemotaxins can induce a positive movement toward and a negative movement away from a chemotactic response. Antigens function as chemoattractants; when antigenic material is present in the body, phagocytes are attracted to its source by moving up its concentration gradient.

Phagocytes detect antigens using various cell surface receptors. The speed of phagocytosis can be greatly increased by recruiting the following two attachment devices present on the surface of phagocytic cells:

- Fc receptor—binds the Fc portion of antibody molecules, chiefly immunoglobulin G (IgG). The IgG attaches to the organism through its Fab site.
- **Complement receptor**—the third component of complement, C3, also binds to organisms and then attaches to the complement receptor.

This coating of the organisms by molecules that speed up phagocytosis is termed *opsonization;* the Fc portions of antibody and C3 are called opsonins. The steps in opsonization are as follows:

1. Antibody attached to the surface of a bacterium minimally binds the Fc phagocyte receptor.
2. Complement C3b is attached to the surface of the bacterium and binds loosely to the phagocyte C3b receptor.
3. Both antibody and C3b are attached to the surface of the bacterium and bound tightly to the phagocyte, allowing greater opportunity for the phagocyte to engulf the bacterium.

Necrotic cells release an independent chemoattractant of necrotaxis signal, which directs PMN migration beyond the intravascular chemokine gradient. This intravascular danger sensing and recruitment mechanisms have evolved to limit the collateral damage during a response to sterile injury. In this process, PMNs are allowed to migrate intravascularly as they

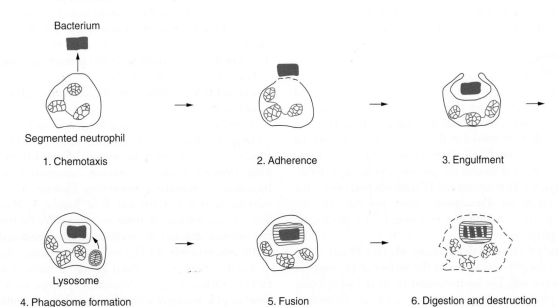

Bacterium

Segmented neutrophil

1. Chemotaxis   2. Adherence   3. Engulfment

Lysosome

4. Phagosome formation   5. Fusion   6. Digestion and destruction

Figure 3-2 **Process of phagocytosis.** *(Adapted from Turgeon ML: Clinical hematology: theory and procedures, ed 5, Philadelphia, 2012, Lippincott-Williams & Wilkins.)*

navigate through healthy tissue to sites of injury. Necrotaxis signals promote localization of neutrophils directly into existing areas of injury to focus the innate immune response on damaged areas and away from healthy tissue, which provides an additional safeguard against collateral damage during sterile inflammatory responses. The innate immune system can clean up the dead by killing the living.

Adherence

The leukocyte adhesion cascade is a sequence of adhesion and activation events that ends with the cell exerting its effects on the inflamed site (see later, "Acute Inflammation"). At least five steps appear to be necessary for effective leukocyte recruitment to the site of injury—capture, rolling, slow rolling, firm adhesion, and transmigration.

The process known as capture (tethering) represents the first contact of a leukocyte with the activated endothelium. Capture occurs after margination, which allows phagocytes to move in a position close to the endothelium. P-selectin on endothelial cells is the primary adhesion molecule for capture and the initiation of rolling. Functional E-selectin ligands include CD44.

In addition, many studies have suggested that L-selectin also has an important role in capture. Other **cell adhesion molecules (CAMs)** have been implicated in capture (e.g., PECAM-1, ICAM-1, VE-cadherin, LFA-1 [CD11a/CD18], IAP [CD47], VLA-4 [$4\beta_1$–integrin]), although their level of actual involvement varies.

The inflammatory response begins with a release of inflammatory chemicals into the extracellular fluid. Sources of these inflammatory mediators, the most important of which are histamine, prostaglandins, and cytokines, are injured tissue cells, lymphocytes, mast cells, and blood proteins. The presence of these chemicals promotes the reactions to inflammation (redness, heat, swelling, pain).

The transit time through the microcirculation and, more specifically, the contact time during which the leukocyte is close to the endothelium, appears to be a key parameter in determining the success of the recruitment process, as reflected in firm adhesion.

Engulfment

On reaching the site of infection, phagocytes engulf and destroy the foreign matter (Fig. 3-3). Eosinophils can also undergo this process, except that they kill parasites. After the phagocytic cells have arrived at the site of injury, the bacteria can be engulfed through active membrane invagination. Pseudopodia are extended around the pathogen, pulled by interactions between the Fc receptors and Fc antibody portions on the opsonized bacterium. Pseudopodia meet and fuse, thereby internalizing the bacterium and enclosing it in a phagocytic vacuole, or phagosome.

The principal factor in determining whether phagocytosis can occur is the physical nature of the surface of the bacteria and phagocytic cell. The bacteria must be more hydrophobic than the phagocyte. Some bacteria, such as *Diplococcus pneumoniae*, possess a hydrophilic capsule and are not normally phagocytized. Most nonpathogenic bacteria are easily

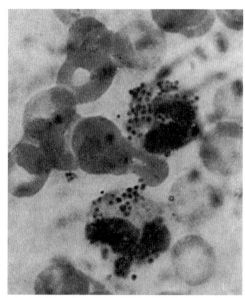

Figure 3-3 Two phagocytic cells have engulfed numerous *Staphylococcus aureus* cells. *(From Barrett JT: Textbook of immunology, ed 5, St Louis, 1988, Mosby.)*

phagocytized because they are very hydrophobic. The presence of certain soluble factors such as complement, a plasma protein, coupled with antibodies and chemicals such as acetylcholine enhance the phagocytic process. Enhancement of phagocytosis through opsonization can speed up the ingestion of particles. If the surface tensions are conducive to engulfment, the phagocytic cell membrane invaginates. This invagination leads to the formation of an isolated vacuole (phagosome) within the cell.

Digestion

Digestion follows the ingestion of particles, with the required energy primarily provided by anaerobic glycolysis. Granules in the phagocyte cytosol then migrate to and fuse with the phagosome to form the phagolysosome. These granules contain degradatory enzymes of the following three types:

1. Primary, or azurophilic, granules containing enzymes (e.g., lysozyme, myeloperoxidase)
2. Secondary, or specific, granules containing substances such as lactoferrin
3. Tertiary granules containing substances such as caspases

Degranulation of the neutrophil releases antibacterial substances (e.g., lactoferrin, lysozyme, defensin) from the granules; released enzymes promote bactericidal activity by increasing membrane permeability. Elastase, one of several substances that can damage host tissues, is also released. The myeloperoxidase granules are responsible for the action of the oxygen-dependent, myeloperoxidase-mediated system. Hydrogen peroxide (H_2O_2) and an oxidizable cofactor serve as major factors in the actual killing of bacteria within the vacuole. Other oxygen-independent systems, such as alterations in pH, lysozymes, lactoferrin, and the granular cationic proteins, also participate in the bactericidal process. Monocytes are particularly effective as phagocytic cells because of the large amounts of lipase in their cytoplasm. Lipase is able to attack bacteria with a lipid capsule, such as *Mycobacterium tuberculosis*. Monocytes are further able to bind and destroy cells coated with complement-fixing antibodies because of the presence of membrane receptors for specific components or types of immunoglobulin.

Release of lytic enzymes results in the destruction of neutrophils and their subsequent phagocytosis by macrophages. Macrophage digestion proceeds without risk to the cell unless the ingested material is toxic. If the ingested material damages the lysosomal membrane, however, the macrophage will also be destroyed because of the release of lysosomal enzymes.

During phagocytosis, cells demonstrate increased metabolic activity, referred to as a respiratory burst. This results in the production by the phagocyte of large quantities of **reactive oxygen species (ROS),** which are released into the phagocytic vesicle. This phenomenon is achieved by the activity of the enzyme known as reduced nicotinamide-adenine dinucleotide phosphate (NADPH) oxidase. Together, the granule-mediated and NADPH oxidase–mediated effects elicit microbicidal results. NADPH oxidase forms the centerpiece of the phagocyte-killing mechanism and is activated in about 2 seconds. The NADPH oxidase generates ROS by generating the superoxide radical (O_2^-); the associated cyanide-insensitive increase in oxygen consumption is the respiratory burst.

The importance of the oxygen-dependent microbicidal mechanism is dramatically illustrated by patients with chronic granulomatous disease (CGD), a severe congenital deficit in bacterial killing that results from the inability to generate phagocyte-derived superoxide and related reactive oxygen intermediates (ROIs). The production of residual ROIs is predicted by the specific NADPH oxidase mutation, regardless of the specific gene affected. CGD results from defects in the genes encoding individual components of the enzyme system responsible for oxidant production. Acquisition of oxidase activity occurs in the course of myeloid cell maturation, and the genes for several of its components have been identified. This system also lends itself to analysis of the transcriptional and translational events that occur during cellular differentiation and under the influence of specific cytokines.

Rather than being discarded by **exocytosis,** some peptides undergo an important separate process at this stage. Instead of being eliminated, they attach to a host molecule called major histocompatibility complex (MHC) class II and are expressed on the surface of the cell within a groove on the MHC molecule (antigen presentation).

Subsequent Phagocytic Activity

If invading bacteria are not phagocytized at entry into the body, they may establish themselves in secondary sites such as the lymph nodes or various body organs. These undigested bacteria produce a secondary inflammation, where neutrophils and macrophages again congregate. If bacteria escape from secondary tissue sites, a **bacteremia** will develop. In patients who are unresponsive to antibiotic intervention, this situation can prove fatal.

Neutrophil Extracellular Traps

In addition to phagocytosis, including the release of antimicrobial molecules at the site of infection, an additional defense mechanism has been discovered. This mechanism is the formation of **neutrophil extracellular traps (NETs),** which are produced following the release of the nuclear contents of the neutrophil into the extracellular space. NETs function in innate immunity. They are composed of chromatin components, including histones, and neutrophil antimicrobial proteins. Microbes are trapped in NETs, where they encounter high concentrations of antimicrobial proteins.

MONOCYTES-MACROPHAGES

In the past, the mononuclear monocyte-macrophage was known only as a scavenger cell. Only recently has its role as a complex cell of the immune system in the host defense against infection been recognized.

Mononuclear Phagocyte System

The macrophage (Fig. 3-4) and its precursors are widely distributed throughout the body. These cells constitute a physiologic system, the mononuclear phagocyte system (previously referred to as the reticuloendothelial system), which includes promonocytes and their precursors in the bone marrow, monocytes in the circulating blood, and macrophages in tissues. This collection of cells is considered to be a system because of the common origin, similar morphology, and shared functions, including rapid phagocytosis mediated by receptors for IgG and the major fragment of C3.

Macrophages and monocytes (see Color Plate 7) migrate freely into the tissues from the blood to replenish and reinforce the macrophage population. Cells of the macrophage system originate in the bone marrow from the multipotential stem cell. This common committed progenitor cell can differentiate into the granulocyte or monocyte-macrophage pathway, depending on the microenvironment and chemical regulators. Maturation and differentiation of these cells may occur in various directions. Circulating monocytes may continue to be multipotential and give rise to different types of macrophages.

Macrophages exist as fixed or wandering cells. Specialized macrophages such as the pulmonary alveolar macrophages are the so-called dust phagocytes of the lung that function as the first line of defense against inhaled foreign particles and bacteria. Fixed macrophages line the endothelium of capillaries and the sinuses of organs such as the bone marrow, spleen, and lymph nodes. Macrophages, along with the network of reticular cells of the spleen, thymus, and other lymphoid tissues, are organized into the mononuclear phagocyte system (Fig. 3-5).

Functionally, the most important step in the maturation of macrophages is the cytokine-driven conversion of the normal resting macrophage to the activated macrophage. Macrophages can be activated during infection by the release of macrophage-activating cytokines such as interferon-gamma (IFN-γ) and granulocyte colony-stimulating factor (G-CSF)

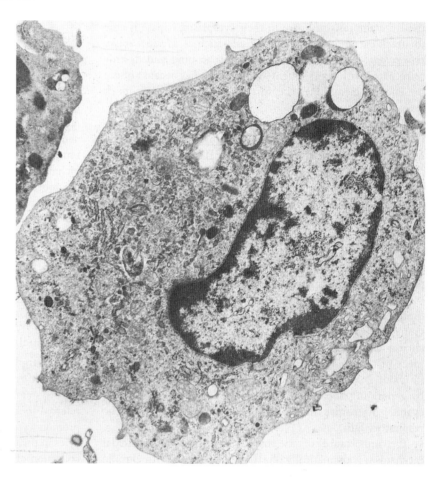

Figure 3-4 Electron micrograph of a macrophage. *(From Barrett JT: Textbook of immunology, ed 5, St Louis, 1988, Mosby.)*

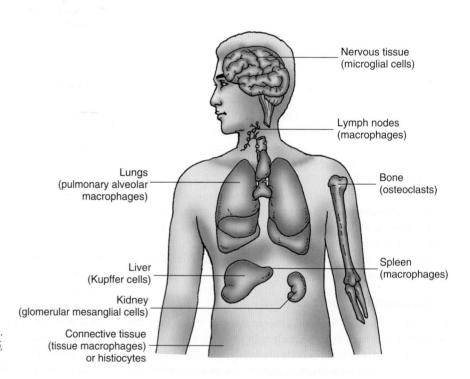

Figure 3-5   Mononuclear phagocyte system. *(Adapted from Roitt IM: Essential immunology, ed 5, Oxford, 1984, Blackwell Scientific.)*

Nervous tissue (microglial cells)

Lymph nodes (macrophages)

Bone (osteoclasts)

Spleen (macrophages)

Lungs (pulmonary alveolar macrophages)

Liver (Kupffer cells)

Kidney (glomerular mesanglial cells)

Connective tissue (tissue macrophages) or histiocytes

from T lymphocytes specifically sensitized to antigens from the infecting microorganisms. This interaction constitutes the basis of cell-mediated immunity. In addition, macrophages exposed to an **endotoxin** release a hormone, tumor necrosis factor α (TNF-α, cachectin), which can activate macrophages itself under certain in vitro conditions.

The terminal stage of development in the mononuclear phagocyte cell line is the multinucleated giant cell, which characterizes granulomatous inflammatory diseases such as tuberculosis. Both monocytes and macrophages can be shown in the lesions in these diseases before the formation of giant cells, thought to be precursors of the multinucleated cells.

Host Defense Functions

Functionally, monocytes-macrophages have phagocytosis as their major role, but these cells perform at least three distinct but interrelated functions in host defense. The categories of host defense functions of monocytes-macrophages include phagocytosis, antigen presentation and induction of the immune response, and secretion of biologically active molecules.

Phagocytosis

The principal functions of mononuclear phagocytes in body defenses result from the changes that take place in these functions when the macrophage is activated (Box 3-1). Macrophages carry out the fundamental function of ingesting and killing invading microorganisms such as intracellular parasites, *M. tuberculosis,* and some fungi. In addition, macrophages remove and eliminate such extracellular pathogens as pneumococci from the blood circulation. The macrophage also has the capacity to phagocytize particulate and aggregated soluble materials. This process is enhanced by the presence of receptors on the surface of the Fc portion of IgG and C3. The ability to internalize soluble substances supports the increased microbicidal and tumoricidal ability of activated macrophages. Activation of macrophages or monocytes can result in the release of parasiticidal mediators and in receptor-mediate phagocytosis during malaria infection. The most likely location for this innate immune response is within the spleen which is crucial for development of immunity to malaria.

Another important phagocytic function of macrophages is their ability to dispose of damaged or dying cells. Macrophages lining the sinusoids of the spleen are particularly important in ingesting aging erythrocytes. They are also involved in removing tissue debris, repairing wounds, and removing debris as embryonic tissues replace one another.

Phagocytic activity increases when there is tissue damage and inflammation, which releases substances that attract macrophages. Activated macrophages migrate more vigorously in response to chemotactic factors and should enter sites of inflammation (e.g., locations of infection or cancer) more efficiently than resting macrophages. Migration of monocytes into different body tissues appears to be a random phenomenon in the absence of localized inflammation. An essential factor in the protective function of monocytes is the capacity of the cell

Box 3-1	**Functions of Mononuclear Phagocytes**

Increased Activity in Activated Macrophages
Antigen presentation
Chemotaxis
Glucose transport and metabolism
Microbicidal activity
Phagocytosis (variable activity, depending on particle)
Phagocytosis-associated respiratory burst
Pinocytosis
Tumoricidal activity

Increased Constituents in Activated Macrophages
Acid hydrolases
Angiogenesis factor
Arginase
Collagenase
Complement components*
Cytolytic proteinase
Fibronectin
Interleukin-1
Interferon (α and β)
Plasminogen activator
TNF-α (cachectin)†

Decreased Constituents in Activated Macrophages
Apolipoprotein E and lipoprotein lipase
Elastase
Prostaglandins, leukotrienes

Constituent Demonstrating No Change in Activated Macrophages
Lysoenzyme

Adapted from Johnston RB: Current concepts: immunology. Monocytes and macrophages, N Engl J Med 318:747–752, 1988.
*Increased or no change.
†When stimulated.

to move through the endothelial wall of blood vessels (diapedesis) to the site of microbial invasion in tissues. The attracting forces for monocytes, chemotactic factors, include complement products and chemoattractants derived from neutrophils, lymphocytes, or cancer cells.

The activity of mononuclear phagocytes against cancer cells in humans is less well understood than the phagocytosis of microorganisms. Phagocytes are thought to suppress the growth of spontaneously arising tumors. The ability of these cells to control malignant cells may not involve phagocytosis but may be related to secreted cellular products such as lysosomal enzymes, oxygen metabolites (e.g., H_2O_2), proteinases, and TNF-α (cachectin). The proteolytic enzymes present on the surface membrane of monocytes also may play a role in tumor rejection.

Antigen Presentation and Induction of the Immune Response

The phagocytic property of the macrophage is particularly important in the processing of antigens as part of the immune response. Macrophages are believed to process antigens and physically present this biochemically modified and more reactive form of antigen to lymphocytes (particularly helper T cells) as an initial step in the immune response. Recognition of

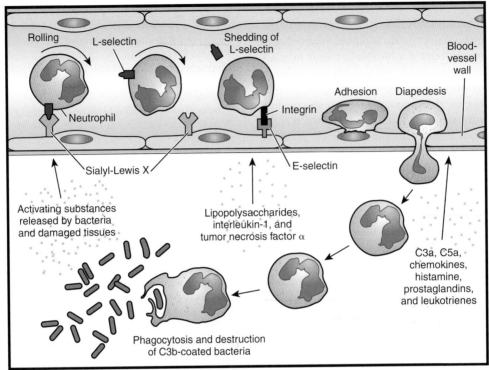

Figure 3-6   Acute inflammatory response. Neutrophils are among the first cells to arrive at the scene of an infection and are important contributors to the acute inflammatory response. As the neutrophil rolls along the blood vessel wall, the L-selectin on its surface binds to carbohydrate structures such as sialyl-Lewis X on the adhesion molecules on the vascular endothelium, and its progress is eventually halted. As the neutrophil becomes activated, it replaces L-selectin with other cell surface adhesion molecules, such as integrins. These molecules bind E-selectin, which is present on the blood vessel wall as a result of the influence of inflammatory mediators such as bacterial lipopolysaccharides and the cytokines IL-1 and TNF-α. The activated neutrophil then enters the tissues, where it is attracted to the infection site by a number of chemoattractants. The neutrophil can then phagocytose and destroy the C3b-coated bacteria. *(Adapted from Delves PJ, Roitt IM: The immune system. First of two parts, N Engl J Med 343:37–49, 2000.)*

antigen on the macrophage surface by T lymphocytes, however, requires an additional match of the surface MHC class II gene product. This gene product is the Ia product in the mouse and D gene region product in humans. With proper recognition, the macrophage secretes a lymphocyte-activating factor (IL-1), lymphocyte proliferation ensues, and the immune response (T cell–B cell response) is facilitated.

Secretion of Biologically Active Molecules

Monocytes-macrophages release many factors associated with host defense and inflammation. These cells serve as supportive accessory cells to lymphocytes, at least partly by releasing soluble factors. In cellular immunity, monocytes assume a killer role in that they are activated by sensitized lymphocytes to phagocytize offending cells or antigen particles. This is important in fields such as tumor immunology.

In addition to their phagocytic properties, monocytes-macrophages are able to synthesize a number of biologically important compounds, including transferrin, complement, **interferon,** pyrogens, and certain growth factors. Approximately 100 distinct substances have been identified as being secreted by monocytes-macrophages.

Blood monocytes and tissue macrophages are primary sources of the polypeptide hormone called IL-1, which has a particularly potent effect on the inflammatory response.

IL-1 also supports B lymphocyte proliferation and antibody production, as well as T lymphocyte production of lymphokines. The increased synthesis of IL-1 by activated macrophages could contribute to enhancement of the immune response. Endotoxin also induces the synthesis of IL-1. This effect is achieved at least partly by stimulation of the macrophages to release TNF-α, which then stimulates the production of IL-1 by endothelial cells and macrophages. Activated macrophages release much more TNF-α than resting macrophages exposed to endotoxin. Both TNF-α and IL-1 can induce the fever and synthesis of acute-phase reactants that characterize inflammation.

ACUTE INFLAMMATION

Tissue damage results in inflammation, a series of biochemical and cellular changes that facilitate the phagocytosis of invading microorganisms or damaged cells (Fig. 3-6). If inflammation is sufficiently extensive, it is accompanied by an increase in the plasma concentration of acute-phase reactants (see Chapter 5). Leukocyte recruitment into inflamed tissue follows a well-defined cascade of events beginning with the capture of free-flowing WBCs to the vessel wall and subsequent leukocyte rolling along and adhesion to the inflamed endothelial layer. During rolling, WBCs come into close contact with the endothelial surface, which allows endothelium-bound chemokines to interact with their specific receptors on the leukocyte surface. This triggers the activation of integrins, which leads to firm leukocyte arrest on the endothelium. In addition, integrin-dependent signaling events induce cytoskeletal rearrangements and cell polarization, modifications necessary to help prepare the attached leukocyte to spread and crawl in search for a way out of the vasculature into tissue.

Celsus, a practitioner of Greek medicine who was born in 25 BCE, is credited with recording the cardinal signs of inflammation—rubor (redness), calor (heat), dolor (pain), and tumor (swelling). The primary objective of inflammation is to localize and eradicate the irritant and repair the surrounding tissue. The inflammatory response involves the following three major stages:

1. Dilation of capillaries to increase blood flow
2. Microvascular structural changes and escape of plasma proteins from the bloodstream
3. Leukocyte transmigration through endothelium and accumulation at the site of injury

Hypoxia can induce inflammation. Inflammation in response to hypoxia is clinically relevant. Ischemia in organ grafts increases the risk of inflammation and graft failure or rejection. Hypoxia has multiple effects on the innate and adaptive immune systems.

Once inflammation is triggered, it must be appropriately resolved or pathologic tissue damage will occur. In some diseases, the body's defense system (immune system) inappropriately triggers an inflammatory response when no foreign substances are present. In these autoimmune disorders, the body's normally protective immune system causes damage to its own tissues (see Chapter 28).

SEPSIS

If an inflammation overwhelms the whole body, systemic inflammatory response syndrome (SIRS) is diagnosed. Sepsis, severe sepsis, and septic shock are progressively severe stages of SIRS. The criteria for SIRS require two or more conditions: alteration of body temperature ($>38°C$ or $<36°C$), increased heart rate, increased respiratory rate, and a total leukocyte count of $>12.0 \times 10(9)/L$ (or $>10\%$ immature forms). Sepsis is defined as SIRS + infection; severe sepsis is defined as sepsis + evidence of organ dysfunction. Patients with severe sepsis are considered to have defective adaptive immunity.

Sepsis begins when the innate immune system responds aggressively to the presence of bacteria. Toll-like receptors (TLR) cause the antigen presenting cell (APC) to produce proinflammatory cytokines. Biochemical markers associated with sepsis include tumor necrosis factor (TNF) and interleukins (ILs) IL-1 and IL-6, a proinflammatory cytokine. Other proteins produced in response infection and/or inflammation include procalcitonin and chemokine production. Another consequence of inflammation is that the liver is stimulated to produce C-reactive protein (C-RP) (see Chapter 5).

These cytokines produce systemic inflammation by activating circulating polymorphonuclear leukocytes (PMNs). APCs involve the adaptive immune system by presenting bacterial antigen to T-cell receptor using a Class II major histocompatibility complex (MHC) protein and co-stimulation of CD28.

CELL SURFACE RECEPTORS

Cellular communication is essential to the development, tissue organization, and function of all multicellular organisms. Cells communicate with each other and their environment through soluble mediators and during direct contact (e.g., phagocytosis). An immunologic response is a result of the interactions of various leukocytes with each other and other cells in the body. These interactions occur through **cell surface receptors** that mediate cell-cell binding, or adhesion, of leukocytes.

The discovery of several cell surface receptors involved in cellular communication has been a key factor in understanding the mechanisms underlying inflammatory and immune phenomena. Three protein families—the immunoglobulin (Ig) family, integrin family, and the rather recently designated **selectin** family—form a network of cellular interactions in the immune system. Neutrophil tether to and roll on P- and E-selectin expressed on activated endothelial cells. Rolling neutrophils encounter immobilized chemokines. **Chemokines** activate integrins to their high-affinity states that enable interactions with intercellular adhesion molecule-1 (ICAM-1), which promote arrest, adhesion strengthening, intraluminal crawling, and transendothelial migration. E-selectin directly triggers signals in rolling PMN that cooperate with chemokine signals to minimize neutrophil recruitment during inflammation.

Members of the Ig superfamily include antigen-specific receptors (e.g., T cell receptor [TCR] and surface immunoglobulin [sIg]), as well as antigen-independent receptors and their counterreceptors, such as CD2 and lymphocyte function–associated antigen-3. Ig superfamily members function in cell activation, differentiation, and cell-cell interaction. In some cases, both an adhesion receptor and the counterreceptor to which it binds are members of the Ig superfamily.

Three selectin family molecules—endothelial cell adhesion molecule-1, leukocyte adhesion molecule (LAM-1, Mel-14), and CD62, also known as platelet activation–dependent granule–external membrane protein and granule membrane protein of 140 kDa (GMP-140)—have been implicated in a number of leukocyte adhesion phenomena, including leukocyte homing to lymphoid tissue. Selectins are expressed on leukocytes and endothelial cells. Mel-14 functions early in neutrophil-endothelium adhesion.

The integrin family consists of at least 14 alpha-beta heterodimers divided into subfamilies with distinct structural and functional characteristics. The subfamily of **leukocyte integrins** contains three members—LFA-1, Mac-1, and p150,95. These molecules are glycoproteins composed of noncovalently associated alpha and beta subunits. LFA-1 is expressed on all leukocytes, whereas Mac-1 and p150,95 are found primarily on granulocytes and monocytes.

The integrin family is phylogenetically ancient. Integrin family members engage in interactions with cell surface ligands and **extracellular matrix (ECM)** components. ECM components, including fibronectin, collagen, and laminin, have been shown to be ligands for members of the beta-1 and beta-3 subfamilies. Members of these subfamilies are of great significance in embryogenesis, growth and repair, and hemostasis. The leukocyte integrins, or beta-2 subfamily, have been shown to be involved in a diverse number of leukocyte adhesion–dependent phenomena, giving them a critical role in inflammatory and immune responses. The term *integrin* was initially used to emphasize that these receptors integrate signals from the extracellular environment with the intracellular cytoskeleton. A signal is transduced from outside to inside the cell.

In addition to the involvement of these receptors in a variety of immune functions, integrin molecules play a role in the spread of malignant cells. The major cause of death in malignant disease is not the primary tumor but rather the metastasis of tumor cells to distant sites within the body. Metastasis is a complex multistep process that begins with the detachment of a few tumor cells from the primary tumor. The tumor cells then move into the circulatory system, where they can be transported to other organs. While in the circulatory system, tumor cells must survive the natural defense system of the body before attaching to and invading the tissues of another organ. A better understanding of the metastatic process could provide the basis for diagnostic and therapeutic strategies.

DISORDERS OF NEUTROPHILS

Noninfectious Neutrophil-Mediated Inflammatory Disease

Although neutrophils provide the major means of defense against bacterial and fungal infections, they can also be destructive to host tissues. The same oxidative and nonoxidative processes that destroy microorganisms can affect adjacent host tissues. A number of disease states correspond to inappropriate phagocytosis (Box 3-2), as with prolonged activation of NADPH oxidase. This process occurs when phagocytes attempt to engulf particles that are too large. The phagocyte releases oxygen radicals and granule contents onto the particle, but these escape into the surrounding tissues, generating tissue damage. This is often observed in response to dust inhalation and smoking (e.g., nicotine) and in persistent infections such as cystic fibrosis. In addition, many autoimmune diseases are thought to be caused by inappropriate activation of the process of phagocytosis, whereby the body attacks its own cells and tissues. Examples include rheumatoid arthritis, multiple sclerosis, and Graves' disease.

Abnormal Neutrophil Function

Patients with quantitative or qualitative defects of neutrophils have a high rate of infection, which illustrates the importance of the neutrophil to body defenses. Individuals with a marked decrease of neutrophils (neutropenia) or severe defects in neutrophil function frequently have recurrent systemic bacterial infections (e.g., pneumonia), disseminated cutaneous pyogenic lesions, and other types of life-threatening bacterial and fungal infections.

Leukocyte mobility may be impaired in some diseases (e.g., rheumatoid arthritis, cirrhosis, CGD). Defective locomotion

or leukocyte immobility can also be seen in patients receiving steroids and in those with lazy leukocyte syndrome. A marked defect in the cellular response to chemotaxis, an important step in phagocytosis, can be seen in patients with diabetes mellitus, Chédiak-Higashi anomaly (syndrome), or sepsis, as well as in those with high levels of antibody immunoglobulin E (IgE), as in Job's syndrome.

Congenital Neutrophil Abnormalities

A small number of patients have congenital abnormalities of neutrophil structure and function (Box 3-3).

Chédiak-Higashi Syndrome

The **Chédiak-Higashi syndrome** represents a qualitative disorder of neutrophils. It is a rare familial disorder inherited as an autosomal recessive trait and expressed as an abnormal granulation of neutrophils. Neutrophils having giant granules display impaired chemotaxis and delayed killing of ingested bacteria.

Chronic Granulomatous Disease

The **chronic granulomatous diseases (CGDs)** are a genetically heterogeneous group of disorders of oxidative metabolism affecting the cascade of events required for H_2O_2 production by phagocytes. Patients with X-linked CGD (X-CGD) have a mutation in CYBB encoding the transmembrane gp91^{phox} subunit of phagocyte NADPH oxidase

Box 3-2	Noninfectious Neutrophil-Mediated Diseases*

Autoimmune arthritides
Autoimmune vasculitis
Dermatophytic disorders
    Autoimmune bullous dermatoses
    Behçet's disease
    Psoriasiform dermatoses
    Pyoderma gangrenosum
    Sweet's syndrome
Glomerulonephritis
Gout
Inflammatory bowel disease
Malignant neoplasms at site of chronic inflammation
Myocardial infarction
Respiratory disorders
    Adult respiratory distress syndrome
    Asthma and allergic asthma
    Emphysema

*Signs, symptoms, and injury may be partly mediated by neutrophils.

Box 3-3	Congenital Neutrophil Abnormalities

Chédiak-Higashi syndrome (anomaly)
Chronic granulomatous disease (CGD)
Complement receptor 3 (CR3) deficiency
Myeloperoxidase deficiency
Specific granule deficiency

required for microbicidal ROS production by neutrophils and monocytes. As a result, patients have life-threatening infections and granulomatous complications. If a suitable hematopoietic stem cell donor is available, it can cure X-CGD, but graft-versus-host disease (see Chapter 31) is a significant risk.

A number of types of inheritance of the disorder have been described, including sex-linked (X chromosome–linked) in 66%, autosomal recessive in 34%, and autosomal dominant in less than 1% of cases. Patients with the autosomal recessive form may have a less severe clinical course than patients with the X-linked form. CGD is a defect of neutrophil microbicidal ROS generation resulting from gp91phox deficiency. CGD is caused by a missense, nonsense, frameshift, splice, or deletion mutation in the genes for p22 phox, p40 phox, p47 phox, p67 phox (autosomal CGD), or gy91phox (X-linked CGD), which results in variable production of neutrophil-derived ROIs.

The onset of CGD is during infancy, with one third of patients dying before the age of 7 years because of infections. It was observed that in the presence of normal or elevated leukocyte counts, the neutrophilic granulocytes in vitro ingested and destroyed only streptococci, not staphylococci. Subsequent testing revealed that cells from patients with CGD can phagocytize non–H_2O_2-producing bacteria such as *Staphylococcus aureus* and gram-negative rods (e.g., Enterobacteriaceae), but cannot destroy them. In the X-linked form, the defective leukocytes fail to exhibit increased anaerobic metabolism during phagocytosis because of a cytochrome b558 deficiency (which expresses itself as a defect in the 91,000-Da glycoprotein membrane anchor of the cytochrome complex), or these defective leukocytes produce H_2O_2 because of a myeloperoxidase deficiency.

Patients with CGD have infections with catalase-positive bacteria and fungi affecting the skin, lungs, liver, and bones. They also develop granulomas, resulting from a lack of resolution of inflammatory foci, even after the infection has been eliminated. This leads to extensive granuloma formation and, in some circumstances, impairment of physiologic processes (e.g., obstruction of the esophagus or urinary tract).

Laboratory evaluation of CGD begins with non-specific testing to rule out other disorders. These assays include serum quantitative immunoglobulin, complement activity enzyme immunoassay, CBC with differential, myeloperoxidase stain and a neutrophil receptor profile. The evaluation of neutrophil phagocytic function is best determined by the neutrophil oxidative burst assay (DHR) via flow cytometry (see Appendix C) that can indicate CGD by the absence or significant alteration of activity. Other, less-reliable tests include measurement of superoxide production, ferrocytochrome reduction, and the classic nitroblue tetrazolium test (NBT).

Complement Receptor 3 Deficiency

The complement receptor 3 (CR3) deficiency is a rare condition inherited as an autosomal recessive trait. A deficiency of CR3 on phagocytic cells presents as a leukocyte adhesion deficiency. Leukocyte adhesion deficiency type 1 (LAD-1) is caused by a deficiency of CD18. LAD-2 is caused by the absence of sialyl–Lewis X (CD15s) blood group antigen.

A CR3 deficiency in neutrophils is associated with marked abnormalities of adherence-related functions, including decreased aggregation of neutrophils to each other after activation, decreased adherence of neutrophils to endothelial cells, poor adherence and phagocytosis of opsonized microorganisms, defective spreading, and decreased diapedesis and chemotaxis. Patients may also lack an intravascular marginating pool of neutrophils. Defects in T lymphocytes are characterized by faulty lymphocyte-mediated cytotoxicity, with poor adherence to target cells. Abnormalities of B lymphocytes have also been observed.

Clinically, a deficiency can manifest as delayed separation of the umbilical cord. Other signs and symptoms include early onset of bacterial infections, including skin infections, mucositis, otitis, gingivitis, and periodontitis. A depressed inflammatory response and neutrophilia can be observed.

Myeloperoxidase Deficiency

A deficiency of myeloperoxidase is inherited as an autosomal recessive trait on chromosome 17. Myeloperoxidase is an iron-containing heme protein responsible for the peroxidase activity characteristic of azurophilic granules; it accounts for the greenish color of pus. Human neutrophils contain many granules of various sizes that are morphologically, biochemically, and functionally distinct. The azurophilic granules normally contain myeloperoxidase. In this disorder, azurophilic granules are present, but myeloperoxidase is decreased or absent. If phagocytes are deficient in myeloperoxidase, the patient's phagocytes manifest a mild to moderate defect in bacterial killing and a marked defect in fungal killing in vitro.

Persons with a myeloperoxidase deficiency are generally healthy and do not have an increased frequency of infection, probably because of other microbicidal mechanisms compensating for the deficiency. Patients with diabetes and myeloperoxidase deficiency, however, may have deep fungal infections caused by *Candida* spp.

Specific Granule Deficiency

Specific granule deficiency is believed to be an autosomal recessive disease. It is caused by a failure to synthesize specific granules and some contents of other granules during differentiation of neutrophils in the bone marrow. Patients with specific granule deficiency have recurrent, severe bacterial infections of the skin and deep tissues, with a depressed inflammatory response.

MONOCYTE-MACROPHAGE DISORDERS

Monocytes-macrophages have been shown to be abnormal in a variety of diseases (Table 3-2). The abnormality is partial and no related association with increased susceptibility to infection has been established. In cases of severely depressed migration of monocytes, however, it is likely that this dysfunction

Table 3-2	Primary and Secondary Abnormalities of Monocyte-Macrophage Function
Abnormality	**Condition/Group**
Defect in phagocyte killing	Chronic granulomatous disease, corticosteroid therapy, newborn infants, viral infections
Defective monocyte cytotoxicity	Cancer, Wiskott-Aldrich syndrome
Defective release of macrophage-activating factors	Acquired immunodeficiency syndrome (AIDS), intracellular infections (e.g., lepromatous leprosy, tuberculosis, visceral leishmaniasis)
Depressed migration	AIDS, burns, diabetes, immunosuppressive therapy, newborn infants
Impaired phagocytosis	Congenital deficiency of CD11 to CD18, monocytic leukemia, systemic lupus erythematosus

predisposes a patient to infection because other defects of host defense coexist in these disorders.

The signs and symptoms of abnormalities of monocyte-macrophage function are extremely evident in some conditions. The profound defect of phagocytic killing exhibited by patients with CGD results in the formation of subcutaneous abscesses and abscesses in the liver, lungs, spleen, and lymph nodes. Cancer patients with a defective monocyte cytotoxicity may develop this defect because tumors have the ability to release factors that suppress the generation of toxic oxygen metabolites by macrophages. In newborn infants, depressed chemotaxis, killing, and decreased synthesis of the phagocytosis-promoting factors fibronectin, C3, and complement factor B have been observed. In addition, the newborn's macrophages may not respond effectively to infection because the lymphocytes have impaired the production of the macrophage activator IFN-γ.

Qualitative disorders of monocytes-macrophages manifest as lipid storage diseases, including a number of rare autosomal recessive disorders. The expression in macrophages of a systemic enzymatic defect permits the accumulation of cell debris normally cleared by macrophages. The macrophages are particularly prone to accumulate undegraded lipid products. Resistance to infection can be impaired, at least partially, because of a defect in macrophage function. Disorders of this type include Gaucher's disease and Niemann-Pick disease.

Gaucher's Disease

An inherited disease caused by a disturbance in cellular lipid metabolism, **Gaucher's disease** most frequently affects children. The prognosis varies; with mild disease, the patient may live a relatively normal life, whereas with severe disease the patient may die prematurely.

The disorder represents a deficiency of β-glucocerebrosidase, the enzyme that normally splits glucose from its parent sphingolipid, glucosylceramide. As a result of this enzyme deficiency, cerebroside accumulates in histiocytes (macrophages). Gaucher's cells are rarely found in the circulating blood; the typical cell is large, with one to three eccentric nuclei and a characteristically wrinkled cytoplasm. These cells are found in the bone marrow, spleen, and other organs of the mononuclear phagocyte system. Production of erythrocytes and leukocytes decreases as these abnormal cells infiltrate the bone marrow.

Niemann-Pick Disease

Niemann-Pick disease is similar to Gaucher's disease, also an inherited abnormality of lipid metabolism. Niemann-Pick disease affects infants and children, with an average life expectancy of 5 years.

This disorder represents a rare autosomal recessive deficiency of the enzyme sphingomyelinase, characterized by massive accumulation of sphingomyelin in the mononuclear phagocytes. The characteristic cell in this disorder, Pick's cell, is similar in appearance to Gaucher's cell, although the cytoplasm of the cell is foamy.

DISEASE STATES INVOLVING LEUKOCYTE INTEGRINS

Leukocyte adhesion deficiency (LAD) ultimately leads to recurrent and often fatal bacterial and fungal infections. The cause of this very rare condition is mutations in the gene or chromosome; about 300 cases have been diagnosed worldwide.

There are several types of LAD based on genotypes and phenotypes. Two genotypes have been identified, LAD-1 and LAD-2. LAD-1 can affect people of all racial groups. LAD-2 has been reported only in people from the Middle East and Brazil. LAD-1 patients have a deficiency of the β_2-integrin subunit (CD18). The phenotypes are severe, moderate, and novel or variant. LAD-2 is described as the failure to convert guanosine diphosphate (GDP) mannose to fructose.

Patients have a history of delayed separation of the umbilical cord, gingivitis, recurrent and persistent bacterial or fungal skin infections, and impaired wound healing. A lack of pus formation has also been noted. Patients frequently develop severe life-threatening infections, although their neutrophil counts are usually elevated (25.0×10^9/L). Affected individuals do not have increased susceptibility to viral infections or malignant neoplasms. Patients with LAD-2 have a characteristic facial appearance, short stature, limb malformations, and severe developmental delay.

Adhesion defects can also be caused by two common drugs, epinephrine and corticosteroids. Both demarginate neutrophils from the peripheral vasculature, although the mechanism is not understood. Epinephrine acts by causing endothelial cells to release cyclic adenosine monophosphate (cAMP), which in turn interrupts adherence.

CASE STUDY 1

History and Physical Examination

This family had a son who had died at age 2 weeks because of overwhelming bacterial infection. When their newborn daughter began developing recurrent infections, she was immediately taken to a pediatrician.

Laboratory Data

Hemoglobin and hematocrit—within normal range
Total WBC count—62.0×10^9/L
Absolute leukocyte counts—above normal for each leukocyte type
Leukocyte differential—neutrophils 76%, lymphocytes 22%, eosinophils 2%
Flow cell cytometry
    T lymphocytes—normal proportions of CD4+ and CD8+ cells
    B lymphocytes (X∆19+)—elevated
    Natural killer (NK) cells—elevated
    CD15+ lymphocytes—absent
Serum Ig fractions—within reference ranges

Treatment

The infant was given busulfan cyclophosphamide and antithymocyte serum for 10 days. She received mature T lymphocyte–depleted bone marrow transplanted from her mother. This was followed by a short period of immuno-suppressive therapy.

She recovered from the procedures and did well clinically.

Questions

1. What significant finding in flow cytometry suggests an immune deficiency?
    a. Elevated B-lymphocytes (CD19+) count.
    b. Normal CD4+ and CD8+ lymphocyte counts
    c. Elevated NK cell count
    d. Absence of CD15+ cells
2. What does the patient's family history suggest?
    a. Acute leukemia
    b. Immune antibody dysfunction
    c. Genetic leukocyte disorder
    d. Hereditary anemia

See Appendix A for the answers to these questions.

Critical Thinking Group Discussion Questions

1. What laboratory test is of the greatest diagnostic value in diagnosing this patient?
2. What value in the reported flow cytometry results is diagnostic?
3. Can leukocyte adhesion deficiency be misdiagnosed?

See instructor site on ⊖volve for discussion of the answers to these questions.

CASE STUDY 2

History and Physical Examination

This 6-year-old white male patient was taken to a pediatrician because of recurring abscesses since the age of 1 month. The current abscesses were lanced and he was placed on antibiotic therapy.

The patient had two brothers who had died in infancy of infections. His parents and two sisters are healthy.

Laboratory Data

Hemoglobin and hematocrit—slightly decreased
Total leukocyte count—elevated
Differential leukocyte count—increased percentage of segmented neutrophils
Immunoglobulin profile—polyclonal elevation of all Ig classes
Neutrophil oxidative burst assay (DHR) activity absent
Nitroblue tetrazolium (NBT) test (automated)—reduction of unstimulated and stimulated neutrophils
Culture of abscess revealed *S. aureus*

Questions

1. What does the patient's family history suggest?
    a. A genetic disorder in male offspring
    b. A genetic disorder in female offspring
    c. Lack of leukocyte production
    d. Anemia producing an immune dysfunction
What laboratory assay is the most helpful in the diagnosis of this case?
    a. Percentage of segmented neutrophils
    b. Immunoglobulin profile
    c. Neutrophil oxidative burst assay (DHR)
    d. Nitroblue tetrazolium (NBT) test (automated)

See Appendix A for the answers to these questions.

Critical Thinking Group Discussion Questions

1. Does this boy's condition appear to be gender-related?
2. Why are the bacteria not killed?

See instructor site ⊖volve for discussion of the answers to these questions.

⁜ Screening Test for Phagocytic Engulfment

Principle

A mixture of bacteria and phagocytes is incubated and examined for the presence of engulfed bacteria. This simple procedure may be useful in supporting the diagnosis of impaired neutrophilic function in conjunction with clinical signs and symptoms (Fig. 3-7).

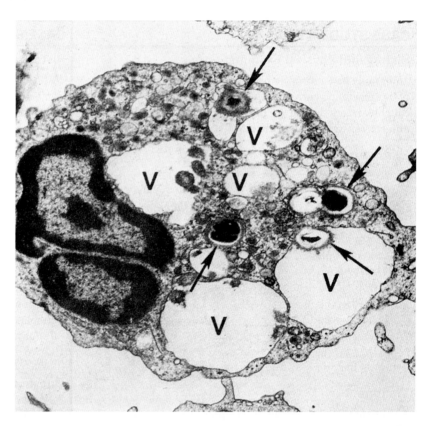

Figure 3-7 Electron photomicrograph of polymorphonuclear leukocyte from normal control patient incubated with staphylococci for 30 minutes. Many bacteria *(arrows)* in various stages of destruction are evident within the cell. Note the cytoplasmic vacuoles (V) around and adjacent to degenerating bacteria. *(From Bauer JD: Clinical laboratory methods, ed 9, St Louis, 1982, Mosby.)*

See **volve** website for information related to performing the procedure.

Reporting Results

- Positive—demonstration of the engulfment of bacteria
- Negative—no engulfment of bacteria

Sources of Error

This procedure may produce false-negative results if the blood specimen is not fresh or if a coagulase-positive *S. aureus* specimen is used. It is important to distinguish between granules and cocci. In addition, the bacteria must be intracellular and not extracellular for the test result to be positive.

Clinical Applications

The failure of phagocytes to engulf bacteria can support the diagnosis of neutrophilic dysfunction; however, these results must be used in conjunction with patient signs and symptoms.

Limitations

This is a simple screening procedure for engulfment. The presence of engulfed bacteria does not demonstrate that the bacteria have been destroyed.

CHAPTER HIGHLIGHTS

- The entire leukocytic cell system is designed to defend the body against disease. Each cell type has a unique function and behaves independently and, in many cases, in cooperation with other cell types.

- The primary phagocytic cells are the neutrophilic leukocytes and the mononuclear monocytes-macrophages.
- The neutrophilic leukocyte provides an effective host defense against bacterial and fungal infections. Although the monocytes-macrophages and other granulocytes are also phagocytic cells, the neutrophil is the principal leukocyte associated with phagocytosis and a localized inflammatory response.
- Phagocytosis can be divided into movement of cells, engulfment, and digestion.
- Cells communicate with each other and their environment through soluble mediators and during direct contact (e.g., phagocytosis). These interactions occur through cell surface receptors that mediate cell-cell binding (adhesion) of leukocytes.
- Three protein families (immunoglobulin, integrin, selectin) are associated in a network of cellular interactions in the immune system.
- Qualitative monocyte-macrophage disorders manifest as lipid storage diseases, including a number of rare autosomal recessive disorders.
- Leukocyte adhesion deficiency ultimately leads to recurrent and often fatal bacterial and fungal infections.

REVIEW QUESTIONS

1. The site of hematopoiesis in the first month of gestation is the:
    a. Yolk sac
    b. Spleen
    c. Liver
    d. Bone marrow

2. The principal type of leukocyte in the process of phagocytosis is the:
   a. Eosinophil
   b. Basophil
   c. Monocyte
   d. Neutrophil

3. Chronic granulomatous disease represents a defect of:
   a. Oxidative metabolism
   b. Abnormal granulation of neutrophils
   c. Diapedesis
   d. Chemotaxis

4. A primary function of the eosinophil is:
   a. Phagocytosis
   b. Suppression of the inflammatory response
   c. Reacting in acute, systemic hypersensitivity reactions
   d. Antigen recognition

5. The cells of the mononuclear phagocyte system include:
   a. Monocytes and promonocytes
   b. Monocytes and macrophages
   c. Lymphocytes and monocytes
   d. Both a and b

6. The host defense function(s) of monocytes-macrophages include(s):
   a. Antigen presentation
   b. Phagocytosis
   c. Secretion of biologically active molecules
   d. All of the above

7. The surface MHC class II gene product is important in:
   a. Antigen recognition by T lymphocytes
   b. Antigen recognition by B lymphocytes
   c. Synthesis of antibody by plasma cells
   d. Phagocytosis

8-12. Match the appropriate monocyte-macrophage abnormality with its respective condition.

8. _D_ Defect in phagocytic killing

9. _A_ Defective monocyte cytotoxicity

10. _E_ Defective release of macrophage-activating factors

11. _B_ Depressed migration

12. _C_ Impaired phagocytosis
   a. Wiskott-Aldrich syndrome
   b. Burns or diabetes
   c. Systemic lupus erythematosus
   d. Corticosteroid therapy
   e. Intracellular infections

13-16. Arrange the steps of phagocytosis in the proper sequence.

13. _B_

14. _D_

15. _C_

16. _A_
   a. Digestion of bacteria
   b. Increase in chemoattractants at site of tissue damage
   c. Ingestion of bacteria
   d. Movement of phagocytic cells

17-20. Match the following cell types to their respective functions. (An answer can be used more than once.)

17. _A_ Polymorphonuclear neutrophil (PMN) leukocytes

18. _C_ Lymphocytes

19. _A_ Mononuclear monocytes-macrophages

20. _B_ Plasma cells
   a. Primary phagocytic cells
   b. Antibody-synthesizing cells
   c. Recognition of foreign antigen and production of antibody

21-23. Arrange the sites of blood cell development (hematopoiesis) in the embryo and fetus in the correct sequence of development.

21. _B_ Site of initial red blood cell production

22. _A_ Predominant site from 2 to 5 months of fetal life

23. _C_ Ultimate site of primary hematopoiesis
   a. Liver and spleen
   b. Yolk sac
   c. Bone marrow

24. Patients with a marked decrease in neutrophils or severe defects in neutrophil function have:
   a. A high rate of infection
   b. Recurrent systemic bacterial infections
   c. Recurrent life-threatening fungal infections
   d. All of the above

25-28. Match each disorder or deficiency to its characteristics.

25. _B_ Chronic granulomatosus disease

26. _D_ Lazy leukocyte syndrome

27. _A_ Chédiak-Higashi anomaly (syndrome)

28. _C_ Myeloperoxidase deficiency
   a. Marked defect in cellular response to chemotaxis
   b. Failure to exhibit increased anaerobic metabolism during phagocytosis
   c. Mild to marked defect in bactericidal ability of neutrophils
   d. Defective leukocyte locomotion

29. Which statement about eosinophils is false?
   a. They are homeostatic regulators of inflammation.
   b. They attempt to suppress an inflammatory reaction.
   c. They participate in hypersensitivity reactions.
   d. They interact with the larval stages of some helminth parasites.

30. Which statement about basophils is false?
    a. They have a high concentration of heparin in the granules.
    b. They have a high concentration of histamine in the granules.
    c. They react with two adjacent IgA molecules on mast cells.
    d. They are associated with anaphylactic shock.

31. The cells that constitute the physiologic, mononuclear phagocyte system do not include:
    a. Promonocytes and their precursors
    b. Monocytes in circulating blood
    c. Macrophages in tissues
    d. Polymorphonuclear neutrophils

32-36. Identify the types of mononuclear phagocytic cells found in the various locations shown in the illustration. Choose from the following answers:
    a. Kupffer cells
    b. Macrophages
    c. Microglial cells
    d. Histiocytes (tissue macrophages)

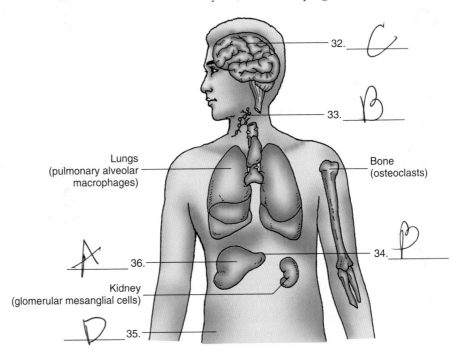

32. C
33. B
34. B
35. D
36. A

Lungs (pulmonary alveolar macrophages)

Bone (osteoclasts)

Kidney (glomerular mesanglial cells)

(From Turgeon ML: Clinical hematology: theory and procedures, ed 5, Philadelphia, 2012, Lippincott Williams & Wilkins)

37-40. Name the steps in the process of phagocytosis shown in the illustration. Choose from the following answers:
    a. Engulfment
    b. Chemotaxis
    c. Phagosome formation
    d. Adherence

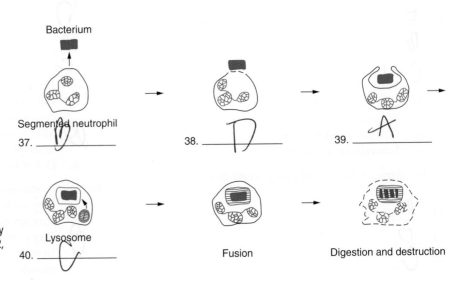

Bacterium

Segmented neutrophil

37. ____   38. D ____   39. A ____

Lysosome

40. ____   Fusion   Digestion and destruction

(From Turgeon ML: Clinical hematology: theory and procedures, ed 5, Philadelphia, 2012, Lippincott Williams & Wilkins)

BIBLIOGRAPHY

Abbas AK, Lichtman AH: Basic immunology: functions and disorders of the immune system, updated edition, ed 3, Philadelphia, 2011, Saunders.

Aiuti A, Roncarolo MG: Ten years of gene therapy for primary immune deficiencies, Hematology Am Soc Hematol Educ Program 682–689, 2009.

Camous L, Roumenina L, Bigot S, et al: Complement alternative pathway acts as a positive feedback amplification of neutrophil activation, Blood 117:1340–1349, 2011.

Charo IF, Ransohoff RM: The many roles of chemokines and chemokine receptors in inflammation, N Engl J Med 354:610–621, 2006.

Danese S, Vetrano S, Zhang L, et al: The protein C pathway in tissue inflammation and injury: pathogenic role and therapetutic implications, Blood 115:1121–1130, 2010.

Eltzschig HK, Carmeliet P: Hypoxia and inflammation, N Engl J Med 364:656–665, 2011.

Etzion A: Integrins: the molecular glue of life, Hosp Pract 35:102, 2000.

Faix J: Sepsis: new approaches to diagnosis and treatment, Cl Lab News 38:12–14, 2012.

Frenette PS: Locking a leukocyte integrin with statins, N Engl J Med 345:1419–1421, 2001.

Frommhold D, Kamphues A, Hepper I, et al: RAGE and ICAM-1 cooperate in mediating leukocyte recruitment during acute inflammation in vivo, Blood 116:841–849, 2010.

Green CE, Schaff UY, Sarantos MR, et al: Dynamic shifts in LFA-1 affinity regulate neutrophil rolling, arrest, and transmigration on inflamed endothelium, Blood 107:2101–2110, 2006.

Grosser T, Fries S, Fitzgerald GA: Biological basis for the cardiovascular consequences of COX-2 inhibition: therapeutic challenges and opportunities, J Clin Invest 116:4–15, 2006.

Hansson G: Inflammation, atherosclerosis, and coronary artery disease, N Engl J Med 352:1685–1695, 2005.

Harvey RA, Champe PC: Immunology, Philadelphia, 2008, Lippincott Williams & Wilkins.

Hotchkiss RS, Karl IE: The pathophysiology and treatment of sepsis, N Engl J Med 348:138–150, 2003.

Johnston RB: Monocytes and macrophages, N Engl J Med 318:747–752, 1988.

Katz P: Clinical and laboratory evaluation of the immune system, Med Clin North Am 69:453–459, 1985.

Klinke A, Nussbaum C, Kubala L, et al: Myeloperoxidase attracts neutrophils by physical forces, Blood 117:1350–1358, Jan 27, 2011.

Kuhns D, Alvord WG, Heller T, et al: Residual NADPH oxidase and survival in chronic granulomatous disease, N Engl J Med 363:2600–2610, 2010.

Larson RS, Springer TA: Structure and function of leukocyte integrins, Immunol Rev 114:181–217, 1990.

Ledue TB, Neveux LM, Palomaki GE, et al: The relationship between serum levels of lipoprotein (a) and proteins associated with the acute-phase response, Clin Chim Acta 223:73–82, 1993.

Lieschke G: Fluorescent neutrophils throw the spotlight on inflammation, Blood 108:3961–3962, 2006.

Luscinskas FW: Neutrophil CD44 rafts and rolls, Blood 116:314–315, 2010.

Malech HL, Malech JI: Neutrophils in human diseases, N Engl J Med 317:687–692, 1987.

Meissner F, Seger RA, Moshous D, et al: Inflammasome activation in NADPH oxidase defective mononuclear phagocytes from patients with chronic granulomatous disease, Blood 116:1570–1573, 2010.

Peakman M, Vergani D: Basic and clinical immunology, ed 2, Edinburgh, 2009, Churchill Livingstone.

Pillay J, den Braber I, Vrisekoop N, et al: In vivo labeling with 2H2O reveals a human neutrophil lifespan of 5.4 days, Blood 116:625–627, July 29, 2010.

Serhan CN, Chiang N: Putting the brakes on neutrophils, Blood 107:1742–1743, 2006.

Turgeon ML: Fundamentals of immunohematology, ed 2, Baltimore, 1995, Williams & Wilkins.

Turgeon ML: Clinical hematology, ed 5, Philadelphia, 2012, Lippincott Williams & Wilkins.

Yago T, Shao B, Miner JJ, et al: E-selectin engages PSGL-1 and CD44 through a common signaling pathway to induce integrin αLβ2-mediated slow leukocyte rolling, Blood 116:485–494, 2010.

Zou J, Sweeney CL, Chou BK, et al: Oxidase-deficient neutrophils from X-linked chronic granulomatous disease iPS cells: functional correction by zinc finger nuclease-mediated safe harbor targeting, Blood 117:5561–5572, 2011.

Cells and Cellular Activities of the Immune System: Lymphocytes and Plasma Cells

Learning Objectives

At the conclusion of this chapter, the reader should be able to:
- Differentiate and compare the function of primary and secondary lymphoid tissues.
- Describe the structure and function of a lymph node.
- Explain the role of the thymus in T lymphocyte maturation.
- Describe the maturation of a B lymphocyte from origination to plasma cell development.
- Compare the function of T lymphocytes and B lymphocytes in immunity.
- Explain the function of natural killer (NK) cells.
- Define the term *cluster of differentiation* (CD) and explain the purpose of detecting this marker.
- Differentiate the characteristics of T lymphocyte subsets on the basis of antigen structures and function.
- Describe the evaluation of suspected lymphocytic or plasma cell defects.
- Name and compare disorders of immunologic (lymphocytic or plasma cell) origin.
- Compare various categories of immunodeficiency disorders.
- Analyze and apply knowledge from this chapter to a representative case study.
- Correctly answer case study–related multiple choice questions.
- Be prepared to participate in a discussion of critical thinking questions.
- Describe the assessment of the cellular immune status.
- Correctly answer end of chapter review questions.

Key Terms

allograft
anergy
antigen-presenting cells (APCs)
B lymphocytes
cell surface markers
cluster of differentiation (CD)
cytotoxic
double-negative lymphocytes
double-negative thymocytes
double-positive thymocytes
dyscrasias
dysplastic
effector T cells
endogenous pathway

exogenous pathway
granzyme A-B
gut-associated lymphoid tissue (GALT)
immune senescence
immunodeficiency syndromes
immunoproliferative
immunoregulatory cells
immunosuppression
interleukin (IL)
lymphocyte recirculation
macrophages
memory cells
monoclonal gammopathies

monocytes
natural killer cells
natural Treg cells
negative selection
neoantigen
plasma cells
positive selection
primary immunodeficiency disorders
suppressor-cytotoxic lymphocytes
surface immunoglobulin (sIg)
T cell receptor (TCR)
T lymphocytes
thymus
T-independent antigens

LYMPHOCYTES AND PLASMA CELLS

The adaptive immune system is comprised of the humoral and cellular systems. Each of the two arms of the adaptive immune system has fundamental mechanisms allowing the body to attack an invading pathogen. The immunologically specific cellular component of the immune system is organized around two classes of specialized cells, **T lymphocytes** and **B lymphocytes.** Lymphocytes recognize foreign antigens, directly destroy some cells, or produce antibodies as **plasma cells.** The total immune response involves the interaction of many different cell types and cell-mediated and antibody-mediated responses. Recent studies have shown that T cells are not just the latecomers in inflammation, but might also play a key role in the early phase of this response. T cell subsets, including NK cells, together with classic innate immune cells, contribute significantly to the development and establishment of acute and chronic inflammatory diseases.

LYMPHOID AND NONLYMPHOID SURFACE MEMBRANE MARKERS

Before 1979, human lymphocytes could be classified as T or B cells based on observation of these cells with electron microscopy (Fig. 4-1). T lymphocytes have a relatively smooth surface compared with the rough pattern of the B lymphocytes.

The introduction of monoclonal antibody (MAb) testing (see Chapter 2) led to the present identification of surface membrane markers on lymphocytes and other cells. In practical terms, surface markers are used to identify and enumerate various lymphocyte subsets, establish lymphocyte maturity, classify leukemias, and monitor patients on immunosuppressive therapy.

Cell surface molecules recognized by MAbs are called antigens, because antibodies can be produced against them, or markers, because they identify and discriminate between, or "mark," different cell populations. Originally, surface markers

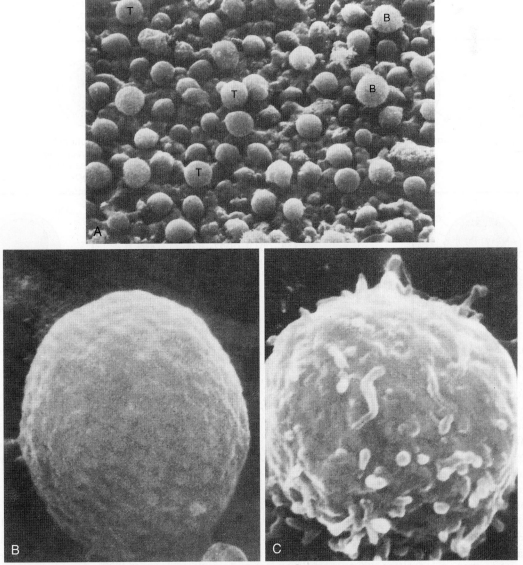

Figure 4-1   Scanning electron photomicrographs of lymphocyte cell surface membranes. **A,** T and B lymphocytes. **B,** T lymphocyte. **C,** B lymphocyte. *(From Polliack A, Lampen N, Clarkson BD, et al: Identification of human B and T lymphocytes by scanning electron microscopy, J Exp Med 138:607–624, 1973.)*

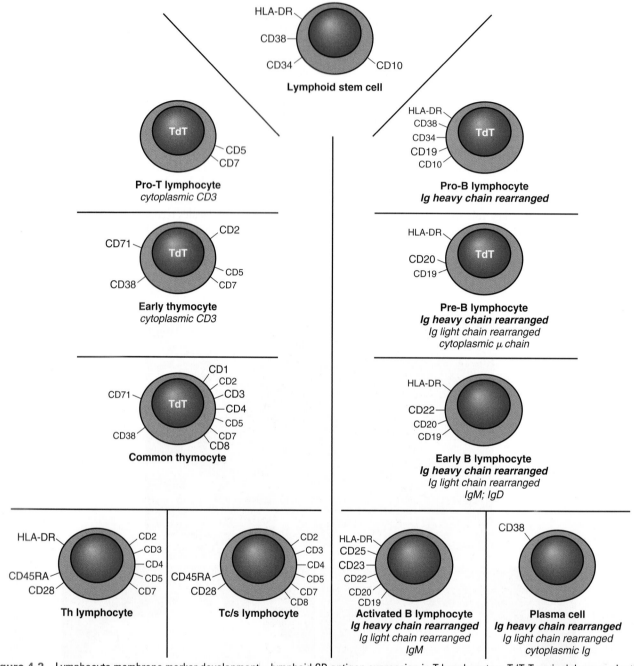

Figure 4-2 Lymphocyte membrane marker development—lymphoid CD antigen expression in T lymphocytes. *TdT,* Terminal deoxynucleotidyl transferase. *CD,* cluster of differentiation; *HLA,* human leukocyte antigen; *Ig,* immunoglobulin.

were named according to the antibodies that reacted with them, but a uniform nomenclature system has now been adopted.

In this system, a surface marker that identifies a particular lineage or differentiation stage with a defined structure, and that can be identified with a group or cluster of MAbs, is called a member of a **cluster of differentiation** (CD; Fig. 4-2). Markers can be categorized as follows:

- Some markers are specific for cells of a particular lineage or maturational pathway.
- Some markers vary in expression, depending on the state of activation or differentiation of the same cells—for example, when CD antigen identification is used to classify lymphocyte subsets (e.g., CD4 and CD8).

In addition to using CD classification for the identification and separation of lymphocytes, CD antigens are involved in various lymphocyte functions, usually the following:

- Promotion of cell to cell interactions and adhesion
- Transduction of signals that lead to lymphocyte activation

Sites of Lymphocyte Development

In mammalian immunologic development, the precursors of lymphocytes arise from progenitor cells of the yolk sac and liver (Fig. 4-3). Later in fetal development, and throughout the life cycle, the bone marrow becomes the sole provider of undifferentiated progenitor cells, which can further develop into lymphoblasts. Continued cellular development and proliferation of

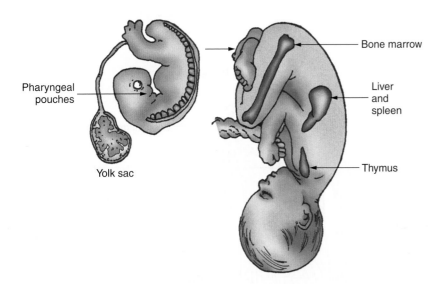

Bone marrow

Liver and spleen

Pharyngeal pouches

Thymus

Yolk sac

Figure 4-3   Development of immunologic organs. The anatomy of the human fetus illustrates the development of the mammalian immune system. Cells of the pharyngeal pouches migrate into the chest and form the thymus. Precursors of lymphocytes originate early in embryonic life in the yolk sac and eventually migrate to the bone marrow via the spleen and liver.

lymphoid precursors occur as the cells travel to the primary and secondary lymphoid tissues.

Primary Lymphoid Tissue

In mammals, both the bone marrow (and/or fetal liver) and thymus are classified as primary or central lymphoid organs (Fig. 4-4). **Thymus.** Early in embryonic development, the stroma and nonlymphoid epithelium of the **thymus** are derived from the third and fourth pharyngeal pouches. The characteristics of the thymus gland change with aging. Older persons are immunologically challenged because aging causes a reduction in the production of naïve T cells by the thymus. Intrinsic defects in mature T cell function, alterations in the life span of naïve T cells and in naïve or memory T cell ratios in the peripheral lymphoid tissues, occur as the result of the decline of the T cell response in older persons.

The thymus, located in the mediastinum, exercises control over the entire immune system. It is believed that the development of diversity occurs mainly in the thymus and bone marrow, although clonal expansion can occur anywhere in the peripheral lymphoid tissue.

Progenitor cells that migrate to the thymus proliferate and differentiate under the influence of the humoral factor, thymosin. These lymphocyte precursors with acquired surface membrane antigens are referred to as thymocytes.

The reticular structure of the thymus allows a significant number of lymphocytes to pass through it to become fully immunocompetent (able to function in the immune response), thymus-derived T cells. The thymus also regulates immune function by the secretion of multiple soluble hormones.

Many cells die in the thymus and apparently are phagocytized, a mechanism to eliminate lymphocyte clones reactive against self. It is estimated that approximately 97% of the cortical cells die in the thymus before becoming mature T cells. Viable cells migrate to the secondary tissues. The absence or abnormal development of the thymus results in a T lymphocyte deficiency.

Involution of the thymus is the first age-related change occurring in the human immune system. In postnatal life, the thymus

is the primary organ that produces naïve T cells for the peripheral T cell pool but production of cells declines as early as 3 months of age. The thymus gradually loses up to 95% of its mass during the first 50 years of life (Fig. 4-5). The accompanying functional changes of decreased synthesis of thymic hormones and the loss of ability to differentiate immature lymphocytes are reflected in an increased number of immature lymphocytes within the thymus and as circulating peripheral blood T cells. Most changes in immune function, such as dysfunction of T and B lymphocytes, elevated levels of circulating immune complexes, increases in autoantibodies, and **monoclonal gammopathies** are correlated with involution of the thymus (see Chapter 27). **Immune senescence** may account for the increased susceptibility of older adults to infections, autoimmune disease, and neoplasms.

Bone Marrow. The bone marrow is the source of progenitor cells. These cells can differentiate into lymphocytes and other hematopoietic cells (e.g., granulocytes, erythrocytes, megakaryocyte populations). In mammals, the bone marrow also supports eventual differentiation of mature T and B lymphocytes, probably from a common lymphoid cell progenitor. It is believed that the bone marrow and **gut-associated lymphoid tissue (GALT)** may also play a role in the differentiation of progenitor cells into B lymphocytes.

Secondary Lymphoid Organs

Secondary lymphoid organs provide a unique microenvironment for the initiation and development of immune responses. The secondary lymphoid tissues include lymph nodes, spleen, GALT, thoracic duct, bronchus-associated lymphoid tissue (BALT), skin-associated lymphoid tissue, and blood. Mature lymphocytes and accessory cells (e.g., antigen-presenting cells) are found throughout the body, although the relative percentages of T and B cells vary in different locations (Table 4-1).

The highly sophisticated structure of secondary lymphoid organs allows migration and interactions between antigen-presenting cells, T and B lymphocytes, and follicular dendritic cells (FDCs) and other stromal cells. The cooperative activities of lymphoid cells within secondary organs dramatically increase

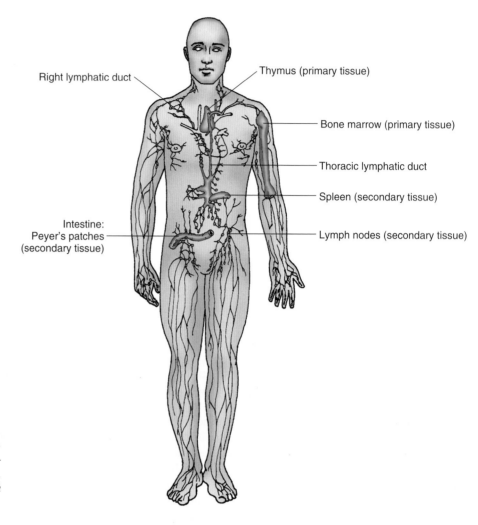

Right lymphatic duct

Thymus (primary tissue)

Bone marrow (primary tissue)

Thoracic lymphatic duct

Spleen (secondary tissue)

Intestine: Peyer's patches (secondary tissue)

Lymph nodes (secondary tissue)

Figure 4-4 Human primary and secondary tissues. *(Adapted from Turgeon ML: Clinical hematology: theory and procedures, ed 4, Philadelphia, 2005, Lippincott Williams & Wilkins.)*

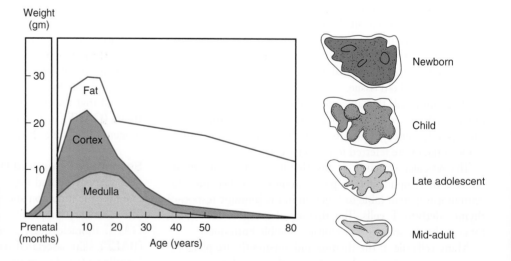

Figure 4-5 Thymic development. Histology of the thymus changes with age. The main feature of these changes is a loss of cellularity with increasing age.

the probability of interactions of rare B, T, and APCs that results in effective generation of humoral immune responses.

Tumor necrosis factor (TNF) and lymphotoxin are essential to the formation and maintenance of secondary organs. These cytokines are produced by B and T lymphocytes. Proliferation of the T and B lymphocytes in the secondary or peripheral lymphoid tissues (Fig. 4-6) is primarily dependent on antigenic stimulation.

The T lymphocytes or T cells populate the following:
1. Perifollicular and paracortical regions of the lymph nodes
2. Medullary cords of the lymph nodes

Table 4-1	Approximate Percentage of Lymphocytes in Lymphoid Organs	
Lymphoid Organ	**T Lymphocytes (%)**	**B Lymphocytes (%)**
Thymus	100	0
Blood	80	20
Lymph nodes	60	40
Spleen	45	55
Bone marrow	10	90

Adapted from Claman HN: The biology of the immune response, JAMA 268:2790–2796, 1992.

3. Periarteriolar regions of the spleen
4. Thoracic duct of the circulatory system

The B lymphocytes or B cells multiply and populate the following:

1. Follicular and medullary (germinal centers) of the lymph nodes
2. Primary follicles and red pulp of the spleen
3. Follicular regions of GALT
4. Medullary cords of the lymph nodes

Lymph Nodes. Lymph nodes act as lymphoid filters in the lymphatic system. Lymph nodes respond to antigens introduced distally and routed to them by afferent lymphatics (Fig. 4-7). Generalized lymph node reactivity can occur after systemic antigen challenge (e.g., serum sickness).

Spleen. The spleen acts as a lymphatic filter within the blood vascular tree. It is an important site of antibody production in response to IV particulate antigens (e.g., bacteria). The spleen is also a major organ for the clearance particles.

Gut-Associated Lymphoid Tissue. GALT includes lymphoid tissue in the intestines (Peyer's patches) and the liver. GALT features immunoglobulin A (IgA) production and involves a unique pattern of **lymphocyte recirculation.** Pre–B cells develop in Peyer's patches and, after meeting antigen from the gut, many enter the general circulation and then return back to the gut. GALT is also important for the development of tolerance to ingested antigens.

Thoracic Duct. The thoracic duct lymph is a rich source of mature T cells. Chronic thoracic duct drainage can cause T cell depletion and has been used as a method of **immunosuppression.**

Bronchus-Associated Lymphoid Tissue. BALT includes lymphoid tissue in the lower respiratory tract and hilar lymph nodes. It is mainly associated with IgA production in response to inhaled antigens.

Skin-Associated Lymphoid Tissue. Antigens introduced through the skin are presented by epidermal Langerhans cells, which are bone marrow–derived accessory cells. These epidermal cells then interact with lymphocytes in the skin and in draining lymph nodes.

Blood. The blood is an important lymphoid organ and immunologic effector tissue. Circulating blood has enough mature T cells to produce a graft-versus-host reaction. In addition, blood transfusions have been responsible for inducing acquired immunologic tolerance in kidney **allograft** patients.

Blood is the most frequently sampled lymphoid organ. It is assumed that what is found in blood samples represents what is present in other lymphoid tissues. Although this may be a true representation, it is not always accurate.

Circulation of Lymphocytes

Mature T lymphocytes survive for several months or years, whereas the average life span of B lymphocytes is only a few days. Lymphocytes move freely between the blood and lymphoid tissues. This activity, termed *lymphocyte recirculation,* enables lymphocytes to come into contact with processed foreign antigens and disseminate antigen-sensitized memory cells throughout the lymphoid system. Clonal expansion may occur regionally, as in lymph nodes draining a contact allergic reaction, and then the whole body becomes susceptible to rechallenge because T cells recirculate, but generally are excluded from returning to the thymus. Research has shown that a pool of T cell clonal elements is developed by a combination of **positive selection** of clones able to recognize and react to foreign antigens, and **negative selection** (purging) of clones able to interact with self-antigens in a damaging way.

Recirculation of lymphocytes back to the blood is through the major lymphatic ducts. Lymphocytes enter the lymph node from the blood circulation via arterioles and capillaries to reach the specialized postcapillary venules. From the venule, the lymphocytes enter the node and remain in the node or pass through the node and return to the circulating blood. Lymphatic fluid, lymphocytes, and antigens from certain body sites enter the lymph node through the afferent lymphatic duct and exit the lymph node through the efferent lymphatic duct (see Fig. 4-7).

VIRGIN OR NAÏVE LYMPHOCYTES

Virgin or naïve lymphocytes are cells that have not encountered their specific antigen. These cells do express high-molecular-weight variants of leukocyte common antigen.

Memory cells are populations of long-lived T or B cells that have been stimulated by antigen. They can make a quick response to a previously encountered antigen. Memory B cells carry surface IgG as their antigen receptor; memory T cells express the CD45RO variant of the leukocyte common antigen and increased levels of cell-adhesion molecules (CAMs), chemical mediators involved in inflammatory processes throughout the body (Fig. 4-8).

DEVELOPMENT OF T LYMPHOCYTES

Most lymphocytes (see Color Plate 8) found in the circulating blood are T cells derived from bone marrow progenitor cells that mature in the thymus gland (Table 4-2). These cells are responsible for cellular immune responses and are involved in the regulation of antibody reactions in conjunction with B lymphocytes.

During cellular development, T lymphocyte function–associated antigens vary in expression. Some antigens appear

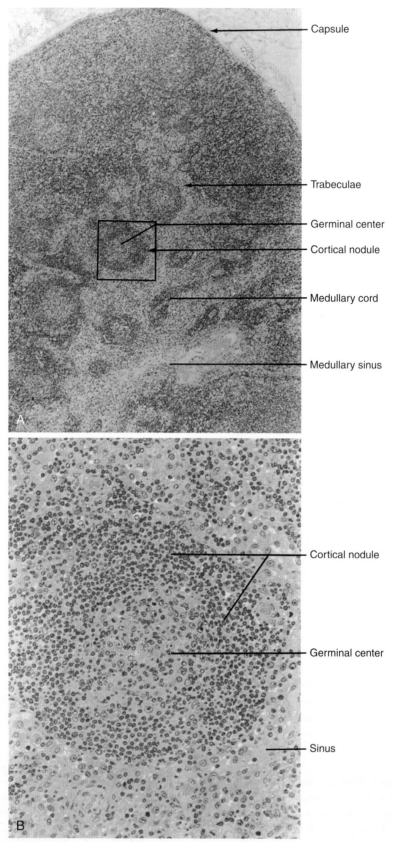

Figure 4-6 **A,** Lymph node (×90). **B,** Enlargement of cortical nodule seen in **A** (×450). *(From Anthony CP, Thibodeau GA: Textbook of anatomy and physiology, ed 12, St Louis, 1987, Mosby.)*

early in cellular development and remain on mature T cells. Others appear at an early or intermediate stage of cellular maturation and are lost before maturity.

Early Cellular Differentiation and Development

Differentiation of a lymphocyte begins in the thymus as a thymocyte. Early surface markers on thymocytes that are committed to becoming T cells include CD44 and CD25. As thymocytes develop, there is an orderly rearrangement of the genes coding for an antigen receptor.

Maturation is a complicated process that lasts for a period of 3 weeks. During this period, cells filter through the cortex to

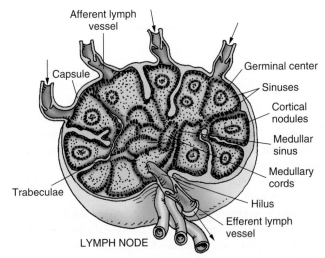

Figure 4-7 **Structure of a lymph node.** Several valved afferent lymphatics bring lymph to the node. An efferent lymphatic leaves the node at the hilus. Note that the artery and vein enter and leave at the hilus. *(Adapted from Anthony CP, Thibodeau GA: Textbook of anatomy and physiology, ed 12, St Louis, 1987, Mosby.)*

the medulla of the thymus. Thymic stromal cells include fibroblasts, macrophages, epithelial cells, and dendritic cells; all these cell types play a role in T cell development.

Double-Negative Thymocytes

Early thymocytes lacking CD4 and CD8 surface membrane markers are referred to as **double-negative thymocytes.** These cells proliferate in the outer cortex of the thymus under the influence of interleukin-7 (IL7). IL-7 is critical for this growth and differentiation.

Rearrangement of the genes that code for the antigen receptor, the **T cell receptor (TCR)**, begin at this developmental stage. CD3 constitutes the main part of the T cell antigen receptor. The configuration of two of the eight chains of the receptor have variable regions that recognize specific antigens. These are coded for by selecting gene segments and deleting others.

Rearrangement of the beta (β) chain occurs first; the appearance of a functional β chain on the cell surface sends a signal to suppress any further β chain gene rearrangements. The combination of the β chain with the CD3 forms the pre–T-cell antigen receptor (TRC). Signaling by the β chain promotes the development of a CD4+ and CD8+ thymocyte.

Thymocytes that express gamma (γ) and delta (δ) chains follow a different developmental pathway. Cells expressing gamma-delta (γδ) chains typically remain both CD4– and CD8–. These double-negative cells represent most of the population of T lymphocytes in the skin and intestinal and pulmonary epithelium.

Circulating CD3+ **double-negative lymphocytes** are phenotypically and functionally distinct from single-positive CD3+CD4+ and CD3+CD8+ lymphocytes and are thought to represent a distinct T cell lineage. The presence of low numbers

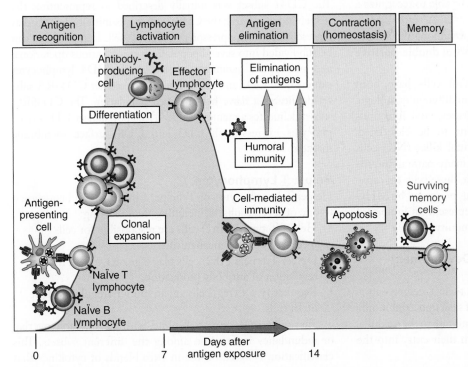

Figure 4-8 **Phases of an adaptive immune response.** An adaptive immune response consists of distinct phases; the first three are the recognition of antigen, activation of lymphocytes, and elimination of antigen (effector phase). The response declines as antigen-stimulated lymphocytes die by apoptosis, restoring homeostasis, and the antigen-specific cells that survive are responsible for memory. The duration of each phase may vary in different immune responses. The y-axis represents an arbitrary measure of the magnitude of the response. These principles apply to humoral immunity (measured by B lymphocytes) and cell-mediated immunity (mediated by T lymphocytes). *(From Abbas AK, Lichtman AH: Basic immunology: functions and disorders of the immune system, updated edition, ed 3, Philadelphia, 2011, Saunders.)*

Table 4-2	Lymphocyte Characteristics		
Type	**Function(s)**	**Phenotypic Marker**	**Peripheral Blood (% of Total)**
Helper T (Th) cells	Stimulate B cell growth and differentiation (humoral immunity); macrophage activation by secreted cytokines (cell-mediated immunity)	CD3+, CD4+, CD8−	50-60
Cytotoxic T (Tc) cells	Lysis of virus-infected cells, tumor cells, and allografts (cell-mediated immunity); macrophage activation by secreted cytokines (cell-mediated immunity)	CD3+, CD4−, CD8+	20-25
Natural killer (NK) cells	Lysis of virus-infected cells, (antibody-dependent cellular cytotoxicity)	Fc receptor for IgG or cells CD16	~10
B cells	Antibody production (humoral immunity)	Fc receptors, MHC class II, CD19, CD21	10-15

of double-negative T cells in healthy individuals and the increase observed in association with lymphoproliferative disorders, graft-versus-host disease, and autoimmune diseases suggest a pathogenic or immunoregulatory role for this population of T lymphocytes.

Double-Positive Thymocytes

Cells with both CD4+ and CD8+, or double-positive, surface markers represent the second stage of thymocyte development. These thymocytes begin to demonstrate rearranged genes coding for the alpha (α) chain. When the CD3-αβ receptor complex (TCR) is expressed on the cell surface, a process known as positive selection permits only double-positive cells with functional TCR receptors to survive. T cells must recognize foreign antigen in association with class I or II major histocompatibility complex (MHC) molecules. Any thymocyte that is unable to recognize self-MHC dies without ever leaving the thymus gland. Functioning T lymphocytes must be able to recognize a foreign antigen along with MHC molecules. A second selection process, negative selection, takes place among the surviving double-positive T cells. Only 1% to 3% of **double-positive thymocytes** survive in the cortex.

Double-positive (DP) CD4CD8 Tαβ cells have been reported in normal individuals as well as in different pathologic conditions, including inflammatory diseases, viral infections and cancer, but their function remains to be elucidated. Double-negative cells may act like natural killer (NK) cells because they are capable of binding to many natural, unprocessed cell surface molecules. In addition, these cells are capable of recognizing antigens without being presented by MHC proteins. Consequently, NK cells may represent an important bridge between natural and adaptive immunity.

Later Cellular Differentiation and Development of T Lymphocytes

When mature T cells leave the thymus, their T cell receptors (TCRs) are CD4+ or CD8+. Survivors of selection exhibit only one type of marker, CD4+ or CD8+ and migrate to the medulla. These cells gain functional maturity with their entry into the peripheral blood circulation.

T cells develop into a variety of clones. Each lymphocyte displays a single type of structurally unique receptor. The repertoire of antigen receptors in the entire population of lymphocytes is extremely large and diverse. This increases the probability that an individual lymphocyte will encounter an antigen that binds to its receptor, thereby triggering activation and proliferation of the cell. This process, clonal selection, accounts for most of the basic properties of the adaptive immune system.

Antigen receptors for common pathogens need to be reinvented by every generation of cells. Because the binding sites of antigen receptors arise from random genetic mechanisms, the receptor repertoire contains binding sites that can react not only with infectious microorganisms, but also with innocuous environmental antigens and self antigens.

T-Lymphocyte Subsets

The CD4+ subset was initially described as representing the helper-inducer T cell; the CD8+ subset was initially described as representing the suppressor-cytotoxic T cell. Lymphocytes can be subdivided into several populations using various operational and phenotypic parameters. For example, CD4 lymphocytes express both CD3 and CD4. The surface marker CD45RA subset delineates a naïve helper T cell population. The CD45RO subset delineates a memory helper T cell population. CD8+ lymphocytes express both CD3 and CD8 surface membrane markers.

Helper T Lymphocytes

Helper T lymphocytes, or T-helper (Th) cells, can be assigned to one of several subsets, including the following:
- Helper T type 1 (Th1) cells are responsible for cell-mediated effector mechanisms.
- Helper T type 2 (Th2) cells play a greater role in the regulation of antibody production.
- Regulatory T (Treg) cells are an immunoregulatory type of Th cells.

These divisions are not absolute, with considerable overlap or redundancy in function among the different subsets. This classification is based on the in vitro blends of cytokines that

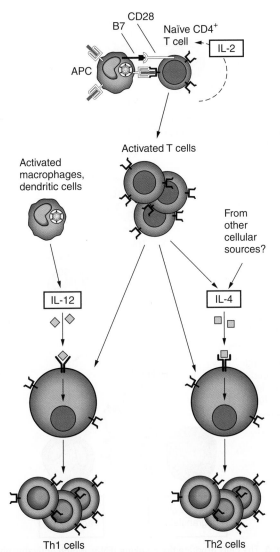

Figure 4-9 Differentiation of naïve CD4+ helper T (Th) cells into Th1 and Th2 effector cells. After their activation by antigen and costimulators, naïve helper T cells may differentiate into Th1 and Th2 cells under the influence of cytokines. IL-12 produced by microbe-activated macrophages and dendritic cells stimulates differentiation of CD4+ T cells into Th1 effectors. In the absence of IL-12, the T cells themselves (and perhaps other cells) produce IL-4, which stimulates their differentiation into Th2 effectors. *(Adapted from Abbas AK, Lichtman AH: Basic immunology: functions and disorders of the immune system, ed 3, Philadelphia, 2008, Saunders.)*

they produce. Th1 and Th2 cells can promote the development of **cytotoxic** cells and are believed to develop from Th0 cells. Th1 cells interact most effectively with mononuclear phagocytes; Th2 cells release cytokines that are required for B cell differentiation (Fig. 4-9).

Characterized by high interferon-gamma (IFN-γ) production, Th1 responses promote the elimination of intracellular pathogens (Fig. 4-10, *A*). Characterized by IL-4 and IL-5, Th2 responses promote a different type of effector response that involves immunoglobulin E (IgE) production and eosinophils capable of eliminating larger extracellular pathogens, such as helminths (see Fig. 4-10, *B*). In situations of repeated pathogen

exposure or persistent infection, the polarization of T cell responses serves to focus the antigen-specific response on a specific effector pathway.

The following factors can influence the terminal differentiation of lymphocytes:
- Type of antigen-presenting cell (APC)
- Affinity of the specific antigenic peptide
- Types of costimulatory molecules expressed by APCs
- Cytokines acting on T cells during primary activation through TCRs

A hierarchy is apparent among these factors and is determined by how they influence T cell differentiation. Certain cytokines acting directly on T cells during primary activation appear to be the most proximal or direct mediators of CD4+ T cell differentiation. The presence of IL-12 during primary T cell activation leads to strong development of Th1 responses, and IL-4 promotes Th2 development. Activation through the TCR is a requirement for initiating terminal differentiation, but the signals from the TCR appear to be phenotype-neutral.

Certain T cells carry out delayed hypersensitivity reactions. These T cells react with antigen MHC class II on APCs and create their effects mainly through cytokine production. These cells generally are of the CD4+ phenotype.

T cells can also be differentiated into two populations depending on whether they use an αβ (TCR2) or γδ (TCR1) antigen receptor. The TCR consists of a heterodimer and a number of associated polypeptides that form the CD3 complex. The dimer recognizes processed antigen associated with an MHC molecule. The CD3 complex is required for receptor expression and is involved in signal transduction. TCR1 cells constitute less than 5% of total lymphocytes but appear in greater proportions in some sites (e.g., skin, vagina). TCR1 cells appear to recognize different antigens than TCR2 cells, including carbohydrate and intact protein antigens. In addition, some TCR1 cells do not require antigen to be processed or presented by MHC molecules.

T Regulatory Lymphocytes

Treg cells are immunoregulatory Th cells that control autoimmunity in the peripheral blood through dominant tolerance. Types of Treg cells include the following:
- Natural CD4+ Treg cells
- Th3 cells
- Tr1 cells
- CD8+ Treg cells

Natural Treg cells, characterized by constitutive expression of CD25, are developed primarily in the thymus from positively selected thymocytes with a relatively high avidity for self antigens. Natural Treg cells represent approximately 5% to 10% of the total CD4+ T cell population. The signal to develop into Treg cells is thought to come from interactions between the TCR and MHC class II self-peptide complex expressed on the thymic stroma. In humans, natural Treg cells express CD4 and CD25.

Other types of Treg cells that can develop in the periphery are Tr1 and Th3 cells. Tr1 cells are CD4+ and are functionally

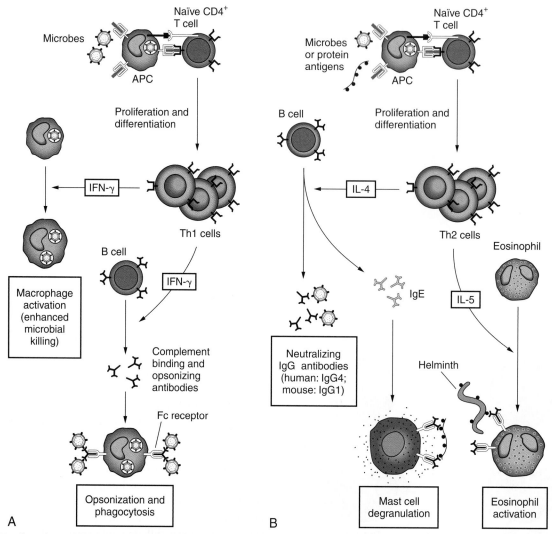

Figure 4-10   Functions of Th1 and Th2 subsets of CD4+ helper T lymphocytes. A, Th1 cells produce the cytokine IFN-γ, which activates phago-cytes to kill ingested microbes and stimulates the production of antibodies that promote the ingestion of microbes by the phagocytes. **B,** Th2 cells specific for microbial or nonmicrobial protein antigens produce the cytokines IL-4, which stimulates the production of IgE antibody, and IL-5, which activates eosinophils. IgE participates in the activation of mast cells by protein antigens and coats helminths for destruction by eosinophils. Th2 cells also stimulate the production of other antibodies (IgG4 in humans) that neutralize microbes and toxins but do not bind to Fc receptors or activate complement efficiently. *(Adapted from Abbas AK, Lichtman AH: Basic immunology: functions and disorders of the immune system, ed 3, Philadelphia, 2008, Saunders.)*

induced by IL-10. These Treg cells, in turn, secrete IL-10 and regulate the immune system. Th3 progenitor cells are also CD4+. In vitro CD4+ cells have been shown to secrete transforming growth factor β (TGF-β). CD8+ Treg cells are less well characterized and are reportedly capable of suppressing CD4+ cells in vitro.

Cytotoxic T Lymphocytes

Cytotoxic T lymphocytes, or T cytotoxic (Tc) cells, are effector cells found in the peripheral blood that are capable of directly destroying virally infected target cells. Most Tc cells are CD8+ and recognize antigen on the target cell surface associated with MHC class I molecules (e.g., human leukocyte antigen [HLA] types A, B, and C) or MHC class I alone. This process is demonstrated by the immune response to virus-infected cells or tumor cells (Fig. 4-11).

In a primary viral infection, naïve CD8+ T cells are primed in secondary lymph nodes and consequently proliferate and differentiate into effector CD8+ T cells to eliminate virus-infected cells. After clearance of the virus, most effector CD8+ T cells contract because of apoptosis but a small number of these CD8+ T cells form a memory T cell pool.

Studies have demonstrated that human CD8+ T cells undergo a change in the expression of costimulatory molecules (e.g., CD27, CD28, and CD45RA) on their surface, according to their differentiation and maturation. Cytolytic effector molecules, perforin, and **granzyme A-B,** are considered to be markers for effector CD8+ T cells because they are the actual functional molecules for killing target cells.

Naïve and central memory CD8+ T cells express the membrane marker, CCR7, for homing to secondary lymph nodes, but effector memory and effector CD8+ T cells express the

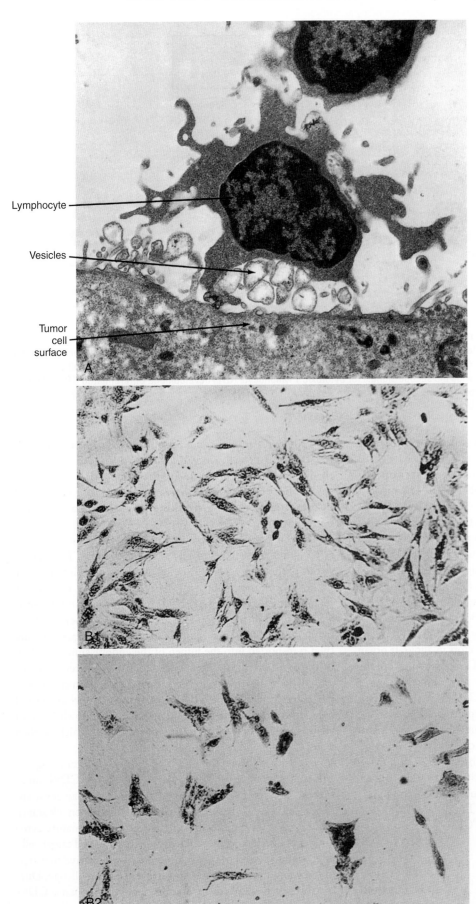

Lymphocyte

Vesicles

Tumor
cell
surface

Figure 4-11   A, Transmission electron photomicrograph demonstrating the initial stages of the attack of a cytotoxic lymphocyte on a tumor cell, only a portion of which is seen. Note vesicles and blebs of cytoplasm being shed by the lymphocyte. **B,** Effects of cytotoxic lymphocytes on tumor cells. *1,* Tumor cells before contact with immune lymphocytes. *2,* Tumor cells after contact. Note that many cells have detached from the surface, some cells are swollen, and a few cells exhibit the morphology of normal cells. *(From Barrett JT: Textbook of immunology, ed 5, St Louis, 1988, Mosby.)*

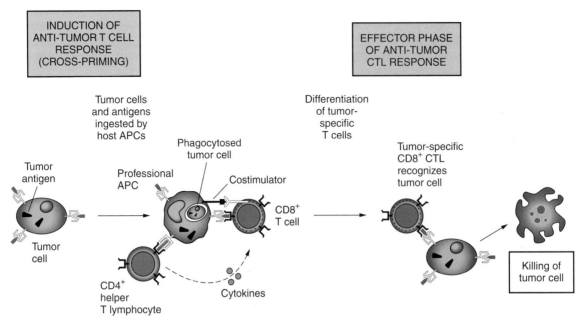

Figure 4-12   Induction of CD8+ T cell responses against tumors. Responses to tumors may be induced by cross-priming (or cross-presentation), in which the tumor cells and tumor antigens are taken up by specialized (so-called professional) APCs, processed, and presented to T cells. In some cases, B7 costimulators expressed by the APCs provide the second signals for the differentiation of the CD8+ T cells. APCs may also stimulate CD4+ helper T cells, which provide the second signals for cytotoxic T lymphocyte (CTL) development. Differentiated CTLs kill tumor cells without a requirement for costimulation or T cell assistance. *(From Abbas AK, Lichtman AH: Basic immunology: functions and disorders of the immune system, ed 3, Philadelphia, 2008, Saunders.)*

chemokine receptors for inflammatory cytokines, which enable the cells to migrate toward infected and inflamed sites. A unique subset of the effector CD8+ T cell population expresses CXCR1. These CXCR1 CD8+ T cells possess chemotactic activity toward the CDCR1 ligand IL-8, a potent inflammatory cytokine produced in inflamed tissues and in tissues infected with some viruses, such as human cytomegalovirus (HCMV) or influenza A. This suggests that these CXCR1+ effector CD8+ T cells immediately migrate to inflamed and infected sites to exert their effector function in the initial stage of an immune response. It is possible that effector CD8+ T cell subsets are functionally distinct populations of T lymphocytes.

In addition to destruction of virally infected, MHC class I–bearing targets, Tc cells are major effectors in allograft organ rejection. Tc cells express CD4 or CD8, depending on the MHC antigen restriction that governs their antigen recognition (i.e., class I or II antigens; Fig. 4-12).

Suppressor T lymphocytes, or T suppressor (Ts) cells, are functionally defined T cells that downregulate the actions of other T and B cells. Ts cells have no unique markers. Although antigen-specific suppression was described in 1970, and many investigators believe that Ts cells are critical in various phases of immunoregulation, peripheral tolerance, and autoimmunity, their mode of action is unclear. Many Ts cells are CD8+ and may operate through secretion of free TCRs.

Antigen Processing and Antigen Presentation to T Cells

Antigen-presenting cells (APCs) are a group of functionally defined cells capable of taking up antigens and presenting them to lymphocytes in a form that they can recognize.

APCs take up antigens (e.g., dendritic cells, macrophages, B cells, even tissue cells) in various ways. Some are collected in the periphery and transported to the secondary lymphoid tissues; other APCs normally reside in lymphoid tissues and intercept antigen as it arrives. B cells recognize antigen in a native form.

There are two major pathways of antigen processing for the APC and target cell, endogenous and exogenous. The **endogenous pathway** processes proteins that have been internalized, processed into fragments, and reexpressed at the cell surface membrane in association with MHC molecules. In this pathway, proteins in the cytoplasm are cleaved into peptide fragments about 20 amino acids in length. These fragments are then transported into the lumen of the endoplasmic reticulum by the transporter associated with the antigen-processing complex, where the fragments encounter newly formed, heavy-chain molecules of MHC class I and their associated beta$_2$-microglobulin (β_2m) light chains. The heavy chain, light chain, and peptide form a trimeric complex, which is then transported to and expressed on the cell surface.

T cells that express the CD8+ cell surface marker recognize antigens presented by MHC class I molecules. CD8+ functions as a coreceptor in this process, binding to an invariant region of the MHC class I molecule. Pathogen clearance requires that CD8+ effector cells produce inflammatory cytokines and develop cytolytic activity against infected target cells, after which a small number of memory cells survive that rapidly regain effector function in the event of rechallenge. During this process, a relatively homogeneous pool of naïve CD8+ T cells differentiates into heterogeneous pools of effector and memory CD8+ T cells.

In the **exogenous pathway,** soluble proteins are taken up from the extracellular environment, generally by specialized or so-called professional APCs. The antigens are then processed in a series of intracellular acidic vesicles called endosomes. During this process, the endosomes intersect with vesicles that are transporting MHC class II molecules to the cell surface. CD4+ T cells recognize antigens that are presented by MHC class II molecules. As with CD8, the CD4 molecule functions as a coreceptor, increasing the strength of the interaction between the T cell and APC.

For both systems of antigen presentation, recognition of the antigen by the T cells is described as being MHC-restricted, a process whereby T cells recognize only antigen presented by self MHC molecules.

Antigen Recognition by T Cells

T cells are clonally restricted, so that each T cell expresses a receptor that can interact with a given peptide. Each lymphocyte makes only one type of antigen receptor and can recognize only a very limited number of antigens. Because receptors differ on each clone of cells, the entire lymphocyte population has an enormous number of different, specific antigen receptors.

The TCR of most T lymphocytes is composed of an alpha and beta polypeptide chain, with constant regions located close to the cell surface and the part that binds to the antigenic peptide of appropriate fit located away from the cell surface. The difference in structure of the distal regions of the alpha and beta chains allows the development of different clones of T cells. The TCR reacts with antigen in the context of MHC class I or II molecules on an APC (Fig. 4-13).

T cells recognize protein antigens in the form of peptide fragments presented at the cell surface by MHC I or II molecules. When the antigen-specific TCR on the T cell surface (specifically the zeta-beta chains) of the CD3 complex interacts with the appropriate peptide-MHC complex, it triggers phosphorylation of the intracellular domains of the CD3 zeta chains. Subsequently, the zeta-associated protein 70 (ZAP-70) binds to the phosphorylated zeta chains and is activated.

Simultaneous colligation of the cell marker CD4 (or CD8) with the MHC class II (or I) molecule results in the phosphorylation of particular kinases. These events stimulate the activation of at least three intracellular signaling cascades. T cell activation also requires a second costimulatory signal (e.g., interaction between marker CD28 on T cells and marker CD80 on APCs). This interaction also triggers several intracellular signaling pathways.

T Cell Activation

T cell activation requires a minimum of two signals:
- Signal 1 is delivered by the TCR-CD3 complex through interaction of the TCR α and β chains as they recognize peptide presented by a class I CD8+ T cell or a class II CD4+ T cell MHC molecule.
- Signal 2 is usually provided by the engagement of CD28 on the T cell with the costimulatory molecule CD80 or CD86 on the APC. The surface markers CD 137 and CD134 also provide costimulation to T cells.

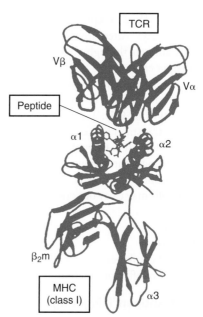

Figure 4-13 Recognition of peptide-MHC by TCR. This ribbon diagram is drawn from the crystal structure of the extracellular portion of a peptide-MHC bound to a T cell antigen receptor (TCR) that is specific for the peptide displayed by the MHC molecule. The peptide can be seen attached to the cleft at the top of the MHC molecule, and one residue of the peptide contacts the variable (V) region of a TCR. *(Adapted from Bjorkman PJ: MHC restriction in three dimensions: a view of T cell receptor/ligand interactions, Cell 89:167-170, 1997.)*

BOX 4-1	Screening for Congenital Immunodeficiencies
Components	
CD2	
CD3	
HLA-DR	
CD4	
CD45RA	
CD45RO	
CD 8	
CD4/CD8 ratio	
CD19	
NK cells	

Adapted from Associated Regional and University Pathologists (ARUP): Lymphocyte subset panel 7: congenital immunodeficiencies, 2012 (http://www.aruplab.com/guides/ug/tests/0095899.jsp).

The optimal combination of effector function, proliferation, and survival requires both signals. Delivery of signal 1 without costimulation, which often occurs in tumor-infiltrating lymphocytes, leads to **anergy** and apoptosis, which limits the antitumor response of the cells.

Activation of T cells can lead to the following:
- Cell division
- Cytokine secretion by T cells
- Expression by T cells of antigens associated with activated state

Activated T cells frequently express activation antigens (Box 4-1). Expression of CD69 occurs within 12 hours of activation, followed by CD25 (IL-2 receptor) and CD71 (transferrin receptor) in 1 to 3 days. Alternatively, in the case of Tc cells, interaction with antigen through the specific TCR leads to destruction of target cells.

If a cell does not receive a full set of signals, it will not divide and may even become anergic. Peripheral T cells generally exist in a resting state (G0 or G1). T cell activation is a complex reaction involving transmembrane signaling and intracellular enzyme activation steps. It is through soluble cytokines that T cell regulation influences the action of other T cells, accessory cells, and nonimmune constituents. When activated by the proper signals, T cells may carry out one or more of the following functions:

1. Proliferation
2. Differentiation
3. Production of cytokines
4. Development of effector function

T-Independent Antigen Triggering

Some antigens, particularly polysaccharide polymers (e.g., dextran), can trigger B cells without help from T cells. These **T-independent antigens** generally are not strong, provoke mainly IgM responses, and induce minimal immunologic memory.

NATURAL KILLER AND K-TYPE LYMPHOCYTES

A subpopulation of circulating lymphocytes (≈10%), NK and K-type lymphocytes, lack conventional antigen receptors of T or B cells. These cells are classified as effector lymphocytes that produce mediators (e.g., IL-2).

Although these cells were previously classified as null cells, MAbs demonstrate that NK and K-type cells express a variety of surface membrane markers (Table 4-3). Most of these cells lack CD3 but express CD2, CD16, CD56, CD57 and, occasionally, CD8.

Natural Killer Cells *APPear LGL Clean lymph.*

Natural killer (NK) **cells** are essential mediators of virus immunity. Their deficiency in humans lead to uncontrolled

Table 4-3	Natural Killer Cell Profile
Components	**Reference Interval (% Positive)**
CD2	75-92
CD3	63-84
CD5	61-88
CD7	73-94
CD8	14-39
CD16	1-12
CD56	7-27
CD57	1-26

Data from Associated Regional and University Pathologists (ARUP): Interpretive data guide, ed 2, Salt Lake City, Utah, 1999, Associated Regional and University Pathologists, p 473.

Tumor killer

viral replication and poor clinical outcome. MHC class I (MCH I) is essential to NK and T cell effector and surveillance functions. A total of 70% to 80% of NK cells have the appearance of large granular lymphocytes (LGLs). Up to about 75% of LGLs function as NK cells and LGLs appear to account fully for the NK activity in mixed cell populations.

NK cells destroy target cells through an extracellular non-phagocytic mechanism referred to as a cytotoxic reaction, MHC-unrestricted cytolysis. Target cells include tumor cells, some cells of the embryo, cells of the normal bone marrow and thymus, and microbial agents. Studies have suggested that a considerable number of NK cells may be present in other tissues, particularly in the lungs and liver, where they may play important roles in inflammatory reactions and in host defense, including defense against certain viruses (e.g., cytomegalovirus, hepatitis). NK cells will actively kill virally infected target cells and, if this activity is completed before the virus has time to replicate, a viral infection may be stopped.

Several cytokines affect NK cell activation and proliferation. NK cells are highly responsive to IL-2, IL-7, and IL-12. These cytokines generate high cytokine-activated killer activity in these cells. In addition, NK cells synthesize a number of cytokines involved in the modulation of hematopoiesis and immune responses and in the regulation of their own activities.

Target cell recognition and the molecular identification and analysis of the involved NK cell receptors are undergoing intensive research. These molecules are mainly classified under the family of cell adhesion molecules (CAMs). The main class of effector CAMs shown to mediate NK cell functions is the leukocyte integrins—more specifically, the β_2 class of integrins.

Several NK cell surface molecules involved in target cell recognition and binding have been identified. NK cells recognize targets using several cell surface molecular receptors (e.g., CD2, CD69, NKR-P1) and a high density of the Fc receptor CD16 of IgG (FC-R III). They also receive inhibitory signals from MHC class I on potential target cells, transduced by a killer inhibitory receptor on the NK cell. CD56 may mediate interactions between effector and target cells. NK cells are able to bind and lyse antibody-coated nucleated cells through a membrane Fc receptor that can recognize part of the heavy chain of immunoglobulins. This enables NK cells to mediate antibody-dependent, cell-mediated cytotoxic (ADCC) activities. Some, if not all, of the activation of NK cells is mediated by CD16, which exerts a regulatory role in their cytolytic function. NK cells respond to cross-linking of CD16 and CD69 as follows:

- Increasing the rate of proliferation of NK cells
- Elevating the levels of TNF production within 4 hours of stimulation
- Increasing the expression of CD69 on the cell surface of NK cells
- Increasing the cytotoxicity activity against a normally resistant cell line (P815)

K-Type Lymphocytes *Ress small lymph*

K-type killer cells are mononuclear cells that can kill target cells sensitized with antibody, which they engage through their

Fc receptors. Most K-type cells are non-T, non-B lymphocytes, but macrophages and eosinophils can also have K cell activity.

K-type cells exhibit a different cytotoxic mechanism than NK cells. The target cell must be coated with low concentrations of IgG antibody, referred to as an ADCC reaction. An ADCC reaction may be exhibited by both K cells and phagocytic and nonphagocytic myelogenous-type leukocytes. K cells are capable of lysing tumor cells. Although morphologically similar to a small lymphocyte, the precise lineage of the K cell is uncertain.

DEVELOPMENT AND DIFFERENTIATION OF B LYMPHOCYTES

B cells represent a small proportion of the circulating peripheral blood lymphocytes. The unfavorable image of B lymphocytes in the pathogenesis of immune disease has been associated mainly with their capacity to produce harmful antibodies after differentiation into plasma cells.

Other roles have been discovered for B lymphocytes, including an antibody-independent pathogenic role of B cells (e.g., capability to present antigen). On recognition of a specific antigen, the B cell membrane is reorganized, resulting in an aggregation of B cell receptors in an immunologic synapse that functions as a platform for internalization of the complex. Internalized antigen is degraded and subsequently exposed to the B cell surface in association with MHC complex molecules for presentation to T cells. This surface presentation of antigen, in the presence of various costimulatory molecules, elicits the assistance of T cells required to assist B cell maturation, which in turns allows B cells to drive optimal T cell activation and differentiation into memory subsets.

B cells also have the capacity to expand clonally, which allows them to become the numerically dominant APCs. Activated B cells also produce a wide range of cytokines and chemokines that modulate the maturation, migration, and function of other immune effector cells.

B LYMPHOCYTE SUBSETS

B1 and B2 cells are B cell subsets. B1 cells are distinguished by the CD5 marker, appear to form a self-renewing set, respond to a number of common microbial antigens, and occasionally generate autoantibodies. B2 cells account for most of the B lymphocytes in adults. This subset generates a greater diversity of antigen receptors and responds effectively to T-dependent antigen.

B cells are derived from progenitor cells through an antigen-independent maturation process occurring in the bone marrow and GALT. Participation of B cells in the humoral immune response is accomplished by reacting to antigenic stimuli through division and differentiation into plasma cells. Plasma cells or antibody-forming cells are terminally differentiated B cells. These cells are entirely devoted to antibody production, a primary host defense against microorganisms.

The specific antibodies produced are able to bind to infected cells, free organisms bearing the antigen, and then inactivate those cells or organisms and destroy them. The condition of hyperacute rejection of transplanted organs is also mediated by B cells. In addition, antigenic stimulation prompts B cells to multiply.

Cell Surface Markers

B lymphocytes are best known to express CD19 but not CD3 surface membrane markers. During B-cell differentiation in the bone marrow, the surface molecule CD19 appears early and remains on the B cell unit until it differentiates into a plasma cell. Four proteins on the surface of mature B cells-CD19, CD21, CD81, and CD225—from the CD19 complex.

Primitive B cell precursors have δ chains in their cytoplasm and no Ig on their surface. More differentiated (but still immature) B cells have intact cytoplasmic IgM and surface IgM. Mature B cells lose their cytoplasmic IgM and add surface IgD to the surface IgM. These changes appear to occur in the absence of antigen and depend on cytokines.

In humans, there is evidence of four types of B **cell surface markers:**

1. Ig receptor is the best studied B cell surface marker. This receptor is actually an antibody molecule with antigenic specificity. According to the clonal selection theory, B cells exist in the body with Ig receptors specific for antigen before exposure to the antigenic substances. When specific antigen exposure does occur, the antigen will select the B cell having an Ig receptor with the best fit.

After binding and cooperative interaction with T cells, B cells undergo transformation into plasma cells. The secreted antibody, in turn, has the same specificity as the Ig receptor on the B cell. Almost all the antibody produced by plasma cells is secreted (plasma cells have few Ig receptors), but 90% of the antibody produced by B cells is expressed as surface Ig receptors. Some antigens (e.g., lipopolysaccharides from some gram-negative organisms) can bind to the Ig receptor and also stimulate an antibody response independent of T cell cooperation (T-independent antigens). This type of response is generally of low intensity and is class-restricted to the production of IgM antibody.

B cells have **surface immunoglobulin (sIg),** except for very immature lymphocytes and mature plasma cells, that are normally polyclonal (i.e., kappa and lambda light chains are present on the cytoplasmic membrane of B cells). Mu and delta heavy chains are usually found with kappa or lambda chains on any one cell surface. Gamma and alpha chains are rarely found on the surface of properly prepared, normal lymphocytes.

2. An Fc receptor that specifically binds the Fc portion of IgG antibody may function to aid B cells in binding to antigen already bound to antibody.
3. Receptors that bind fragments of the cleaved complement component C3 have been reported on the surface of approximately 75% of B cells. This receptor binds C3b, iC3b (inactivated C3b), and C3d, but the function of these receptors is not completely understood.
4. B cell surface antigens coded by the MHC class II genes are a fourth type of human B cell marker.

B Cell Activation

B cells can be stimulated in their resting state to enlarge, develop synthetic machinery, divide, mature, and secrete antibody. The proper signals for this sequence depend on the type of triggers, which can be specific or nonspecific and polyclonal. Specific activation involves the antigen that is complementary to the particular Ig on the surface. Nonspecific activation occurs with B cell mitogens.

Efficient antibody production to complex protein antigens requires T cell help, which in turn develops from APCs presenting antigen to the T cell. Activated T cells secrete a variety of cytokines that together with the specific antigen, trigger the B cell to develop into an antibody-secreting cell. This process also involves class switching.

In the immune response to a foreign protein, the first antibodies to appear are of the IgM class (or isotype). As the response proceeds, other isotypes (IgG, IgA, and IgE) emerge from Ig class switching. The isotype switch has considerable clinical importance because each of the four major isotypes has specialized biologic properties. IgG is the principal class of antibody in interstitial fluids and IgA is the protective antibody of mucosal surfaces. Isotype switching requires collaboration between antibody-synthesizing B cells and helper CD4+ T cells. The B cell uses IgM molecules on its surface to capture the antigen and present the antigen to the T cell. Contact between the collaborating lymphocytes is enhanced by complementary pairs of CAMs. Some CAMs (e.g., CD4, MHC class II antigens) are constitutively expressed on the surface of T and B cells, whereas others are induced. For example, contact between B and T cells induces the T cell to express a ligand for the B cell surface molecule CD40. In turn, CD40 interacts with the newly expressed CD40 ligand on the T cell, which leads to the expression of another B cell surface molecule, B7. The latter's partner on the surface of the T lymphocyte is CD28. These cooperative and synergistic interactions between T and B cells induce the secretion of cytokines such as IL-2 and IL-4.

Isotype switching requires two signals. The first is delivered by an interleukin and the second by the binding of CD40 to its ligand on the T cell. In the process of switching from IgM synthesis to IgE synthesis, IL-4 makes the IgE gene in the B cell accessible to the switch machinery initiated when CD40 binds to its ligand. In this process, the gene that encodes the variable region (the part of the antibody molecule that contains the antigen-binding site) moves from its position near the gene that encodes for IgM to a position near the gene that encodes for IgE.

PLASMA CELL BIOLOGY

The function of **plasma cells** (see Color Plate 9) is the synthesis and excretion of immunoglobulins. Plasma cells are not normally found in the circulating blood but are found in the bone marrow in concentrations that do not normally exceed 2%. Plasma cells arise as the end stage of B cell differentiation into a large, activated plasma cell.

The pathway from the B lymphocyte to the antibody-synthesizing plasma cell forms when the B cell is antigenically stimulated and undergoes transformation because of the stimulation of various **interleukins.** The immune antibody response begins when individual B lymphocytes encounter an antigen that binds to their specific Ig surface receptors. After receiving an appropriate second signal provided by interaction with helper T cells, these antigen-binding B cells undergo transformation and proliferation to generate a clone of mature plasma cells that secretes a specific type of antibody.

An increase in plasma cells can be seen in a variety of nonmalignant disorders, such as viral disease (e.g., rubella, infectious mononucleosis), allergic conditions, chronic infections, and collagen diseases. In plasma cell **dyscrasias,** the plasma cells can be greatly increased or infiltrate the bone marrow completely (e.g., multiple myeloma, Waldenström's macroglobulinemia).

Antibody molecules secreted by plasma cells consist of four chains—two light chains and two heavy chains, based on molecular weight—and can be enzymatically cleaved into Fab (antigen-binding) and Fc (crystallizable) fragments. The Fab portion binds antigen and contains the light chains and their antigenic markers (kappa, lambda), as well as heavy chains.

The Fc fragment contains the markers that distinguish the different classes of antibody and sites that will bind and activate complement and bind to Fc receptors on cells. The amino acid sequence for most of the antibody protein is constant, except for the antigen-binding portion of the molecule, which has a hypervariable region and accounts for the various antigenic specificities that the antibody is programmed to recognize.

ALTERATIONS IN LYMPHOCYTE SUBSETS

The normal functioning of helper cells and suppressor cells in the immune response can be reversed under certain conditions. For example, the target cell for human T cell leukemia or human immunodeficiency virus (HIV) is phenotypically a helper cell but functionally a suppressor cell. Functionally, the helper-inducer subset of cells signals B cells to generate antibodies, control production and switching of types of antibodies formed, and activate suppressor cells. The **suppressor-cytotoxic lymphocytes** control and inhibit antibody production by suppressing helper cells or by turning off B cell differentiation. The normal ratio of helper cells and suppressor cells ($\approx$2:1) can be reversed under certain conditions.

Changes With Aging

Except for inconsistent values seen in extremely old adults, the total number of T cells in the peripheral blood is relatively stable throughout adult life. However, there is a change in the distribution of T cell subpopulations. A decrease in the number of suppressor cells and an increase in the helper cell population are demonstrated in older adults.

The effect of aging on the immune response is highly variable, but the ability to respond immunologically to disease is age-related. Faulty immunologic reactions (e.g., aberrant functioning of **immunoregulatory cells, effector T cells,** and antibody-producing B cells) may contribute to poor immunity in older adults. Functional deficits of T lymphocytes have been identified with aging, causing impairment of cell-mediated immunity. In addition, skin testing reveals decreases in the intensity of delayed hypersensitivity in older adults. The proliferative response of T lymphocytes to mitogens or antigens such as *Mycobacterium tuberculosis* or varicella-zoster virus is impaired.

A decrease in Th cells is the primary cause of the impaired humoral response in older adults. Although the total number of B cells and total Ig concentration remain unchanged, the serum concentration of IgM is decreased and IgA and IgG concentrations are increased.

EVALUATION OF IMMUNODEFICIENCY SYNDROMES

Although more than 50 genetically determined **immunodeficiency syndromes** have been reported since 1952, defects in immunity were considered rare until acquired immunodeficiency syndrome (AIDS) emerged more than 30 years ago. This growing list of primary and secondary diseases now encompasses all major components of the immune system, including lymphocytes, phagocytic cells, and complement proteins.

Older children and adults with recurrent upper and lower respiratory tract infections and/or diarrhea, abscesses, sepsis, or meningitis should be evaluated for immunodeficiency. Before proceeding with laboratory testing, primary care providers need to rule out the following:

- Anatomic or physical causes (e.g., foreign bodies, indwelling catheters)
- Cancer
- Connective tissue disease
- Diabetes
- Renal disease

Laboratory testing can then proceed with a complete blood cell (CBC) count, including a platelet count and erythrocyte sedimentation rate (ESR). These are among the most cost-effective screening tests. If the ESR is normal, chronic bacterial infection is unlikely. If the absolute neutrophil count is normal, congenital and acquired neutropenias and severe chemotactic defects are eliminated. If the absolute lymphocyte count is normal, the patient is not likely to have a severe T cell defect. The absolute lymphocyte count is the number of lymphocytes in the total white blood cell (WBC) population (Box 4-2).

Laboratory tests to screen for more common immunodeficiencies include immunoglobulin testing, complement testing, cell-mediated immunity testing, and the neutrophil function test. Additional laboratory testing should include a general metabolic panel to assess overall general health, HIV types 1 and 2, protein electrophoresis, sweat chloride, and pneumococcal antibody IgG titers pre- and postvaccine in patients with only recurrent sinopulmonary infections. Follow-up testing based on any initially abnormal results is presented in Tables 4-4 and 4-5. If all initial test results are normal, IL-1 receptor-associated kinase-4 (IRAK-4) deficiency screening or a Toll-like receptor function assay should be performed. If abnormal results are subsequently found, the diagnosis is an innate immune deficiency.

Cell-Mediated Immune System

Deficiencies of cell-mediated immunity are often suspected in individuals with recurrent viral, fungal, parasitic, and protozoal infections. Patients with AIDS exhibit some of the most severe manifestations of cell-mediated immunity (see Chapter 25).

One avenue of testing involves delayed hypersensitivity skin testing to determine the integrity of the patient's cell-mediated immune response. More than 90% of normal adults will react to one of the following antigens within 48 hours after antigen exposure: *Candida albicans*, *Trichophyton*, tetanus toxoid, mumps, and streptokinase-streptodornase. Reactivity to histoplasmin or purified protein derivative (PPD) is positive in patients with active infection or previous exposure to histoplasmosis or tuberculosis, respectively; therefore these tests are not useful for the assessment of anergy.

The number of T lymphocytes, the primary effector cells in cell-mediated reactions, can be determined by several techniques. Previously, the gold standard was the E rosette technique (erythrocyte rosette formation), but the development of flow cytometry with MAbs has replaced this technique. Testing for the functionality of lymphocytes is just as important as a quantitative count of CD4+ and CD8+ cells.

Box 4-2	Determination of Absolute Lymphocyte Count
Absolute number of lymphocytes = total leukocyte count × percentage (%) of lymphocytes	
Total leukocyte count = 25×10^9/L	
Relative percentage (%) of lymphocytes = 76%	
Absolute number = 19×10^9/L	

Table 4-4	Next Steps in Laboratory Evaluation of Suspected Immunodeficiency
Abnormal Initial Laboratory Result	**Follow-Up Testing**
Protein electrophoresis	Immunofixation electrophoresis monoclonal protein detection; quantitation and characterization of IgA, IgG and IgM, and Bence Jones protein; depending on individual results, additional testing may be needed
Sweat chloride	Cystic fibrosis (CFTR)—32 mutations with reflex to sequencing
Positive for HIV-1, HIV-2	HIV-1 antibody confirmation by Western blot
Pneumococcal antibodies absent after vaccination	Specific antibody deficiency

Adapted from Associated Regional and University Pathologists (ARUP) Consult: Immunodeficiency evaluation for chronic infections in adults and older children testing algorithm, 2012 (http://www.arupconsult.com/Algorithms/ChronicInfections Adults.pdf).

The in vitro diagnostic test (IVD; see later, "Assessment of Cellular Immune Status") is the newest approach to testing the functionality of T lymphocytes. It is important to recognize that CD4 counts do not always reflect the actual status of the patient's immune system. ImmuKnow (Cylex, Columbia, Md) is the first U.S. Food and Drug Administration (FDA)–approved immune function test. It is widely considered to be the gold standard of immune function testing.

The QuantiFERON-CMI kit (Cellestis, Valencia, Calif) is an in vitro assay for measuring cell-mediated immune functionality. The procedure is a single-step enzyme-linked immunosorbent assay (ELISA) to determine T cell responses by measuring IFN-γ levels in plasma. This is a specific marker cytokine for a cell-mediated or inflammatory immune response (e.g., bacterial, parasitic, or viral).

Research-Based Tests

Various procedures are research-based, including a lymphocyte antigen and mitogen proliferation panel. This type of procedure measures cytokine production by mononuclear cells in response to mitogen stimulation by IL-1β types 6 and 8 and TNF-α. Another method includes flow cytometry and the enzyme-linked immunosorbent spot assay (ELISPOT). Flow cytometry can be used in conjunction with intracellular cytokine staining with ³H-thymidine to detect the T cell response to specific antigenic stimulation by multianalyte fluorescence detection. In addition, peptide–MHC complex tetramer or pentamer staining is used to quantify the number of T cells with a particular antigenic epitope based on the expression of a specific T cell receptor. A multiplex cytokine analysis (e.g., multiplex bead-based Luminex assay [Life Technologies, Grand Island, NY]) is being used to detect multiple cytokines in serum, plasma, or tissue culture supernatants.

Humoral System

The humoral system can be screened for abnormalities by quantitating the concentrations of IgM, IgG, and IgA. An initial simple screening can be determined by the presence and titer of antibodies to type A and B red blood cell (RBC) antigens.

IMMUNOLOGIC DISORDERS

A breakdown in any part of the immune mechanism can lead to disease. Disorders with an immunologic origin can involve progenitor cells, phagocytosis (see Chapter 3), T cells, B cells, or complement (see Chapter 5).

Immunologic disorders can be divided into primary processes (dysfunction in the immune organ itself) and acquired, or secondary, processes (disease or therapy causing an immune defect). A third category, diseases mediated through immune mechanisms, can also be included. Because of its complexity and contemporary importance, AIDS is discussed separately in Chapter 25. Other immunoproliferative and autoimmune disorders are discussed in Chapters 27 to 30.

Table 4-5	Next Steps in Evaluation of Suspected Immunodeficiency Based on Physical Findings	
Physical Manifestations	**Follow-Up Laboratory Assays**	**Differential Diagnosis**
Recurrent severe viral or fungal infections (e.g., candidiasis, herpes)	Lymphocyte subset for congenital immunodeficiencies, lymphocyte antigen and mitogen proliferation panel, proliferation panel with cytokine responses to mitogens; testing for 12 cytokines	T cell deficiency, HIV, CD4 deficiency, adenosine deaminase deficiency, nucleoside phosphorylase deficiency, chronic mucocutaneous candidiasis
Recurrent severe sepsis, Neisseria spp., Streptococcus pneumoniae infections	Rule out previous splenectomy and immunoglobulin abnormality; then order a total CAEI. If abnormal (low) activity, analyze C2-C5 components.	Complement deficiency
Abscesses, pneumonia, recurrent respiratory infections with or without diarrhea	Order quantitative IgM, IgG and IgA, IgE, CAEI, neutrophil oxidative burst assay (DHR), leukocyte adhesion deficiency panel, and myeloperoxidase stain.	Low IgM– or IgG–hypogammaglobulinemia Low complement—complement defect Abnormal DHR—chronic granulomatous disease Decreased CD11b/CD18—LAD-1, Decreased CD15—LAD-2 Increased IgE—Possible hyper-IgE syndrome (Job syndrome) but must be followed by Candida-specific IgE neutrophil chemotaxis and subsequent genetic testing Positive neutrophil antibody—autoimmune neutropenia, Absence of myeloperoxidase—myeloperoxidase deficiency

Adapted from Associated Regional and University Pathologists (ARUP) Consult: Immunodeficiency evaluation for chronic infections in adults and older children testing algorithm, 2012 (http://www. arupconsult.com/Algorithms/ChronicInfections Adults.pdf).
CAEI, Complement activity enzyme immunoassay; *DHR,* neutrophil oxidative burst assay; *LAD-1,* leukocyte adhesion deficiency, type 1; *LAD-2,* leukocyte adhesion deficiency, type 2.

Immunodeficiency disorders may be caused by defects in the quality (defects) or quantity (deficiencies) of lymphocytes and may be congenital or acquired. These conditions may be combined disorders or may involve T cells or B cells (Table 4-6).

Primary Immunodeficiency Disorders

Primary immunodeficiencies (PID) are rare genetic disorders of the innate and adaptive immune system. Classic **primary immunodeficiency disorders (PIDs)** are usually monogenic (mendelian) disorders affecting host defenses (Box 4-3). More than 200 clinical phenotypes of PID have been described. Over 120 different gene mutations have been identified which cause impairment in the differentiation and/or function of immune cells with different degrees of severity. Diseases associated with a primary defect in the immune response are comprised of about 40% T cell disorders, 50% B cell disorders, 6% phagocytic abnormalities, and 4% complement alterations (Fig. 4-14). The most common T cell deficiency states are those associated with a concurrent B cell abnormality. Primary immunodeficiency disorders are predominantly seen (75%) in children younger than 5 years.

Gene therapy with hematopoietic stem cells (HSC) is a therapeutic strategy for the treatment of several forms of primary immunodeficiency. Current approaches use gene transfer of the therapeutic gene into autologus HSC by retroviral vector-mediated gene transfer. This method has been successful in severe combined immunodeficiencies (SCID-1) and chronic granulomatous disease (CGD). Wiskott-Aldrich syndrome is another good candidate for gene therapy treatment.

T Cell and Combined Immunodeficiency Disorders
DiGeorge's Syndrome   ZINC

Cause. This T cell defect is a congenital anomaly that represents faulty embryogenesis of the endodermal derivation of the third and fourth pharyngeal pouches, which results in aplasia of the parathyroid and thymus glands. At autopsy, parathyroid and vestigial thymus glands may be found in ectopic locations. The newborn may exhibit various facial and vascular anomalies, collectively referred to as pharyngeal pouch syndrome. In addition to the established embryonic cause of DiGeorge's syndrome,

a nutrient (zinc) deficiency in utero has been suggested as a cause of this process.

Signs and Symptoms. DiGeorge's syndrome is present at birth. Initial manifestations can include hypocalcemic tetany, unusual facies, and congenital heart defects. An increased susceptibility to viral, fungal, and disseminated bacterial infections (e.g., acid-fast

Box 4-3	Primary Immunodeficiency Diseases

T Cells
Combined immunodeficiency
Thymic alymphoplasia
Swiss type
Adenosine deaminase deficiency
Nezelof syndrome
DiGeorge's syndrome (thymic hypoplasia)
Wiskott-Aldrich syndrome
Chronic mucocutaneous candidiasis
Immunodeficiency associated with nucleoside
    phosphorylase deficiency
Short-limbed dwarfism
Ataxia-telangiectasia
Thymoma
Leukocyte adhesion deficiency (LAD)

B Cells
Selected IgA deficiency associated with:
Normal state
Allergy
Autoimmune disease
Central nervous system disease
Gastrointestinal disorders
Malignancy
Pulmonary infections
X-linked infantile agammaglobulinemia
X-linked immunodeficiency with hyper-IgM
Common variable hypogammaglobulinemia
Selective IgM deficiency
IgG subclass deficiency

Adapted from Graziano FM, Bell CL: The normal immune response and what can go wrong. A classification of immunologic disorders, Med Clin North Am 69:439–452, 1985.

Table 4-6	T Cell and B Cell Disorders
T Cell Disorder	**B Cell Disorder**
Congenital	
Thymic hypoplasia (DiGeorge's syndrome)	Bruton's agammaglobulinemia
Acquired	
Acquired immunodeficiency syndrome	Autoimmune disorders
Hodgkin's disease	Multiple myeloma
Chronic lymphocytic leukemia	
Systemic lupus erythematosus SLE	

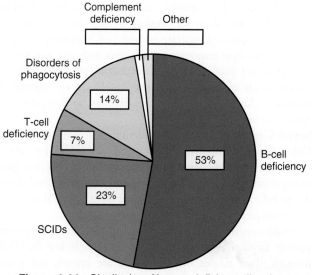

Figure 4-14   Distribution of immunodeficiency disorders.

bacilli, *Listeria monocytogenes*, *Pneumocystis jiroveci* [formerly known as *P. carinii*]) result from the defect of T cells normally controlled by cell-mediated immunity. Infants usually die of sepsis during the first year of life.

Immunologic Manifestations. Peripheral lymphoid tissue appears to be normal except for the depletion of T cells in thymus-dependent zones, such as subcortical region of the lymph nodes and perifollicular and periarteriolar lymphoid sheaths of the spleen. Lymph node paracortical areas and thymus-dependent regions of the spleen show variable degrees of depletion.

In the circulating blood, lymphopenia is generally present, although in some cases the concentration of lymphocytes is normal. However, an abnormally high CD4+/CD8+ ratio is present because of a decrease in CD8+ cells. Most patients with DiGeorge's syndrome have a decreased percentage of cells expressing the CD3+ (mature T cell) antigen. Because patients do demonstrate lymphocytes capable of differentiating to the more mature surface markers, such as CD4+, a small rudimentary thymus is believed to be present in these patients. Lymphocytic responsiveness to antigenic and mitogenic stimulation can be absent, reduced, or normal, depending on the degree of thymic deficiency. Cell-mediated immune reactions such as delayed hypersensitivity and skin allograft rejections, however, are absent or feeble.

Serum Ig concentrations are near normal. Levels of IgA may be diminished and of IgE may be elevated. Antibody response to primary antigenic stimulation may be unimpaired.

Nezelof Syndrome (Cellular Immunodeficiency With Immunoglobulins)

Cause. An autosomal recessive pattern of inheritance is often seen. The defect appears to exist on chromosome 14q13.1.

Signs and Symptoms. Nezelof syndrome is the PID most likely to be confused with AIDS in the pediatric age group. Infants have failure to thrive, recurrent or chronic pulmonary infections, oral or cutaneous candidiasis, chronic diarrhea, recurrent skin infections, gram-negative sepsis, urinary tract infections, and severe varicella.

Immunologic Manifestations. Nezelof syndrome is characterized by lymphopenia, neutropenia, and eosinophilia. In addition, diminished lymphoid tissue and abnormal thymus architecture are observed. Peripheral lymphoid tissues are hypoplastic and demonstrate paracortical lymphocyte depletion. Lymphocyte responses to mitogens, antigens, and allogeneic cells are profoundly depressed but not totally absent. Serum levels of most of the five Ig classes are normal or increased. Antibody-forming capacity has been reported as normal in one third of cases.

Severe Combined Immunodeficiency

Cause. Severe combined immunodeficiency (SCID) is caused by the inappropriate development of progenitor cells into lymphocyte precursors. This hereditary and invariably fatal disorder in infants results from the lack of both T and B cells and the consequent inability to synthesize antibody.

Mutations in the IL-2 receptor complex, a hematopoietic growth factor, have been shown to cause X-linked SCID in humans. Two modes of inheritance are known, autosomal recessive and X-linked recessive. X-linked recessive SCID is

thought to be the most common form of SCID in the United States, which accounts for the 3:1 male-to-female ratio with the disorder.

Of patients with autosomal SCID, 50% have a concomitant deficiency of adenosine deaminase (ADA), an aminohydrolase that converts adenosine to inosine. Analysis by complementary (copy) DNA (cDNA) probe has revealed that the deficiency results from a hereditable point mutation in the ADA gene. Another variant with a severe deficiency in T cell immunity but normal B cell concentrations is associated with purine nucleotide phosphorylase deficiency.

There are two main forms of defective expression of MHC antigens. In a less common form of SCID, known as bare lymphocyte syndrome, an MHC class I antigen deficiency is present. In another form of defective expression, MHC class I antigen deficiency plus the absence of class II antigens is present. Patient lymphocytes cannot be typed by standard serologic cytotoxicity tests.

Signs and Symptoms. No important differences in signs and symptoms exist between the two major genetic types of SCID. Initial manifestations of SCID are repeated debilitating infections beginning within the first 6 months of life. These are dominated by bacterial, viral, and fungal infections of the respiratory and intestinal systems and skin. Infants with SCID usually die within 3 years of birth from lung abscesses, *Pneumocystis* pneumonitis, or a common viral disorder such as chickenpox or measles.

Immunologic Manifestations. The thymus and other lymphoid organs are severely hypoplastic. The bone marrow is devoid of lymphoblasts, lymphocytes, and plasma cells. Lymphocytes are also absent from lymphoid tissues such as the spleen, tonsils, appendix, and intestinal tract. Variable hypogammaglobulinemia with decreased serum IgM and IgA levels and poor to absent antibody production are representative features. Moderate lymphocytopenia is detectable early in infancy. T cell functions are decreased. The circulating blood contains no CD4+, CD8+, or CD3+ cells. The percentage of B cells is usually normal.

Patients with the X-linked form of SCID usually appear similar to those with the autosomal recessive form, except that they tend to have an increased percentage of B cells. However, the defect affects B-lineage cells as well as T-lineage cells.

Chronic Mucocutaneous Candidiasis

Cause. Chronic mucocutaneous candidiasis (CMC) results from a primary defect in cell-mediated immunity. T cells specifically fail to recognize only the *Candida* antigen.

Signs and Symptoms. Patients with CMC usually survive to adulthood. The characteristic manifestation is *Candida* infection of the mucous membranes, scalp, skin, and nails. Endocrine abnormalities, often polyendocrinopathies, are frequently associated with fungal manifestations. Sudden death from adrenal insufficiency has been reported in patients with CMC.

Immunologic Manifestations. Patients demonstrate normal skin reactions to testing with all antigens except *Candida*.

B Cell and Antibody Deficiency Disorders

Because the primary function of B cells is to produce antibody, the major clinical manifestation of a B cell deficiency is an increased susceptibility to severe bacterial infections. Selective

IgA deficiency is the most common B cell disorder, affecting 1 in 400 to 800 persons. Because IgA is the primary immunoglobulin in secretions, a deficiency contributes to pulmonary infections, gastrointestinal (GI) disorders, and allergic respiratory disorders. Most cases (50% of reported cases are associated with Ig deficiencies) are autoimmune in nature, including rheumatoid arthritis (RA), systemic lupus erythematosus (SLE), thyroiditis, and pernicious anemia.

Bruton's X-Linked Agammaglobulinemia

Cause. This is a classic example of an X-linked agammaglobulinemia, in which a disease-causing variant in the gene coding for Bruton's tyrosine kinase (BTK) leads to the arrest of B cell development at the pre–B cell stage.

Signs and Symptoms. X-linked agammaglobulinemia occurs primarily in young boys, but scattered cases have been identified in girls. Manifestations begin in the first or second year of life. Hypersusceptibility to infection does not develop until 9 to 12 months after birth because of passive protection by residual maternal immunoglobulin. Thereafter, patients repeatedly acquire infections with high-grade extracellular pyogenic organisms such as streptococci. This disorder is characterized by sinopulmonary and central nervous system (CNS) infectious episodes and severe septicemia, but patients are not abnormally susceptible to common viral infections (excluding fulminant hepatitis), enterococci, or most gram-negative organisms. Chronic fungal infections are not usually present.

An autoimmune phenomenon, especially a juvenile RA type of disease, has also been associated with X-linked agammaglobulinemia. In addition, patients are highly vulnerable to a malignant form of dermatomyositis that eventually involves destructive T cell infiltration surrounding the small vessels of the CNS. In addition to infections and connective tissue disorders, agammaglobulinemic patients also have hemolytic anemia, drug eruptions, atopic eczema, allergic rhinitis, and asthma.

Immunologic Manifestations. The diagnosis of X-linked agammaglobulinemia is suspected if serum concentrations of IgG, IgA, and IgM are notably below the appropriate level for the patient's age. Tests for natural antibodies to blood group substances and for antibodies to antigens given during standard courses of immunization (e.g., diphtheria) are useful in distinguishing this disorder from transient hypogammaglobulinemia of infancy (see later).

B cells are almost absent from bone marrow and lymphoid tissues. A deficiency or absence of peripheral B lymphocytes is usually noted. If present, B cells are unresponsive to T cells and incapable of antibody synthesis or secretion. Surface immunoglobulins are absent. However, patients have normal numbers of CD3+ and CD8+ cells and many have normal CD4+ cells. Male children possess normal T cell function; therefore, homograft rejection mechanisms are intact and delayed-hypersensitivity reaction for both tuberculin and skin contact types can be elicited.

Common Variable Immunodeficiency

Cause. Common variable immunodeficiency (CVID) is a form of primary acquired agammaglobulinemia, occurring equally in males and females. The cause of CVID seems to be heterogeneous, with abnormalities of B cell maturation, antibody production, antibody secretion, or T cell regulation. Family clusters have been reported in which first-degree relatives of patients with selective IgA deficiency have a high incidence of abnormal Ig concentration, autoantibodies, autoimmune disease, and malignant neoplasms. Findings of rare alleles or deletions of MHC class III genes in patients with IgA deficiency of CVID have suggested that the susceptibility gene(s) is (are) on chromosome 6.

Signs and Symptoms. CVID usually manifests in the second or third decade of life. Signs and symptoms include frequent sinopulmonary infections, diarrhea, endocrine and autoimmune disorders, and malabsorption (e.g., of vitamin B_{12}). Intestinal giardiasis is also prevalent.

Immunologic Manifestations. Both the decreased concentration of immunoglobulins and near absence of serum and secretory IgA are thought to represent the most common and well-defined type of PID. The pattern of inheritance suggests that an autosomal function of antibodies is usually compromised. The number of B cells is typically normal or mildly depressed. Despite a normal number of circulating Ig-bearing B lymphocytes and the presence of lymphoid cortical follicles, blood lymphocytes do not differentiate into Ig-producing cells. In most patients the defect appears to be intrinsic to the B cell. The primary defect in Ig synthesis may be caused by the absence or dysfunction of CD4+ cells or by increased CD8+ supressor cell activity. Therefore, cellular immunity and Ig production are impaired by the interaction between helper and suppressor T cell subsets. Lymph nodes lack plasma cells, but may show striking follicular hyperplasia.

The total IgG level may be normal, but a subclass (usually IgG2 or IgG3) is deficient. Both IgA and IgM may be detectable, but IgM levels may be elevated. In addition, some patients may have thymoma and refractory anemia.

Immunoglobulin Subclass Deficiencies

Some patients have deficiencies of one or more subclasses of IgG despite a normal total IgG serum concentration. Most of those with absent or very low concentrations of IgG2 have been patients with selective IgA deficiency.

Selective Immunoglobulin A Deficiency

Cause. An isolated absence mode is often seen in pedigrees of individuals with CVID. IgA deficiency has been noted to evolve into CVID, and rare alleles and deletions of MHC class III genes in both conditions suggest a common basis.

Signs and Symptoms. IgA deficiency is typically associated with poor health. Infections occur predominantly in the respiratory, GI, and urogenital tracts. There is no clear evidence that patients have any increased susceptibility to viral agents. IgA deficiency has been noted in patients treated with phenytoin, sulfasalazine, penicillamine, and gold, suggesting that environmental factors may lead to expression of the defect.

Immunologic Manifestations. As many as 44% of patients with selective IgA deficiency demonstrate antibodies to IgA. Severe or fatal anaphylactic reactions after IV administration of blood products containing IgA and anti-IgA antibodies (particularly IgE anti-IgA antibodies) have occurred.

Immunodeficiency With Elevated Immunoglobulin M (Hyper-IgM)

Cause. A sex-linked mode of inheritance has been noted in some pedigrees. The abnormal gene in the X-linked type has been localized to Xq24-Xq27. However, more than one genetic cause is suspected.

Signs and Symptoms. Patients with hyper-IgM defect become symptomatic during the first or second year of life, with recurrent pyogenic infections, including otitis media, sinusitis, pneumonia, and tonsillitis. Hemolytic anemia and thrombocytopenia have been observed. Transient, persistent, or cyclic neutropenia is a common feature.

Immunologic Manifestations. This disorder is characterized by extremely low concentrations of IgG and IgA and, most frequently, greatly elevated concentrations of polyclonal IgM. Normal or slightly reduced numbers of IgM and IgD B lymphocytes have been observed.

Transient Hypogammaglobulinemia of Infancy

Unlike patients with Bruton's X-linked agammaglobulinemia or CVID, patients with transient hypogammaglobulinemia of infancy can synthesize antibodies to A and B erythrocyte antigens, if they lack the antigen(s), and to diphtheria and tetanus toxoids. Antibody production usually occurs by 6 to 11 months of age. This antibody production occurs before Ig levels become normal.

X-Linked Lymphoproliferative Disease (Duncan's Disease)

Cause. Duncan's disease is caused by a recessive trait. The defective gene has been localized to the Xq26-Xq27 region.

Signs and Symptoms. The disease is characterized by an inadequate immune reaction to infection with Epstein-Barr virus (EBV). Infected patients are apparently healthy until they experience infectious mononucleosis (see Chapter 22). Two thirds of more than 100 patients studied died of overwhelming EBV-induced B cell proliferation during mononucleosis. Most patients surviving the primary infection developed hypogammaglobulinemia and/or B cell lymphomas.

Immunologic Manifestations. A marked impairment in the production of antibodies to the EBV nucleus has been noted in affected patients. In contrast, titers of antibodies to the viral capsid antigen range from zero to extremely elevated.

Antibody-dependent, cell-mediated cytotoxicity against EBV-infected cells has been low in many patients. NK cell function is also depressed. There is also a deficiency in long-lived T cell immunity to EBV.

Partial Combined Immunodeficiency Disorders

Wiskott-Aldrich Syndrome (Immunodeficiency With Thrombocytopenia and Eczema)

Cause. The primary defect in this uncommon X-linked recessive pediatric disease is caused by a mutation of the gene encoding Wiskott-Aldrich syndrome protein (WASp), which plays a critical role in actin polymerization in blood cells. The mutated gene is expressed uniquely in hematopoietic cells. The effects of WAS gene mutation on this process are of interest particularly, because the actin cytoskeleton has a prominent role in the basic mechanisms of cell adhesion and migration.

Signs and Symptoms. Wiskott-Aldrich syndrome is characterized by the triad of thrombocytopenic purpura, increased susceptibility to infection, and eczema (atopic dermatitis). Affected boys rarely survive beyond 10 years of age. Thrombocytopenia and bleeding are common. Platelets are small, with an intrinsic defect. Patients usually die from sepsis, hemorrhage, or malignancy.

Immunologic Manifestations. There is a tendency toward the development of autoimmune disease. Progressive deterioration of the thymus leads to a defect in cellular immunity and the attrition of T cell populations from the lymph nodes and spleen. Decreased numbers of T cells and alteration in the normal T4:T8 ratio of lymphocytes are manifested. Serum levels of IgM are low, but IgG concentrations are usually normal. IgA levels are normal or elevated, and IgE levels are usually elevated.

The lymph nodes and spleen of WAS patients show relative depletion of lymphocytes from T cell areas. Depletion of the splenic and circulating marginal zone B cells is characteristic and may explain the defective antibody responses, particularly to polysaccharide antigens.

Hereditary Ataxia-Telangiectasia

Cause. This autosomal recessive disorder apparently results from the coexistence of a T cell deficiency with a defect in DNA repair, which leads to extreme, nonrandom chromosomal instability. The sites of chromosomal breakage involve chromosomes 7 and 14 in more than 50% of patients.

Signs and Symptoms. Ataxia-telangiectasia is characterized by ataxia and choreoathetosis in infancy. Multiple telangiectases appear on exposed oculocutaneous surfaces during childhood. A high incidence of malignancy (e.g., lymphoma) is also seen. Children with this disorder eventually die of respiratory insufficiency and sepsis.

Immunologic Manifestations. The thymus is hypoplastic or **dysplastic,** and the thymus-dependent zones of the lymph nodes are void of cells. About 80% of patients lack serum and secretory IgA and some develop IgG antibodies to injections of IgA. The signs and symptoms of the disease appear to result from a concomitant T cell deficiency, deficiency of DNA repair, and disordered IgG synthesis.

Hyperimmunoglobulinemia E Syndrome

Cause. This disorder has a presumed autosomal dominant pattern of inheritance.

Signs and Symptoms. Hyperimmunoglobulinemia E syndrome is a relatively rare PID characterized by recurrent severe staphylococcal abscesses. From infancy, patients have histories of staphylococcal abscesses involving the skin, lungs, joints, and other sites; persistent pneumatoceles develop as a result of the recurrent pneumonias. Pruritic dermatitis also occurs.

Immunologic Manifestations. Patients have elevated levels of serum IgE and IgD; usually, normal concentrations of IgG, IgA, and IgM are present. Poor antibody and cell-mediated responses to **neoantigens** are demonstrated. In addition, a decreased percentage of T cells with the memory receptor CD45RO has been noted.

T Cell Activation Defects

Some patients with defective activation of T cells have experienced the following:

- Defective surface expression of the CD3-TCR complex caused by mutation in the gene encoding the CD3 γ subunit
- Defective signal transduction from the TCR to intracellular metabolic pathways
- Pretranslational defect in IL-2 or other cytokine production

These conditions are characterized by the presence of T cells that appear phenotypically normal but fail to proliferate or produce cytokines in response to stimulation with mitogens, antigens, or other signals delivered to the T cell antigen receptor. Patients' symptoms are similar to those of other T cell–deficient individuals; some patients with severe T cell activation defects may clinically resemble patients with SCID.

Other Primary Immunodeficiencies

In addition to hereditary or congenital disorders of lymphocytes, several PIDs involve the complement system and phagocytic cells. **Complement Deficiency.** Deficiencies in all of the components of the complement system have been described (see Chapter 5). These deficiencies are genetic in origin. Unusual susceptibility to infection is characteristic of some of these components, particularly deficiencies involving C3, C5, C6, and C7 (Table 4-7).

A functional deficiency of polymorphonuclear neutrophil (PMN) leukocytes is chronic granulomatous disease (CGD; see Chapter 3). This fatal syndrome usually begins with the onset of symptoms during the first year of life.

Secondary Immunodeficiency Disorders

A secondary immunodeficiency can result from a disease process that causes a defect in normal immune function, which leads to a temporary or permanent impairment of one or multiple components of immunity in the host (Box 4-4). Patients with secondary immunodeficiencies, which are much more common than primary deficiencies, have an increased susceptibility to infections, as seen in the PIDs.

Immunosuppressive agents and burns are major causes of secondary immunodeficiencies. In varying degrees, immunosuppressive agents have been demonstrated to affect every component of the immune response. In burn patients, septicemia is a common complication in those who survive the initial period of hemodynamic shock. The mechanism that seems most critical in thermal injury is disruption of the skin; however, interference with phagocytosis and deficiencies of serum Ig and complement levels have also been observed.

Immune-Mediated Disease

The immune system is normally efficient in eliminating foreign antigens. The nature of the antigen or the genetic makeup of the host, however, can cause alterations of the immune response that can be injurious and lead to immune-mediated disease (Table 4-8). In these disorders, the immune response is normal but the reactivity is heightened, prolonged, or inappropriate.

A major concern is allergic reactions, characterized by an immediate response on exposure to an offending antigen and the release of mediators (e.g., histamine, leukotrienes, prostaglandins) capable of initiating signs and symptoms (see Chapter 26). Although allergic reactions are associated with IgE, not all allergic reactions are IgE-mediated. Complement activation by immune complexes or through the alternative complement pathway has been shown to release complement C3a and C5a anaphylatoxins, which are capable of producing similar reactions.

Table 4-7	Complement Deficiencies
Deficient Component	**Common Types of Infections**
C1 (r/q)	Gram-positive, mainly respiratory
C2	Gram-positive, recurrent respiratory; meningitis, sepsis, tuberculosis
C3	Gram-positive, recurrent
C4	Gram-positive; sepsis, meningitis
C5	Meningitis (*Neisseria meningitidis*), disseminated gonococcal infection
C6	Meningitis (*N. meningitidis*), disseminated gonococcal infection
C7	Meningitis (*N. meningitidis*)
C8	Meningitis (*N. meningitidis*), disseminated gonococcal infection
C9	Meningitis (*N. meningitidis*)

Box 4-4	Secondary Immunodeficiencies

Hematologic Lymphoproliferative Disorders
Hodgkin's disease and lymphoma
Leukemia, myeloma, macroglobulinemia
Agranulocytosis and aplastic anemia
Sickle cell disease

Other Systemic Processes and Metabolic Disorders
Nephrotic syndrome
Protein-losing enteropathy
Diabetes mellitus
Malnutrition
Hepatic disease
Uremia
Aging

Viral Infection
AIDS

Surgical Procedures and Trauma
Splenectomy
Burns

Immunosuppressive Agents
Antimetabolites
Corticosteroids
Radiation

Adapted from Graziano FM, Bell CL: The normal immune response and what can go wrong. A classification of immunologic disorders, Med Clin North Am 69:439–452, 1985.

Table 4-8	Immune-Mediated Disease
Type	**Cause, Disease**
Allergic hypersensitivity	Foods, drugs, aeroallergens (dust, pollens, molds)
Contact hypersensitivity	Poison ivy, nickel, cosmetics
Transfusion Reactions	
Autoimmune disease	Systemic lupus erythematosus, rheumatoid arthritis, vasculitis syndromes, hemolytic anemia, idiopathic thrombocytopenia, pernicious anemia, Goodpasture's syndrome, myasthenia gravis, Graves' disease

Autoimmune disease is thought to be caused by antibody or T cell sensitization with autologous self-antigens (see Chapter 28). Postulated mechanisms of this process include the following:

- Altered antigen or neoantigen. These antigens may be created by chemical, physical, or biologic processes. Hemolytic anemia caused by a drug interaction is an example of this process occurring in RBCs.
- Shared or cross-reactive antigens. Evidence has suggested that poststreptococcal disease occurs through this mechanism.

Autoimmune Lymphoproliferative Syndrome

Autoimmune lymphoproliferative syndrome (ALPS) is a disease in which a genetic defect in programmed cell death, or apoptosis, leads to breakdown of lymphocyte homeostasis and normal immunologic tolerance. ALPS is the first pediatric syndrome described in which the primary defect is in apoptosis.

Defective apoptosis in lymphocytes (and, in ALPS type II, dendritic cells) leads to accumulation of these cells in the lymphoid organs after they would normally be eliminated. As a result, cells with autoimmune potential are unchecked and can induce a variety of autoimmune diseases; the risk for malignant transformation to lymphoma is increased.

Patients with ALPS have chronic enlargement of the spleen and lymph nodes, various manifestations of autoimmunity, and elevation of a normally rare population of double-negative T cells (DNTs). When lymphocytes from ALPS patients are cultured in vitro, they are resistant to apoptosis, as compared with cells from healthy controls.

Most ALPS patients have mutations in a TNF receptor gene that is a member of a superfamily (TNFRSF6). This gene, previously known as *APT1*, encodes the cell surface receptor for the major apoptosis pathway in mature lymphocytes. This receptor has many names, including Fas. The Fas apoptotic pathway is important for eliminating excess T cells after they have been activated and also eliminating antigen-driven and autoreactive T cell clones. Fas is a functional trimer residing at the cell membrane that when engaged by trimeric Fas ligand (FasL), initiates a proteolytic cascade leading to chromosomal DNA degradation and cell death.

CASE STUDY

History and Physical Examination

A 33-year-old man, the child of unrelated parents of Mexican descent, was examined because of a history of frequent sore throats and sinus headaches. Recently, he had a severe bout of pneumonia and was just diagnosed with bacterial conjunctivitis and chronic gastritis caused by *Helicobacter pylori.*

Laboratory Data

Assay	Patient's Result	Reference Range
Total leukocytes	7.2×10^9/L	4.5-9.0×10^9/L
Total lymphocytes	3.2×10^9/L	2.7-5.4×10^9/L
T lymphocytes	3.15×10^9/L	2.7-5.3×10^9/L
B lymphocytes	Too low to count, almost undetectable	
Serum Immunoglobulins		
IgM	0.03g/L	3.0-15.8g/L
IgG	0.31g/L	0.4-2.2g/L
IgA	Not detectable	0.15-1.3g/L
IgE	Not detectable	<100IU/mL

Assay	Patient
Blood group	O
Anti-A and anti-B titer	1:2, very low
Serum immunoglobulin (mg/dL)	
IgM	45, low
IgG	200, very low
IgA	23, very low

Questions

1. A laboratory result of significance to the diagnosis of this patient is:
   a. Low or absent immunoglobulin levels
   b. Extremely low B-lymphocyte count
   c. Low T-lymphocyte count
   d. Both a and b
2. When vaccinated, this boy's immune system should:
   a. Recognize the vaccine as a foreign antigen
   b. Mount a weak antibody response to a vaccine
   c. Fail to recognize the vaccine as a foreign antigen
   d. Both a and b

See Appendix A for the answers to these questions.

Continued

CASE STUDY—Cont'd

Critical Thinking Group Discussion Questions
1. What abnormalities are evident in the laboratory assay results?
2. Does the patient's history suggest a genetic abnormality?
3. What kind of response would be expected from a vaccination?

See Instructor ⊜volve for discussion of the answers to these questions.

Procedural Protocol

*See ⊜volve for a complete description of the method.

Results

ATP Level Results	Risk of Infection	Risk of Rejection
Low	Increased	Decreased
Moderate	Normal	Decreased
Strong	Normal	Increased

Adapted from Associated Regional and University Pathologists (ARUP) Laboratories, 2012 (http://www.aruplab.com).

Assessment of Cellular Immune Status*

Transplantation Immune Cell Function Assay ImmuKnow, Cylex Inc., Columbia, MD

Principle

Phytohemagglutinin (PHA) is a nonspecific mitogen that can be used to stimulate cell division in CD4 T lymphocytes, regardless of their antigenic specificity or memory status. Therefore, PHA is considered to be a global stimulator of the immune system. The production of intracellular adenosine triphosphate (ATP) is one of the first steps in cellular activation following stimulation with mitogens such as PHA. ATP is a multifunctional nucleotide that plays an indispensable role in the transfer of intracellular chemical energy.

When a sample of patient blood is incubated with PHA, increased ATP production (see figure below) occurs within PHA-activated CD4 T cells. These cells are then isolated by the addition of magnetic beads coated with anti-CD4 monoclonal antibody. The isolated CD4 cells are washed on a magnetic tray and lysed to release intracellular ATP. The amount of measured light emitted following the addition of a luminescence reagent is proportional to the amount of ATP present. An established calibration curve is used to characterize the cellular immune function of the sample.

CHAPTER HIGHLIGHTS

- Lymphocytes represent the cellular components of the specific system of body defense. These cells function cooperatively in cell-mediated or humoral immunity.
- The primary lymphoid organs in mammals are the bone marrow (and/or fetal liver) and thymus.
- The secondary lymphoid tissues include the lymph nodes, spleen, and Peyer's patches in the intestine. Proliferation of the T and B lymphocytes in the secondary or peripheral lymphoid tissues is primarily dependent on antigenic stimulation.
- Several major categories of lymphocytes are recognized by the presence of cell surface membrane markers. These categories are T and B cells and natural killer (NK) and K-type lymphocytes.
- The function of plasma cells is the synthesis and excretion of immunoglobulins.
- Monoclonal antibody (MAb) testing led to the present identification of surface membrane markers. Relating MAbs to cell surface antigens now provides a method for classifying and identifying specific cellular membrane characteristics. The current method of testing uses flow cytometry with immunofluorescence.

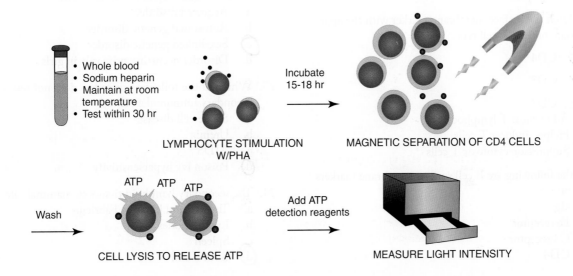

- Whole blood
- Sodium heparin
- Maintain at room temperature
- Test within 30 hr

LYMPHOCYTE STIMULATION W/PHA

Incubate 15-18 hr

MAGNETIC SEPARATION OF CD4 CELLS

Wash

ATP ATP ATP

CELL LYSIS TO RELEASE ATP

Add ATP detection reagents

MEASURE LIGHT INTENSITY

- Immunologic disorders can be divided into primary, secondary (acquired), and those mediated through immune mechanisms. Diseases associated with a primary immunodeficiency are comprised of 40% T cell disorders, 50% B cell disorders, 6% phagocytic abnormalities, and 4% complement alterations. The most common T cell deficiency states are those associated with a concurrent B cell abnormality.

REVIEW QUESTIONS

1. A function of the cell-mediated immune response not associated with humoral immunity is:
   a. Defense against viral and bacterial infection
   b. Initiation of rejection of foreign tissues and tumors
   c. Defense against fungal and bacterial infection
   d. Antibody production

2. The primary or central lymphoid organs in humans are the:
   a. Bursa of Fabricius and thymus
   b. Lymph nodes and thymus
   c. Bone marrow and/or fetal liver and thymus
   d. Lymph nodes and spleen

3. All the following are a function of T cells except:
   a. Mediation of delayed-hypersensitivity reactions
   b. Mediation of cytolytic reactions
   c. Regulation of the immune response
   d. Synthesis of antibody

4-7. Match the type of lymphocyte with its function (use an answer only once).

4. ___B___ T cells

5. ___D___ B cells

6. ___A___ K-type lymphocytes

7. ___C___ Natural killer (NK) cells
   a. Antibody-dependent, cell-mediated cytotoxicity (ADCC) reaction
   b. Cellular immune response
   c. Cytotoxic reaction
   d. Humoral response
   e. Phagocytosis

8-10. Match the surface membrane marker with the appropriate normal T cell type.

8. ___B___ CD4

9. ___C___ CD8

10. ___A___ CD3
    a. All or most T lymphocytes
    b. Helper-inducer T cells
    c. Suppressor-cytotoxic T cells

11. All the following are B cell surface membrane markers except:
    a. sIg
    b. Fc receptor
    c. C3 receptor
    d. CD4

12-17. Match the following congenital or acquired disorders with the major type of lymphocyte affected.

12. ___A___ Thymic hypoplasia

13. ___C___ AIDS

14. ___C___ Chronic lymphocytic leukemia

15. ___C___ Systemic lupus erythematosus

16. ___d___ Multiple myeloma

17. ___B___ Bruton's agammaglobulinemia
    a. Congenital T cell disorder
    b. Congenital B cell disorder
    c. Acquired T cell disorder
    d. Acquired B cell disorder

18. Most diseases associated with a primary defect are ___B cell___ disorders.
    a. T cell
    b. B cell
    c. Complement
    d. Phagocytic

19. Severe combined immunodeficiency is caused by:
    a. T cell depletion
    b. B cell depletion
    c. Inappropriate development of stem cells
    d. Phagocytic dysfunction

20. DiGeorge's syndrome is caused by:
    a. Faulty embryogenesis
    b. Deficiency of calcium in utero
    c. Inappropriate stem cell development
    d. Autosomal recessive disorder

21. The major clinical manifestation of a B cell deficiency is:
    a. Impaired phagocytosis
    b. Diminished complement levels
    c. Increased susceptibility to bacterial infections
    d. Increased susceptibility to parasitic infections

22. Bruton's agammaglobulinemia is a(n):
    a. Acquired disorder
    b. Autosomal genetic disorder
    c. Sex-linked genetic disorder
    d. Disorder occurring primarily in girls

23. Which of the following disorders does not result in a secondary immunodeficiency?
    a. Sickle cell disease
    b. Uremia
    c. AIDS
    d. Poison ivy hypersensitivity

24. The secondary lymphoid tissues in mammals are:
    a. Thymus and bursa of Fabricius
    b. Lymph nodes
    c. Spleen
    d. Both b and c

25. In mammalian immunologic development, the precursors of lymphocytes arise from progenitor cells of the:
    a. Yolk sac
    b. Lymph nodes
    c. Spleen
    d. Both b and c

26. The thymus is embryologically derived from the:
    a. Yolk sac
    b. Pharyngeal pouches

    c. Lymphoblasts
    d. Bone marrow

27. Identify the sites of secondary tissue on the body diagram.
    a. A, B, and C
    b. B, C, and D
    c. B, D, and E
    d. C, D, and E

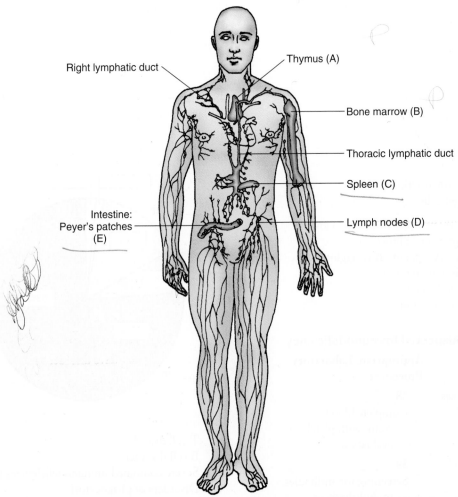

Right lymphatic duct

Thymus (A)

Bone marrow (B)

Thoracic lymphatic duct

Spleen (C)

Lymph nodes (D)

Intestine: Peyer's patches (E)

See question 31. *(Adapted from Turgeon ML: Clinical hematology: theory and procedures, ed 4, Philadelphia, 2005, Lippincott Williams & Wilkins.)*

28. The process of aging causes the thymus to:
    a. Decrease in size
    b. Not change over time
    c. Lose cellularity
    d. Both a and c

29. T lymphocytes can also be referred to as:
    a. Mast cells
    b. Memory cells
    c. Phagocytic cells
    d. Short-lived cells

30. Which of the following characteristics of T lymphocytes is false?
    a. Can form a suppressor-cytotoxic subset
    b. Can be helpers-inducers
    c. Can be CD4+ or CD8+
    d. Can synthesize and secrete immunoglobulin

31. and 32. Match each type of lymphocyte to the appropriate function.

31. _A_ T lymphocytes

32. _B_ B lymphocytes
    a. Cellular immune response
    b. Humoral antibody response

33-35. Match each to the appropriate function.

33. _b_ Cytotoxic or effector T cells

34. _a_ Helper or regulator T cells

35. _c_ Suppressor T cells
    a. Secrete a variety of cytokines
    b. Recognize antigens associated with MHC class I
    c. Inhibit response of helper T cells

36. Natural killer cells:
    a. Produce interferon
    b. Produce IL-2
    c. Were previously called null cells
    d. All of the above

37. K-type cells:
    a. Synthesize antibody
    b. Secrete antibody
    c. Destroy by cytotoxic reaction
    d. Phagocytize target cells

38-41. Complete the chart, choosing from the following answers for the appropriate procedures:
    a. Screening for anti-A and anti-B isoagglutinins
    b. Erythrocyte sedimentation rate
    c. Absolute neutrophil count
    d. Absolute lymphocyte count

Initial Evaluation of Suspected Immunodeficiency

Suspected Immunodeficiency	Appropriate Laboratory Procedures
All suspected deficiencies	38. _____ Complete blood count with platelet evaluation
Antibody deficiency	39. _____ Screening for antibodies to diphtheria or tetanus toxoids
T cell deficiency	40. _____ Intradermal skin test
Phagocytic cell deficiency	41. _____

42. Calculate the absolute lymphocyte count when the following conditions exist:
    Total leukocyte count = 20 × 10^9/L
    Relative percentage of lymphocytes = 50%
    a. 5 × 10^9/L
    b. 10 × 10^9/L
    c. 15 × 10^9/L
    d. 20 × 10^9/L

43-44. Select an appropriate B cell disorder for each category (may use an answer more than once):
    a. Chronic lymphocytic leukemia
    b. Bruton's agammaglobulinemia
    c. Autoimmune disorder

T Cell Disorder	B Cell Disorder
Congenital	
DiGeorge's syndrome	43. _____
Acquired	
Hodgkin's disease	44. _____
Systemic lupus erythematosus	Systemic lupus erythematosus

45-48. Identify the distribution of immunodeficiencies shown in the illustration.

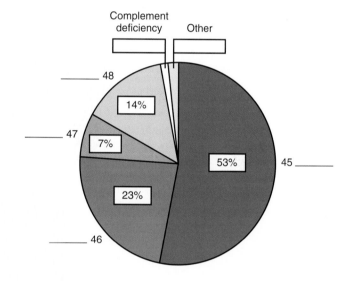

a. T cell disorder
b. B cell disorder
c. Severe combined immunodeficiencies (SCIDs)
d. Disorders of phagocytosis

BIBLIOGRAPHY

Abbas AK, Lichtman AH: Basic immunology: functions and disorders of the immune system, updated edition, ed 3, Philadelphia, 2011, Saunders.

Aiuti A, Roncarolo MG: Ten years of gene therapy for primary immune deficiencies, Am Soc of Hematology 682–688, 2009.

Alanio C, Lemaitre F, Law HKW, et al: Enumeration of human antigen-specific naïve CD8+ T cells reveals conserved precursor frequencies, Blood 115:3718–3725, 2010.

Associated Regional and University Pathologists (ARUP) Consult: Immunodeficiency evaluation for chronic infections in adults and older children testing algorithm, 2012, http://www.arupconsult.com/Algorithms/ChronicInfectionsAdults.pdf.

Boztug K, Schmidt M, Schwarzer A, et al: Stem-cell gene therapy for the Wiskott-Aldrich syndrome, N Engl J Med 363:1918–1927, 2010.

Buckley RH: Immunodeficiency diseases, JAMA 268:268–2797, 1992.

Busby J, Caranasos GJ: Immune function, autoimmunity, and selective immunoprophylaxis in the aged, Med Clin North Am 69:465–474, 1985.

Claman HN: The biology of the immune response, JAMA 268:2790–2796, 1992.

Cooper MD, Lawton AR Jr: The development of the immune system, Sci Am 231:59–70, 1974.

D'Acquisto F, Crompton T: CD3+CD4-CD8- (double negative) T cells: saviours or villains of the immune response? Biochem Pharmacol 82:333–340, 2011.

D'Andrea AD: Cytokine receptors in congenital hematopoietic disease, N Engl J Med 330:330–839, 1994.

Denny T, Yogev R, Gelman R, et al: Lymphocyte subsets in healthy children during the first 5 years of life, JAMA 267:267–1484, 1992.

Desfrançois J, Moreau-Aubry A, Vignard V, et al: Double positive CD4CD8 αβ T cells: a new tumor-reactive population in human melanomas, PLoS One 5:e8437, 2010.

Filipovich A, Zhang K, Snow AL, Marsh RZ: X-linked lymphoproliferative syndromes: brothers or distant cousins? Blood 116:3398–3408, 2010.

Geha RS, Rosen FS: The genetic basis of immunoglobulin-class switching, N Engl J Med 330:330–1008, 1994.

Graziano FM, Bell CL: The normal immune response and what can go wrong. In Corman LC, Katz P, editors: Medical Clinics of North America: Symposium on Clinical Immunology I, Philadelphia, 1985, Saunders.

Heinzel FP: Infections in patients with humoral immunodeficiency, Hosp Pract 24:97–123, 1989. (Off Ed.)

Hester JD: Cellular immunity, Adv Med Lab Professionals 22:24–25, 2010.

Jackson CE, Fischer RE, Hsu AP, et al: Autoimmune lymphoproliferative syndrome with defective Fas: genotype influences penetrance, Am J Hum Genet 64:1002–1014, 1999.

Jiang H, Chess L: Regulation of immune response by T cells, N Engl J Med 354:354–1166, 2006.

Kindt TJ, Goldsby RA, Osborne BA: Kuby immunology, ed 6, New York, 2007, WH Freeman, pp 45–270.

Medzhitov R, Janeway C Jr: Innate immunity, N Engl J Med 343:343–338, 2000.

National Primary Immunodeficiency Resource Center: Primary immunodeficiency syndromes—leukocyte adhesion deficiency, 2004, http://npi.jmfworld.org.

Peakman M, Vergani D: Basic and clinical immunology, ed 2, London, 2009, Elsevier.

Schejbel L, Garred P: Primary immunodeficiency: complex genetics disorders? Clin Chem 53:159, 2007.

Sneller MC: New insights into common variable immunodeficiency, Ann Intern Med 118:118–720, 1993.

Stadnisky MD, Xie X, Coats ER, et al: Self MHC class I-licensed NK cells enhance adaptive CD8 T cell viral immunity, Blood 117:5133–5141, 2011.

Takata H, Naruto T, Takiguchi, M. Functional heterogeneity of human effector CD8+ T cells, Blood 119:1390-1398.

Thaunat O, Morelon E, Defrance T: Am"B" valent: anti-CD20 antibodies unravel the dual role of B cells in immunopathogenesis, Blood 116:515–521, 2010.

Thrasher AJ: New insights into the biology of Wiskott-Aldrich syndrome (WAS), Hematology Am Soc Hematol Educ Program 132–138, 2010.

Tumanov A, Grivennikov SI, Kruglov AA, et al: Cellular source and molecular form of TNF specify its distinct functions in organization of secondary lymphoid organs, Blood 116:3456–3464, 2010.

Turgeon ML: Fundamentals of immunohematology, ed 2, Baltimore, 1995, Williams & Wilkins.

Turgeon ML: Clinical hematology, ed 5, Philadelphia, 2012, Lippincott Williams & Wilkins.

Van Zelm MC, et al: An antibody-deficiency syndrome due to mutations in the CD19 Gene, NEJM 354:1901–1912, 2006. May 4.

Yocum MW, Kelso JM: Common variable immunodeficiency: the disorder and treatment, Mayo Clin Proc 66:6–83, 1991.

Zook EC, Krishack PA, Zhang S, et al: Overexpression of FOXn1 attenuates age-associated thymic involution and prevents the expansion of peripheral Cd4 memory T cells, Blood 118:5723–5731, 2011.

CHAPTER 5

Soluble Mediators of the Immune System

complement

Learning Objectives

At the conclusion of this chapter, the reader should be able to:

- Name and compare the three complement activation pathways.
- Describe the mechanisms and consequences of complement activation.
- Explain the biological functions of the complement system.
- Name and describe alterations in complement levels.
- Briefly describe the assessment of complement levels.
- Compare other types of nonspecific mediators of the immune system, including cytokines, interleukins, tumor necrosis factor, hematopoietic growth factors, and chemokines.

- Discuss the clinical applications of C-reactive protein.
- Compare acute-phase reactant methods.
- Analyze an acute-phase protein case study.
- Correctly answer case study related multiple choice questions.
- Be prepared to participate in a discussion of critical thinking questions.
- Describe the principle, reporting results, sources of error, limitations, and clinical applications of the C-reactive protein procedure.
- Correctly answer end of chapter review questions.

Key Terms

acute-phase proteins (acute-phase reactants)
agglutination
antineoplastic agents
ceruloplasmin
colony-stimulating factors (CSFs)
complement cascade
convertase
effector cells
factor H
febrile

haptoglobin
hemolysis
hydrophilic
hydrophobic
immunomodulators
integrins
ligands
lipemic
lysis
malignant neoplasia
membrane attack complex

natural immune system
nephelometry
osmotic cytolytic reaction
peptide
polymerize
properdin
proteinases
proteolytic
pyogenic
tumor necrosis factor
zymosan

The immune system is composed of the phylogenetically oldest, highly diversified innate immune system and the adaptive immune system. Some components of the innate or **natural immune system** (e.g., phagocytosis) are discussed in previous chapters. This chapter discusses the other components of the innate immune system: the complement system and other circulating effector proteins of innate immunity, including cytokines and acute-phase reactants.

Regulatory mechanisms of complement are finely balanced. The activation of complement is focused on the surface of invading microorganisms, with limited complement deposited on normal cells and tissues. If the mechanisms that regulate this delicate balance malfunction, the complement system may cause injury to cells, tissues, and organs, such as destruction of the kidneys in systemic lupus erythematosus or hemolytic anemias.

THE COMPLEMENT SYSTEM

Complement is a heat-labile series of 18 plasma proteins, many of which are enzymes or **proteinases.** Collectively, these proteins are a major fraction of the beta-1 and beta-2 globulins.

The complement system proteins are named with a capital C followed by a number. A small letter after the number indicates that the protein is a smaller protein resulting from the cleavage of a larger precursor by a protease. Several complement proteins are cleaved during activation of the complement system; the fragments are designated with lower case suffixes, such as C3a and C3b. Usually, the larger fragment is designated as "b" and the smaller fragment as "a." The exception is the designation of the C2 fragments; the larger fragment is designated C2a and the smaller fragment is C2b.

Proteins of the alternative activation pathway are called factors and are symbolized by letters such as B. Control proteins include the inhibitor of C1 (C1 INH), factor I, and factor H.

The complement system displays three overarching physiologic activities (Table 5-1). These are initiated in various ways through the following three pathways (Table 5-2):

1. Classic pathway
2. Alternative pathway
3. Mannose-binding lectin pathway

The three pathways (Fig. 5-1) converge at the point of cleavage of C3 to C3b, the central event of the common final pathway, which in turn leads to the activation of the lytic complement sequence, C5 through C9, and cell destruction (Fig. 5-2).

Activation of Complement

Normally, complement components are present in the circulation in an inactive form. In addition, the control proteins C1 INH, factor I, factor H, and C4-binding protein (C4-bp) are normally present to inhibit uncontrolled complement activation. Under normal physiologic conditions, activation of one pathway probably also leads to the activation of another pathway, as follows:

- The classic pathway is initiated by the bonding of the C1 complex, consisting of C1q, C1r, and C1s, to antibodies bound to an antigen on the surface of a bacterial cell.

- The alternative pathway is initiated by contact with a foreign surface such as the polysaccharide coating of a microorganism and the covalent binding of a small amount of C3b to hydroxyl groups on cell surface carbohydrates and proteins. The pathway is activated by low-grade cleavage of C3 in plasma.

- The mannose-binding lectin pathway is initiated by binding of the complex of mannose-binding lectin and

Table 5-1	**Three Main Physiologic Activities of the Complement System**
Activity	**Responsible Complement Protein**
Host Defense Against Infections	
Opsonization	Covalently bonded fragments of C3 and C4
Chemotaxis and leukocyte activation	C5a, C3a, and C4a; anaphylatoxin leukocyte receptors
Lysis of bacterial and mammalian cells	C5-C9 membrane attack complex
Interface Between Innate and Adaptive Immunity	
Augmentation of antibody	C3b and C4b bound to immune complexes and to antigen
Responses	C3 receptors on B cells and antigen-presenting cells
Enhancement of immunologic memory	C3b and C4b bound to immune complexes and to antigen; C3 receptors on follicular dendritic cells
Disposal of Waste	
Clearance of immune complexes from tissues	C1q; covalently bonded fragments of C3 and C4
Clearance of apoptotic cells	

Adapted from Walport MJ: Complement, N Engl J Med 344:1058–1065, 2001.

Table 5-2	**Initiators of Three Complement Activation Pathways**
Pathway	**Initiators**
Classic	Immune complexes Apoptotic cells Certain viruses and gram-negative bacteria C-reactive protein bound to ligand
Alternate	Various bacteria, fungi, viruses, or tumor cells
Mannose-binding lectin	Microbes with terminal mannose groups

Adapted from Walport MJ: Complement, N Engl J Med 344:1058–1065, 2001.

associated serine proteases (MASP1 and MASP2) to arrays of mannose groups on the surface of a bacterial cell.

Enzyme Activation

After complement is initially activated, each enzyme precursor is activated by the previous complement component or complex, which is a highly specialized proteinase. This converts the enzyme precursor to its catalytically active form by limited proteolysis.

The pathways leading to the cleavage of C3 are triggered enzyme cascades. During this activation process, a small peptide fragment is cleaved, a membrane-binding site is exposed, and the major fragment binds. As a consequence, the next active enzyme of the sequence is formed. Because each enzyme can activate many enzyme precursors, each step is amplified until the C3 stage; therefore, the whole system forms an amplifying cascade.

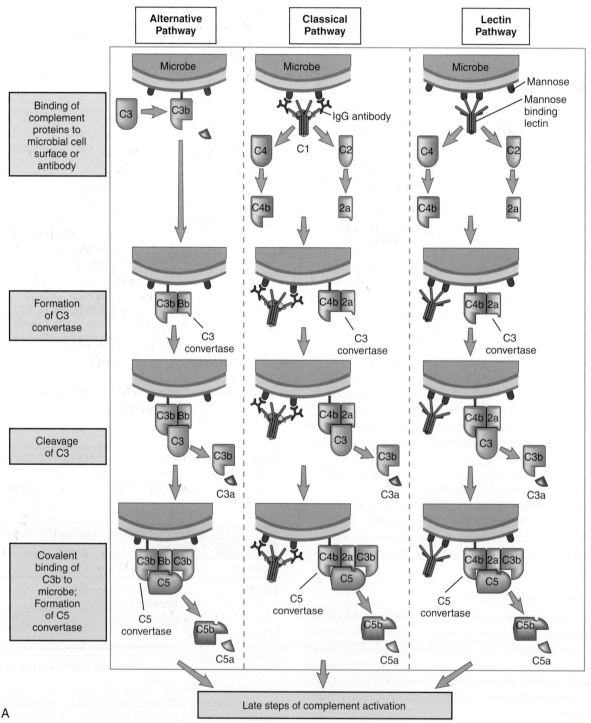

Figure 5-1   Early steps of complement activation. The steps in the activation of the alternative, classical, and lectin pathways are shown. Note the sequence of events is similar in all three pathways, although they differ in their requirement for antibody and in the proteins used. *(From Abbas AK, Lichtman AH: Basic immunology: functions and disorders of the immune system, updated edition, ed 3, Philadelphia, 2011, Saunders.)*

Continued

Protein	Serum conc. (µg/mL)	Function
C3	1000-1200	C3b binds to the surface of a microbe where it functions as an opsonin and as a component of C3 and C5 convertases C3a stimulates inflammation
Factor B	200	Bb is a serine protease and the active enzyme of C3 and C5 convertases
Factor D	1-2	Plasma serine protease which cleaves Factor B when it is bound to C3b
Properdin	25	Stabilizes the C3 convertase (C3bBb) on microbial surfaces

B

Protein	Serum conc. (µg/mL)	Function
C1 (C1qr2s2)		Initiates the classical pathway; C1q binds to Fc portion of antibody; C1r and C1s are proteases that lead to C4 and C2 activation
C4	300-600	C4b covalently binds to surface of microbe or cell where antibody is bound and complement is activated C4b binds to C2 for cleavage by C1s C4a stimulates inflammation
C2	20	C2a is a serine protease functioning as an active enzyme of C3 and C5 convertases
Mannose binding lectin (MBL)	0.8-1	Initiates the lectin pathway; MBL binds to terminal mannose residues of microbial carbohydrates. An MBL-associated protease activates C4 and C2, as in the classical pathway.

C

Figure 5-1, cont'd

Complement Receptors

Various cell types express surface membrane glycoproteins that react with one or more of the fragments of C3 produced during complement activation and degradation. The functions of these receptors depend on the type of cell and often are incompletely understood. Complement receptor 1 (CR1) is important in enhancing phagocytosis and CR3 is also important in these host defense mechanisms.

Plasmodium falciparum adhesin PfRh4 binds to complement receptor type-1 (CR1) on human erythrocytes. CR1 is a complement regulator and immune adherence receptor on erythrocytes required for shuttling C3bC4b-opsonized particles to the liver and spleen for phagocytosis.

Effects of Complement Activation

The activation of complement and the products formed during the **complement cascade** have a variety of physiologic and cellular consequences. Physiologic consequences include blood vessel dilation and increased vascular permeability. The cellular consequences include the following:
- Cell activation, such as production of inflammatory mediators.
- Cytolysis or **hemolysis,** if the cells are erythrocytes. The most important biologic role of complement in blood group serology is the production of cell membrane lysis of antibody-coated targets.

- Opsonization, which renders cells vulnerable to phagocytosis.

In addition to the function of complement as a major effector of antigen-antibody interaction, physiologic concentrations of complement have been found to induce profound alterations in the molecular weight, composition, and solubility of immune complexes. The activation of complement may also play a role in mediating hypersensitivity reactions. This process may occur from direct alternative pathway activation by immunoglobulin E (IgE)–antigen complexes or through a sequence initiated by the activated Hageman coagulation factor that causes the generation of plasmin, which subsequently activates the classic pathway. In either case, activation of complement components from C3 onward leads to the generation of anaphylatoxins in an immediate-hypersensitivity reaction.

CLASSIC PATHWAY

The classic complement pathway is one of the major effector mechanisms of antibody-mediated immunity. The principal components of the classic pathway are C1 through C9. The sequence of component activation—C1, 4, 2, 3, 5, 6, 7, 8, and 9—does not follow the expected numeric order.

C3 is present in the plasma in the largest quantities; fixation of C3 is the major quantitative reaction of the complement cascade. Although the principal source of synthesis of complement in vivo is debatable, the majority of the plasma complement components are made in hepatic parenchymal cells, except for C1 (a calcium-dependent complex of the three glycoproteins C1q, C1r, and C1s), which is primarily synthesized in the epithelium of the gastrointestinal and urogenital tracts.

The classic pathway has three major stages:
1. Recognition
2. Amplification of proteolytic complement cascade
3. Membrane attack complex (MAC)

Recognition

The recognition unit of the complement system is the C1 complex—C1q, C1r, and C1s, an interlocking enzyme system. In the classic pathway, the first step is initiation of the pathway triggered by recognition by complement factor C1 of antigen-antibody complexes on the cell surface. When C1 complex interacts with aggregates of immunoglobulin G (IgG) with antigen on a cell's surface, two C1-associated proteases, C1r and C1s, are activated. A single IgM molecule is potentially able to fix C1, but at least two IgG molecules are required for this purpose. The amount of C1 fixed is directly proportional to the concentration of IgM antibodies, although this is not true of IgG molecules. C1s is weakly proteolytic for free intact C2, but is highly active against C2 that has complexed with C4b molecules in the presence of magnesium (Mg^{2+}) ions. This reaction will occur only if the C4bC2 complex forms close to the C1s.

The resultant C2a fragment joins with C4b to form the new C4bC2a enzyme, or classic pathway C3 **convertase.** The catalytic site of the C4bC2a complex is probably in the C2a **peptide.** A smaller C2b fragment from the C2 component is lost to the surrounding environment.

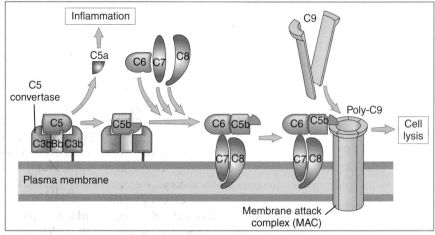

Figure 5-2 **Late steps of complement activation. A,** The late steps of complement activation start after the formation of the C5 convertase and are identical in the alternative and classical pathways. Products generated in the late steps induce inflammation (C5a) and cell lysis (the membrane attack complex [MAC]). **B,** The properties of the proteins of the late steps of complement activation are listed. *(From Abbas AK, Lichtman AH: Basic immunology: functions and disorders of the immune system, updated edition, ed 3, Philadelphia, 2011, Saunders.)*

Protein	Serum conc. (µg/mL)	Function
C5	80	C5b initiates assembly of the MAC C5a stimulates inflammation
C6	45	Component of the MAC: binds to C5b and accepts C7
C7	90	Component of the MAC: binds C5b, 6 and inserts into lipid membranes
C8	60	Component of the MAC: binds C5b, 6, 7 and initiates binding and polymerization of C9
C9	60	Component of the MAC: binds C5b, 6, 7, 8 and polymerizes to form membrane pores

Amplification of Proteolytic Complement Cascade

Once C1s is activated, the **proteolytic** complement cascade is amplified on the cell membrane through sequential cleavage of complement factors and recruitment of new factors until a cell surface complex containing C5b, C6, C7, and C8 is formed.

The complement cascade reaches its full amplitude at the C3 stage, which represents the heart of the system. The C4bC2a complex, the classic pathway C3 convertase, activates C3 molecules by splitting the peptide, C3 anaphylatoxin, from the N-terminal end of the peptide of C3. This exposes a reactive binding site on the larger fragment, C3b. Consequently, clusters of C3b molecules are activated and bound near the C4bC2a complex. Each catalytic site can bind several hundred C3b molecules, even though the reaction is very efficient because C3 is present in high concentration. Only one C3b molecule combines with C4bC2a to form the final proteolytic complex of the complement cascade.

Membrane Attack Complex

The **membrane attack complex** (MAC) is a unique system that builds up a lipophilic complex in cell membranes from several plasma proteins. To initiate C5b fixation and the MAC, C3b splits C5a from the alpha chain of C5. No further proteinases are generated in the classic complement sequence. Other bound C3b molecules not involved in the C4b2a3b complex form an opsonic macromolecular coat on the erythrocyte or other target, which renders it susceptible to immune adherence by C3b receptors on phagocytic cells.

When fully assembled in the correct proportions, C7, C6, C5b, and C8 form the MAC (see Fig. 5-2, *inset*). The C5bC6 complex is **hydrophilic** but, with the addition of C7, it has additional detergent and phospholipid-binding properties as well. The presence of **hydrophobic** and hydrophilic groups within the same complex may account for its tendency to **polymerize** and form small protein micelles (a packet of chain molecules in parallel arrangement). It can attach to any lipid bilayer within its effective diffusion radius, which produces the phenomenon of reactive lysis on innocent so-called bystander cells. Once membrane bound, C5bC6C7 is relatively stable and can interact with C8 and C9.

The C5bC6C7C8 complex polymerizes C9 to form a tubule (pore), which spans the membrane of the cell being attacked, allowing ions to flow freely between the cellular interior and exterior. By complexing with C9, the **osmotic cytolytic reaction** is accelerated. This tubule is a hollow cylinder with one end inserted into the lipid bilayer and the other projecting from the membrane. A structure of this form can be assumed to disturb the lipid bilayer sufficiently to allow the free exchange of ions and water molecules across the membrane. Ions flow out, but large molecules stay in, causing water to flood into the cell. The consequence in a living cell is that the influx of sodium (Na^+) ions and H_2O leads to disruption of osmotic balance, which produces cell lysis.

ALTERNATIVE PATHWAY

The alternative pathway shows points of similarity with the classic sequence. Both pathways generate a C3 convertase that activates C3 to provide the pivotal event in the final common pathway of both systems. However, in contrast to the classic pathway, which is initiated by the formation of antigen-antibody reactions, the alternate complement pathway is predominantly a non–antibody-initiated pathway.

Microbial and mammalian cell surfaces can activate the alternative pathway in the absence of specific antigen-antibody complexes. Factors capable of activating the alternative pathway include inulin, **zymosan** (polysaccharide complex from surface of yeast cells), bacterial polysaccharides and endotoxins, and the aggregated IgG2, IgA, and IgE. In paroxysmal nocturnal hemoglobinuria (PNH), the patient's erythrocytes act as an activator and result in excessive **lysis** of these erythrocytes. This nonspecific activation is a major physiologic advantage because host protection can be generated before the induction of a humoral immune response.

A key feature of the alternative pathway is that the first three proteins of the classic activation pathway—C1, C4, and C2—do not participate in the cascade sequence. The C3a component is considered to be the counterpart of C2a in the classic pathway. C2 of the classic pathway structurally resembles factor B of the alternative pathway. The omission of C1, C4, and C2 is possible because activators of the alternative pathway catalyze the conversion of another series of normal serum proteins, which leads to the activation of C3. It was previously believed that **properdin,** a normal protein of human serum, was the first protein to function in the alternative pathway; thus, the pathway was originally named after this protein.

The uptake of factor B onto C3b occurs when C3b is bound to an activator surface. However, C3b in the fluid phase or attached to a nonactivator surface will preferentially bind to and therefore prevent C3b,B formation. C3b and factor B combine to form C3b,B, which is converted into an active C3 convertase, C3b,Bb. This results from the loss of a small fragment, Ba (glycine-rich α_2-globulin believed to be physiologically inert), through the action of the enzyme, factor D. The C3b,Bb complex is able to convert more C3 to C3b, which binds more factor B and the feedback cycle continues.

The major controlling event of the alternative pathway is **factor H,** which prevents the association between C3b and factor B. Factor H blocks the formation of C3b,Bb, the catalytically active C3 convertase of the feedback loop. Factor H (formerly β_1-H) competes with factor B for its combining site on C3b, eventually leading to C3 inactivation. Factors B and H apparently occupy a common site on C3b. The factor that is preferentially bound to C3b depends on the nature of the surface to which C3b is attached. Polysaccharides are called activator surfaces and favor the uptake of factor B on the chain of C3b, with the corresponding displacement of factor H. In this situation, binding of factor H is inhibited, and consequently factor B will replace H at the common binding site. When factor H is excluded, C3b is thought to be formed continuously in small amounts. Another controlling point in the amplification loop depends on the stability of the C3b,Bb convertase. Ordinarily, C3b,Bb decays because of the loss of Bb, with a half-life of approximately 5 minutes. However, if properdin (P) binds to C3b,Bb, forming C3b,BbP, the half-life is extended to 30 minutes.

The association of numerous C3b units, factor Bb, and properdin on the surface of an aggregate of protein or the surface of a microorganism has potent activity as a C5 convertase. With the cleavage of C5, the remainder of the complement cascade continues as in the classic pathway.

MANNOSE-BINDING LECTIN PATHWAY

Mannose-binding lectin is a member of a family of calcium-dependent lectins, the collectins (collagenous lectins), and is homologous in structure to C1q. Mannose-binding lectin, a pattern recognition molecule of the innate immune system, binds to arrays of terminal mannose groups on a variety of bacteria.

A deficiency of mannose-binding lectin is caused by one of three point mutations in its gene, each of which reduces levels of the lectin. After the discovery that the binding of mannose-binding lectin to mannose residues can initiate complement activation, the mannose-binding lectin–associated serine protease (MASP) enzymes were discovered. MASP activates complement by interacting with two serine proteases called MASP1 and MASP2. These components make up the mannose-binding lectin pathway.

BIOLOGICAL FUNCTIONS OF COMPLEMENT PROTEINS

The biological functions of the complement system fall into the following two general categories:
1. Cell lysis by the membrane attack complex (MAC)
2. Biological effects of proteolytic fragments of complement

The first category is the situation in which the MAC leads to osmotic lysis of a cell. The second category encompasses other effects of complement in immunity and inflammation that are mediated by the proteolytic fragments generated during complement activation. These fragments may remain bound to the same cell surfaces at which complement has been activated or may be released into the blood or extracellular fluid. In either situation, active fragments mediate their effects by binding to specific receptors expressed on various types of cells, including phagocytic leukocytes and the endothelium (Table 5-3).

In contrast, the absence of an integral component of the classic, alternative, or terminal lytic pathways can lead to decreased complement activation and a lack of complement-mediated biological functions.

Alterations in Complement Levels

The complement system can cause significant tissue damage in response to abnormal stimuli. Biological effects of complement activation can occur as a reaction to persistent infection or an autoantibody response to self antigens. In these infectious or autoimmune conditions, the inflammatory or lytic effects of complement may contribute significantly to the pathology of the disease.

Complement activation is also associated with intravascular thrombosis, which leads to ischemic injury to tissues. Complement levels may be abnormal in certain disease states (e.g., rheumatoid arthritis, systemic lupus erythematosus [SLE]) and in some genetic disorders.

Elevated Complement Levels

The complement level can be elevated in many inflammatory conditions. Increased complement levels are often associated with inflammatory conditions, trauma, or acute illness such as myocardial infarction because separate complement components

(e.g., C3) are acute-phase proteins. However, these elevations are common and nonspecific. Therefore, increased levels are of limited clinical significance.

Decreased Complement Levels

Low levels of complement suggest one of the following biological effects:

- Complement has been excessively activated recently.
- Complement is currently being consumed.
- A single complement component is absent because of a genetic defect.

Specific component deficiencies are associated with a variety of disorders (Table 5-4). Deficiencies of complement account for a small percentage of primary immunodeficiencies (<2%), but depression of complement levels frequently coexists with SLE and other disorders associated with an immunopathologic process (Box 5-1).

Deficiencies in any of the protein components of complement are usually caused by a genetic defect that leads to abnormal patterns of complement activation. If regulatory components are absent, excess activation may occur at the wrong time or at the wrong site. The potential consequences of increased activation are excess inflammation and cell lysis and consumption of complement components.

Hypocomplementemia can result from the complexing of IgG or IgM antibodies capable of activating complement. Depressed values of complement are associated with diseases that give rise to circulating immune complexes. Because of the rapid normal turnover of the complement proteins—within 1

Table 5-3	Selected Complement Components and Functions
Complement Component(s)	**Function**
C5-C9	Lysis of cells
C3B, IC3B	Opsonization in phagocytosis
C5A >C3A >>C4A	Anaphylatoxins/inflammation (vascular responses)
C5A	Polymorphonuclear leukocyte activation
Classic complement pathway, C3B, ?iC3b, C3dg	Immune complex removal B-lymphocyte activation

Table 5-4	Complement Deficiency in Human Beings
Deficiency	**Associated Disease**
C1q	SLE-like syndrome; decreased secondary to agammaglobulinemia
C1r	SLE-like syndrome; dermatomyositis, vasculitis, recurrent infections and chronic glomerulo-nephritis, necrotizing skin lesions, arthritis
C1s	SLE, SLE-like syndrome
C1 INH	Hereditary angioedema, lupus nephritis
C2	Recurrent pyogenic infections, SLE, SLE-like syndrome, discoid lupus, membranoproliferative glomerulonephritis, dermatomyositis, synovitis, purpura, Henoch-Schönlein purpura, hypertension, Hodgkin's disease, chronic lymphocytic leukemia, dermatitis herpetiformis, polymyositis
C3	Recurrent pyogenic infections, SLE-like syndrome, arthralgias, skin rash
C3 inactivator	Recurrent pyogenic infections, urticaria
C4	SLE-like syndrome, SLE, dermatomyositis-like syndrome, vasculitis
C5	*Neisseria* infections, SLE
C5 dysfunction	Leiner's disease, gram-negative skin and bowel infection
C6	*Neisseria* infections, SLE, Raynaud's phenomenon, scleroderma-like syndrome, vasculitis
C7	*Neisseria* infections, SLE, Raynaud's phenomenon, scleroderma-like syndrome, vasculitis
C8	*Neisseria* infections, xeroderma pigmentosa, SLE-like syndrome

Modified from Colten HR, Rosen FS: Complement deficiencies annual review of immunology, 10:809-834, 1992 and Nusinow SR, Zuraw BL, Curd JG: The hereditary and acquired deficiencies of complement, Med Clin North Am 69:487-504, 1985.

Box 5-1	Diseases Associated With Hypocomplementemia

Rheumatic Diseases With Immune Complexes
Systemic lupus erythematosus
Rheumatoid arthritis (with extraarticular disease)
Systemic vasculitis
Essential mixed cryoglobulinemia
Glomerulonephritis
Poststreptococcal type
Membranoproliferative type

Infectious Diseases
Subacute bacterial endocarditis
Infected atrioventricular shunts
Pneumococcal sepsis
Gram-negative sepsis
Viremias (e.g., hepatitis B surface antigenemia, measles)
Parasitic infections (e.g., malaria)

Deficiency of Control Proteins
C1 inhibitor deficiency: hereditary angioedema
Factor I deficiency
Factor H deficiency

or 2 days of the cessation of complement activation by immune complexes—complement levels return to normal rapidly.

The following three types of complement deficiency can cause increased susceptibility to pyogenic infections:

1. Deficiency of the opsonic activities of complement
2. Any deficiency that compromises the lytic activity of complement
3. Deficient function of the mannose-binding lectin pathway

Increased susceptibility to **pyogenic** bacteria (e.g., *Haemophilus influenzae, Streptococcus pneumoniae*) occurs in patients with defects of antibody production, complement proteins of the classic pathway, or phagocyte function. The sole clinical association between inherited deficiency of MAC components and infection is with neisserial infection, particularly *Neisseria meningitidis*. Low levels of mannose-binding lectin in young children with recurrent infections suggest that the mannose-binding lectin pathway is important during the interval between the loss of passively acquired maternal antibody and the acquisition of a mature immunologic repertoire of antigen exposure.

DIAGNOSTIC EVALUATION

During immune complex reactions, certain complement proteins become physically bound to the tissue in which the immunologic reaction is occurring. These proteins can be demonstrated in tissue by appropriate immunopathologic stains. The most frequent evaluation of complement is by serum or plasma assay (Table 5-5). Complement components (e.g., C3 and C4) can be assessed by **nephelometry.** These assays are useful for the diagnosis and monitoring of patients.

Assessment of Complement

The procedures discussed next can be used in diagnostic immunology.

C1 Esterase Inhibitor (C1 Inhibitor)

C1 measures the activity and concentration of C1 inhibitor in serum. A deficiency of this protein is characteristic of hereditary angioedema (HAE; see later). Some patients demonstrate catalytically inactive protein.

C1r, C1s, C2, C3, C4, C5, C6, C7, C8

Homozygous deficiencies predispose a patient to autoimmune disease (especially SLE) and to arthritis, chronic glomerulonephritis, infections, and vasculitis.

C1q

The complement component C1q is evaluated in serum. Decreased levels can be demonstrated in patients with hypocomplementemic urticarial vasculitis, severe combined immunodeficiency (SCID), or X-linked hypogammaglobulinemia.

C1q Binding

This procedure measures the binding of immune complexes containing IgG1, IgG2, or IgG3 and IgM to the complement component C1q. High values of C1q binding are associated with the presence of circulating immune complexes of the type that interacts with the classic pathway of complement activation. This test can be useful as a prognostic tool at diagnosis and during remission of acute myelogenous leukemia.

C2

The most common complement deficiency is of C2. It is an autosomal recessive disorder; the C2 gene is on chromosome 6 in the major histocompatibility complex (MHC). The incidence is 1:28,000 to 1:40,000; the carrier state is 1.2% in the general population.

Half of patients with homozygous C2 deficiency have no symptoms; those with symptoms have infections with *S. pneumoniae, N. meningitidis,* and *H. influenzae.* Of symptomatic patients, 50% exhibit a lupus-like disorder with photosensitivity and rash.

C3

Also an acute-phase protein, elevated C3 levels can indicate an acute inflammatory disease. Although C3 lies at the junction of the two pathways, it is much more severely depressed when activation occurs via the alternative pathway. Extremely decreased levels are seen in patients with poststreptococcal glomerulonephritis and in those with inherited (C3) complement deficiency. This component is also decreased in cases of severe liver disease and in SLE patients with renal disease.

C3b Inhibitor (C3b Inactivator)

The C3b component of complement causes low complement C3 levels, the absence of C3PA in serum, and high C3b levels. A deficiency of C3b inhibitor is associated with an increased predisposition to infection.

C3PA (C3 Proactivator, Properdin Factor B)

The factor B component is consumed by activation of the alternative complement pathway. Assessment of C3PA indicates

Table 5-5	Interpretation of Complement Activation by Individual Components			
Complement Determination	**Classic Pathway**	**Alternative Pathway**	**Improper Specimen***	**Inflammation**
C3	Decreased	Decreased	Normal	Increased
C4	Decreased	Normal	Decreased	Increased

*Results if specimen is improperly stored or too old.

whether a decreased level of C3 results from the classic or alternative pathways of complement activation. Decreased levels of C3 and C4 demonstrate activation of the classic pathway. Decreased levels of C3 and C3PA with a normal level of C4 indicate complement activation via the alternative pathway (Table 5-5).

Activation of the classic pathway (and sometimes with accompanying alternative pathway activation) is associated with disorders such as immune complex diseases, various forms of vasculitis, and acute glomerulonephritis. Activation of the alternative pathway is associated with many disorders, including chronic hypocomplementemic glomerulonephritis, disseminated intravascular coagulation (DIC), septicemia, subacute bacterial endocarditis, PNH, and sickle cell anemia.

In SLE, both the classic and alternative pathways are activated.

C4

The C4 level often provides the most sensitive indicator of disease activity. C4 is also an acute-phase reactant. Elevated C4 levels can indicate an acute inflammatory reaction or a malignant condition. Measurement of C4 may demonstrate inflammation or infection long before it is clinically evident by standard assessment methods (e.g., total white blood count [WBC] and leukocyte differential, **febrile** response, or elevated erythrocyte sedimentation rate [ESR]).

C4 is destroyed only when the classic pathway is activated. A decreased C4 level with elevated anti–n-DNA and antinuclear antibody (ANA) titers confirm the diagnosis of SLE in a patient. In these cases of SLE, the periodic assessment of C4 can be useful for monitoring the progress of the disorder. Patients with extremely low C4 levels in the presence of normal levels of the C3 component may be demonstrating the effects of a genetic deficiency of C1 inhibitor or C4. Reduction of C3 and C4 components implies that activation of the classic pathway has been initiated.

C4 Allotypes

The antigenically distinct forms of C4A and C4B are located on chromosome 6 in the MHC. C4 allotypes in conjunction with specific human leukocyte antigens (HLAs) are markers for disease susceptibility.

C5

A genetic deficiency of the C5 component is associated with increased susceptibility to bacterial infection and is expressed as an autoimmune disorder (e.g., SLE). Patients with dysfunction

of C5 (Leiner's disease) are predisposed to infections of the skin and bowel, characterized by eczema. Their C5 level is normal, but the C5 component fails to promote phagocytosis.

C6

A decreased quantity of C6 predisposes an individual to significant neisserial (bacterial) infections.

C7

A decreased level of C7 is associated with Raynaud's phenomenon, sclerodactyly, telangiectasia, and severe bacterial infections caused by *Neisseria* spp.

C8

A decreased quantity of C8 is associated with SLE. A C8 deficiency makes patients highly susceptible to *Neisseria* infections.

Select Complement Deficiencies

Properdin Deficiency

Properdin acts to stabilize the alternative pathway C3 convertase (C3bBb). A deficiency leads to bacterial infections, often meningococcemia. This disorder is an X-linked recessive trait.

Hereditary Angioedema

This disorder is a deficiency in a complement protein. Infections are not usually a significant problem. HAE is autosomal dominant, unlike other complement deficiencies. Two types exist, type 1 (low antigen level and low functional protein) and type 2 (normal antigen level with low function).

Familial Mediterranean Fever

This defect in protease in peritoneal and synovial fluid is transmitted as an autosomal recessive trait on chromosome 16. Patients with this defect experience recurrent episodes of fever and inflammation in the joints and pleural and peritoneal fluids.

OTHER SOLUBLE IMMUNE RESPONSE MEDIATORS

Biological Response Modifiers

Biological response modifiers (BRMs) modulate an individual's own immune response. There are four main sources of major BRMs secreted by mononuclear leukocytes:

1. B lymphocytes that secrete specific antibodies
2. T lymphocytes that secrete soluble mediators, such as interleukin-2 (IL-2) and other ILs, granulocyte-monocyte

colony-stimulating factor (GM-CSF), interferon-γ (IFN-γ) and tumor necrosis factor-β (TNF-β)
3. Natural killer (NK) lymphocytes that secrete IFN-α
4. Monocytes and macrophages that secrete IFN-α, IL-1, and other ILs, TNF-α, and GM-CSF and monocyte colony-stimulating factor (M-CSF)

Biological response modifiers can be used therapeutically. The classes of immunotherapy are as follows:
- Active—use of microbial or chemical immunomodulators (adjuvants) in a specific or nonspecific form
- Adoptive—use of soluble mediators, such as ILs, to regulate components of the immune system
- Passive—transfer of preformed antibodies to tumorous recipients, such as monoclonal antibodies

Table 5-6	Examples of Cytokines of Innate and Adaptive Immunity
Innate Immunity	**Adaptive Immunity**
Chemokines	IFN-γ
IFN type 1 (IFN-α, IFN-β)	IL-2
IL-1	IL-4
IL-6	IL-5
IL-10	IL-13
IL-12	Lymphotoxin (Lt)
IL-15	TGF-β
IL-18	
TNF	

IFN, Interferon; *IL,* interleukin; *TGF,* transforming growth factor; *TNG,* tumor necrosis factor.

- Restorative—application of soluble substances, such as interferons, for a wide range of diseases

Cytokines

Migratory inhibitory factor (MIF) was the first cytokine activity to be described. MIF performs a T cell–derived activity that immobilizes macrophage migration, which may cause retention and accumulation of phagocytes at sites of inflammation.

Research is ongoing and the list of individual cytokines steadily increases. Cytokines are synthesized and secreted by the cells associated with innate and adaptive immunity in response to microbial and other antigen exposures (Tables 5-6 and 5-7).

The generic term *cytokines* has become the preferred name for this class of mediators. Lymphokines is another term used to describe cytokines produced by activated lymphocytes. Cytokines produced by leukocytes that act on other leukocytes are also referred to by the imperfect but descriptive term *interleukins* (ILs). As cytokines are discovered and characterized, they are assigned a number using a standard nomenclature (e.g., IL-1).

Cytokines are polypeptide products of activated cells that control a variety of cellular responses and thereby regulate the immune response. Many cytokines are released in response to specific antigens; however, cytokines are nonspecific in that their chemical structure is not determined by the stimulating antigen. Most cytokines have multiple activities and act on numerous cell types. Hematopoietic and lymphoid cell compartments are regulated by a complex network of interacting cytokines. The **colony-stimulating factors (CSFs)** and ILs have been shown to play important roles in normal proliferation, differentiation, and activation of several hematopoietic and lymphoid lineages (Tables 5-8 and 5-9).

Cytokines have a variety of roles in host defense. In innate immunity, cytokines mediate early inflammatory reactions to microbial organisms and stimulate adaptive immune responses. In contrast, in adaptive immunity, cytokines stimulate proliferation

Table 5-7	Comparative Features of Innate and Adaptive Immunity	
	Type of Immunity	
	Innate	**Adaptive**
Examples	TNF-α, IFN-β, IL-1, IL-12	IFN-γ, IL-2, IL-4, IL-5
Major cell source	Macrophages, NK cells	T lymphocytes
Major physiologic function	Mediators of innate immunity and inflammation (local and systemic)	Regulation of lymphocyte growth and differentiation Activation of effector cells (macrophages, eosinophils, mast cells)
Stimuli	LPS (endotoxin), bacterial peptidoglycans, viral RNA, T cell–derived cytokines (e.g., IFN-β)	Protein antigens
Quantity produced	Possibly high, detectable in serum	Usually low, usually undetectable in serum
Effects on body	Local and systemic	Usually local
Roles in disease	Systemic diseases	Local tissue injury
Inhibitors	Corticosteroids	Cyclosporine, FK-506

Adapted from Abbas AK, Lichtman AH, Pober JS: Cellular and molecular immunology, ed 4, Philadelphia, 2000, Saunders.

IFN, Interferon; *IL,* interleukin; *LPS,* lipopolysaccharides; *TNF,* tumor necrosis factor.

Table 5-8	Origin and Immunoregulatory Activity of Cytokines	
Cytokines	**Origin**	**Prominent Biological Activities**
Interleukins (ILs)		
IL-1 superfamily	Both IL-1α and IL-1β are produced by monocytes-macrophages and dendritic cells.	Original members: IL-1α, IL-1β, and IL-1 receptor antagonist (IL-1RA). IL-1α and IL-1β are proinflammatory cytokines involved in immune defense against infection. IL-1RA is a molecule that competes for receptor binding with IL-1α and IL-1β, blocking their role in immune activation. Principal function of IL-1—mediator of host inflammatory response to infections and other inflammatory stimuli. These cytokines increase the expression of adhesion factors on endothelial cells to enable transmigration of leukocytes to sites of infection and reset the hypothalamic thermoregulatory center, leading to increased body temperature (fever), which helps the immune system fight infection. IL-1 also important in regulation of hematopoiesis.
IL-2 (formerly "T-cell growth factor")	Helper T cells	Has high capacity to induce activation of almost all clones of cytotoxic cells. Increases cytotoxic functions of T killer and NK cells; promotes production of perforins and IFN-γ by these cells. Activates monocytes-macrophages to synthesize and secrete TNF-α, IL-1β, IL-6, IL-8, G-CSF, and GM-CSF.
IL-3 (formerly "multicolony colony-stimulating factor")	Activated T cells	Promotes expansion of early blood cells (hematopoiesis) that differentiate into all known mature cell types. Supports growth and differentiation of T cells from bone marrow through immune response.
IL-4	T cells, mast cells	Induces differentiation of naive helper T cells (Th0 cells) to Th2 cells. On activation by IL-4, Th2 cells subsequently produce additional IL-4. Cell that initially produces IL-4 and induces Th0 differentiation has not been identified. Early activation of resting B cells—upregulates MHC class II production (induces HLA-DR molecules on B cells, macrophages) and governs B cell isotype switching to IgG1 and IgE. Key regulator in humoral and adaptive immunity.
IL-5	Helper T cells type 2 (Th2) and mast cells	Principal function—activate eosinophils and serve as link between T cell activation and eosinophilic inflammation. Stimulates growth and differentiation of eosinophils and activates mature eosinophils (IL-5 expressed on eosinophils). Growth and differentiation–inducing factor for activated T and B cells; induces class-specific B cell differentiation (IgA production).
IL-6	Macrophages, T cells, osteoblasts	Functions in innate immunity and adaptive immunity; in the latter, stimulates growth of B cells that have differentiated into antibody producers. IL-1, TNF, and IL-6 appear to be major factors that induce the acute-phase response.
IL-7	Stromal cells of red bone marrow and thymus	Stimulates proliferation of lymphoid progenitors; important for proliferation during certain stages of B cell maturation and in T cell and NK survival, development, and homeostasis. IL-7 has recently been shown to have therapeutic potential and safety in several clinical trials designed to demonstrate T cell restoration in immunodeficient patients.
IL-8	Macrophages and certain types of epithelial cells (e.g., endothelium)	Potent stimulator of neutrophils in chemotaxis. Activates "respiratory burst" and release of specific and azurophilic granular contents.
IL-9	T cells (specifically by CD4+ helper cells)	Promotes proliferation of T cells, thymocytes, and mast cells. Supports proliferation of some T cell lines and of bone marrow–derived mast cell progenitors; supports growth of erythroid blast-forming units.
IL-10	Monocytes, Th2 cells, B cells	Inhibits activated macrophages; displays potent abilities to suppress antigen-presenting capacity of APCs. Released by cytotoxic T (Tc) cells to inhibit the actions of NK cells during immune response to viral infection. IL-10 is stimulatory toward certain T cells, mast cells, and B cells. It can downregulate the synthesis of other ILs.

Table 5-8	**Origin and Immunoregulatory Activity of Cytokines—cont'd**	
Cytokines	**Origin**	**Prominent Biological Activities**
IL-11	Bone marrow stroma	Acts in a manner similar to IL-6 on hematopoietic progenitor cells. IL-11 has been shown to synergize with IL-3 to stimulate production of megakaryocyte and myeloid progenitors and to increase number of Ig-secreting B lymphocytes in vivo and in vitro.
IL-12 (NK stimulatory factor)	B cells, macrophages	Although it shares functional properties of enhancing cytotoxic function of NK cells and activated T cells with IL-2, IL-12 appears to act through a distinct mechanism independent of IL-2. Biological actions of IL-12 include stimulating production of IFN-γ by NK and T cells, stimulating differentiation of naive T cells into Th1 cells, and enhancing cytolytic functions of activated NK cells and CD8+ Tc cells. Growth factor for activated NK-LAK cells.
IL-13	T cells	Possesses many biological effects similar to IL-4 but appears to have less effect on T or B cells than IL-4. Major action of IL-13 on macrophages is to inhibit their activation and to antagonize IFN-γ. Important mediator of allergic inflammation and disease. Functions of IL-13 overlap considerably with those of IL-4, especially changes induced on hematopoietic cells, but these effects are probably less important given the more potent role of IL-4. IL-13 acts more prominently as a molecular bridge linking allergic inflammatory cells to nonimmune cells, altering physiologic function. It is associated primarily with induction of airway disease and also has antiinflammatory properties.
IL-14 (high-molecular-weight B cell growth factor [HMW-BCGF])	T cells and malignant B cells	Acts as B-cell growth factor (BCGF) in proliferation of normal and cancerous B cells. Hyperproduction of IL-14 enables progression of B-cell non-Hodgkin's lymphoma (NHL-B); conversely, its antibodies slow down growth of NHL-B.
IL-15	T cells	Biologically similar to IL-2; acts as synergist, particularly in LAK cell induction process; increases antitumoral activities of T-killer and NK cells and can be chemoattractant for T lymphocytes; endogenous IL-15 is key condition for IFN-γ synthesis. IL-15 produced in response to viral infection and other signals that trigger innate immunity; homologous to IL-2. Function of IL-15 is to promote proliferation of NK cells. Maintenance of memory cells does not appear to require persistence of the original antigen; instead, survival signals for memory lymphocytes are provided by cytokines such as IL-15.
IL-16	Monocytes, CD8+ lymphocytes, B lymphocytes	Acts as a T-cell chemoattractant; increases mobility of CD8+ and CD4+ T cells and, with IL-2, promotes their activation. IL-16 is found in B lymphocytes. Recruits and activates many other cells expressing CD4 molecule, including monocytes, eosinophils, and dendritic cells.
IL-17	CD4+ lymphocytes	Induces granulopoiesis through G-CSF; can reinforce antibody-dependent tumor cell destruction; participates in regulation of many cytokines (IL-1, IL-4, IL-6, IL-10, IL-12, IFN-γ). Histamine and serotonin increase production of IL-17. IL-17 mimics many proinflammatory actions of TNF-α and TNF-β.
IL-18	Macrophages	Acts as synergist with IL-12 in some effects, especially induction of IFN-γ production and inhibition of angiogenesis; high IFN-γ production under integrated effect of IL-18 and IL-12 suppresses tumor growth. IL-18 stimulates production of IFN-γ by NK cells and T cells, synergistic with IL-12.
IL-19	Monocytes	Lipopolysaccharides (LPS) and GM-CSF stimulate synthesis of IL-19, which is then upregulated in monocytes. Biological function similar to that of IL-10; regulates functions of macrophages and suppresses activities of Th1 and Th2.

Continued

Table 5-8	Origin and Immunoregulatory Activity of Cytokines—cont'd	
Cytokines	**Origin**	**Prominent Biological Activities**
IL-20	Activated keratinocytes, monocytes	Biological activities similar to those of IL-10 and can stimulate tumor growth. Regulates proliferation and differentiation of keratocytes during inflammation, particularly inflammation associated with the skin. Causes expansion of multipotential hematopoietic progenitor cells.
IL-21	Various lymphocytes	Regulates hematopoiesis and immune response and influences development of lymphocytes; similar to IL-2 and IL-15 in antitumor defense system; promotes high production of T lymphocytes, fast growth and maturation of NK cells, and fast growth of B lymphocytes. Has potent regulatory effects on immune cells, interacting with cell surface IL-21 receptor, expressed in bone marrow cells and various lymphocytes.
IL-22	Activated T cells	Similar to IL-10, but does not prohibit production of proinflammatory cytokines through monocytes in response to LPS; somewhat similar to IFN-α, -β, and -γ.
IL-23	—	Newly discovered cytokine that shares some in vivo functions with IL-12. IL-23 is important part of inflammatory response against infection; as proinflammatory cytokine, it enhances T cell priming and stimulates production of proinflammatory molecules (IL-1, IL-6, TNF-α, NOS-2, chemokines), resulting in inflammation.
IL-24	Activated monocytes-macrophages, Th2 cells	Appears to participate in cell survival and proliferation by inducing rapid activation of particular transcription factors called STAT-1 and STAT-3; predominantly released by and acts on nonhematopoietic (skin, lung, reproductive) tissues. Performs important roles in wound healing and cancer; cell death occurs in cancer cells and cell lines after exposure to IL-24.
IL-25	Th2 cells, mast cells	Biologically characterized as a member of IL-17 cytokine family. Supports proliferation of cells in lymphoid lineage. Induces production of other cytokines (IL-4, IL-5, IL-13) in multiple tissues, which stimulate the expansion of eosinophils. Important molecule in controlling immunity of the gut; implicated in chronic inflammation associated with gastrointestinal tract; identified in chromosomal region associated with autoimmune diseases such as inflammatory bowel disease (IBD), although no direct evidence suggests that IL-25 plays a role in IBD.
IL-26	Expressed in certain herpesvirus-transformed T cells, but not in primary stimulated T cells	Induces rapid phosphorylation of transcription factors STAT-1 and STAT-3, which enhance IL-10 and IL-8 secretion and expression of CD54 molecule on surface of epithelial cells.
IL-27	—	Has important function in regulating activity of B and T lymphocytes; belongs to the IL-12 family.
IL-28	—	Plays role in immune defense against viruses.
IL-29	—	Plays important role in host defenses against microbes; its gene is highly upregulated in cells infected with virus.
IL-30 (also IL27p28)	New name of p28, a subunit of IL27	Interleukin 30 (IL-30), a member of the long-chain four-helix bundle cytokine family, and EBI3 form the IL-27 heterdimer, which is expressed by APCs. IL-27 triggers expansion of antigen-specific naive CD4-positive T cells and promotes polarization toward a Th1 phenotype with expression of IFN-γ. IL-27 acts in synergy with IL-12 and binds to WSX1.
IL-31	Produced preferentially by Th2 cells. Receptor subunits expressed in activated monocytes and unstimulated epithelial cells.	Believed to play role in skin inflammation.

Table 5-8	Origin and Immunoregulatory Activity of Cytokines—cont'd	
Cytokines	**Origin**	**Prominent Biological Activities**
IL-32	Monocytes-macrophages	Can induce cells of immune system (e.g., monocytes-macrophages) to secrete TNF-α in addition to chemokines such as IL-8.
		Induces expression of TNF-α and IL-8 in THP-1 monocytic cells. Expression of IL-32 is induced in human peripheral lymphocyte cells after mitogen stimulation, in human epithelial cells by IFN-γ, and in NK cells after exposure to IL-12–IL-18 combination.
		Involved in activation induced cell death. Expression of IL-32 is upregulated in T killer and NK-cells after cell activation, and IL-32β is predominant isoform in activated T cells. IL-32 is expressed specifically in T cells undergoing cell death; enforced expression of IL-32 induces apoptosis; downregulation rescues the cells from apoptosis.
IL-33	Helper T cells	Induces type 2 cytokine production from Th cells.
		Mediates biological effects by interacting with orphan IL-1 receptor, activating intracellular molecules in certain signaling pathways that drive production of type 2 cytokines (e.g., IL-4, IL-5, IL-13) from polarized Th2 cells.
		Constitutive expression of IL-33 is found in smooth muscle cells and bronchial epithelial cells. Expression in primary lung or dermal fibroblasts and keratinocytes is inducible by treatment with TNF-α and IL-1β; these two cytokines only induce low-level expression in dendritic cells and macrophages.
Interferons (IFNs)		
IFN-α	Leukocytes	Antiviral, increased MHC class I expression.
IFN-β	Fibroblasts, epithelial cells	Antiviral, increased MHC class I expression.
IFN-γ	T cells, NK cells	Major macrophage activator; induces MHC class II molecules on many cells and can synergize with TNF; augments NK cell activity; antagonist to IL-4.

From Abbas AK, Lichtman AH: Basic Immunology ed 3 Update, Saunders, 2011, pp. 258-259 and http://www.gene.ucl.ac.uk/nomeclature/genefamily/il.php, 2007.

IFN, Interferon; *TNF,* tumor necrosis factor; *G-CSF,* granulocyte colony-stimulating factor; *GM,* granulocyte-macrophage; *MHC,* major histocompatibility complex; *NK,* natural killer; *APCs,* antigen-presenting cells.

Table 5-9	Immunoregulatory Activity of Other Cytokines	
Factor	**Target Cells**	**Prominent Biological Activities**
Tumor Necrosis Factor (TNF)		
TNF-α (cachectin)	Macrophages, NK cells	Local inflammation, endothelial activation
TNF-β (lymphotoxin)	T cells, B cells	Killing, endothelial activation
Tumor necrosis family	T cells, mast cells	
CD40 ligand		B-cell activation, class switching
TNF Family		
CD27 ligand	T cells	Stimulates T-cell proliferation
CD30 ligand	T cells	Stimulates T- and B-cell proliferation
Chemokines		
Membrane cofactor protein (MCP-1)	Macrophages, others	Chemotactic for monocytes

Adapted from Claman HN: The biology of the immune response, JAMA 268:2790–2796, 1992; Janeway C, Travers P: Immunobiology, ed 3, New York, 1997, Garland; and Abbas AK, Lichtman AH, Pober JS: Cellular and molecular immunology, ed 4, Philadelphia, 2000, Saunders.

and differentiation of antigen-stimulated lymphocytes and activate specialized **effector cells** (e.g., macrophages).

Cytokines are very potent, even in minute concentrations. Their action is usually limited to affecting cells in the local area of their production, but they can also have systemic effects. As

a group, cytokines differ in molecular structure but share the following actions:

- Secrete cytokines in rapid bursts, synthesized in response to cellular activation.
- Bind to specific membrane receptors on target cells.

- Regulate receptor expression in T and B cells, which drives positive amplification or negative feedback.
- Act on different cell types.
- Excite the same functional effects with multiple cytokines (redundancy).
- Act close to the site of synthesis on the same cell or on a nearby cell.
- Influence the synthesis and actions of other cytokines.

Cytokines act on other cells by bonding to cytokine receptors on the surface of cells. Individual cytokines have characteristic functions and differ in how they transduce signals as a result of binding. All cytokine receptors consist of one or more transmembrane proteins whose extracellular portions are responsible for cytokine binding and whose cytoplasmic portions are responsible for initiating the intracellular signaling pathways. These six pathways are as follows:

1. Janus kinase (JAK/STAT) pathway
2. Tumor necrosis factor (TNF) receptor signaling by TRAFs (tumor necrosis receptor–associated factors)
3. TNF receptor signaling by death domains
4. Toll receptor signaling
5. Receptor-associated tyrosine kinases
6. G-protein signaling

Interleukins

Many different individual and superfamilies of ILs have been identified. A characteristic of ILs is that secreted peptides and proteins mediate local interactions between leukocytes but do not bind antigen. ILs include molecules that are made by and act on lymphocytes.

Interleukins have widely overlapping functions. These molecules modulate inflammation and immunity by regulating growth, mobility, and differentiation of lymphoid cells. Each of the ILs has been shown to be a distinct molecule by gene cloning and sequencing. In addition, each IL functions through a separate receptor system.

Interferons

The interferons are a group of cytokines discovered in virally infected cultured cells. This interference with viral replication in the cells by another virus led to the term *interferon.*

The IFNs are one of the body's natural defensive responses to foreign components (e.g., microbes, tumors, antigens). IFNs are among the most broadly active physiologic regulators, enhancing the expression of specific genes, inhibiting cell proliferation, and augmenting immune effector cells. IFNs have been demonstrated to act as antiviral agents, **immunomodulators,** and **antineoplastic agents.**

Type I IFNs mediate the early innate immune response to viral infections. They consist of two distinct groups of proteins, IFN-α and IFN-β that are structurally different but that bind to the same cell surface receptor and induce similar biologic responses.

IFN-γ is the principal macrophage-activating cytokine and serves a critical function in innate immunity and in specific cell-mediated immunity. It stimulates expression of MHC class I and class II molecules and costimulates antigen-presenting cells (APCs), promotes the differentiation of naive CD4+ T cells to the helper T cell type 1 (Th1) subset and inhibits the proliferation of Th2 cells. In addition, IFN-γ acts on B cells to promote switching to certain IgG subclasses, activates neutrophils, and stimulates the cytolytic activity of natural killer (NK) cells. It is also antagonistic to IL-4. IFN-γ is of most immunologic interest because of its diverse effects on the immune response. Its ability to augment the activity of many cytokines has resulted in clinical trials in a number of different diseases.

Tumor Necrosis Factor

Tumor necrosis factor is the principal mediator of the acute inflammatory response to gram-negative bacteria and other infectious microbes. TNF is responsible for many of the systemic complications of severe infections. The TNF receptor family stimulates gene transcription or induces apoptosis in a variety of cells. The gene-encoding TNF-α is located in the HLA region between the HLA-DR and HLA-B loci.

TNF-α and TNF-β share similar activities. The principal physiologic functions of TNF are as follows: (1) to stimulate the recruitment of neutrophils and monocytes to sites of infection; and (2) to activate these cells to eradicate microbes.

In low concentrations, TNF acts on leukocytes and endothelium to induce acute inflammation. At moderate concentrations, TNF mediates the systemic effects of inflammation. In severe infections, TNF is produced in large amounts and causes clinical and pathologic abnormalities (e.g., septic shock). When TNFs gain access to the circulation during infection, they mediate a series of reactions that induce shock and can result in death. The syndrome known as septic shock is a complication of severe gram-negative bacterial sepsis.

HEMATOPOIETIC STIMULATORS

Stem Cell Factor (c-kit Ligand)

Stem cell factor is a cytokine that interacts with a tyrosine kinase membrane receptor, the protein product of the cellular oncogene *c-kit.* The cytokine that interacts with this receptor is called c-kit ligand, or stem cell factor, because it acts on immature stem cells.

Stem cell factor is needed to make bone marrow stem cells responsive to other CSFs but it does not cause colony formation itself. Stem cell factor may also play a role in sustaining the viability and proliferative capacity of immature T cells in the thymus and mast cells in mucosal tissues.

Colony-Stimulating Factors

A variety of CSFs, such as granulocyte-CSF (G-CSF) and GM-CSF, are also made by T cells. These pathways provide a link between the lymphoid and hematopoietic systems. For example, G-CSF and GM-CSF regulate the production of granulocytes and monocytes, thus enabling the T cell system to promote the inflammatory response.

The biological activity of CSF is measured by its ability to stimulate hematopoietic progenitor cells to form colonies in semisolid medium. These proteins are necessary for the survival, proliferation, and differentiation of precursor cells of the immune system.

CSFs are potentially important in the treatment of human disease. GM-CSF has been used in a number of clinical trials to increase circulating leukocytes in patients with AIDS, other immunocompromised patients (e.g., those recovering from chemotherapy), and bone marrow transplant recipients.

Transforming Growth Factors

As with the IFNs, transforming growth factors (TGFs) were identified as products of virally transformed cells. These factors were found to induce phenotypic transformation in non-neoplastic cells and subsequently were termed *transforming growth factors.* TGF-β is a group of five cytokines released by many cell types, including macrophages and platelets. TGF-β is known to be a potent inhibitor of IL-1–induced T cell proliferation.

The principal action of TGF-β in the immune system is to inhibit the proliferation and activation of lymphocytes and other leukocytes. It inhibits the proliferation and differentiation of T cells and the activation of macrophages.

Chemokines

Chemokines are a large family of structurally homologous cytokines that stimulate transendothelial leukocyte movement from the blood to the tissue site of infection and regulate the migration of polymorphonuclear leukocytes (PMNs) and mononuclear leukocytes within tissues (see Chapter 3). The largest family consists of CC chemokines that attract mononuclear cells to sites of chronic inflammation, such as monocyte chemoattractant protein 1 (MCP-1). A second family of chemokines consists of CXC chemokines, of which IL-8 (CXCL8) is the prototype. CXCL8 attracts PMNs to sites of acute inflammation, activates monocytes, and may direct the recruitment of these cells to vascular lesions. The third family, CX3, forms a cell adhesion receptor capable of arresting cells under physiologic flow conditions. TNF-α–converting enzyme can cleave CX3CL1 from the cell membrane.

Other functions of various chemokines include the following:
- Increasing the affinity of leukocyte **integrins** for their **ligands** on endothelium (e.g., intercellular adhesion molecule-1 [ICAM-1], ICAM-2, vascular cell adhesion molecule-1 [VCAM-1])
- Regulating the traffic of lymphocytes and other leukocytes through peripheral lymphoid tissues
- Maintaining normal migration of immune cells into lymphoid organs or other specialized cells to particular sites

Assessment of Cytokines

Defects in cytokine production can lead to autoimmunity (Table 5-10). Traditional methods for assessment of cytokines include the following:
- Bioassays
- Enzyme-linked immunosorbent assay (ELISA)
- Intracellular staining
- Ribonuclease protection assay
- Polymerase chain reaction (PCR)

Table 5-10	Defects in Cytokine Production that Can Lead to Autoimmunity	
Cytokine or Protein	**Defect**	**Disorder**
IL-1 receptor antagonist	Underexpression	Arthritis
IL-2 IL-7 IL-10	Overexpression	IBD
IL-2 receptor	Overexpression	IBD
IL-10 receptor	Overexpression	IBD
IL-3	Overexpression	Demyelinating syndrome
TNF-α	Overexpression	IBD, arthritis, vasculitis
	Underexpression	SLE
IFN-γ	Overexpression in skin	SLE
TGF-β	Underexpression	Systemic wasting syndrome, IBD
TGF-β receptor in T cells	Underexpression	SLE

Adapted from Davidson A, Diamond B: Autoimmune diseases, N Engl J Med 345:340–350, 2001.

IL, interleukin; *IBD,* inflammatory bowel disease; *TNF,* tumor necrosis factor; *SLE,* systemic lupus erythematosus; *IFN,* interferon; *TGF,* transforming growth factor.

Newer methods of measurement include the following:
- Multiplexed assay using the FlowMetrix; quantifies multiple cytokines simultaneously
- Intracellular staining using flow cytometry
- Cord blood mononuclear cells stimulated by allergens (celELISA).
- Real-time PCR for lymph nodes or spleen
- Enzyme-linked immunosorbent spot (ELISPOT) assays
- Enhanced immunoassays for cytokines
- Biotrak assay—high-sensitivity ELISA

ACUTE-PHASE PROTEINS

The acute-phase response is an innate body defense. This response is a nonspecific indicator of an inflammatory process.

Overview

A group of glycoproteins associated with the acute-phase response are collectively called **acute-phase proteins** or **acute-phase reactants.** The various acute-phase proteins rise at different rates and in varying levels in response to tissue injury (e.g., inflammation, infection, **malignant neoplasia,** various diseases or disorders, trauma, surgical procedures, drug response). The increased synthesis of these proteins takes place shortly after a trauma and is initiated and sustained by proinflammatory cytokines.

The main biological sign of inflammation is an increase in the ESR. In addition to the ESR, measurement of the plasma

- Monitoring the progress of diagnosed disease activity
- Assessing response to therapy in inflammatory diseases (e.g., rheumatoid arthritis, juvenile chronic arthritis, ankylosing spondylitis, Reiter's syndrome, psoriatic arthropathy, vasculitis, rheumatic fever)
- Detection of complications of a known disease (e.g., immune complex deposition, postsurgical infection)

Table 5-11	Examples of Clinically Useful Acute-Phase Proteins		
Protein	Normal Concentration (g/L)	Concentration in Acute Inflammation (g/L)	Response Time (hr)
C-reactive protein	0.0008-0.004	0.4	6-10
α_1-Antichymotrypsin	0.3-0.6	3.0	10
α_1-Antitrypsin	2.0-4.0	7.0	24
Orosomucoid	0.5-1.4	3.0	24
Haptoglobin	1.0-3.0	6.0	24
Fibrinogen	2.0-4.5	10.0	24
C3	0.55-1.2	3.0	48-72
C4	0.2-0.5	1.0	48-72
Ceruloplasmin	0.15-0.6	2.0	48-72

concentration of acute-phase reactants is usually a good indicator of local inflammatory activity and tissue damage. More than 20 acute-phase proteins have a definable role in inflammation (Box 5-2). These reactants constitute most of the serum glycoproteins (Table 5-11).

Acute-phase reactants include C-reactive protein (CRP), inflammatory mediators (e.g., complement components C3 and C4), fibrinogen, transport proteins such as **haptoglobin**, inhibitors (e.g., α_1-antitrypsin), and α_1-acid glycoprotein. Profiles of inflammatory changes yield detailed information but rarely provide major evidence for diagnosis or treatment.

Produced by the liver under the control of IL-6, CRP is a parameter of inflammatory activity. Serum concentrations can increase 1000-fold with an acute inflammatory reaction. Persistent increases in CRP can also occur in chronic inflammatory disorders (e.g., autoimmune disease, malignancy).

CRP is prominent among the acute-phase proteins because its changes show great sensitivity. Changes in CRP are independent of those of ESR and parallel the inflammatory process. CRP is a direct and quantitative measure of the acute-phase reaction and, as a result of its fast kinetics, provides adequate information about the actual clinical situation (see later). In contrast, ESR is an indirect measure of the acute-phase reaction. It reacts much slower to changes of inflammatory activity

and is influenced by other factors. ESR can be falsely normal in conditions such as polyglobulinemia, cryoglobulinemia, and hemoglobinopathy. ESR may also be spuriously high in the absence of inflammation in patients with anemia or hypergammaglobulinemia.

Synthesis and Catabolism

All the acute-phase proteins are synthesized rapidly in response to tissue injury. The elevation is twofold to fivefold in certain disease states. In addition, strenuous exercise triggers an inflammatory response similar to that in sepsis. Indices of the inflammatory response, especially to exercise, include leukocytosis, release of inflammatory mediators and acute-phase reactants, tissue damage, priming of various white blood cell lines, production of free radicals, activation of complement, coagulation, and fibrinolytic cascades.

Acute-phase proteins have different kinetics and various degrees of increase. Some, the negative acute-phase proteins, actually decrease, possibly resulting from a loss of protein from the vascular space. In addition, acute-phase proteins can be modified by causes other than inflammation (e.g., low fibrinogen level in DIC, very low haptoglobin level in hemolysis, elevated α_1-acid glycoprotein [orosomucoid] in renal insufficiency, elevated transferrin level in iron deficiency). In addition, liver insufficiency or leakage through the kidney or gut lesions can lower these reactants.

The rate of change and peak concentration of separate acute-phase reactants vary with the component and the clinical situation. In acute inflammation, CRP and α_1-antichymotrypsin levels become elevated within the first 12 hours. The levels of complement components, C3 and C4, and ceruloplasmin do not rise for several days.

Acute-phase proteins do not always change in parallel. This mismatch in acute-phase protein levels is most often the result of increased catabolism and elimination from the circulation of certain proteins. Differences may also be caused by discrepancies in rates of synthesis. Most acute-phase proteins have half-lives of 2 to 4 days, but CRP has a half-life of 5 to 7 hours. Thus, the CRP level falls much more rapidly than that of the other acute-phase proteins when the patient recovers.

C-Reactive Protein

Traditionally, CRP has been used clinically for monitoring infection, autoimmune disorders and, more recently, healing after a myocardial infarction (MI). Levels of CRP parallel the course of the inflammatory response and return to lower undetectable levels as the inflammation subsides. CRP demonstrates a large incremental change, with as much as a 100-fold increase in concentration in acute inflammation, and is the fastest responding and most sensitive indicator of acute inflammation. CRP increases faster than ESR in responding to inflammation, whereas the leukocyte count may remain within normal limits despite infection. An elevated CRP level can signal infection many hours before it can be confirmed by culture results; therefore, treatment can be prompt. Because of these characteristics, CRP is the method of choice for screening for inflammatory and malignant organic diseases and monitoring therapy in inflammatory diseases.

Elevations of the CRP level occur in about 70 disease states, including septicemia and meningitis in neonates, infections in immunosuppressed patients, burns complicated by infection, serious postoperative infections, MI, malignant tumors, and rheumatic disease. Measurement of CRP may add to the diagnostic procedure in select cases (e.g., differentiation between bacterial and a viral infection). An extremely elevated CRP level suggests a possible bacterial infection (see later, procedure description). In general, CRP is advocated as an indicator of bacterial infection in at-risk patients in whom the clinical assessment of infection is difficult to make, but a lack of specificity rules out CRP as a definitive diagnostic tool.

Levels of CRP rise after tissue injury or surgery. In uncomplicated cases, the CRP level peaks about 2 days after surgery and gradually returns to normal levels within 7 to 10 days. If the CRP level is persistently elevated or returns to an increased level, it may indicate underlying sepsis preceding clinical signs and symptoms and should alert the clinician to postoperative complications.

In clinical practice, CRP is particularly useful when serial measurements are performed. The course of the CRP level may be useful for monitoring the effect of treatment and for early detection of postoperative complications or intercurrent infections. In rheumatoid arthritis (RA), the CRP level reflects short-term and long-term disease activity. Monitoring of CRP levels allows for early prediction of response to a particular drug, often months before clinical and radiologic confirmation are possible. In disorders such as RA, CRP can be used to assess the effect of antiinflammatory drugs (e.g., aspirin) and the nature of their action. Aspirin-like drugs do not suppress acute-phase proteins in inflammation, allowing optimal therapy in the shortest time and minimizing ongoing inflammation and joint damage. Assessment of CRP is also valuable in monitoring therapy and disease activity in other arthritides. Rheumatic fever and Crohn's disease can also be monitored by CRP. In addition, CRP level assessment has been found to enhance the value of traditional enzyme measurements in MI.

In a number of chronic inflammatory diseases, however, CRP is an unreliable indicator. CRP values may be normal when other acute-phase proteins are altered in disorders such as SLE, dermatomyositis, and ulcerative colitis. SLE shows little or no CRP response, despite apparently active inflammation.

Both CRP and low-density lipoprotein (LDL) cholesterol levels are known to be elevated in persons at risk for cardiovascular disease. CRP level may be a stronger predictor of cardiovascular events than LDL cholesterol, an established benchmark of cardiovascular risk.

Other Acute-Phase Reactants

α_1-Antitrypsin is an acute-phase protein that increases in acute inflammatory reactions. Generalized vasculitis, such as in immune complex disease, may result in inappropriately low levels of α_1-antitrypsin, probably resulting from increased elimination of complexes with leukocyte lysosomal enzymes.

Defects in the complement components C3a and C5a and the opsonin C3b result in serious infections. In addition, immune complex disease and gram-negative bacteremia result in low levels of complement components, particularly C3 and C4, because the components are consumed during complement activation. Acute inflammation leads to normal or slightly elevated levels. If both disorders are present, complement consumption may be masked, making it deceptive to use complement measurement as the only index of immune complex deposition in disease. The detection of complement breakdown products is more useful than the measurement of total complement component concentrations. It is more desirable to measure C3 breakdown products than total C3 in conditions such as peritonitis or pancreatitis.

Lymphomas may result in a marked increase in C1 esterase inhibitor, with little other change. **Ceruloplasmin,** often measured as serum copper, is used to monitor Hodgkin's disease; increases are considered specific indicators of relapse. Although not definitely established, ceruloplasmin monitoring may provide similar information in non-Hodgkin's lymphoma.

Assessment Methods

Inflammation almost always follows acute tissue damage. Diagnostic categories of acute inflammation can include bacterial causes and nonbacterial causes such as trauma, chronic inflammation, and viral disease. Many laboratory tests have been advocated for the early diagnosis of acute inflammation: total WBC count (including the absolute count and percentage of band and segmented neutrophils, as determined by a 100-cell differential count on a peripheral blood smear), acute-phase proteins, and the ESR.

The ESR ("sed rate") is a nonspecific indicator of disease, with increased sedimentation of erythrocytes seen in acute and chronic inflammation and malignancies. Although nonspecific, the ESR is one of the most frequently performed laboratory tests.

In addition to these hematologic tests, several tests are of direct value in immunologic testing. These procedures include a simple phagocytic cell function test and the determination of CRP.

CASE STUDY

Signs and Symptoms

A 39-year-old woman was admitted for a cholecystectomy. She had a history of chronic cholecystitis; recent x-ray studies revealed stones in the gallbladder and a large stone in the biliary duct (Fig. 5-3). During surgery, a large stone was removed from the duct, and a cholangiogram showed no further obstructions of the hepatic or common bile ducts.

The patient became febrile 1 day after surgery. A 48-hour postoperative complete blood count (CBC) and CRP were ordered (Fig. 5-4). On the seventh postoperative day, she had abdominal pain and began vomiting. A CBC, ESR, CRP, and blood culture were ordered at that

CASE STUDY—Cont'd

time. Immediately after drawing the blood work, the patient was started on a broad-spectrum antibiotic and discharged on hospital day 15.

Laboratory Data

At 48 hours after surgery, the CBC was within normal limits and the CRP was 7.5 g/L.

Results after the episode of abdominal pain showed a CRP of 8.4 g/L and a subsequently positive blood culture for *Pseudomonas* spp.

Questions

1. The patient's C-Reactive Protein (C-RP) was elevated at 7 days post-operatively because:
   a. It reflects the leukocyte (WBC) response.
   b. It is a sensitive indicator of inflammation.
   c. It is diagnostic of sepsis.
   d. It is normal to manifest an extremely elevated C-RP 7 days after surgery.
2. In an uncomplicated cholecystectomy:
   a. The highest level of C-RP is at 48 hours postoperatively.
   b. The highest level of C-RP is at 72 hours postoperatively.
   c. The lowest level of C-RP is at 5 days postoperatively.
   d. The lowest level of C-RP is at 7 days postoperatively.

See Appendix A for the answers to these questions.

Critical Thinking Group Discussion Questions

1. Which test was the most rapid and sensitive indicator of infection?
2. Is the CRP diagnostic?
3. Why was the CRP level elevated immediately after surgery?

See instructor ⊜volve for discussion of the answers to these questions.

C-Reactive Protein Rapid Latex Agglutination Test

Principle

The C-reactive protein rapid latex **agglutination** test is based on the reaction between patient serum containing CRP as the antigen and the corresponding antihuman (CRP) antibody coated to the treated surface of latex particles. The coated particles enhance the detection of an agglutination reaction when antigen is present in the serum being tested. The clinical applications of CRP evaluation include detecting inflammatory diseases, particularly infections. It is also a useful indicator in screening for organic disease, inflammatory and malignant disease, and monitoring therapy in inflammatory diseases. Because CRP is more rapidly synthesized than other acute-phase proteins, assays of CRP are the measurement of choice in suspected inflammatory conditions.

See instructor ⊜volve for the procedural protocol.

Reporting Results

In patients who are free of inflammation and tissue necrosis, CRP is absent from the serum or present in concentrations below 0.5 mg/dL. Reference range mean values are 0.01 mg/dL in newborns and less than 0.05 mg/dL in adult men and nonpregnant women.

Positive Reaction

Agglutination of the latex suspension is a positive result. A positive reaction is reported when the undiluted specimen or the 1:5 diluted specimen demonstrates agglutination, or when both exhibit agglutination.

Negative Reaction

The absence of visible agglutination and the presence of opaque fluid constitute a negative reaction. A negative reaction is reported only when both the undiluted specimen and the 1:5 diluted specimen exhibit no visible agglutination.

Comments

Specimen collection and handling are important to the quality of the test. Strict adherence must be paid to technique, with a special emphasis on drop size, complete mixing, reaction time, and temperature of reagents.

The strength of a positive reaction may be graded as follows:

1+ Very small clumping with an opaque fluid background
2+ Small clumping with a slightly opaque fluid background
3+ Moderate clumping with a fairly clear fluid background
4+ Large clumping with a clear fluid background

Sources of Error

False-positive results may be observed if serum specimens are **lipemic,** hemolyzed, or heavily contaminated with bacteria. If the reaction time is longer than 2 minutes, a false-positive result may also be produced from a drying effect.

False-negative results may be observed in undiluted serum specimens because of high levels of CRP (antigen excess). A 1:5 dilution of serum is also tested for this reason.

Limitations

Because the latex slide agglutination test is a qualitative and semiquantitative procedure, other methods such as nephelometry should be used for the quantitative determination of the CRP level when indicated. The strength of the agglutination reaction is not always indicative of the CRP concentration. Weak reactions may be produced in samples with elevated or low CRP values. Results may vary, depending on the patient's condition.

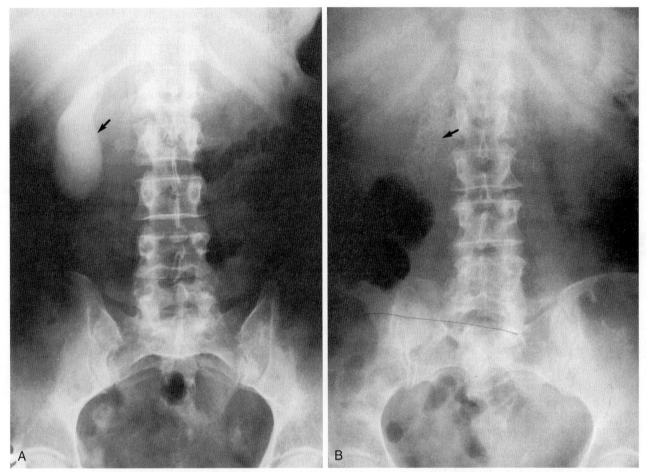

Figure 5-3   Radiographs of gallbladder (contrast dye). A, Normal gallbladder *(arrow).* **B,** Gallbladder filled with stones *(arrow).*

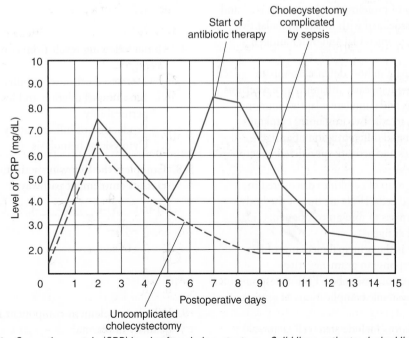

Figure 5-4   C-reactive protein (CRP) levels after cholecystectomy. *Solid lines,* patients; *dashed line,* example.

This 2-minute slide latex agglutination test has a detection level of 1 mg CRP/dL; therefore, patients with CRP values less than 1 mg/dL may go undetected. The sensitivity of the procedure has been assessed at 93%.

Clinical Applications

With the onset of a substantial inflammatory event (e.g., infection, MI, surgery), the CRP level usually increases significantly (>tenfold) above the reference range values for healthy individuals. The test is clinically useful for the early detection of inflammatory diseases (particularly infections), as an indicator in screening for organic diseases, and in monitoring patient progress.

CHAPTER HIGHLIGHTS

- The complement system is a heat-labile series of 18 plasma proteins, many of which are enzymes or proteinases. Normally, complement components are present in the circulation in an inactive form.
- Complement is composed of three interrelated enzyme cascades—the classic, alternate, and mannose-binding lectin pathways.
- Complement levels may be abnormal in certain disease states. Increased complement levels are often associated with inflammatory conditions, trauma, and acute illness. Separate complement components (e.g., C3) are acute-phase proteins.
- The biological functions of the complement system fall into two general categories, cell lysis by the membrane attack complex or biological effects of proteolytic fragments of complement.
- Cytokines are a family of proteins that are synthesized and secreted by the cells associated with innate and adaptive immunity in response to microbial and other antigen exposure.
- Cytokines also participate in host defense. In innate immunity, cytokines mediate early inflammatory reactions to microbial organisms and stimulate adaptive immune responses. In contrast, in adaptive immunity, cytokines stimulate proliferation and differentiation of antigen-stimulated lymphocytes and activate specialized effector cells (e.g., macrophages).
- The interferons are a group of cytokines discovered in virally infected cultured cells. IFNs are one of the body's natural defensive responses to foreign components (e.g., microbes, tumors, and antigens).
- Tumor necrosis factor is the principal mediator of the acute inflammatory response to gram-negative bacteria and other infectious microbes. TNF is responsible for many of the systemic complications of severe infections.
- Hematopoietic stimulators include stem cell factor, a cytokine that acts on immature stem cells.
- Chemokines are a large family of structurally homologous cytokines that stimulate transendothelial leukocyte movement from the blood to tissue site of infection and regulate the migration of polymorphonuclear leukocytes and mononuclear leukocytes within tissues. Chemokines appear to control the phased arrival of different cell populations at sites of inflammation.
- The acute-phase response is an innate body defense. This response is a nonspecific indicator of an inflammatory process.
- C-reactive protein is used clinically for monitoring infection, autoimmune disorders and, more recently, healing after a myocardial infarction. CRP levels parallel the course of the inflammatory response and return to lower undetectable levels as the inflammation subsides.

REVIEW QUESTIONS

1. The complement system is:
   a. A heat-labile series of plasma proteins
   b. Composed of many proteinases
   c. Composed of three interrelated pathways
   d. All of the above

2. All the following are complement-controlling proteins except:
   a. C1 (INH)
   b. Factor I
   c. Factor H
   d. C3

3. The three complement activation pathways converge at the point of cleavage of complement component _____.
   a. C3
   b. C5
   c. C7
   d. C8

4. All the following result from complement activation except:
   a. Decreased cell susceptibility to phagocytosis
   b. Blood vessel dilation and increased vascular permeability
   c. Production of inflammatory mediators
   d. Cytolysis or hemolysis

5-8. Complete the following activation sequence of the classic complement pathway:
   C1 to C_(5)-C__(6)-__-C3-_C(7)___-C6-C7-C_(8)_-C9
   a. 2
   b. 4
   c. 5
   d. 8

9. Which complement component is present in the greatest quantity in plasma?
   a. 2
   b. 3
   c. 4
   d. 8

10-12. Arrange the three stages of the classic complement pathway in their correct sequence.

10. __C__

11. __a__

12. __b__
    a. Enzymatic activation
    b. Membrane attack
    c. Recognition

13. Fixation of the C1 complement component is related to each of the following factors except:
    a. Molecular weight of the antibody
    b. The presence of IgM antibody
    c. The presence of most IgG subclasses
    d. Spatial constraints

14. At which stage does the complement system reach its full amplitude?
    a. C1q, C1r, C1s complex
    b. C2
    c. C3
    d. C4

15. Which of the following is not a component of the membrane attack complex?
    a. C3b
    b. C6
    c. C7
    d. C8

16. The final steps (C8 and C9) in complement activation lead to:
    a. Cell lysis
    b. Phagocytosis
    c. Immune opsonin adherence
    d. Virus neutralization

17-20. Select the appropriate pathway response.

17. __A__ Activated by antigen-antibody complexes

18. __b__ Generates an active (C3b, Bb) C3 convertase

19. __b__ Activated by microbial and mammalian cell surfaces

20. _____ Terminates in a membrane attack complex
    a. Classic pathway
    b. Alternative pathway
    c. Both a and b

21. The alternate complement pathway is(can be):
    a. Initiated by the formation of antigen-antibody reactions
    b. Predominantly a non–antibody-initiated pathway
    c. Activated by factors such as endotoxins
    d. Both b and c

22. Which of the following conditions can be associated with hypercomplementemia?
    a. Myocardial infarction
    b. Systemic lupus erythematosus
    c. Glomerulonephritis
    d. Subacute bacterial endocarditis

23-26. Match the following complement deficiency states in humans with their respective deficient components. (Use an answer only once.)

23. __D__ C2

24. __b__ C5 dysfunction

25. __C__ C6 and C7

26. __a__ C8
    a. Xeroderma pigmentosa
    b. Leiner's disease
    c. Raynaud's phenomenon
    d. Recurrent pyogenic infections

27. A (the) nonspecific component(s) of the immune system is (are):
    a. Complement
    b. T cells
    c. B cells
    d. Both a and b

28-31. Match the following:

28. __B__ Interleukin-1 (IL-1) *lympho act.*

29. __A__ Interleukin-2 (IL-2) *T ce Sruth.*

30. __D__ Interleukin-3 (IL-3) *Multi col-stimfctor.*

31. __C__ Interleukin-5 (IL-5) *Bcell grawt*
    a. T cell growth factor
    b. Lymphocyte-activating factor
    c. B cell growth factor 2
    d. Multicolony colony-stimulating factor

32-35. Match the following:

32. __C__ Interleukin-6 (IL-6) *acutephose resp.*

33. __D__ Interleukin-7 (IL-7) *Exp. T+B cells*

34. __B__ Interleukin-8 (IL-8) *neutrophils-chemo.*

35. __A__ Interleukin-12 (IL-12) *NK.*
    a. NK cell stimulatory factor
    b. Stimulates neutrophils in chemotaxis
    c. Induce acute phase response
    d. Stimulates expansion of immature T and B cells

36-39. Match the following:

36. __b__ Interleukin-1 (IL-1)

37. __a__ Interleukin-2 (IL-2) *lanc*

38. __C__ Interleukin-3 (IL-3)

39. __a__ Interleukin-4 (IL-4)
    a. Enhances cytolytic activity of lymphokine-activated killer cells (LAK)
    b. Potent mediator in acute-phase response
    c. Stimulates hematopoietic cells
    d. Enhances production of IgG and inhibits production of IgE by activated B cells

40-43. Match the following:

40. __a__ Interleukin-5 (IL-5) *eosinophil*
41. __a__ Interleukin-6 (IL-6) *Secretion Ig*
42. __c__ Interleukin-7 (IL-7) *Bcell prog.*
43. __b__ Interleukin-8 (IL-8) *respiratory burst.*
    a. Induction of secretion of Ig
    b. Activates the respiratory burst
    c. Stimulates early B cell progenitor cells
    d. Activates eosinophils

44-47. Match the following:

44. __c__ Interleukin-9 (IL-9) *T cells*
45. __a__ Interleukin-10 (IL-10)
46. __b__ Interleukin-11 (IL-11)
47. __d__ Interleukin-12 (IL-12)
    a. Inhibits cytokine synthesis
    b. Increases the number of IgG-secreting B lymphocytes
    c. Stimulates proliferation of T cells and mast cells
    d. Enhances the activity of cytotoxic effector T cells

48-51. Match the following:

48. __a__ Interleukin-13 (IL-13)
49. __d__ Interleukin-14 (IL-14)
50. __b__ Interleukin-15 (IL-15)
51. __c__ Interleukin-16 (IL-16}
    a. Inhibits activation of macrophages
    b. Produced in response to viral infection
    c. Acts as a T cell chemoattractant
    d. Acts as a B cell growth factor

52-55. Match the following:

52. __d__ Interleukin-17 (IL-17)
53. __a__ Interleukin-18 (IL-18)
54. __b__ Interleukin-19 (IL-19)
55. __c__ Interleukin-20 (IL-20)
    a. Acts as a synergist with IL-12
    b. Suppresses activities of Th1 and Th2
    c. Associated with skin inflammations
    d. Induces granulopoiesis

56-59. Match the following:

56. __a__ Interleukin-21 (IL-21)

57. __b__ Interleukin-22 (IL_22)
58. __a__ Interleukin-23 (IL-23)
59. __c__ Interleukin-25 (IL-25)
    a. Promotes increased production of T cells
    b. Somewhat similar to IFN-α, IFN-β, and IFN-γ
    c. A member of the IL-17 cytokine family
    d. Shares some in vivo functions with IL-12

60-63. Indicate true statements with the letter A and false statements with the letter B.

60. __A__ Cytokines secreted by lymphocytes are also called lymphokines.
61. __A__ Cytokines are polypeptide products of activated cells.
62. __B__ Cytokines are released only in response to specific antigens.
63. __A__ Most cytokines have multiple activities and act on numerous cell types.

64-67. Match each term to its appropriate description. (Use each answer only once.)

64. __b__ Interleukins
65. __c__ Interferons
66. __a__ Tumor necrosis factor
67. __d__ Colony-stimulating factors
    a. Unable to stimulate T cell proliferation
    b. Act(s) between leukocytes
    c. Discovered in virally infected cells
    d. Provide(s) a link between the lymphoid hematopoietic system

68. Transforming growth factors:
    a. Are products of virally transformed cells
    b. Can be a potent inhibitor of IL-1–induced T cell proliferation in their beta form
    c. Are important in inflammation, tumor defense, and cell growth
    d. All of the above

69. Which activity is associated with interferon?
    a. Enhances phagocytosis
    b. Retards expression of specific genes
    c. Promotes complement-mediated cytolysis
    d. Interferes with viral replication

70. Tumor necrosis factor (TNF) differs from IL-1 in that TNF is not able to:
    a. Mediate an acute inflammatory reaction
    b. Increase the expression of IL-2 receptors
    c. Enhance the proliferation and differentiation of B lymphocytes
    d. Stimulate T cell proliferation

71-73. Match the following:

71. _____ Tumor necrosis factor

72. __A__ Colony-stimulating factors

73. __C__ Transforming growth factors

   a. Stimulates hematopoietic growth factor

   b. Encoding gene located in the HLA region between the HLA-DR and HLA-B loci

   c. Induce phenotypic transformation in non-neoplastic cells

BIBLIOGRAPHY

Aziz H: Biological response modifiers, 2010 (laboratory-manager.advanceweb.com/Features/Articles/Biological-Response-Modifiers.aspx).

Charo IF, Ransohoff RM: The many roles of chemokines and chemokine receptors in inflammation, N Engl J Med 354:610–621, 2006.

Fort MM, Cheung J, Yen D, et al: IL-25 induces IL-4, IL-5, and IL-13 and Th2-associated pathologies in vivo, Immunology 15:985–995, 2001.

Frank MM: Complement in the pathophysiology of human disease, N Engl J Med 316:1525, 1987.

Frucht DM: IL-23: a cytokine that acts on memory T cells, Sci STKE(114):pe1, 2002.

Gabay C, Kushner I: Acute-phase proteins and other systemic responses to inflammation, N Engl J Med 340:448–454, 1999.

Hansson GK: Inflammation, atherosclerosis, and coronary artery disease, N Engl J Med 352:1685–1695, 2005.

Human Gene Nomenclature Committee (HUGO): 2007 (www.gene.ucl.ac.uk).

Hurst SD, Muchamuel T, Gorman DM, et al: New IL-17 family members promote Th1 or Th2 responses in the lung: in vivo function of the novel cytokine IL-25, J Immunol 169:443–453, 2002.

Ibelgaufts H: COPE cytokines and cells online pathfinder encyclopedia, version 29.0, 2012 (www.copewithcytokines.de).

Kelleher K, Bean K, Clark SC, et al: Human interleukin-9: genomic sequence, chromosomal location, and sequences essential for its expression in human T-cell leukemia virus (HTLV)-I-transformed human T cells, Blood 77:1436–1441, 1991.

Larchmann PJ, Rosen FS: Genetic defects of complement in man, Springer Semin Immunopathol 1:339–353, 1978.

Larson RS, Springer TA: Structure and function of leukocyte integrins, Immunol Rev 18:181–217, 1990.

Liblau RS, Fugger L: Tumor necrosis factor-alpha and disease progression in multiple sclerosis, N Engl J Med 326:272, 1992.

MacKay IR, Rosen RS: Allergy and allergic diseases, N Engl J Med 344:109–113, 2001.

Marsik C, Sunder-Plassmann R, Jilma B, et al: The C-reactive protein +1444C/T alteration modulates the inflammation and coagulation response in human endotoxemia, Clin Chem 52:1952–1957, 2006.

Medzhitov R, Janeway C Jr: Innate immunity, N Engl J Med 343:338–344, 2000.

Muller-Eberhardt HJ: Complement abnormalities in human disease, Hosp Pract 13:65–76, 1978.

Parham C, Chirica M, Timans J, et al: A receptor for the heterodimeric cytokine IL-23 is composed of IL-23Rb1 and a novel cytokine receptor subunit, IL-23R, J Immunol 168:5699–5708, 2002.

Parker R, Dutrieux J, Beq S, et al: Interleukin-7 treatment counteracts IFN-α therapy-induced lymphopenia and stimulates SIV-specific cytotoxic T lymphocyte responses in SIV-infected rhesus macaques, Blood 116:5589–5599, 2010.

Pedrazzi AH: Acute phase proteins: clinical and laboratory diagnosis: a review, Ann Pharm Fr 56:108–114, 1998.

Rhen T, Cidlowski JA: Antiinflammatory action of glucocorticoids: new mechanisms for old drugs, N Engl J Med 353:1711–1723, 2005.

Ridker PM, Rifai N, Rose L, et al: Comparison of C-reactive protein and low-density lipoprotein cholesterol levels in the prediction of first cardiovascular events, N Engl J Med 347:1557–1565, 2002.

Roberts WL, Sedrick R, Moulton L, et al: Evaluation of four automated high-sensitivity C-reactive protein methods: implications for clinical and epidemiological applications, Clin Chem 46:461–468, 2000.

Soiffer R, Robertson MJ, Murray C, et al: Interleukin-12 augments cytolytic activity of peripheral blood lymphocytes from patients with hematologic and solid malignancies, Blood 82:2790–2796, 1993.

Taga K, Mostowski H, Tosato G: Human interleukin-10 can directly inhibit T cell growth, Blood 81:2964–2971, 1993.

Tagaya Y: Time to restore individual rights for IL-2 and IL-15? Blood 108:409, 2006.

Tham W, Schmidt CQ, Hauhart RE, et al: Plasmodium falciparum uses a key functional site in complement receptor type-1 for invasion of human erythrocytes, Blood 118:1923–1933, 2011.

Tulin EE, Onoda N, Nakata Y, et al: SF20/IL-25, a novel bone marrow stroma-derived growth factor that binds to mouse thymic shared antigen-1 and supports lymphoid cell proliferation, J Immunol 167:6338–6347, 2001.

Turgeon ML: Fundamentals of immunohematology, ed 3, Baltimore, 1999, Williams & Wilkins.

Van Leeuwen MA, van Rijswijk MH: Acute phase proteins in the monitoring of inflammatory disorders, Baillieres Clin Rheumatol 8:531–552, 1994.

Waldmann TA: The multichain interleukin-2 receptor, JAMA 263:272–274, 1990.

Walport MJ: Complement, N Engl J Med 344:1058–1065, 2001.

CHAPTER 6

Safety in the Immunology-Serology Laboratory

Safety Standards and Agencies
Prevention of Transmission of Infectious Diseases
Safe Work Practices for Infection Control
Protective Techniques for Infection Control
    Selection and Use of Gloves
    Facial Barrier Protection and Occlusive Bandages
    Laboratory Coats or Gowns as Barrier Protection
Handwashing
Specimen-Processing Protection
Additional Laboratory Hazards
Decontamination of Work Surfaces, Equipment, and Spills
Disposal of Infectious Laboratory Waste
    Containers for Waste
    Final Decontamination of Waste Materials

Disease Prevention
    Immunization
    Screening Tests
    Postexposure Prophylaxis
Basic First Aid and Procedures
Case Study in Safety
    Questions
    Critical Thinking Group Discussion Questions
Procedure: Test Your Safety Knowledge
Chapter Highlights
Review Questions
Bibliography

Learning Objectives

At the conclusion of this chapter, the reader should be able to:
- Name the federal or national agencies responsible for safety issues.
- Discuss the occupational transmission of hepatitis B virus (HBV) and human immunodeficiency virus (HIV).
- Describe the practice of Standard Blood and Body Fluid Precautions.
- Explain the proper handling of hazardous material and waste management, including infectious waste, chemicals, and radioactive waste.
- Describe the basic aspects of infection control policies, including the use of personal protective equipment or devices (gowns, gloves, goggles) and the purpose of Standard Precautions.
- Compare preexposure and postexposure prophylactic measures for handling potential occupational transmission of certain pathogens (HBV, HCV, HIV).

- Demonstrate the proper decontamination of a work area at the start and completion of work and after a hazardous spill.
- Explain the process of properly segregating and disposing of various types of waste products generated in the clinical laboratory.
- Analyze a safety case study to identify violations and remediations for the violations.
- Correctly answer case study related multiple choice questions.
- Be prepared to participate in a discussion of critical thinking questions.
- Identify items essential to safety in the clinical laboratory.
- Correctly answer end of chapter review questions.

Key Terms

autoclaving
autodilutor
biohazard
biosafety policies
enzyme immunoassay (EIA)
immunocompromised
immunoprophylaxis
infectious waste

nonintact
nosocomial transmission
occlusive
percutaneous (parenteral)
personal protective equipment (PPE)
phlebotomy
pipetting
seroconversion

seronegative
sharps
skin lesions
Standard Precautions
Western blot (WB)
window period

In the immunology-serology laboratory, precautions must be taken to prevent accidental exposure to infectious diseases and other laboratory hazards. Clinical laboratory personnel are routinely exposed to potential hazards in their daily activities. The importance of safety and correct first aid procedures cannot be overemphasized. Many accidents do not just happen; they are caused by carelessness or lack of proper communication. For this reason, the practice of safety should be uppermost in the mind of any worker in a clinical laboratory. This chapter presents safety issues that are applicable to the immunology-serology laboratory.

SAFETY STANDARDS AND AGENCIES

Safety standards for clinical laboratories are initiated, governed, and reviewed by several agencies or committees. These include the following:

- U.S. Department of Labor, Occupational Safety and Health Administration (OSHA)
- Clinical and Laboratory Standards Institute (CLSI), a nonprofit educational organization that provides a forum for the development, promotion, and use of national and international standards
- Centers for Disease Control and Prevention (CDC), part of the U.S. Department of Health and Human Services Public Health Service
- College of American Pathologists (CAP)
- The Joint Commission (TJC)

The primary purpose of OSHA standards is to ensure safe and healthful working conditions for every U.S. worker. To ensure that workers have safe and healthful working conditions, the federal government passed the Occupational Safety and Health Act of 1970 and, in 1988, expanded the Hazard Communication Standard to apply to hospital staff. Occupational Safety and Health Act regulations apply to all businesses with one or more employees and are administered by the U.S. Department of Labor through OSHA. The programs deal with many aspects of safety and health protection, including compliance arrangements, inspection procedures, penalties for noncompliance, complaint procedures, duties and responsibilities for administration and operation of the system, and how the standards are set. Responsibility for compliance is placed on the administration of the institution and the employee.

OSHA standards, where appropriate, include provisions for warning labels or other appropriate forms of warning to alert all workers to potential hazards, suitable protective equipment, exposure control procedures, and implementation of training and education programs. In 1991, OSHA mandated that all clinical laboratories must implement a chemical hygiene plan and an exposure control plan. As part of the chemical hygiene plan, a copy of the material safety data sheet (MSDS) must be on file and readily accessible and available to all employees at all times. The MSDS describes hazards, safe handling, storage, and disposal of hazardous chemicals. Information is provided by chemical manufacturers and suppliers about each chemical and accompanies the shipment of each chemical. Each MSDS contains basic information about the specific chemical or product, including its trade name, chemical name and synonyms, chemical family, manufacturer's name and address, emergency telephone number for further information about the chemical, hazardous ingredients, physical data, fire and explosion data, and health hazard and protection information. The MSDS describes the effects of overexposure or exceeding the threshold limit value of allowable exposure for an employee in an 8-hour day. The MSDS also describes protective personal clothing and equipment requirements, first aid practices, spill information, and disposal procedures.

In 2006, the CDC introduced the National Healthcare Safety Network (NHSN). This voluntary system integrates a number of surveillance systems and provides data on devices, patients, and staff. Many hospitals have reorganized the physical layout of handwashing stations (see later, "Handwashing") to prevent the spread of pathogens.

Adherence to general safety practices will reduce the risk of inadvertent contamination with blood or body fluids, as follows:

1. Staff must wear laboratory coats and be additionally protected from contamination by infectious agents.
2. Food and drinks should not be consumed in work areas or stored in the same area as specimens. Containers, refrigerators, or freezers used for specimens should be marked as containing a **biohazard.**
3. Specimens needing centrifugation are capped and placed into a centrifuge with a sealed dome.
4. A gauze square is used when opening rubber-stoppered test tubes to minimize aerosol production (introduction of substances into the air).

5. **Autodilutors** or safety bulbs are used for pipetting. **Pipetting** of any clinical material by mouth is strictly forbidden.

Each laboratory must have an up to date safety manual. This manual should contain a comprehensive listing of approved policies, acceptable practices, and precautions, including Standard Blood and Body Fluid Precautions. Specific standards that conform to current state and federal requirements (e.g., OSHA regulations) must be included in the manual.

PREVENTION OF TRANSMISSION OF INFECTIOUS DISEASES

According to the CDC concept of **Standard Precautions,** all human blood and other body fluids are treated as potentially infectious for human immunodeficiency virus (HIV), hepatitis B virus (HBV), and other blood-borne microorganisms that can cause disease in human beings. Compliance with the OSHA Bloodborne Pathogens Standard and the Occupational Exposure Standard is required to provide a safe work environment. OSHA mandates that the employer do the following:

- Educate and train all health care workers in Standard Precautions and in preventing bloodborne infections.
- Provide proper equipment and supplies (e.g., gloves).
- Monitor compliance with protective **biosafety policies.**

Blood is the most important source of HIV, HBV, and other bloodborne pathogens in the occupational setting. HBV can be present in extraordinarily high concentrations in blood, but HIV is usually found in lower concentrations. HBV may be stable in dried blood and blood products at 25° C for up to 7 days. HIV retains infectivity for more than 3 days in dried specimens at room temperature and for more than 1 week in an aqueous environment at room temperature.

Both HBV and HIV may be transmitted indirectly. Viral transmission can result from contact with inanimate objects, such as work surfaces or equipment contaminated with infected blood or certain body fluids. If the virus is transferred to the skin or mucous membranes by hand contact between a contaminated surface and **nonintact** skin or mucous membranes, it can produce viral exposure.

Medical personnel must remember that HBV and HIV are different diseases caused by unrelated viruses. The most feared hazard of all, the transmission of HIV through occupational exposure, is among the least likely to occur. The modes of transmission for HBV and HIV are similar, but the potential for transmission in the occupational setting is greater for HBV than HIV.

The transmission of hepatitis B can also be fatal and it is more probable than transmission of HIV. The number of cases of acute hepatitis among health care workers because of occupational exposure has sharply declined since hepatitis B vaccine became available in 1982. The likelihood of infection in health care workers after exposure to blood infected with HBV or HIV depends on the following factors:

- Concentration of HBV or HIV; viral concentration is higher for HBV than HIV
- Duration of the contact

- Presence or **skin lesions** or abrasions on the hands or exposed skin of the health care worker
- Immune status of the health care worker for HBV

Both HBV and HIV may be directly transmitted by various portals of entry. In the occupational setting, however, the following situations may lead to infection:

- **Percutaneous (parenteral)** inoculation of blood, plasma, serum, or certain other body fluids from accidental needlesticks
- Contamination of the skin with blood or certain body fluids without overt puncture, caused by scratches, abrasions, burns, weeping, or exudative skin lesions
- Exposure of mucous membranes (oral, nasal, or conjunctival) to blood or certain body fluids, as the direct result of pipetting by mouth, splashes, or spattering
- Centrifuge accidents or the improper removal of rubber stoppers from test tubes, producing droplets. If these aerosol products are infectious and come into direct contact with mucous membranes or nonintact skin, direct transmission of virus can result.

Most exposures do not result in infection. The risk varies not only with the type of exposure but also with the amount of infected blood in the exposure, the length of contact with the infectious material, and the amount of virus in the patient's blood or body fluid or tissue at exposure. Studies have reported that the average risk of HIV transmission is approximately 0.3% after percutaneous exposure to HIV-infected blood and 0.09% after mucous membrane exposure.

SAFE WORK PRACTICES FOR INFECTION CONTROL

The use of CDC Standard Precautions is an approach to infection control that prevents occupational exposures to bloodborne pathogens. It eliminates the need for separate isolation procedures for patients known or suspected to be infectious. The application of Standard Precautions also eliminates the need for warning labels on specimens.

OSHA requires laboratories to have a **personal protective equipment (PPE)** program. The components of this regulation include the following:

- A workplace hazard assessment, with a written hazard certification
- Proper equipment selection
- Employee information and training, with written competency certification
- Regular reassessment of work hazards

Laboratory personnel should not rely solely on PPE to protect themselves against hazards. They should also apply PPE standards when using various forms of safety protection.

A clear policy on institutionally required Standard Precautions is needed. For usual laboratory activities, PPE consists of gloves and a laboratory coat or gown; other equipment such as masks would normally not be needed. Standard Precautions are intended to supplement rather than replace handwashing recommendations for routine infection control. The risk of

nosocomial transmission of HBV, HIV, and other blood-borne pathogens can be minimized if laboratory personnel are aware of and adhere to essential safety guidelines.

PROTECTIVE TECHNIQUES FOR INFECTION CONTROL

Selection and Use of Gloves

Gloves for medical use are sterile surgical or nonsterile examination gloves made of vinyl or latex. There are no reported differences in barrier effectiveness between intact latex and intact vinyl gloves. Tactile differences have been observed between the two types of gloves, with latex gloves providing more tactile sensitivity; however, either type is usually satisfactory for **phlebotomy** and as a protective barrier during technical procedures. Latex-free gloves should be available for personnel with sensitivity to usual glove material. Rubber household gloves may be used for cleaning procedures.

General guidelines related to the selection and general use of gloves include the following:

1. Use sterile gloves for procedures involving contact with normally sterile areas of the body or during procedures in which sterility has been established and must be maintained.
2. Use nonsterile examination gloves for procedures that do not require the use of sterile gloves. Gloves must be worn when receiving phlebotomy training. The National Institute of Occupational Safety and Health mandates the use of gloves for phlebotomy.
3. Gloves should be changed between each patient contact.
4. Wear gloves when processing blood specimens, reagents, or blood products, including reagent red blood cells.
5. Gloves should be changed frequently and immediately if they become visibly contaminated with blood or certain body fluids or if physical damage occurs.
6. Do not wash or disinfect latex or vinyl gloves for reuse. Washing with detergents may cause increased penetration of liquids through undetected holes in the gloves. Rubber gloves may be decontaminated and reused, but disinfectants may cause deterioration. Rubber gloves should be discarded if they have punctures, tears, or evidence of deterioration or if they peel, crack, or become discolored.
7. Using items potentially contaminated with human blood or certain body fluids (e.g., specimen containers, laboratory instruments, countertops)

Care must be taken to avoid indirect contamination of work surfaces or objects in the work area. Gloves should be properly removed (Fig. 6-1) or covered with an uncontaminated glove or paper towel before answering the telephone, handling laboratory equipment, or touching doorknobs.

Facial Barrier Protection and Occlusive Bandages

Facial barrier protection should be used if there is a potential for splashing or spraying of blood or certain body fluids. Masks and facial protection should be worn if mucous membrane contact with blood or body fluids is anticipated. All disruptions of exposed skin, including defects on the arms, face, and neck, should be covered with a water-impermeable **occlusive** bandage.

Laboratory Coats or Gowns as Barrier Protection

A color-coded, two–laboratory coat or equivalent system should be used whenever laboratory personnel are working with potentially infectious specimens. The garment worn in the laboratory must be changed or covered with an uncontaminated coat when leaving the immediate work area. Garments should be changed immediately if grossly contaminated with blood or body fluids to prevent seepage through to street clothes or skin. Contaminated coats or gowns should be placed in an appropriately designated biohazard bag for laundering. Disposable plastic aprons are recommended if blood or certain body fluids may be splashed. Aprons should be discarded into a biohazard container.

The introduction of water-retardant gowns has been the greatest change in many PPE practices.

HANDWASHING

Frequent handwashing is an important safety precaution. It should be performed after contact with patients and laboratory specimens (Box 6-1). Gloves should be used as an adjunct to, not a substitute for, handwashing.

The efficacy of handwashing in reducing the transmission of microbial organisms has been demonstrated. At the very minimum, hands should be washed with soap and water (if visibly soiled) or by hand antisepsis with an alcohol-based handrub (if not visibly soiled) in the following situations:

1. After completing laboratory work and before leaving the laboratory
2. After removing gloves. The Association for Professionals in Infection Control and Epidemiology has reported that extreme variability exists in the quality of gloves, with leakage in 4% to 63% of vinyl gloves and in 3% to 52% of latex gloves.
3. Before eating, drinking, applying makeup, and changing contact lenses, and before and after using the bathroom
4. Before all activities that involve hand contact with mucous membranes or breaks in the skin
5. Immediately after accidental skin contact with blood, body fluids, or tissues
   a. If the contact occurs through breaks in gloves, the gloves should be removed immediately and the hands thoroughly washed.
   b. If accidental contamination occurs to an exposed area of the skin or because of a break in gloves, wash first with a liquid soap, rinse well with water, and then apply a 1:10 dilution of bleach (Table 6-1) or 50% isopropyl or ethyl alcohol. The bleach or alcohol is left on skin for at least 1 minute before final washing with liquid soap and water.

Two important points in the practice of hand hygiene technique follow (see Box 6-1):

When the hand hygiene indication occurs before a contact requiring glove use, perform hand hygiene by rubbing with an alcohol-based handrub or by washing with soap and water.

I. How to don gloves:

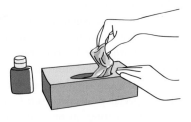

1. Take out a glove from its original box

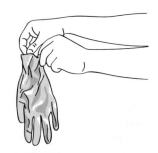

2. Touch only a restricted surface of the glove corresponding to the wrist (at the top edge of the cuff)

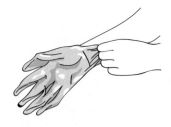

3. Don the first glove

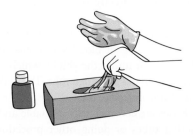

4. Take the second glove with the bare hand and touch only a restricted surface of glove corresponding to the wrist

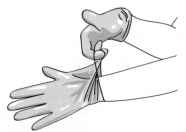

5. To avoid touching the skin of the forearm with the gloved hand, turn the external surface of the glove to be donned on the folded fingers of the gloved hand, thus permitting to glove the second hand

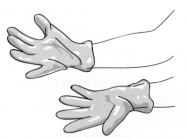

6. Once gloved, hands should not touch anything else that is not defined by indications and conditions for glove use

II. How to remove gloves:

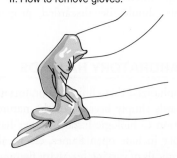

1. Pinch one glove at the wrist level to remove it, without touching the skin of the forearm, and peel away from the hand, thus allowing the glove to turn inside out

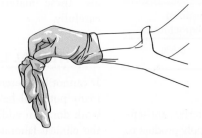

2. Hold the removed glove in the gloved hand and slide the fingers of the ungloved hand inside between the glove and the wrist. Remove the second glove by rolling it down the hand and fold into the first glove

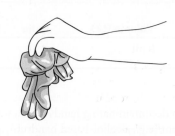

3. Discard the removed gloves

4. Then, perform hand hygiene by rubbing with an alcohol-based handrub or by washing with soap and water.

Figure 6-1   Technique for donning and removing nonsterile examination gloves. *(From World Health Organization: Glove use information leaflet, Geneva, Switzerland, 2009, WHO.)*

| Box 6-1 | Guidelines for Handwashing and Hand Antisepsis in Health Care Settings |

- Wash hands with a nonantimicrobial soap and water or an antimicrobial soap and water when hands are visibly dirty or contaminated with proteinaceous material.
- If hands are not visibly soiled, use an alcohol-based waterless antiseptic agent for routinely decontaminating hands in all other clinical situations.
- Waterless antiseptic agents are highly preferable, but hand antisepsis using an antimicrobial soap may be considered in settings in which time constraints are not an issue and easy access to hand hygiene facilities can be ensured, or in rare cases when a caregiver is intolerant of the waterless antiseptic product used in the institution.
- Decontaminate hands after contact with a patient's intact skin.
- Decontaminate hands after contact with body fluids or excretions, mucous membranes, nonintact skin, or wound dressings, as long as hands are not visibly soiled.
- Decontaminate hands if moving from a contaminated body site to a clean body site during patient care.
- Decontaminate hands after contact with inanimate objects in the immediate vicinity of the patient.
- Decontaminate hands before caring for patients with severe neutropenia or other forms of severe immune suppression.
- Decontaminate hands after removing gloves.

Adapted from Boyce JM, Pittet D; Healthcare Infection Control Practices Advisory Committee; HICPAC/SHEA/APIC/IDSA Hand Hygiene Task Force: Guideline for Hand Hygiene in Health-Care Settings. Recommendations of the Healthcare Infection Control Practices Advisory Committee and the HICPAC/SHEA/APIC/IDSA Hand Hygiene Task Force. Society for Healthcare Epidemiology of America/Association for Professionals in Infection Control/Infectious Diseases Society of America., MMWR Recomm Rep 51(RR-16):1–45, 2002.

Table 6-1	Preparation of Diluted Household Bleach		
Volume Bleach	Volume H$_2$O	Ratio	Sodium Hypochlorite
1 mL	9 mL	1:10	0.5%

- When decontaminating hands with a waterless antiseptic agent (e.g., alcohol-based handrub), apply product to the palm of one hand and rub hands together, covering all surfaces of hands and fingers, until hands are dry. Follow the manufacturer's recommendations on the volume of product to use. If an adequate volume of an alcohol-based handrub is used, it should take 15 to 25 seconds for hands to dry.
- When washing with a nonantimicrobial or antimicrobial soap, wet hands first with warm water, apply 3 to 5 mL of detergent to hands, and rub hands together vigorously for at least 15 seconds, covering all surfaces of the hands and fingers. Rinse hands with warm water and dry thoroughly with a disposable towel. Use the towel to turn off the faucet.

SPECIMEN-PROCESSING PROTECTION

Specimens should be transported to the laboratory in plastic leakproof bags. Protective gloves should always be worn for handling any type of biological specimen.

Substances can become airborne when the stopper (cap) is popped off a blood-collecting container, a serum sample is poured from one tube to another, or a serum tube is centrifuged. When the cap is being removed from a specimen tube or a blood collection tube, the top should be covered with a disposable gauze pad or special protective pad. Gauze pads with an impermeable plastic coating on one side can reduce contamination of gloves. The tube should be held away from the body and the cap gently twisted to remove it. Snapping off the cap or top can cause some of the contents to aerosolize. When not in place on the tube, the cap should still be kept in the gauze and not placed directly on the work surface or countertop.

Specially constructed plastic splash shields are used in many laboratories for the processing of blood specimens. The tube caps are removed behind or under the shield, which acts as a barrier between the worker and specimen tube. This is designed to prevent aerosols from entering the nose, eyes, or mouth. Laboratory safety boxes are commercially available and can be used for unstoppering tubes or doing other procedures that might cause spattering. Splash shields and safety boxes should be periodically decontaminated.

When specimens are being centrifuged, the tube caps should always be kept on the tubes. Centrifuge covers must be used and left on until the centrifuge stops. The centrifuge should be allowed to stop by itself and should not be manually stopped by the worker.

Another step to lessen the hazard from aerosols is to exercise caution in handling pipettes and other equipment used to transfer human specimens, especially pathogenic materials. These materials should be discarded properly and carefully.

ADDITIONAL LABORATORY HAZARDS

It cannot be overemphasized that clinical laboratories present many potential hazards simply because of the nature of the work done. In addition to biologic hazards, other hazards in the clinical laboratory include open flames, electrical equipment, glassware, chemicals of varying reactivity, flammable solvents, and toxic fumes.

In addition to the safety practices common to all laboratory situations, certain procedures are mandatory in a medical laboratory. Proper procedures for the handling and disposal of toxic, radioactive, and potentially carcinogenic materials must be included in the safety manual. Information regarding the hazards of particular substances must be included as a safety practice and to comply with the legal right of workers to know about the hazards associated with these substances. Some chemicals (e.g., benzidine) previously used in the laboratory are now known to be carcinogenic and have been replaced with safer chemicals.

DECONTAMINATION OF WORK SURFACES, EQUIPMENT, AND SPILLS

Sodium hypochlorite solutions are inexpensive and effective broad-spectrum germicidal solutions. Generic sources of sodium hypochlorite include household chlorine bleach. Concentrations of 1:10 to 1:100 free chlorine are effective, depending on the amount of organic material present on the surface to be cleaned and disinfected. Many chlorine bleaches (available at grocery stores) are not registered by the U.S. Environmental Protection Agency (EPA) for use as surface disinfectants and are unacceptable surface disinfectants. The EPA encourages the use of registered products because the agency reviews them for safety and performance when the products are used according to label instructions. When unregistered products are used for surface disinfection, users do so at their own risk. EPA-registered chemical germicides may be more compatible with certain materials that could be corroded by repeated exposure to sodium hypochlorite, especially the 1:10 dilution.

While wearing gloves, all work surfaces should be cleaned and sanitized at the beginning and end of the shift with a 1:10 dilution of household bleach. Instruments such as scissors or centrifuge carriages should be sanitized daily with a diluted solution of bleach. It is equally important to clean and disinfect work areas frequently during the workday and before and after each shift. Studies have demonstrated that HIV is inactivated rapidly after being exposed to common chemical germicides at concentrations much lower than used in practice. Diluted household bleach prepared daily inactivates HBV in 10 minutes and HIV in 2 minutes. Disposable materials contaminated with blood must be placed in containers marked "Biohazard" and properly discarded.

Hepatitis C virus (HCV), HBV, and HIV have never been documented as being transmitted from a housekeeping surface (e.g., countertops). However, an area contaminated by blood or body fluids needs to be treated as potentially hazardous and requires prompt removal and surface disinfection.

Strategies differ for decontaminating spills of blood and other body fluids, based on the setting. The cleanup procedure depends on the porosity of the surface and volume of the spill. The following protocol is recommended for managing spills in a clinical laboratory:

1. Wear gloves and a laboratory coat.
2. Absorb the blood with disposable towels. Bleach solutions are less effective in the presence of high concentrations of protein. Remove as much liquid blood or serum as possible before decontamination.
3. Using a diluted bleach (1:10) solution, clean the spill site of all visible blood.
4. Wipe down the spill site with paper towels soaked with diluted bleach.
5. Place all disposable materials used for decontamination into a biohazard container.

Decontaminate nondisposable equipment by soaking overnight in a dilute (1:10) bleach solution and rinsing with methyl alcohol and water before reuse. Disposable glassware or supplies that have come into contact with blood should be autoclaved or incinerated. Staff should receive training in environmental surface and infection control strategies and procedures as part of an overall infection control and safety program.

DISPOSAL OF INFECTIOUS LABORATORY WASTE

The control of infectious, chemical, and radioactive waste is regulated by a variety of government agencies, including OSHA and the U.S. Food and Drug Administration (FDA). Legislation and regulations that affect laboratories include the Resource Recovery and Conservation Act, the Toxic Substances Control Act, clean air and water laws, right to know laws, and HazCom (chemical hazard communication). Laboratories should implement applicable federal, state, and local laws that pertain to hazardous material and waste management by establishing safety policies. Laboratories with multiple agencies should follow the guidelines of the most stringent agency. Safety policies should be reviewed and signed annually or whenever a change is instituted. Employers are responsible for ensuring that personnel follow the safety policies.

OSHA has defined **infectious waste** as blood and blood products, contaminated **sharps,** pathologic wastes, and microbiological wastes. Infectious waste is packaged for disposal in color-coded containers and labeled as such with the standard symbol for a biohazard (Fig. 6-2).

Infectious waste (e.g., contaminated gauze squares and test tubes) must be discarded into proper biohazard containers with the following features:

1. Conspicuously marked "Biohazard" with the universal biohazard symbol
2. Universal color—orange, orange and black, or red

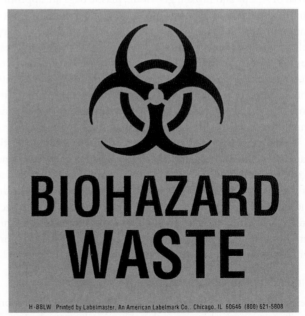

H-BBLW Printed by Labelmaster, An American Labelmark Co., Chicago, IL 60646 (800) 621-5808

Figure 6-2   Biohazard symbol. *(From Rodak BF, Fritsma GA, Keohane EM: Hematology: clinical principles and applications, ed 4, St Louis, 2012, Saunders.)*

3. Rigid, leakproof, and puncture resistant. (Cardboard boxes lined with leakproof plastic bags are available.)
4. Used for blood and other potentially infectious body fluids, as well as disposable materials contaminated with blood or fluid

Containers for Waste

Containers must be easily accessible to personnel needing them and must be located in the laboratory areas in which they are typically used. They should be constructed so that their contents will not spill out if the container is tipped over accidentally.

Biohazard Containers

Body fluid specimens, including blood, must be placed in well-constructed biohazard containers with secure lids to prevent leakage during transport and for future disposal. Contaminated specimens and other materials used in laboratory tests should be decontaminated before reprocessing for disposal or should be placed in special impervious bags for disposal, in accordance with established waste removal policies. If outside contamination of the bag is likely, a second bag should be used.

Hazardous specimens and potentially hazardous substances should be tagged and identified as such. The tag should read "Biohazard," or the biological hazard symbol should be used. All persons working in the laboratory area must be informed about the meaning of these tags and precautions to take for each.

Contaminated equipment must be placed in a designated area for storage, washing, decontamination, or disposal. With the increased use of disposable PPE (e.g., gloves), the volume of waste for disposal will increase.

Biohazard Bags

Although rigid impermeable containers are used for the disposal of sharps and broken glassware, plastic bags are appropriate for the disposal of most infectious waste materials. Plastic bags with the biohazard symbol and lettering prominently visible can be used in secondary metal or plastic containers. These containers can be decontaminated or disposed of regularly, or immediately when visibly contaminated. These biohazard bags should be used for all blood, body fluids, tissues, and other disposable materials contaminated with infectious agents and should be handled with gloves.

If the primary infectious waste containers are red plastic bags, they should be kept in secondary metal or plastic cans. Extreme care should be taken not to contaminate the exterior of these bags. If they do become contaminated on the outside, the entire bag must be placed into another red plastic bag. Secondary plastic or metal cans should be decontaminated regularly, and immediately after any grossly visible contamination, with an agent such as a 1:10 solution of household bleach.

Final Decontamination of Waste Materials

Terminal disposal of infectious waste should be by incineration; an alternate method is terminal sterilization by **autoclaving.** If incineration is not done in the health care facility or by an outside contractor, all contaminated disposables should be autoclaved before leaving the facility for disposal with routine waste. Disposal of medical waste should be done by licensed organizations to ensure that no environmental contamination or aesthetic problem occurs. Congress has passed various acts and regulations regarding the proper handling of medical waste to assist the EPA to carry out this process in the most prudent manner.

DISEASE PREVENTION

Immunization

A well-planned and implemented immunization program is an important component of a health care organization's infection prevention and control program. When planning these programs, valuable resources are available from the Advisory Committee on Immunization Practices (ACIP) and the Hospital Infection Control Practices Advisory Committee (HICPAC). The characteristics of the health care workers employed and the individuals served should be considered, as well as the requirements of regulatory agencies and local, state, and federal regulations.

In their recommendations for the immunization of health care workers, ACIP and HICPAC identify those health care workers whose maintenance of immune status is especially important, which includes laboratory staff. Other individuals are recognized as being at risk for exposure to and possible transmission of diseases that can be prevented by immunizations. The ACIP-HICPAC recommendations are divided into the following three categories:

1. Immunizing agents strongly recommended for health care workers
2. Other immunologic agents that are or may be indicated for health care workers
3. Other vaccine-preventable diseases

All health care organizations should include the strongly recommended immunizations. To determine whether to include other immunologic agents, the incidence of the vaccine-preventable diseases in the community served needs to be reviewed. Also, comparing the demographics of the workforce pool with the disease pattern in the community will determine which of these immunologic agents is (are) indicated for the specific organization's program. Other vaccines may not be routinely administered but may be considered after an injury or exposure incident or for **immunocompromised** or older health care workers.

The ACIP-HICPAC recommendations determine which vaccines to include based on documented nosocomial transmission and significant risk for acquiring or transmitting the following vaccine-preventable diseases:

- Hepatitis B
- Influenza
- Measles
- Mumps
- Rubella
- Varicella

Optional immunizations include hepatitis A, diphtheria, pneumococcal disease, and tetanus. Because health care workers are not at greater risk for acquiring these diseases than the general population, they should seek recommendations for these immunizations from their primary care provider.

Screening Tests

Purified Protein Derivative Tuberculin Skin Test

If recently exposed to an individual with active tuberculosis (TB) infection, a health care worker may not yet have a positive TB skin test reaction. The worker may need a second skin test 10 to 12 weeks after the last exposure to the infected person. It can take several weeks after infection for the immune system to react to this purified protein derivative (PPD, Mantoux) tuberculin skin test. If the reaction to the second test is negative, the worker probably does not have latent TB infection. Strongly positive reactors, with a skin test diameter more than 15 mm and symptoms suggestive of TB, should be evaluated clinically and microbiologically. Two sputum specimens, collected on successive days, should be investigated for TB by microscopy and culture.

QuantiFERON-TB Gold

QuantiFERON-TB Gold (QFT) is a blood test used to detect infection with TB bacteria. The QFT measures the response to TB proteins when they are mixed with a small amount of blood. Currently, few health departments offer the QFT. If your health department does offer the QFT, only one visit is required, at which time your blood is drawn for the test.

Rubella

All phlebotomists and laboratory staff need to demonstrate immunity to rubella. If antibodies are not demonstrable, vaccination is necessary.

Hepatitis B Surface Antigen

All phlebotomists and laboratory staff need to demonstrate immunity to hepatitis B. If a positive test is not demonstrable, vaccination is necessary.

Postexposure Prophylaxis

Although the most important strategy for reducing the risk of occupational HIV transmission is to prevent occupational exposures, plans for postexposure management of health care personnel should be in place. The U.S. Public Health Service has issued guidelines for the management of health care personnel exposure to HIV and recommendations for postexposure prophylaxis (PEP).*

These guidelines outline considerations in determining whether health care personnel should receive PEP and in choosing the type of PEP regimen. For most HIV exposures that warrant PEP, a basic 4-week, two-drug regimen is recommended. For HIV exposures that pose an increased risk of transmission, a three-drug regimen may be recommended.

Special circumstances are also discussed in the guidelines, including delayed exposure report, unknown source person, pregnancy in an exposed woman, resistance of the source virus

to antiviral agents, and toxicity of PEP regimens. Occupational exposures should be considered urgent medical concerns.

Hepatitis B Virus Exposure

After occupational exposure to Hepatitis B virus (HBV), appropriate and timely prophylaxis can prevent HBV infection and subsequent development of chronic infection or liver disease. The mainstay of postexposure prophylaxis (PEP) is Hepatitis B vaccine. In certain circumstances, Hepatitis B immune globulin is recommended in addition to vaccine for added protection.

After skin or mucosal exposure to blood, the ACIP recommends **immunoprophylaxis,** depending on several factors. If an individual has not been vaccinated, hepatitis B immune globulin (HBIG) is usually given for temporary protection, i.e., 3 to 6 months. It should be administered within 24 hours if practical, and concurrently with hepatitis B vaccine postexposure injuries. Recommendations for HBV postexposure management include initiation of the hepatitis B vaccine series to any susceptible, unvaccinated person who sustains an occupational blood or body fluid exposure. Both passive-active PEP with HBIG and hepatitis B vaccination and active PEP with hepatitis B vaccination alone have been demonstrated to be highly effective in preventing transmission after exposure to HBV.

PEP with HBIG and hepatitis B vaccine series should be considered for occupational exposures after evaluation of the hepatitis B surface antigen (HBsAg) status of the source and the vaccination and vaccine-response status of the exposed person. The specific protocol for these measures is determined by the institution's infection control division. Postvaccination testing for the development of antibody to HBsAg (anti-HBsAg) for persons at occupational risk who may have had needlestick exposures necessitating PEP should be done to ensure that the vaccination has been successful.

In cases of non-occupational exposure* to hepatitis B virus (HBV) through a discrete, identifiable exposure to blood or body fluids, the suggested CDC protocol is as follows:

HBsAg-Positive Exposure Source

- Persons who have written documentation of a complete hepatitis B vaccine series and who did not receive postvaccination testing should receive a single vaccine booster dose.
- Persons who are in the process of being vaccinated but who have not completed the vaccine series should receive the appropriate dose of hepatitis B immune globulin (HBIG) and should complete the vaccine series.
- Unvaccinated persons should receive both HBIG and hepatitis B vaccine as soon as possible after exposure (preferably within 24 hours). Hepatitis B vaccine may be administered simultaneously with HBIG in a separate injection site. The hepatitis B vaccine series should be

*U.S. Public Health Service: Updated U.S. Public Health Service guidelines for the management of occupational exposures to HBV, HCV, and HIV and recommendations for postexposure prophylaxis, MMWR Recomm Rep 50(RR-11):1–52, 2001.

*U.S. Department of Health and Human Services, Centers for Disease Control and Prevention (CDC): MMWR Appendix B PostExposure Guidelines, 55(RR16):30-31, 2006.

completed in accordance with the age-appropriate vaccine dose and schedule (see Table 2 and Box 5).*

Exposure Source With Unknown HBsAg Status

- Persons with written documentation of a complete hepatitis B vaccine series require no further treatment.
- Persons who are not fully vaccinated should complete the vaccine series.

Unvaccinated persons should receive the hepatitis B vaccine series with the first dose administered as soon as possible after exposure, preferably within 24 hours. The vaccine series should be completed in accordance with the age-appropriate dose and schedule.

Hepatitis C Virus Exposure

Immune globulin and antiviral agents (e.g., interferon, with or without ribavirin) are not recommended for PEP of hepatitis C. For HCV postexposure management, the HCV status of the source and the exposed person should be determined; for health care personnel exposed to an HCV-positive source, follow-up HCV testing should be performed to determine whether infection develops. After exposure to the blood of a patient infected or suspected of being infected with HCV, immune globulin should be given as soon as possible. No vaccine is currently available.

In addition, special circumstances (see earlier PEP section) should be addressed during consultation with local experts or the National Clinicians' Post-Exposure Prophylaxis Hotline ([PEPline] 1-888-448-4911).

Human Immunodeficiency Virus

Transmission of HIV is believed to result from intimate contact with blood and body fluids from an infected person. Casual contact with infected persons has not been documented as a mode of transmission. If there has been occupational exposure to a potentially HIV-infected specimen or patient, the antibody status of the patient or specimen source should be determined, if it is not already known. If the source is a patient, voluntary consent should be obtained, if possible, for testing for HIV antibodies as soon as possible. High-risk exposure prophylaxis includes the use of a combination of antiretroviral agents to prevent **seroconversion.**

The CDC bases PEP guidelines on the determined risks of transmission, stratified as highest risk, increased risk, and no risk. Highest risk exists when there has been occupational exposure to a large volume of blood (e.g., a deep percutaneous injury or cut with a large-diameter hollow needle previously used in source patient's vein or artery) and to blood containing a high titer of HIV (known as a high viral load), to fluids containing visible blood, or to specific other potentially infectious fluids or tissue, including semen, vaginal secretions, and cerebrospinal, peritoneal, pleural, pericardial, and amniotic fluids.

If a known or suspected parenteral exposure takes place, a technician or technologist may request follow-up monitoring for HBV or HIV antibodies. This monitoring and follow-up

counseling must be provided free of charge. If voluntary informed consent is obtained, the source of the potentially infectious material and the technician or technologist should be tested immediately. The laboratory technologist should also be tested at intervals after exposure. An injury report must be filed after parenteral exposure.

An **enzyme immunoassay (EIA)** screening test is used to detect antibodies to HIV. Before any HIV result is considered positive, the result is confirmed by **Western blot (WB)** analysis. A negative antibody test for HIV does not confirm the absence of virus. There is a **window period** after HIV infection during which detectable antibody is not present. In these patients, detection of antigen is important; a polymerase chain reaction (PCR) assay for HIV DNA can be used for this purpose and a p24 antigen test is used for screening blood donors for HIV antigen.

If the source patient is **seronegative,** the exposed worker should be screened for antibody again at 3 and 6 months. If the source patient is at high risk for HIV infection, more extensive follow-up of both the worker and source patient may be needed.

If the source patient or specimen is HIV-positive (HIV antibodies, WB, HIV antigen, or HIV DNA by PCR), the blood of the exposed worker should be tested for HIV antibodies within 48 hours, if possible. Exposed workers who are initially seronegative for the HIV antibody should be tested again 6 weeks after exposure. If this test is negative, the worker should be tested again at 12 weeks and 6 months after exposure. Most reported seroconversions have occurred between 6 and 12 weeks after exposure. PEP should be started immediately and according to policies set by the institution's infection control program. A policy of "hit hard, hit early" should generally be in place.

During the early follow-up after exposure, especially the first 6 to 12 weeks, the worker should follow the recommendations of the CDC regarding the transmission of acquired immunodeficiency syndrome (AIDS), as follows:

1. Refrain from donating blood or plasma.
2. Inform potential sex partners of the exposure.
3. Avoid pregnancy.
4. Inform health care providers of their potential exposure so they can take necessary precautions.
5. Do not share razors, toothbrushes, or other items that could become contaminated with blood.
6. Clean and disinfect surfaces on which blood or body fluids have spilled.

The exposed worker should be advised of and alerted to the risks of infection and evaluated medically for any history, signs, or symptoms consistent with HIV infection. Serologic testing for HIV antibodies should be made available to all health care workers who are concerned that they may have been infected with HIV.

Occupational exposures should be considered urgent medical concerns to ensure timely postexposure management and administration of HBIG, hepatitis B vaccine, and HIV PEP.

BASIC FIRST AID PROCEDURES

Because there are so many potential hazards in a clinical laboratory, knowledge of basic first aid should be an integral part of any educational program. A key rule in dealing with laboratory emergencies is to keep calm, which may not always be easy but

---

*Table 2 and Box 5 can be found in U.S. Department of Health and Human Services, Centers for Disease Control and Prevention (CDC): MMWR Appendix B PostExposure Guidelines, 55(RR16):30-31, 2006.

is important to the victim's well-being. Keep crowds of people away, and give the victim plenty of fresh air. Because injuries can be extreme and immediate care is critical, application of the proper first aid procedures must be thoroughly understood by every person in the medical laboratory.

In serious laboratory accidents, medical assistance should be summoned while first aid is being administered. For general accidents, competent medical help should be sought as soon as possible after the first aid treatment has been completed. In cases of chemical burns, especially involving the eyes, rapid treatment is essential.

Remember that first aid is useful not only in your working environment, but also at home and in your community. It deserves your earnest attention and study.

CASE STUDY IN SAFETY

Ms. MM was a new employee in a rural laboratory. When she started to work, she wiped down the work bench with 5% bleach and donned latex gloves that she had rinsed off the night before. When she opened up a specimen (a red top tube), a small amount of serum spilled out of the tube. She promptly wiped it up with a sterile paper towel and discarded the paper towel into a cardboard box marked "Biohazard." When it was lunchtime, she removed her gloves, discarded them in the biohazard container and left the laboratory to go to the cafeteria. Her lab coat was clean, so she did not remove it to go to lunch. On returning from lunch, MM put on clean gloves and worked until the end of the shift. She discarded her gloves into the biosafety box and hung her lab coat on a hook in the laboratory.

Questions
1. A safety violation in the case study is:
   a. Use of freshly prepared 10% bleach on the countertops
   b. Use of new latex-free gloves
   c. Washing hands before applying gloves
   d. Not washing hands after removing gloves
2. Wearing a laboratory coat to do testing and then back home to wash it is:
   a. Acceptable if coat is washed when stained
   b. Always acceptable
   c. Never acceptable
   d. OK, if only done once in awhile

See Appendix A for the answers to these questions.

Critical Thinking Group Discussion Questions
1. Name all the safety violations that occurred in this case study.
2. State the corrective action for each of the violations.
3. How can these violations be avoided?

See instructor's site on ⊖volve for discussion of answers to these questions.

Test Your Safety Knowledge

Using the clues provided, fill in the puzzle for objects found in a laboratory.
ACROSS
1. Used to handle concentrated acids
3. Used to clean the surface of a laboratory bench
4. Used for chemical or heat burns on the skin
5. Indicates flammability and is red in color
6. Used to discard sharp objects, such as used needles
8. Can have a rating of a, b, c, or a combination rating
9. Used for emergencies, such as lab coat catching on fire
10. Used for handling specimens that generate infectious aerosols
DOWN
2. Alcohol-based; used to reduce transmission of microbial organisms
7. Used for alkali or acid burns in the eye

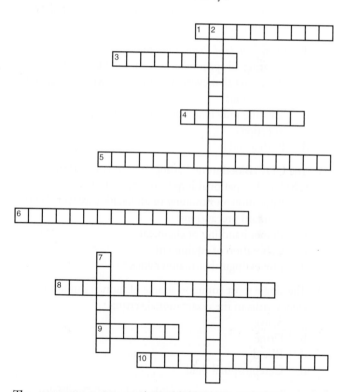

The answers are given in Appendix B.

CHAPTER HIGHLIGHTS

- Clinical laboratories have instituted Standard Blood and Body Fluid Precautions, or Standard Precautions, to prevent parenteral, mucous membrane, and nonintact skin exposures of health care workers to bloodborne pathogens such as HIV and HBV.
- Although HIV has been isolated from blood, semen, vaginal secretions, saliva, tears, breast milk, cerebrospinal fluid, amniotic fluid, and urine, only blood, semen, vaginal secretions, and possibly breast milk have been implicated in the transmission of HIV to date.

- Medical personnel should be aware that HBV and HIV are different diseases caused by unrelated viruses. The most feared hazard of all, the transmission of HIV through occupational exposure, is among the least likely to occur if proper safety practices are followed.
- The control of infectious, chemical, and radioactive waste is regulated by various governmental agencies (e.g., OSHA, FDA).

REVIEW QUESTIONS

1. Which of the following is the government agency primarily responsible for safeguards and regulations to ensure a safe and healthful workplace throughout the United States?
   a. Occupational Safety and Health Administration (OSHA)
   b. Clinical Laboratory Improvement Amendments of 1988 (CLIA '88)
   c. Centers for Disease Control and Prevention (CDC)
   d. City ordinances

2. The term *Standard Precautions* refers to:
   a. Treating all specimens as if they are infectious
   b. Assuming that every direct contact with a body fluid is infectious
   c. Treating only blood or blood-tinged specimens as infectious
   d. Both a and b

3. The CDC Bloodborne Pathogen Standard and the OSHA Occupational Exposure Standard mandate:
   a. Education and training of all health care workers in standard precautions
   b. Proper handling of chemicals
   c. Calibration of equipment
   d. Fire extinguisher maintenance

4. The single most common source of human immunodeficiency virus in the occupational setting is:
   a. Saliva
   b. Urine
   c. Blood
   d. Cerebrospinal fluid

5-8. Indicate true statements with the letter "a" and false statements with the letter "b."

5. _____ Sterile gloves need to be worn for all laboratory procedures.

6. _____ Hands should be washed after removing gloves.

7. _____ Hands should be washed before leaving the laboratory.

8. _____ Hands should be washed before and after using the bathroom.

9. Gloves for medical use may be:
   a. Sterile or nonsterile
   b. Latex or vinyl
   c. Used only once
   d. All of the above

10. and 11. Diluted bleach for disinfecting work surfaces, equipment, and spills should be prepared daily by preparing a (10) _____ dilution of household bleach. This dilution requires (11) _____ mL of bleach diluted to 100 mL with H_2O.

10. a. 1:5
    b. 1:10
    c. 1:20
    d. 1:100

11. a. 1
    b. 10
    c. 25
    d. 50

12. Infectious waste must be discarded into containers with all the following features except:
    a. Marked "Biohazard"
    b. Has standard biohazard symbol
    c. Orange, orange and black, or red
    d. Made of sturdy cardboard for landfill disposal

13. Clinical laboratory personnel need to have demonstrable immunity to:
    a. Rubella
    b. Polio
    c. Hepatitis B
    d. Both a and c

BIBLIOGRAPHY

Centers for Disease Control and Prevention (CDC): Hospital Infection Control Practices Advisory Committee (HICPAC): guidelines for isolation precautions in hospitals, Atlanta, 1996, CDC.

Centers for Disease Control and Prevention (CDC): Update: provisional public health service recommendations for chemoprophylaxis after occupational exposure to HIV, MMWR Morb Mortal Wkly Rep 45:468–472, 1996.

Centers for Disease Control and Prevention (CDC): Surveillance of healthcare personnel with HIV/AIDS, as of December 2002, http://www.thebody.com/content/art17253.html.

Centers for Disease Control and Prevention (CDC): Guidelines for environmental infection control in health-care facilities, Atlanta, 2003, CDC.

Centers for Disease Control and Prevention (CDC): Hand hygiene in healthcare settings: training, 2011, http://www.cdc.gov/handhygiene/training.html.

Miller LE: Recommended concentrations of bleach, Lab Med 21:116, 1990.

National Committee for Clinical Laboratory Standards: Clinical laboratory waste management: approved guideline, Villanova, Pa, 1993, NCCLS Document GP5-A.

Occupational Safety and Health Administration (OSHA): Occupational exposure to hazardous chemicals in laboratories: final rule, Fed Regist 55:3327–3335, 1990.

Occupational Safety and Health Administration (OSHA): Occupational exposure to bloodborne pathogens: final rule, Fed Regist 56:64004–64182, 1991.

Protection against viral hepatitis: Recommendations of the Immunization Practices Advisory Committee (ACIP), MMWR Morb Mortal Wkly Rep 39:1–23, 1990.

Sebazcp S: Considerations for immunization programs, 2005, http://www.infectioncontrol today.com/articles/0a1feat4.html.

Turgeon ML: Linné & Ringsrud's clinical laboratory science, ed 6, St Louis, 2012, Mosby.

CHAPTER 7

Quality Assurance and Quality Control

Learning Objectives

At the conclusion of this chapter, the reader should be able to:

- Identify the regulatory and accrediting organizations that influence quality assessment in clinical laboratories.
- Describe the eight nonanalytical factors related to testing accuracy.
- Identify and give examples of the three categories of errors related to the phase of testing.
- Define the terms *accuracy, precision, reproducibility,* and *reliability.*
- Describe the use of the coefficient of variation and give the formula.
- Define true positive, true negative, false positive, and false negative.
- Provide the equations for calculating percentage sensitivity and percentage specificity.
- Define positive predictive value and negative predictive value.

- Describe the process of proficiency testing.
- Explain the use of control specimens.
- Cite seven causes for a control value being out of the acceptable range or out of control.
- Define the terms *mean, median, mode, standard deviation,* and *reference range.*
- Discuss issues related to testing outcomes.
- Describe parallel testing of test kits.
- Describe how a new procedure is validated.
- Write and evaluate a procedural write-up using CLSI requirements.
- Correctly answer case study–related multiple choice questions.
- Be prepared to participate in a discussion of critical thinking questions.
- Correctly answer end of chapter review questions.

Key Terms

accuracy
aliquots
biometrics
coefficient of variation (CV)
confidence limits
control specimen
Gaussian curve
hemolyzed specimens
mean

median
mode
nonwaived assays
normal values
precision
predictive value (PV)
proficiency testing (PT)
quality assurance (QA)
quality control (QC)

reference range
reliability
reproducibility
sensitivity
specificity
standard deviation (SD)
systematic

The introduction of routine **quality assurance (QA)** programs and **quality control (QC)** in the clinical laboratory was a major advance in improving the accuracy and reliability of testing. This process ensures the clinician ordering the test that the testing method has been done in the best possible way to provide the most useful information in diagnosing or managing a patient. QA indicators and QC are tools to ensure that reported laboratory results are of the highest quality.

CLINICAL LABORATORY REGULATORY AND ACCREDITING ORGANIZATIONS

The U.S. Congress enacted the Clinical Laboratory Improvement Amendments of 1988 (CLIA '88) in response to the concerns about laboratory testing errors. The final CLIA rule, Laboratory Requirements Relating to Quality Systems and Certain Personnel Qualification, was published in the *Federal Register* in January 2003. Enactment of the CLIA established a minimum threshold for all aspects of clinical laboratory testing.

Voluntary standards have been set by The Joint Commission (TJC), the Commission on Office Laboratory Accreditation (COLA), and the College of American Pathologists (CAP).

A more recent development in voluntary accreditation aimed at improving quality was the introduction of ISO 15189. The International Organization for Standardization (ISO) is the world's largest nongovernmental developer and publisher of international standards. ISO standards and certification are widely used by industry, but ISO 15189 has now been formulated for clinical laboratories. ISO 15189 has gained some standing abroad as a mandatory accreditation, such as in Australia, Ontario, and many European countries. In the United States, ISO 15189 accreditation remains optional. Requirements for quality and competence in ISO 15189 are unique because it takes into consideration the specific requirements of the medical environment and the importance of the medical laboratory to patient care. CAP 15189 is a voluntary nonregulated accreditation to the ISO 15189:2007 standard as published by ISO. CAP 15189 does not replace CAP's CLIA-based Laboratory Accreditation Program, but complements CAP accreditation and other quality systems by optimizing processes to improve patient care, strengthen the deployment of quality standard, reduce errors and risk, and control costs.

NONANALYTICAL FACTORS RELATED TO TESTING ACCURACY

Qualified Personnel

The competence of personnel is an important determinant of the quality of the laboratory result. Only properly certified personnel can perform **nonwaived assays** (see Chapter 9 for levels of laboratory testing).

Established Laboratory Policies

Laboratory policies should be included in a laboratory reference manual that is available to all hospital personnel. Each laboratory must have an up-to-date safety manual. This manual contains a comprehensive listing of approved policies, acceptable practices, and precautions, including Standard Blood and Body Fluid Precautions. Specific regulations that conform to current state and general requirement, such as Occupational Safety and Health Administration (OSHA) regulations, must be included in the manual.

Laboratory Procedure Manual

A complete laboratory procedure manual for all analytical procedures performed in the laboratory must be provided. The manual must be reviewed regularly, in some cases annually, by the supervisory staff and updated as needed.

A complete laboratory procedure manual for all procedures performed in the laboratory must be provided. The Clinical and Laboratory Standards Institute (CLSI) recommends that these manuals follow a specific pattern for how procedures are organized (Box 7-1).

Test Requisitioning

A laboratory test request must include the following: (1) patient identification data; (2) time and date of specimen collection; (3) source of the specimen; and (4) analyses to be performed. The information on the accompanying specimen container must exactly match the patient identification on the test request.

Patient Identification, Specimen Procurement, and Labeling

Patients must be carefully identified. For outpatients, identification may be validated with two forms of identification. Using established specimen-processing information, the clinical specimens must be properly labeled or identified once obtained from the patient. An important rule is that the analytical result can only be as good as the specimen. Specimens must be efficiently transported to the laboratory.

For elimination of the most frequent source of pretesting error, a patient must be positively identified when a blood specimen is obtained. This specimen must be properly collected and labeled. In general, **hemolyzed specimens** should not be used for serologic testing.

Box 7-1	Written Procedural Protocol

- Procedure name
- Name of the test method
- Principle and purpose of the test
- Specimen collection and storage
- Quality control
- Reagents, supplies, and equipment
- Procedural protocol
- Expected or normal (reference) values
- Procedural notes:
  Sources of error
  Limitations
  Clinical applications

Adapted from Clinical and Laboratory Standards Institute: Clinical laboratory technical procedure manual: approved guideline, ed 4, Wayne, Pa, 2002, CLSI Document GP2-A4.

Preventive Maintenance of Equipment

Microscopes, centrifuges, and other pieces of equipment need to be cleaned and checked for accuracy. A preventive maintenance schedule should be followed for all automated equipment. Failure to monitor equipment regularly can produce inaccurate test results and lead to expensive repairs.

Appropriate Testing Methods

Each laboratory must have an assessment routine for all procedures, performed on a daily, weekly, or monthly basis, to detect problems. When such problems are indicated, they must be corrected as soon as possible.

Another part of a quality control program concerns the way new procedures are validated before they are included in the methods routinely used by the laboratory. Each laboratory must determine the reproducibility (or **confidence limits**) for each procedure used and establish acceptable limits of variation for control specimens.

Inaccurate Results

Inaccuracies in testing can be systematic or sporadic. **Systematic** errors can be eliminated by a program that monitors equipment, reagents, and other supplies. Sporadic or isolated errors in technique can produce false-positive and false-negative results, depending on the technique used for testing (Box 7-2).

An important aspect of quality is documentation of results. CLIA regulations mandate that any problem or situation that might affect the outcome of a test result be recorded and reported. These incidents can involve specimens that are improperly collected, labeled, or transported to the laboratory or problems concerning prolonged turnaround times for test results. There must be a reasonable attempt to correct the problems or situation and all steps in this process must be documented.

ERRORS RELATED TO PHASE OF TESTING

The Institute for Quality Laboratory Medicine has developed measures to evaluate quality in the laboratory based on the preanalytical, analytical, and postanalytical phases of testing.

Errors occurring during the analytical phase of testing in clinical laboratories are now relatively rare. Currently, most laboratory errors are related to the preanalytical and postanalytical phases of testing. To guarantee the highest quality laboratory results and to comply with CLIA regulations, various preanalytical factors need to be considered (Boxes 7-3 and 7-4).

QUALITY DESCRIPTORS

Quality control activities include monitoring the performance of laboratory instruments, reagents, other testing products, and equipment. A written record of QC activities for each procedure or function should include details of deviation from the usual results, problems, or failures in functioning or in the analytical procedure and any corrective action taken in response to these problems. All solutions and kits used in testing must be carefully checked before actually being used for testing patient samples.

Definitions

Quality control consists of procedures used to detect errors that result from test system failure, adverse environmental conditions, and differences between technologists, as well as the monitoring of the accuracy and precision of test performance over time. Accrediting agencies require monitoring and documentation of quality assessment records. Documentation of QC includes preventive maintenance records, temperature charts, and QC charts for specific assays.

Quality control monitors the accuracy and reproducibility of results through the use of control specimens. The diagnostic usefulness of a test and its procedure is assessed by using statistical evaluations, such as descriptions of the accuracy and **reliability** of the test and its methodology.

The terms *accuracy* and *precision* are often used to describe quality. **Accuracy** describes how close a test result is to the true value. **Precision** describes how close the test results are to one another when repeated analyses of the same specimen are performed. It is possible to achieve great precision, with all laboratory personnel who perform the same procedure arriving at the

Box 7-2	Possible Causes of Technical Errors

False-Positive Errors
Overcentrifugation of serum cell mixture
Dirty glassware
Hemolyzed patient serum
Inadequate dispersal of centrifuged serum cell mixture
Extended incubation

False-Negative Errors
Omitting patient serum from test mixture
Omitting reagent from test mixture
Undercentrifugation of serum cell mixture
Vigorous shaking of centrifuged serum cell mixture

False-Positive or False-Negative Errors
Incorrect labeling of test tubes
Addition of wrong reagent to test tube
Erroneously reading or interpreting results
Inaccurately recording results
Expired or improperly stored reagents

Box 7-3	Preanalytical Errors

Incorrect test request
Specimen obtained from wrong patient
Specimen procured at wrong time
Specimen collected in wrong tube or container
Blood specimens collected in wrong order
Incorrect labeling of specimen
Improper processing of specimen

Box 7-4	Postanalytical Errors

Recording results inaccurately
Verbally reporting results for wrong patient

same answer, but without accuracy if the answer does not represent the actual value being tested. Accuracy can be improved by the following:

- Use of properly standardized procedures
- Statistically valid comparisons of new methods with established reference methods
- Use of samples of known values (controls)
- Participation in proficiency testing programs

The precision of a test, its **reproducibility,** may be expressed as the **standard deviation (SD)** or derived **coefficient of variation (CV).** A procedure may be extremely accurate, yet so difficult to perform that individual laboratory personnel are unable to arrive at values that are close enough to be clinically meaningful.

Precision can be ensured by the proper inclusion of standards, reference samples, and/or control solutions, statistically valid, replicate determinations of a single sample, or duplicate determinations of sufficient numbers of unknown samples. Day-to-day and between-run precision are measured by the inclusion of blind samples and control specimens.

Coefficient of Variation

The CV can be used to compare the standard deviations of two samples. Standard deviations cannot be compared directly without considering the mean. The CV can be used to compare a day's work with that of a similar day or to compare test results from one laboratory with the same type of test results from another laboratory. The coefficient of variation (%) is equal to the standard deviation divided by the mean, as follows:

$$CV(\%) = \frac{SD}{Mean} \times 100$$

Sensitivity and Specificity

Laboratory results should provide medically useful information, including the specificity and sensitivity of the tests being ordered and reported. Both specificity and sensitivity are desirable characteristics for a test, but in different clinical situations, one is generally preferred over the other.

Assessing the sensitivity and specificity of a test requires four factors: tests positive, tests negative, disease present (positive), and disease absent (negative). True positives are subjects who have a positive test result and who also have the disease in question. True negatives represent those who have a negative test result but do not have the disease. False positives are those who have a positive test result but do not have the disease. False negatives are those who have a negative test result but do have the disease.

Sensitivity

The **sensitivity** of a test is defined as the proportion of subjects with the specific disease or condition who have a positive test result (i.e., assay correctly predicts with a positive result):

$$\text{Sensitivity (\%)} = \frac{\text{True positives}}{\text{True positives} + \text{False negatives}} \times 100$$

Practically, sensitivity represents how much of a given substance is measured; the more sensitive the test, the smaller the amount of assayed substance that is measured.

Specificity

The **specificity** of a test is defined as the proportion of subjects without the specific disease or condition who have a negative test result (i.e., assay correctly excludes with a negative result):

$$\text{Sensitivity (\%)} = \frac{\text{True negatives}}{\text{False positives} + \text{True negatives}} \times 100$$

Practically, specificity represents what is being measured. A highly specific test measures only the assay substance in question; it does not measure interfering or similar substances.

Predictive Values

To assess the **predictive value (PV)** for a test, the sensitivity, specificity, and prevalence of the disease in the population being studied must be known. The prevalence of a disease is the proportion of a population who have the disease. The incidence is the number of subjects found to have the disease within a defined period, such as 1 year, in a population of 100,000.

A positive predictive value for a test indicates the number of patients with an abnormal test result who have the disease compared with all patients with an abnormal result:

$$\text{Positive PV} = \frac{\text{Number of patients with disease and with abnormal test results}}{\text{Total number of patients with abnormal test results}}$$

$$\text{Positive PV} = \frac{\text{True positives}}{\text{True positives} + \text{False positives}}$$

A negative predictive value for a test indicates the number of patients with a normal test result who do not have the disease compared with all patients with a normal (negative) result:

$$\text{Negative PV} = \frac{\text{True negatives}}{\text{True negatives} + \text{False negatives}}$$

MONITORING QUALITY

Proficiency Testing

Proficiency testing (PT) is incorporated into the CLIA requirements. In addition to the use of internal QC programs, each laboratory should participate in an external PT program as a means of verification of laboratory accuracy. Periodically, a laboratory tests a specimen that has been provided by a government agency, professional society, or commercial company. Identical samples are sent to a group of laboratories participating in the PT program. Each laboratory analyzes the specimen, reports the results to the agency, and is evaluated and graded on those results compared with results from other laboratories. In this way, quality control between laboratories is monitored.

Control Specimens

A QC program for the laboratory uses a **control specimen,** a specimen with a known value that is similar in composition to the patient's blood. A control specimen must be carried through the entire test procedure and treated in exactly the same way as any unknown specimen; it must be affected by all the variables that affect the unknown specimen. Control specimens are used because repeated determinations on the same or different portions (or **aliquots**) of the same sample will not give identical values. Many factors can produce variations in laboratory analyses. With a properly designed control system, it is possible to monitor testing variables.

If the control value in a determination is out of the acceptable range (out of control), one or more of the following factors may be responsible:
1. Deterioration of reagents or standards
2. Faulty instrument or equipment
3. Dirty glassware
4. Lack of attention to timing or incubation temperature
5. Use of a method not suited to the needs and facilities of the laboratory
6. Use of poor technique by the technologist doing the test
7. Statistics: a certain percentage of all determinations will be statistically out of control.

REFERENCE RANGE STATISTICS

In analytical immunology and serology testing using methods such as enzyme immunoassay, quantitative reference range statistics can be used. Statistically, the **reference range** for a particular measurement is usually related to a normal, bell-shaped curve (Fig. 7-1). This **Gaussian curve** has been shown to be correct for almost all types of biological, chemical, and physical measurements. A statistically valid series of individuals who are thought to represent a normal healthy group are measured and the average value is calculated. This mathematical average is defined as the mean ($\overline{X}$, called the X-bar). The distribution of all values around the average for the particular group measured is described statistically by SD.

Mean Mathematical average calculated by dividing the sum of all individual values by the number of values

Median Middle value in a body of data; if all the variables are arranged in order of increasing magnitude, the median is the variable that falls halfway between the highest and lowest variables.

Mode Value that occurs most frequently in a mass of data

Use of the mean, median, and mode is explained in the following example:

A series of results reported for a laboratory test on seven different specimens = 7, 2, 3, 6, 5, 4, and 2

The mean is the mathematical average and is calculated by taking the sum of the values (29) and dividing by the number of values (7) in the list. The mean is 4.1 (rounded off to 4).

The median equals the middle value. To find the median, the list of numbers must first be ranked according to magnitude: 2, 2, 3, 4, 5, 6, 7. There are seven values in the list, and the median is the middle value, 4.

The mode is the value most frequently occurring value, or 2 in this example.

The standard deviation is the square root of the variance of the values in any one observation or in a series of test results. In a normal population, 68% of the values will be clustered above and below the average and defined statistically as falling within the first standard deviation (±1 SD; see Fig. 8-1). The second standard deviation (±2 SD) represents 95% of the values falling equally above and below the average, and 99.7% is included within the third standard deviation (±3 SD). (Again, variations occur equally above and below the average value [or mean] for any measurement.) Thus, in determining reference values for a particular measurement, a statistically valid series of people are chosen and assumed to represent a healthy population. These people are then tested and the results are averaged.

The reference range is the range of values that includes 95% of the test results for a healthy reference population. The term replaces **normal values,** or normal range. The limits (or range) of normal are defined in terms of the standard deviation from the average value. Thus, normal or reference values are stated as a range of values in terms of SD units.

TESTING OUTCOMES

Before physicians can determine whether a patient has a disease, they must know what is acceptable for a representative population of similar patients (e.g., same age, same gender, same ethnicity), as well as the analytical method used for an assay. Furthermore, an individual may show daily, circadian, and physiologic variations.

Biometrics, the science of statistics applied to biologic observations, has been a rapidly expanding field that attempts to describe these variations. The selection of a group on whom to base reference groups is another problem confronting the individual laboratory. To develop reference values (normal values), the proper statistical tools of sampling, selection of the comparison group, and analysis of data must be used by the manufacturer of testing kits or individual laboratories.

Although generally accepted values are published, reference values will vary, especially between laboratories and between

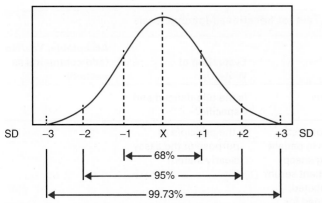

Figure 7-1   Normal, bell-shaped Gaussian curve. *SD,* Standard deviation. *(From Turgeon ML: Linné and Ringsrud's clinical laboratory science: the basics and routine techniques, ed 6, St Louis, 2012, Mosby.)*

geographic locations. Each laboratory must give the physician information concerning the range of reference values for that particular laboratory.

VALIDATING NEW PROCEDURES

The QC program also determines how new procedures are validated before being included as one of the methods routinely used by the laboratory. Each laboratory must determine the reproducibility (or confidence limits) for each procedure used and establish acceptable limits of variation for control specimens. The QC program includes calculation of the mean (or average value) and standard deviation and the preparation of control charts for each procedure.

Parallel Testing of Test Kits

The requirements for the parallel testing of test kits differ depending on your accreditation agency. For example, the CAP and Clinical Laboratory Improvement Acts (CLIAs) have slightly different requirements. There is also a difference in the requirements, depending on the circumstances. Are you changing manufacturers and tests kits, or are you only changing lot numbers for the same kit?

The CAP asserts that CLIA-waived assays are not recognized and the laboratory must treat all tests the same way. It is best to check the immunology checklist at www.cap.org for the latest revisions to questions related to kits. Currently, CAP checklist question IMM.33150 (phase II) is "Are new reagent lots checked against old reagent lots, or with suitable reference material before, or concurrently with, being placed in service?"

A CLIA inspection focuses on the following:

- If the test is moderate or of high complexity and the change is to a new kit manufacturer, the new test kit must be validated for accuracy and precision. This can be done with controls, other known samples, or comparison with an old kit. If the laboratory is receiving a new lot shipment of the same test kit, only controls need to be done, or whatever the manufacturer requires.
- If the test is a waived test, a laboratory only needs to follow the manufacturer's directions if a new test is put into use or if there is a lot change of a current test. This

rule is also applicable if the waived test is being performed in a moderate- or high-complexity laboratory. If an assay is waived anywhere, it is performed under CLIA requirements.

CASE STUDY

A new employee was asked to exam a CLSI procedural protocol worksheet and rate the write up. She noted the following entries:

Title	Entry
Title	Test for Staphylococcus
Quality Control	No positive or negative controls available

Questions

1. Is the title acceptable as written?
   a. Yes
   b. No
2. Is the quality control requirement acceptable?
   a. Yes
   b. No

See Appendix A for the answers to these questions.

Critical Thinking Group Discussion Question

1. Why are positive and negative control essential to the accuracy of a test result?

See ⊖volve instructor site for the discussion of these questions.

Validation of a New Procedure Write-Up

Each student should develop a procedure checklist following the CLSI procedural format. A manufacturer's package insert or book should be used as a source of information. After completing the CLSI procedural protocol, a fellow student should rate the write-up.

Procedure Validation Checklist Example: Traditional Screening Test for Infectious Mononucleosis

Format	Procedure Details	Evaluation of Write-Up	Acceptable: Yes/No (add comments as needed)
Title	Paul-Bunnell Screening Test for Infectious Mononucleosis	Is the title defined and specific?	
Purpose or principle of assay	The Paul-Bunnell test is a hemagglutination test designed to detect heterophil antibodies in patient serum when mixed with antigen-bearing sheep erythrocytes. Dilutions of inactivated patient serum are mixed with sheep erythrocytes, incubated, centrifuged, and macroscopically examined for agglutination. Positive reactions are preliminarily associated with the manifestation of infectious mononucleosis.	Is the principle or purpose of the assay clearly stated?	

Format	Procedure Details	Evaluation of Write-Up	Acceptable: Yes/No (add comments as needed)
Specimen Collection and Preparation			
Preliminary specimen preparation	No special preparation of the patient is required before specimen collection. The patient must be positively identified when the specimen is collected. The specimen should be labeled at the bedside and include the patient's full name, date the specimen is collected, patient's hospital identification number, and phlebotomist's initials. Blood should be drawn by aseptic technique. The required specimen is a minimum of 2 mL of clotted blood (red-topped evacuated tube). Centrifuge the tube of blood and remove an aliquot of clear serum. The presence of hemolysis makes the specimen unsuitable for testing. Inactivate the serum at 56° C for 30 min before testing.	Are the specimen collection requirements clearly stated? Are there any special specimen processing requirements stated?	
Reagents, supplies, and equipment	2% suspension of washed sheep cells in normal saline (prepared by pipetting 0.2 mL of packed erythrocytes into 9.8 mL of saline) 0.9% sodium chloride (normal physiologic saline) 12- × 75-mm test tubes Note: The cell should be no more than 1 wk old. Graduated serologic pipettes Centrifuge 37° C incubator (optional)	Are all of the necessary reagents, supplies, and equipment listed?	
Quality Control			
Positive control serum; negative control serum	A known positive control should be run concurrently.	Are the QC requirements stated?	
Procedural steps	1. Label two sets of test tubes. Each set should consist of 10 tubes. 2. Pipette 0.5 mL of saline into tube 1 and 0.25 mL of saline into each of the remaining nine tubes. 3. To the first set of tubes, add 0.1 mL of patient's inactivated serum to the first tube; mix and transfer 0.25 mL of the dilution to the second tube; mix and transfer 0.25 mL of the dilution to the third tube. Repeat this process to tube 10. Discard 0.25 mL from the final tube, tube 10. 4. To the second set of tubes, add 0.1 mL of the control serum and proceed to dilute it as in step 3. 5. Add 0.1 mL of 2% sheep cells to each tube. 6. Gently shake the tubes until mixed. 7. Incubate the tubes at 37° C for 1 hr or overnight at room temperature. 8. Centrifuge the tubes for 1 min at 1500 rpm. 9. Gently shake each tube and examine macroscopically for agglutination. 10. Record the results.	Are the steps in the procedure understandable? Can the procedure be performed as described?	
Reporting Results			
Positive reaction	A titer >1:56 is considered to be a positive presumptive test.		
Negative reaction	The antigens on sheep erythrocytes are associated with infectious mononucleosis, serum sickness, and the Forssman antigen.		

Continued

Procedure Validation Checklist Example: Traditional Screening Test for Infectious Mononucleosis—cont'd

Format	Procedure Details	Evaluation of Write-Up	Acceptable: Yes/No (add comments as needed)
Reporting Results—cont'd			
Procedural notes		Are the criteria for acceptable results clearly defined?	
Sources of error	False-positive reactions have been observed in conditions such as hepatitis infection and Hodgkin's disease. An improperly inactivated serum will produce hemolysis.		
Limitations	The test is only indicative of the presence or absence of heterophil antibodies. Demonstrating agglutination by using sheep erythrocytes does not make a distinction between antibodies associated with infectious mononucleosis, serum sickness, or the Forssman antigen. Heterophil antibody assay lacks sensitivity as a diagnostic criterion for infectious mononucleosis. Sheep erythrocytes are less sensitive than erythrocytes from other species such as the horse. A patient may take as long as 3 mo to develop a detectable heterophil titer.		
Clinical applications	The Paul-Bunnell test is a useful screening test for the presence of heterophil antibodies because it is simple and inexpensive. Although the specificity of the heterophil assay is rated as good, negative results are demonstrated in individuals who do not produce infectious mononucleosis heterophil antibody. If negative results are displayed, however, Epstein-Barr virus (EBV) serology may be indicated.		

General question: Are all necessary fields of the CLSI format addressed?

Additional general comments:

Evaluation of write-up validation by: _____ Date _____

Supervisory reviewer: _____ Date _____

Adapted from Paul JR, Bunnell WW: The presence of heterophil antibodies in infectious mononucleosis, Am J Med Sci 183:90–104, 1932; and Sumaya CV: Infectious mononucleosis and other EBV infections: diagnostic factors, Lab Manage 24:37–45, 1986.

CHAPTER HIGHLIGHTS

- Quality assurance indicators and quality control (QC) are tools to ensure that reported laboratory results are of the highest quality.
- The Clinical Laboratory Improvement Amendments of 1988 (CLIA '88) established a minimum threshold for all aspects of clinical laboratory testing.
- Voluntary QC standards have been set by TJC, COLA, and CAP.
- Nonanalytical factors related to testing accuracy include the following: qualified personnel; established policies; procedure manual; test requisitioning; patient identification, specimen procurement, and labeling; preventive maintenance of equipment; appropriate testing methods; and inaccurate results.
- The Institute for Quality Laboratory Medicine has developed measures to evaluate quality in the laboratory based on the phase of testing: preanalytical, analytical, and postanalytical.

- Quality control monitors the accuracy and reproducibility of results through control specimens. Accuracy describes how close a test result is to the true value. Precision describes how close the test results are to one another when repeated analyses of the same specimen are performed. It is possible to have great precision, but without accuracy if the answer does not represent the actual value tested.
- The precision of a test, its reproducibility, may be expressed as a standard deviation (SD) or the derived coefficient of variation (CV); it is used to compare SDs of two samples. A procedure may be extremely accurate but so difficult that values are not clinically meaningful.
- Assessing sensitivity and specificity of a test involves tests positive, tests negative, disease present (positive), and disease absent (negative). Sensitivity is the proportion of subjects with a specific disease or condition who have a positive test result. Specificity is the proportion of subjects

without the specific disease or condition who have a negative test result.

- Assessing the predictive value (PV) requires knowledge of the sensitivity, specificity, and disease prevalence. Prevalence is the proportion of a population who has the disease. Incidence is the number of subjects who have the disease within a defined period per 100,000 population.
- Proficiency testing (PT) is incorporated into the CLIA requirements. In addition to internal QC programs, each laboratory should participate in an external PT program to verify laboratory accuracy.
- A control specimen has a known value and is similar in composition to the patient's blood. A control value out of the acceptable range (out of control) may result from the deterioration of reagents, faulty equipment, dirty glassware, lack of attention to timing or temperature, use of inappropriate methods, or poor technique.
- Reference range for a particular measurement is usually a normal bell-shaped curve.
- Mean is the mathematical average of the values. Median is the middle value. Mode is the most frequently occurring value. Standard deviation (SD) is the square root of the variance of the values.
- Reference range is the range of values that includes 95% of the test results for a healthy reference population, formerly referred to as normal values or normal range.
- Biometrics attempts to describe statistical variations in biological observation.
- Each laboratory must determine the reproducibility for each new procedure and establish acceptable limits of variation for control specimens.

REVIEW QUESTIONS

1-3. Match the factors (a-c) with the three phases of testing.

1. ____ Preanalytical

2. ____ Analytical

3. ____ Postanalytical
   a. Accuracy in testing
   b. Patient identification
   c. Critical value reporting

4-6. Match the errors with the phase of testing. (An answer may be used more than once.)

4. ____ Blood from the wrong patient

5. ____ Specimen collected in wrong tube

6. ____ Quality control outside of acceptable limits
   a. Preanalytical
   b. Analytical
   c. Postanalytical

7-9. Match the terms with the definitions.

7. ____ Accuracy

8. ____ Control

9. ____ Precision
   a. How close results are to one another when repeatedly analyzed
   b. Describes how close a test result is to the true value
   c. Specimen similar to patient's blood; known concentration of constituent
   d. Comparison of an instrument measure or reading to a known physical constant

10. and 11. Match the terms with the definitions.

10. ____ Sensitivity

11. ____ Specificity
    a. Subjects with specific disease or condition produce a positive result.
    b. Subjects without a specific disease or condition produce a negative result.

12-16. Indicate the type of error for the following causes of technical errors.

12. ____ Omitting patient serum or reagent from the test mixture

13. ____ Dirty glassware

14. ____ Addition of the wrong reagent

15. ____ Inaccurately recording results

16. ____ Hemolyzed patient serum
    a. False-positive error
    b. False-negative error
    c. False-positive or false-negative error

17-20. Insert the missing elements in the list below, choosing from the following answers:
    a. Quality control
    b. Sources of error
    c. Principle and purpose of the test
    d. Procedural protocol

A written procedural protocol should contain this information in the following order:

Procedure name

Name of test method

17. ____

Specimen collection and storage

18. ____

Reagents, supplies, and equipment

19. ____

Expected or normal (reference) values

Procedural notes

20. ____

Limitations

BIBLIOGRAPHY

Astion ML, Shojania KG, Hamill TR, et al: Classifying laboratory incident reports to identify problems that jeopardize safety, Am J Clin Pathol 120:18–26, 2003.

Burtis CA, Ashwood ER, Bruns DB, editors: Tietz fundamentals of clinical chemistry, ed 6, St Louis, 2008, Saunders.

Campbell JB, Campbell JM: Laboratory mathematics: medical and biological applications, ed 5, St Louis, 1997, Mosby.

Centers for Disease Control and Prevention: Clinical Laboratory Improvement Amendments (CLIA): equivalent quality control procedures, Brochure no. 4, 2004.

Centers for Disease Control and Prevention (CDC) (2) Centers for Medicare & Medicaid Services (CMS)HHSCenters for Disease Control and Prevention (CDC) (2) Centers for Medicare & Medicaid Services (CMS)HHS: Medicare, Medicaid, and CLIA Programs. Laboratory requirements relating to quality systems and certain personnel qualifications: final rule, Fed Regist 68:3639–3714, 2003.

Clinical and Laboratory Standards Institute: Training and competence assessment: approved guideline, ed 2, Wayne, 2004, Pa. CLSI Document GP21–A2.

Clinical and Laboratory Standards Institute: Clinical laboratory technical procedure manual: approved guideline, ed 4, Wayne, 2002, Pa. CLSI Document GP2–A4.

Committee on Quality of Health Care in America; Institute of Medicine; Kohn LT, Corrigan JM, Donaldson MS, editors: To err is human: building a safer health system, Washington, DC, 2000, National Academy Press.

Lasky FD: Technology variations: strategies for assuring quality results, 2005, http://labmed. ascpjournals.org/content/36/10/617.full.pdf+html.

National Committee for Clinical Laboratory Standards: Continuous quality improvement: essential management approaches and their use in proficiency testing: approved guideline, ed 2, Wayne, 2004, Pa. NCCLS Document GP22–A2.

Turgeon ML: Linné and Ringsrud's clinical laboratory science: the basics and routine techniques, ed 6, St Louis, 2012, Mosby.

Yost J, Mattingly P: CLIA and equivalent quality control: options for the future, 2005, http://labmed.ascpjournals.org/content/36/10/614.full.pdf.

CHAPTER 8

Basic Serologic Laboratory Techniques

Learning Objectives

At the conclusion of this chapter, the reader should be able to:

- Identify and explain the parts of a procedure.
- Describe the preparation of blood specimens for testing.
- Provide examples of the types of specimens that can be tested using immunologic procedures.
- Explain how complement is inactivated in a serum sample.
- Compare the differences between the two types of pipettes typically used in the immunology-serology laboratory.
- Describe and demonstrate pipetting techniques using manual and automatic pipettes.
- Define the term *dilution*.
- Calculate the concentration of a substance using the dilution factor.

- Calculate the concentration of a single dilution.
- Compare the characteristics of the acute and chronic phases of illness.
- Define the term *antibody titer*.
- Analyze a case study with the interpretation of the assay results.
- Correctly answer case study related multiple choice questions.
- Be prepared to participate in a discussion of critical thinking questions.
- Correctly answer end of chapter review questions.
- Explain and prepare a serial dilution.

Key Terms

acute phase	hemagglutination	meniscus
aliquot	hemagglutination assays	microbial antigens
antibody titer	hematology	microbiology
chyle	icteric	passive agglutination assays
colorimetric reactions	immunohematology	serial dilutions
convalescent phase	immunologic	serologic
cytopathology	in vitro	spectrophotometrically
diluent	inactivation	toxicology
dilution	lipemia	turbid

Serologic testing has long been an important part of diagnostic tests in the clinical laboratory for viral and bacterial diseases. **Immunologic** testing is done in many areas of the clinical laboratory—**microbiology,** chemistry, **toxicology,** immunology, **hematology,** surgical pathology, **cytopathology,**

immunohematology (blood banking)—and a great variety of specimens are tested. Rapid testing is typically used in the laboratory as well as in home-testing kits.

The advent of monoclonal antibody (MAb) technology has led to the development of highly specific and sensitive immunoassays. Common serologic and immunologic tests include pregnancy tests for human chorionic gonadotropin (hCG) and tests for infectious mononucleosis and syphilis.

PROCEDURES MANUAL

The procedures manual must be a complete document of current techniques and approved policies that is available at all times in the immediate bench area of laboratory personnel. It is extremely important that all personnel review this manual periodically. The manual should comply with the CLSI format for a procedure (see Box 7-1). The procedural format found in this text generally follows these guidelines.

Alternate techniques can be included with each procedure if more than one technique is acceptable. New pages must be dated and initialed when inserted and removed pages must be retained for 5 years, with the date of removal and the reason for removal indicated. It may be legally necessary to identify the procedure followed for a particular reason.

Procedures used in immunology apply many techniques common to other scientific disciplines, such as chemistry. In the field of immunology, different serologic techniques are used to detect the interaction of antigens with antibodies. These methods are suitable for the detection and quantitation of antibodies to infectious agents, as well as **microbial antigens** and nonmicrobial antigens (see Part III of this text).

BLOOD SPECIMEN PREPARATION

After blood has been obtained from a patient, in a plain evacuated tube, without anticoagulant, it should be allowed to clot and the serum should be promptly removed for testing. Clotting and clot retraction should take place at room temperature or in the refrigerator, depending on the protocol for the specific procedure. Complete clot retraction normally takes about 1 hour. After clot retraction, the clot should be loosened from the sides of the test tube with an applicator stick and centrifuged for 10 minutes at a moderate speed.

After centrifugation, serum can be transferred to a labeled tube with a Pasteur pipette and rubber bulb. If the serum is contaminated with erythrocytes, it should be recentrifuged. The serum-containing tube should be sealed.

Excessive heat and bacterial contamination are avoided. Heat coagulates the proteins and bacterial growth alters protein molecules. If the test cannot be performed immediately, the serum should be refrigerated. In most cases, if the testing cannot be done within 72 hours, a serum specimen must be frozen at −20° C. Standard Precautions must be followed when blood specimens are handled.

For some testing, the serum complement must first be inactivated (see following discussion). If the protein complement is not inactivated, it will promote lysis of the red blood cells and other types of cells and can produce invalid results. Complement is also known to interfere with certain tests for syphilis.

TYPES OF SPECIMENS TESTED

Most immunology tests are done on serum, although body fluids may also be tested. **Lipemia,** hemolysis, or any bacterial contamination can make the specimen unacceptable. **Icteric** or **turbid** serum may yield valid results for some tests but may interfere with others. Blood specimens should be collected before a meal to avoid the presence of **chyle,** an emulsion of fat globules that often appears in serum after eating, during digestion. Contamination with alkali or acid must be avoided because these substances have a denaturing effect on serum proteins and make the specimens useless for serologic testing.

Other specimens include urine for pregnancy tests and tests for urinary tract infection. It is important that the urine specimen be collected after thorough cleaning of the external genitalia to prevent contamination of microbiological assays. Urine for the hCG assay (pregnancy test) must be collected at a suitable time interval after fertilization to allow the concentration of the hCG hormone to rise to a significantly detectable level.

Any specimen must be collected into a suitable container to prevent **in vitro** changes that could affect the assay results. Proper handling and storage of the specimen until testing are essential. Immunologic assays are also done on cerebrospinal fluid (CSF), other body fluids, and swabs of various body exudates and discharges. The established protocol for each specific assay must be followed in terms of specimen collection requirements and conditions for the assay itself.

INACTIVATION OF COMPLEMENT

Some procedures require the use of inactivated serum. **Inactivation** is the process that destroys complement activity. Complement is known to interfere with the reactions of certain syphilis tests and complement components (e.g., C1q). It can agglutinate latex particles and cause a false-positive reaction in latex **passive agglutination assays.** Complement may also cause lysis of the indicator cells in **hemagglutination assays.**

Complement in body fluids can be inactivated by heating to 56° C for 30 minutes. When more than 4 hours has elapsed since inactivation, a specimen can be reinactivated by heating it to 56° C for 10 minutes.

PIPETTES

Pipettes are used in the immunology-serology laboratory for the quantitative transfer of reagents and the preparations of serial dilutions of specimens such as serum (Fig. 8-1). Although semiautomated micropipettes have replaced traditional glass pipettes in the laboratory, traditional methods may still be needed at times.

Graduated Pipettes

A method for delivering a particular amount of liquid is to deliver the amount of liquid contained between two calibration marks on a cylindrical tube, or pipette. Such a pipette is called a graduated pipette, or measuring pipette. It has several graduation, or calibration, marks. Graduated pipettes are used when great accuracy is not required, although these pipettes should not be used with any less care than volumetric pipettes. Graduated pipettes are used primarily for measuring reagents but are not calibrated with sufficient tolerance for measuring standard or control solutions, unknown specimens, or filtrates.

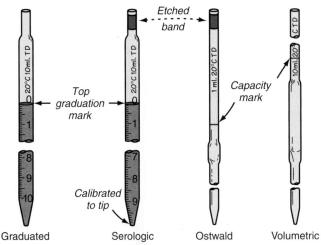

Figure 8-1   Types of manual pipettes. *TD,* To deliver. *(From Turgeon ML: Linné & Ringsrud's clinical laboratory science: the basics and routine techniques, ed 6, St Louis, 2012, Mosby.)*

A graduated pipette is a straight piece of glass tubing with a tapered end and graduation marks on the stem separating it into parts. Depending on the size used, graduated pipettes can be used to measure parts of a milliliter or many milliliters. These pipettes come in various sizes, or capacities, including 0.1, 0.2, 1.0, 2.0, 5.0, 10, and 25 mL. If 4 mL of deionized water is to be measured into a test tube, a 5-mL graduated pipette would be the best choice.

Because graduated pipettes require draining between two marks, they introduce one more source of error compared with volumetric pipettes, which have only one calibration mark. This makes measurements with the graduated pipette less precise. Because of this relatively poor precision, the graduated pipette is used when speed is more important than precision (e.g., measurement of reagents) and is generally not considered accurate enough for measuring samples and standard solutions.

Serologic Pipettes

Another pipette used in the laboratory, the serologic pipette, looks similar to the graduated pipette. However, the orifice, or tip opening, is larger in the serologic pipette than in other pipettes. The rate of fall of liquid is much too fast for great accuracy or precision.

The serologic pipette is recognized by a frosted ring at the noncalibrated end, with calibrations extending to the tip. The letters TD (to deliver) appear on the pipette and, for quick recognition, each size of pipette has an imprinted, color-coded band that indicates the volume. The serologic pipette is usually allowed to empty by gravity. Depending on the calibration, the remaining drop needs to be expelled to deliver the full volume.

Each serologic pipette is marked with identifying numerals (e.g., 10 mL in 1/10). The first of these numbers represents the total capacity of the pipette. The second number represents the smallest gradation into which the pipette is divided. In the example cited, therefore, the total pipette volume is 10 mL. Markings then divide it into 1-mL sections and each milliliter is further divided into tenths. Sizes of serologic pipettes most frequently used are 10 mL in 1/10 , 5 mL in 1/10, 2 mL in 1/10, 2 mL in 1/100, 1 mL in 1/10, and 1 mL in 1/100. For greatest accuracy, the smallest pipette that will hold the desired volume should be used.

Inspection and Use

Before use, glass pipettes should be inspected for broken or chipped ends or contamination. A safety bulb must be used to aspirate liquid into the pipette and to dispense it.

- Aspirate liquid to about 1 inch (2.5 cm) above the top (zero) line of the pipette.
- Raise the pipette vertically to avoid the introduction of air bubbles and wipe off the exterior surface with a clean gauze or tissue square.
- Working at eye level, slowly lower the liquid so that the meniscus is at zero.
- Aspirate the contents of the pipette into the appropriate test tube or vessel.
- Wear gloves during pipetting procedures in compliance with Standard Precautions.

PIPETTING TECHNIQUES

Manual Pipettes

With practice, it is important to develop a good technique for handling pipettes (Fig. 8-2). The same general steps apply to pipetting with all manual pipettes (Box 8-1), with few exceptions.

Laboratory accidents frequently result from improper pipetting techniques. The greatest potential hazard is when mouth pipetting is done instead of mechanical suction. *Mouth pipetting is never acceptable in the clinical laboratory.*

After the pipette has been filled above the top graduation mark, removed from the vessel, and held in a vertical position, the meniscus must be adjusted. The **meniscus** is the curvature in the top surface of a liquid (Fig. 8-3). The pipette should be held so that the calibration mark is at eye level. All readings must be made with the eye at the level of the meniscus. The delivery tip is touched to the inside wall of the original vessel, not the liquid, and the meniscus of the liquid in the pipette is eased, or adjusted, down to the calibration mark.

Before the measured liquid in the pipette is allowed to drain into the receiving vessel, any liquid adhering to the outside of the pipette must be wiped off with a clean piece of gauze or tissue. If this is not done, any drops present on the outside of the pipette might drain into the receiving vessel along with the measured volume. This would make the volume more than that specified and an error would result.

Automatic Pipettes

Automatic pipettes allow fast, repetitive measurement and delivery of solutions of equal volumes. The sampling type measures the substance in question. The sampling-diluting type measures the substance and then adds the desired **diluent.** The sampling type of automatic pipette is mechanically operated and uses a piston-operated plunger. These are adjustable so that varying amounts of reagent or sample can be delivered with the same device. Disposable and exchangeable tips are available for these pipettes. Automatic pipettes and micropipettors must be calibrated before use.

Micropipettors

Automatic micropipetting devices allow rapid repetitive measurements and delivery of predetermined volumes of reagents

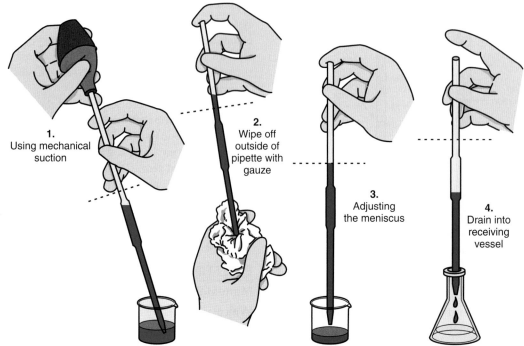

Figure 8-2   Pipetting technique. *(From Turgeon ML: Linné & Ringsrud's clinical laboratory science: the basics and routine techniques, ed 6, St Louis, 2012, Mosby.)*

Box 8-1	Pipetting With Manual Pipettes

1. Check the pipette to ascertain its correct size, being careful also to check for broken delivery or suction tips.
2. Wearing protective gloves, hold the pipette lightly between the thumb and the last three fingers, leaving the index finger free.
3. Place the tip of the pipette well below the surface of the liquid to be pipetted.
4. Using mechanical suction or an aspirator bulb, carefully draw the liquid up into the pipette until the level of liquid is well above the calibration mark.
5. Quickly cover the suction opening at the top of the pipette with the index finger.
6. Wipe the outside of the pipette dry with a piece of Kim-Wipe tissue to remove excess fluid.
7. Hold the pipette in a vertical position with the delivery tip against the inside of the original vessel. Carefully allow the liquid in the pipette to drain by gravity until the bottom of the meniscus is exactly at the calibration mark. To do this, do not entirely remove the index finger from the suction hole end of the pipette; rather, by rolling the finger slightly over the opening, allow slow drainage to take place.
8. While still holding the pipette in a vertical position, touch the tip of the pipette to the inside wall of the receiving vessel. Remove the index finger from the top of the pipette to permit free drainage. Remember to keep the pipette in a vertical position for correct drainage. In TD (to deliver) pipettes, a small amount of fluid will remain in the delivery tip.
9. To be certain that the drainage is as complete as possible, touch the delivery tip of the pipette to another area on the inside wall of the receiving vessel.

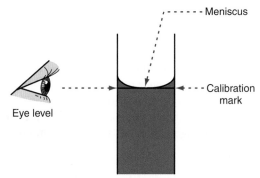

Figure 8-3   Reading the meniscus. *(From Turgeon ML: Linné & Ringsrud's clinical laboratory science: the basics and routine techniques, ed 6, St Louis, 2012, Mosby.)*

or specimens. The most common type of micropipette used in many laboratories is one that is automatic or semiautomatic, called a micropipettor. These are piston-operated devices that allow repeated, accurate, reproducible delivery of specimens, reagents, and other liquids requiring measurement in small amounts. Many micropipettors are continuously adjustable so that variable volumes of liquids can be dispensed with the same device. Delivery volume is selected by adjusting the settings. Different types or models are available, which allow volume delivery ranging, for example, from 0.5 to 5000 µL. The calibration of these micropipettes should be checked periodically.

The piston, usually in the form of a thumb plunger, is depressed to a stop position on the pipetting device. The tip is placed in the liquid to be measured, and then the plunger is slowly allowed to rise back to the original position (Fig. 8-4). This will fill the tip with the desired volume of liquid. The tips are usually drawn along the inside wall of the vessel from

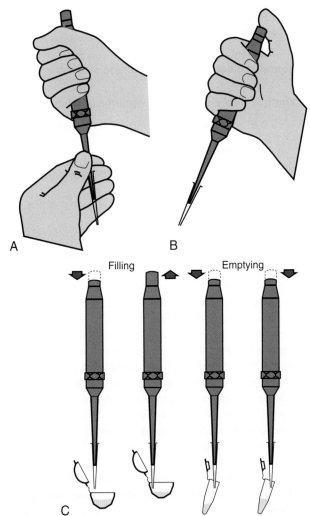

Figure 8-4 Steps in using piston-type automatic micropipette. A, Attaching proper tip size for range of pipette volume, and twisting tip as it is pushed onto pipette to give an airtight, continuous seal. **B,** Holding pipette before use. **C,** Follow instructions for filling and emptying pipette tip. *(From Kaplan LA, Pesce A: Clinical chemistry: theory, analysis, correlation, ed 5, St Louis, 2010, Mosby.)*

which the measured volume is drawn, so that any adhering liquid is removed from the end of the tip. These pipette tips are not usually wiped, as is done with the manual pipettes, because the plastic surface is considered nonwettable. The tip of the pipette device is then placed against the inside wall of the receiving vessel and the plunger is depressed. When the manufacturer's directions for the device being used are followed, sample delivery volume is judged to be extremely accurate.

The pipette tips are usually made of disposable plastic, so no cleaning is necessary. Various types of tips are available. Some pipetting devices automatically eject the tip after use. These will also allow the user to insert a new tip and remove the used tip without touching it, minimizing infectious biohazard exposures.

The problems encountered with automatic pipetting depend largely on the nature of the solution to be pipetted. Some reagents cause more bubbles than others and some are more

viscous. Bubbles and viscous solutions can cause problems with the measurement and delivery of samples and solutions.

Micropipettors contain or deliver 1 to 500 μL of solution. It is important to follow the individual manufacturer's instructions for the device being used; each may be slightly different. In general, the following steps apply for use of a micropipettor:

1. Attach the proper tip to the pipettor and set the delivery volume.
2. Depress the piston to a stop position on the pipettor.
3. Place the tip into the solution and allow the piston to rise back slowly to its original position (this fills the pipettor tip with the desired volume of solution).
4. Some tips are wiped with a dry gauze at this step and some are not. Follow the manufacturer's directions.
5. Place the tip on the wall of the receiving vessel and depress the piston, first to a stop position where the liquid is allowed to drain and then to a second stop position where the full dispensing of the liquid takes place.
6. Dispose of the tip in the waste disposal receptacle. Some pipettors automatically eject the used tips, minimizing biohazard exposure.

Automatic Dispensers or Syringes

Many types of automatic dispensers or syringes are used in the laboratory for repetitively adding multiple doses of the same reagent or diluent. These devices are used for measuring serial amounts of relatively small volumes of the same liquid. The volume to be dispensed is determined by the pipettor setting. Dispensers are available with a variety of volume settings. Some are available as syringes and others as bottle top devices. Most of these dispensers can be cleaned by autoclaving.

Diluter-Dispensers

In automated instruments, diluter-dispensers are used to prepare a number of different samples for analysis. These devices pipette a selected aliquot of sample and diluent into the instrument or receiving vessel. They are primarily of the dual-piston type, with one used for the sample and the other for the diluent or reagent.

DILUTIONS

It is often necessary to make dilutions of specimens being analyzed or to make weaker solutions from stronger solutions in various laboratory procedures. Clinicians must be able to work with various dilution problems and dilution factors. They often need to determine the concentration of antibody in each solution, the actual amount of material in each solution, and the total volume of each solution. All dilutions are a form of ratio. **Dilution** is an indication of relative concentration.

Diluting Specimens

In most laboratory determinations, a small sample is taken for analysis and the final result is expressed as concentration per some convenient standard volume. In a certain procedure, 0.5 mL of blood is diluted to a total of 10 mL with various reagents, and 1 mL of this dilution is then analyzed for a particular chemical constituent. The final result is to be expressed in terms of the concentration of that substance per 100 mL of blood.

Dilution Factor

A dilution factor is used to correct for having used a diluted sample in a determination rather than the undiluted sample. The result (answer) using the dilution must be multiplied by the reciprocal of the dilution made. For example, a dilution factor by which all determination answers are multiplied to give the concentration per 100 mL of sample (blood) may be calculated as follows.

First, determine the volume of blood that is actually analyzed in the procedure. Using a simple proportion, it is evident that 0.5 mL of blood diluted to 10 mL is equivalent to 1 mL of blood diluted to 20 mL:

$$\frac{0.5 \text{ mL blood}}{10 \text{ mL solution}} = \frac{1 \text{ mL blood}}{x \text{ mL solution}}$$

$$x = \frac{1 \text{ mL blood} \times 10 \text{ mL}}{0.5 \text{ mL}} = 20 \text{ mL}$$

The concentration of specimen (blood) in each milliliter of solution may be determined by the use of another simple proportion to be 0.05 mL of blood per milliliter of solution:

$$\frac{1 \text{ mL blood}}{20 \text{ mL solution}} = \frac{x \text{ mL blood}}{1 \text{ mL solution}}$$

$$x = \frac{1 \text{ mL} \times 1 \text{ mL}}{20 \text{ mL}} = 0.05 \text{ mL}$$

Because 1 mL of the 1:20 dilution of blood is analyzed in the remaining steps of the procedure, 0.05 mL of blood is actually analyzed (1 mL of the dilution used × 0.05 mL/mL = 0.05 mL of blood analyzed).

To relate the concentration of the substance measured in the procedure to the concentration in 100 mL of blood (the units in which the result is to be expressed), another proportion may be used:

$$\frac{\frac{100 \text{ mL}}{(\text{volume of blood desired})}}{\frac{0.05 \text{ mL}}{(\text{volume of blood used})}} = \frac{\text{concentration desired}}{\text{concentration used or determined}}$$

$$\text{Concentration desired} = \frac{100 \text{ mL} \times \text{concentration determined}}{0.05 \text{ mL}}$$

$$\text{Concentration desired} = 2000 \times \text{value determined}$$

The concentration of the substance being measured in the volume of blood actually tested (0.05 mL) must be multiplied by 2000 to report the concentration per 100 mL of blood.

The preceding material may be summarized by the following statement and equations. In reporting results obtained from laboratory determinations, one must first determine the amount of specimen actually analyzed in the procedure and then calculate the factor that will express the concentration in

the desired terms of measurement. Thus, in the previous example, the following equations may be used:

$$\frac{\frac{0.5 \text{ mL}}{(\text{volume of blood used})}}{\frac{10 \text{ mL}}{(\text{volume of total dilution})}} = \frac{\frac{x \text{ mL}}{(\text{volume of blood analyzed})}}{\frac{1 \text{ mL}}{(\text{volume of dilution used})}}$$

$$x = 0.05 \text{ mL (volume of blood actually analyzed)}$$

$$\frac{\frac{100 \text{ mL (volume of blood}}{\text{required for expression of result)}}}{\frac{0.05 \text{ mL (volume of}}{\text{blood actually analyzed)}}} = 2000 \text{ (dilution factor)}$$

Single Dilutions

When the concentration of a particular substance in a specimen is too great to be determined accurately, or when there is less specimen available for analysis than the procedure requires, it may be necessary to dilute the original specimen or further dilute the initial dilution (or filtrate). These single dilutions are usually expressed as a ratio, such as 1:2, 1:5, or 1:10, or as a fraction, ½, ⅕, or ⅒. These ratios or fractions refer to 1 unit of the original specimen diluted to a final volume of 2, 5, or 10 units, respectively. A dilution, therefore, refers to the volume or number of parts of the substance to be diluted in the total volume, or parts, of the final solution. A dilution is an expression of concentration, not volume; it indicates the relative amount of substance in solution. Dilutions can be made singly or in series.

To calculate the concentration of a single dilution, multiply the original concentration by the dilution expressed as a fraction.

Example of Calculation of Concentration of a Single Dilution

A specimen contains 500 mg of substance per deciliter of blood. A 1:5 dilution of this specimen is prepared by volumetrically measuring 1 mL of the specimen and adding 4 mL of diluent. The concentration (C) of substance in the dilution is calculated as follows:

$$C = 500 \text{ mg/dL} \times \tfrac{1}{5} = 100 \text{ mg/dL}$$

Note that the concentration of the final solution (or dilution) is expressed in the same units as that of the original solution.

To obtain a dilution factor that can be applied to the determination answer and express it as a concentration per standard volume, proceed as follows. Rather than multiply by the dilution expressed as a fraction, multiply the determination value by the reciprocal of the dilution fraction. In the case of a 1:5 dilution, the dilution factor applied to values obtained in the procedure would be 5, because the original specimen was five times more concentrated than the diluted specimen tested in the procedure.

Use of Dilution Factors

A 1:5 dilution of a specimen is prepared and an **aliquot** (one of a number of equal parts) of the dilution is analyzed for a

Table 8-1	**Example of Preparation of a Serial Dilution**									
	Tube									
	1	**2**	**3**	**4**	**5**	**6**	**7**	**8**	**9**	**10**
Saline (mL)	1	1	1	1	1	1	1	1	1	1
Patient serum or preceding dilution (mL)	1	1 of 1:2	1 of 1:4	1 of 1:8	1 of 1:16	1 of 1:32	1 of 1:64	1 of 1:128	1 of 1:256	1 of 1:512
Final dilution	1:2	1:4	1:8	1:16	1:32	1:64	1:128	1:256	1:512	1:1024

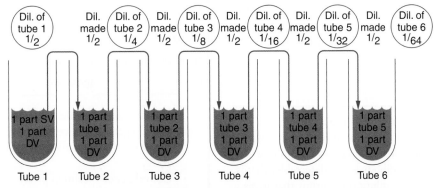

SV = Sample volume (e.g., serum)
DV = Diluent volume (e.g., saline)

Figure 8-5   Schematic of a twofold serial dilution. *(From Turgeon ML: Linné & Ringsrud's clinical laboratory science: the basics and routine techniques, ed 6, St Louis, 2012, Mosby, p. 166.)*

particular substance. The concentration of the substance (C) in the aliquot is multiplied by 5 to determine its concentration in the original specimen. If the concentration of the dilution is 100 mg/dL, the concentration of the original specimen is:

$$C = 100 \text{ mg/dL} \times 5 \text{ (dilution factor)} = 500 \text{ mg/dL in blood}$$

Serial Dilutions

Dilutions can also be made in series, in which the original solution is further diluted. A general rule for calculating the concentrations of solutions obtained by dilution in series is to multiply the original concentration by the first dilution (expressed as a fraction), this by the second dilution, and so on, until the desired concentration is known.

Several laboratory procedures, especially serologic methods, make use of a dilution series in which all dilutions, including or following the first one, are the same. Such dilutions are referred to as **serial dilutions** (Table 8-1). A complete dilution series usually contains 5 or 10 tubes, although any single dilution may be made directly from an undiluted specimen or substance. In calculating the dilution or concentration of a substance or serum in each tube of the dilution series, the rules previously discussed apply.

A twofold dilution may be prepared as follows (Fig. 8-5). A serum specimen is diluted 1:2 with buffer. A series of five tubes are prepared, in which each succeeding tube is rediluted 1:2. This is accomplished by placing 1 mL of diluent into each of four tubes (tubes 2 to 5). Tube 1 contains 1 mL of undiluted serum. Tube 2 contains 1 mL of undiluted serum plus 1 mL of diluent, resulting in a 1:2 dilution of serum. A 1-mL portion of the 1:2 dilution of serum is placed in tube 3, resulting in a 1:4 dilution of serum ($\frac{1}{2} \times \frac{1}{2} \times \frac{1}{4}$). A 1-mL portion of the 1:4 dilution from tube 3 is placed in tube 4, resulting in a 1:8 dilution ($\frac{1}{4} \times \frac{1}{2} \times \frac{1}{8}$). Finally, 1 mL of the 1:8 dilution from tube 4 is added to tube 5, resulting in a 1:16 dilution ($\frac{1}{8} \times \frac{1}{2} \times \frac{1}{16}$). One milliliter of the final dilution is discarded so that the volumes in all the tubes are equal.

Note that each tube is diluted twice as much as the previous tube, and that the final volume in each tube is the same. The undiluted serum may also be given a dilution value, 1:1.

The concentration of serum in terms of milliliters in each tube is calculated by multiplying the previous concentration (mL) by the succeeding dilution. In this example, tube 1 contains 1 mL of serum, tube 2 contains 1 mL × ½ × 0.5 mL of serum, and tubes 3 to 5 contain 0.25, 0.125, and 0.06 mL of serum, respectively.

Other serial dilutions might be fivefold or tenfold; that is, each succeeding tube is diluted 5 or 10 times. A fivefold series would begin with 1 mL of serum in 4 mL of diluent and a total volume of 5 mL in each tube. A tenfold series would begin with 1 mL of serum in 9 mL of diluent and a total volume of 10 mL in each tube. Other systems might begin with a 1:2 dilution and then dilute five succeeding tubes 1:10. The dilutions in such a series would be 1:2, 1:20 ($\frac{1}{2} \times \frac{1}{10} \times \frac{1}{20}$), 1:200 ($\frac{1}{20} \times \frac{1}{10} \times \frac{1}{200}$), 1:2000, 1:20,000, and 1:200,000.

ANTIBODY TESTING

In obtaining specimens for serologic testing, it is important to consider the phase of the disease and the condition of the patient at the time of specimen collection. This is especially important in assays for diagnosis of infectious diseases. If serum is being tested for antibody levels with a specific infectious organism, generally the blood should be drawn during the **acute phase** of the illness—when the disease is first discovered or suspected—and another sample drawn during the **convalescent phase,** usually about 2 weeks later. Accordingly, these samples are called acute and convalescent serum. A difference in the amount of antibody present, or the antibody titer, may be noted when the two different samples are tested concurrently. Some infections, such as Legionnaires' disease or hepatitis, may not manifest a rise in titer until months after the acute infection.

ANTIBODY TITER

A central concept of serologic testing is the manifestation of a rise in titer, or concentration, of an antibody. The **antibody titer** is defined as the reciprocal of the highest dilution of the patient's serum in which the antibody is still detectable. That is, the titer is read at the highest dilution of serum that gives a positive reaction with the antigen. If a serum sample has been diluted 1:64 and reacts positively with the antigen suspension used in the testing process, and if the next highest dilution of 1:128 does not give a positive reaction, the titer is read as 64. A high titer indicates that there is a relatively high concentration of the antibody present in the serum.

Determination of the concentration of antibody (titer) for a specific antigen involves the following two steps:

1. Preparing a serial dilution of the antibody-containing solution (e.g., serum)
2. Adding an equal volume of antigen suspension to each dilution

A high titer indicates that a considerable amount of antibody is present in the serum. For most pathogenic infections, an increase in the patient's titer of two doubling dilutions, or from a positive result of 1:8 to a positive result of 1:32 over several weeks, is an indication of a current infection. This is known as a fourfold rise in the antibody titer.

CASE STUDY

JJ, a 9-year-old boy, was taken to the emergency department with a sore throat. On examination, he had redness of the throat and slightly swollen glands. The physician assistant ordered a throat culture and blood drawn for an antistreptolysin-O antibody (ASO). An antibiotic was prescribed for a 10-day period. His mother was told to make an appointment with his pediatrician for a follow-up.

At the follow-up visit 2 weeks later, the results of the laboratory test revealed a throat culture with a few colonies of β-streptococci. The qualitative ASO test result was reported as positive. The acute serum was frozen at the time of testing. The pediatrician ordered a convalescent specimen to be tested semiquantitatively in parallel with the acute specimen for an ASO titer.

The acute and convalescent specimens were prepared as twofold serial dilutions of each specimen (see table).

	Tube					
	1	2	3	4	5	6
Saline (μL)	—	50	50	50	50	50
Serum (μL)	50	50	**50 (1:2)**	**50 (1:4)**	50	50
Mix and transfer to next tube		**50**	**50**	**50**	**50**	**50**
Dilution/titer	1:1	1:2	1:4	1:8	1:16	1:32
IU/mL	200	4008	800	1600	3200	6400

The results of the parallel testing of the acute and convalescent specimens revealed the following:
- Acute specimen positive, 1:1 dilution/titer (IU/mL 200)
- Convalescent specimen positive, 1:4 dilution/titer (IU/mL 800)

Questions
1. The convalescent specimen demonstrated:
   a. No evidence of streptococci infection
   b. A possibility of streptococci infection
   c. Significant evidence of streptococci infection
   d. Evidence of a chronic streptococci infection
2. Comparing acute and chronic patient specimens can:
   a. Distinguish acute from chronic infection.
   b. Diagnose the cause of the infection.
   c. Demonstrate at least a two-fold dilution rise that is significant for an acute infection.
   d. Demonstrate at least a two-fold dilution rise that is significant for a chronic infection.

See Appendix A for the answers to these questions.

Critical Thinking Group Discussion Questions
1. Is the difference between the acute and convalescent titers significant?
2. What does a rise in titer mean?

See instructor site ⊖volve for the discussion of the answers to these questions.

⠿ Serial Dilution

Principle

Serial dilutions are a method for determining the concentration of a substance (e.g., antibody). The greatest dilution of the sample that yields a positive result is the end point. This end point dilution can be expressed as a fraction. The reciprocal of that fraction is called the titer of the antibody.

A series of dilutions of a sample is necessary for determining an antibody titer. In serial dilution, each dilution is prepared from the previous dilution. Dilutions can be in large test tubes, macrotitration, or in a miniaturized version, microtitration.

Microtitration is valuable for any procedure in which dilutions are made and red blood cells (RBCs) are used as indicator cells (e.g., **hemagglutination**). **Colorimetric reactions** can be performed (e.g., enzyme immunoassay) and quantitated **spectrophotometrically** with specialized instruments for microtiter plates.

Interpretation of Results

In clinical immunology, the titer of an antibody in an individual's serum can have clinical significance, depending on the antibody in question. Antibody titers are sometimes used to evaluate a person's immune status. Titers may be obtained over time, as with acute and convalescent specimens for infectious diseases or monitoring a mother's titer for blood group antibodies during pregnancy.

CHAPTER HIGHLIGHTS

- Traditional serologic tests have been done for viral and bacterial diseases. Other common tests include pregnancy tests for human chorionic gonadotropin (hCG) and immunologic tests for infectious mononucleosis and syphilis.
- The procedures manual describes current techniques (in CLSI format) and approved policies and is always available to laboratory personnel.
- After a blood sample has clotted, serum should be promptly removed for testing or frozen at –20° C. Standard Precautions must be followed when blood specimens are handled.
- Lipemia, hemolysis, and bacterial contamination can make the specimen unacceptable. Icteric or turbid serum may give valid results or may interfere. Blood specimens should be collected before a meal to avoid chyle. Contamination with alkali or acid must be avoided.
- Some procedures require inactivated serum. Complement can be inactivated by heating to 56° C for 30 minutes or, after 4 hours, reinactivated by heating for 10 minutes.
- A graduated pipette delivers the liquid between two calibration marks. A serologic pipette resembles the graduated pipette, but has a frosted ring and enlarged tip opening.
- Automatic pipettes allow fast repetitive measurement and delivery of solutions of equal volumes.
- All dilutions are a ratio. Dilution is an indication of relative concentration.
- A dilution factor is used to correct for having used a diluted sample in a determination rather than the undiluted sample. The result (answer) using the dilution must be multiplied by the reciprocal of the dilution made.
- When the concentration is too high or less specimen is available for analysis, the original specimen may be diluted or the initial dilution (or filtrate) further diluted. These

single dilutions are usually expressed as a ratio (1:2, 1:5, 1:10) or a fraction (½, ⅕, ⅒).

- A dilution is the volume or number of parts of the substance to be diluted in the total volume, or parts, of the final solution. A dilution is an expression of concentration, the relative amount of substance in solution. Dilutions can be made singly or in series.
- In a dilution series, all dilutions, including or following the first one, are the same, called serial dilutions.
- A complete dilution series usually contains 5 or 10 tubes, although any single dilution may be made directly from an undiluted specimen or substance.
- When testing antibody levels for a specific infectious organism, blood should be drawn during both the acute and convalescent phases.
- A difference in the amount of antibody present, or the antibody titer, may be noted when two different samples are tested concurrently. A rise in titer is central to serologic testing.
- The antibody titer is defined as the reciprocal of the highest dilution of the patient's serum in which the antibody is still detectable.

REVIEW QUESTIONS

1. A written procedural protocol should contain the following information, in the correct order: ____, ____, ____, ____. Choose from (A) to (D).
   A. Specimen collection and storage
   B. Reference values
   C. Reagents, supplies, and equipment
   D. Procedural method
   a. A, B, C, D
   b. B, C, A, D
   c. A, C, D, B
   d. D, C, B, A

2. Factors that can denature, coagulate, or alter protein molecules include:
   a. Heat
   b. Strong acid solution
   c. Strong alkali solution
   d. All of the above

3. If testing cannot be done within _____ hours of collection, a serum specimen should be frozen at –20° C.
   a. 24
   b. 48
   c. 72
   d. 96

4. Complement can be inactivated in human serum by heating to _____ ° C.
   a. 25
   b. 37
   c. 45
   d. 56

5. A specimen should be reinactivated when more than
   _____ hour(s) has (have) elapsed since inactivation.
   a. 1
   b. 2
   c. 4
   d. 8

6. A graduated pipette can be used when:
   a. Extreme accuracy is not needed.
   b. Very precise accuracy is needed.
   c. Precision is more important than speed.
   d. Precision and speed are important.

7. A meniscus is the:
   a. Curvature in the top surface of a liquid
   b. Zero mark on a pipette
   c. Last marking on a serologic pipette
   d. Flat line of liquid in a pipette

8. Automatic pipettes have the advantage of:
   a. Being fast
   b. Allowing repetitive measurement of solutions
   c. Delivering equal volumes of solutions
   d. All the above

9. A dilution is a(n):
   a. Ratio of volume or number of parts of the substance
      to be diluted in the total volume, or parts, of the final
      solution
   b. Indication of relative concentration
   c. Frequently used measure in serologic testing
   d. All the above

10. If a serial dilution is prepared in 1:2 dilutions, the final
    dilution in tube 6 is:
    a. 1:25
    b. 1:32
    c. 1:64
    d. 1:256

11. and 12. To prepare 10 mL of a diluted serum specimen 1:10,

11. _____ part of serum is needed.
    a. 1.0
    b. 0.75
    c. 0.50
    d. 0.20

and

12. _____ parts of distilled water is (are) needed to reach the
    total volume.
    a. 10
    b. 9
    c. 4.5
    d. 0.1

13. Serum for detection of antibodies should be drawn
    during the:
    a. Acute phase of illness only
    b. Acute and convalescent phases of illness
    c. Convalescent phase of illness only
    d. Acute and convalescent phases, as well as 6 months
       after an illness

14. A central concept of serologic testing is:
    a. Antigen-antibody interaction
    b. Determination of antibody composition
    c. Quantitation of antigen titer
    d. Manifestation of a rise in antibody titer

BIBLIOGRAPHY

Bishop ML, Fody EP, Schoeff L: Clinical chemistry: principles, procedures,
    correlations, ed 6, Philadelphia, 2010, Lippincott Williams & Wilkins.
Burtis CA, Ashwood ER, Bruns DB, editors: Tietz fundamentals of clinical
    chemistry, ed 6, St Louis, 2008, Saunders.
Campbell JM, Campbell JB: Laboratory mathematics: medical and biological
    applications, ed 5, St Louis, 1997, Mosby.
Kaplan LA, Pesce AJ: Clinical chemistry: theory, analysis, correlation, ed 5,
    St Louis, 2010, Mosby.
Turgeon ML: Linné & Ringsrud's clinical laboratory science: the basics and
    routine techniques, ed 6, St Louis, 2012, Mosby.

CHAPTER 9

Point-of-Care Testing

Learning Objectives

At the conclusion of this chapter, the reader should be able to:
- Define point-of-care testing (POCT).
- Cite some advantages and disadvantages of POCT.
- Differentiate among the four different types of testing categories.
- Analyze a POCT case study.

- Correctly answer case study related multiple choice questions.
- Be prepared to participate in a discussion of critical thinking questions.
- Describe the principle and clinical application of one POCT assay.
- Correctly answer end of chapter review questions.

Key Terms

ectopic pregnancy
follicle-stimulating hormone (FSH)
human chorionic gonadotropin
   (hCG)

immunochromatographic
luteinizing hormone
monoclonal
nontrophoblastic neoplasms

point-of-care testing (POCT)
preanalytic
sandwich-format
trophoblastic neoplasms

Point-of-care testing (POCT) is defined as laboratory assays performed near the patient. The development of new POCT assays has been increasing at a rapid rate. POCT testing can include home test kits and handheld monitors. The major advantage is the rapidity of obtaining quality results if the procedure is performed by an appropriately patient or health care provider. The major drawback is cost, particularly if a large volume of testing is done. Other areas of concern include maintenance of quality control (QC) and quality assurance (QA).

TESTING CATEGORIES

Diagnostic testing that is not performed within a traditional laboratory is called waived testing by The Joint Commission (TJC, formerly known as the Joint Commission on Accreditation of Healthcare Organizations [JCAHO]). The Clinical Laboratory Improvement Acts of 1988 (CLIA '88) subjects all clinical laboratory testing to federal regulation and inspection. According to CLIA '88, test procedures are grouped into one of four following categories:
1. Waived tests. Simple procedures with little chance of negative outcomes if performed inaccurately.
2. Moderately complex tests. More complex than waived tests but usually automated (e.g., enzyme immunoassays).

3. Highly complex tests. Usually nonautomated or complicated tests requiring considerable judgment (e.g., serum protein electrophoresis).
4. Provider-performed microscopy tests. Slide examinations of freshly collected body fluids.

Test complexity is determined by criteria that assess knowledge, training, reagent and material preparation, operational technique, QC-QA characteristics, maintenance and troubleshooting, and interpretation and judgment. Any over-the-counter test approved by the U.S. Food and Drug Administration (FDA) is automatically placed into the "waived" category. POCT falls within the "waived" or "moderately complex" category.

QUALITY CONTROL STANDARDS

All laboratory testing must meet the same quality standards regardless of where it is performed. State and city governments may enact mandatory regulations, including qualifications of personnel performing the test, which may be more (but not less) stringent than federal regulations. Voluntary participation in QA programs is also available.

The Centers for Disease Control and Prevention (CDC; www.cdc.gov) has invited providers to participate in a new performance evaluation program (HIV Rapid Testing MPEP) that offers the external evaluation of rapid tests for human immunodeficiency virus (e.g., OraQuick Rapid HIV-1 Antibody Test) and other licensed tests (e.g., MedMira Reveal Rapid HIV-1 Test).

Ultimate responsibility and control of POCT reside within the CLIA-certified laboratory and require a minimum of one laboratory staff member to be responsible for each POCT program. Written policies and procedures must be available to all laboratory personnel for patient preparation, specimen collection and preservation, instrument calibration, policies for QC and remedial actions, equipment performance evaluations, procedures for test performance, result report, and recording. The greatest source of error is **preanalytic** error, such as patient identification and specimen collection.

NON–INSTRUMENT-BASED TESTING

In immunology and serology testing, most POCT testing is done by manual rapid test methods, such as pregnancy testing. More rapid tests are being developed for the identification of infectious organisms, such as group A streptococci and HIV, in emergency rooms, in hospital settings, and even at home. Numerous POCT tests are referenced throughout this book in various chapters. The card pregnancy test is presented as an example in this chapter.

CASE STUDY

MM, a 28-year-old woman, has been trying to get pregnant for the last 6 months. Although she has no health problems, conceiving a child is proving to be difficult. She is considering fertility treatment. Her period is now 10 days late and she has been experiencing pain in her side. She performed an at-home pregnancy test but it was negative.

Questions
1. A false-negative hCG test can be the result of:
   a. hCG concentration being below the sensitivity threshold of the assay
   b. Delayed ovulation
   c. Delayed implantation
   d. All of the above
2. The earliest marker of fertilization is:
   a. Early pregnancy factor (EPF)
   b. hCG latex agglutination procedure
   c. Serum progesterone
   d. Serum estrogen

See Appendix A for the answers to these questions.

Critical Thinking Group Discussion Questions
1. Is a negative test result conclusive for the lack of conception?
2. Would a serum progesterone level be helpful in determining her status?

---

3. What is early pregnancy factor? Would it be helpful in establishing a diagnosis?

See Instructor site ⊖volve for the discussion of the answers to these questions.

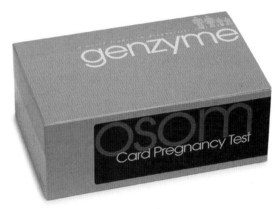

Figure 9-1   Pregnancy test kit, an example of POCT. *(From Turgeon ML: Linné & Ringsrud's clinical laboratory science, ed 6, St Louis, 2012, Mosby.)*

✚ Card Pregnancy Test*

Principle

The OSOM Card Pregnancy Test (Fig. 9-1) is a solid-phase, **sandwich-format**, **immunochromatographic** assay for the qualitative detection of **human chorionic gonadotropin (hCG)**.

Urine is added to the sample well and the sample migrates through reaction pads, where hCG, if present in the sample, binds to a **monoclonal** anti-hCG dye conjugate. The sample then migrates across a membrane toward the "results window," where the labeled hCG complex is captured at a test line region containing immobilized rabbit anti-hCG. Excess conjugate will flow past the test line region and will be captured at a control line region containing an immobilized antibody directed against the anti-hCG dye conjugate (with or without hCG complexed to it).

The appearance of two black bands in the results window, one at T (test) and the other at C (control), indicates the presence of hCG in the sample. If a detectable level of hCG is not present, only the control band will appear in the results window.

See ⊖volve website for the procedural protocol.

Reporting Results

Positive

Two separate black or gray bands, one at T and the other at C, are visible in the results window, indicating that the specimen contains detectable levels of hCG. Although the intensity of

---

*Adapted from product directional insert for Genzyme Diagnostics OSOM Card Pregnancy Test.

the test band may vary with different specimens, the appearance of two distinct bands should be interpreted as a positive result.

Negative

If no band appears at T and a black or gray band is visible at the C position, the test can be considered negative, indicating that a detectable level of hCG is not present.

Invalid

If no band appears at C or incomplete or beaded bands appear at the T or C position, the test is invalid. The test should be repeated using another OSOM Card Pregnancy Test device.

Note: The test is valid if the control line appears by the stated read time, regardless of whether the sample has migrated all the way to the end of the sample window.

Clinical Applications

Human CG is not normally detected in the urine specimens of healthy men and nonpregnant women.

In normal pregnancy, 20 mIU/mL hCG is reported to be present in urine 2 to 3 days before the first missed menstrual period. The levels of hCG continue to increase up to 200,000 mIU/mL at the end of the first trimester.

Limitations

- This assay is capable of detecting only whole-molecule (intact) hCG. It cannot detect the presence of free hCG subunits. Therefore, this test should only be used for the qualitative detection of hCG in urine for the early determination of pregnancy.
- For diagnostic purposes, hCG test results should always be used with other methods and in the context of the patient's clinical information (e.g., medical history, symptoms, results of other tests, clinical impression). An **ectopic pregnancy** cannot be distinguished from normal pregnancy by hCG measurements alone.
- If the hCG level is inconsistent with or unsupported by clinical evidence, results should also be confirmed by an alternative hCG method. Test results should be confirmed using a quantitative hCG assay before any critical medical procedure.
- Interfering substances may falsely depress or falsely elevate results. These interfering substances may cause false results over the entire range of the assay, not only at low levels, and may indicate the presence of hCG when there is none. As with any immunochemical reaction, unknown interferences from medications or endogenous substances may affect results.
- Infrequently, hCG levels may appear consistently elevated and could be caused by, but are not limited to, the following:
  - **Trophoblastic neoplasms** or **nontrophoblastic neoplasms.** These abnormal physiologic states may falsely elevate hCG levels and should not be diagnosed with this test.
  - Human CG–like substances.

- Because of the high degree of sensitivity of the assay, specimens tested as positive during the initial days after conception may later be negative because of natural termination of the pregnancy.
- Overall, natural termination occurs in 22% of clinically unrecognized pregnancies and 31% of other pregnancies. In the presence of weakly positive results, it is good laboratory practice to sample and test again after 48 hours.
- If the test band appears very faint, it is recommended that a new sample be collected 48 hours later and tested again using another OSOM Card Pregnancy Test device.
- Dilute urine specimens may not have representative levels of hCG.
- Detection of very low levels of hCG does not rule out pregnancy; low levels of hCG can occur in apparently healthy nonpregnant subjects. Additionally, postmenopausal specimens may elicit weak positive results because of low hCG levels unrelated to pregnancy. In a normal pregnancy, hCG values double approximately every 48 hours. Patients with very low levels of hCG should be sampled and tested again after 48 hours, or tested with an alternative method.
- Some antipsychotic drugs are known to cause false-positive results in pregnancy tests.

Cross-Reactivity

The addition of **luteinizing hormone** (300 mIU/mL of LH), **follicle-stimulating hormone** (FSH; 1000 mIU/mL of FSH), or thyroid-stimulating hormone (1000 µIU/mL of TSH) to negative urine serum specimens gives negative results in the OSOM Card Pregnancy Test.

The following substances were added to urine specimens containing 0 or 20 mIU/mL hCG. The substances at the concentrations listed below were not found to affect the performance of the test.

Interfering Substance	Concentration
Acetaminophen	20 mg/dL
Acetoacetic acid	2000 mg/dL
Acetylsalicylic acid	20 mg/dL
Amitriptyline	100 mg/dL
Amphetamines	10 µg/mL
Ascorbic acid	20 mg/dL
Atropine	20 mg/dL
Benzoylecgonine	10 mg/dL
Bilirubin	2 mg/dL
Caffeine	20 mg/dL
Cannabinol	10 mg/dL
Chlorpromazine	5 mg/dL
Codeine	10 mg/dL

Continued

Interfering Substance	Concentration
Desipramine	20 mg/dL
Diazepam	2 mg/dL
Ephedrine	20 mg/dL
Estradiol	25 ng/mL
Estriol	1 mg/dL
Ethanol	200 mg/dL
Gentisic acid	20 mg/dL
Glucose	2000 mg/dL
Hemoglobin	250 mg/dL
Human albumin	2000 mg/dL
β-Hydroxybutyrate	2000 mg/dL
Ibuprofen	40 mg/dL
Imipramine	100 mg/dL
Lithium	3.5 mg/dL
Methadone	10 mg/dL
Mesoridazine	1 mg/dL
Morphine	6 µg/mL
Nortriptyline	100 mg/dL
Phenobarbital	15 mg/dL
Phenylpropanolamine	20 mg/dL
Pregnanediol	1500 µg/dL
Progesterone	40 ng/mL
Proteins	2000 mg/dL
Salicylic acid	20 mg/dL
Tetracycline	20 mg/dL
Thioridazine	2 mg/dL

Adapted from OSOM Card Pregnancy Test, Philadelphia, 2007, Genzyme Diagnostics.

CHAPTER HIGHLIGHTS

- Point-of-care testing (POCT) involves laboratory assays performed near the patient and includes home test kits and handheld monitors.
- The major advantage of POCT is the rapidity of assay results; the major drawback is cost.
- Testing can be divided into waived, moderately complex, highly complex, and provider-performed microscopy tests. POCT is in the waived or moderately complex category.
- State and city governments may enact mandatory POCT regulations that are more stringent than federal regulations.
- Written POCT policies and procedures must be available to all laboratory personnel.
- The greatest source of POCT error is preanalytic errors.
- Most POCT is done by manual rapid tests (e.g., pregnancy testing).

REVIEW QUESTIONS

1. A major advantage of POCT is:
   a. Faster turnaround time
   b. Lower cost
   c. Better quality than traditional testing
   d. Both a and c

2. POCT assays are usually in the _____ CLIA category.
   a. Waived
   b. Provider-performed microscopy
   c. Moderately complex
   d. Highly complex

3. Over-the-counter test kits are in the _____ CLIA category.
   a. Waived
   b. Provider-performed microscopy
   c. Moderately complex
   d. Highly complex

4-7. Indicate whether each characteristic is true with the letter A or false with the letter B.

Important characteristics to consider when selecting a POCT kit are:

4. _____ Rapid turnaround time

5. _____ Easy to perform protocol

6. _____ Storage of temperature reagents

7. _____ Length of time until expiration

BIBLIOGRAPHY

Burtis CA, Ashwood ER, Bruns DB, editors: Tietz fundamentals of clinical chemistry, ed 6, St Louis, 2008, Saunders.

Kaplan LA, Pesce AJ: Clinical chemistry: theory, analysis, correlation, ed 5, St Louis, 2010, Mosby.

Joint Commission on Accreditation of Healthcare Organizations: 2005-2006, Comprehensive accreditation manual for laboratory and point-of-care testing, Oak Brook Terrace, Ill, 2005, Department of Communications Laboratory Accreditation Program, JCAHO.

National Committee for Clinical Laboratory Standards (NCCLS): Physician's office laboratory guidelines: tentative guidelines, ed 3, Villanova, Pa, 1995, NCCLS Document POL 1/2-T3 and POL 3-R.

Turgeon ML: Linné & Ringsrud's clinical laboratory science, ed 6, St Louis, 2012, Mosby.

CHAPTER 10

Agglutination Methods

Learning Objectives

At the conclusion of this chapter, the reader should be able to:

- Describe the principles of agglutination.
- Identify and compare the characteristics of agglutination methods.
- Explain methods for enhancing agglutination.
- Describe the characteristics of graded agglutination reactions.
- Discuss the principles of pregnancy testing, including sources of error.
- Analyze a case study.

- Correctly answer case study related multiple choice questions.
- Be prepared to participate in a discussion of critical thinking questions.
- Explain agglutination reactions of the ABO blood group procedure.
- Describe the principle and sources of error of the ABO blood group procedure.
- Correctly answer end of chapter review questions.

KEY TERMS

agglutination
antigenic determinants
antihuman globulin (AHG)
antisera
chimerism
coagglutination
conjugated
elution
flocculation tests

hemagglutination
human chorionic gonadotropin (hCG)
in vitro agglutination inhibition
isoagglutinins
lattice hypothesis
liposome-enhanced
postzone phenomenon
precipitation
precipitins

prozone phenomenon
pseudoagglutination
reagent
rouleaux formation
steric hindrance
zeta potential
zone of equivalence

PRINCIPLES OF AGGLUTINATION

Precipitation and agglutination are the visible expression of the aggregation of antigens and antibodies through the formation of a framework in which antigen particles or molecules alternate with antibody molecules (Fig. 10-1). **Precipitation** is the term for the aggregation of soluble test antigens. Precipitation is the combination of soluble antigen with soluble antibody to produce a visible insoluble complex. **Agglutination** is the process whereby specific antigens (e.g., red blood cells) aggregate to form larger visible clumps when the corresponding specific antibody is present in the serum.

Artificial carrier particles may be needed to indicate visibly that an antigen-antibody reaction has taken place; examples include latex particles and colloidal charcoal. Cells unrelated to the antigen, such as erythrocytes coated with antigen in a constant amount, can be used as biological carriers. Whole bacterial cells can contain an antigen that will bind with antibodies produced in response to that antigen when it is introduced into the host (Table 10-1).

The quality of test results depends on the following technical factors:

- Time of incubation with the antibody source (e.g., patient serum)

- Amount and avidity of an antigen **conjugated** to the carrier
- Conditions of the test environment (e.g., pH, protein concentration)

Agglutination tests are easy to perform and, in some cases, are the most sensitive tests currently available. It is important to note that quality results are dependent on the proper training of the person performing the assay and adherence to strict quality control regulations (e.g., positive and negative control sera). Agglutination-type tests have a wide range of applications in the clinical diagnosis of noninfectious immune disorders and infectious disease.

LATEX AGGLUTINATION

In latex agglutination procedures (Box 10-1), antibody molecules can be bound to the surface of latex beads. Many antibody molecules can be bound to each latex particle, increasing the potential number of exposed antigen-binding sites. If an antigen is present in a test specimen such as C-reactive protein, the antigen will bind to the combining sites of the antibody exposed on the surface of the latex beads, forming visible cross-linked aggregates of latex beads and antigen (Fig. 10-2). In some procedures (e.g., pregnancy testing, rubella antibody testing), latex particles can be coated with antigen. In the presence of serum antibodies, these particles agglutinate into large visible clumps.

Procedures based on latex agglutination must be performed under standardized conditions. The amount of antigen-antibody binding is influenced by factors such as pH, osmolarity, and ionic concentration of the solution. A variety of conditions can produce false-positive or false-negative reactions in agglutination testing (see Table 10-4).

Coagglutination and **liposome-enhanced** testing are variations of latex agglutination (Fig. 10-3). Coagglutination uses antibodies bound to a particle to enhance the visibility of agglutination. It is a highly specific method but may not be as sensitive as latex agglutination for detecting small quantities of antigen.

PREGNANCY TESTING

The principle of antigen and antibody interaction has been applied to pregnancy testing since the first agglutination tests were developed in the 1960s. These assays have replaced animal testing.

Human Chorionic Gonadotropin

Pregnancy tests are designed to detect minute amounts of **human chorionic gonadotropin (hCG)**, a glycoprotein hormone secreted by the trophoblast of the developing embryo that rapidly increases in the urine or serum during the early stages of pregnancy.

This glycoprotein hormone consists of two noncovalently linked subunits, alpha (α) and beta (β). The α unit is identical to that found in luteinizing hormone (LH), follicle-stimulating hormone (FSH), and thyroid-stimulating hormone (TSH). The β subunit has a unique carboxy-terminal region. Using antibodies made against the β subunit will cut down on

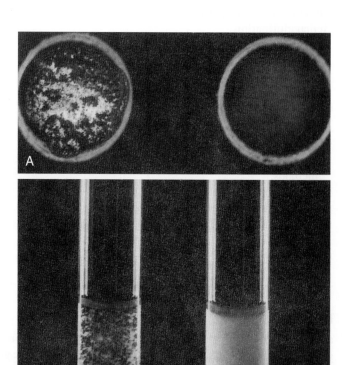

Figure 10-1 Agglutination patterns. A, Slide agglutination of bacteria with known antisera or known bacteria. *Left,* Positive reaction; *right,* negative reaction. **B,** Tube agglutination. *Left,* Positive reaction; *right,* negative reaction. *(From Barrett JT: Textbook of immunology, ed 5, St Louis, 1988, Mosby.)*

Table 10-1	Examples of Carriers		
Type (Reagent)	**Type of Assay**	**Principle**	**Result**
Latex particles	C-reactive protein (CRP)	A suspension of polystyrene latex particles of uniform size is coated with the IgG fraction of an antihuman CRP-specific serum.	If CRP is present in the serum, an antigen-antibody reaction takes place. This reaction causes a change in the uniform appearance of the latex suspension and a clear agglutination results.
Stabilized sheep erythrocytes sensitized with rabbit gamma globulin suspended in buffer solution	Rheumatoid factor (RF)	RF acts like antibodies against gamma globulin that acts as the antigen.	If gamma globulin is attached to a particular carrier (e.g., RBCs or latex particles), the reaction of RF with gamma globulin becomes a visible agglutination.

- C-reactive protein
- Immunoglobulin G rheumatoid factors
- Immunoglobulin M rheumatoid factors
- Rubella antibody

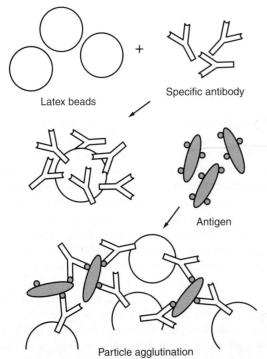

Figure 10-2   Alignment of antibody molecules bound to surface of a latex particle and latex agglutination reaction. *(Adapted from Forbes BA, Sahm DF, Weissfeld AS: Bailey and Scott's diagnostic microbiology, ed 12, St Louis, 2007, Mosby.)*

Latex beads

Specific antibody

Antigen

Particle agglutination

cross-reactivity with the other three hormones. Accordingly, many pregnancy test kits contain monoclonal antibody (MAb) directed against the β subunit to increase the specificity of the reaction.

For the first 6 to 8 weeks after conception, hCG helps maintain the corpus luteum and stimulate the production of progesterone. As a general rule, the level of hCG should double every 2 to 3 days. Pregnant women usually attain serum concentrations of 10 to 50 mIU/mL of hCG in the week after conception. If a test is negative at this stage, the test should be repeated within a week. Peak levels are reached approximately 2 to 3 months after the last menstrual period (LMP).

Agglutination Inhibition

The determination of **in vitro agglutination inhibition** depends on the incubation of the patient's specimen with anti-hCG, followed by the addition of latex particles coated with hCG. If hCG is present, it neutralizes the antibody; thus, no agglutination of latex particles is seen. If no hCG is present, agglutination occurs between the anti-hCG and hCG-coated latex particles.

Pregnancy Latex Slide Agglutination

Principle

The rapid, direct, monoclonal latex slide agglutination test for detection of hCG is based on the principle of agglutination between latex particles coated with anti-hCG antibodies and hCG, if present, in the test specimen.

See **evolve** for the procedural protocol.

Results

- Agglutination within 2 minutes represents a positive reaction.
- No agglutination represents a negative reaction.

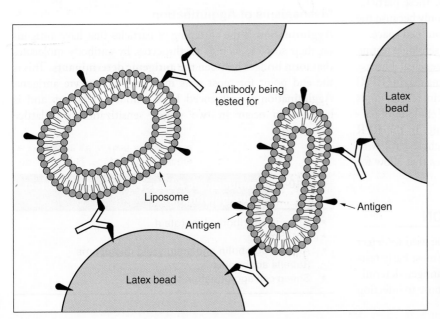

Antibody being tested for

Latex bead

Liposome

Antigen

Antigen

Latex bead

Figure 10-3 Diagram of liposome-enhanced latex agglutination reactions. *(Adapted from Neo-Planotest Ducoclox slide test, Organon Teknika, Durham, NC.)*

Technical Sources of Error

Reagents should never be expired; latex reagent must be well shaken and agglutination should be read within 3 minutes to avoid erroneous results caused by evaporation.

False-Positive Results

If a patient has been given an hCG injection (e.g., Pregnyl) to trigger ovulation or lengthen the luteal phase of the menstrual cycle, trace amounts can remain in the patient's system for as long as 10 days after the last injection. This will produce a false-positive result. Two consecutive quantitative hCG blood assays can circumvent this problem. If the hCG level increases by the second test, the patient is probably pregnant. Chorioepithelioma, hydatidiform mole, or excessive ingestion of aspirin may give false-positive results.

In men, a test identical to that used for pregnancy may be performed to detect the presence of a testicular tumor. If MAb against the β subunit is not used, other hormones with the same α unit may cross-react and cause a false-positive reaction.

False-Negative Results

Testing before reaching detectable levels of hCG will yield false-negative results.

Alternate Procedural Protocols

Latex agglutination slide tests have been replaced in many situations (e.g., home testing; see Chapter 9) by one-step chromatographic color-labeled immunoassays for the qualitative detection of hCG in urine (e.g., Clearview hCG II and Clearview hCG Easy, Wampole Laboratories, Princeton, NJ). Another variation is a one-step chromatographic color-labeled immunoassay for use with urine or serum (e.g., Wampole PreVue hCG Stick or Cassette, Status hCG).

FLOCCULATION TESTS

Flocculation tests for antibody detection are based on the interaction of soluble antigen with antibody, which results in the formation of a precipitate of fine particles. These particles are macroscopically or microscopically visible only because the precipitated product is forced to remain in a confined space.

Flocculation testing can be used in syphilis serologic testing (see Chapter 18). These tests are the classic Venereal Disease Research Laboratories (VDRL) and rapid plasma reagin (RPR) tests. In the VDRL test, an antibody-like protein, reagin, binds to the test antigen, cardiolipin-lecithin–coated cholesterol particles, and produces the particles that flocculate. In the RPR test, the antigen, cardiolipin-lecithin–coated cholesterol with choline chloride, also contains charcoal particles that allow for macroscopically visible flocculation.

DIRECT BACTERIAL AGGLUTINATION

Direct agglutination of whole pathogens can be used to detect antibodies directed against the pathogens. The most basic tests measure the antibody produced by the host to antigen determinants on the surface of a bacterial agent in response to infection with that bacterium. In a thick suspension of the bacteria, the binding of specific antibodies to surface antigens of the bacteria causes the bacteria to clump together in visible aggregates. This type of agglutination is called bacterial agglutination.

The formation of aggregates in solution is influenced by electrostatic and other forces; therefore, certain conditions are usually necessary for satisfactory results. The use of sterile physiologic saline with free positive ions in the agglutination procedure enhances the aggregation of bacteria because most bacterial surfaces exhibit a negative charge that causes them to repel each other. Because it allows more time for the antigen-antibody reaction, tube testing is considered more sensitive than slide testing. The small volume of liquid used in slide testing requires rapid reading before the liquid evaporates.

HEMAGGLUTINATION

The **hemagglutination** method of testing detects antibodies to erythrocyte antigens. The antibody-containing specimen can be serially diluted and a suspension of red blood cells (RBCs) added to the dilutions. If a sufficient concentration of antibody is present, the erythrocytes are cross-linked and agglutinated. If nonreacting antibody or an insufficient quantity of antibody is present, the erythrocytes will fail to agglutinate.

By binding different antigens to the RBC surface in indirect hemagglutination or passive hemagglutination (PHA), the hemagglutination technique can be extended to detect antibodies to antigens other than those present on the cells (Box 10-2). Chemicals such as chromic chloride, tannic acid, and glutaraldehyde can be used to cross-link antigens to the cells.

Some antibodies (e.g., immunoglobulin G [IgG]) do not directly agglutinate erythrocytes. This incomplete or blocking type of antibody may be detected by using an enhancement medium such as **antihuman globulin (AHG)** reagent (also known as Coombs reagent). If AHG reagent is added, this second antibody binds to the antibody present on the erythrocytes (see procedure in Chapter 26).

Mechanisms of Agglutination

Agglutination is the clumping of particles that have antigens on their surface, such as erythrocytes, by antibody molecules that form bridges between the **antigenic determinants**. This is the end point for most tests involving erythrocyte antigens. Agglutination is influenced by a number of factors and is believed to occur in two stages, sensitization and lattice formation.

Box 10-2	Immunologic Assays Performed by Indirect Hemagglutination

- Antinuclear ribonucleoprotein
- Anti-Sm
- Antithyroglobulin and antithyroid microsome
- Rubella antibodies
- Sheep cell agglutination titer

Sensitization

The first phase of agglutination, sensitization, represents the physical attachment of antibody molecules to antigens on the erythrocyte membrane. The combination of antigen and antibody is a reversible chemical reaction. Altering the physical conditions can result in the release of antibody from the antigen-binding site. When physical conditions are purposely manipulated to break the antigen-antibody complex, with subsequent release of the antibody into the surrounding medium, the procedure is referred to as an **elution.**

The amount of antibody that will react is affected by the equilibrium constant, or affinity constant, of the antibody. In most cases, the higher the equilibrium constant, the higher is the rate of association and the slower the rate of dissociation of antibody molecules. The degree of association between antigen and antibody is affected by a variety of factors and can be altered in some cases in vitro by altering some of the factors that influence antigen-antibody association, including the following:

- Particle charge
- Electrolyte concentration and viscosity
- Antibody type
- Antigen-to-antibody ratio
- Antigenic determinants
- Physical conditions (e.g., pH, temperature, duration of incubation)

Particle Charge. Inert particles such as latex, RBCs, and bacteria have a net negative surface charge called the **zeta potential** (Fig. 10-4). The concentration of salt in the reaction medium has an effect on antibody uptake by the membrane-bound erythrocyte antigens. Sodium (Na^+) and chloride (Cl^-) ions in a solution have a shielding effect. These ions cluster around and partially neutralize the opposite charges on antigen and antibody molecules, which hinders antibody-antigen association. By reducing the ionic strength of a reaction medium (e.g., using low ionic strength saline [LISS]), antibody uptake is enhanced. Charges can be overcome by centrifugation, addition of charged molecules (e.g., albumin, LISS), or enzyme pretreatment to permit the cross-linking that results in agglutination (Table 10-2).

Antibody Type. Immunoglobulin M (IgM) antibodies are more efficient at agglutination because their large size and multivalency permit more effective bridging of the space between cells caused by zeta potential. IgG antibodies are too small to overcome electrostatic forces between cells. The use of AHG forms cross-links between antibody molecules that have bound to the surface of RBCs. This promotes this formation of agglutination and allows for visual observation of an antigen-antibody reaction.

Antigen-Antibody Ratio. Under conditions of antibody excess, there is a surplus of molecular antigen-combining sites not bound to antigenic determinants. Precipitation reactions depend on a **zone of equivalence,** the zone in which optimum precipitation occurs, because the number of multivalent sites of antigens and antibodies are approximately equal. For a precipitation reaction to be detectable, the reaction must occur in the zone of equivalence. In this zone, each antibody or antigen

binds to more than one antigen or antibody, respectively, forming a stable lattice or network (see later). This **lattice hypothesis** is based on the assumptions that each antibody molecule must have at least two binding sites and that an antigen must be multivalent.

On either side of the zone of equivalence, precipitation is prevented because of an excess of antigen or antibody. If excessive antibody concentration is present, the phenomenon known as the **prozone phenomenon** occurs, which can result in a false-negative reaction. In this case, antigen combines with only one or two antibody molecules and no cross-linkages are formed. This phenomenon can be overcome by serially diluting the antibody-containing serum until optimum amounts of antigen and antibody are present in the test system.

If an excess of antigen occurs, the **postzone phenomenon** occurs, in which small aggregates (clumps) are surrounded by

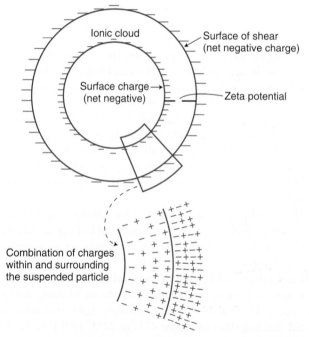

Figure 10-4 Zeta potential. Difference in electrostatic potential between net charge at cell membrane and charge at surface of shear. *(From Turgeon ML: Fundamentals of immunohematology, ed 2, Baltimore, 1995, Williams & Wilkins.)*

Table 10-2	Techniques to Reduce Zeta Potential	
Technique	**Action**
Enzyme pretreatment of red blood cells	Removes negatively charged sialic acid residues from cell surface membrane
Addition of colloids (e.g., albumin)	Increases electrical conductivity of environment
Centrifugation	Mechanical process to force red blood cells closer together

Adapted from Lehman CA: Saunders manual of clinical laboratory science, Philadelphia, 1998, WB Saunders, p 391.

excess antigen and no lattice formation is established. Excess antigen can block the presence of a small amount of antibody. To correct the postzone phenomenon, a repeat blood specimen should be collected 1 or more weeks later. If an active antibody reaction is occurring in vivo, the titer of antibody will increase and should be detectable. Repeated negative results generally suggest that the patient has the specific antibody being tested for by the procedure.

Antigenic Determinants. The placement and number of antigenic determinants both affect agglutination. For example, the A blood group antigen has more than 1.5 million sites/RBC, whereas the Kell blood group antigen has about 3500 to 6000 sites/RBC. If the number of antigenic sites is small or if the antigenic sites are buried deeply in the cell membranes, antibodies will be unable physically to contact antigenic sites.

Steric hindrance is an important physiochemical effect that influences antibody uptake by cell surface antigens. If dissimilar antibodies with approximately the same binding constant are directed against antigenic determinants located close to each other, the antibodies will compete for space in reaching their specific receptor sites. The effect of this competition can be mutual blocking, or steric hindrance, and neither antibody type will be bound to its respective antigenic determinant. Steric hindrance can occur whenever there is a conformational change in the relationship of an antigenic receptor site to the outside surface. In addition to antibody competition, competition with bound complement, other protein molecules, or the action of agents that interfere with the structural integrity of the cell surface can produce steric hindrance.

pH. The pH of the medium used for testing should be near physiologic conditions, or an optimum pH of 6.5 to 7.5. At a neutral pH, high electrolyte concentrations act to neutralize the net negative charge of particles.

Temperature and Length of Incubation. The optimum temperature needed to reach equilibrium in an antibody-antigen reaction differs for different antibodies. IgM antibodies are cold-reacting (thermal range, 4° C to 22° C [39° F to 72° F]), and IgG antibodies are warm-reacting, with an optimum temperature of reaction at 37° C (98.6° F).

The duration of incubation required to achieve maximum results depends on the rate of association and dissociation of each specific antibody. In laboratory testing, incubation times range from 15 to 60 minutes. The optimum time of incubation varies, depending on the class of immunoglobulin and how tightly an antibody attaches to its specific antigen.

Lattice Formation

Lattice formation, or the establishment of cross-links between sensitized particles (e.g., erythrocytes) and antibodies, resulting in aggregation, is a much slower process than the sensitization phase. The formation of chemical bonds and resultant lattice formation depend on the ability of a cell with attached antibody on its surface to come close enough to another cell to permit the antibody molecules to bridge the gap and combine with the antigen receptor site on the second cell. As antigens and antibodies combine, a multimolecular lattice increases in size until it precipitates out of solution as a solid particle. Cross-linking is influenced by factors such as the zeta potential.

Methods of Enhancing Agglutination

Techniques used to enhance agglutination include the following:
- Centrifugation
- Treatment with proteolytic enzymes
- Use of colloids
- AHG testing

Treatment with proteolytic enzymes and the use of colloids or AHG techniques could be applied in the immunology laboratory.

Centrifugation attempts to overcome the problem of distance by subjecting sensitized cells to a high gravitational force that counteracts the repulsive effect and physically forces the cells together.

Enzyme treatment alters the zeta potential or dielectric constant to enhance the chances of demonstrable agglutination. Mild proteolytic enzyme treatment can strip off some of the negative charges on the cell membrane by removing surface sialic acid residues (cleaving sialoglycoproteins from the cell surface), which reduces the surface charge of cells, lowers the zeta potential, and permits cells to come closer together for chemical linking by specific antibody molecules.

Some IgG antibodies will agglutinate if the zeta potential is carefully adjusted by the addition of colloids and salts.

In some cases, antigens may be so deeply embedded in the membrane surface that the previous techniques will not bring the antigens and antibodies close enough to cross-link. The AHG test is frequently incorporated into the protocol of many laboratory techniques to facilitate agglutination. The direct AHG test can be used to detect disorders such as hemolytic disease of the newborn, transfusion reactions, and differentiation of immunoglobulin from complement coating of erythrocytes.

Graded Agglutination Reactions

Observation of agglutination is initially made by gently shaking the test tube containing the serum and cells and viewing the lower portion, the button, with a magnifying glass as it is dispersed. Because agglutination is a reversible reaction, the test tube must be treated delicately, and hard shaking must be avoided; however, all the cells in the button must be resuspended before an accurate observation can be determined. Attention should also be given to whether discoloration of the fluid above the cells, the supernatant, is present. Rupture or hemolysis of erythrocytes is as important a finding as agglutination.

The strength of agglutination (Table 10-3; Fig. 10-5), called grading, uses a scale of 0, or negative (no agglutination), to 41 (all erythrocytes clumped). Table 10-4 describes false-positive and false-negative reactions. **Pseudoagglutination,** or the false appearance of clumping, may rarely occur because of **rouleaux formation.** Rouleaux formation can be encountered in

Table 10-3	**Grading Agglutination Reactions**
Grade	**Description**
Negative	No aggregates
Mixed field	A few isolated aggregates; mostly free-floating cells; supernatant appears red
Weak (±)	Tiny aggregates barely visible macroscopically; many free erythrocytes; turbid and reddish supernatant
1+	A few small aggregates just visible macroscopically; many free erythrocytes; turbid and reddish supernatant
2+	Medium-sized aggregates; some free erythrocytes; clear supernatant
3+	Several large aggregates; some free erythrocytes; clear supernatant
4+	All erythrocytes are combined into one solid aggregate; clear supernatant.

Table 10-4	**Causes of False-Positive and False-Negative Agglutination Test Reactions**	
Cause		**Correction**
False-Positive Reactions		
Contaminated equipment or reagents may cause particles to clump.		Store equipment and reagent in clean, dust-free environment, and handle with care. Use negative quality control (QC) steps.
Autoagglutination		Use a control with saline and no antibody as a negative control. If positive, patient's result is invalid.
Delay in reading slide reactions results in drying out of mixture.		Follow procedural directions and read reactions exactly as specified.
Overcentrifugation causes cells or particles to clump too tightly.		Calibrate centrifuge to proper speed and time.
False-Negative Reactions		
Inadequate washing of red blood cells in antihuman globulin (AHG) testing* may result in unbound immunoglobulins neutralizing the reagent.		Wash cells according to directions. Use positive and negative QC steps.
Failure to add AHG reagent		Use positive QC steps.
Contaminated or expired reagents		Use positive and negative QC steps.
Improper incubation		Follow procedural protocol exactly. Use positive and negative QC steps.
Delay in reading slide reactions		Follow procedural protocol exactly. Use positive and negative control steps.
Undercentrifugation		Calibrate centrifuge to proper speed and time.
Prozone phenomenon		Dilute patient serum containing antibody, and repeat the procedure.

*See Chapter 26.

patients with high or abnormal types of globulins in their blood, such as in multiple myeloma or after receiving dextran as a plasma expander. On microscopic examination, the erythrocytes appear as rolls resembling stacks of coins. To disperse the pseudoagglutination, a few drops of physiologic NaCl (saline) can be added to the reaction tube, remixed, and reexamined. This procedure, saline replacement, should be performed carefully after pseudoagglutination is suspected. It should never be done before the initial testing protocol is followed; a false-negative result may occur from the dilutional effect of the saline.

Microplate Agglutination Reactions

Serologic testing has usually been performed by slide or test tube techniques, but the increased emphasis on cost containment has stimulated interest in microtechniques as an alternative to conventional methods. Micromethods for RBC antigen and antibody testing include hemagglutination and solid-phase adherence assays. These methods are also considered to be easier to perform. The use of microplates allows for the performance of a large number of tests on a single plate, which eliminates time-consuming steps such as labeling test tubes.

A microplate is a compact plate of rigid or flexible plastic with multiple wells. The wells may be U-shaped or have a flat bottom configuration. The U-shaped well has been used most often in immunohematology. The volume capacity of each well is approximately 0.2 mL, which prevents spilling during mixing. Samples and reagents are dispensed with small-bore Pasteur pipettes. These pipettes are recommended because they deliver 0.025 mL, which prevents splashing. After the specimens and reagents are added to the wells, they are mixed by gentle agitation of the plates. The microplate is then centrifuged for an immediate reading.

Countertop or floor model centrifuges are suitable if they are equipped with special rotors that can accommodate microplate centrifuge carriers and are capable of speeds of 400 to 2000 rpm. Smaller plates can be centrifuged in serologic centrifuges with an appropriate adapter.

After centrifugation, the cell buttons are resuspended by gently tapping the microplate or by using a flat-topped

READING AGGLUTINATION

GRADE	DESCRIPTION		APPEARANCE	
	Cells	Supernate	Macroscopic*	Microscopic†
0	No agglutinates	Dark, turbid, homogeneous	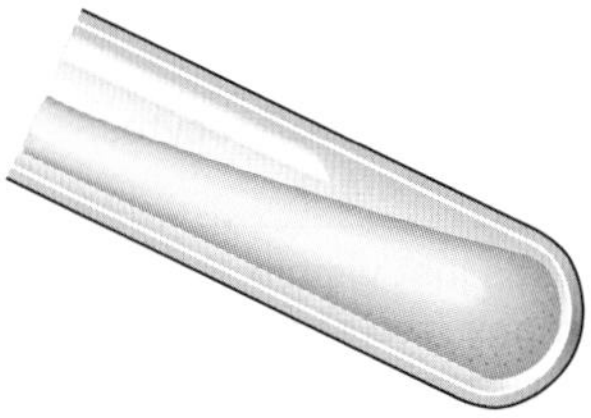	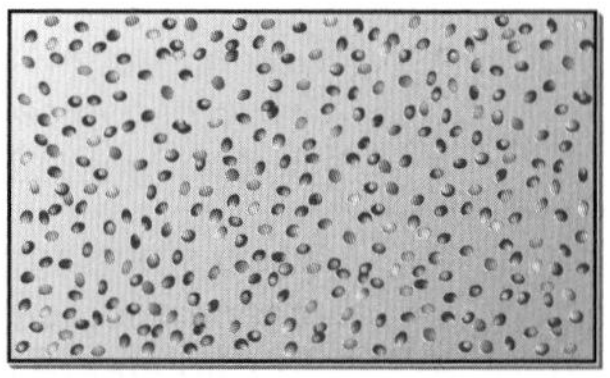
w+	Many tiny agglutinates Many free cells May not be visible without microscope	Dark, turbid	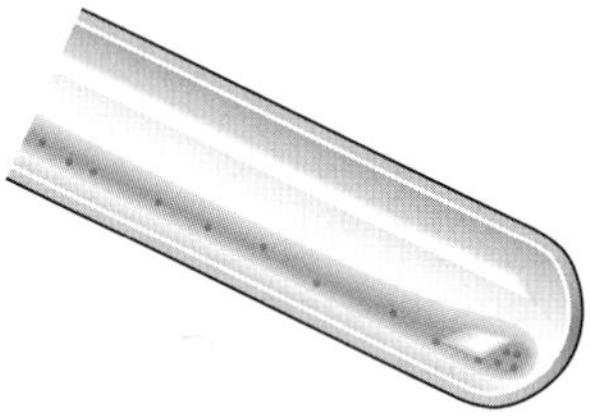	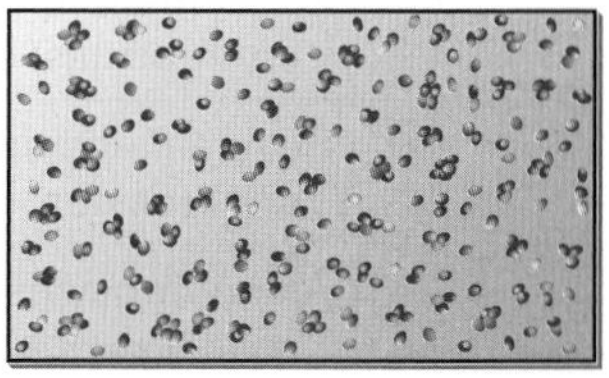
1+	Many small agglutinates Many free cells	Turbid	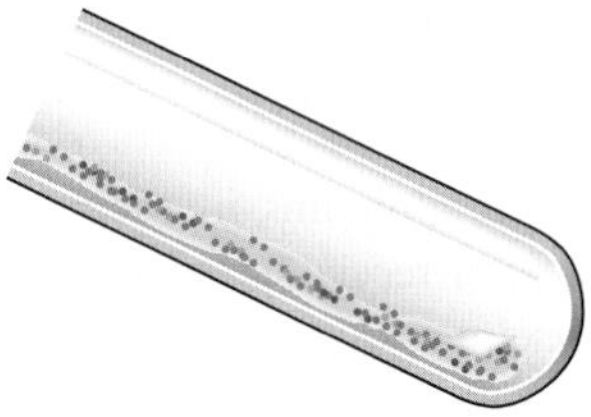	
2+	Many medium-sized agglutinates Moderate number of free cells	Clear	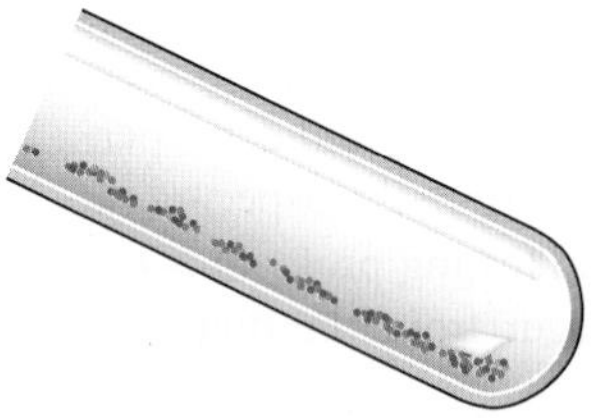	
3+	Several large agglutinates Few free cells	Clear	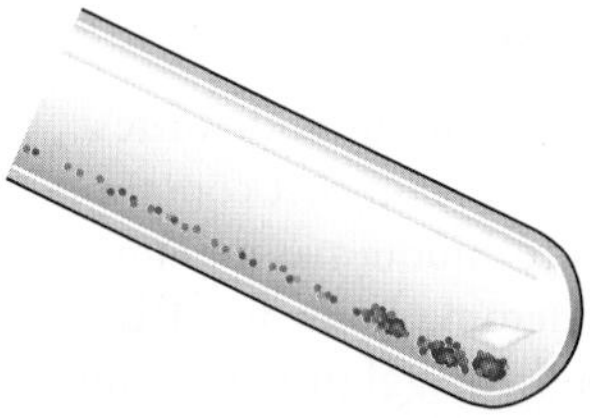	
4+	One large, solid agglutinate No free cells	Clear	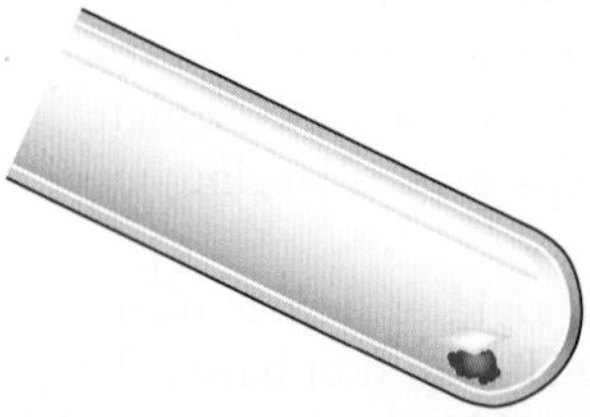	

*For any one grade, readings can be on a scale from weak+ to strong+ (e.g., grade 2 can be scored as 2+w, 2+, or 2+s, depending on the number and size of agglutinates).
†Microscopic readings are generally performed to differentiate pseudoagglutination (rouleaux) from true agglutination, to detect mixed-field reactions, and to confirm a negative reaction.

Figure 10-5   Reading red blood cell agglutination reactions. *(From Lehman CA: Saunders manual of clinical laboratory science, Philadelphia, 1998, Saunders, pp 394-395.)*

mechanical shaker. A shaker provides a more consistent and standard resuspension of the cells than manual tapping. After the cells are resuspended, the wells are examined with an optical aid or over a well-lit surface. A positive reaction will settle in a diffuse uneven button; negative reactions are manifested by a smooth compact button. Detection of weakly positive reactions is enhanced by allowing the RBCs to settle.

CASE STUDY

JR, an 85-year-old man, has a discrepancy between his forward grouping (ABO antigens) and reverse grouping (ABO antibodies).

ABO Testing Results

	Patient RBCs	Patient Serum
Anti-A typing sera	Negative	
Anti-B typing sera	Negative	
A1 RBCs		2+
B RBCs		Negative

Questions
1. The discrepancy between ABO antigen and antibody (forward and reverse testing) can be caused by:
   a. Too much A antigen on RBCs
   b. Too much B antigen on RBCs
   c. False positive antibody to A antigen
   d. False negative antibody to B antigen
2. The cause of the discrepancy between this patient's ABO antigen and antibody testing can be due to:
   a. Deteriorated regent RBCs
   b. Hypogammaglobulinemia
   c. Age of the patient
   d. All of the above

See Appendix A for the answers to these questions.

Critical Thinking Group Discussion Questions
1. What is the most likely cause of the discrepancy between ABO antigens and antibodies in this patient?
2. How can the discrepancy be resolved?

See instructor site ⊖volve for the discussion of the answers to these questions.

⠿ ABO Blood Grouping (Reverse Grouping)

Principle

The reverse (serum) typing procedure to confirm ABO blood grouping is based on the presence or absence of the antibodies,

anti-A and anti-B, in serum. If these antibodies are present in serum, agglutination should be demonstrated when the serum is combined with reagent erythrocytes expressing A or B antigens.

Reverse typing is a cross-check for forward typing (see Chapter 2 procedure). Because of the lack of synthesized immunoglobulins in newborn and very young infants, this procedure is not performed on specimens from these patients.

See ⊖volve for the procedural protocol.

Reporting Results

Agglutination indicates that an antibody specific for the A or B antigen is present in the serum or plasma being tested. Grade all positive reactions.

Reactions of Patient Serum and Reagent Erythrocytes

A1 Cells	B Cells	Antibody	Blood Group
+	+	Anti-A and anti-B	O
0	+	Anti-B	A
+	0	Anti-A	B
0	0	Neither	AB

Procedure Notes

A hemolyzed specimen is unsuitable for this test. As in forward typing, testing must be conducted at room temperature or colder. If the expected results of both forward and reverse typing are not demonstrated, a variation in the patient or a technical error may exist.

Biological Sources of Error

If a patient has been recently transfused with non–group-specific blood, mixed-field agglutination may be observed. If large quantities of non–group-specific blood have been transfused, determination of the correct ABO grouping may be impossible.

Discrepancies in forward typing can result from conditions such as weak antigens, altered expression of antigens caused by disease, **chimerism,** or excessive blood group substances. Excess amounts of blood group–specific soluble substances present in the plasma in certain disorders (e.g., carcinoma of stomach or pancreas) neutralize the reagent anti-A or anti-B, leaving no unbound antibody to react with the patient's erythrocytes. This excess of blood group–specific substance produces a false-negative or weak reaction in the forward grouping. If the patient's erythrocytes are washed with saline, the substance should be removed and a correct grouping can be observed.

Incorrect typing can also result from additional antigens, caused by the following:
- Polyagglutinable RBCs
- Acquired B-like antigen; acquired A-like antigen
- Complexes attached to RBCs
- Agents causing nonspecific erythrocyte agglutination

- Antibody-sensitized RBCs: effect of colloids and antiantibodies (e.g., hemolytic disease of the newborn, incompatible transfusion, autoimmune process)

Discrepancies in serum (reverse) grouping can result from additional or missing antibodies caused by the following:

- Passively acquired **isoagglutinins**
- Alloantibodies
- Rouleaux formation
- Auto–anti-I; iso–anti-I
- Anti-A1 in Ax, A2, and A2B blood
- Anti-H in A1B, A1, B, and Bombay blood
- Anti-IA and IA

Causes of weak or missing antibodies include the following:

- Deteriorated reagent erythrocytes
- Hypogammaglobulinemic
- **Elderly** patients
- Newborn infants
- Chimerism
- Rare variants of A or B

Technical Sources of Error

Each manufacturer provides, with each package of antiserum, detailed instructions for the use of anti-A and anti-B. Because the details vary, it is important to follow the directions for the specific antiserum in use.

Procedures that apply to all tests for ABO grouping include the following:

1. Do not rely on the color of dyes to identify reagent **antisera.** All tubes must be properly labeled.
2. Do not perform tests at temperatures higher than room temperature (20° C to 24° C [68° F to 75° F]).
3. Perform observations of agglutination with a well-lit background, not a warm view box.
4. Record results immediately after observation.
5. Remember that contaminated blood specimens, reagents, or supplies may interfere with the test results.

Limitations

Antisera prepared from human sources are capable of detecting A1 and A2 groups. Except in the case of newborn and very young infants, a reverse cell typing should also be performed to verify the results of forward typing.

CHAPTER HIGHLIGHTS

- Agglutination of particles to which soluble antigen has been adsorbed is a serum method of demonstrating **precipitins.** Examples of artificial carriers include latex particles and colloidal charcoal. Cells unrelated to the antigen, such as erythrocytes coated with antigen in a constant amount, can be used as biological carriers.
- In latex agglutination procedures, antibody molecules can be bound to the surface of latex beads. If an antigen is present in a test specimen, the antigen will bind to the combining sites of the antibody exposed on the surface of the latex beads, forming visible cross-linked aggregates of latex beads and antigen.

- Flocculation tests for antibody detection are based on the interaction of soluble antigen with antibody, which results in the formation of a precipitate of fine particles.
- Direct bacterial agglutination can be used to detect antibodies directed against pathogens.

REVIEW QUESTIONS

1. The quality of test results in an agglutination reaction depends on all the following except:
   a. Duration of incubation
   b. Amount of antigen conjugated to the carrier
   c. Avidity of antigen conjugated to the carrier
   d. Whether the carrier is artificial or biological

2. Flocculation procedures differ from latex agglutination procedures because:
   a. Antigen is bound to a carrier.
   b. Antibody is bound to a carrier.
   c. Soluble antigen reacts with antibody.
   d. Flocculation procedures are only qualitative.

3. In the hemagglutination technique, antihuman globulin is used as an enhancement medium to detect _____ antibodies.
   a. IgM
   b. IgG
   c. IgD
   d. IgE

4. The prozone phenomenon can result in a (an):
   a. False-positive reaction
   b. False-negative reaction
   c. Enhanced agglutination
   d. Diminished antigen response

5. The effect of competing antibodies seeking to attach to antigen sites is called:
   a. Prozone phenomenon
   b. Ionic strength
   c. Steric hindrance
   d. Sensitization

6. All the following are methods that can be used to enhance the agglutination of IgG antibodies except:
   a. Centrifugation
   b. Treatment with proteolytic enzymes
   c. Acidifying the mixture
   d. Using colloids

7-10. Match the following grades of agglutination with the appropriate description.

7. _b_ Mixed field

8. _d_ 1+

9. _c_ 2+

10. _a_ 4+
   a. All the erythrocytes are combined into one solid aggregate; clear supernatant.

b.   Few isolated aggregates; supernatant appears red.

c.   Medium-sized aggregates; clear supernatant

d.   A few small aggregates; turbid and reddish supernatant

e.   Several large aggregates; clear supernatant

11. A classic technique for the detection of viral antibodies is:
a.   Passive hemagglutination
b.   Indirect hemagglutination
c.   Hemagglutination inhibition
d.   Latex particle agglutination

12-16. Match each term to its definition.

12. _b_   Precipitation

13. _a_   Agglutination

14. _c_   Coagglutination

15. _e_   Flocculation

16. _d_   Hemagglutination
a.   Aggregation of particulate test antigens
b.   Aggregation of soluble test antigens
c.   Uses antibodies bound to a particle to enhance visibility of agglutination
d.   Agglutination of erythrocytes in tests for antibody detection
e.   Based on the interaction of soluble antigen with antibody, resulting in formation of a precipitate of fine particles

17. Artificial or biological carriers that can be used in an agglutination reaction include:
a.   Latex particles
b.   Colloidal charcoal
c.   Erythrocytes coated with antigen in a constant amount
d.   All of the above

18. and 19. Identify the components (a and b) of a latex agglutination reaction in the figure.

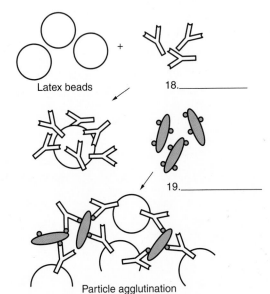

Latex beads   +   18._____

19._____

Particle agglutination

(Adapted from Forbes BA, Sahm DF, Weissfeld AS: Bailey and Scott's diagnostic microbiology, ed 12, St Louis, 2007, Mosby.)

a.   Antigen
b.   Specific antibody

20. Sensitization:
a.   Is the first phase of agglutination
b.   Represents the physical attachment of antibody molecules to antigens on the RBC membrane
c.   Is an irreversible reaction
d.   Both a and b

21. Agglutination can be used to enhance reactions by all the following means except:
a.   Decreasing ionic strength of the reaction
b.   Centrifugation
c.   Increasing pH of the reaction
d.   Using colloids and antihuman globulin

22-24. Match each grade of agglutination with its respective description.

22. _____ Negative

23. _____ Weak (1+ or 2+)

24. _____ 3+
a.   Tiny aggregates that are barely visible macroscopically
b.   Several large aggregates
c.   All erythrocytes combined into one solid aggregate
d.   No aggregates

25. All the following statements are correct regarding human pregnancy testing except:
a.   Tests detect human chorionic gonadotropin (hCG).
b.   The hCG is secreted by the trophoblast of the developing embryo.
c.   The presence of hCG rapidly increases in urine or serum.
d.   The presence of hCG in maternal urine or serum persists throughout pregnancy.

26. All the following statements are correct regarding hCG except:
a.   It helps maintain the corpus luteum.
b.   It stimulates production of progesterone.
c.   It is detectable within 102 hours after the last expected menstrual period.
d.   It reaches peak levels at 2 to 3 months after the last menstrual period.

27. The most common laboratory method for detecting hCG is:
a.   Latex agglutination
b.   Enzyme-linked immunosorbent assay
c.   Immunofluorescence
d.   Antibody titration

28. In the latex agglutination method for the detection of hCG, no agglutination indicates the:
a.   Absence of hCG
b.   Presence of hCG
c.   Absence of hCG, a positive test
d.   Presence of hCG, a negative test

29. A urine specimen for pregnancy testing _____ be frozen.
    a. May
    b. May not

30. A false-positive reaction in a latex agglutination test for hCG can be caused by all the following except:
    a. Chorioepithelioma
    b. Hydatidiform mole
    c. Taking oral contraceptives
    d. Excessive ingestion of aspirin

BIBLIOGRAPHY

Aloisi RM: Principles of immunology and immunodiagnostics, Philadelphia, 1988, Lea & Febiger.

Baines W, Noble P: Sensitivity limits of latex agglutination tests, Am Clin Lab 12:14–18, 1993.

Forbes BA, Sahm DF, Weissfeld AS: Bailey and Scott's diagnostic microbiology, ed 12, St Louis, 2007, Mosby.

Kaplan LA, Pesce AJ, Kazmierczak SC: Clinical chemistry: theory, analysis, correlation, ed 5, St Louis, 2010, Mosby.

Lehman CA: Saunders manual of clinical laboratory science, Philadelphia, 1988, WB Saunders.

Mahon CR, Lehman DC, Manuselis G: Textbook of diagnostic microbiology, ed 4, St Louis, 2011, Mosby.

McPherson RA, Pincus MR: Henry's clinical diagnosis and management by laboratory methods, ed 22, Philadelphia, 2012, Saunders.

Turgeon ML: Fundamentals of immunohematology, ed 2, Baltimore, 1998, Williams & Wilkins.

CHAPTER 11

Electrophoresis Techniques

Learning Objectives

At the conclusion of this chapter, the reader should be able to:
- Define the term *electrophoresis*.
- Describe the electrophoresis technique.
- Identify the fractions into which serum proteins can be divided by electrophoresis.
- Describe the characteristics of immunoelectrophoresis.
- Explain the features of immunofixation electrophoresis.
- Discuss the clinical applications of immunoelectrophoresis.
- Compare immunoelectrophoresis and immunofixation electrophoresis.
- Compare capillary electrophoresis and microchip capillary electrophoresis.

- Describe two electrophoresis separation methods.
- Analyze a case study related to the results of serum protein electrophoresis.
- Correctly answer case study related multiple choice questions.
- Be prepared to participate in a discussion of critical thinking questions.
- Describe the principle of the immunofixation electrophoresis procedure.
- Correctly answer end of chapter review questions.

Key Terms

antigen-antibody precipitin arcs
Bence Jones (BJ) protein
circulating immune complexes
cryoglobulinemia
double immunodiffusion systems
dysgammaglobulinemias
electrophoresis
immunodiffusion
immunoelectrophoresis (IEP)

immunofixation
immunofixation electrophoresis (IFE)
isoelectric focusing
M protein
macroglobulinemia
monoclonal gammopathy
monoclonal protein
monovalent antiserum
multiple myeloma

paraprotein
polyclonal gammopathy
polyvalent antiserum
precipitin lines
prozone phenomenon
pyroglobulinemia
zone electrophoresis

ELECTROPHORESIS

Electrophoresis is the migration of charged solutes or particles in an electrical field. Using this principle, charged molecules can be made to move and different molecules can be separated if they have different velocities in an electrical field.

The electrical field is applied to a solution with oppositely charged electrodes. Charged particles in this solution begin to migrate. Positively charged particles (cations) move to the negatively charged (−) electrode; negatively charged particles (anions) migrate to the positively charged (+) electrode (Fig. 11-1).

Serum proteins are often separated by electrophoresis. Serum electrophoresis results in the separation of proteins into five fractions using cellulose acetate as a support medium (Fig. 11-2). This separation is based on the rate of migration of these individual components in an electrical field.

Electrophoresis is a versatile analytic technique. Immunoglobulins are separated by electrophoresis using agarose as a support medium. The immunologic applications of electrophoresis include identification of monoclonal proteins in serum or urine, immunoelectrophoresis, and various blotting techniques (see Chapter 14).

IMMUNOELECTROPHORESIS

Immunoelectrophoresis (IEP) involves the electrophoresis of serum or urine followed by immunodiffusion.

Passive Immunodiffusion Procedures

Immunodiffusion is a laboratory method for the quantitative study of antibodies (e.g., radial immunodiffusion [RID]) and rocket electrophoresis or for identifying antigens (e.g., Ouchterlony technique). Single diffusion preceded radial immunodiffusion. In the single diffusion procedure, antigen was layered on top of a gel medium and, as the antigen moved

down into the gel, precipitation occurred and migrated down a tube in proportion to the amount of antigen present. In radial immunodiffusion (RID) (Fig. 11-3), antibody is uniformly distributed in the gel medium and antigen is added to a well cut into the gel. As the antigen diffuses from the well, the antigen-antibody combination occurs in changing proportions until the zone of equivalence is reached and a stable lattice network is formed in the gel. The area of the visible ring is compared with standard concentrations of antigens. A variation of this principle is rocket immunoelectrophoresis (Fig. 11-4).

The classic Ouchterlony double diffusion technique (Fig. 11-5). performed on a gel medium is used to detect the presence of antibodies and determine their specificity by visualization of lines of identity, or precipitin lines. The reaction of antigen-antibody combination occurs by means of diffusion. The size and position of precipitin bands provide information regarding equivalence or antibody excess. Proteins are differentiated not only by their electrophoretic mobility, but also by their diffusion coefficient and antibody specificity. Although double immunodiffusion produces a separate precipitation band for each antigen-antibody system in a mixture, it is often difficult to determine all the components in a complex mixture.

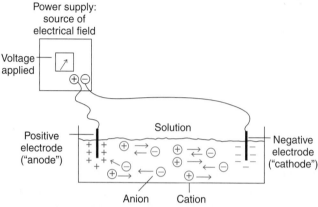

Figure 11-1   Application of electrical field to a solution of ions makes the ions move. *(From Kaplan LA, Pesce AJ: Clinical chemistry: theory, analysis, correlation, ed 5, St Louis, 2010, Mosby.)*

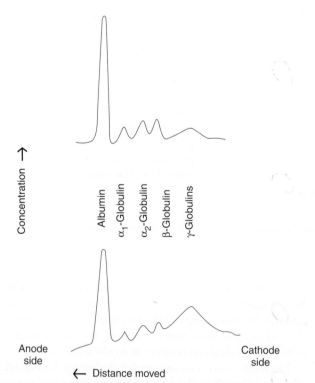

Figure 11-2   Example of the effect of disease (hepatic cirrhosis) on serum protein electrophoresis pattern. *Upper profile,* Distribution characteristic of healthy people. *(From Kaplan LA, Pesce AJ: Clinical chemistry: theory, analysis, correlation, ed 5, St Louis, 2010, Mosby.)*

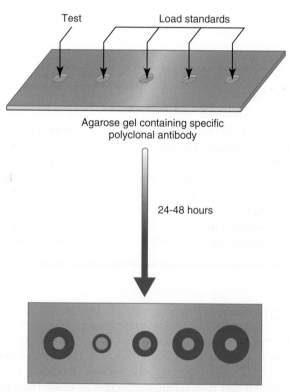

Figure 11-3   Measurement of immune-related proteins by a radial immunodiffusion. *(From Peakman M, Vergani D: Basic and clinical immunology, ed 2, Edinburgh, 2009, Churchill Livingstone.)*

Principle

Immunoelectrophoresis is a combination of the techniques of electrophoresis and double immunodiffusion. IEP separates the antigen mixture by electrophoresis before performing immunodiffusion. In the first phase, electrophoresis, serum is placed in an appropriate medium (e.g., cellulose acetate or agarose) and then electrophoresed to separate its constituents according to their electrophoretic mobility—albumin; α_1-, α_2-, β-, and γ-globulin fractions

After electrophoresis, in the second phase, immunodiffusion, the fractions are allowed to act as antigens and to interact with their corresponding antibodies. Antiserum (polyvalent or monovalent) is deposited in a trough cut into the gel to one side and parallel to the line of separated proteins. Incubation allows double immunodiffusion of the antigens and antibodies. Each antiserum diffuses outward, perpendicular to the trough, and each serum protein diffuses outward from its point of electrophoresis. When a favorable antigen-to-antibody ratio exists (equivalence), the antigen-antibody complex becomes visible as precipitin lines or bands. Diffusion is halted by rinsing the plate in 0.85% saline. Unbound protein is washed from the agarose with saline and the **antigen-antibody precipitin arcs** are stained with a protein-sensitive stain.

Each line represents one specific protein (Fig. 11-6). Proteins are thus differentiated by their diffusion coefficient and antibody specificity as well as electrophoretic mobility. Antibody diffuses as a uniform band parallel to the antibody trough. If the proteins are homogeneous or of like composition, the antigen diffuses in a circle and the antigen-antibody precipitation line resembles a segment, or arc, of a circle. If the antigen is heterogeneous or not uniform in composition, the antigen-antibody line assumes an elliptical shape. One arc of precipitation forms for each constituent in the antigen mixture. This technique can be used to resolve the protein of normal serum into 25 to 40 distinct precipitation bands. The exact number depends on the strength and specificity of the antiserum used.

Normal Appearance of Precipitin Bands

Immunoprecipitation bands should be of normal curvature, symmetry, length, position, intensity, and distance from the antigen well and antibody trough. In normal serum, immunoglobulin G (IgG), IgA, and IgM are present in sufficient concentrations of 10 mg/mL, 2 mg/mL, and 1 mg/mL, respectively, to produce precipitin lines. The normal concentrations of IgD and IgE are too low to be detected by IEP.

A normal IgG precipitin band is elongated, elliptical, slightly curved, and clearly visible in undiluted serum and 1:10 diluted serum. An IgG band is located cathodic to the antigen well in the alpha (α) area of the electrophoretogram. If monospecific serum is used, it is fused with a thin precipitin line positioned midway between the antigen well and antibody trough and extending into the beta (β) area. The IgM and IgA bands are visible in undiluted serum but disappear at a 1:10 dilution of serum. The IgA band is a flattened, thin arc, slightly cathodic to the well in the α-β position. The IgM line is a barely visible thin line, slightly cathodic to the antigen well.

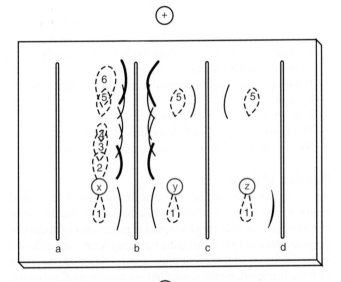

Figure 11-4 Configuration for immunoelectrophoresis. Sample wells are punched in the agar-agarose, sample is applied, and electrophoresis is carried out to separate the proteins in the sample. Antiserum is loaded into the troughs and the gel is incubated in a moist chamber at 4° C (39° F) for 24 to 72 hours. Track *x* represents the shape of the protein zones after electrophoresis; tracks *y* and *z* show the reaction of proteins *5* and *1* with their specific antisera in troughs *c* and *d*. Antiserum against proteins *1* through *6* is present in trough *b*. *(From Burtis CA, Ashwood ER, Bruns DB: Tietz fundamentals of clinical chemistry, ed 6, St Louis, 2008, Saunders.)*

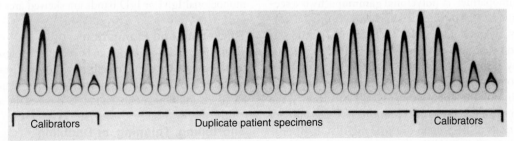

Figure 11-5 Rocket immunoelectrophoresis of human serum albumin. Patient samples were applied in duplicate. Calibrators were placed at opposite ends of the plate. *(From Burtis CA, Ashwood ER, Bruns DB: Tietz fundamentals of clinical chemistry, ed 6, St Louis, 2008, Saunders.)*

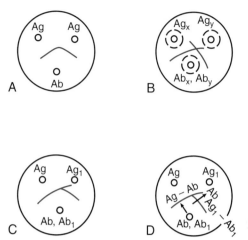

Figure 11-6 Double immunodiffusion in two dimensions by the Ouchterlony technique. A, Reaction of identity. **B,** Reaction of non-identity. **C,** Reaction of partial identity. **D,** Scheme for spur formation. *Ab,* Antibody; *Ag,* antigen. *(From Burtis CA, Ashwood ER, Bruns DB: Tietz fundamentals of clinical chemistry, ed 6, St. Louis, 2008, Saunders.)*

Clinical Applications

Immunoelectrophoresis is most often used to determine qualitatively the elevation or deficiency of specific classes of immunoglobulins. Also, IEP is a reliable and accurate method for detecting structural abnormalities and concentration changes in proteins. It is possible to identify the absence of a normal serum protein (e.g., congenital deficiency of complement component) or alterations in serum proteins. This method can be used to screen for circulating immune complexes, characterize **cryoglobulinemia** and **pyroglobulinemia,** and recognize and characterize antibody syndromes and the various **dysgammaglobulinemias.**

The most common application of IEP is in the diagnosis of a **monoclonal gammopathy,** a condition in which a single clone of plasma cells produces elevated levels of a single class and type of immunoglobulin. The elevated immunoglobulin is referred to as a **monoclonal protein, M protein,** or **paraprotein.** Monoclonal gammopathies may indicate a malignancy such as **multiple myeloma** or **macroglobulinemia.** Antikappa (anti-κ) and antilambda (anti-λ) antisera are necessary for complete typing of the immunoglobulin in the evaluation of the ratio and for the diagnosis of M proteins. The class (heavy [H] chain) and type (light [L] chain) must be established because a patient's prognosis and treatment may differ, depending on the immunoglobulin identified.

Differentiation must also be made between monoclonal and polyclonal gammopathies. A **polyclonal gammopathy** is a secondary condition caused by disorders such as liver disease, collagen disorders, rheumatoid arthritis, and chronic infection. It is characterized by elevation of two or more (often all) immunoglobulins by several clones of plasma cells. Polyclonal increases of proteins are usually twice the normal levels.

The most important application of IEP of urine is the demonstration of **Bence Jones (BJ) protein.** IEP detects very low concentrations of BJ protein (≈1 to 2 mg/dL). If BJ protein is present in a urine specimen, **precipitin lines** will form with κ or λ anti–L chain antisera because BJ protein is

composed of homogeneous L chains of a single antigen type, either κ or λ. Normal L chains are heterogeneous and include equal concentrations of κ and λ.

Sources of Error

The **prozone phenomenon** is an incomplete precipitin reaction caused by antigen excess (antigen-to-antibody ratio too high). Prozoning should be suspected if a precipitin arc appears to run into a trough, if an L chain appears fuzzy when an H chain is increased, or if an arc appears to be incomplete.

Abnormal Appearance of Precipitin Bands

The size and position of precipitin bands provide the same type of information regarding equivalence or antigen-antibody excess as **double immunodiffusion systems.** The position and shape of precipitin bands in the IEP assay of serum are relatively stable and reproducible; almost any deviation is abnormal (Fig. 11-7). These abnormalities can be detected by evaluating the following features of the precipitin bands:

- Position of the band in relation to electrophoretically identified protein fractions
- Position of the band between the antigen well and antibody trough
- Distortion of the curvature or arc formation
- Thickening (density) and elongation of a band
- Shortening (inhibition), thinning, or doubling of a band

Position of Band

The precipitin band may be displaced compared with its normal position in the control serum because molecular charges in the abnormal protein may affect its speed of migration in the electrophoresis phase of IEP. A precipitin band may form a line of fusion or partial fusion with another protein, indicating the presence of proteins immunologically similar but electrophoretically distinct.

A distinct abnormality in the position of the band is seen in cases of monoclonal IgA gammopathy. The monoclonal IgA band is closer to the antibody trough than normal IgA.

Distortion of Curvature or Arc

An abnormal curvature of the precipitin band can be observed with M proteins because of an antigen excess. The monoclonal IgG band shows an arc of a circle rather than the elongated elliptical shape of a normal band. This distortion of IgG reflects its homogeneous nature and limited electrophoretic mobility of the abnormal protein.

Normal IgM and IgD bands are hardly visible, but the monoclonal IgM or IgD bands are skewed arcs of a circle.

Thickening and Elongation

Thickening and elongation can be seen in the presence of M proteins because excess antigen diffuses a greater distance. Monoclonal IgM, IgG, IgD, and IgA all demonstrate denser than normal bands. In addition, monoclonal IgG touches the antisera trough.

Shortening, Thinning, or Doubling

A band may be shortened and incomplete because of inhibition of a segment, resulting from the antibody's reacting with

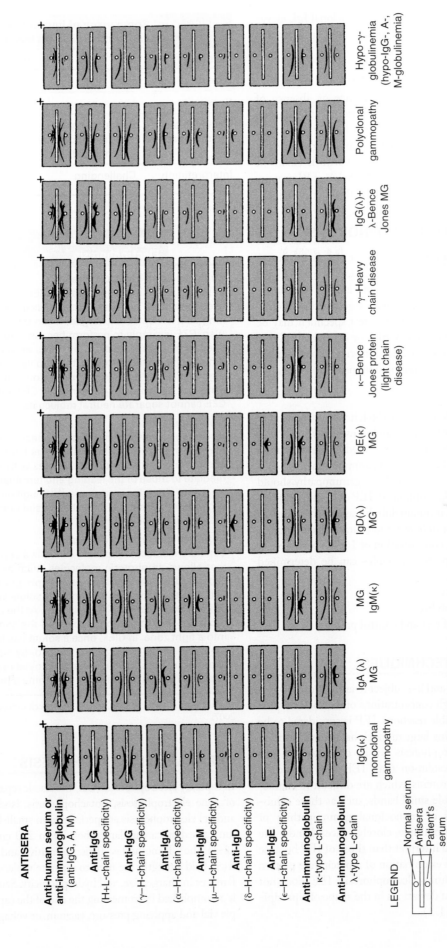

Figure 11-7 **Example of immunoglobulin (Ig) profile on immunoelectrophoresis showing abnormal Ig pattern.** *(Adapted from Ritzman SE, Daniels JC: Laboratory notes—serum proteins, No. 3, Somerville, NJ, 1973, Behring Diagnostics—Hoechst Pharmaceuticals.)*

only a portion of the abnormal protein. Monoclonal IgE elevation leads to a short thick arc in the antigen well area, extending to the anodal side.

Polyvalent and Monovalent Antisera

Polyvalent antiserum confirms the presence or absence of major protein fractions. Monovalent antiserum for specific individual immunoglobulins identifies only the corresponding proteins. If the nonspecific antisera have combining sites for H and L chains, the combining sites will react with L chains of other immunoglobulins or with the free L chains of BJ protein. H-chain–specific sera do not cross-react with other proteins.

IMMUNOFIXATION ELECTROPHORESIS

Immunofixation electrophoresis (IFE), or simply **immunofixation**, has replaced IEP in the evaluation of monoclonal gammopathies because of its rapidity and ease of interpretation. IFE is a two-stage procedure, agarose gel protein electrophoresis and immunoprecipitation. The test specimen may be serum, urine, cerebrospinal fluid (CSF), or other body fluids. The primary use of IFE in clinical laboratories is for the characterization of monoclonal immunoglobulins.

Clinical Applications

Although IFE was first described in 1964, it was introduced as a procedure for the study of immunoglobulins in 1976. IEP and IFE are complementary techniques best used in the workup of a patient with a suspected monoclonal gammopathy. The laboratory protocol for ruling out monoclonal gammopathy should include high-resolution electrophoresis, IEP of both serum and urine, and a quantitative immunoglobulin assay. These procedures are usually sufficient to detect and characterize monoclonal proteins with a serum concentration of 1 g/dL or more.

The following three protein variables can be determined using IFE:

1. Antigenic specificity
2. Electrophoretic mobility
3. Quantity or ratio of test and control proteins

COMPARISON OF TECHNIQUES

IEP is technically simpler and less subject to antigen excess phenomenon than IFE. If high concentrations of monoclonal protein with IFE give no visible reactions, IEP is considered to be a better technique for typing large monoclonal gammopathies.

Immunofixation electrophoresis can be optimized to give greater sensitivity and resolution than IEP. IFE should be reserved for anomalous proteins, which are difficult to characterize by IEP. These include small bands, such as those exhibited in the early stages of monoclonal gammopathies or L-chain disease, and any multiple, closely spaced bands. The results of IFE are easier to interpret than those of IEP because interpretation is based on examination of a precipitate pattern directly analogous to routine electrophoresis; IFE does not depend on detecting slight deviations in the shape of a precipitin arc (Fig. 11-8; Table 11-1).

Table 11-1	Comparison of Immunoelectrophoresis and Immunofixation Electrophoresis	
Feature	**IEP**	**IFE**
Ease of use	Easy	More complex
Sensitivity	Less sensitive	More sensitive
Monoclonal gammopathies	Better for typing large monoclonal gammopathies	Used for difficult to characterize anomalous proteins
Interpretation	Challenging	Easier

Box 11-1	Separation Techniques Used in Capillary Electrophoresis

Capillary Zone Electrophoresis
Capillary zone electrophoresis (CZE) is the most widely used type of CE because of its simplicity and versatility. As long as a molecule is charged, it can be separated by CZE. Also, CZE is simple to perform because the capillary is only filled with buffer. Separation occurs as solutes migrate at different velocities through the capillary. Another advantage of CZE is that it separates anions and cations in the same run, which is not done in other CE methods. However, CZE cannot separate neutral molecules.

Isotachophoresis
Isotachophoresis (ITP) is a focusing technique based on the migration of the sample components between the leading and terminating electrolytes. Solutes with mobilities intermediate to those of the leading and terminating electrolytes stack into sharp focused zones. Although used as a mode of separation, transient ITP has been used primarily as a sample concentration technique.

Capillary Isoelectric Focusing
Capillary isoelectric focusing (CIEF) is a separation method that allows amphoteric molecules, such as proteins, to be separated by electrophoresis in a pH gradient generated between the cathode and anode. A solute will migrate to a point at which its net charge is zero. At the solute's isoelectric point (pI), migration stops, and the sample is focused into a tight zone. In CIEF, once a solute has focused at its pI, the zone is mobilized past the detector by either pressure or chemical means. CIEF is often employed in protein characterization as a mechanism to determine a protein's pI.

Modified from www.chemsoc.org and www.beckmancoulter.com, November 2007.

CAPILLARY ELECTROPHORESIS

In capillary electrophoresis (CE) the classic separation techniques of zone electrophoresis, isotachophoresis, **isoelectric focusing**, and gel electrophoresis are performed in small-bore (10- to 100-μm), fused silica capillary tubes, 20 to 200 cm in length (Box 11-1). The CE method is efficient, sensitive, and rapid. High electrical field strengths are used to separate molecules based on differences in charge, size, and hydrophobicity. Sample introduction is accomplished by immersing the end of the capillary into a sample vial and applying pressure, vacuum, or voltage.

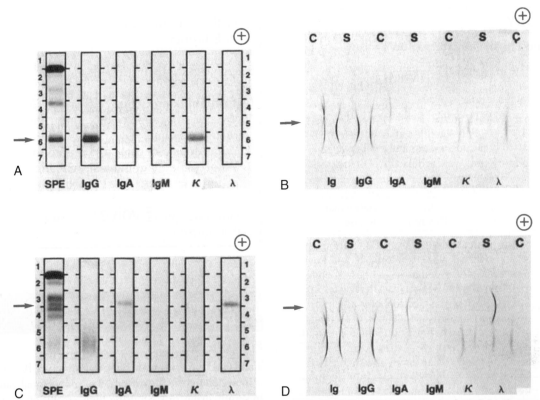

Figure 11-8 **Comparison of immunofixation electrophoresis (IFE) and immunoelectrophoresis (IEP) for two patients with monoclonal gammopathies. A,** Patient specimen with an IgG (κ) monoclonal protein, as identified by IFE. Note the position of the monoclonal protein *(arrow)*. After electrophoresis, each track except serum protein electrophoresis (SPE) is reacted with its respective antiserum; then, all tracks are stained to visualize the respective protein bands. Immunoglobulins G, A, and M (IgG, IgA, IgM); kappa (κ); and lambda (λ) indicate antiserum used on each track. **B,** Same specimen as in **A,** with proteins identified by IEP. Note the position of the monoclonal protein *(arrow)*. Normal control (C) and patient sera (S) are alternated. After electrophoresis, antiserum is added to each trough, as indicated by the labels Ig, IgG, IgA, IgM, κ, and λ. The antisera react with separated proteins in the specimens to form precipitates in the shape of arcs. The IgG and κ arcs are shorter and thicker than those in the normal control, showing the presence of the IgG (κ) monoclonal protein. The concentrations of IgA, IgM, and λ light chains also are reduced. **C,** Patient specimen with an IgA (λ) monoclonal protein identified by the IFE procedure, as described in **A. D,** Same specimen as in **C,** with proteins identified by IEP, as described in **B.** The abnormal IgA and λ arcs for the patient specimen indicate an elevated concentration of a monoclonal IgA (λ) protein. All separations were performed with the Beckman paragon system. *(From Burtis CA, Ashwood ER, Bruns DB: Tietz fundamentals of clinical chemistry, ed 6, St Louis, 2008, Saunders.)*

Table 11-2	Comparison of Traditional Capillary Electrophoresis and Microchip Capillary Electrophoresis	
Feature	**Conventional CE**	**Microchip CE**
Separation channels	Mainly silica, single capillary or capillary array	Glass or polymer
Separation media	Buffers, gels, sieving polymers, microparticles	Buffers, sieving polymers, microparticles
Speed of analysis	Fast (typically minutes)	Very fast (typically seconds)
Integration	Difficult to connect capillaries	Easy to integrate multiple functions (e.g., PCR CE)
Potential for growth	Relatively mature	Emerging technology with potential for new designs and applications

Adapted from Li SFY, Kricka LJ: Clinical analysis by microchip capillary electrophoresis, Clin Chem 52:42, 2006.

PCR, Polymerase chain reaction.

Microchip CE was developed in the early 1990s. The advantages of microchip CE include high speed, reduced reagent consumption, integration analysis, and miniaturization. The applications of microchip CE are diverse and include immune disorders.

Conventional CE revolutionized DNA analysis and was vital to the Human Genome Project. Microchip CE is still in the early stages of development but has demonstrated distinct advantages compared with traditional CE (Table 11-2).

CASE STUDY

History and Physical Examination

MA is a 40-year-old woman with a long history of alcohol abuse. She came to the emergency department complaining of difficulty breathing.

Physical examination revealed a slightly jaundiced appearance, icteric sclera, hepatomegaly, and splenomegaly. She had decreased breathing sounds and swollen legs (edema). Laboratory tests were ordered.

Case Study Laboratory Data

Hematology	Patient's Results	Reference Range
Hemoglobin	12.5 g/dL	12-16.0 g/dL
Hematocrit	42%	36%-45%
Mean corpuscular volume	100 fL	80-96 fL
Total leukocyte count	13.5×10^9/L	$4.5-11.0 \times 10^9$/L
Platelets	95.0×10^9/L	$150-450 \times 10^9$/L
Coagulation—Prothrombin Time	17 sec	10-14 sec
Urinalysis		
Occult blood	1+	Negative
Bilirubin	Moderate	Negative
Clinical Chemistry		
Bilirubin	2.5 mg/dL	0.3-1.2 mg/dL
Liver enzymes (alanine aminotransferase [ALT])	55 IU/L	10-35 IU/L
Total protein	5.5 g/dL	6.4-8.3 g/dL
Albumin	2.5 g/dL	3.9-5.g/dL

Laboratory Results

- Serum protein electrophoresis interpretation—normal electrophoretic migration
- Decreased prealbumin, alpha lipoprotein, and transferrin levels
- α_2-Macroglobulin level—markedly increased
- Questionable increase in IgG and IgA because of a diffuse increase in background staining in the beta and gamma immunoglobulin regions

Questions

1. The organ system dysfunction in this patient is:
   a. Renal
   b. Hepatic
   c. Respiratory
   d. Urinary
2. The acute-phase reactant that is the most sensitive indicator of hepatocellular disease is:
   a. C-Reactive Protein (C-RP)
   b. α_1 –Antitrypsin
   c. Prothrombin time
   d. Bilirubin

See Appendix A for the answers to these questions.

Critical Thinking Group Discussion Questions

1. What is the cause of the abnormal laboratory results?
2. What does a decrease in prealbumin suggest?
3. What is the diagnostic significance of α_1-antitrypsin?

See instructor site ⊖**volve** for discussion of the answers to these questions.

Immunofixation Electrophoresis Procedure

Principle

Titan Gel ImmunoFix (Helena Laboratories, Beaumont, Texas) is intended for the identification of monoclonal gammopathies in serum, urine, or CSF using high-resolution protein electrophoresis and immunofixation.

In the first step of the IFE procedure, a single specimen is applied to six different positions on an agarose plate and the proteins are separated according to their net charge by electrophoresis. In the second phase, monospecific antisera are applied to five of the electrophoresis patterns: IgG, IgA, IgM, and κ and γ antisera. A protein fixative solution is applied to the sixth pattern to produce a complete protein reference pattern. The plate is incubated for 10 minutes.

If complementary antigen is present in the proper proportions in the test sample, antigen-antibody complexes form and precipitate. The formation of a stable antigen-antibody precipitate fixes the protein in the gel. After fixation, the gel is washed in deproteinization solution (e.g., dilute NaCl) and nonprecipitated proteins are washed out of the agarose, leaving only the antigen-antibody complex. The protein reference pattern and the antigen-antibody precipitation bands are stained with a protein-sensitive stain.

See instructor site ⊖**volve** for the procedural protocol, sources of error, and clinical applications.

CHAPTER HIGHLIGHTS

- Serum electrophoresis results in the separation of proteins into five fractions on cellulose acetate based on the rate of migration of these individual components in an electrical field.
- Immunoelectrophoresis (IEP) involves the electrophoresis of serum or urine, followed by immunodiffusion. Proteins are differentiated by electrophoretic mobility and by their diffusion coefficient and antibody specificity.

- Immunofixation electrophoresis (IFE) has two stages, agarose gel protein electrophoresis and immuno-precipitation.
- Capillary electrophoresis (CE) and microchip CE are important techniques for the study of various immunoglobulins.

REVIEW QUESTIONS

1. Protein can be separated into _____ fractions by use of serum electrophoresis.
   a. Three
   b. Four
   c. Five
   d. Six

2. Which of the following is the most common application of immunoelectrophoresis (IEP)?
   a. Identification of the absence of a normal serum protein
   b. Structural abnormalities of proteins
   c. Screening for circulating immune complexes
   d. Diagnosis of monoclonal gammopathies

3. Abnormalities of precipitin bands in an IEP assay can be evaluated by all the following features except:
   a. Position of the band between antigen well and antibody trough
   b. Position of the band in relationship to electrophoretically identified protein fractions
   c. General location of the band
   d. Distortion of the arc formation

4. Immunofixation electrophoresis (IFE) is best used in the:
   a. Workup of a polyclonal gammopathy
   b. Workup of a monoclonal gammopathy
   c. Screening for circulating immune complexes
   d. Identification of hypercomplementemia

5-9. Indicate true statements with A and false statements with B.

5. _____ IEP is technically simpler and less subject to antigen excess phenomenon than IFE.

6. _____ IFE is considered to be a better technique than IEP for typing large monoclonal gammopathies.

7. _____ IFE can be optimized to give greater sensitivity and resolution than IEP.

8. _____ IFE should be reserved for anomalous proteins that are difficult to characterize by IEP.

9. _____ IEP is easier to interpret than IFE.

10. Immunoelectrophoresis (IEP) involves:
    a. Separation of proteins based on the rate of migration of individual components in an electrical field
    b. Electrophoresis of serum or urine
    c. Double immunodiffusion following electrophoresis
    d. All of the above

11. In IEP, proteins are differentiated by:
    a. Electrophoresis
    b. Diffusion coefficient
    c. Antibody specificity
    d. All of the above

12. IEP can divide the proteins of normal serum into _____ distinct precipitation bands.
    a. 5 to 10
    b. 15 to 20
    c. 25 to 40
    d. 45 to 100

13. IEP is useful for clinically detecting:
    a. Structural abnormalities
    b. Concentration changes in proteins
    c. Congenital deficiency of some complement components
    d. All of the above

14. The most common application of IEP of serum is for the:
    a. Diagnosis of monoclonal gammopathy
    b. Diagnosis of polyclonal gammopathy
    c. Diagnosis of autoimmune hemolysis
    d. Demonstration of Bence Jones (BJ) protein

15. Immunofixation electrophoresis (IFE) can test:
    a. Serum and urine
    b. Cerebrospinal fluid
    c. Whole blood
    d. Both a and b

16. The primary use of IFE is:
    a. Characterization of monoclonal immunoglobulins
    b. Characterization of polyclonal immunoglobulins
    c. Identification of monoclonal immunoglobulins
    d. Identification of polyclonal immunoglobulins

BIBLIOGRAPHY

Burtis CA, Ashwood ER, Bruns DB: Tietz fundamentals of clinical chemistry, ed 6, St Louis, 2008, Saunders.

Helena Laboratories: Protein electrophoresis; protein electrophoresis and IFE; immunofixation for identification of monoclonal gammopathies, 2011, http://www.helena.com/ educaslides.html.

Kaplan LA, Pesce AJ: Clinical chemistry: theory, analysis, correlation, ed 5, St Louis, 2010, Mosby.

Killingsworth LM, Warren BM: Immunofixation for the identification of monoclonal gammopathies, Beaumont, Texas, 1986, Helena Laboratories.

Li SFY, Kricka LJ: Clinical analysis by microchip capillary electrophoresis, Clin Chem 52:42, 2006.

Ritzmann EE: Immunoglobulin abnormalities. In Ritzman S, editor: Serum protein abnormalities: diagnostic and clinical aspects, Boston, 1976, Little, Brown.

Sun T: Immunofixation electrophoresis procedures. Protein abnormalities. Physiology of immunoglobulins: diagnostic and clinical aspects, vol 1, New York, 1982, Alan R Liss.

CHAPTER 12

Labeling Techniques in Immunoassay

Learning Objectives

At the conclusion of this chapter, the reader should be able to:

- Compare heterogeneous and homogeneous immunoassays.
- Name and cite applications of at least three types of labels that can be used in an immunoassay.
- Describe chemiluminescence.
- Describe and compare chemiluminescence, enzyme immunoassay (EIA), and immunofluorescence techniques.
- Briefly compare direct immunofluorescent, inhibition immunofluorescent, and indirect immunofluorescent assays.
- Describe the advantages, disadvantages, and application of Q dots, SQUID technology, luminescent oxygen-channeling

immunoassay, fluorescent in situ hybridization, signal amplification technology, and magnetic labeling technology.
- Analyze a case study related to immunoassay.
- Correctly answer case study related multiple choice questions.
- Be prepared to participate in a discussion of critical thinking questions.
- Describe the principle of the solid-phase immunosorbent assay for pregnancy testing.
- Describe the direct fluorescent antibody test for *N. gonorrhea*.
- Correctly answer end of chapter review questions.

Key Terms

antinuclear antibodies (ANAs)
capture enzyme immunoassay
chemiluminescence
competitive enzyme immunoassay
competitive immunoassay
conjugated antibody
direct fluorescent antibody (DFA)
enzyme immunoassay (EIA)
fluorescence in situ hybridization
  (FISH)

fluorescence polarization
  immunoassay
fluorescent antibody (FA)
immunofluorescent assay
immunohistochemistry (IHC)
indirect fluorescent assay (IFA)
inhibition immunofluorescent
  assay
luminescent oxygen-channeling
  immunoassay (LOCI)

noncompetitive enzyme
  immunoassay
photomultiplier tube
radioimmunoassay (RIA)
sandwich immunoassay
superconducting quantum
  interference device (SQUID)
time-resolved fluoroimmunoassay
tyramide signal amplification (TSA)

IMMUNOASSAY FORMATS

Immunoassays can be divided into two types, heterogeneous and homogeneous immunoassays. Heterogeneous immuno-assays involve a solid phase (microwell, bead) and require washing steps to remove unbound antigens or antibodies.

Heterogeneous immunoassays can have a competitive or non-competitive format.

Homogeneous immunoassays consist only of a liquid phase and do not require washing steps. Homogeneous immu-noassays are faster and easier to automate than heterogeneous

Table 12-1	Types of Immunoassays	
Type	Antibody	Comments
Enzyme immunoassay (EIA; enzyme-linked immunosorbent assay, ELISA)	Enzyme-labeled antibody (e.g., horseradish peroxidase)	Competitive ELISA Noncompetitive (e.g., direct ELISA, indirect ELISA)
Chemiluminescence	Chemiluminescent molecule–labeled antibody (e.g., isoluminol or acridinium ester labels)	Competitive or sandwich immunoassay
Electrochemiluminescence	Electrochemiluminescent molecule–labeled antibody (e.g., ruthenium label)	—
Fluoroimmunoassay	Fluorescent molecule–labeled antigen (e.g., europium or fluorescein label)	Heterogeneous (e.g., time-resolved immunofluoroassay) Homogeneous (e.g., fluorescence polarization immunoassay)

immunoassays. In addition, homogeneous immunoassays have competitive formats.

TYPES OF LABELS

The principles and applications of enzyme immunoassays, chemiluminescence, and fluorescent substances as labels are presented in this chapter (Table 12-1).

The original technique of using antigen-coated cells or particles in agglutination techniques may be considered as the earliest method for labeling components in immunoassays. Ideal characteristics of a label include the quality of being measurable by several methods, including visual inspection. The properties of a label used in an immunoassay determine how detection is possible. For example, coated latex particles can be detected by various methods—visual inspection, light scattering (nephelometry), and particle counting. The conversion of a colorless substrate into a colored product in enzyme immunoassay allows for two methods of detection, colorimetry and visual inspection.

Yalow and Berson developed the **radioimmunoassay (RIA)** method in 1959 using a radioactive label that could identify an immunocomponent at very low concentrations. In the 1960s, researchers began to search for a substitute for the successful RIA method because of the inherent drawbacks of using radioactive isotopes as labels (e.g., radioactive waste, short shelf life). Currently, chemiluminescent reactions have replaced most RIAs in the clinical laboratory. Relatively simple and cost-effective, chemiluminescence technology has sensitivity at least as good as that of an RIA.

ENZYME IMMUNOASSAY

There are two general approaches to diagnosing condition, diseases or conditions by immunoassay, testing for specific antigens or for antigen-specific antibodies. The enzyme-linked immunosorbent assay (ELISA), also known as an **enzyme immunoassay (EIA),** is designed to detect antigens or antibodies by producing an enzyme-triggered color change.

The EIA method uses a nonisotopic label that offers the advantage of safety. EIA is usually an objective measurement that provides numerical results. Some EIA procedures provide

Box 12-1	Enzyme Immunoassays

- *Borrelia burgdorferi* (IgG and IgM)
- Cytomegalovirus (IgG and IgM)
- Cytomegalovirus (Ag)
- Hepatitis A virus (total Ab)
- Hepatitis B virus (HBV)
  Anti-HBs
  Anti-HBc
  Anti-HBe
  Anti-HBc (IgM)
  HBs Ag
  HBe Ag
- Hepatitis delta virus (total Ab)
- HIV Ab
- HIV Ag
- HTLV-I Ab
- HTLV-II Ab
- Human B-lymphotropic virus Ab
- Rubella virus (IgG and IgM)
- *Toxoplasma gondii* (IgG and IgM)

Ab, Antibody; *Ag,* antigen; *HIV,* human immunodeficiency virus; *HTLV,* human T-lymphotropic (leukemia-lymphoma) virus; *Ig,* immunoglobulin.

diagnostic information and measure immune status (e.g., detect total antibody IgM or IgG).

The EIA method uses the catalytic properties of enzymes to detect and quantitate immunologic reactions. An enzyme-labeled antibody or enzyme-labeled antigen conjugate is used in immunologic assays (Box 12-1). The enzyme, with its substrate, detects the presence and quantity of antigen or antibody in a patient specimen. In some tissues, an enzyme-labeled antibody can identify antigenic locations.

Various enzymes are used in enzyme immunoassay (Table 12-2). Common enzyme labels are horseradish peroxidase, alkaline phosphatase, glucose-6-phosphate dehydrogenase, and beta-galactosidase. To be used in an EIA, an enzyme must fulfill the following criteria:

- High degree of stability
- Extreme specificity
- Absence from the antigen or antibody
- No alteration by inhibitor within the system

Table 12-2	Enzymes Used in Enzyme Immunoassays
Enzyme	**Source**
Acetylcholinesterase	*Electrophorous electicus*
Alkaline phosphatase	*Escherichia coli*
β-Galactosidase	*Escherichia coli*
Glucose oxidase	*Aspergillus niger*
Glucose-6-phosphate dehydrogenase (G6PD)	*Leuconostoc mesenteroides*
Lysozyme	Egg white
Malate dehydrogenase	Pig heart
Peroxidase	Horseradish

In a representative EIA test, a plastic bead or plastic plate is coated with antigen (e.g., virus; Fig. 12-1). The antigen reacts with antibody in the patient's serum. The bead or plate is then incubated with an enzyme-labeled antibody conjugate. If antibody is present, the conjugate reacts with the antigen-antibody complex on the bead or plate. The enzyme activity is measured spectrophotometrically after the addition of the specific chromogenic substrate. For example, peroxidase cleaves its substrate, *o*-dianisidine, causing a color change. In some cases, the test can be read subjectively.

The results of a typical test are calculated by comparing the spectrophotometric reading of the patient's serum to that of a control or reference serum. The advantage of an objective enzyme test is that results are not dependent on a technician's interpretations. In general, the EIA procedure is faster and requires less laboratory work than comparable methods.

Antigen Detection

EIAs for antigen detection (e.g., hepatitis B surface antigen [HBsAg]) have four steps. Antigen-specific antibody is attached to a solid-phase surface (e.g., plastic beads). The patient's serum that may contain the antigen is added. Next, an enzyme-labeled antibody specific to the antigen (conjugate) is added. Finally, a chromogenic substrate is added, which changes color in the presence of the enzyme. The amount of color that develops is proportional to the amount of antigen in the patient specimen.

Antibody Detection

There are three types of EIAs for antibody detection—noncompetitive, competitive, and capture.

Noncompetitive Enzyme Immunoassay

The **noncompetitive enzyme immunoassay** takes place when a specific antigen is attached to a solid-phase surface, such as a plastic bead or microtiter well. The patient's serum that could contain antibody (e.g., cytomegalovirus [CMV] immunoglobulin G [IgG], HIV antibody) is added to the solid-phase surface, followed by an enzyme-labeled antibody specific to the test antibody. The added chromogenic substrate changes color if the enzyme is present. The amount of color that develops is proportional to the amount of antibody in the patient's serum.

Competitive Enzyme Immunoassay

Competitive enzyme immunoassay involves using a solid-phase surface to which specific antigen is attached. The patient's potentially containing antibody (e.g., hepatitis B core antibody) and an enzyme-labeled antibody specific to the test antibody (conjugate) are mixed. Chromogenic substrate is then added, which changes color in the presence of the enzyme. The amount of color that develops is inversely proportional to the amount of antibody in the patient's serum.

Capture Enzyme Immunoassay

Capture enzyme immunoassay is designed to detect a specific type of antibody, such as IgM or IgG, CMV IgM, rubella IgM, or *Toxoplasma* IgM. Antibody specific for IgM or IgG is attached to a solid-phase surface (plastic bead, microtiter well). The patient specimen potentially containing IgM or IgG is added. Specific antigen is then added. Finally, chromogenic substrate is added, which changes color in the presence of the enzyme. The amount of color that develops is proportional to the amount of antigen-specific IgM or IgG in the patient's serum.

CHEMILUMINESCENCE

Chemiluminescence refers to light emission produced during a chemical reaction; it is used extensively in automated immunoassays (see Chapter 13). This methodology has excellent sensitivity and dynamic range. It does not require sample radiation and nonselective excitation and source instability are eliminated. Most chemiluminescent reagents and conjugates are stable and relatively nontoxic.

In immunoassays, chemiluminescent labels can be attached to an antigen or antibody. Acridinium esters are highly specific activity labels that can be used to label antibodies and haptens. Chemiluminescent labels are used to detect proteins, viruses, oligonucleotides, and genomic nucleic acid sequences in an immunoassay. Two formats are used, competitive and sandwich immunoassays.

In a **competitive immunoassay,** a fixed amount of labeled antigen competes with unlabeled antigen from a patient specimen for a limited number of antibody-binding sites (Fig. 12-2). The amount of light emitted is inversely proportional to the amount of analyte (antigen) measured.

In a **sandwich immunoassay,** the sample antigen binds to an antibody fixed onto a solid phase; a second antibody, labeled with a chemiluminescent label, binds to the antigen-antibody complex on the solid phase (Fig. 12-3). In the sandwich assay, the emitted light is directly proportional to the analyte concentration. The detection device for analyses is a simple **photomultiplier tube** used to detect the emitted light.

Chemiluminescent labels can be divided into five major groups: (1) luminol; (2) acridinium esters; (3) peroxyoxalates; (4) dioxetanes; and (5) tris(2,2′-bipyridyl)-ruthenium (II). Direct labels include luminol, acridinium ester, and electrogenerated luminescent chelate from ruthenium and tripropylamine (TPA) complex [$Ru(bpy)^{3+}$]. These labels are attached directly to antigens, antibodies, or deoxyribonucleic acid (DNA) probes, depending on the assay format.

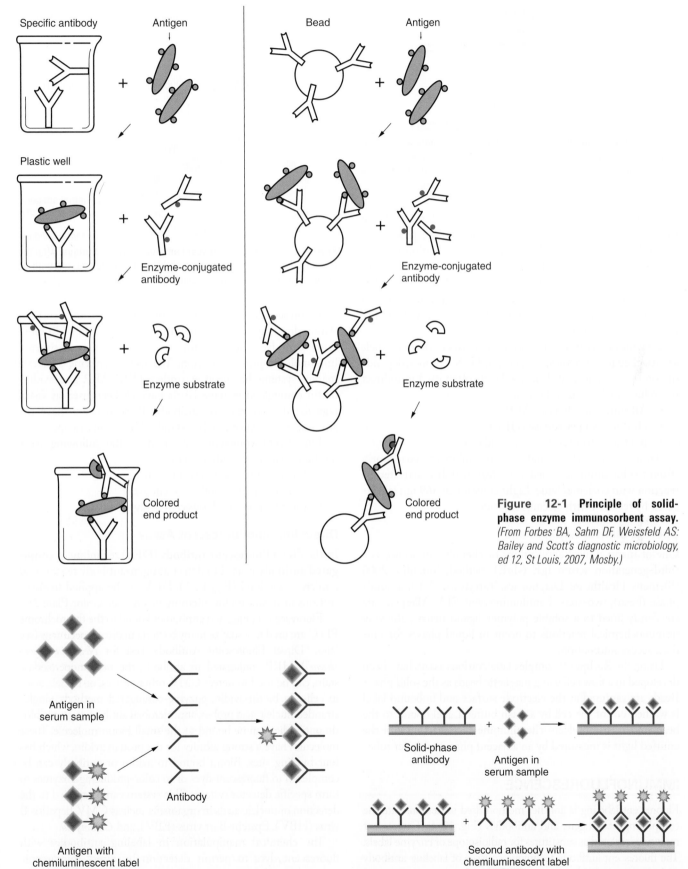

Specific antibody   Antigen

Plastic well

Enzyme-conjugated antibody

Enzyme substrate

Colored end product

Bead   Antigen

Enzyme-conjugated antibody

Enzyme substrate

Colored end product

Figure 12-1 Principle of solid-phase enzyme immunosorbent assay. *(From Forbes BA, Sahm DF, Weissfeld AS: Bailey and Scott's diagnostic microbiology, ed 12, St Louis, 2007, Mosby.)*

Antigen in serum sample

Antigen with chemiluminescent label

Antibody

Figure 12-2 Format for competitive immunoassays. *(Adapted from Jandreski MA: Chemiluminescence technology in immunoassays, Lab Med 29:555, 1998.)*

Solid-phase antibody   Antigen in serum sample

Second antibody with chemiluminescent label

Figure 12-3 Format for sandwich immunoassays. *(Adapted from Jandreski MA: Chemiluminescence technology in immunoassays, Lab Med 29(9):555, 1998.)*

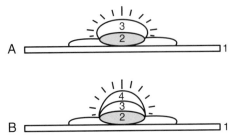

Figure 12-4 **Principles of direct and indirect fluorescent techniques.** **A**, Direct fluorescence. **B**, Indirect fluorescence. *1,* Microscopic slide; *2,* cell (cytoplasm and nucleus); *3,* antiserum (conjugate in **A**, unconjugate in **B**); *4,* conjugated antiglobulin serum.

Oxidation of isoluminol by hydrogen peroxide (H_2O_2) in the presence of a catalyst (e.g., microperoxidase) produces a relatively long-lived emission at 425 nm. Oxidation of acridinium ester by alkaline H_2O_2 in the presence of detergent produces a rapid flash of light lasting from 1 to 5 seconds at 429 nm. Peak intensity can be used for the measurement. An alternate method is to use an integrator to measure the entire light output for greater sensitivity.

Enzymes are typically used for indirect labels. Indirect labels are attached to antibodies, antigens, and DNA probes, depending on the assay format. Enzyme labels often used in indirect procedures include the following:

- Alkaline phosphatase (ALP)
- Horseradish peroxidase (HRP)
- Beta-galactosidase (β-galactosidase)

An interesting label is native or recombinant apoaequorin (from the bioluminescent jellyfish, *Aequorea*). It is activated by reaction with coelenterazine. Light emission at 469 nm is triggered by reaction with calcium chloride.

Specific Clinical Applications

One of many clinical applications of chemiluminescence is a third-generation serum IgE (sIgE) method, Immulite 2000 (Siemens Healthcare Diagnostics, Tarrytown, NY), a solid-phase (bead), two-step chemiluminescent EIA. Allergens are covalently lined to a soluble polymer-ligand matrix, allowing immunochemical reactions to occur in liquid phases for random access automation.

Using the Ru(bpy)$^{3+}$ complex label, various assays have been developed in a flow cell using magnetic beads as the solid phase. Beads are captured at the electrode surface and unbound label is washed out of the cell by a wash buffer. Label bound to the bead undergoes an electrochemiluminescent reaction and the emitted light is measured by an adjacent photomultiplier tube.

IMMUNOFLUORESCENCE

Fluorescent labeling is another method used to demonstrate the complexing of antigens and antibodies (Fig. 12-4). Fluorescent molecules are used as substitutes for radioisotope or enzyme labels. The fluorescent antibody technique consists of labeling antibody with fluorescein isothiocyanate (FITC), a fluorescent compound with an affinity for proteins, to form a complex (conjugate). This conjugate is able to react with antibody-specific antigen.

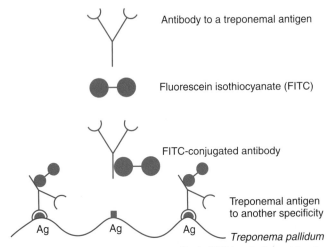

Figure 12-5 **Direct fluorescent antibody (DFA) technique.** After the labeling of a specific antibody with FITC, it can be reacted with its antigen and identified microscopically.

Fluorescent techniques are extremely specific and sensitive. Antibodies may be conjugated to other markers in addition to fluorescent dyes; the use of these markers is called colorimetric immunologic probe detection. The use of enzyme-substrate marker systems has been expanded. HRP, ALP, and avidin-biotin conjugated enzyme labels have all been used as visual tags for the presence of antibody. These reagents have the advantage of requiring only a standard light microscope.

Fluorescent conjugates are used in the following basic methods, which are widely used:

- Direct immunofluorescent assay
- Inhibition immunofluorescent assay
- Indirect immunofluorescent assay

Direct Immunofluorescent Assay

In the **direct fluorescent antibody (DFA)** technique, a **conjugated antibody** is used to detect antigen-antibody reactions at a microscopic level (Fig. 12-5). DFA can be applied to tissue sections or in smears for microorganisms (see Color Plate 2).

Fluorescein-conjugated antibodies bound to the fluorochrome FITC are used to visualize many bacteria in direct specimens (see later, "Direct Fluorescent Antibody Test for *Neisseria gonorrhoeae*"). HRP conjugated to antibody, the immunoperoxidase stain, can be used to detect CMV, other viruses, or nucleic acids in cells. In biotin-avidin, enzyme-conjugated methods, single-stranded nucleic acid probes, antimicrobial antibodies, or antibiotin antibodies can be bound to the small biotin molecule. These molecules have a strong affinity for the protein avidin, which has four binding sites. Biotin bound to avidin or antibody can be complexed to fluorescent dyes or to color-producing enzymes to form specific detector systems. This system can be applied to the detection of nucleic acids in organisms such as CMV, hepatitis B virus (HBV), Epstein-Barr virus (EBV), and *Chlamydia*.

The chemical manipulation in labeling antibodies with fluorescent dyes to permit detection by direct microscopic examination does not seriously impair antibody activity, the ability of fluorescent antibody conjugate to react specifically with its homologous antigen. Monoclonal antibodies (MAbs) have also been successfully conjugated to fluorescein for the detection of chlamydiae, rabies virus, and other pathogens in directly stained specimens.

When absorbing light of one wavelength, a fluorescent substance emits light of another (longer) wavelength. In **fluorescent antibody (FA)** microscopy, the incident or exciting light is often blue-green to ultraviolet. The light is provided by a high-pressure mercury arc lamp with a primary (e.g., blue-violet) filter between the lamp and the object that passes only fluorescein-exciting wavelengths. The color of the emitted light depends on the nature of the substance. Fluorescein gives off yellow-green light and the rhodamines fluoresce in the red portion of the spectrum. The color observed in the fluorescence microscope depends on the secondary or barrier filter used in the eyepiece. A yellow filter absorbs the green fluorescence of fluorescein and transmits only yellow. Fluorescein fluoresces an intense apple-green color when excited.

Inhibition Immunofluorescent Assay

The **inhibition immunofluorescent assay** is a blocking test in which an antigen is first exposed to unlabeled antibody and then to labeled antibody, and is finally washed and examined. If the unlabeled and labeled antibodies are both homologous to the antigen, there should be no fluorescence. This result confirms the specificity of the FA technique. Antibody in an unknown serum can also be detected and identified by the inhibition test.

Indirect Immunofluorescent Assay

The basis for **indirect fluorescent assay (IFA)** is that antibodies (immunoglobulins) not only react with homologous antigens, but also can act as antigens and react with antiimmunoglobulins (Box 12-2). IFA is the serologic method most widely used for the detection of diverse antibodies. Immunofluorescence is used extensively in the detection of autoantibodies and antibodies to tissue and cellular antigens. For example, **antinuclear antibodies (ANAs)**—a heterogeneous group of circulating immunoglobulins that react with the whole nucleus or nuclear components (e.g., nuclear proteins, DNA, histones) in host tissues—are frequently assayed by indirect fluorescence. By using tissue sections that contain a large number of antigens, it is possible to identify antibodies to several different antigens in a single test. The antigens are differentiated according to their different staining patterns.

Immunofluorescence can also be used to identify specific antigens on live cells in suspension (flow cytometry). When a live stained cell suspension is put through a fluorescence-activated cell sorter (FACS), which measures its fluorescent intensity, the cells are separated according to their particular fluorescent brightness. This technique permits the isolation of different cell populations with different surface antigens (e.g., CD4+ and CD8+ lymphocytes; see Chapter 4).

In the IFA, the antigen source (e.g., whole *Toxoplasma* microorganism, virus in infected tissue culture cells) to the specific antibody being tested is affixed to the surface of a microscope slide. The patient's serum is diluted and placed on the slide to cover the antigen source. If antibody is present in the serum, it will bind to its specific antigen. Unbound antibody is then

Box 12-2	**Immunologic Assays Performed by Indirect Fluorescent Antibody Technique**

Antiadrenal antibodies
Antibody (histone-reactive [HR]–ANA)
Anticentriole antibodies
Anticentromere antibodies
Anti–glomerular basement membrane antibodies
Anti–islet cell antibodies
Anti–liver-kidney microsomal (LKM) antibodies
Antimitochondrial
Antimyelin
Antimyocardial
Antinuclear antibody
Anti–parietal cell
Antiplatelet
Antireticulin
Antiribosome
Antiskin (dermal-epidermal)
Antiskin (interepithelial)
Anti–smooth muscle
Antistriational
Cytomegalovirus (IgM antibody)
Histone-reactive antinuclear antibody (HR-ANA)
Human immunodeficiency virus (total and IgM antibody)
Immunoglobulin M (IgM) antibodies (antigen specific)
Lymphocyte typing
Rubella virus antibody
Toxoplasma gondii antibody

removed by washing the slide. In the second phase, antihuman globulin (AHG, directed specifically against IgM or IgG) conjugated to a fluorescent substance that will fluoresce when exposed to ultraviolet light is placed on the slide. This conjugated marker for human antibody will bind to the antibody already bound to the antigen on the slide and will serve as a marker for the antibody when viewed under a fluorescence microscope.

A major problem in interpreting IFA results is background staining. For most IFAs, laboratories must choose a screening dilution because undiluted specimens will show background staining resulting from nonspecific binding or clinically insignificant levels of circulating autoantibodies. The screening dilution plays a critical role; the more dilute the specimen becomes, the less sensitive but more specific the procedure.

An example of a changing clinical situation is that many laboratories have replaced indirect immunofluorescence, once the standard for ANA testing, with the EIA. Less labor and technical experience are cited as reasons for switching from indirect immunofluorescence. However, the trade-off may not be valuable if patients have antibody titers of less than 1:160.

EMERGING LABELING TECHNOLOGIES
Quantum Dots (Q dots)

An advanced labeling technique, quantum dots are semiconductor nanocrystals used as fluorescent labeling reagents for biological imaging. A valuable property of Q dots is that different sizes of crystals produce different signals with a single laser excitation. This seemingly simple physical property implies

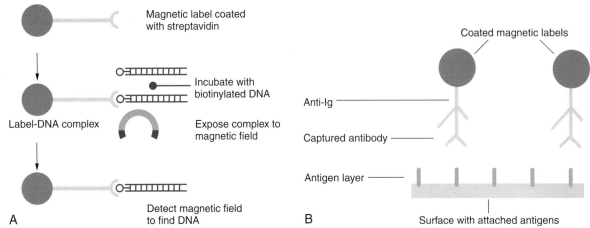

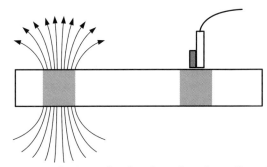

Figure 12-6   **Magnetic labeling techniques. A,** Detection of deoxyribonucleic acid. **B,** Detection of antibodies. *(Adapted from Adelman L: Laboratory technology: magnetic labeling technology, Adv Med Lab Admin 11:131, 1999.)*

that different-sized Q dots could be directed against different analyte targets, and the Q dots would fluoresce with different colors in a size-dependent manner. This allows for the detection of multiple analytes with a single assay. Q dots are the next step in the evolution of luminescence-based assays.

SQUID Technology

A novel method of target labeling is to tag antibodies with superparamagnetic particles, allow the tagged antibodies to bind with the target antigen, and use a **superconducting quantum interference device (SQUID)** to detect the tagged antigen-antibody complex. The amplitude of the signal is proportional to the number of bound particles and correspondingly to the amount of target. A current application of this technology is its use in the detection of *Listeria monocytogenes*.

Luminescent Oxygen-Channeling Immunoassay

This novel detection technology is based on two different 200-nm latex particles, a sensitizer particle that absorbs energy at 680 nm with the generation of singlet oxygen (donor bead) and a chemiluminescer molecule that shifts the emission wavelength to 570 nm (receptor bead). When these particles are in proximity during excitation, singlet oxygen moves from the donor bead to the receptor bead, where it triggers the generation of a luminescent signal. **Luminescent oxygen-channeling immunoassay (LOCI)** technology is broadly applicable to any molecule that can be determined in a binding assay. The production of end point ribonucleic acid (RNA) determination by LOCI has been investigated.

Signal Amplification Technology

Tyramide signal amplification (TSA) can be used in various fluorescent and colorimetric detection applications. TSA protocols are simple and require few changes to standard operating procedures. TSA provides a messenger RNA (mRNA) in situ hybridization protocol that is effective in detecting B cell clonality in plastic-embedded tissue specimens. Immunoglobulin light-chain mRNA molecules can be detected directly in paraffin-embedded tissue using fluorescein-labeled oligonucleotide probes. TSA amplification enables B cells to be detected

Figure 12-7 Cross-sectional schematic of small region of sequencing gel or nylon membrane with magnetic labels bound to DNA, separated into two bands. *Left,* Arrows on band represent the magnetic field resulting from the magnetized labels. *Right,* Band has a sensor near the surface. *(Adapted from Adelman L: Laboratory technology: magnetic labeling technology, Adv Med Lab Admin 11:131, 1999.)*

in tissue sections without additional processing steps and specially prepared sections. Similar in situ hybridization technology can also be used for the detection of cytokines, such as interferon gamma (IFN-γ) and interleukin-4 (IL-4).

Magnetic Labeling Technology

Magnetic labeling technology is an application of the high-resolution magnetic recording technology developed for the computer disk drive industry. Increased density of microscopic, magnetically labeled biological samples (e.g., nucleic acid on a biochip) translates directly into reduced sample-processing times. Magnetic labeling can be applied to automated DNA sequences, DNA probe technology, and gel electrophoresis (Fig. 12-6). Compared with other nonradioactive labeling systems, magnetic labels are inherently safe, instrumentation is less expensive, signals are almost permanent, and spatial resolution is increased.

In a magnetic label–based gel electrophoresis application sphere, DNA is analyzed. DNA is separated into bands using electrophoresis and magnetic labels are bound to the DNA in each band. By applying and then removing a magnetic field, the magnetic domains in each label are oriented in the same direction, resulting in a net magnetic field near the bands in the direction of the applied field (Fig. 12-7).

Time-Resolved Fluoroimmunoassay

In a time-resolved assay, fluorescence is measured after a certain period to exclude background interference fluorescence. This form of immunoassay is heterogeneous with a direct format (sandwich assay), similar to direct ELISA. The **time-resolved fluoroimmunoassay** uses europium-labeled antibodies. If excited at 340 nm, europium fluoresces at 620 nm. The fluorescence is measured and is directly proportional to the concentration of the substance.

Fluorescence Polarization Immunoassay

In the **fluorescence polarization immunoassay,** a homogeneous competitive fluoroimmunoassay, the polarization of the fluorescence from a fluorescein-antigen conjugate is determined by its rate of rotation during the lifetime of the excited state in solution. Binding to a large antibody molecule slows down the rate of rotation and increases the degree of polarization, and the fluorescence emitted is polarized.

Fluorescence in Situ Hybridization

Fluorescence in situ hybridization (FISH) uses fluorescent molecules to brightly "paint" genes or chromosomes. The rapid expansion in the availability of polyclonal and monoclonal antibodies has fostered a dramatic increase in light microscopic **immunohistochemistry (IHC)** and in situ hybridization.

The FISH molecular cytogenetic technique uses recombinant DNA technology. Probes are short sequences of single-stranded DNA that are complementary to the DNA sequences to be examined. Probes hybridize, or bind, to the complementary DNA (cDNA) and labeled fluorescent tags indicate the location of the sequences. Probes can be locus-specific, centromeric repeat probes, or whole-chromosome probes.

In metaphase FISH, a specific nucleic acid sequence (probe) is bound to the homologous segment on a metaphase chromosome affixed to a glass slide. Uniquely, the existence of a region-specific DNA sequence in a nondividing cell can be detected using interphase FISH.

Clinical applications of FISH for the detection of inherited and acquired chromosomal abnormalities include hematopathology and oncology. Many genetic syndromes have been recognized by geneticists, but laboratory tests often are unavailable for confirmation. The DiGeorge syndrome is an example of a chromosomal deletion leading to the loss of several genes.

A simple sensitive method for in situ amplified chemiluminescent detection of sequence-specific DNA and IgG immunoassay has been developed. This immunoassay uses highly active gold nanoparticles as the label and can be confirmed by clinical testing. The method has many desirable features, including rapid detection, selectivity, and minimal instrumentation. The protocol has potentially broad applications for clinical immunoassays and DNA hybridization analysis.

Case Study

A 25-year-old woman had a missed menstrual period 3 weeks ago. She suspected pregnancy and went to her primary care provider for confirmation.

Questions
1. Failure to develop a colored line with a quality control specimen in a lateral flow chromatographic immunoassay for pregnancy indicates:
   a. Weakly positive result
   b. Strongly positive result
   c. Invalid test result
   d. Negative result
2. A negative hCG level can be observed in a lateral flow chromatographic immunoassay for pregnancy, if:
   a. The specimen contains hCG at a level close to or greater than 24 mIU/mL
   b. hCG in the specimen binds to sites on the anti-hCG antibody-gold conjugate to form a complex, the complex binds to the capture antibody coated on the test line, and a burgundy red colored band develops
   c. No color develops at the test line of the test strip
   d. Both a and b

See Appendix A for the answers to these multiple choice questions.

Critical Thinking Group Discussion Questions
1. When she reads the test result after the specified limit of 7 minutes, no colored lines appeared on the strip. What does this mean?
2. If the test had resulted in a negative result, should the test be repeated?
3. Can a woman have a positive pregnancy test after delivering a baby?

See instructor site ⊖volve for the discussion of the answers to these questions.

Pregnancy Testing

Solid-Phase Immunosorbent Assay Principle

Most commercially developed EIA applications require physical separation of the specific antigens from nonspecific complexes found in clinical samples. If the antibody directed toward the agent being assayed is fixed firmly to a solid matrix, either to the inside of the wells of a microdilution tray or to the outside of a spherical plastic or metal bead or some other solid matrix, the system is termed a *solid-phase immunosorbent assay* (SPIA). A modification of SPIA uses a disposable plastic cassette consisting of the antibody-bound membrane and a small chamber to which the specimen can be added. An absorbent material is placed below the membrane to wick the liquid reactants through the membrane. This helps separate nonreacted components from the antigen-antibody complexes being studied.

A Clinical Laboratory Improvement Amendments (CLIA)–waived pregnancy test uses monoclonal antibody specific to human chorionic gonadotropin (hCG) in a one-step, lateral flow chromatographic immunoassay. The test strip includes a conjugate pad containing mouse monoclonal anti-hCG antibody conjugated to colloidal gold and a nitrocellulose membrane containing a test line and control line. When a specimen is applied to the testing pad, hCG in the specimen binds to sites on the anti-hCG antibody-gold conjugate in the conjugate pad to form a complex, which it migrates along the membrane strip. If the specimen contains hCG at a level of approximately 24 mIU/mL or higher, the complex will bind to the capture antibody coated on the test line and a burgundy red colored band will develop. If the specimen does not contain hCG or is below a detectable level, the test line will not develop a color.

See ⊖volve for the complete procedural protocol and information related to the procedure.

Direct Fluorescent Antibody Test for *Neisseria gonorrhoeae*

Principle

Immunofluorescence is a reliable, simple, rapid test used extensively in the clinical laboratory. The demonstration of microbial antigens is one of the many applications of the direct immunofluorescence procedure; the microbes are incubated with fluorescent-labeled antibodies. Under appropriate conditions, the labeled antibodies bind to specific antigens. Any unbound antibodies are washed off and the bound antibodies are visualized with a fluorescence microscope.

N. gonorrhoeae is a gram-negative diplococcus that causes urogenital infections. The Syva Microtrak *N. gonorrhoeae* culture confirmation test is a direct fluorescent antibody (FA) assay that uses fluorescein-labeled MAbs that react specifically with *N. gonorrhoeae*. The test is performed on primary culture isolates and requires only a small inoculum. Culture isolates presumptively identified as *N. gonorrhoeae* are transferred to a slide well and stained with fluorescein-labeled anti–*N. gonorrhoeae* reagent antibody (anti-GC/FITC). The antibodies bind specifically to gonococcal antigen. Unbound antibodies are then removed by a rinse step. Under a fluorescence microscope, cultures positive for *N. gonorrhoeae* show apple-green fluorescent staining of the kidney-shaped diplococci.

See ⊖volve for procedural protocol.

CHAPTER HIGHLIGHTS

- Heterogeneous immunoassays have a solid phase (microwell, bead) and require washing steps to remove unbound antigens or antibodies. Faster and easier to automate, homogeneous immunoassays have only a liquid phase and do not require washing steps.
- The ideal label should be measurable by several methods, including visual inspection.
- Enzyme immunoassay (EIA) uses a nonisotopic label and is safer than but shares the specificity, sensitivity, and rapidity of radioimmunoassay (RIA).
- In EIA antibody detection, the antigen in question is firmly fixed to a solid matrix (microplate well, outside of bead); this is called solid-phase immunosorbent assay.
- Chemiluminescence is the technology of choice of most immunodiagnostics manufacturers. In competitive and sandwich immunoassays, chemiluminescent labels can be attached to an antigen or antibody.
- Fluorescent labeling (direct and indirect) also demonstrates the complexing of antigens and antibodies. Fluorescent antibodies are used as substitutes for radioisotope or enzyme labels.
- Fluorescent conjugates are used in the basic methods of direct, inhibition, and indirect immunofluorescent assay. In direct immunofluorescence, a conjugated antibody is used to detect antigen-antibody reactions. In the indirect method, antibodies react with homologous antigens but also can act as antigens.
- Emerging labeling technologies include Q dots, SQUID, LOCI, signal amplification, and magnetic labeling.
- Fluorescence in situ hybridization (FISH) is often applied in immunology, hematopathology, and oncology.

REVIEW QUESTIONS

1. Chemiluminescence:
   a. Has excellent sensitivity and dynamic range
   b. Does not require sample radiation
   c. Uses unstable chemiluminescent reagents and conjugates
   d. Both a and b

2 and 3. Match the descriptions (a and b) to the assays.

2. _____ Competitive immunoassay

3. _____ Sandwich immunoassay
   a. Fixed amount of labeled antigen competes with unlabeled antigen from patient specimen for a limited number of antibody-binding sites.
   b. Sample antigen binds to antibody fixed onto solid phase; chemiluminescent-labeled antibody binds to antigen-antibody complex.

4. Enzyme labels often used in indirect procedures are:
   a. Alkaline phosphatase
   b. Horseradish peroxidase
   c. Beta-galactosidase
   d. All of the above

5 and 6. Match the following:

5. _____ Enzyme immunoassay (EIA)

6. _____ Immunofluorescent technique
   a. Uses a nonisotopic label
   b. Uses antibody labeled with fluorescein isothiocyanate (FITC)
   c. Uses colloidal particles consisting of a metal or insoluble metal compound

7-9. Match the assays and definitions.

7. _____ Direct immunofluorescent assay

8. _____ Inhibition immunofluorescent assay

9. _____ Indirect immunofluorescent assay
   a. Based on antibodies acting as antigens and reacting with antiimmunoglobulins
   b. Uses conjugated antibody to detect antigen-antibody reactions
   c. Antigen first exposed to unlabeled antibody, then labeled antibody

10. For an enzyme to be used in an EIA, it must meet all the following criteria except:
    a. High amount of stability
    b. Extreme specificity
    c. Presence in antigen or antibody
    d. No alteration by inhibitor with the system

11. and 12. Fill in the blanks below, choosing from the answers for each.

A fluorescent substance is one that while (11) _____ light of one wavelength, (12) _____ light of another (longer) wavelength.

11.
a. Emitting
b. Absorbing
c. Generating bright
d. Generating dull

12.
a. Emits
b. Absorbs
c. Reduces
d. Increases

13-16. Match the following.

13. _____ Quantum dots (Q dots)

14. _____ SQUID technology

15. _____ Luminescent oxygen-channeling immunoassay (LOCI)

16. _____ Fluorescent in situ hybridization (FISH)
    a. Semiconductor nanocrystals
    b. Method of tagging antibodies with superparamagnetic particles
    c. Technology based on two different 200-nm latex particles
    d. Molecular cytogenetic technique

BIBLIOGRAPHY

Adelman L: Laboratory technology: magnetic labeling technology, Adv Med Lab Admin 11:131, 1999.

Forbes BA, Sahm DF, Weissfeld AS: Bailey and Scott's diagnostic microbiology, ed 12, St Louis, 2007, Mosby.

Hyde A: Enzyme-linked immunosorbent assay (ELISA): an overview, 2006, http://laboratorian.advanceweb.com/Article/Enzyme-Linked-mmunosorbent-Assay-ELISA-An-Overview.aspx.

Jandreski MA: Chemiluminescence technology in immunoassays, Lab Med 29(9):555, 1998.

Mark HFL: Fluorescent in situ hybridization as an adjunct to conventional cytogenetics, Ann Clin Lab Sci 24:153, 1994.

McDowell J: Beyond ANA testing, Clin Lab News October 25:1, 2005.

Sainato D: The coming revolution in assay technologies, Clin Lab News 20:26, 2000.

Van Den Berg F: Applications of a signal amplification technique for light microscopy, Clin Lab News 15:8, 1996.

Wang Z, Hu J, Jin Y, Yao X, Li J: In situ amplified chemiluminescent detection of DNA and immunoassay of IgG using special-shaped gold nanoparticles as label, Clin Chem 52:1958, 2006.

CHAPTER 13

Automated Procedures

Learning Objectives

At the conclusion of this chapter, the reader should be able to:

- Identify and give examples of the three phases in automated testing.
- Describe the principle, advantages, and disadvantages of nephelometry.
- Discuss the analysis and clinical implications of cryoglobulins.
- Explain the principle of flow cell cytometry and cite clinical applications.
- Discuss current trends in immunoassay.

- List at least three potential benefits of automated immunoassay.
- Analyze a case study related to immunoassay.
- Correctly answer case study related multiple choice questions.
- Be prepared to participate in a discussion of critical thinking questions.
- View and discuss questions related to videos about flow cytometry.
- Correctly answer end of chapter review questions.

Key Terms

antibovine antibodies
cryoglobulins
cuvette
denaturation
electromagnetic spectrum
flow cell cytometry
fluorescent polarization immunoassay

fluorochrome
harmonization
Heidelberger curve
immunofluorescence
immunophenotyping
laser
leukocyte

lysing
macromolecular complex
photometrically
photon
seronegative spondyloarthropathies

CHARACTERISTICS OF AUTOMATED TESTING

Laboratory automation can be separated into preanalytic, analytic, and postanalytic phases. Accuracy in each of these phases is critical to quality results. The preanalytic phase includes specimen labeling (bar coding preferred), accessioning, and tracking, along with proper test ordering.

The analytic phase involves the following areas:

- Automated results entry
- Quality control
- Validation of results
- Networking to laboratory information systems

Automated analyzers link each specimen to its specific test request. Any results generated must be verified (approved or reviewed) by the operator before the data are released to the patient report. Useful data for this verification process include flags, signifying results outside the reference range, critical or panic values (possibly life-threatening), values that are out of the technical range for the analyzer, and failures in other checks and balances built into the system.

The postanalytic phase includes adding to patient cumulative reports, workload recording, and networks to other systems. Quality assurance (QA) procedures, including the use of

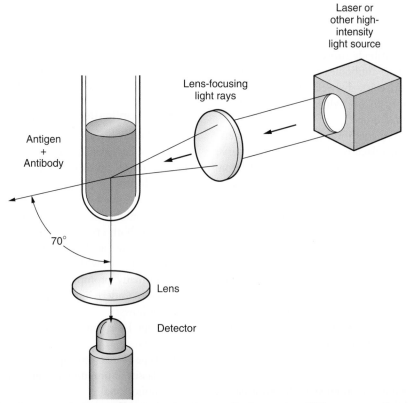

Figure 13-1 Principle of nephelometry for the measurement of antigen-antibody reactions. Light rays are collected in a focusing lens and can ultimately be related to the antigen or antibody concentration in a sample.

quality control (QC) solutions, are part of the analytic functions of the analyzer and its interfaced computer. The Clinical Laboratory Improvement Amendments of 1988 (CLIA '88) regulations require the documentation of all QC data associated with any test results reported (see Chapter 7). **Harmonization** of analytes has been gaining momentum as an essential component of the outcomes of analysis. In the future, harmonized or normalized results may be mapped together and presented numerically and graphically to reduce data output.

NEPHELOMETRY

Nephelometry has become increasingly more popular in diagnostic laboratories and depends on the light-scattering properties of antigen-antibody complexes (Fig. 13-1).

The quantity of cloudiness or turbidity in a solution can be measured **photometrically.** When specific antigen-coated latex particles acting as reaction intensifiers are agglutinated by their corresponding antibody, the increased light scatter of a solution can be measured by nephelometry as the macromolecular complex form. The use of polyethylene glycol (PEG) enhances and stabilizes the precipitates, thus increasing the speed and sensitivity of the technique by controlling the particle size for optimal light angle deflection. The kinetics of this change can be determined when the photometric results are analyzed by computer.

In immunology, nephelometry is used to measure complement components, immune complexes, and the presence of a variety of antibodies (Box 13-1).

Box 13-1	**Immunologic Assays Performed by Nephelometry**
Acid α_1-glycoprotein	Ceruloplasmin
Albumin	Complement components
α_1-Antitrypsin	(C1r, C1s, C2, C3, C4, C5,
α_2-Macroglobulin	C6, C7, C8)
C1 esterase inhibitor (C1	C-reactive protein (CRP)
inhibitor)	Cryofibrinogen
C3	Cryoglobulins
C3b inhibitor (C3b	Haptoglobin
inactivator)	Hemopexin
C3PA (C3 proactivator,	Immunoglobulins
properdin factor B)	Properdin factor B
C4	Transferrin
C6	
C7	
C8	

Principle

Formation of a **macromolecular complex** is a fundamental prerequisite for nephelometric protein quantitation. The procedure is based on the reaction between the protein being assayed and a specific antiserum. Protein in a patient's specimen reacts with specific nephelometric antiserum to human proteins and forms insoluble complexes. When light is passed through such a suspension, the resulting complexes of insoluble precipitants scatter incident light in solutions. The scattered light can be detected with a photodiode. The amount of scattered light is proportional to the number of insoluble complexes and can be quantitated by comparing the unknown patient values with standards of known protein concentration.

The relationship between the quantity of antigen and measuring signal at a constant antibody concentration is expressed by the **Heidelberger curve.** If antibodies are present to excess, a proportional relationship exists between the antigen and resulting signal. If the antigen overwhelms the quantity of antibody, the measured signal drops.

By optimizing the reaction conditions, the typical antigen-antibody reactions as characterized by the Heidelberger curve are effectively shifted in the direction of high concentration. This ensures that these high concentrations will be measured on the ascending portion of the curve. At concentrations higher than the reference curve, the instrument will transmit an out of range warning.

Physical Basis

Nephelometry is based on the principle that light is scattered by a homogeneous particulate solution at a variety of angles. Three types of scatter can occur: (1) scatter around the particles; (2) forward scatter caused by out of phase backscatter; and (3) forward scatter exceeding backscatter.

Optical System

In the nephelometric method, an infrared high-performance, light-emitting diode (LED) is used as the light source. Because an entire solid angle is measured after convergence of this light through a lens system, an intense measuring signal is available when the primary beam is blocked off. In connection with the lens system, this produces a light beam of high colinearity. The wavelength is 840 nm. Light scattered in the forward direction in a solid angle to the primary beam ranges between 13 and 24 feet and is measured by a silicon photodiode with an integrated amplifier. The electrical signals generated are digitized, compared with reference curves, and converted to protein concentrations.

Measuring Methods

A fixed-time method is used routinely for precipitation reactions. Ten seconds after all reaction components have been mixed, a **cuvette** reading (initial blank measurement) is taken. A second measurement is taken 6 minutes later and, after subtraction of the original 1-second blanking value, a final answer is calculated against the multiple-point or single-point calibration in the computerized program memory for the assay.

Advantages and Disadvantages

Nephelometry represents an automated system that is rapid, reproducible, relatively simple to operate, and common in higher volume laboratories. It has many applications in the immunology laboratory. Currently, instruments using a rate method and fixed-time approach are commercially available with tests for immunoglobulin G (IgG), IgA, IgM, C3, C4, properdin, C-reactive protein (CRP), rheumatoid factor, ceruloplasmin, α_1-antitrypsin, apolipoproteins, and haptoglobins.

The disadvantages of nephelometry include high initial equipment cost and interfering substances such as microbial contamination, which may cause protein **denaturation** and erroneous test results. Intrinsic specimen turbidity or lipemia may exceed the preset limits. In these cases, a clearing agent may be needed before an accurate assay can be performed. In addition, low-molecular-weight immunoglobulins, monoclonal immunoglobulins, and **antibovine antibodies** also may produce spurious results in nephelometry.

Clinical Application: Cryoglobulins

Cryoglobulin analysis is frequently requested when patient symptoms such as pain, cyanosis, Raynaud's phenomenon, and skin ulceration on exposure to cold temperatures are present. **Cryoglobulins** are proteins that precipitate or gel when cooled to 0° C (32° F) and dissolve when heated. In most cases, monoclonal cryoglobulins are IgM or IgG. Occasionally, the macroglobulin is both cryoprecipitable and capable of cold-induced anti-i–mediated agglutination of red blood cells.

Cryoglobulins with a detected monoclonal protein component normally prompt a clinical investigation to determine whether an underlying disease exists. Cryoglobulins are classified as follows:

- Type I—cryoprecipitate is a monoclonal IgG, IgA, or IgM.
- Type II—cryoprecipitate is mixed, containing two classes of immunoglobulins, at least one of which is monoclonal.
- Type III—cryoprecipitate is mixed and no monoclonal protein is found.

To test for the presence of cryoglobulins, blood is collected, placed in warm water, and centrifuged at room temperature. The serum is then put into a graduated centrifuge tube and placed in a 4° C (39° F) environment for 7 days. If a gel or precipitate is observed, the tube is centrifuged and the precipitate is washed at 4° C (39° F), redissolved at 37° C (98.6° F), and evaluated by double diffusion and immunoelectrophoresis for the content of the cryoglobulin. Newer methods use nephelometry with cold treatment for analysis.

FLOW CELL CYTOMETRY

Fundamentals of Laser Technology

In 1917, Einstein speculated that under certain conditions, atoms or molecules could absorb light or other radiation and then be stimulated to shed this gained energy. Lasers have been developed with numerous medical and industrial applications.

The **electromagnetic spectrum** ranges from long radio waves to short, powerful gamma rays (Fig. 13-2). Within this spectrum is a narrow band of visible or white light, composed of red, orange, yellow, green, blue, and violet light. **Laser** (*l*ight *a*mplification by *s*timulated *e*mission of *r*adiation) light ranges from the ultraviolet (UV) and infrared (IR) spectrum through all the colors of the rainbow. In contrast to other diffuse forms of radiation, laser light is concentrated. It is almost exclusively of one wavelength or color, and its parallel waves travel in one direction. Through the use of fluorescent dyes, laser light can occur in numerous wavelengths. Types of lasers include glass-filled tubes of helium and neon (most common), yttrium-aluminum-garnet (YAG; an imitation diamond), argon, and krypton.

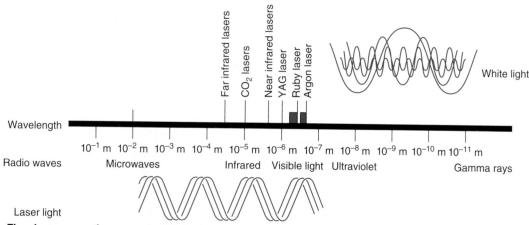

Figure 13-2 **The electromagnetic spectrum.** *YAG,* Yttrium-aluminum-garnet. *(From Turgeon ML: Clinical hematology: theory and procedures, ed 5, Philadelphia, 2012, Lippincott, Williams & Wilkins.)*

Lasers sort the energy in atoms and molecules, concentrate it, and release it in powerful waves. In most lasers, a medium of gas, liquid, or crystal is energized by high-intensity light, an electrical discharge, or even nuclear radiation. When an atom extends beyond the orbits of its electrons or when a molecule vibrates or changes its shape, it instantly snaps back, shedding energy in the form of a photon. The **photon** is the basic unit of all radiation. When a photon reaches an atom of the medium, the energy exchange stimulates the emission of another photon in the same wavelength and direction. This process continues until a cascade of growing energy sweeps through the medium.

Photons travel the length of the laser and bounce off mirrors. First, a few and eventually countless photons synchronize themselves until an avalanche of light streaks between the mirrors. In some gas lasers, transparent disks referred to as Brewster windows are slanted at a precise angle, which polarizes the laser's light. The photons, which are reflected back and forth, finally gain so much energy that they exit as a powerful beam. The power of lasers to transmit energy and information is rated in watts.

Principles of Cell Cytometry

Flow cell cytometry, developed in the 1960s, combines fluid dynamics, optics, laser science, high-speed computers, and fluorochrome-conjugated monoclonal antibodies (MAbs) that rapidly classify groups of cells in heterogeneous mixtures. The principle of flow cytometry is based on cells being stained in suspension with an appropriate **fluorochrome**—an immunologic reagent, a dye that stains a specific component, or some other marker with specific reactivity. Fluorescent dyes used in flow cytometry must bind or react specifically with the cellular component of interest (e.g., reticulocytes, peroxidase enzyme, DNA content). Fluorescent dyes include acridine orange and thioflavin T. Pygon is preferred for fluorescein isothiocyanate (FITC) labeling. Krypton is often used as a second laser in dual-analysis systems and serves as a better light source for compounds labeled by tetramethyl-rhodamine isothiocyanate and tetramethylcyclopropyl-rhodamine isothiocyanate.

A suspension of stained cells is pressurized using gas and transported through plastic tubing to a flow chamber within the instrument (Fig. 13-3). In the flow chamber, the specimen is injected through a needle into a stream of physiologic saline called the sheath. The sheath and specimen both exit the flow chamber through a 75-µm orifice. This laminar flow design confines the cells to the center of the saline sheath, with the cells moving in single file.

The stained cells then pass through the laser beam. The laser activates the dye and the cell fluoresces. Although the fluorescence is emitted throughout a 360-degree circle, it is usually collected by optical sensors located 90 degrees relative to the laser beam. The fluorescence information is then transmitted to a computer, which controls all decisions regarding data collection, analysis, and cell sorting.

Flow cytometry performs fluorescence analysis on single cells. The major applications of this technology are as follows:

- Identification of cells
- Cell sorting before further analysis

Immunophenotyping

Monoclonal antibodies, identified by a cluster designation (CD), are used in most flow cytometry immunophenotyping (Table 13-1). Cell surface molecules recognized by monoclonal antibodies are called antigens because antibodies can be produced against them or are called markers because they identify and discriminate between (mark) different cell populations. Markers can be grouped into several categories. Some are specific for cells of a particular lineage (e.g., CD4+ lymphocytes) or maturational pathway (e.g., CD34+ progenitor stem cells); the expression of others can vary, according to the state of activation or differentiation of the same cells.

In flow cytometry, cells can be sorted from the main cellular population into subpopulations for further analysis (Fig. 13-4). Any fresh specimen that can be placed into a single-cell suspension is a valid candidate for **immunophenotyping** (e.g., T cells, B cells, CD34+ stem cells; detection of minimal residual disease in leukemia). Sorting is accomplished using stored computer information.

When the laser strikes a stained cell, the dye creates distinctive colored light that the cytometer recognizes. This fluorescent intensity is recorded and analyzed by the computer and

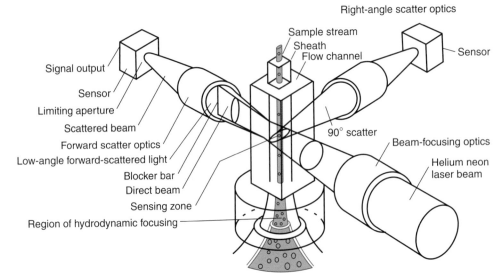

Figure 13-3 Laser flow cytometry. (Courtesy Ortho Diagnostics, Raritan, NJ.)

cells are sorted according to a preprogrammed selection. If the particular cell in the laser beam is of interest, the computer waits the appropriate time for the cell to reach the droplet break-off point within the charging collar. At that point, the computer signals the charging collar to administer an electrostatically positive or negative charge to the stream containing the target cell. A droplet containing this cell is then removed from the main stream before the charge has time to redistribute.

This action produces the cell of interest within a liquid drop that has an electrostatic charge on its surface (only the droplet is charged). The droplet falls between a set of deflection plates, which creates an electrical field. The charged droplets are deflected to the left or right, depending on their polarity, and collected for further analysis.

Multicolor Immunofluorescence

Current fluorescent methods (e.g., BD FACSCanto II flow cytometer; BD, Franklin Lakes, NJ) can perform up to eight-color analysis. The BD LSRII flow cytometer, with up to four lasers, can measure up to 16 colors. It can use four MAbs, each directly conjugated to a distinct fluorochrome, per tube of patient cell suspension. The four most common fluorochromes are FITC, phycoerythrin (PE), peridinin chlorophyll protein (PerCP), and allophycocyanin (APC). The first three fluorochromes are excited by the 488-nm line of an argon laser; the fourth fluorochrome is excited by the 633-nm line of a helium-neon or diode laser.

Eight-color **immunofluorescence** offers the advantages of greater sensitivity and specificity, with increased ability to identify and subclassify individual cells. Improvements in methods and probes may lead to fluorescence in situ hybridization (FISH) in suspension as a routine protocol (see Chapter 12) and enable flow cytometry to operate on a molecular level simultaneously to identify chromosomal abnormalities.

A system that uses a flow cytometer, specific data analysis software, and fluorescent latex particles, the Luminex 100 Total System, has been developed by Luminex Technology (Austin,

Table 13-1	Commonly Used Monoclonal Antibodies in Flow Cytometry
CD Designation	**Cell Type**
CD2	Thymocytes, T lymphocytes, natural killer (NK) cells
CD3	Thymocytes, T lymphocytes
CD4	T lymphocytes (helper subset), monocytes (dimly expressed), macrophages
CD5	Mature T lymphocytes, thymocytes, subset of B lymphocytes (B1)
CD8	T lymphocytes (cytotoxic), macrophages
CD10	T and B lymphocyte precursors, bone marrow stromal cells
CD19	B lymphocytes, follicular dendritic cells
CD21	B cells, follicular dendritic cells, subset of immature thymocytes
CD23	B cells, monocytes, follicular dendritic cells
CD25	Activated T lymphocytes, B cells, monocytes
CD34	Progenitor (hematopoietic stem cells)
CD44	Most leukocytes
CD45	All hematopoietic cells
CD56	Subsets of T lymphocytes, NK cells
CD94	Subsets of T lymphocytes, NK cells

Texas). This system combines advances in computing and optics with a new concept in color coding to create a simple, cost-effective analysis system (Fig. 13-5). Latex beads are coupled to various amounts of two different fluorescent dyes, which are analyzed by the flow cytometer and software to allow the distinct separation of up to 64 slightly different colored bead sets. The color-coded microspheres identify each unique

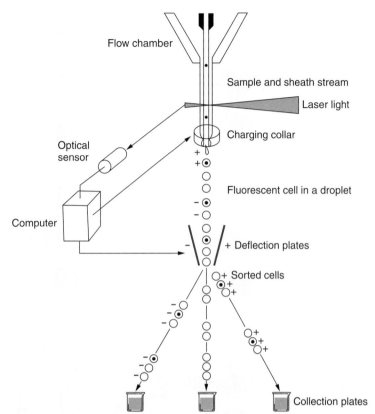

Figure 13-4   Laser and cell-sorting schematic.

reaction. Hundreds of microsphere sets can be identified at once in a single sample. Optical technology recognizes each microsphere and provides a precise, quantitative measure simply and in real time.

Currently, up to 64 microsphere sets are recognized. The current FlowMetrix system is compatible with the BD FACS Vantage SE System and BD FACSCalibur, the most widely used flow cytometers for cellular analysis. Because Luminex technology requires fewer steps to assess multiple parameters, with a high level of sensitivity and accuracy, it is significantly more cost-effective than current methods of analysis. Some immunologic applications already demonstrated with Flow-Metrix are human immunodeficiency virus (HIV) and hepatitis B seroconversion, multicytokine measurement, multiplexed allergy testing, DNA-based tissue typing, herpes simplex viral load, IgG, IgA, and IgM assays, IgG subclassification, autoimmunity panel, epitope mapping, human chorionic gonadotropin (hCG) and α-fetoprotein, HIV viral load, and the TORCHS (*t*oxoplasmosis, *o*ther [viruses], *r*ubella, *c*ytomegalovirus, *h*erpesviruses, *s*yphilis) panel.

Sample Preparation

Specimens that can be used for flow cell analysis include whole blood, bone marrow, and aspirates of body fluids. Whole blood, collected in ethylenediaminetetraacetic acid (EDTA), is the preferred anticoagulant if specimens are processed within 30 hours of collection. Heparin is an alternative anticoagulant for whole blood and bone marrow and can provide stability of specimens more than 24 hours old.

Blood specimens should be stored at room temperature (20° C to 25° C [68° F to 77° F]) before processing. Specimens need to be well mixed prior to delivery into staining tubes. Unsuitable specimens included hemolyzed or clotted samples. For the efficient analysis of white blood cells, whole blood, bone marrow, or aspirates should have the bulk of red blood cells removed prior to analysis. Tissue specimens (e.g., lymph nodes) should be collected and transported in a tissue culture medium at room temperature or at 4° C (39° F) if analysis is delayed. Such a specimen requires disaggregation by enzymatic or mechanical methods to form a single-cell suspension. After proper specimen processing, antibodies are added to the cellular preparation and analyzed. MAbs, tagged with different fluorescent tags, are used for analysis.

Clinical Immunology Applications

Lymphocyte Subsets

A six-color flow cytometry diagnostic application uses the BD FACSCanto II flow cytometer and BD Multitest six-color TBNK with BD Trucount tubes to determine the absolute counts of mature T, B, and natural killer (NK) lymphocytes (Fig. 13-6), as well as CD4+ and CD8+ T cell subsets in human peripheral blood, in a single tube.

Other Cellular Applications

Measuring T Cells for Acquired Immunodeficiency Syndrome Analysis. The quantitation of T and B cells using monoclonal surface markers can be performed using flow cytometry. With the flow cytometer, 10,000 cells can be assayed

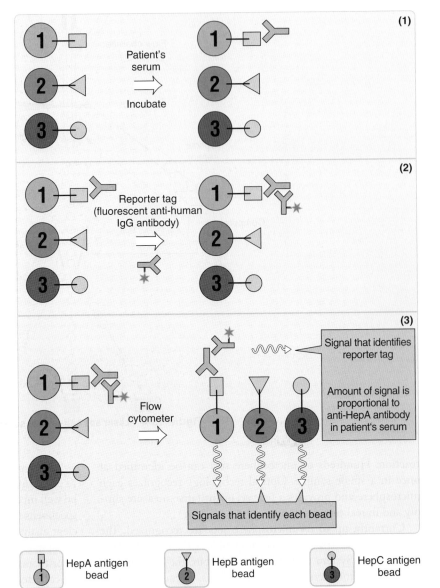

Figure 13-5 Fluorescent microsphere–based immunoassay for antibodies to hepatitis virus (Luminex xMAP technology). This approach is especially valuable when multiple tests must be done. It uses aspects of enzyme-linked immunosorbent assay (ELISA) and flow cytometry. A small amount of sample is known. Polystyrene microspheres are internally color-coded with two fluorescent dyes that can be detected after laser illumination. *(From Nairn R, Helbert M: Immunology for medical students, ed 2, St Louis, 2007, Mosby.)*

into subsets in 1 minute with multiparameter analysis. Using MAbs, T and B cell populations can be divided into subpopulations with specific functions. T cells are divided into two functional subpopulations, helper T (Th) cells and suppressor T (Ts) cells.

Normal individuals have a TH/TS ratio of 2:1 to 3:1. This ratio is inverted in certain disorders and diseases, including the acute phase of cytomegalovirus (CMV) mononucleosis, following bone marrow transplantation, and acquired immunodeficiency syndrome (AIDS).

CD4/CD8 Ratio. The CD4 (helper subset) T lymphocyte cell count is one of the standard measures for diagnosing AIDS and the management of disease progress in patients with HIV infection. The analysis of the T cell and B cell ratio is clinically useful in evaluating the immune system status of patients who may be at an increased risk of opportunistic infections. In addition, the absolute number of CD4+ lymphocytes is reflective of the degree of immunodeficiency in HIV-infected individuals

and may be used as a guide for initiating antiretroviral therapy and monitoring therapy.

In these cases, two cell surface antigens—CD3, which is present on mature T lymphocytes, and CD4, which is only present on the helper subset of T lymphocytes—are used. The percentage of CD4 lymphocytes is determined by using a fluorochrome-conjugated CD3 antibody (e.g., FITC-CD3) together with a CD4 antibody conjugated to a second fluorochrome (e.g., PE-CD4). The absolute CD4 count can be determined. The absolute number of CD4 lymphocytes is reflective of the degree of immunodeficiency in HIV-infected patients and may be used as a guide for timing the administration of antiretroviral therapy and for monitoring the level of immune reconstitution following the initiation of therapy.

Basic Lymphocyte Screening Panel. A basic immune screening panel typically consists of the detection and quantitation of CD3, CD4, CD8, CD19, and CD16/56. Anti–CD45/CD14 is included to assist in distinguishing lymphocytes from

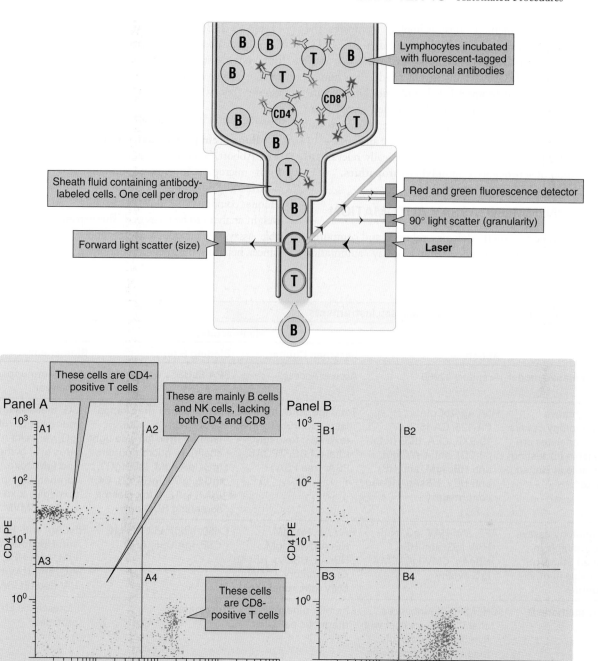

Figure 13-6   Flow cell cytometry dot plots. *Panel A,* Cells stained with the red CD4 antibody account for 59% of all lymphocytes; this is a normal sample. *Panel B,* There is a reduction in the number of red-staining CD4+ T cells; this sample is from a patient with HIV infection. *FITC,* Fluorescein isothiocyanate (emits green light); *PE,* phycoerythrin (emits red light); *(From Nairn R, Helbert M: Immunology for medical students, ed 2, St Louis, 2007, Mosby.)*

monocytes. This panel reveals the frequency of T cells (CD3+), B cells (CD19+), and natural killer cells (CD3–, CD16+, CD56+). It also provides the frequency of Th inducer cells (CD3+, CD4+) and T suppressor or cytotoxic cells (CD3+, CD8+). Typical percentage ranges for lymphocyte subsets in adult donors are as follows: CD3, 56% to 86%; CD4, 33% to 58%; CD8, 13% to 39%; CD16+ CD56, 5% to 26%; and CD19, 5% to 22%.

However, this panel does not provide information on cell activation or signaling pathway receptors, frequency of T subsets (e.g., Th1 or Th2), stem or blast cells, B lymphocytes (e.g., immunoblasts or plasma cells), or nonlymphoid elements.

HLA-B27 Antigen. The automated BD FACSCanto, BD FACSCalibur, BD FACSort, and BD FACScan flow cytometers can rapidly detect HLA-B27 antigen expression in erythrocyte-lysed whole blood (LWB) using a qualitative two-color direct immunofluorescence method. This technology compares the intensity of T lymphocytes stained with anti–HLA-B27 FITC to a predetermined decision marker during analysis. When anti–HLA-B27 FITC/CD3 PE MAb reagent is added to human whole blood, the fluorochrome-labeled antibodies bind specifically to **leukocyte** surface antigens. The stained samples are treated with BD FACS **lysing** solution to lyse erythrocytes and are then washed and fixed before flow cytometric analysis.

This application of flow cytometry is clinically relevant to the evaluation of **seronegative spondyloarthropathies.**

TRENDS IN IMMUNOASSAY AUTOMATION

Technical advances in methodologies, robotics, and computerization have led to expanded immunoassay automation (Table 13-2; Box 13-2). Newer systems use chemiluminescent labels and substrates rather than fluorescent labels and detection systems, such as enzyme immunoassays (see Chapter 12). Immunoassay systems have the potential to improve turnaround time, with enhanced cost-effectiveness (Box 13-3).

Fluorescent Polarization Immunoassay

The **fluorescent polarization immunoassay** IMX System (Biostad-Abbott, Quebec) is an automated analyzer designed to perform microparticle enzyme immunoassay and fluorescence polarization immunoassay using ion capture technology. This unique combination allows both high- and low-molecular-weight analytes to be measured. This expands the range of available assays to include tests for endocrine function, fertility, cancer, hepatitis, transplantation, rubella, and congenital disease.

Table 13-2	**Representative Immunoassay Instruments**			
	Manufacturer			
	Abbott	**Beckman Coulter**	**Binding Site**	**Biomérieux**
Representative model	Architect ii2000	Access/Access2	SPA-PLUS	VIDAS Immunoassay Analyzer
Representative immunology assays (other analytes are available for testing) available in United States*	HIV, Ag/AbCombo, HE-4, CA-125, CA 15-3, CA 19-9XR, CEA, hCG (total β-hCG), anti-HAV IgM, anti-HBc IgM, anti-HBs, anti-HCV, HBsAg, HBsAg confirmatory	Total IgE, EPO, intrinsic factor ab, rubella IgG, toxo IgG, toxo IgM, total β-hCG, TPOAb, PSA, free PSA	Freelite kappa (free kappa light chain), freelite lambda (free lambda light chain), β$_2$-microglobulin, IgG, IgA, IgM, IgD, IgG1, IgG2, IgG3, IgG4, C3, C4, IgA1, IgA2, t. tox plasma screening RUO only	HCG, measles IgG, mumps IgG, rubella IgG, varicella zoster virus IgG, Lyme IgG and IgM, toxo competition, toxo IgG, toxo IgM, toxo IgG avidity, CMVM, CMVG
Immunology assays not available in United States but available in other countries	AFP, anti-HAV IgG, anti-HAV IgG, anti-HBe, HBeAg, CMV IgG, CMV IgG avidity	HAV Ab, HA IgM, HBcAb, HBc IgM, HBsAb, HBsAg, HBsAg confirmatory, CMV IgG, CMV IgM, rubella IgM	CH50, albumin CSF, IgG CSF, IgA CSF, ASO	HBs Ag, anti- HBs total, anti-HBc total, anti-HBc IgM, anti- HBe, HAV IgG, anti-HAV total, HIV duo (ELISA IV)
Assay method(s)*	CHEMIFLEX (enhanced chemiluminescence) with five flexible protocols; magnetic microparticles	Chemiluminescence; magnetic particles	Turbidimetry	Fluorescence EIA, solid particles

	Manufacturer			
	BioRad	**DiaSorin**[†]	**iNova**	**Ortho**
Representative model	Bioplex 2200	LIAISON XL	DSX	VITROS 3600
Immunology assays (other analytes are available for testing) available in United States*	—	EBV IgM, EBNA IgG, VCAIgG, EA IgG, toxo IgG, toxo IgM, CMV IgG, CMV IgM, *Treponema* IgG-IgM, VZV IgG, hGH, HAV IgM, HAV total antibodies, rubella IgG, HSV-1 type specific IgG, HSV-2 type specific IgG, measles IgG, mumps IgG	Autoimmune, infectious diseases	Total β-hCG, CEA, AFP, CA-125 II, CA 15-3, HBsAg, a-HCV, HBsAg (conf), aHBc, aHBc IgM, aHBs, CA 19-9, aHAV total, aHAV IgM, rubella IgG, HIV-1 and -2

Table 13-2	Representative Immunoassay Instruments—cont'd			
	Manufacturer			
	BioRad	**DiaSorin†**	**iNova**	**Ortho**
Immunology assays not available in United States but available in other countries	ANA screen, ENA Plus Screen, anti-dsDNA, anti-Jo-1, anti–SS-A, anti–SS-B, anti–Scl-70, anti-Sm, anti–SM-RNA, anti-centromere, antiphospholipid tests, toxo IgG	HSV-1 and -2 IgM, HSV-1 and -2 IgG, HCG, β_2-microglobulin, AFP, hCG, rubella IgM	Any ELISA	aHBe, HBeAg, rubella IgM, toxo IgG, toxo IgM, CMV IgG, CMV IgM
Assay method(s)	EIA, microwell	Chemiluminescence, magnetic particle	EIA, coated microwell	Chemiluminescence, enhanced chemiluminescence/coated microwell

	Manufacturer		
	Roche	**Siemens**	**TOSOH**
Representative model	Cobas 8000/2010	Dimension Vista 500 Intelligent Lab System	AIA-900/2011
Immunology assays (other analytes are available for testing) available in United States*	Anti-CCP, anti-HAV IgM, anti-HAV total, CA125, CA 15-3, CA 19-9, CEA, hCG II state, HCF and + beta, hGH, IgE, rubella IgG	20 immunoassays including CA 19-9	AFP, CEA, CA 125, CA 19, 27, 29, β_2-microglobulin, IgE II
Immunology assays not available in United States but available in other countries	Anti-HCV, free β-hCG, anti-HBc IgM, HBeAg, anti-HBe, HIV Ag, HIV Ag confirmatory test, HIV combi, toxo IgM, CMV IgG, CMV IgM, CA 72-4	CA 15-3, CA 19-9	HBsAg, ABsAb, HBcAb, HBeAv, HCVAb, hCG
Assay method(s)	Electrochemiluminescence, magnetic particle	Chemiluminescence, LOCI advanced chemiluminescence, EMIT, PETINIA, nephelometry, magnetic particle, homogeneous immunoassay	Fluorescence, enzyme immunoassay, bead

Adapted from CAP TODAY: Automated immunoassay analyzers, Vol. 26, No. 7, July, 2012, pp. 18-54.

AbsAb, Surface antibody; *aHBc,* anti-hepatitits B core antibody; *aHCV,* anti-hepatitis C virus antibody; *AFP,* alpha fetoprotein; *ANA,* antinuclear antibody; *anti-CCP,* anti-cyclic citrullinated peptide antibody; *CA 125,* cancer antigen 125; *CEA,* carcinoembryonic antigen; *EA,* enzyme assay; *EBNA,* major nuclear antigen of Epstein-Barr virus; *EBV,* Epstein-Barr virus; *EMIT,* enzyme-multiplied immunoassay technique; *HbcAb,* hepatitis B core antigen; *HBeAg,* hepatitis B e antigen; *HBsAg,* hepatitis B surface antibody; *HCF,* human growth factor; *HCVAb,* hepatitis C virus antibody; *HSV-1, HSV-2,* herpes simplex virus 1 and 2; *HGH,* human growth hormone; *PETINIA,* particle-enhanced turbidimetric inhibition immunoassay; *RUO,* research use only; *toxo,* toxoplasmosis; *VCA,* viral capsid antigen; *VZV,* varicella zoster virus.

*This is a partial list of immunology assays. It includes autoimmune, cancer-related, and infectious disease antibodies and/or antigens. Other analytes are not included in the list.

†DiaSorin tests not available on other manufacturers' analyzers: *Borrelia burgdorferi,* VZV IgG, HSV-1 type-specific IgG, HSV-2 type-specific IgG, EBV IgM, EBNA IgG, VCA IgG, EA IgG.

Box 13-2	Types of Automated Immunoassays

- Chemiluminescence
- Fluorescent ELISA
- FPIA
- Kinetic fluorescence
- Latex EIA, ELISA
- MEIA

Adapted from CAP Today 21:24–72, 2007.
EIA, Enzyme immunoassay; *ELISA,* enzyme-linked immunosorbent assay; *FPIA,* fluorescent polarization immunoassay; *MEIA,* microparticle enzyme immunoassay.

Box 13-3	Potential Benefits of Immunoassay Automation

- Ability to provide better service with less staff
- Savings on controls, duplicates, dilutions, and repeats
- Elimination of radioactive labels and associated regulations
- Better shelf life of reagents, with less disposal of outdated supplies
- Better sample identification with bar code labels and primary tube sampling
- Automation of sample delivery possible

Adapted from Blick K: Current trends in automation of immunoassays, J Clin Ligand Assay 22:6–12, 1999.

Case Study

History and Physical Examination

BB is a 6-year-old boy. His parents brought him to the hospital complaining of back pain and refusal to walk since falling a week earlier. Consequently, he walked less and slept more than usual; 3 days earlier, after taking a few steps, he had fallen. Consequently, his family took him to see his pediatrician. His temperature was normal. No organomegaly was detected. He had tenderness in the lower back region, with more tenderness on the left side than on the right side. Pain increased with sitting and leg flexion. The neurologic examination was normal. He was prescribed aspirin for pain. A radiograph of his hips was ordered, which was subsequently reported as normal.

One day ago, he was found lying on the bathroom floor crying. He refused to walk or stand and needed assistance because of the lower back pain. The pediatrician advised his parents to take him to the local hospital. He was admitted. Laboratory assays and a repeat hip radiograph, chest film, and magnetic resonance imaging (MRI) studies were ordered.

Admission Laboratory Data

Assay	Patient Results
Hematology	
Hemoglobin	N (negative)
Hematocrit	N
White blood cell count (WBC)	N
Differential WBC	90% immature mononuclear cells; reference range, no immature mononuclear cells
Erythrocyte sedimentation rate (ESR)	High
Chemistry	
Glucose	N
Total protein	N
Albumin	N
Globulin	N
Bilirubin (total)	N
Alkaline phosphatase	High
Lactic dehydrogenase (LDH)	High
Calcium (total)	High
Phosphorus	High
Serology	
C-reactive protein	High
Urinalysis	
Dipstick	All results within normal limits

Follow-Up
Diagnostic Imaging

Radiographs of the chest were normal. MRI scans of the lumbar spine with the administration of gadolinium were considered to be normal. MRI studies of the brain, without gadolinium, were interpreted as normal. MRI scans of the spine and pelvis revealed deformities of several vertebral bodies of the thoracic and lumbar spine.

Hematology

A bone marrow biopsy was ordered. Samples of the bone marrow aspirate were sent for morphologic examination, flow cytometry, and cytogenetic analysis.

Hematology (4 days after admission)

Assay	Patient Results
Peripheral Blood	
Hemoglobin	Low
Hematocrit	Low
White blood cell count (WBC)	Low
Differential WBC	90% immature mononuclear cells; reference range, no immature mononuclear cells
Bone Marrow	
Microscopic examination	Predominant population of small to medium size immature mononuclear cells; nucleoli present

Flow Cytometry (4 days after admission)

Cell Surface Markers	Reactivity
CD34	Positive
Terminal deoxynucleotidyl transferase (TdT)	Positive
CD19	Positive
CD10	Positive
CD45	Weakly positive

Cytogenetic Analysis

A normal male karyotype (46,XY) was found. Fluorescence in situ hybridization showed normal numbers of chromosomes 4, 10, and 17 and no evidence of rearrangements involving *TEL, AML1, BCR, ABL1,* or *MLL,* normal leukocytes, platelets, and red cells.

Questions
1. The CD34+ surface membrane marker is exhibited by:
    a. Stem cells
    b. Mature T lymphocytes
    c. Mature B lymphocytes
    d. Mature plasma cells

2. The classic marker for mature B-lymphocytes is:
   a. CD4
   b. CD8
   c. CD10
   d. CD20

Answers to these questions can be found in Appendix A.

Critical Thinking Group Discussion Questions
1. What is the significance of positive reactivity of CD45?
2. What is the significance of positive reactivity of CD34?
3. What is the significance of positive reactivity of CD19 and CD20?
4. What is the significance of a normal cytogenetic profile?

See instructor site ⊖volve for the discussion of the answers to these questions.

Procedure Laboratory Activities

This laboratory activity consists of viewing two videos produced by the Beckman Coulter, Inc. company. After watching these videos, be prepared to answer the group discussion questions.

http://www.coulterflow.com/bciflow/flowanimations/principles/a001_flowprinciples_content_objectives.html

Animated Flow Cytometry Theory—Theory #1

After completing this presentation you will be able to:
- Define the terms: sheath, hydrodynamic focusing, forward scatter, side scatter, fluorescence, peak, integral, amplification, noise discrimination, analog to digital, histogram, dotplot, gating, TOF (Gallios only), and analysis.
- Identify the hardware components: flow cell, laser beam, filters, and photomultiplier tubes.
- Identify the sequence of events in the sensing process.
- Describe the effect that pressure, high voltage, gains, and noise discrimination have on the signals.
- Identify region types and the use of regions for gating and analysis.

Animated Flow Cytometry Theory—Theory #5

After completing this presentation you will be able to:
- Describe the basic concepts involved in the application(s) of interest.
- Recognize the basic plots representing the application(s) of interest.

Discussion Questions

Theory #1
1. What is the sequence of events in the cell separation and identification process?

2. What types of regions exist in cell flow analysis?
3. What is the use of regions for gating and analysis?

Theory #5
1. Name at least six clinical laboratory applications of flow cytometry.
2. What is the basic concept associated with the applications named in question #1?
3. Describe the basic plots representing the applications of interest.

CHAPTER HIGHLIGHTS

- When specific antigen-coated latex particles acting as reaction intensifiers are agglutinated by their corresponding antibody, the increased light scatter of a solution can be measured by nephelometry as the macromolecular complex form.
- Nephelometry is a rapid and highly reproducible automated method.
- Cryoglobulins are proteins that precipitate or gel when cooled to $0°$ C ($32°$ F) and dissolve when heated. In most cases, monoclonal cryoglobulins are IgM or IgG.
- Flow cytometry is based on cells being stained in suspension with an appropriate fluorochrome (immunologic reagent, dye that stains specific component, other marker with specified reactivity).
- Laser light is the most common light source used in flow cytometers.
- Color immunofluorescence uses monoclonal antibodies, each directly conjugated to a distinct fluorochrome, per tube of patient cell suspension. Eight-color immunofluorescence offers the advantages of greater sensitivity and specificity.
- Newer systems in immunoassay automation use chemiluminescent labels and substrates rather than fluorescent labels and detection systems.

REVIEW QUESTIONS

1. Nephelometry measures the light scatter of:
   a. Ions
   b. Macromolecules
   c. Antibodies
   d. Soluble antigens

2. Nephelometry can be used to assay all the following except:
   a. IgM
   b. IgG
   c. IgD
   d. IgA

3. Cryoglobulins are proteins that precipitate or gel when cooled to:
   a. $−18°$ C ($−0.4°$ F)
   b. $0°$ C ($32°$ F)
   c. $4°$ C ($39°$ F)
   d. $18°$ C ($64°$ F)

4-6. Match the following types of cryoglobulin with their respective descriptions.

4. _____ Type I

5. _____ Type II

6. _____ Type III
   a. Contains two classes of immunoglobulins, at least one of which is monoclonal
   b. Mixed, no monoclonal protein found
   c. Monoclonal IgG, IgA, or IgM

7. Cryoglobulin analysis can be useful in the diagnosis of:
   a. Hypothermia
   b. Raynaud's phenomenon
   c. Hepatitis C
   d. Rheumatoid arthritis

8. Laser is an acronym for:
   a. Light amplification by stimulated emission of radiation
   b. Light augmentation by stimulated emitted radiation
   c. Light amplified by stimulated energy radiation
   d. Large angle stimulation by emitted radiation

9. All the following are descriptive characteristics of laser light except:
   a. Intensity
   b. Stability
   c. Polychromaticity
   d. Monochromaticity

10. A photon is a:
    a. Basic unit of light
    b. Basic unit of all radiation
    c. Component of an atom
    d. Component of laser light

11. The major application of flow cell technology is:
    a. Identification of cells
    b. Cell sorting before further analysis
    c. Diagnosis of autoimmune disease
    d. Both a and b

12. Four-color immunofluorescence typically uses:
    a. Fluorescein isothiocyanate (FITC)
    b. Phycoerythrin (PE)
    c. Peridinin chlorophyll protein (PerCP)
    d. All of the above

BIBLIOGRAPHY

Bakke AC: The principles of flow cytometry, Lab Med 32:207–211, 2001.

Behring nephelometer system folder, Branchburg, NJ, 1987, Behring Diagnostics.

Blick KE: Current trends in automation of immunoassays, J Clin Ligand Assay 22:6–12, 1999.

Hoffman EG: Laboratory evaluation of monoclonal gammopathies, Can J Med Technol 49:99–115, 1987.

Kaplan LA, Pesce AJ: Clinical chemistry: theory, analysis, correlation, ed 5, St Louis, 2010, Mosby.

Kelliher AS, Keele B, McBreen M, Preffer FI: Multiparameter flow cytometry in the clinical lab: present capacities and future projections, 2001, (laboratorian.advanceweb.com/Article/Multiparameter-Flow-Cytometry-in-the-Clinical-Lab-Present-Capacities–Future-Projections.aspx).

Lovett EJ 3rd, Schnitzer B, Keren DF, et al: Application of flow cytometry to diagnostic pathology, Lab Invest 50:115–140, 1984.

Smalley D, Aller RD: Picturing tomorrow's system, Cap Today 15:53–84, 2001.

Turgeon ML: Clinical hematology: theory and procedures, ed 5, Philadelphia, 2012, Lippincott, Williams & Wilkins.

CHAPTER 14

Molecular Techniques

Learning Objectives

At the conclusion of this chapter, the reader should be able to:

- Describe the composition of DNA and RNA.
- Compare the functions of DNA and various forms of RNA.
- Describe the polymerase chain reaction (PCR) amplification technique.
- Compare various PCR modifications.
- Identify and briefly describe other amplification techniques.
- Describe the gold standard of genetic analysis.
- Compare DNA sequencing and branched DNA protocols.
- Identify and compare three hybridization techniques.
- Explain how microarrays are applied to immunologic testing.
- Discuss the general concept of nucleic acid blotting.
- Compare the characteristics and clinical applications of Southern, Northern, and Western blotting techniques.
- Analyze a case study related to immunoassay.
- Correctly answer case study related multiple choice questions.
- Be prepared to participate in a discussion of critical thinking questions.
- Describe a molecular testing procedure.
- Correctly answer end of chapter review questions.

Key Terms

amplicon
anneal
autologous
clonality
cryptic plasmid
deoxynucleotide
deoxyribonucleic acid (DNA)
DNA ligase
hematopathology
hybridize

immunosorbent
low-density lipoprotein receptor (LDLR)
nucleic acid probe
nucleotides
oligonucleotide
polymerase chain reaction (PCR)
primers
proto-oncogenes
purine

pyrimidine
radiolabeled
reverse transcriptase (RT)
ribonucleic acid (RNA)
single-base mutations
thermocycler
transcription
translation
tumorigenesis
tumor suppressor genes

Molecular genetic testing is a diagnostic discipline in the clinical laboratory. In industry, molecular diagnostics can also be referred to as biotechnology. Industrial applications include the pharmaceutical and agricultural industries.

Since the complete human genome (sequence) became available in 2003, molecular genetic testing has been expanded extensively. It is important to remember, however, that even with highly standardized molecular methods, these tests are as susceptible to laboratory errors as any other laboratory procedure.

CHARACTERISTICS OF NUCLEIC ACIDS

Nucleic acids are of two main types, **deoxyribonucleic acid (DNA)** and **ribonucleic acid (RNA).** Human beings have 46 chromosomes arranged in 23 pairs of **autologous** chromosomes and one pair of sex chromosomes. Genes are sequences of DNA carried on chromosomes that encode information for the translation of nucleic acid sequences into amino acid sequences that result in the production of proteins. Although the human genome has more than 3 billion DNA bases, the number of encoded genes is approximately 30,000. In comparison, RNA acts as an intermediate nucleic acid structure that helps convert the DNA-encoded genetic information into proteins. DNA is the template for the synthesis of RNA.

DNA and RNA are polymers made up of repeating **nucleotides** or bases that are linked together (Fig. 14-1). DNA and RNA have the same two **purine** bases, adenine (A) and guanine (G), but the **pyrimidine** bases differ. DNA has cytosine (C) and thymine (T); RNA substitutes uracil (U) for T. DNA is predominantly a double-stranded molecule with specific base pairs linked together (Fig. 14-2). Nucleotides are bonded together and two strands are twisted into an alpha helix (Fig. 14-3).

How Does DNA Replicate?

DNA is a very stable molecule and replication is straightforward. The process of replication (Fig. 14-4) involves one strand of the molecule acting as a template for the creation of a complementary strand. As a result of this process, two identical daughter molecules are produced. In the laboratory, the hydrogen bonds that hold the strands of the double helix can be broken apart or denatured. If complementary strands of DNA are denatured in the laboratory, they can spontaneously rejoin, or **anneal.** The process of denaturation and annealing (see later discussion) can be used effectively in molecular testing.

Production of functional protein from genetically encoded DNA is achieved by two processes, transcription and translation. **Transcription** is a process of generating a strand of messenger RNA (mRNA) that encodes for the gene and is expressed as a protein. **Translation** occurs when the mRNA moves from the nucleus of a cell into the cellular cytoplasm to the ribosomes. mRNA is translated into an amino acid

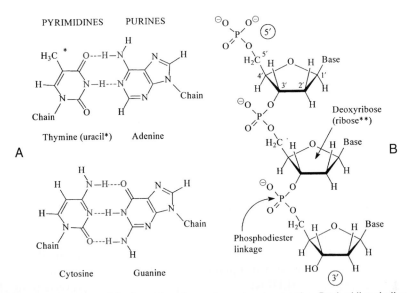

Figure 14-1   A, Purine and pyrimidine bases and the formation of complementary base pairs. *Dashed lines* indicate the formation of hydrogen bonds. **B,** A single-stranded DNA chain. Repeating nucleotide units are linked by phosphodiester bonds that join the 5′ carbon of one sugar to the 3′carbon of the next. Each nucleotide monomer consists of a sugar moiety, a phosphate residue, and a base. *In RNA, thymine is replaced by uracil, which differs from thymine only in its lack of the methyl group. **In RNA, the sugar is ribose, which adds a 2′-hydroxyl to deoxyribose. *(Adapted from Piper MA, Unger ER: Nucleic acid probes: a primer for pathologists, Chicago, 1989, ASCP Press.)*

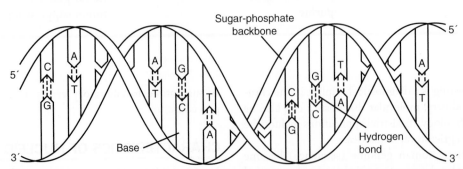

Figure 14-2   Structure of DNA. The DNA molecule is a double helix that consists of two sugar-phosphate backbones with four bases—cytosine *(C),* guanine *(G),* adenine *(A),* and thymine *(T)*—attached. *C* and *G* residues and *A* and *T* residues on opposite strands pair through hydrogen bonding. *(From LeGrys V, Leinbach SS, Silverman L: Clinical applications of DNA probes in the diagnosis of genetic diseases, Crit Rev Clin Lab Sci 25:255, 1987.)*

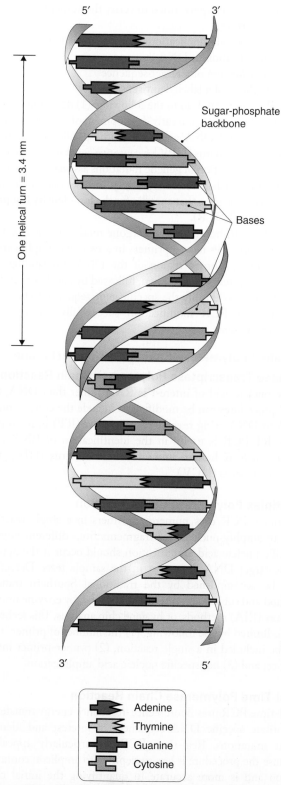

Figure 14-3 **The DNA double helix, with sugar-phosphate backbone and pairing of the bases in the core forming planar structures.** *(From Jorde CB, Carey JC, Bamshead MJ et al, editors: Medical genetics, ed 3, St Louis, 2006, Mosby.)*

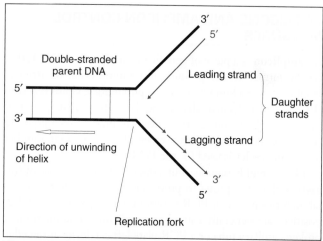

Figure 14-4 **DNA replication.** Double-stranded DNA is separated at the replication fork. The leading strand is synthesized continuously, whereas the lagging strand is synthesized discontinuously but joined later by DNA ligase. *(From Burtis CA, Ashwood ER, Bruns DB: Tietz fundamentals of clinical chemistry, ed 6, St Louis, 2008, Saunders.)*

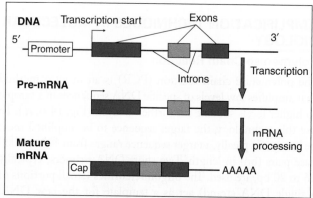

Figure 14-5 **DNA transcription and mRNA processing.** A gene that encodes for a protein contains a promoter region with a variable number of introns and exons. Transcription commences at the transcription start site. Pre-mRNA is processed by capping, polyadenylation, and intron splicing and becomes a mature mRNA. *(From Burtis CA, Ashwood ER, Bruns DB: Tietz fundamentals of clinical chemistry, ed 6, St Louis, 2008, Saunders.)*

sequence on the ribosome. This process manufactures a protein that was originally encoded in DNA in the cellular nucleus.

Forms of RNA

RNA can be easily replicated and is used in molecular laboratory testing. RNA exists in three forms, mRNA, tRNA, and rRNA. All the forms of RNA exist as single-stranded polymers and are longer than DNA. The function of each form of RNA differs, as follows :

- mRNA—translates DNA coding into functional proteins (Fig. 14-5)
- tRNA—transports various amino acids to manufacture proteins
- rRNA—site of protein synthesis directed by mRNA

AMPLICONS AND AMPLICON CONTROL MEASURES

An **amplicon** is a piece of genetic material, such as DNA, that can be formed as the product of a natural event or artificial amplification technique, such as a **polymerase chain reaction (PCR)**. A molecular diagnostic laboratory that performs in vitro amplification reactions needs to practice techniques to control contamination. This is especially true if a high number of thermal cycles is used for the PCR.

PCR is highly sensitive but a disadvantage to the use of this assay is that it is prone to producing false-positive results. In laboratories in which PCR is performed frequently, any false-positives are generally caused by amplicon contamination. A broken capillary tube or a PCR plate left carelessly at the edge of a table can aerosolize those amplicons, which can then adhere to lab coats and objects in the room.

A simple and effective way to combat amplicon contamination is to wipe down everything—equipment, workstations, and pipettes—with bleach. Generously spray with 10% bleach and then let it sit for 15 to 30 minutes.

AMPLIFICATION TECHNIQUES IN MOLECULAR BIOLOGY

Polymerase Chain Reaction

The polymerase chain reaction (PCR) is an in vitro method that amplifies low levels of specific DNA sequences in a sample to higher levels suitable for further analysis (Fig. 14-6, *A*). To use this technology, the target sequence to be amplified must be known. Typically, a target sequence ranges from 100 to 1000 base pairs (bp) in length. Two short DNA **primers,** typically 16 to 20 bp, are used. The **oligonucleotides** (small portions of a single DNA strand) act as a template for the new DNA. These primer sequences are complementary to the 3′ ends of the sequence to be amplified.

This enzymatic process is carried out in cycles. Each repeated cycle consists of the following:

- DNA denaturation. Separation of the double DNA strands into two single strands through the use of heat.
- Primer annealing. Recombination of the oligonucleotide primers with the single-stranded original DNA.
- Extension of primed DNA sequence. The enzyme DNA polymerase synthesizes new complementary strands by the extension of primers.

Each cycle theoretically doubles the amount of specific DNA sequence present and results in an exponential accumulation of the DNA fragment being amplified (amplicons). In general, this process is repeated approximately 30 times. At the end of 30 cycles, the reaction mixture should contain about 2^{30} molecules of the desired product.

After cycling is complete, the amplification products can be analyzed in various ways. Typically, the contents of the reaction vessel are subjected to gel electrophoresis. This allows visualization of the amplified gene segments (e.g., PCR products, bands) and determination of their specificity. Additional product analysis by probe hybridization or direct DNA sequencing is often performed to verify the authenticity of the amplicon further.

Three important applications of PCR are as follows:
1. Amplification of DNA
2. Identification of a target sequence
3. Synthesis of a labeled antisense probe

PCR analysis can lead to the following: (1) detection of gene mutations that signify the early development of cancer; (2) identification of viral DNA associated with specific cancers (e.g., human papillomavirus [HPV], a causative agent in cervical cancer); and (3) detection of genetic mutations associated with various diseases, such as coronary artery disease associated with mutations of the gene that encodes for the **low-density lipoprotein receptor (LDLR).**

The PCR technique has undergone modifications (see Fig. 14-6, *B*). One uses nested primers in a two-step amplification process. First, a broad region of the DNA surrounding the sequence of interest is amplified, followed by another round of amplification to amplify the specific gene sequence to be studied. Another PCR modification successfully differentiates alleles of the same gene.

Modified Polymerase Chain Reaction Techniques

Reverse Transcriptase Polymerase Chain Reaction

If the nucleic acid of interest is RNA rather than DNA, the PCR procedures can be modified to include the conversion of RNA to DNA using **reverse transcriptase (RT)** in the initial steps. RT-PCR is useful in the identification of RNA viral agents, such as human immunodeficiency virus (HIV) and hepatitis C virus (HCV).

Multiplex Polymerase Chain Reaction

Multiplex PCR uses numerous primers in a single reaction tube to amplify nucleic acid fragments from different targets. Specific nucleic acid amplification should occur if the appropriate target DNA is present in the sample tests. Detection may be accomplished by the traditional Southern transfer method and subsequent **nucleic acid probe,** by enzyme immunoassay (EIA) methods, or by gene chip analysis. This technology is limited by the following: (1) the number of primers that can be included in a single reaction; (2) primer-primer interference; and (3) nonspecific nucleic acid amplification.

Real-Time Polymerase Chain Reaction

Real-time PCR uses fluorescence-resonance energy transfer to quantitate specific DNA sequences of interest and identify point mutations. Real-time PCR is particularly appealing because the procedure is less susceptible to amplicon contamination and is more accurate in quantifying the initial copy number.

Other Amplification Techniques

Strand Displacement Amplification

Strand displacement amplification (SDA) is a fully automated method that amplifies target nucleic acid without the use of a **thermocycler.** A double-stranded DNA fragment is created and becomes the target for exponential amplification.

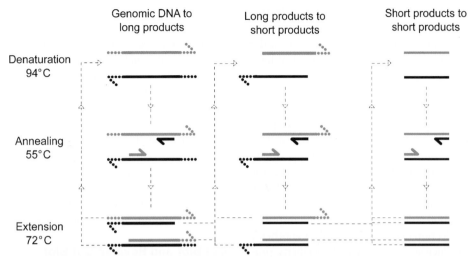

Figure 14-6 Schematic diagram of polymerase chain reaction. Repetitive cycles of denaturation, annealing, and extension are paced by temperature cycling of the reaction. Two primers indicated as short segments anneal to opposite template strands *(long line)* to define the region to be amplified. Extension occurs from the 3′ ends *(half-arrowheads)*. In each cycle, genomic DNA is denatured and annealed to primers that extend in opposite directions across the same region, producing long products of undefined length. Long products generated by extension of one of the primers anneal to the other primer during the next cycle, producing short products of defined length. Any short products present also produce more short products. After *n* cycles, up to 2*n* new copies of the amplified region are present—*n* long products and (2*nn* − *n*) short products plus one original genomic copy. A similar approach can be used to amplify RNA targets by initial reverse transcription of the RNA template to produce the DNA template. *(From Burtis CA, Ashwood ER, Bruns DB: Tietz fundamentals of clinical chemistry, ed 6, St Louis, 2008, Saunders.)*

Transcription-Mediated Amplification

Transcription-mediated amplification (TMA) is another isothermal assay that targets DNA or RNA, but generates RNA as its amplified product. TMA is used to detect microorganisms (e.g., *Mycobacterium tuberculosis*).

Nucleic Acid Sequence–Based Amplification

Nucleic acid sequence–based amplification (NASBA) is similar to TMA, but only RNA is targeted for amplification. Its applications include the detection and quantitation of HIV and detection of cytomegalovirus (CMV).

Ligase Chain Reaction Nucleic Acid Amplification

Oligonucleotide pairs **hybridize** to target sequences within the gene or the **cryptic plasmid**. The bound oligonucleotides are separated by a small gap at the target site. The enzyme DNA polymerase uses nucleotides in the ligase chain reaction (LCR)–nucleic acid amplification reaction mixture to fill in this gap, creating a ligatable junction. Once the gap is filled, **DNA ligase** joins the oligonucleotide pairs to form a short, single-stranded product that is complementary to the original target sequence. This product can itself serve as a target for hybridization and ligation of a second pair of oligonucleotides present in the LCR reaction mixture.

Subsequent rounds of denaturation and ligation lead to the geometric accumulation of amplification product. The amplified products can be detected in an LCx analyzer (Abbott Laboratories, Abbott Park, Ill) by microparticle EIA.

Target Enrichment Strategies

In the last 10 years, next generation sequencing (NGS) technologies have been developed. This approach overcomes the limitations of traditional Sanger sequencing by providing highly parallel sequencing with a separate sequence result for every sequence of interest. This has positioned NGS as the method of choice for targeted re-sequencing of regions of the human genome. Two main technologies have been used to enable target enrichment: PCR and hybridization.

ANALYSIS OF AMPLIFICATION PRODUCTS

Many of the revolutionary changes that have occurred in research in the biological sciences, particularly the Human Genome Project, can be directly attributed to the ability to manipulate DNA in defined ways. Molecular genetic testing focuses on the examination of nucleic acids (DNA or RNA) by special techniques to determine whether a specific nucleotide base sequence is present.

The applications of nucleic acid testing have expanded, despite higher costs associated with testing, in various areas of the clinical laboratory. These include genetic testing, **hematopathology** diagnosis and monitoring, and identification of infectious agents. Molecular testing has the following advantages:
- Faster turnaround time
- Smaller required sample volumes
- Increased specificity and sensitivity

Conventional Analysis

Detection of DNA products by PCR assay can be conventionally analyzed using agarose gel electrophoresis after ethidium bromide staining. This technique is simply an extra step after a PCR assay has been run. DNA and other biomolecules can be separated based on charge, size, and shape. DNA has a net negative charge and will migrate toward the anode (positive pole). PCR products are loaded into an agarose gel and electrophoresed. Ethidium bromide is a dye that intercalates into nucleic acids and will fluoresce with an orange color under ultraviolet (UV) irradiation. An image analyzer uses UV light to capture computer images of the PCR products.

Other Techniques

Other techniques are used to enhance the sensitivity and specificity of amplification techniques. Probe-based DNA detection systems have the advantage of providing sequence specificity and lower detection limits. Other techniques include the hybridization protection assay, DNA EIA, automated DNA sequencing technology, single-strand conformational polymorphism, and restriction fragment length polymorphism (RFLP) analysis. The selection of one technique over another is often based on factors such as sensitivity and specificity profiles, cost, turnaround time, and local experience.

DNA Sequencing

DNA sequencing is considered to be the gold standard to which other molecular methods are compared. DNA sequencing displays the exact nucleotide or base sequence of a fragment of DNA that is targeted. The Sanger method, which uses a series of enzymatic reactions to produce segments of DNA complementary to the DNA being sequenced, is the most frequently used method for DNA sequencing. Automated sequencing techniques use primers with four different fluorescent labels.

1. The first step in sequencing a target is usually to amplify it by cloning or in vitro amplification, usually PCR. Once the amplified DNA is purified from the clinical specimen (the target DNA), it is heat-denatured to separate the double-stranded DNA (dsDNA) into single strands (ssDNA).
2. The second step involves adding primers to the ssDNA. Primers are short synthetic segments of ssDNA that contain a nucleotide sequence complementary to a short strand of target DNA. The patient's DNA serves as a template to copy. DNA polymerase catalyzes the addition of the appropriate nucleotides to the preexisting primer. DNA synthesis is terminated when the **deoxynucleotide** is incorporated into a growing DNA chain.

Branched DNA

Branched DNA (bDNA) is another quantitative test that uses signal amplification instead of target amplification. Target DNA or RNA is hybridized at different sites by two types of probes. Branched DNA assays are used to measure the viral load of hepatitis B virus (HBV), HCV, HIV-1, CMV, and microbial organisms (e.g., *Trypanosoma brucei*).

The Versant HIV-1 RNA 3.0 assay (bDNA; Bayer, Berkeley, Calif), uses bDNA technology. It is the only viral load assay specifically designed to target multiple sequences of the HIV-1 genome with more than 80 nucleic acid probes.

Hybridization Techniques

Many forms of probe hybridization assays involve the complementary pairing of a probe with a DNA or RNA strand derived from the patient's specimen. The common feature of probe hybridization assays is the use of a labeled nucleic acid probe to examine a specimen for a specific, homologous DNA or RNA sequence. Clinical probes are usually labeled with nonradioisotopic molecules such as digoxigenin, alkaline phosphatase, biotin, or a fluorescent compound. The detection systems are conjugate-dependent and include chemiluminescent, fluorescent, and calorimetric methodologies.

Liquid-Phase Hybridization

In the liquid-phase hybridization (LPH) assay, the target nucleic acid and labeled probe interact in solution. Specific homologous hybrids are subsequently separated from the remaining nucleic acid component and the hybrids are identified by an appropriate detection system.

Dot Blot and Reverse Dot Blot

These hybridization methods are used in the clinical laboratory for the detection of disorders in which the DNA sequence of the mutated region has been identified (e.g., sickle cell anemia, cystic fibrosis). These techniques are capable of distinguishing the homozygous or heterozygous state of a mutation.

Dot Blot. The dot blot hybridization method detects **single-base mutations** using allele-specific oligonucleotides (ASOs). Unlike other assays, dot blot does not require enzyme digestion or electrophoretic separation of DNA fragments. The procedure uses labeled oligonucleotide probes of about 15 to 19 bp. DNA is amplified in the region of a known mutation, denatured, and applied to separate areas of a membrane or filter. A probe designed to detect a normal DNA sequence is added to one area; a second probe for the detection of a sequence with the single-base mutation is applied to a second area. Ideally, only the labeled probe whose base sequences perfectly match those of the patient will hybridize.

Reverse Dot Blot. In this variation of the dot blot procedure, the ASO probes are bound to a filter and denatured DNA from the patient is added to the immobilized ASO. Hybridization occurs only if the patient's DNA contains base sequences that are 100% complementary to those of the probe. A common variation of the reverse dot blot procedure is to bind oligonucleotide probes of a slightly longer length than usual to a 96-well microtiter plate. Biotin is used to label copies of the target sequence. The labeled copies are hybridized in the wells to the bound probes and detected using avidin conjugated to horseradish peroxidase. Subsequent addition of substrate produces a colored reaction that can be read photometrically.

Blotting Protocols

The Southern blot and Northern blot techniques are used to detect DNA and RNA, respectively. These procedures share the following steps:

1. Electrophoretic separation of the patient's nucleic acid
2. Transfer of nucleic acid fragments to a solid support (e.g., nitrocellulose)
3. Hybridization with a labeled probe of known nucleic acid sequence
4. Autoradiographic or colorimetric detection of the bands created by the probe–nuclei acid hybrid

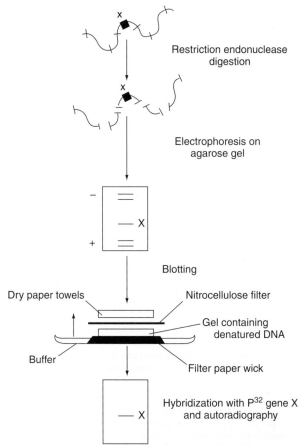

Restriction endonuclease digestion

Electrophoresis on agarose gel

Blotting

Dry paper towels — Nitrocellulose filter

— Gel containing denatured DNA

Buffer — Filter paper wick

Hybridization with P³² gene X and autoradiography

Figure 14-7 Identification by Southern blot hybridization of DNA fragment containing gene X. DNA was digested with restriction endonuclease, and resulting fragments were fractionated according to size by electrophoresis in agarose gel. DNA fragments in gel were denatured and blotted to nitrocellulose filter as a result of flow of buffer through gel and nitrocellulose filter to dry paper towels. Subsequent hybridization of DNA on filter to ³²P-labeled gene X probe and autoradiography revealed single DNA fragment containing gene X. *(Reprinted with permission from LeGrys V, Leinbach SS, Silverman L: CRC Crit Rev Clin Lab Sci 25:255, 1987. Copyright CRC Press, Boca Raton, FL.)*

Southern Blot. Specimen DNA is denatured and treated with restriction enzymes to create DNA fragments; then the ssDNA fragments are separated by electrophoresis (Figure 14-7). The electrophoretically separated fragments are then blotted to a nitrocellulose membrane, retaining their electrophoretic position and hybridized with **radiolabeled** single-stranded DNA fragments with sequences complementary to those being sought. The resulting dsDNA bearing the radiolabel, if present, is then detected by radiography.

The Southern blot procedure has clinical diagnostic applications for disorders associated with significant changes in DNA, a deletion or insertion of at least 50 to 100 bp (e.g., fragile X syndrome), and determination of **clonality** in lymphomas of T or B cell origin. If a single-base mutation changes an enzyme restriction site on the DNA, resulting in an altered band or fragment size, the Southern blot procedure can detect these changes in DNA sequences, referred to as RFLPs. Single-base mutations that can be determined by the Southern blot technique include sickle cell anemia and hemophilia A.

Northern Blot. mRNA from the specimen is separated by electrophoresis and blotted to a specially modified paper support; this results in covalent fixing of the mRNA in the electrophoretic positions. Radiolabeled, ssDNA fragments complementary to the specific mRNA being sought are then hybridized to the bound mRNA. If the specific mRNA is present, its radioactivity is detected by autoradiography.

The derivation of this technique from the Southern blot technique used for DNA detection has led to the common usage of the term *Northern blot* for the detection of specific mRNA. However, the Northern blot technique is not routinely used in clinical molecular diagnostics.

Western Blot. Compared with the Southern blot technique, which separates and identifies RNA fragments and proteins, and the Northern blot technique, which concentrates on isolating mRNA, in the Western blot technique proteins are separated electrophoretically, transferred to membranes, and identified through the use of labeled antibodies specific for the protein of interest (Fig. 14-8).

The Western blot technique detects antibodies to specific epitopes of antigen subspecies. Electrophoresis of antigenic material results in the separation of the antigen components by molecular weight (MW). Blotting the separated antigen to nitrocellulose, retaining the electrophoretic position, and causing it to react with patient specimen will result in the binding of specific antibodies, if present, to each antigenic band. Electrophoresis of known MW standards allows for the determination of the MW of each antigenic band to which antibodies may be produced. These antibodies are then detected using EIA reactions that characterize antibody specificity.

The Western blot technique is often used to confirm the specificity of antibodies detected by enzyme-linked **immunosorbent** assay (ELISA) screening procedures.

Microarrays

Microarray (DNA chip) technology has helped accelerate genetic analysis, just as microprocessors accelerated computation (Fig. 14-9). Microarrays are basically the product of bonding or direct synthesis of numerous specific DNA probes on a stationary, often silicon-based support. The chip may be tailored to particular disease processes. The technique is easily performed and readily automated.

Microarrays are miniature gene fragments attached to glass chips. These chips are used to examine the gene activity of thousands or tens of thousands of gene fragments and to identify genetic mutations using a hybridization reaction between the sequences on the microarray and a fluorescent sample. After hybridization, the chips are scanned with high-speed fluorescent detectors and the intensity of each spot is quantitated (Fig. 14-10).

The identity and amount of each sequence are revealed by the location and intensity of fluorescence displayed by each spot. Computers are used to analyze the data (Fig. 14-11).

The applications of microarrays in clinical medicine include the analysis of gene expression in malignancies (e.g., mutations in the breast cancer 1 gene *[BRCA-1]*, mutations of the *p53* tumor suppressor gene, genetic disease testing, viral resistance mutation detection).

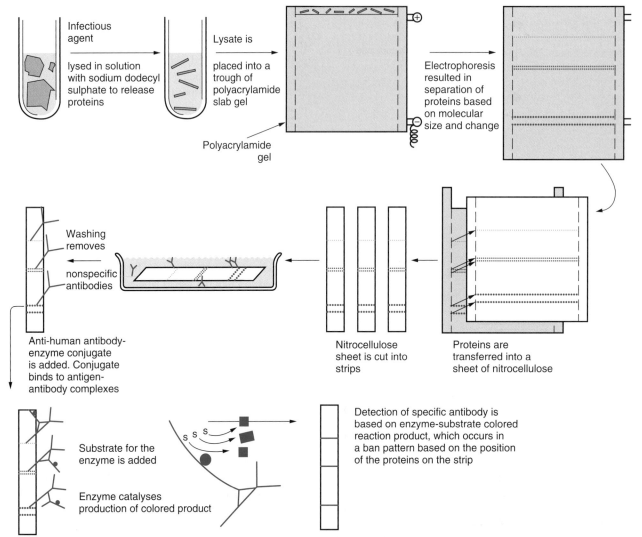

Figure 14-8 **Western blot immunoassay.** *(Adapted from Forbes BA, Sahm DF, Weissfeld AS: Bailey & Scott's diagnostic microbiology, ed 12, St Louis, 2007, Mosby.)*

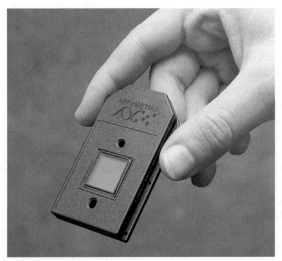

Figure 14-9 **Affymetrix GeneChip probe array.** *(Courtesy Affymetrix, Santa Clara, Calif.)*

The Human Genome GeneChip set (HG-U133 Set; Affymetrix, Santa Clara, Calif), consisting of two GeneChip arrays, contains almost 45,000 probe sets representing more than 39,000 transcripts derived from approximately 33,000 well-substantiated human genes. The sequence clusters were created from the UniGene database and then refined by analysis and comparison with a number of other publicly available databases (e.g., Washington University EST trace repository and University of California, Santa Cruz, Golden Path human genome database).

The HG-U133A array includes representation of the Ref-Seq database sequences and probe sets related to sequences previously represented on the Human Genome U95Av2 array. The HG-U133B array contains primarily probe sets representing expressed sequence tag (EST) clusters. The applications of this array include defining tissue and cell type–specific gene expression and investigating cellular and tissue responses to the environment (e.g., heat shock, interactions with other cells, exposure to chemical compounds, growth factors, or other signaling molecules). In addition, this array helps elucidate human

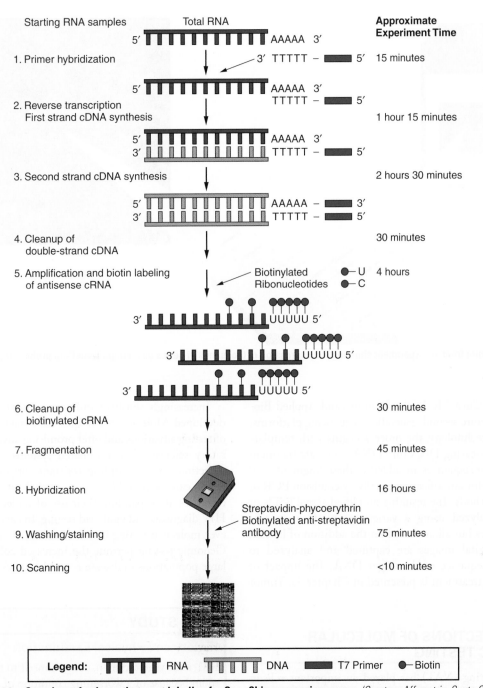

Starting RNA samples	Total RNA	Approximate Experiment Time

1. Primer hybridization — 15 minutes

2. Reverse transcription First strand cDNA synthesis — 1 hour 15 minutes

3. Second strand cDNA synthesis — 2 hours 30 minutes

4. Cleanup of double-strand cDNA — 30 minutes

5. Amplification and biotin labeling of antisense cRNA — Biotinylated Ribonucleotides ●—U ●—C — 4 hours

6. Cleanup of biotinylated cRNA — 30 minutes

7. Fragmentation — 45 minutes

8. Hybridization — 16 hours

9. Washing/staining — Streptavidin-phycoerythrin Biotinylated anti-streptavidin antibody — 75 minutes

10. Scanning — <10 minutes

Legend: RNA   DNA   T7 Primer   ●—Biotin

Figure 14-10   Overview of eukaryotic target labeling for GeneChip expression arrays. *(Courtesy Affymetrix, Santa Clara, Calif.)*

cell differentiation by the following: (1) determining which transcripts are increased or decreased during distinct stages in cellular differentiation; and (2) detecting which genes are uniquely expressed during different stages of **tumorigenesis.**

Another genomic microarray, GenoSensor (Tempe, Ariz), enables researchers to screen for abnormal gene amplifications and deletions with the sensitivity to detect single-gene copy change in a variety of specimens. The GenoSensor system simultaneously screens for gene copy number changes in 287 targets spotted in triplicate. This permits the screening of **proto-oncogenes, tumor suppressor genes,** microdeletion syndrome, gene regions, and subtelomeric regions.

NEXT GENERATION SEQUENCING TECHNOLOGY

Molecular characterization of tumors typically include Sanger sequencing (described previously) of a limited number of genes known to harbor mutations with well-described clinical appearances. If several genes need to be studied, Sanger sequencing can be costly and time-consuming. Next Generation Sequencing (NGS) technologies have the potential to be more cost-effective and be able to simultaneously sequence complete genomes of patients to deliver personalized medicine. NGS can produce thousands to millions of genome sequences at one compared to the 96 sequences processed by the traditional

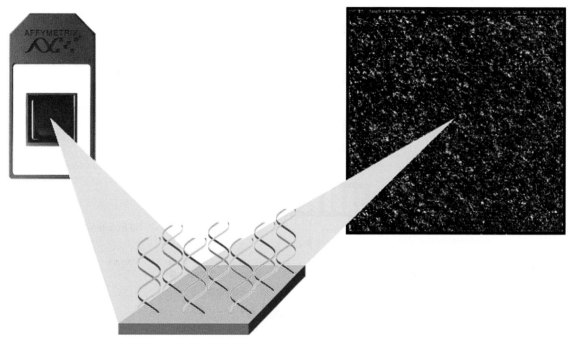

Figure 14-11   **Data from an experiment showing the expression of thousands of genes on a single GeneChip probe array.** *(Courtesy Affymetrix, Santa Clara, Calif.)*

Sanger method. Currently, Roche, Illumina, and Applied Biosystems manufacture second-generation sequencing platforms.

With NGS technology, the process begins with template preparation by shearing DNA (or cDNA) to create fragment libraries. Adaptor sequences are added to these fragments and serve as primers for amplification usually by emulsion PCR or bridge PCR methods. The resulting amplified signal beads or clusters are analyzed using a variety of platform-specific chemical analyses but all are based on the addition of labeled nucleotides. Digital images are captured and analyzed to determine the sequence of the target DNA. The impact of NGS on cancer treatment is presented in Chapter 33, Tumor Immunology.

FUTURE DIRECTIONS OF MOLECULAR DIAGNOSTIC TESTING

Nucleic acid testing (NAT) has played an important role in reducing transfused transmitted infections. NAT testing has been adopted in the United States, Canada, France, Australia, New Zealand, and South Africa. Additional countries in Europe and the Far East continue to be added to the list of NAT testing countries. NAT testing includes PCR assays and TMA.

Molecular testing is no longer confined to high-volume reference laboratories. Molecular diagnostics has advanced in precision, accuracy, speed, detection, and cost. Applications range from detection of infectious diseases to cellular and tissue antigens. Molecular diagnostic testing using nucleic acid–based assays provides rapid and accurate diagnosis and identification of infectious diseases that previously involved a long waiting period for pathogen identification. Past challenges, such as contamination, have become less of a problem because of the use of these new techniques.

Increasingly sensitive and specific methods continue to be developed. Molecular techniques are attractive in a wide variety of testing situations and offer promising advancements in laboratory science. New automated systems focus on pathogen detection and multidrug-resistant organisms, particularly health care–acquired (e.g., nosocomial) infections. Developing countries are expanding their use of molecular diagnostics in HIV diagnosis and viral load testing. In cancer detection, however, molecular testing is still considered an immature industry. Genomic testing permits the increased collection of data on large populations in disease research studies.

CASE STUDY

History and Physical Examination

KM, a 38-year-old man, drove himself to the emergency room because of a worsening condition of shortness of breath. He had a sore throat, felt tired, and had a fever, nonproductive cough, and mild chest pain. He had no history of serious medical conditions and was a lifelong nonsmoker.

During the last 5 years, he had been diagnosed with genital herpes and gonorrhea. He reported having persistent diarrhea for the past several months. He also noted a weight loss during the same period. He and his male partner had been having unprotected intercourse for several years. There was no history of IV drug use.

Physical examination revealed an underweight man with palpable lymph nodes. Plaques of *Candida albicans* were seen in the back of his throat. His chest sounds had diffuse crackles in both lungs.

Laboratory assays and a chest x-ray were ordered. He was also referred to counseling because of his high risk status for HIV-AIDS.

Laboratory Results

Assay	Patient's Results	Reference Range
Hemoglobin	10.5 g/dL	13.5-16.5 g/dL
Hematocrit	29%	40%-50%
Total leukocyte count	7.0×10^9/L	$4.5\text{-}10.0 \times 10^9$/L
Total lymphocyte count	0.80×10^9/L	$1.\text{-}3.5 \times 10^9$/L
CD4+ T cells	0.04×10^9/L	$0.7\text{-}1.1 \times 10^9$/L
CD8+ T cells	0.41×10^9/L	$0.5\text{-}0.9 \times 10^9$/L
B lymphocytes	0.09×10^9/L	$0.2\text{-}0.5 \times 10^9$/L
ELISA HIV test	Positive	Negative

- Chest x-ray: Bilateral diffuse interstitial shadowing was seen.

Follow-Up

A bronchoscopy with bronchoalveolar lavage was performed. Microscopic examination revealed the presence of *Pneumocystis jiroveci* (formerly called *Pneumocystis carinii*).

Review Questions

1. Diagnosis of suspected HIV infection is:
    a. Real-time PCR Western Blot
    b. Antibody to HIV-1
    c. Antibody to HIV-2
    d. CD4 and CD8 cell counts
2. Monitoring the course of HIV infection includes:
    a. Viral load monitoring
    b. CD4+ absolute lymphocyte count
    c. Monitoring CD 34+ cell counts
    d. Both a and b

Answers to these questions are in Appendix A.

Critical Thinking Group Discussion Questions

1. Which molecular assays can be used to diagnose a suspected HIV infection?
2. Which serologic or cellular assays can be used to monitor the course of an HIV infection?
3. Which molecular assays could be used to monitor drug therapy?

See instructor site ⊖volve for discussion of the answers to these questions.

Molecular Testing Procedure: Group A *Streptococcus* Direct Test

Principles

Nucleic acid hybridization tests are based on the ability of complementary nucleic acid strands to align and associate specifically to form stable, double-stranded complexes. The Gen-Probe DNA Probe assay (Gen-Probe, San Diego, Calif) uses an ssDNA probe with a chemiluminescent label that is complementary to the ribosomal RNA of the target organism. After the ribosomal RNA is released, the labeled DNA probe combines with the target organism's ribosomal RNA to form a stable DNA-RNA hybrid. The selection reagent differentiates nonhybridized from hybridized probes. The labeled DNA-RNA hybrids are measured in a luminometer. A positive result is a luminometer reading greater than or equal to the cutoff value. A value below this cutoff is a negative result.

See ⊖volve website for the complete procedural protocol.

Clinical Application

This test offers a method for definitively identifying *Streptococcus pyogenes* from throat swabs. Identification is based on the detection of specific ribosomal RNA sequences that are unique to *S. pyogenes*.

CHAPTER HIGHLIGHTS

- The polymerase chain reaction (PCR) is an in vitro method that amplifies low levels of specific DNA sequences in a sample to higher levels suitable for further analysis.
- PCR, an enzymatic process, is carried out in cycles. Each repeated cycle consists of DNA denaturation, primer annealing, and extension of the primed DNA sequence. Each cycle theoretically doubles the amount of specific DNA sequence present and results in an exponential accumulation of the DNA fragment being amplified (amplicons).
- PCR analysis can lead to the detection of gene mutations, identification of viral DNA associated with specific cancers, and detection of genetic mutations.
- Adaptations of the PCR technique include nested primers. Modifications include RT-PCR, multiplex PCR, and real-time PCR.
- Conventional analysis uses agarose gel electrophoresis after ethidium bromide staining.
- Probe-based DNA detection systems provide sequence specificity and lower detection limits.
- Selection of technique is based on sensitivity and specificity profiles, cost, turnaround time, and local experience.
- Probe hybridization assays involve the complementary pairing of a probe with DNA or RNA from the patient's specimen; these include liquid-phase, dot blot, and reverse dot blot assays.
- The Southern blot technique can determine single-base mutations (e.g., sickle cell anemia, hemophilia A).

- The Northern blot technique can be used for the detection of specific mRNA. This procedure is not routinely used in clinical molecular diagnostics.
- In the Western blot technique, proteins are separated electrophoretically, transferred to membranes, and identified through labeled antibodies. It is used to detect antibodies to specific epitopes of antigen subspecies and confirm the specificity of antibodies detected by ELISA screening.
- Microarrays (DNA chips) are the product of bonding or synthesis of specific DNA probes on a stationary support. These chips are used to examine gene activity and identify genetic mutations in malignancies, test for genetic disease test, and detect virally resistant mutations.

REVIEW QUESTIONS

1. In comparison to serologic assays, nucleic acid testing offers all the following benefits except:
   a. Reduced cost
   b. Enhanced specificity
   c. Increased sensitivity
   d. All of the above

2. Polymerase chain reaction (PCR) testing is useful in:
   a. Forensic testing
   b. Genetic testing
   c. Disease diagnosis
   d. All of the above

3. The traditional PCR technique:
   a. Extends the length of the genomic DNA
   b. Alters the original DNA nucleotide sequence
   c. Copies the target region of DNA
   d. Amplifies the target region of RNA

4. For the PCR reaction to occur, the clinician must provide which of the following?
   a. Oligonucleotide primers
   b. Individual deoxynucleotides
   c. Thermostable DNA polymerase
   d. All of the above

5. The enzyme reverse transcriptase converts:
   a. mRNA to cDNA
   b. tRNA to DNTP
   c. dsDNA to ssDNA
   d. Mitochondrial to nuclear DNA

6. DNA polymerase catalyzes:
   a. Primer annealing
   b. Primer extension
   c. Hybridization of DNA
   d. Hybridization of RNA

7. The figure below depicts:
   a. Polymerase chain reaction (PCR)
   b. Nested primer PCR
   c. Western blot analysis
   d. Southern blot analysis

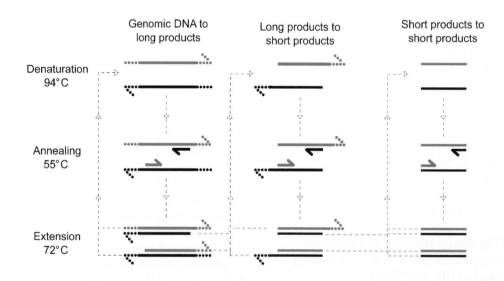

(From Burtis CA, Ashwood ER, Bruns DB: Tietz fundamentals of clinical chemistry, ed 6, St Louis, 2008, Saunders.)

8 to 10. Match the method with the appropriate description.

8. _____ Southern blot immunoassay

9. _____ Northern blot immunoassay

10. _____ Western blot immunoassay
   a. Messenger RNA is studied.
   b. Called immunoblot, it is used to detect antibodies to subspecies of antigens.
   c. Single-stranded DNA is studied.

11. Which of the following techniques uses signal amplification?
    a. bDNA
    b. TMA
    c. NASBA
    d. RT-PCR

12. Which of the following nucleic acid amplification techniques does not require the use of a thermocycler?
    a. PCR
    b. SDA
    c. NASBA
    d. TMA

BIBLIOGRAPHY

Bakker E: Is the DNA sequence the gold standard in genetic testing? Quality of molecular genetic tests assessed, Clin Chem 52:557, 2006.

Branca M: One genome—two chips, Bio-IT World 1:12, 2002.

Capetandes A: Polymerase chain reaction: the making of something big, Med Lab Observer 31:26, 1999.

Doty A: Monitoring the quality of nucleic acid testing for infectious disease, 2001, http://laboratorian.advanceweb.com/Article/Monitoring-the-Quality-of-Nucleic-Acid-Testing-for-Infectious-Disease.aspx.

Forbes BA, Sahm DF, Weissfeld AS: Bailey and Scott's diagnostic microbiology, ed 12, St Louis, 2007, Mosby.

Kazmi S, Krull IS: Proteonomics and the current state of protein separations, PharmaGenomics 1:14, 2001.

Miyake K: Olympus develops DNA computer, Bio-IT World 1:2, 2002.

Nadder TS: The new millennium laboratory: molecular diagnostics goes clinical, Clin Lab Sci 14:252, 2001.

Rhea JM, Singh HV, Molinaro RJ: Next generation sequencing in the clinical molecular diagnosis of cancer: advantages and challenges to clinical laboratory implementation, Med Lab Observer vol. 43:8–10, Dec 2011, no 12.

Sandhu R, Parker JS, Jones WD, Livasy CA: Microarray-based gene expression profiling for molecular classification of breast cancer and identification of new targets for therapy, Lab Med 41:364, 2010.

Schena M: Microarray biochip technology, Natick, Mass, 2000, Eaton.

Strobl F: NAT in blood screening around the world, MLO Med Lab Obs 43:12, 2011.

Tang Y, Procop GW, Persing DH: Molecular diagnostics of infectious diseases, Clin Chem 43:2021, 1997.

Turgeon ML: Clinical hematology: theory and procedures, ed 5, Philadelphia, 2012, Lippincott, Williams & Wilkins.

Uphoff TS: Basic concepts and innovations in molecular diagnosis, 2002, http://laboratorian.advanceweb.com/Article/Basic-Concepts-and-Innovations-in-Molecular-Diagnosis.aspx.

Warden BA, Thompson E: Apolipoprotein E and the development of atherosclerosis, Lab Med 25:449, 1994.

Weiss RL: Interpretive data guide, Salt Lake City, Utah, 1999, ARUP Laboratories.

Weiss RL, editor: ARUP's guide to molecular diagnostics clinical laboratory testing, ed 2, Salt Lake City, Utah, 2001, ARUP Laboratories.

Wisecarver J: Amplification of DNA sequences, Lab Med 28:191, 1997.

PART III

Immunologic Manifestations of Infectious Diseases

CHAPTER 15

The Immune Response in Infectious Diseases

Characteristics of Infectious Diseases
Development of Infectious Diseases
Bacterial Diseases
Parasitic Diseases
Fungal Diseases
  Histoplasmosis
  Aspergillosis
  Coccidioidomycosis
  North American Blastomycosis
  Sporotrichosis
  Cryptococcosis
Viral, Rickettsial, and Mycoplasmal Diseases
  Dengue Fever
  Herpesviruses

Herpes Simplex Virus
Varicella-Zoster Virus
Human Herpesvirus 6
Laboratory Detection of Immunologic Responses
  Antibody Significance
  TORCH Testing
Case Study
  Questions
  Critical Thinking Group Discussion Questions
Procedure: Latex-Cryptococcus Antigen Detection System
Chapter Highlights
Review Questions
Bibliography

Learning Objectives

At the conclusion of this chapter, the reader should be able to:

- Describe important characteristics in the acquisition and development of infectious diseases.
- Compare how the body develops immunity to bacterial; parasitic; fungal; and viral, rickettsial, and mycoplasmal diseases.
- Briefly describe the laboratory detection of immunologic responses.

- Analyze a case study related to the immune response in infectious diseases.
- Correctly answer case study related multiple choice questions.
- Be prepared to participate in a discussion of critical thinking questions.
- Describe the principle and results of the latex *Cryptococcus* antigen detection system.
- Correctly answer end of chapter review questions.

Key Terms

complement fixation (CF)
cytomegalovirus (CMV)
Dengue fever
endotoxins
enzyme immunoassay (EIA)
Epstein-Barr virus (EBV)
etiologic agent

exotoxins
hepatosplenomegaly
immunoCAP
immunocompromised
immunoperoxidase
neurologic sequelae
pathogenicity

prodromal
serodiagnostic tests
seropositivity
TORCH
varicella-zoster virus (VZV)
zoonoses

CHARACTERISTICS OF INFECTIOUS DISEASES

The acquisition of an infectious disease (e.g., viral, bacterial, parasitic, fungal) is influenced by factors related to the microorganism and host. The following factors can influence exposure to and development of an infectious disease:

- The immune status of an individual (Immunocompromised individuals have a much higher rate of microbial disease.)
- Overall incidence of an organism in the population
- **Pathogenicity** or virulence of the agent
- Presence of a sufficiently large dose of the agent or organism to produce an infection
- Appropriate portal of entry

In many cases, the successful dissemination of a microorganism results from spread of the microorganism over long distances by insect vectors or rapidly from country to country by global travelers. Also, some microorganisms are able to multiply in an intracellular habitat, such as in macrophages, and others can display antigen variation, which makes normal immune mechanism control difficult.

Host factors, such as the general health and age of an individual, influence the likelihood of developing an infectious disease and are important determinants of its severity. The very young and older populations develop infectious diseases more frequently than individuals in other age groups. In addition, a history of previous exposure to a disease or harboring of an organism such as a virus in a dormant condition is also a determining factor in disease development.

DEVELOPMENT OF INFECTIOUS DISEASES

For an infectious disease to develop in a host, the organism must penetrate the skin or mucous membrane barrier (first line of defense) and survive other natural and adaptive body defense mechanisms (see Chapter 1). These mechanisms include phagocytosis, antibody and cell-mediated immunity or complement activation, and associated interacting effector mechanisms. Phagocytosis and complement activation may be initiated within minutes of invasion by a microorganism; however, unless primed by previous contact with the same or similar antigen, antibody and cell-mediated responses do not become activated for several days. Complement and antibodies are the most active constituents against microorganisms free in the blood or tissues, whereas cell-mediated responses are most active against microorganisms associated with cells.

The most effective mechanism of body defense in a healthy host depends on factors such as an appropriate portal of entry and the characteristics of each microorganism. The routes of infection or portals of entry can include transmission through oral routes (e.g., foodborne or water-borne contamination), maternal-fetal transmission, insect vectors, sexual transmission, parenteral routes (e.g., injection or transfusion of infected blood), and respiratory transmission. Development of an infectious disease occurs only if a microorganism can evade, overcome, or inhibit normal body defense mechanisms.

BACTERIAL DISEASES

The presence of key substances (e.g., lysozyme) and the process of phagocytosis represent major immunologic defense mechanisms against bacteria. A microorganism, however, can survive phagocytosis if it possesses a capsule that impedes attachment or a cell wall that interferes with the digestion and release of **exotoxins,** which damage phagocytic and other cells. Most capsules and toxins are strongly antigenic, but antibodies can overcome many of their effects; this is the basis of most antibacterial vaccines.

Examples of representative bacterial diseases of importance in the study of immunology and serology are presented in Chapters 17 and 18.

PARASITIC DISEASES

Parasites are relatively large, may have resistant body walls, and may avoid being phagocytized because of their ability to migrate away from an inflamed area. These differences set parasitic infections apart from bacterial and viral infections to which some forms of natural and adaptive immunity afford protection. (Toxoplasmosis, a representative disease, is discussed in Chapter 20.)

Immune responses (effectors) to parasitic infections include immunoglobulins, complement, antibody-dependent, cell-mediated cytotoxicity, and cellular defenses such as eosinophils and T cells. Some cestodes, especially in their larval stages, may be eradicated by complement-fixing immunoglobulin G (IgG) antibodies. In addition, some antibodies may cross-react with other parasitic antigens. Increased levels of IgE may be noted in many helminth infections. Activation of the classic and alternate complement pathways may occur in some cases of schistosomiasis, and the alternate pathway of complement activation may kill larvae in the absence of antibody (see Chapter 5).

Phagocytosis may have some direct activity against parasitic organisms, but the most effective protection in some parasitic infections is provided by antibody-dependent, cell-mediated cytotoxicity. Macrophages, neutrophils, and eosinophils may demonstrate direct toxicity or phagocytosis toward parasites. The actual attachment of the cytotoxic cells is usually mediated by IgG, although IgE may be effective. The role of eosinophils is complex. They may phagocytize immune complexes and act as effector cells in mediating local (type I) reactions, primarily in tissue stage parasites. T cells are frequently involved in body defenses against parasites. Sequestration of microorganisms is a classic T-cell–dependent hypersensitivity response. In addition, helper T cells may sensitize B cells to specific parasitic antigens.

Other nonspecific factors (e.g., nonstimulated monocytes) are a major protective mechanism against parasites such as *Giardia* spp. Natural killer (NK) cells also have a direct activity against cancer cells and some parasites. Delayed hypersensitivity may be helpful in preventing some parasitic infections but may cause disease in other cases. Deposition of antigen-antibody complexes, demonstrated by Raji cell assays, is responsible for severe pathologic lesions in some parasitic infections. In addition, high levels of circulating IgE may cause hypersensitivity reactions in helminth and cestode infections. Anaphylaxis is a clear risk in echinococcal infections, especially with spontaneous or surgical rupture of a hydatid cyst.

FUNGAL DISEASES

Fungal, or mycotic, infections are normally superficial, but a few fungi can cause serious systemic disease, usually entering through the respiratory tract in the form of spores. Disease manifestation depends on the degree and type of immune response elicited by the host. Fungi are common and harmless inhabitants of skin and mucous membranes under normal conditions (e.g., *Candida albicans*). In immunocompromised hosts, *Candida* spp. and other fungi become opportunistic agents that take advantage of the host's weakened resistance. Manifestations of fungal disease may range from unnoticed respiratory episodes to rapid, fatal dissemination of a violent hypersensitivity reaction.

Survival mechanisms of fungi that successfully invade the body are similar to bacterial characteristics and include the following: (1) presence of an antiphagocytic capsule; (2) resistance to digestion within macrophages; and (3) destruction of phagocytes (e.g., neutrophils). Some types of yeast activate complement through the alternative pathway, but it is unknown whether this activation has any effect on the microorganism's survival.

Fungal infections are increasing worldwide for a variety of reasons, including the use of immunosuppressive drugs and the development of diseases that result in an immunocompromised host (e.g., acquired immune deficiency syndrome [AIDS]). Serologic tests often play an important role in the diagnosis of these fungal infections (Table 15-1).

Several species of fungi are associated with respiratory disease in human beings. These diseases are acquired by inhaling spores from exogenous reservoirs, including dust, bird droppings, and soil.

Histoplasmosis

Histoplasma capsulatum can be found in soil contaminated with chicken, bird, or bat excreta. Spore-laden dust is the source of histoplasmosis, caused by inhalation.

Histoplasmosis can be difficult to diagnose and can range from asymptomatic to chronic pulmonary disease. In addition, a disseminated form manifesting **hepatosplenomegaly** with diffuse lymphadenopathy is usually present in varying degrees of severity because of the propensity of the fungus to invade the cells of the mononuclear phagocyte system. Disseminated disease is characterized by fever, anemia, leukopenia, weight loss, and lassitude.

Definitive diagnosis requires isolation in culture and microscopic identification of the fungus, as well as serologic evidence. If an immunodiffusion technique is used, H and M bands appearing together indicate active infection. If only an M band is present, it indicates early infection, chronic infection, or a recent reactive skin test. An H band appears later than the M

Table 15-1	Testing Methods for Fungal Disease
Disease	**Procedure**
Aspergillosis	Gel immunodiffusion, EIA; IgG to *Aspergillus fumigatus* (≤110 mg/L), 85% of farmers and some persons with no evidence of disease
Blastomycosis	Complement fixation (>50% positive in proven cases); immunodiffusion (test is positive in about 80% of cases)
Coccidioidomycosis	Complement fixation using coccidioidin (blood, CSF)
Cryptococcosis	Latex agglutination (serum, CSF), EIA, immunofluorescence assay
Histoplasmosis	Complement fixation, immunodiffusion, PCR (sputum, blood, tissue); *Histoplasma capsulatum* antigen by EIA (urine); nucleic acid probe
Sporotrichosis	Latex particle agglutination

EIA, Enzyme immunoassay; *CSF*, cerebrospinal fluid; *PCR*, polymerase chain reaction.

band and disappears earlier. Disappearance of an H band suggests regression of the infection.

Delayed hypersensitivity skin testing is confirmed by a rise in complement-fixing antibodies to *Histoplasma* antigens. Titers of 8 and 16 (dilutions of 1:8 and 1:16) are highly suggestive of infection. A titer of 32 or higher usually indicates active infection. A rising titer indicates progressive infection; a decreasing titer suggests regression. Some disseminated infections are nonreactive in **complement fixation (CF)** tests. In addition, recent skin tests in individuals with prior exposure to *Histoplasma capsulatum* will produce a rise in the CF titer in 17% to 20% of patients. Cross-reactions in the CF test occur in patients with aspergillosis, blastomycosis, or coccidioidomycosis, but the titers are usually lower. Several follow-up serum samples should be tested at 2- to 3-week intervals.

Aspergillosis

Another opportunistic mycotic infection occurring in human beings is aspergillosis, which can be allergic, invasive, or disseminating, depending on pathologic findings in the host. Aspergillosis is usually secondary to another disease. Allergic bronchopulmonary aspergillosis is characterized by allergic reactions to the toxins and **endotoxins** of *Aspergillus* spp.

Species identification of aspergillosis can be made microscopically. Serologically, skin reactions and immunodiffusion are useful tools for identification, especially if the culture is negative.

Immunodiffusion antibody test with reference antisera and known antigen is a frequently used test for the identification of *Aspergillus* spp. in almost all clinical types of aspergillosis. Precipitin formation by immunodiffusion is useful for identifying patients with pulmonary eosinophilia, severe allergic aspergillosis, and aspergillomas. The presence of one or more precipitin bands suggests active infection. The precipitin bands correlate with CF titers. In this test, the greater the number of bands, the higher is the titer. In general, immunodiffusion measures IgG and a positive result may suggest past infection. The test is positive in about 90% of sera from patients with aspergilloma and 50% to 70% of patients with allergic bronchopulmonary aspergillosis. A negative test does not exclude aspergillosis.

In addition, the **enzyme immunoassay (EIA)** can be used to detect IgE and IgG antibodies. **ImmunoCAP** is a newer method used to detect *Aspergillus niger* IgE in serum.

Enzyme immunoassay is used to detect *Aspergillus* galactomannan antigen in serum. Negative results do not exclude the diagnosis of invasive aspergillosis. A single positive test result should be confirmed by testing a separate serum specimen. Many agents (e.g., antibiotics, food) can cross-react with the assay. The false-positive rate is higher in children than in adults. If invasive aspergillosis is suspected in high-risk patients, serial sampling is recommended.

Hypersensitivity testing is characterized by immediate and delayed-type hypersensitivity reactions as a result of the presence of *Aspergillus*-specific immunoglobulin. IgE titers are greatly increased in allergic bronchopulmonary aspergillosis.

Coccidioidomycosis

Coccidioidomycosis is also known as desert fever, San Joaquin fever, or valley fever. The disease may assume several forms, including primary pulmonary, primary cutaneous, and disseminated. The disease is contracted from inhalation of soil or dust containing the arthrospores of *Coccidioides immitis*.

Hypersensitivity testing using intradermal injections is useful in screening for *C. immitis*. It is usually the first immunologic test to be positive in asymptomatic and symptomatic cases. Skin testing does not differentiate between recent and past exposures to *C. immitis*. A positive skin test should be followed by other serodiagnostic tests. A negative test in a previously positive person can indicate a disseminated infection and a state of anergy.

The fluorescent antibody (FA) test can be applied directly to clinical specimens. This procedure is invaluable for making a rapid and specific identification of fungal structures. In addition to culturing the organism, serologic tests used to confirm the diagnosis of coccidioidomycosis include the tube precipitin test, immunodiffusion, CF, and latex agglutination. The CF test is the most widely used quantitative serodiagnostic test to identify infection with *C. immitis*. It is very effective in detecting disseminated disease. The tube precipitin test is positive in more than 90% of primary symptomatic cases.

Immunodiffusion is equivalent to CF; it can be used as a screening test, but the results should be confirmed by CF. Latex agglutination is not usually a recommended method because it lacks specificity, which leads to many false-positive results.

Two antigens have been developed for the serologic identification of circulating antibodies to *C. immitis*. IgM appears 1 to 3 weeks after infection in 90% of symptomatic patients. IgG develops 3 to 6 months after the onset of symptoms.

Titers of 1:2 to 1:4 are presumptive evidence of an early infection and should be repeated in 3 to 4 weeks. Titers of 1:8 to 1:16 are evidence of active infection, particularly when accompanied by a positive immunodiffusion test. Titers higher than 1:16 occur in 90% to 95% of patients with disseminated coccidioidomycosis.

North American Blastomycosis

Blastomycosis is a chronic fungal disease that is usually secondary to pulmonary involvement. *Blastomyces dermatitidis* causes tumors in the skin or lesions in the lungs, bones, subcutaneous tissues, liver, spleen, and kidneys.

Serologic diagnosis is problematic because of high cross-reactivity with antigenic components of the organism. Although immunodiffusion and CF are used, immunodiffusion is considered the better method. CF titers of 8 and 16 are highly suggestive of active infection and titers of 32 or higher are diagnostic. A decreasing titer indicates regression; however, most patients with blastomycosis have negative CF tests.

Sporotrichosis

This chronic, progressive, subcutaneous lymphatic mycosis is caused by *Sporothrix schenckii*. The disease takes three forms—lymphatic (which is the most common), disseminated, and respiratory. It is characterized by a sporotrichotic chancre at the site of inoculation, followed by the development and formation of subcutaneous nodules along the lymphatics draining the primary lesions. Infection is associated with injuries caused by thorns or splinters. Handlers of peat moss are particularly susceptible to the disease, especially when working in rose gardens.

Laboratory methods of identification include cultures, serologic techniques, and the FA staining technique. Two of the most sensitive tests are yeast cell and latex agglutination. Titers of 80 or higher usually indicate active infection.

Skin testing is also available. Patients with cutaneous infection usually demonstrate negative tests; patients with extracutaneous infections have positive tests.

Cryptococcosis

Cryptococcus neoformans is the **etiologic agent** of this disease. Infected pigeons are the chief vector. Cryptococcosis is acquired by inhaling the fungus, which grows in culture as yeast. It may initially be asymptomatic or may develop as a symptomatic pulmonary infection. Any organ or tissue of the body may be infected, but localization outside the lungs or brain is relatively uncommon. The disease can be serious in **immunocompromised** or debilitated patients.

Antigen tests take less time to perform and are more specific than antibody detection. Latex agglutination antigen tests can be performed on serum or cerebrospinal fluid (CSF). Titers of 1:2 suggest infection, although such findings have been found in individuals with no evidence of cryptococcosis. Titers of 1:4 or higher are evidence of an active infection. Higher titers also indicate more severe infections. Positive titers are found in CSF in 95% of patients with involvement of the central nervous system.

The indirect FA test detects antibodies to *C. neoformans*. It is most valuable when antigen tests are negative and can even be combined with an antigen test to determine a patient's prognosis. A positive test suggests a present or recent infection.

Complement fixation is the most specific antibody detection test but is very insensitive. Tube agglutination, using serum or CSF that demonstrates a titer of 1:2 or higher, suggests a current or recent infection with *C. neoformans*.

As cryptococcosis progresses, antigens begin to appear, along with a decrease in antibody production. After treatment, a decrease in antigen titer and reappearance of antibodies indicate a good prognosis.

VIRAL, RICKETTSIAL, AND MYCOPLASMAL DISEASES

The characteristic process associated with viral infections is cellular replication, which may or may not lead to cell death. Interferon plays a major role in body defenses against viral infections. Antibodies are valuable in preventing the entry and bloodborne spread of some viruses, but the ability of other viruses to spread from cell to cell places the burden of adaptive immunity on the T cell system, which specializes in recognizing altered self histocompatibility antigens (histocompatibility leukocyte antigen [HLA]). Macrophages may also play a role in immunity. Some of the most virulent viruses for human beings are **zoonoses** (e.g., rabies). Other viruses, however, can persist for years without symptoms and can then be reactivated to cause serious disease, possibly including tumors.

New viruses can cause old diseases, and old viruses can cause new diseases (see Chapters 21 to 25 for representative examples of immunologically important viral diseases). The mutation rates of viruses, especially ribonucleic acid (RNA) viruses such as human immunodeficiency virus (HIV), are extraordinarily high. Consequently, RNA viruses evolve much more rapidly under selective conditions than their hosts and contemporary RNA viruses may have descended from a common ancestor only relatively recently. The survival of influenza A and B viruses as new viruses depends on a continual evolution of mutants. These mutant forms are not recognized by the body as being variations of past viral exposures. The most frequent cause of new viral infections is old viruses that are not natural infections of human beings, but rather are accidentally transmitted from other species as zoonoses.

Organisms intermediate between viruses and bacteria are obligatory intracellular organisms with cell walls (e.g., rickettsiae) and without cell walls but capable of extracellular replication (e.g., *Mycoplasma*). Immunologically, the former are closer to viruses and the latter are closer to bacteria.

Dengue Fever

The rapidly expanding global footprint of **Dengue fever** is a public health challenge. An estimated 50 million infections occur every year in about 100 countries with the potential to spread to further. According to the World Health Organization and the Centers for Disease Control and Prevention, Florida and the coastal areas of Texas are included in the geographic areas that have high suitability for Dengue transmission. The major areas of disease are endemic tropical and subtropical latitudes (e.g. India, Southeast Asia). The primary vector is the urban-adapted *Aedes aegypti* mosquito. Global trade, with the unintentional transport of mosquitoes, and increased travel by viremic people, urban crowding, and ineffective mosquito control are all factors in this modern pandemic.

Dengue can be caused by one of four single-stranded, positive-sense RNA viruses (serotypes dengue virus type 1 to dengue virus type 4) of the *Flavivirus* genus. After an incubation period of 3 to 7 days, signs and symptoms start suddenly and follow three phases—initial febrile phase, a critical phase at about the time that the fever subsides (defervescence), and the final spontaneous recovery phase.

Most dengue virus infections are asymptomatic, with a wide variety of clinical manifestations. Signs and symptoms range from mild febrile illness to severe and fatal disease.

Laboratory diagnostic testing is by detection of viral components in serum or directly by serologic testing. Diagnostics tests are as follows:

- Viral component testing
  - Detection of viral nucleic acid in serum by reverse-transcriptase polymerase-chain reaction (RT-PCR)
  or
  - Detection of soluble nonstructural protein 1 (NS1) by enzyme-linked immunosorbent assay (ELISA) or lateral-flow rapid testing
- Serologic testing
  - Detection of IgM seroconversion by ELISA
  or
  - Lateral flow methods
  or
  - Detection of IgG in secondary infections by ELISA or lateral flow methods

Currently, no effective antiviral agents are available to treat dengue infection. Treatment is supportive. If patients have severe bleeding, a blood transfusion can be lifesaving. Clinical research with potential drugs or vaccines is ongoing.

Herpesviruses

Two members of the human herpesviruses, **cytomegalovirus (CMV)** and **Epstein-Barr virus (EBV),** are described in detail in Chapters 21 and 22. The following sections briefly describe other members of the human herpesvirus family, including herpes simplex, varicella-zoster, and human herpesvirus-6.

All the human herpesviruses are large, enveloped DNA viruses that replicate within the cell's nucleus. The virus gains an envelope when the virus buds through the nuclear membrane, which has been altered to contain specific viral proteins.

The herpesviruses cause a number of clinical diseases, although they share the basic characteristic of being cell-associated, which may partly account for their ability to produce subclinical infections that can be reactivated under appropriate stimuli.

Herpes Simplex Virus

Herpes simplex virus (HSV) can be cultured from the oropharynx in about 1% of healthy adults and from the genital tract of slightly less than 1% of asymptomatic adult women who are not pregnant. HSV is widespread. Human beings are the only natural hosts or known reservoir of infection. The incubation period is 2 to 12 days. The incidence of **seropositivity** rises to almost 100% in some populations by the age of 45 years. Antibody prevalence in adults varies greatly with socioeconomic class; 30% to 50% of upper socioeconomic class adults have detectable antibody to HSV compared with 80% to 100% of adults in lower socioeconomic groups.

The most frequent manifestation of HSV infection is the common cold sore or fever blister. HSV has been shown to be related to a wide variety of clinical syndromes and to subclinical infection, occurring with primary or recurrent disease. Recurrent HSV disease usually results from the reactivation of latent virus resting in paraspinal or cranial nerve ganglia that innervate the site of primary infection. Distant sites may be involved. Activated virus presumably travels down the axon to the skin (or other site) and induces disease. In some cases, exogenous reinfection can occur. Recurrence with cell-to-cell spread of virus occurs in the presence of serum-neutralizing antibodies.

Two cross-reacting antigen types of HSV have been identified, type 1 (HSV-1) and type 2 (HSV-2). HSV-1 is generally found in and around the oral cavity and in skin lesions that occur above the waist. HSV-2 is isolated primarily to the genital tract and skin lesions below the waist.

Congenital and Neonatal Infection

Malnutrition, severe illness, many acute childhood illnesses, and prematurity predispose infants and young children to disseminated primary infection. Neonatal HSV infections may be acquired in the antenatal or perinatal period. Active lesions in the mother's genital tract at birth present the greatest risk of infection to the newborn. The spectrum of disease in an infected newborn varies from subclinical to severe. In cases of overwhelming generalized infection, the infant may develop encephalitis and respiratory failure; hepatic failure, with increasing jaundice and adrenal insufficiency, may occur. Infants who survive severe infection are frequently left with some neurologic damage and may have recurrent vesicular skin lesions for many years.

Laboratory Diagnosis

Methods for the laboratory diagnosis of HSV include isolation of the virus and direct detection of antigen in tissues or cytologic preparation through the use of immunofluorescence or immunoenzyme methods. In addition, detection of the virus in body fluids (using monoclonal antibodies) can be performed with immunoassays or immunoblot techniques. Serologic diagnosis of primary infections can be demonstrated when a fourfold or higher positive-sense RNA viruses rise in titer occurs. Titers may rise significantly in early recurrent infection but usually become stable at moderately high levels after multiple recurrences.

Varicella-Zoster Virus

Varicella-zoster virus (VZV) is the cause of two different types of clinical diseases resulting from the same virus infection. Primary infection with the virus results in the clinical manifestations of chickenpox. After a primary infection, the virus enters a latent phase, presumably within nuclei in the dorsal root ganglia. Reactivation of the virus results in the characteristic clinical manifestation of (zoster), known as shingles.

Epidemiology and Etiology

Human beings are the only natural hosts of VZV. Varicella primarily affects children age 2 to 5 years. The virus is endemic and highly contagious. Periodic epidemics do occur. The presumed route of transmission is through the respiratory tract.

Zoster is less communicable than varicella. This sporadic disease occurs most frequently in older individuals. Antibodies to varicella do not protect against reactivation or clinical zoster. The reactivation of VZV is associated with a depressed immune response. Patients with AIDS, older adults, and immunocompromised persons are at high risk of developing disease. In addition, manipulation of the spinal cord, local radiation therapy, and therapy that suppresses cellular immunity have been associated with triggering the onset of zoster.

Varicella has an incubation period of 14 to 17 days. There may be a 1- to 3-day **prodromal** period of fever, headache, and malaise. This precedes the eruption of the characteristic red macular rash, which progresses to papules, vesicles, and pustules that crust over and shed without scarring. Successive crops of lesions continue to appear for 2 to 6 days; therefore, multiple lesions in various stages of development are present at any one time.

The name of the virus reflects two associated diseases—varicella (chickenpox) and zoster (shingles). Primary infection with the virus results in the clinical manifestation of chickenpox. After this, the virus enters a latent phase, presumably within nuclei of neurons in dorsal root ganglia or cranial nerve sensory ganglia. The reactivity of the virus results in the clinical manifestations characteristic of zoster.

Signs and Symptoms

Complications of VZV include pneumonitis, encephalitic conditions, nephritis, hepatitis, myocarditis, arthritis, and Reye's syndrome. Susceptible individuals who are immunosuppressed have a greater risk of complications after VZV exposure. Another complication can include febrile purpura, which can occur a few days after the onset of the rash and is seen in children and adults. This complication is characterized by thrombocytopenia and hemorrhage into the vesicles. Postinfection purpura, which begins 1 to 2 weeks after the appearance of the rash, is characterized by thrombocytopenia with gastrointestinal, genitourinary, cutaneous, and mucous membrane hemorrhage. More severe hemorrhagic complications include malignant varicella with purpura and purpura fulminans.

Zoster Infection. Zoster infection is characterized by vesicular eruptions, typically confined to one or two adjacent dermatomes. The viral replication follows the nerve fiber. Neuralgia accompanies the skin eruptions and can last for months after the skin heals. Persistent neuralgia can be severe and can last months or longer.

Neonatal Varicella Infection. Neonatal varicella may be acquired in utero or in the perinatal period and can result in congenital abnormalities. The infant is at greatest risk if the mother's illness occurs 4 days or less before delivery.

Laboratory Diagnosis

The laboratory diagnosis of VZV is similar to HSV methods. Serologic methods include indirect immunofluorescence, which detects antibodies to specific membrane antigens, and EIA.

Rapid preliminary diagnosis can also be made by direct immunofluorescence to detect viral antigens in vesicular lesions. A smear of cells taken from lesions enables direct examination. A presumptive diagnosis can be made by examining scrapings from the base of a vesicular lesion and histologically observing multinucleated giant cells containing intranuclear inclusion bodies, or by observing virus particles on electron microscopy. The best way to confirm VZV infection is to recover the virus in human diploid fibroblast cell cultures.

Antibodies to varicella are detectable within several days of the onset of rash and peak at 2 to 3 weeks. Antibodies to zoster increase more rapidly and are detectable at the onset of clinical symptoms. Because of the rapid turnaround time and correlation with clinical symptoms, serologic methods are preferable to viral isolation methods. In addition, ELISA methods are valuable for assessing the immune status of adults.

Prevention

A vaccine is available for those in high-risk groups. The vaccine can be administered prior to an infection or to prevent reinfection because of waning immunity.

Human Herpesvirus 6

A new virus classified as a herpesvirus because of its shape, size, and in vitro behavior has been identified. Genomic analysis shows the virus to be molecularly unrelated to other human herpesviruses. Initially the virus was called B-lymphotropic virus, but subsequent studies indicated that T cells are the primary target of infection. This viral agent is classified as human herpesvirus 6 (HHV-6).

Patients with serologic evidence of acute HHV-6 infection are reported to experience mild nonspecific symptoms and cervical lymphadenopathy. The same agent has been implicated as the cause of roseola infantum (exanthema subitum). Up to 75% of infants develop antibody to HHV-6 by age 10 to 11 months, which suggests a high rate of seropositivity in the general population.

Laboratory methods include direct examination by immunofluorescence or **immunoperoxidase** staining of cells taken from lesions. In addition, PCR, DNA probes, and serologic methods (e.g., ELISA, radioimmunoassay, indirect immunofluorescence, latex agglutination) can be used.

Culture methods include the cocultivation of the patient's peripheral blood cells with cord blood mononuclear cells and examination of these cultures after 5 to 10 days by electron microscopy. Anticomplement immunofluorescence of infected cell culture has also been used for antibody detection and titration.

LABORATORY DETECTION OF IMMUNOLOGIC RESPONSES

Because immunoglobulin M (IgM) is usually produced in significant quantities during the first exposure of a patient to an infectious agent, the detection of specific IgM can be of diagnostic significance (see Chapter 2). This immunologic characteristic is particularly important in diseases that do not manifest decisive clinical signs and symptoms (e.g., toxoplasmosis) or under conditions in which a rapid therapeutic decision may be required (e.g., rubella).

Antibody Significance

In many diseases, infected individuals show a spectrum of responses. Some patients may develop and manifest antibodies from a subclinical infection or after colonization of an agent without actually developing disease. In these patients, the presence of antibody in a single serum specimen or a comparative titer of antibody in paired specimens may merely indicate past contact with the agent; the presence of antibodies cannot be used for the accurate diagnosis of a recent disease. In comparison, some patients may respond to an antigenic stimulus by producing antibodies that can cross-react with other antigens. These antibodies are nonspecific and may lead to misinterpretation of serologic tests.

Serologic diagnosis of recent infection using acute and convalescent specimens is the method of choice. Except for the detection of IgM or in diseases with no chance of developing an immune response (e.g., rabies virus, botulism toxin), testing a single specimen is usually not recommended. In a number of circumstances, when only one specimen is tested to determine immune status, antibody to past infection or to immunization can be determined.

The testing protocols described in this chapter for the immunologic detection of representative infectious diseases are examples of the types of procedures typically encountered in the immunology-serology laboratory.

TORCH Testing

Procedures that specifically evaluate the presence of IgM or IgG are frequently used to detect CMV, herpesviruses (types 1 and 2), *Toxoplasma gondii*, and rubella. The names of the tests have been grouped under the acronym **TORCH**: *Toxoplasma*, *o*ther (viruses), *r*ubella, *C*MV, and *h*erpes (Tables 15-2 and 15-3).

A spectrum of congenital defects called TORCH syndrome occurs with maternal exposure to rubella (also to *T. gondii*, CMV, and HSV). Congenital defects may be asymptomatic. A TORCH panel is ordered if a pregnant woman is suspected of having any of the TORCH infections. Rubella infection during the first 16 weeks of pregnancy presents major risks for the unborn baby. If a pregnant woman has a rash and other symptoms of rubella, laboratory tests are required to make the diagnosis. Women infected with *Toxoplasma* or CMV may have flulike symptoms that are not easily differentiated from other

Table 15-2	TORCH Antibodies: Immunoglobulin M
Infectious Agent	**Interpretation of Assay**
CMV	Positive—IgM antibody to CMV detected; may indicate current or recent infection; 1:10 IV or greater = positive
HSV-1, HSV-2	Positive (>1.10 IV)—IgM antibody to HSV detected (ELISA); may indicate current or recent infection
Rubella	Positive—1.10 IV or greater; IgM antibody to rubella detected; may indicate current or recent infection or immunization
Toxoplasma gondii	Positive: 1.10 IV or greater; significant level of antibody detected; may indicate current or recent infection

Adapted from Associated Regional and University Pathologists: ARUP test reference guide, 2011 (http://www.aruplab.com/Testing-Information/lab-test-directory.jsp).

TORCH, Toxoplasma, other (viruses), rubella, *CMV*, herpes; *CMV*, cytomegalovirus; *HSV*, herpes simplex virus; *ELISA*, enzyme-linked immunosorbent assay.

Table 15-3	TORCH Antibodies: Immunoglobulin G
Infectious Agent	**Interpretation of Assay**
CMV antibody	Positive—≥1:10; IgG antibody to CMV detected; may indicate current or previous CMV infection.
HSV-1, HSV-2	Positive—≥1:10; IgG antibody to HSV detected (ELISA); may indicate current or previous HSV infection.
Rubella	Positive—10 IU/mL or greater; IgG antibody to rubella detected; may indicate current or previous exposure/immunization to rubella.
Toxoplasma gondii	≥6 IU/mL, negative; ≥9 IU/mL, positive; results may indicate current or past infection.

Adapted from Associated Regional and University Pathologists: ARUP test reference guide, 2011 (http://www.aruplab.com/Testing-Information/lab-test-directory.jsp).

illnesses. Antibody testing will help diagnose an infection that may be harmful to the fetus.

In addition, a TORCH panel may be ordered on the newborn if the infant shows any signs suggestive of these infections, such as exceptionally small size relative to gestational age, deafness, mental impairment, seizures, heart defects, cataracts, enlarged liver or spleen, low platelet level, and/or jaundice.

Toxoplasmosis

Toxoplasmosis infection during pregnancy can cause congenital infection and manifestations, such as mental retardation and blindness. Hydrocephalus, intracranial calcification, and retinochoroiditis are the most common manifestations of tissue damage from congenital toxoplasmosis.

A neonatal screening program based on detecting IgM antibodies against *T. gondii* alone would identify 70% to 80% of congenital toxoplasmosis cases. The prevalence of congenital toxoplasmosis is 1/10,000 live births in the United States, in which 85% of women of childbearing age are susceptible to acute infection with *T. gondii*.

Cytomegalovirus

Cytomegalovirus is the most common congenital virus infection in the world. Both primary and recurrent infection can result in fetal infection. The birth prevalence of congenital CMV infection varies from 0.3% to 2.4% and at least 90% of congenitally infected infants have no clinical signs. CMV causes illnesses ranging from no clinical signs to prematurity, encephalitis, deafness, hematologic disorders, and death.

Congenital CMV infection is described in 30,000 to 40,000 newborns each year in the United States; approximately 9000 of these children have permanent **neurologic sequelae.** The death rate from symptomatic congenital CMV infection is approximately 30%.

Rubella

Rubella virus infection during early pregnancy can lead to severe birth defects known as congenital rubella syndrome. Sequelae of rubella virus infection include three distinct neurologic syndromes:

- Postinfectious encephalitis after acute infection
- Neurologic manifestations after congenital infection
- Rare neurodegenerative disorder, progressive rubella panencephalitis, that can follow congenital or postnatal infection

---

CASE STUDY

Two-year-old SJ had always been a healthy child who lived on a chicken farm in Arkansas with her parents and two sisters. She had no history of contact with bats, recent travel, insect bites, or other suspicious exposures.

She was taken to her pediatrician because she had a 2-week history of fatigue, nonproductive coughing, and occasional vomiting. On examination, her oral temperature was 104° F. She was very pale and had a severely distended abdomen, with a palpable liver and spleen.

SJ was admitted to the hospital. A complete blood count (CBC), screening test for infectious mononucleosis, and a blood culture (×3) were ordered. A chest radiograph was ordered.

Relevant Laboratory Data
- Hemoglobin, 8.9 g/dL (low)
- Platelet count, 60×10^9/L or 60,000 mm³ (low)
- Infectious mononucleosis screen, negative
- Blood cultures, negative

Diagnostic Imaging Data
Her chest x-ray showed a diffuse nodular prominence.

Follow-Up Tests

A computed tomography (CT) scan of the chest was ordered. A sample of lung tissue was obtained by bronchoscopy and submitted for fungal stain and culture and tuberculosis (TB) stain and culture.

Blood was collected for HIV antigen, *Histoplasma* antigen by enzyme immunoassay, *Histoplasma* mycelia antibody, *Histoplasma* yeast antibody by complement fixation, and qualitative immunodiffusion testing. An aliquot of serum was labeled "acute" and frozen if needed for future testing.

Treatment

Pending results of follow-up studies, her pediatrician initiated empirical antibiotic therapy for tuberculosis and histoplasmosis. IV therapy was continued to rehydrate the patient.

Follow-Up Testing Results

Fungal stain, small intracellular budding yeast cells were observed.
Fungal culture, pending
HIV screening, negative
Histoplasma antibody by immunodiffusion, no detectable precipitins to specific *Histoplasma* protein antigens M and H
Histoplasma antibodies by complement fixation, negative
Histoplasma antigen, weakly positive
TB stain, negative
TB culture, pending

The CT scan of the chest revealed diffuse pulmonary infiltrates without lymphadenopathy.

Continuation of Treatment

The patient was responding successfully to antibiotic therapy. This therapy was continued until a definitive diagnosis could be determined. She was discharged from the hospital and scheduled for an office appointment in 3 weeks if no adverse symptoms developed.

Questions

1. The source of histoplasmosis infection can be:
   a. Parakeet cages
   b. Canary cages
   c. Chicken coops
   d. Squirrels
2. Who is at risk for contracting histoplasmosis?
   a. Infants and young children
   b. Teenagers
   c. Middle age adults
   d. Women of any age

See Appendix A for the answers to these questions.

Critical Thinking Group Discussion Questions

1. Does a negative result for histoplasma antibodies rule out a diagnosis of histoplasmosis?
2. If a convalescent specimen is drawn several weeks after discharge from the hospital, what results might be expected?
3. What factors might suggest a diagnosis of histoplasmosis?

See instructor site ⊖volve for the discussion of the answers to these questions.

Latex-Cryptococcus Antigen Detection System

Principle

This is a simple and rapid latex agglutination test (ImmunoMycologics, Norman, Okla) for the qualitative or semiquantitative detection of the capsular polysaccharide antigens of *Cryptococcus neoformans* in serum and cerebrospinal fluid (CSF) to help diagnose cryptococcosis. The assay is based on the principle that anticryptococcal antibody–coated latex particles will agglutinate with specimens containing cryptococcal capsular polysaccharide antigens.

See the ⊖volve website for information related to performing the procedure.

Results

Negative

If the screening test performed on the undiluted patient specimen was negative or a 1+ reaction, the test should be reported as negative. However, 1+ reactions may be suggestive of cryptococcosis. If the clinical symptoms of the patient are suggestive of cryptococcosis, subsequent specimens and culture are strongly recommended. Weakly reactive specimens (e.g., 1+) should be tested for the prozone effect of high titers by using the titration procedure. If prozoning is suspected, repeat the test with both 1:10 and 1:100 dilutions of the specimen.

Positive

If a 2+ or higher reaction is observed in the screening procedure, the specimen is titrated using the titration procedure. The titer is reported as the highest dilution showing a 2+ or higher reaction.

NOTE: A negative test does not exclude the possibility of cryptococcal infection, particularly when a single patient specimen has been tested and the patient has symptoms consistent with those of cryptococcosis. False-negative reactions may be caused by low titers, early infection, presence of immune complexes, prozone effect of high titers, or poorly encapsulated strains with low production of polysaccharide. False-positive reactions can occur because of the presence of rheumatoid factor.

CHAPTER HIGHLIGHTS

- For an infectious disease to be acquired by a host, the microorganism must penetrate the skin or mucous membrane barrier and survive other natural and adaptive body defense mechanisms.

- Phagocytosis and complement activation may be initiated within minutes of the invasion of a microorganism; however, unless primed by previous contact with the same or similar antigen, antibody and cell-mediated responses do not become activated for several days.
- The mechanism of body defense most effective in a healthy host depends on the microorganism. Defenses such as phagocytosis are highly effective in bacterial immunity; T cells are frequently involved in body defenses against parasites.
- Sequestration of microorganisms is a classic T cell–dependent hypersensitivity response.
- IgM is usually produced in significant quantities after the first exposure to an infectious agent. This is important in diseases that do not manifest decisive clinical signs and symptoms or under conditions requiring a rapid therapeutic decision.
- TORCH procedures evaluate the presence of IgM to detect *Toxoplasma,* other viruses, rubella, CMV, and herpes.
- In most cases, serologic diagnosis of recent infection using acute and convalescent specimens is the method of choice. The testing of a single specimen is not recommended.

REVIEW QUESTIONS

1. Factors that influence the development of an infectious disease include all the following except the:
   a. Immune status of the individual
   b. Incidence of an organism in the population
   c. Pathogenicity of the agent
   d. Sole presence of the agent or microorganism

2-5. Match the appropriate immunologic defense mechanism (a-d) with the class of microorganism.

2. ___B___ Bacteria

3. ___D___ Yeast

4. ___A___ Viruses

5. ___C___ Parasites
   a. Interferon
   b. Lysozymes and phagocytosis
   c. Immunoglobulins, complement, antibody-dependent cell-mediated cytotoxicity, and cellular defenses
   d. Possibly the activation of complement

6. The detection of _____ can be of diagnostic significance during the first exposure of a patient to an infectious agent.
   a. IgM
   b. IgG
   c. IgA
   d. IgD

7. Serologic procedures for the diagnosis of recent infection should include:
   a. Only an acute specimen
   b. Only a convalescent specimen
   c. Acute and convalescent specimens

   d. Acute, convalescent, and 6-month postinfection specimens

8. An important factor affecting microbial disease development is the:
   a. Ability of some microorganisms to multiply in an intracellular habitat
   b. Display of antigen variation
   c. Presence of a related microorganism
   d. Both a and b

9. For an infectious disease to develop in a host, the organism must initially:
   a. Survive phagocytosis
   b. Be in the log phase of multiplication
   c. Penetrate the skin or mucous membrane barrier
   d. Be present in the host for 7 to 10 days

10-12. Match each type of infectious disease to the appropriate description.

10. ___B___ Bacterial disease

11. ___C___ Viral disease

12. ___A___ Parasitic disease
   a. Affected by immune responses such as immunoglobulin, complement, and antibody-dependent cell-mediated cytotoxicity
   b. Inhibited by antibiotics, lysozymes, and phagocytosis
   c. Stimulates production of, and is in turn inhibited by, interferon

13. The first type of antibody that may be apparent in the immune response to an infectious disease is:
   a. IgM
   b. IgG
   c. IgD
   d. IgA

14. A distinguishing characteristic of the herpesviruses is that:
   a. They are cell-associated viruses.
   b. They are enveloped RNA.
   c. Human beings are the only known reservoir of infection.
   d. Both a and c

15. Up to _____ of infants develop antibody to HHV-6 by 10 to 11 months of age.
   a. 25%
   b. 50%
   c. 75%
   d. 95%

16. Varicella-zoster virus causes:
   a. Chickenpox
   b. Shingles
   c. Measles
   d. Both a and b

17. Varicella-zoster virus can be reactivated in:
    a. AIDS patients
    b. Older adults
    c. Immunocompromised persons
    d. All of the above

18. Rapid preliminary diagnosis of varicella-zoster virus can be done in the laboratory by:
    a. Direct immunofluorescence
    b. Viral isolation
    c. ELISA method
    d. Complement fixation

19. Histoplasmosis is caused by a:
    a. Bacterium
    b. Parasite
    c. Fungus
    d. Virus

20. Aspergillosis is:
    a. An opportunistic organism
    b. Caused by a parasite
    c. A cause of skin infections
    d. A relatively mild disease

21. The first test to be positive in coccidioidomycosis is:
    a. Fluorescent antibody
    b. Hypersensitivity testing
    c. Complement fixation
    d. Culture of the organism

22-24. Match the following.

22. _C_ Blastomycosis

23. _A_ Sporotrichosis

24. _B_ Cryptococcosis
    a. Subcutaneous lymphatic mycosis
    b. Vector in infected pigeons
    c. Chronic fungal disease

BIBLIOGRAPHY

Associated Regional and University Pathologists: ARUP test reference guide, 2011, http://www.aruplab.com/Testing-Information/lab-test-directory.jsp.

Davidson RA: Immunology of parasitic infections, Med Clin North Am 69:751–757, 1985.

Forbes BA, Sahm DF, Weissfeld AS: Bailey and Scott's diagnostic microbiology, ed 12, St Louis, 2007, Mosby.

Kilbourne ED: New viral diseases, JAMA 264:68–70, 1990.

Neto EC, Rubin R, Schulte J, Giugliani R: Newborn screening for congenital infectious diseases, Emerg Infect Dis 10:1068–1073, 2004.

Pastuszak AL, Levy M, Schick B, et al: Outcome after maternal varicella infection in the first 20 weeks of pregnancy, N Engl J Med 330:901–906, 1994.

Playfair JHL: Immunology at a glance, Oxford, 1979, Blackwell Scientific.

Simmons CP, Farrar JJ, Chau NV, Willis B: Dengue, N Engl J Med 366:1423–1432, 2012.

Turgeon ML: Bloodborne infectious diseases. In Turgeon ML, editor: Fundamentals of immunohematology, ed 2, Baltimore, 1996, Williams & Wilkins.

CHAPTER 16

A Primer on Vaccines

Learning Objectives

At the conclusion of the chapter, the reader should be able to:

- Identify the federal agency that regulates vaccine products.
- Describe vaccine policy and the role of vaccines in public safety.
- Briefly describe the history and use of several specific vaccines.
- Explain some new targets and technologies for vaccines.
- Identify at least three essential characteristics of a vaccine.
- Based on immunologic principles, describe the host response to vaccination.
- Analyze the problems associated with AIDS vaccine development and use.
- Describe the development and application of human papillomavirus vaccine.
- Compare and contrast the applications of at least four vaccines.
- Analyze a case study.
- Correctly answer case study related multiple choice questions.
- Be prepared to participate in a discussion of critical thinking questions.
- Describe the principle and clinical application of the tetanus antibodies assay.
- Correctly answer end of chapter review questions.

Key Terms

antigenic drift
conjugate vaccines
cytotoxic T cell responses
dendritic cells
herd immunity
humoral and cellular immunity

naked DNA vaccines
pathogen
pathogen recognition receptors
pertussis
polysaccharides
subunit vaccines

toll-like receptor (TLR)
vaccination
vaccine
variolation

WHAT IS A VACCINE?

A **vaccine** is a biological suspension of weakened or killed pathogens or their components. It can be purified protein subunits, conjugated and nonconjugated **polysaccharides,** or split virions. The **pathogen** is usually a bacterium or a virus.

Vaccines can be delivered as a nasal spray, orally, or by injection. Humans become immune to microbial antigens through artificial and natural means. The immune system of the body must recognize the pathogen and be able to develop a defense against a specific pathogen.

The goal of administering vaccines, vaccination, is to produce artificially acquired, active immunity to a specific disease.

Of all the public health measures against infections, administering a vaccine is the most cost-effective strategy.

CHARACTERISTICS OF A VACCINE

The purpose of a vaccine is to stimulate active immunity and create an immune memory so that exposure to the active disease microorganism will stimulate an already primed immune system to fight the disease. Most vaccines can be divided into the following two types:

- Live attenuated vaccines
- Nonreplicating vaccines

Traditionally prepared vaccines are preparations of inactivated (killed) or live attenuated (weakened) bacteria or viruses, parts of the microorganisms, or toxoids (inactivated toxins) from the disease-causing agent. Newer synthetic vaccines use subunit vaccines, **conjugate vaccines,** and **naked DNA vaccines.** Critical to the protective effect of **subunit vaccines** (vaccines consisting of components of the pathogens) are additives called adjuvants, which amplify the immune response. Currently, an aluminum salt-based substance called alum and an oil-based substance called MF59 are two adjuvants licensed for clinical use.

HOST RESPONSE TO VACCINATION

Classic preventive vaccines are designed to mimic the effects of natural exposure to microbes. The earliest host response to vaccination is called the innate immune response. This response is an evolutionarily ancient system of host defense that occurs within minutes or hours after vaccination. The dendritic cell is critical to this response. Dendritic cells can sense components of bacteria, viruses, parasites, and fungi through **pathogen recognition receptors.** One class of these receptors is the **toll-like receptor (TLR);** at least 10 have been described. As a group, TLRs can sense a wide variety of microbial stimuli (e.g., lipopolysaccharides, viral or bacterial DNA).

The intracellular TLR signaling within dendritic cells is mediated by at least four adapter proteins. Once dendritic cells decode and integrate the signals generated by sensing microbial molecules with TLRs, the cells convey this information to naïve antigen-specific T cells, which launch an immune response.

Over time, vaccine-induced immunity wanes; this may result in increased susceptibility later in life (e.g., varicella [shingles]). A second dose of vaccine could improve protection from primary vaccine failure and waning vaccine-induced immunity.

HISTORY OF VACCINES

According to the World Health Organization (WHO), immunization is one of the greatest breakthroughs in medical science. This practice saves 3 million lives a year. Vaccines have reduced some preventable infectious diseases to an all-time low; few people now experience the devastating effects of measles, **pertussis,** and other infectious diseases.

The history of vaccination begins as early as 1000 BCE, when the Chinese used smallpox inoculation or **variolation,** a method of scratching the skin and applying pulverized powder from a smallpox scab. By the 18th century, the practice of variolation became known to Europeans and Americans.

In 1796, Edward Jenner, an English physician, used cowpox scabs to create immunity to smallpox. This was a fundamental principle of immunization, which evolved over 200 years ago and has resulted in the eradication of smallpox globally. The first vaccine for chicken cholera was created in the laboratory of Louis Pasteur in 1879. In 1885, Pasteur developed a rabies vaccine. This launched a period of productive development of many other vaccines (e.g., diphtheria, tetanus, typhoid fever).

APPLICATIONS OF VACCINES

The concept of **vaccination,** or deliberately introducing a potentially harmful microbe into a patient, initially met with suspicion and outrage. Widespread vaccination programs against contagious infectious diseases now have a positive influence worldwide.

In 1721, Cotton Mather, a Boston minister, encouraged smallpox variolation as a preventive step subsequent to the Boston smallpox epidemic. Mather was widely criticized by suspicious citizens for his role in promoting variolation. Since the introduction of the first vaccine, there has been opposition to vaccination. In 1910, Sir William Osler expressed his frustration with the antivaccinationist movement. Although fear and mistrust have arisen every time a new vaccine was introduced in the 18th century, the antivaccine movement receded between the 1940s and the early 1980s. Three trends promoted a positive attitude toward vaccines:

- A boom in scientific discovery and the production of vaccines
- A desire to protect children from significant outbreaks of infectious diseases, including polio, measles, mumps, rubella, and pertussis (whooping cough)
- An increase in the birth rate among more educated and affluent parents, who accepted the use of vaccines

An increase in antivaccinationist thinking emerged in the 1970s, when outbreaks of infectious diseases decreased, with more vaccines in the childhood vaccination schedule. When countries dropped pertussis vaccination from the vaccination schedule, the incidence of whooping cough increased 10 to 100 times. Fears grew in the late 1990s, when vaccines were suspected of causing autism. Once again, in 2009 and 2010, the H1N1 influenza pandemic evoked strong public fear of vaccination. Reemergence of a previously controlled disease, such as pertussis, has led to hospitalizations and deaths. The worst pertussis outbreaks in the past 50 years are now occurring in California.

Despite public fears, American children now receive vaccinations to numerous diseases that were once common childhood infectious diseases. In the United States, the recommended childhood immunization schedule now includes vaccines to protect against 15 diseases, including seasonal influenza. Immunization schedules vary by age and by country (Tables 16-1 to 16-3, *A* and *B*).

The latest adult immunization rates in the United States lag behind target levels. The Centers for Disease Control and Prevention (CDC) has reported that in 2010, the pneumococcal vaccination rate for patients at high risk was less than 20%. The hepatitis B vaccination rate for health care personnel was about 60%. In addition, the human papillomavirus (HPV) vaccination rate among young women was slightly more than 20%.

Adults require updates of certain vaccinations (Fig. 16-1). Especially serious diseases for adults age 65 years and older include diphtheria, herpes zoster (shingles), influenza, pneumococcus, and tetanus (lockjaw). In 2006, a vaccine was approved for adults older than 60 years to reduce the risk of shingles (reactivation of varicella virus) in those who had chickenpox in

Table 16-1	Childhood Vaccination Schedule, South Africa, 2011
Age	**Vaccine (No. of Doses)**
At birth	BCG, vaccine against tuberculosis; trivalent oral polio vaccine (TOPV)
6 wk	TOPV (one); rotavirus vaccine (RV) oral (one); DTaP-IPV/Hib vaccine (one); hepatitis B vaccine (one); PCV7 pneumococcal vaccine (one)
10 wk	DTaP-IPV/Hib vaccine (two); DTaP (two); hepatitis B vaccine (two)
14 wk	RV, oral rotavirus vaccine (two); DTaP-IPV/Hib vaccine (three); hepatitis B vaccine (three); PCV_7, pneumococcal vaccine (two)
9 mo	Measles vaccine (one); PCV_7, pneumococcal vaccine (three)
18 mo	DTaP-IPV/Hib vaccine (four); measles vaccine (two)
6 yr	Td vaccine
12 yr	Td vaccine

BCG, Bacillus Calmette-Guérin; *DTaP-IPV/Hib,* Diphtheria and tetanus toxoids and acellular pertussis vaccine; *Hib, Haemophilus influenzae* type b, tetanus; *IPV,* inactivated polio vaccine; *Td,* vaccine against tetanus (lockjaw) with reduced strength of diphtheria.
From South African Vaccination and Immunisation Centre: www.savic.ac.za.

childhood. International travelers frequently require vaccination to endemic diseases in a particular country (e.g., hepatitis A, yellow fever). Health care professionals are now protected against hepatitis B by vaccines. Also, each year, many adults prepare for winter and the flu season by receiving flu vaccine.

The use of vaccines has spread to pets and livestock as well (e.g., rabies, Lyme disease, feline leukemia).

VACCINE APPROVAL

Safety Issues

The safety of vaccines is a controversial public health issue because vaccines are in a unique niche in the marketplace. No vaccine is totally effective or 100% safe. The same components that make them effective may also cause serious adverse effects. It may not be possible to develop safer versions of vaccines without losing essential function.

In 1986, Congress enacted the National Childhood Vaccine Injury Act (NCVIA) to establish a no-fault compensation system for children who were harmed by adverse events following the administration of a vaccine if there was evidence that the vaccine actually caused the problem. Monitoring programs, such as the Vaccine Adverse Events Reporting System (VAERS) and the Clinical Immunization Safety Assessment Network, are essential to ensure tracking of actual but rare adverse events that may be related to vaccination. In 2011, the U.S. Supreme Court ruled that vaccine makers are immune from lawsuits alleging that the design of a vaccine is

Table 16-2	Recommended Immunizations for Children, Birth Through 6 Years Old, United States, 2011
Age	**Vaccine**
Birth	Hepatitis B (HepB) 1[1]
1 mo	HepB 2[2]
2 mo	HepB 2, if not given at 1 mo; rotavirus vaccine (RV)[2]; diphtheria and tetanus toxoids and acellular pertussis vaccine (DTaP)[3]; *Haemophilus influenzae* type b conjugate vaccine (Hib)[4]; pneumococcal vaccine (PCV)[5]; inactivated poliovirus vaccine (IPV)[6]
4 mo	RV[2]; DTaP[3]; Hib[4]; PCV[5]; IPV[6]
6 mo	HepB 3 (6-18 mo)[1]; RV[2]; DTaP[3]; Hib[4]; PCV[5]; IPV (6-18 mo)[6]; influenza yearly[7] (6 mo-6 yr)
12 mo	Hib[4]; PCV[5]; measles, mumps, and rubella (MMR) (12-15 mo)[8]; varicella (12-15 mo)[9]; hepatitis A (HepA)[10] (12-23 mo); second dose should be given 6-18 mo later
15 mo	DTaP[3]
18 mo	Influenza yearly[7]
2-3 yr	Influenza yearly[7]
4-6 yr	Influenza yearly[7]; DTaP[3]; IPV[6]; MMR[8]; varicella[9]

Note: Meningococcal conjugate vaccine, quadrivalent (MCV4), minimum age, 2 yr.
- Administer two doses of MCV4 at least 8 wk apart, children aged 2-10 yr with persistent complement component deficiency and anatomic or functional asplenia, and one dose every 5 yr thereafter.
- Persons with human immunodeficiency virus (HIV) infection who are vaccinated with MCV4 should receive two doses at least 8 wk apart.
- Administer one dose of MCV4 to children aged 2-10 yr who travel to countries with highly endemic or epidemic disease and during outbreaks caused by a vaccine serogroup.
- Administer MCV4 to children at continued risk for meningococcal disease who were previously vaccinated with MCV4 or meningococcal polysaccharide vaccine after 3 yr if first dose was administered at age 2-6 yr.

[1]Hepatitis B vaccine (HepB) (minimum age, birth).

At birth:
- Administer monovalent HepB to all newborns before hospital discharge.
- If mother is hepatitis B surface antigen (HBsAg)-positive, administer HepB and 0.5 mL of hepatitis B immune globulin (HBIG) within 12 hr of birth.
- If mother's HBsAg status is unknown, administer HepB within 12 hours of birth. Determine mother's HBsAg status as soon as possible and, if HBsAg-positive, administer HBIG (no later than age 1 wk).

Doses following the birth dose:
- The second dose should be administered at age 1 or 2 mo. Monovalent HepB should be used for doses administered before age 6 wk .
- Infants born to HBsAg-positive mothers should be tested for HBsAg and antibody to HBsAg 1-2 mo after completion of at least three doses of the HepB series, at age 9-18 mo (generally at the next well-child visit).
- Administration of four doses of HepB-infants is permissible when a combination vaccine containing HepB is administered after the birth dose.
- Infants who did not receive a birth dose should receive three doses of HepB on a schedule of 0, 1, and 6 mo.
- The final (third or fourth) dose in the HepB series should be administered no earlier than age 24 wk.

[2]Rotavirus vaccine (RV) (minimum age, 6 wk).
- Administer first dose at age 6-14 wk (maximum age, 14 wk, 6 days). Vaccination should not be initiated for infants aged 15 wk, 0 days or older.
- The maximum age for the final dose in the series is 8 mo, 0 days.
- If Rotarix is administered at ages 2 and 4 mo, a dose at 6 mo is not indicated.

[3]Diptheria and tetanus toxides and acellular perfusion vaccine (DTaP) (minimum age, 6 wk).
- The fourth dose may be administered as early as age 12 mo, provided at least 6 mo have elapsed since the third dose.

[4]Hemophilus influenzae type b-conjugate vaccine (Hib) (minimum age, 6 wk).
- If PRP-OMP (PedvaxHIB or Comvax [HepB-Hib]) is administered at ages 2 and 4 mo, a dose at age 6 mo is not indicated.
- Hiberix should not be used for doses at ages 2, 4, or 6 mo for the primary series but can be used as the final dose in children aged 12 mo-4 yr.

[5]Pneumococcal vaccine (minimum age, 6 wk for pneumococcal conjugate vaccine [PCV]; 2 yr for pneumococcal polysaccharide vaccine [PPSV]).
- PCV is recommended for all children <5 yr. Administer one dose of PCV to all healthy children aged 24-59 mo who are not completely vaccinated for their age.
- A PCV series begun with 7-valent PCV (PCV7) should be completed with 13-valent PCV (PCV13).
- A single supplemental dose of PCV13 is recommended for all children aged 14-59 mo who have received an age-appropriate series of PCV7.
- A single supplemental dose of PCV13 is recommended for all children aged 60-71 mo with underlying medical conditions who have received an age-appropriate series of PCV7.
- The supplemental dose of PCV13 should be administered at least 8 wk after the previous dose of PCV7. See MMWR 2010:59(No. RR-11).
- Administer PPSV at least 8 wk after last dose of PCV to children aged 2 yr or older with certain underlying medical conditions, including a cochlear implant.

[6]Inactivated poliovirus vaccine (IPV) (minimum age, 6 wk).
- If 4 or more doses are administered prior to age 4 yr an additional dose should be administered at age 4-6 yr.
- The final dose in the series should be administered on or after the fourth birthday and at least 6 mo following the previous dose.

[7]Influenza vaccine (seasonal); (minimum age, 6 mo for trivalent inactivated influenza vaccine [TIV]; 2 yr for live attenuated influenza vaccine [LAIV]).
- For healthy children aged 2 yr and older (i.e., those who do not have underlying medical conditions that predispose them to influenza complications), LAIV or TIV may be used, except that LAIV should not be given to children aged 2-4 yr who have had wheezing in the past 12 mo.
- Administer two doses (separated by at least 4 wk) to children aged 6 mo-8 yr who are receiving seasonal influenza vaccine for the first time or who were vaccinated for the first time during the previous influenza season but only received one dose.
- Children aged 6 mo-8 yr who received no doses of monovalent 2009 H1N1 vaccine should receive two doses of 2010–2011 seasonal influenza vaccine.

[8]Measles, mumps, and rubella vaccine (MMR) (minimum age, 12 mo). See MMWR 2010;59(No. RR-8):33–34.
- The second dose may be administered before age 4 yr, provided at least 4 wk have elapsed since the first dose.

[i]Varicella vaccine (minimum age, 12 mo).
- The second dose may be administered before age 4 yr, provided at least 3 mo have elapsed since the first dose.
- For children aged 12 mo-12 yr, the recommended minimum interval between doses is 3 mo. However, if the second dose was administered at least 4 wk after the first dose, it can be accepted as valid.

[9]Varicella vaccine (minimum age, 12 mo).
- The second dose may be administered before age 4 yr, provided at least 3 mo have elapsed since the first dose.
- For children aged 12 mo-12 yr, the recommended minimum interval between doses is 3 mo. However, if the second dose was administered at least 4 wk after the first dose, it can be accepted as valid.

[10]Hepatitis A vaccine (HepA) (minimum age, 12 mo).
- Administer two doses at least 6 mo apart.
- HepA is recommended for children >23 mo who live in areas in which vaccination programs target older children, who are at increased risk for infection, or for whom immunity against hepatitis A is desired.

From Centers for Disease Control: www.cdc.gov/vaccines
Immunization Schedules (www.cdc.gov/vaccines) Retrieved October 31, 2011.

Centers for Disease Control: _____ **Prevention of Pneumococcal Disease Among Infants and Children --- Use of 13-Valent Pneumococcal Conjugate Vaccine and 23-Valent Pneumococcal Polysaccharide Vaccine**
December 10, 2010 / 59(RR11);1-18 MMWR Morb Mortal Wkly Rep 59(RR-11) 2010; and
Prevention and Control of Influenza with Vaccines
Recommendations of the Advisory Committee on Immunization Practices (ACIP), 2010
August 6, 2010 / 59(rr08);1-62 Centers for Disease Control: MMWR Morb Mortal Wkly Rep 59(RR-8):33–34, 2010.

Table 16-3A	Recommended Immunization Schedule for Persons 7-18 years, United States, 2011		
	Age (yr)		
Vaccine	**7-10**	**11-12**	**13-16**
Tetanus, diphtheria, pertussis (Tdap)[1]	1 dose, if indicated	Tdap[1]	Tdap[1]
Human papillomavirus (HPV)[2]	See footnote.[2]	3 doses	Complete 3-dose series
Meningococcal (MCV4)[3]	See footnote.[3]	1 dose	MCV4[3]

[1]Tetanus and diphtheria toxoids and acellular pertussis vaccine (Tdap, minimum age, 10 yr for Boostrix and 11 yr for Adacel).
- Persons aged 11-18 yr who have not received Tdap should receive a dose followed by Td booster doses every 10 yr thereafter.
- Persons aged 7-10 yr who are not fully immunized against pertussis (including those never vaccinated or with unknown pertussis vaccination status) should receive a single dose of Tdap. Refer to the catch-up schedule if additional doses of tetanus and diphtheria toxoid–containing vaccine are needed.
- Tdap can be administered regardless of the interval since the last tetanus and diphtheria toxoid–containing vaccine.

[2]Human papillomavirus (HPV) vaccine. HPV4 (Gardasil) and HPV2 (Cervarix). (minimum age, 9 yr).
- Either HPV4 or HPV2 is recommended in a three-dose series for females aged 11 or 12 yr. HPV4 is recommended in a three-dose series for males aged 11 or 12 yr.
- The vaccine series can be started beginning at age 9 yr.
- Administer the second dose 1 to 2 mo after the first dose and the third dose 6 mo after the first dose (at least 24 wk after the first dose).
- See MMWR 2010;59:626-32, available at http://www.cdc.gov/mmwr/pdf/wk/mm5920.pdf

[3]Meningococcal conjugate vaccine/*MCV4,* quadrivalent (minimum age, 2 yr).
- Administer MCV4 at age 11-12 yr with a booster dose at age 16 yr.
- Administer one dose at age 13-18 yr if not previously vaccinated.
- Persons who received first dose at age 13-15 yr should receive a booster dose at age 16-18 yr with a minimum interval of at least 8 wk after the preceding dose.
- If the first dose is administered at age 16 yr or older, a booster dose is not needed.
- Administer two doses at least 8 wk apart to previously unvaccinated persons with persistent complement component deficiency and anatomic or functional asplenia, and one dose every 5 yr thereafter.
- Adolescents aged 11-18 with human immunodeficiency virus (HIV) infection should receive a two-dose primary series of MCV4, at least 8 wk apart.
- See MMWR 2011;60:72-76, available at http://www.cdc.gov/mmwr/pdf/wk/mm6003.pdf and Vaccines for Children Program.
Reference: www.cdc.gov/vaccines, retrieved October 1, 2012.
From Centers for Disease Control: Vaccines and immunizations, 2012 (www.cdc.gov/vaccines).

Table 16-3B	Recommended Immunization Schedule for Persons aged 7-18 years, United States, 2012
Vaccine	**Age: 7-18 yr**
Influenza[4]	Yearly for all children
Pneumococcal (PCV13)[5]	See footnote.[5]
Hepatitis A (Hep A)[6]	Complete 2-dose series
Hepatitis (Hep B)[7]	Complete 3-dose series
Inactivated poliovirus (IPV)[8]	Complete 3-dose series
Measles, mumps, rubella (MMR)[9]	Complete 2-dose series
Varicella[10]	Complete 2-dose series

[4]Influenza vaccine (trivalent inactivated influenza vaccine (TIV) and live, attenuated influenza vaccine (LAIV)).
- For most healthy nonpregnant persons, either LAIV or TIV may be used, except LAIV should not be used for some persons, including those with asthma or any other underlying medical conditions that predispose them to influenza complications. For all other contraindications to use of LAIV, see MMWR 59(RR-8), 2010, available at http://www.cedc.gov/mmwr/pdf/rr/rr5908.pdf.
- Administer one dose to persons aged 9 yr and older.
- For children 6 mo-8 yr of age:
  - For the 2011-2012 season, administer two doses (separated by at least 4 wk) to those who did not receive at least one dose of the 2010-2011 vaccine. Those who received at least one dose of the 2010-2011 vaccine require one dose for the 2011-2012 season.
  - For the 2012-2013 season, follow dosing guidelines in the 2012 ACIP influenza vaccine recommendations.

Table 16-3B	Recommended Immunization Schedule for Persons aged 7-18 years, United States, 2012—cont'd

[5]Pneumococcal vaccines (Pneomococcal conjugate vaccine (PCV) and pneumococcal polysaccharide vaccine (PPSV)).
- A single dose of PCV may be administered to children aged 6-18 yr who have functional or anatomic asplenia, HIV infection or other immunocompromising condition, cochlear implant or CSF leak. See MMWR 59(No. RR-11), 2010.
- Administer PPSV at least 8 wk after the last dose of PCV to children aged 2 yr or older with certain underlying medical conditions, including a cochlear implant. A single revaccination should be administered after 5 yr to children with anatomic/functional asplenia or an immunocompromising condition.

[6]Hepatitis A (HepA) vaccine.
- HepA is recommended for children aged older than 23 mo who live in areas where vaccination programs target older children, or who are at increased risk for infection, or for whom immunity against hepatitis A is desired.
- Administer two doses at least 6 mo apart to unvaccinated persons.

[7]Hepatitis B (Hep B) vaccine.
- Administer the three-dose series to those not previously vaccinated. For those with incomplete vaccination, follow the catch-up schedule.
- A two-dose series (separated by at least 4 mo) of adult formulation Recombivax HB is licensed for children aged 11-15 yr.

[8]Inactivated poliovirus vaccine (IPV).
- The final dose in the series should be administered on or after the fourth birthday and at least 6 mo following the previous dose.
- If both oral polio vaccine (OPV) and IPV were administered as part of a series, a total of four doses should be administered, regardless of the child's current age.
- IPV is not routinely recommended for U.S. residents aged 18 yr or older.

[9]Measles, mumps, and rubella (MMR) vaccine.
- The minimum interval between the two doses of MMR is 4 wk.

[10]Varicella (VAR) vaccine.
- For persons without evidence of immunity (see MMWR 56[No. RR-4], 2007), administer two doses if not previously vaccinated or the second dose if only one dose has been administered.
- For persons aged 7–12 yr, the recommended minimum interval between doses is 3 mo. However, if the second dose was administered at least 4 wk after the first dose, it can be accepted as valid.
- For persons aged 13 yr and older, the minimum interval between doses is 4 wk.
Reference: www.cdc.gov/vaccines, retrieved October 1, 2012.

VACCINE ▼ AGE GROUP ▶	19-21 years	22-26 years	27-49 years	50-59 years	60-64 years	≥65 years
Influenza[2,*]	1 dose annually					
Tetanus, diphtheria, pertussis (Td/Tdap)[3,*]	Substitute 1-time dose of Tdap for Td booster; then boost with Td every 10 years					Td/Tdap[3]
Varicella[4,*]	2 doses					
Human papillomavirus (HPV)[5,*] Female	3 doses					
Human papillamavirus (HPV)[5,*] Male	3 doses					
Zoster[6]						1 dose
Measles, mumps, rubella (MMR)[7,*]	1 or 2 doses			1 dose		
Pnemococcal (polysaccharide)[8,9]	1 or 2 doses					1 dose
Meningococcal[10,*]	1 or more doses					
Hepatitis A[11,*]	2 doses					
Hepatitis B[12,*]	3 doses					

*Covered by the Vaccine Injury Compensation Program

For all persons in this category who meet the age requirements and who lack documentation of vaccination or have any evidence of previous infection

Recommended if some other risk factor is present (e.g., on the basis of medical, occupation, lifestyle, or other indications)

Tdap recommended for ≥65 if contact with ≥12-month-old child. Either Td or Tdap can be used if no infant contact

No recommendation

Figure 16-1 Recommended adult immunization schedule, United States, 2012. *(From Centers for Disease Control and Prevention: Recommended adult immunization schedule—United States, 2012. J Midwifery Womens Health 57:188–195, 2012.)*

defective. Many physicians and public health organizations support this ruling because they believe that it will ensure the availability and promote the use of childhood vaccines. Current vaccines are considered safer and more protective than early products.

A U.S. Food and Drug Administration (FDA)–approved vaccine (Table 16-4) must meet specific requirements, as follows:

1. Produce protective immunity with only minimal side effects.
2. Be immunogenic enough to produce a strong and measurable immune response.
3. Be stable during its shelf life, with potency remaining at a proper level.

Inactivated vaccines are stored in powdered form and are reconstituted before administration. Live attenuated vaccines require refrigeration.

The Center for Biologics Evaluation and Research (CBER) regulates vaccine products. Many of these are childhood vaccines that have contributed to a significant reduction of vaccine-preventable diseases. According to the CDC, vaccines have reduced preventable infectious diseases to an all-time low and few people now experience the devastating effects of measles, pertussis, and other illnesses.

Vaccine development is an important focus of research related to acquired immunodeficiency syndrome (AIDS), malaria, and other devastating diseases. Recently recommended vaccines include a new measles-mumps-rubella-varicella vaccine for 1-year-old children and a tetanus-diphtheria-pertussis vaccine for people age 11 to 65 years.

CONCERNS ABOUT VACCINES

Vaccination requirements, even well-accepted laws on so-called classic childhood diseases (e.g., polio, measles, pertussis), have been resisted in recent years based on philosophical, political, scientific, and ideologic issues. In the past 20 years, the number of recommended pediatric vaccines has increased dramatically, despite unproven theories alleging connections between vaccines and illnesses, including autism, diabetes, and multiple sclerosis. An estimated 1% to 3% of U.S. children are excused by their parents from vaccine requirements, with rates as high as 15% to 20% in a few communities.

A vaccine for hepatitis E virus (HEV) vaccine has raised ethical concerns in Nepal. Testing the recombinant protein (rHEV) vaccine in a civilian population led to concerns that residents might not have access to the vaccines after the clinical trials concluded. Hepatitis E is common (endemic) in Nepal.

REPRESENTATIVE VACCINES

Many different vaccines are currently available. Some emphasize public health safety (e.g., anthrax) and others prevent the return of epidemic diseases.

HIV-AIDS

Vaccines such as one that could provide immunity to human immunodeficiency virus (HIV) continue to be a problem because of the enormous genetic diversity and other unique features of the HIV-B viral envelope protein. Today, according to the International AIDs Conference in Vienna, for every two patients who begin receiving treatment for HIV, five people are newly infected. The rate is estimated as at least 7000 new HIV infections daily worldwide.

Currently, no HIV-AIDS vaccines are approved for use, although many are in clinical trials. The problem is that a natural immune response that could adequately control HIV infection does not occur at all, occurs rarely, is too weak, or is too slow to begin. The goal of an effective HIV vaccine is to induce a response in the recipient that is unnatural immunity. The problem with HIV vaccine candidates is that although these vaccines can be modestly protective, they generally do not induce neutralizing antibodies nor reactive **cytotoxic T cell responses** against HIV.

The status of HIV vaccines to date is as follows:

1. There are no proven effective therapeutic or preventive HIV vaccines.
2. There is a lack of knowledge related to the ability of a vaccine to induce HIV-specific immune responses that are effective in preventing or treating HIV infection.
3. Therapeutic HIV vaccine research is still in its early stages.

Vaccine Development

The goal of producing HIV vaccines is to destroy HIV or keep the virus in check so that it causes no further damage. An ideal vaccine would stop progressive immunodeficiency and restore the immune system to a healthy state.

The requirements for a preventive HIV vaccine are to generate **humoral and cellular immunity** against HIV in the host before exposure to the virus. After initial exposure to HIV, the generation of cellular immune responses against HIV may take time to develop, which makes neutralizing antibodies against free virus important to reduce the initial spread of the virus in the body.

In the United States, research is based on the use of subunit proteins found in the envelope of HIV. Vaccine research scientists are trying to develop the following three types of HIV vaccines:

1. Preventive or prophylactic vaccines to protect individuals from HIV infection
2. Therapeutic vaccines to prevent HIV-infected patients from progressing to AIDS
3. Perinatal vaccines for administration to HIV-infected pregnant women to prevent transmission of HIV to the fetus

Scientists hope that therapeutic and perinatal administration of vaccine will reach a high level of success. Challenges associated with HIV vaccine development include the following:

- A high rate of viral mutation and recombination
- No clearly defined natural immunity to HIV
- HIV infects cells that are critical to the immune body defenses, and HIV is transmitted as a free virus and within infected cells.

Table 16-4	Examples of Available Vaccines Licensed for Immunization and Distribution in the United States		
Vaccine Name		**Trade Name**	**Manufacturer**
BCG Live		BCG Vaccine	Organon Teknika Corp LLC
BCG Live		Mycobax	Sanofi Pasteur, Ltd
BCG Live		TICE BCG	Organon Teknika Corp LLC
Diphtheria & tetanus toxoids adsorbed			Sanofi Pasteur, Inc.
Diphtheria & tetanus toxoids & acellular pertussis vaccine adsorbed		Trepedia	Sanofi Pasteur, Inc.
Diphtheria & tetanus toxoids & acellular pertussis vaccine adsorbed		Infanrix	GlaxoSmithKline Biologicals
Diphtheria & tetanus toxoids & acellular pertussis vaccine adsorbed		DAPTACEL	Sanofi Pasteur, Ltd.
Diphtheria & tetanus toxoids & acellular pertussis adsorbed, hepatitis B (recombinant) and inactivated poliovirus vaccine combined		Pediarix	GlaxoSmithKline Biologicals
Diphtheria & tetanus toxoids & acellular pertussis adsorbed and inactivated poliovirus vaccine		KINRIX	GlaxoSmithKline Biologicals
Diphtheria & tetanus toxoids & acellular pertussis adsorbed, inactivated poliovirus and Haemophilus b conjugate (tetanus toxoid conjugate) vaccine		Pentacel	Sanofi Pasteur, Ltd
Haemophilus b conjugate vaccine (meningococcal protein conjugate)		PedvaxHIB	Merck & Co., Inc.
Haemophilus b conjugate vaccine (tetanus toxoid conjugate)		ActHIB	Sanofi Pasteur, SA
Haemophilus b conjugate vaccine (tetanus toxoid conjugate)		Hiberix	GlaxoSmithKline Biologicals, S.A.
Haemophilus b conjugate vaccine (meningococcal protein conjugate) & Hepatits B vaccine (recombinant)		Comvax	Merck & Co., Inc.
Hepatitis A, inactivated		Havrix	GlaxoSmithKline Biologicals
Hepatitis A, inactivated		VAQTA	Merck & Co., Inc.
Hepatitis A inactivated and hepatitis B (recombinant) vaccine		Twinrix	GlaxoSmithKline Biologicals
Hepatitis B vaccine (recombinant)		Recombivax HB	Merck & Co., Inc.
Hepatitis B vaccine (recombinant)		Engerix-B	GlaxoSmithKline Biologicals
Human papillomavirus quadrivalent (types 6, 11, 16, 18) vaccine, recombinant		Gardasil	Merck & Co., Inc.
Human papillomavirus bivalent (types 16, 18) vaccine, recombinant		Cervarix	GlaxoSmithKline Biologicals
Influenza A (H1N1) 2009 monovalent vaccine		No trade name	CSL Limited
Influenza A (H1N1) 2009 monovalent vaccine		No trade name	MedImmune, LLC
Influenza A (H1N1) 2009 monovalent vaccine		No trade name	ID Biomedical Corp of Quebec
Influenza A (H1N1) 2009 monovalent vaccine		No trade name	Novartis Vaccines and Diagnostics Limited
Influenza A (H1N1) 2009 monovalent vaccine		No trade name	Sanofi Pasteur, Inc.
Influenza virus vaccine		Afluria	CSL Limited
Influenza virus vaccine, live, intranasal		FluMist	MedImmune, LLC
Influenza virus vaccine, H5N1		No trade name	Sanofi Pasteur, Inc.
Influenza virus vaccine, trivalent, types A and B		FluLaval	ID Biomedical Corp of Quebec
Influenza virus vaccine, trivalent, types A and B		Fluarix	GlaxoSmithKline Biologicals
Influenza virus vaccine, trivalent, types A and B		Fluvirin	Novartis Vaccines and Diagnostics S.r.l.
Influenza virus vaccine, trivalent, types A and B		Agriflu	Novartis Vaccines and Diagnostics S.r.l.
Influenza virus vaccine, trivalent, types A and B		Fluzone and Fluzone High-Dose	Sanofi Pasteur, Inc.
Japanese encephalitis virus vaccine, inactivated, adsorbed		Ixiaro	Intercell Biomedical
Japanese encephalitis virus vaccine, inactivated		JE-Vax	Research Foundation for Microbial Diseases of Osaka University

Continued

Table 16-4	Examples of Available Vaccines Licensed for Immunization and Distribution in the United States—cont'd	
Vaccine Name	**Trade Name**	**Manufacturer**
Measles virus vaccine, live	Attenuvax	Merck & Co, Inc.
Measles, mumps, and rubella virus vaccine, live	M-M-R-II	Merck & Co, Inc.
Measles, mumps, rubella and varicella virus vaccine, live	ProQuad	Merck & Co, Inc.
Meningococcal (groups A, C, Y, and W-135) Oligosaccharide diphtheria CRM197 conjugate vaccine	Menveo	Novartis Vaccines and Diagnostics, Inc.
Meningococcal polysaccharide (serogroups A, C, Y, and W-135) diphtheria toxoid conjugate vaccine	Menactra	Sanofi Pasteur, Inc.
Meningococcal polysaccharide (serogroups A, C, Y, and W-135 combined		Sanofi Pasteur, Inc.
Mumps virus vaccine, live	Mumpsvax	Merck & Co, Inc.
Pneumococcal vaccine, polyvalent	Pneumovax 23	Merck & Co, Inc.
Pneumococcal 7-valent conjugate vaccine	Prevnar	Wyeth Pharmaceuticals Inc.
Pneumococcal 13-valent conjugate vaccine	Prevnar 13	Wyeth Pharmaceuticals Inc.
Poliovirus vaccine inactivated (monkey kidney cell)	IPOL	Sanofi Pasteur, SA
Rabies vaccine	Imovax	Sanofi Pasteur, SA
Rabies vaccine	RabAvert	Novartis Vaccines and Diagnostics
Rotavirus vaccine, live, oral	ROTARIX	GlaxoSmithKline Biologicals
Rotavirus vaccine, live, oral	RotaTeq	Merck & Co., Inc.
Rubella virus vaccine, live	Meruvax II	Merck & Co., Inc.
Smallpox (vaccinia) vaccine, live	ACAM 2000	Sanofi Pasteur Biologics Co.
Tetanus & diphtheria toxoids adsorbed for adult use	No trade name	MassBiologics
Tetanus & diphtheria toxoids adsorbed for adult use	DECAVAC	Sanofi Pasteur, Inc.
Tetanus toxoid	No trade name	Sanofi Pasteur, Inc.
Tetanus toxoid adsorbed	No trade name	Sanofi Pasteur, Inc.
Tetanus toxoid, reduced diphtheria toxoid and acellular pertussis vaccine, adsorbed	Adacel	Sanofi Pasteur, Inc.
Tetanus toxoid, reduced diphtheria toxoid and acellular pertussis vaccine, adsorbed	Boostrix	GlaxoSmithKline Biologicals
Typhoid vaccine live oral Ty21a	Vivotif	Berna Biotech, Ltd.
Typhoid VI polysaccharide vaccine	TYPHIM VI	Sanofi Pasteur, Inc.
Varicella virus vaccine, live	Varivax	Merck & Co., Inc.
Yellow Fever vaccine	YF-Vax	Sanofi Pasteur, Inc.
Zoster vaccine, live	ZostaVax	Merck & Co., Inc.

Adapted from U.S. Food and Drug Administration: Complete list of vaccines licensed for immunization and distribution in the U.S., 2012 (http://www.fda.gov/BiologicsBloodVaccines/Vaccines/ApprovedProducts/ ucm093833.htm).

*Two doses given at least 4 wk apart are recommended for children aged 6 mo-8 yr of age who are getting a flu vaccine for the first time. Children who only got one dose in their first year of vaccination should get two doses the following year.

†Children ≥2 yr with certain medical conditions may need a dose of pneumococcal vaccine (PPSV) and meningococcal vaccine (MCV4). See vaccine-specific recommendations at http://www.cdc.gov/vaccines/pubs/ACIP-list.htm.

‡Two doses of HepA vaccine are needed for lasting protection. The first dose of HepA vaccine should be given from 12-23 mo of age. The second dose should be given 6-18 mo later. HepA vaccination may be given to any child 12 mo and older to protect against HepA.

Vaccine Problems

Problems associated with HIV vaccine development are plagued by the lack of scientific understanding of HIV infection and the complex biology of HIV infection and AIDS. Once inside a host cell, HIV is capable of integrating itself into the genetic material of infected cells. For a vaccine to be effective, it needs to produce a constant state of immune protection, not only to block viral entry to most cells but also to continue to block newly produced viruses over the infected person's lifetime.

Researchers have identified the following specific problem areas:

- A lack of knowledge related to the critical components in the body's immune response to HIV infection.

- The high risk of using the entire weakened or inactive HIV in a vaccine.
- The extensive rate of viral mutation as HIV replicates. Strains worldwide vary by as much as 35% in terms of the proteins that make up the outer coat of the virus. Even an infected person can experience a change in viral protein by as much as 10% over years. This genetic diversity may require an effective vaccine to be based on multiple viral strains.
- The protective effect of a vaccine may last only a short time and frequent mandatory booster vaccinations would be impractical and expensive.
- Vaccinated persons could become more susceptible to HIV infection because of vaccine-induced enhancement of infection.
- No vaccine clinical trial to date has demonstrated stimulation of the cellular components of the immune system in the way needed to destroy HIV.
- Animal models have severe limitations, including the possibility of integration of DNA into the human genome from monkeys.
- No research studies have successfully demonstrated which immune responses correlate with protection from HIV infection.

In 2000, vaccine research scientists lowered their expectations and settled for a vaccine that would not completely prevent HIV infection. It is estimated that a vaccine with only 30% effectiveness against HIV (versus the usual 85% to 95% effectiveness of other infectious disease vaccines) can begin to eradicate the virus if it is widely administered and accompanied by disease prevention education. Based on this premise, the FDA has indicated that it will approve an HIV-AIDS vaccine at this level of efficacy.

South Africa's first large-scale HIV vaccine efficacy trial of subtype B HIV in predominantly subtype C patients started in 2007. It is difficult to find populations who are at high risk except for so-called sex workers. Rather than destroying an infection before it becomes established in the cells, the vaccine being tested would more likely modify the infection once it did take hold by pushing the viral set point as low as possible. This would delay the onset of symptoms and possibly make the virus less potent. Alternatively, the vaccine might reduce the initial peak point, when the probability of transmission is much greater.

Modest protection has been demonstrated against HIV infection by immunization with a vaccine regimen consisting of a canarypox vector prime plus a protein subunit booster in the RV144 trial in Thailand. In the future, trials will focus on broadening the limited protection of RV144.

Vaccine Expectations

Reasons for optimism about HIV vaccine development include the following:

1. Nonhuman primates vaccinated with products based on HIV or simian immunodeficiency virus have shown complete or partial protection against infection with the wild-type virus.
2. Successful vaccines have been developed against the feline immunodeficiency virus, also a retrovirus.
3. Almost all humans develop some form of immune response that is protective or able to control the viral infection over a long period. Some individuals remain disease-free for up to 25 years, frequently with undetectable viral load levels.
4. Vaccines that present epitopes to the immune system in a conformationally precise manner may induce the body to produce neutralizing antibodies and provide a high level of protection against HIV infection.
5. In the future, microbial and viral genome sequencing will become increasingly rapid and less expensive. One approach, known as reverse vaccinology, involves cloning and expressing all proteins that are predicted based on a complete genome to be secreted or surface-associated, starting with the complete genome sequence. This approach allows for a small group of proteins from microorganisms (e.g., group B meningococcus, group B *Streptococcus,* extraintestinal pathogenic *Escherichia coli*) to be candidates for multivalent subunit vaccines. To date, however, these organisms have eluded vaccine development.

Cytomegalovirus

There is no available vaccine for preventing congenital CMV disease (present at birth). However, a few CMV vaccines have been tested in humans, including live attenuated (weakened) virus vaccines and vaccines that contain only pieces of the virus.

The Institute of Medicine has ranked the development of a CMV vaccine as its highest priority because of the lives it would save and the disabilities it would prevent. An FDA-approved CMV vaccine, however, may take years. Because CMV is not spread as easily as some other diseases, even a partially effective CMV vaccine will have a large impact on the congenital CMV disease epidemic.

Hay Fever

An experimental DNA-based vaccine to protect against hay fever after just six injections has been in development. Patients who received the vaccine experienced an average 60% reduction in allergy symptoms compared with those receiving placebo.

The vaccine lessens the immune system's excessive reactions to inhaled allergens by stimulating protective cells that turn off the Th2 helper cells. The type 2 helper T cells (Th2) send out signals for the body to create more immunoglobulin E (IgE), the protein largely responsible for allergy symptoms. Also, the vaccine may activate **dendritic cells,** keeping inflammation in check over the long term and breaking an otherwise self-sustaining allergic cycle.

DNA-based and cell line–based vaccines appear to be the future of immunology.

Human Papillomavirus

Cancer vaccines such as those for HPV are another form of biological therapy currently under study. Cancer vaccines have already been developed to fight HPV-16, a common strain that causes cervical cancer. More than 6 million people become infected with HPV every year in the United States, and almost 10,000 women are diagnosed with cervical cancer.

These vaccines work by exposing the body's immune cells to weakened forms of an antigen (foreign substance) that form on the surface of an infectious agent. The immune system increases production of cells that make antibodies to fight the infectious agent and T cells that recognize the infectious agent. These immune cells remember the exposure, so the next time the agent enters the body, the immune system is already prepared to respond and stop the infection.

Types 16 (HPV-16) and 18 (HPV-18) cause approximately 70% of cervical cancers worldwide. A major breakthrough in immunology has resulted in the development of the Gardasil vaccine (Merck, Whitehouse Station, NJ), approved by the FDA in June 2006 for girls and women age 9 to 26 years. More than 30 countries had approved the vaccine before the FDA's approval. The vaccine can prevent cervical cancer and vaginal and vulvar precancers caused by HPV-16 and HPV-18, as well as low-grade and precancerous lesions and genital warts caused by HPV types 6, 11, 16, and 18 in women not previously infected by one of the four covered HPV types.

Additional products in development include vaccines covering other high-risk HPV types for broader coverage, as well as therapeutic vaccines designed to treat women who already have precancerous lesions or cancer.

Influenza

The efficacy of influenza vaccines may decline during years when the circulating viruses have drifted antigenically from those included in the vaccine. WHO coordinates global influences and virus surveillance so that appropriate vaccine candidates can be identified by WHO and national authorities, and vaccines can be reformulated each year. Vaccine viruses must be selected every year because genetic mutations arise continuously in influenza viruses, a process termed **antigenic drift** that results in the emergence of immunologically distinct variants. The process is repeated each year, which imposes severe time restrictions on all groups involved.

Influenza A (H3N2) components in the inactive and live attenuated influenza vaccines were not optimally matched to the circulating strains. Researchers have studied the concept of herd immunity (indirect protection from influenza at community level), a different view of promoting immunity, particularly to vulnerable groups (e.g., very young, older adults).

The FDA has approved FluLaval, an influenza vaccine, for immunizing people 18 years and older against flu. Currently, there are five FDA-licensed flu vaccines.

In 2007, universal vaccination of children 6 to 59 months of age with trivalent inactivated influenza vaccine was recommended by U.S. advisory bodies. In a study of the safety and efficacy of intranasally administered live attenuated influenza vaccine to children without a recent episode of wheezing illness or severe asthma, live attenuated virus had significantly better efficacy than inactivated vaccine.

Leukemia

The search for cancer vaccines had a breakthrough with the development of a therapeutic vaccine for patients with acute myelogenous leukemia (AML). A pilot study to demonstrate the effectiveness and safety of an AML vaccine is underway. The phase 1 stage of the clinical trial with AML patients has been aimed at determining whether the PR1 peptide vaccine (a nine–amino acid, HLA-A2–restricted peptide derived from proteinase 3) can elicit T cell immunity in leukemia patients whose disease has been resistant to treatment.

Malaria

There are four types of human malaria:
- *Plasmodium falciparum*
- *Plasmodium vivax*
- *Plasmodium malariae*
- *Plasmodium ovale*

Plasmodium falciparum and *Plasmodium vivax* are the most common. *P. falciparum* is the most deadly. In recent years, some human cases of malaria have also occurred caused by *Plasmodium knowlesi*, a monkey malaria that occurs in certain forested areas of Southeast Asia.

Malaria, a bloodborne parasite, is transmitted exclusively through the bite of *Anopheles* mosquitoes. The intensity of transmission depends on factors related to the parasite, vector, human host, and environment. In many areas, transmission is seasonal, with a peak during and just after the rainy season. All the important vector species of *Anopheles* bite at night. Transmission is more intense in areas in which the mosquito lifespan is longer, and where it prefers to bite humans rather than other animals. This allows the parasite to have time to complete its development inside the mosquito. The long lifespan and strong human-biting habit of the African vector species is the main reason why more than 85% of the world's malaria deaths are in Africa.

Human immunity is another important factor, especially among adults in areas of moderate or intense transmission conditions. Immunity is developed over years of exposure and although it never provides complete protection, it does reduce the risk that malarial infection will cause severe disease. For this reason, most malaria deaths in Africa occur in young children. In 2009, malaria caused an estimated 781,000 deaths, mostly in African children. In areas with less transmission and low immunity, all age groups are at risk.

Malaria Vaccine Development

The complexity of the malaria parasite makes development of vaccine very difficult. Currently, there is no approved commercially available malaria vaccine, despite many decades of intense research and development.

One vaccine candidate, RTS,S/AS01, directed against the deadly *P. falciparum* strain, is being tested in seven sub-Saharan African countries: Burkina Faso, Gabon, Ghana, Kenya, Malawi, Mozambique, and the United Republic of Tanzania.

The phase 3 trial, which started in May 2009, has completed enrollment with more than 15,000 people involved. The children are in two age groups: (1) children aged 5 to 17 months at first immunization, receiving RTS,S/AS01 without coadministration of other vaccines; and (2) infants 6 to 12 weeks of age at first immunization in coadministration with pentavalent vaccines in the routine immunization schedule. Both groups received three doses of RTS,S/AS01 vaccine at 1-month intervals.

Previously, this vaccine had shown 51% efficacy in reducing all episodes of clinical malaria in infants aged 5 to 17 months in a phase 2 trial in Kenya over 15 months. The first of the interim reports of the phase 3 trial became available in October 2011. The efficacy rate was a 55% reduction in frequency of malaria episodes during the 12 months of follow-up in children 5 to 17 months of age at first immunization. The efficacy in children aged 6 to 14 weeks is not yet known. A further interim report is expected in late 2012. According to the current trial schedule, the phase 3 trial data required for WHO to consider making a policy recommendation is expected to become available in early 2015.

Other vaccines with higher efficacy are desirable. Several promising vaccine candidates are currently being studied, but are at least 5 to 10 years behind RTS,S/AS01 in their development. The malaria vaccine FMP2.1/AS02, a recombinant protein based on apical membrane antigen 1 (AMA1) from the 3D7 strain of *P. falciparum,* has been shown to have immunogenicity and acceptable safety in 400 Malian children. On the basis of the primary end point of signs and symptoms of clinical malaria, this vaccine did not provide significant protection against clinical malaria. Based on the secondary end point—clinical malaria caused by parasites with the AMA1 DNA sequence—the vaccine may have strain-specific efficacy.

Another vaccine, merozoite surface protein 3 (MSP3), was in phase 1b clinical trials in 2007. In this trial, 45 children 12 to 24 months of age were given three doses of the vaccine. The study was designed to study safety of the vaccine. The children from Burkina Faso, Africa, demonstrated some resistance against clinical malaria, at least in the short term.

Polio

The incidence of polio has been reduced by more than 99% and the number of countries with endemic transmission has been reduced by more than 96%.

Poliovirus persists in countries in which the virus is endemic. New outbreaks have been occurring in previously polio-free countries, including, most recently, Kenya's first documented wild-type poliovirus infection in 22 years. Four countries in which the virus remains endemic—Nigeria, India, Pakistan, and Afghanistan—account for 93% of polio cases worldwide; unlike all other countries, they have never succeeded in interrupting the transmission of wild poliovirus.

The biological reason is the same regardless of the location—insufficient immunity in the population to interrupt transmission. In almost all cases, the basic cause remains failure to vaccinate enough children with enough doses to ensure that they are immune to disease and infection.

In the past decade, the initiative to eradicate polio has faced substantial challenges. Large outbreaks associated with spread from primary global reservoirs in Nigeria and India affected 25 countries and were controlled only after more than 2 years of effort. At the same time, the belief that wild-type 2 poliovirus was eradicated in 1999 becomes more certain.

Rotavirus

In 2006, U.S. infants began to be vaccinated with pentavalent rotavirus vaccine (RV5). Prior to the introduction of RV5 vaccination, diarrhea caused by rotavirus accounted for an estimated 400,000 visits to primary health care providers, 200,000 emergency department visits, 55,000 hospitalizations, and 20 to 60 deaths annually of U.S. children younger than 5 years.

Since the introduction of rotavirus vaccine, diarrhea-associated health care utilization and medical expenditures for U.S. children have decreased substantially. In 2007-2008, the annual rates of hospitalization for rotavirus-coded diarrhea among children younger than 5 years declined by 75%. The declines were similar across age groups, despite variation in vaccine coverage, with negligible coverage among 2- to 4-year-old children.

Yellow Fever

Yellow fever is a lethal, mosquito-borne, *Flavivirus* disease. The resulting hemorrhagic fever occurs in tropical areas of Africa and South America. Certain South American countries such as Brazil require vaccination for entry into the country. Other countries, such as South Africa, require vaccination if a traveler is entering from an endemic country.

A live attenuated vaccine (17D) was developed in 1936. This highly immunogenic live vaccine (17D) is required for travel to many countries where yellow fever is endemic. Although rare, adverse effects can include viscerotropic disease and anaphylactic shock. Viscerotropic disease resembles naturally acquired yellow fever and is potentially fatal. The rates of reported cases are 0.4/100,000 population for viscerotropic disease and 1.8/100,000 population for anaphylaxis.

Because of safety issues, an inactivated cell culture vaccine against yellow fever has been developed, XRX-001. This vaccine, administered as a two-dose regimen, contains inactivated yellow fever produced in cell culture and adsorbed to an aluminum hydroxide adjuvant. Clinical trial results have indicated that this vaccine induces a high percentage of neutralizing antibodies in trial participants. Preliminary findings have suggested that XRX-001 has the potential to be a safer alternative to live attenuated 17D vaccine.

VACCINES IN BIODEFENSE

In regard to bioterrorism, the goal of the FDA is to foster the development of vaccines. Many products (e.g., FDA-regulated vaccines) could be affected by bioterrorism. Pathogens or pathogen products adapted for biological warfare include the following:

- Smallpox (variola)
- Anthrax *(Bacillus anthracis)*

Smallpox

Threats of bioterrorism with smallpox as a weapon have launched a high-profile discussion of the reintroduction of smallpox into the general U.S. population. Individuals in high-risk occupations and positions have already begun to be vaccinated.

Category A Agents

Smallpox vaccination was stopped in 1972 after the disease was eradicated in the United States. Smallpox is classified as a Category A agent by the CDC. Other Category A agents include anthrax, plague, botulism, tularemia, and viral hemorrhagic fevers. These agents are believed to pose the greatest potential threat for an adverse public health effect and to have a moderate to high potential for large-scale dissemination.

Smallpox Vaccine

Smallpox vaccine, a preventive vaccine, is the only way to prevent smallpox. The vaccine is made from a live virus called vaccinia, which is another pox-type virus related to smallpox but unable to cause smallpox. A live virus vaccine, including measles, mumps, rubella, chickenpox, and smallpox vaccines, is a vaccine that contains a living virus that can provide and produce immunity, usually without causing illness. For most people with a healthy immune system, live virus vaccines are safe and effective, but the live virus can be transmitted to other parts of the body or to other people from the unhealed vaccination site.

Vaccine Administration

The vaccine is not injected like other types of vaccines. It is given using a bifurcated (two-pronged) needle that is dipped into the vaccine solution. The needle is used to prick the skin a number of times in a few seconds. It takes about 3 weeks for the site to heal, with a scar remaining. The first dose of vaccine offers protection from smallpox for 3 to 5 years, with decreasing immunity thereafter. A repeat vaccination offers longer immunity. Vaccination within 3 days of exposure completely prevents or significantly modifies smallpox in the vast majority of persons. Vaccination 4 to 7 days after exposure likely offers some protection from disease or may modify the severity of the disease.

Anthrax

Anthrax is an infectious disease caused by spores of the bacterium *Bacillus anthracis*. *B. anthracis* spores are highly resistant to inactivation and may be present in the soil, for example, for decades, occasionally infecting grazing animals that ingest the spores. Goats, sheep, and cattle are some animals that may become infected.

Human infection may occur by three routes of exposure to anthrax spores—cutaneous, gastrointestinal, and pulmonary. In North America, human cases of anthrax are infrequent. The U.S. military regards anthrax as a potential biological terrorism threat because the spores are so resistant to destruction and can be easily spread by release in the air. The development of anthrax as a biological weapon by several foreign countries has been documented.

The only known effective preexposure prevention against anthrax is vaccination with anthrax vaccine. The only licensed anthrax vaccine, Anthrax Vaccine Adsorbed (AVA), or BioThraxTM, is indicated for active immunization for the prevention of disease caused by *B. anthracis* in those 18 to 65 years of age who are at high risk of exposure. Next generation anthrax vaccines are under development by a number of manufacturers.

CASE STUDY

A 25-year-old female medical student came to the emergency department because of a fever, cough, and shortness of breath. She noticed the shortness of breath after walking up one flight of stairs. She has noticed increased fatigue with a dry cough.

The patient did not smoke, drink alcohol, or use illegal drugs. Eleven months earlier, she had traveled to Nairobi, Kenya, for a month-long volunteer assignment with a medical group. Since then, she had not traveled outside the United States. A tuberculin skin test performed before she went to Africa was negative. She received many vaccinations, including tetanus vaccine, prior to her international trip.

She was admitted to the hospital. A complete blood count and chest x-ray were ordered.

Laboratory Results

The patient's complete blood count was essentially within reference ranges.

The chest x-ray showed a right pleural effusion and a possible infiltrate. A follow-up echocardiogram showed a pericardial effusion.

A cytologic examination of the pericardial fluid showed blood and no malignant cells. Gram stain showed red cells but no neutrophils or organisms and a culture showed no growth of bacteria. A smear and culture were negative for acid-fast bacilli and mycobacteria. A repeat tuberculin skin test was performed during the hospitalization. There was no skin reaction. Smears and cultures of three specimens of sputum were negative for acid-fast bacilli and mycobacteria.

Questions

1. What are this patient's risk factors?
   a Age
   b. Gender
   c. Global travel
   d. Contaminated vaccines
2. What can cause a negative TB skin test 5 months after traveling to Africa, even if TB is contracted?
   a. Technical problems, e.g., subcutaneous TB skin test
   b. HIV infection
   c. Transient specific anergy due to acute infection
   d. All of the above

See Appendix A for the answers to these questions.

Critical Thinking Group Discussion Questions

1. Is this patient at risk for developing an infectious disease?
2. Could this patient have tuberculosis even though the tuberculin skin test was nonreactive 5 months after returning from Africa and when repeated during this hospital admission?

3. What follow-up assay(s) could be ordered to assess the patient's ability to build antibodies in response to a tetanus vaccination?

See instructor site ⊜volve for the discussion of the answers to these questions.

Tetanus Antibodies (IgG)

Principle

This determines IgG antibodies produced in response to vaccination by the method of quantitative multianalyte fluorescent detection.

Clinical Application

It is used for the detection of tetanus antibodies and titer in response to vaccination. A comparison can be made between specimens collected prior to and 1 month after vaccination. A poor or low titer of IgG tetanus antibodies suggests a state of anergy.

Responder status is determined according to the ratio of a 1-month postvaccination specimen to the prevaccination concentration of tetanus IgG antibodies, as follows:

1. If the postvaccination concentration is less than 1.0 IU, the patient is considered a nonresponder.
2. If the postvaccination concentration is 1.0 IU or higher, a patient with a ratio of less than 1.5 is a nonresponder, a ratio of 1.5 to less than 3.0 is a weak responder, and a ratio of 3.0 or higher is a good responder.
3. If the prevaccination concentration is greater than 1.0, it may be difficult to assess the response based on a ratio alone. A postvaccination concentration above 2.5 IU in this case is usually adequate.

CHAPTER HIGHLIGHTS

- Vaccines provide artificially acquired active immunity to a specific disease.
- The CBER regulates vaccine products. According to the CDC, vaccines have reduced preventable infectious diseases to an all-time low. Vaccine development is an important focus of research for AIDS, malaria, and other devastating diseases.
- Pathogens or pathogen products adapted for biological warfare include smallpox, anthrax, plague, tularemia, brucellosis, Q fever, botulinum toxin, and staphylococcal enterotoxin B.
- Jenner discovered a fundamental principle of immunization with smallpox vaccine and paved the way for the development of rabies (Louis Pasteur) and other vaccines (e.g., diphtheria, typhoid).
- Children now receive vaccines for many childhood diseases (e.g., rubella). Adults require boosters (tetanus). A vaccine approved in 2006 for adults reduces the risk of shingles.

- International travelers frequently require vaccination to endemic diseases (e.g., hepatitis A) in a particular country. Health care professionals are now protected against hepatitis B through vaccines. Many adults receive the flu vaccine. Vaccines are also given to pets and livestock.
- A vaccine stimulates active immunity and creates an immune memory so that exposure to the active disease microorganism will stimulate an already primed immune system to fight the disease.
- Most vaccines can be divided into two categories, live attenuated vaccines and nonreplicating vaccines.
- A vaccine must produce protective immunity with minimal side effects, produce a strong immune response, and be stable during its shelf life.
- Classic preventive vaccines are designed to mimic the effects of natural exposure to microbes. The earliest host response to vaccination is called the innate immune response.
- Vaccines emphasize public health safety (anthrax) or prevent the return of epidemic diseases.
- Preventive AIDS vaccines are for HIV-negative individuals to prevent HIV infection. Therapeutic AIDS vaccines are for HIV-positive individuals to improve the immune system.
- Anthrax vaccine is for emergency use in the event of an anthrax-based attack on the U.S. population.
- No available vaccine can prevent congenital CMV disease, although a few CMV vaccines have been tested in humans.
- Experimental DNA-based vaccine to protect against hay fever after just six injections has been in development.
- Cancer vaccines such as Gardasil for HPV work by exposing the body's immune cells to weakened forms of an antigen.
- FluLaval is an influenza vaccine for immunizing people 18 years of age and older. The FDA has licensed five flu vaccines.
- A therapeutic vaccine is directed at patients with AML.
- Polio has been reduced by more than 99% and the number of countries with endemic transmission has been reduced by more than 96%.
- The threat of bioterrorism with smallpox has led to high-risk individuals already being vaccinated.

REVIEW QUESTIONS

1. The Center for Biologics Evaluation and Research CBER regulates:
   a. Laboratory safety
   b. Vaccine products
   c. Personnel qualifications
   d. Research grants

2. Pathogens adapted for biological warfare include:
   (1) Smallpox
   (2) *Bacillus anthracis*
   (3) Chickenpox
   (4) Q fever
   a. 1, 2, 3
   b. 1, 2, 4
   c. 2, 3, 4
   d. 1, 3, 4

3. Vaccines can be divided into _____ vaccines.
   a. Live, attenuated
   b. Nonreplicating
   c. Naked DNA
   d. Both a and b

4. To meet FDA requirements, a vaccine must:
   a. Produce protective immunity with only minimal side effects.
   b. Be immunogenic enough to produce a strong and measurable immune response.
   c. Be stable during its shelf life.
   d. All of the above.

5. The earliest host response to vaccination is a(n):
   a. Innate immune response
   b. Memory response
   c. Anamnestic response
   d. Both a and b

6 and 7. Match the following:

6. A Preventive HIV vaccine

7. B Therapeutic HIV vaccine
   a. Given to HIV-negative individuals
   b. For HIV-positive patients to improve their immune system to prevent progression to AIDS

8-12. Match the following (use an answer only once):

8. A Anthrax vaccine

9. C Cytomegalovirus CMV vaccine

10. D Hay fever vaccine

11. B Human papillomavirus (HPV) vaccine

12. E Influenza vaccine
   a. Protection against bioterrorism
   b. Protection against cervical cancer
   c. Not available for preventing congenital infection
   d. DNA-based vaccine
   e. Annual vaccination required

13-15. Match the following:

13. B Leukemia vaccine

14. A Polio vaccine

15. C Smallpox vaccine
   a. Has reduced disease by 99%
   b. Successful in cats
   c. Given to high-risk individuals

BIBLIOGRAPHY

Agosti JM, Goldie SJ: Introducing HPV vaccine in developing countries: key challenges and issues, N Engl J Med 356:1908–1910, 2007.

Associated Regional and University Pathologists: Tetanus antibody, IgG, 2012, http://www. aruplab.com/guides/ug/tests/0050535.jsp.

Baden LR, Curfman GD, Morrissey S, Drazen JM: Human papillomavirus vaccine: opportunity and challenge, N Engl J Med 356:1990–1991, 2007.

Basu S: Hepatitis E vaccine, N Engl J Med 356:2421, 2007.

Belshe RB, Edwards KM, Vesikari T, et al: Live attenuated virus inactivated influenza vaccine in infants and young children, N Engl J Med 356:685–695, 2007.

Bozzette SA, Boer R, Bhatnagar V, et al: A model for a smallpox-vaccination policy, N Engl J Med 348:416–425, 2003.

Centers for Disease Control and Prevention: Smallpox disease overview, 2004, http://emergency.cdc.gov/agent/smallpox/overview/disease-facts.asp.

Centers for Disease Control and Prevention: Recommended adult immunization schedule—United States, J Midwifery Womens Health 2012(57):188–195, 2012.

Charo A: Politics, parents, and prophylaxis: mandating HPV vaccination in the United States, N Engl J Med 356:1905–1907, 2007.

Chaves S, Gargiullo P, Zhang JX, et al: Loss of vaccine-induced immunity to varicella over time, N Engl J Med 356:1121–1128, 2007.

Cortes JE, Curns AT, Tate JE, et al: Rotavirus vaccine and health care utilization for diarrhea in U.S. children, N Engl J Med 365:1108–1117, 2011.

Dolin R: HIV vaccine trial results—an opening for further research, N Engl J Med 361:2279–2280, 2009.

Fukuda K, Kieny MP: Different approaches to influenza vaccination, N Engl J Med 355:2586–2589, 2006.

Herman D: Large-scale HIV vaccine trials to start in South Africa next year, Immunol News 6:1, 2006.

Hoffmann P, Roumeguère T, van Velthoven R: Use of statins and outcome of BCG treatment for bladder cancer, N Engl J Med 355:2705–2706, 2006.

Johnston MI, Fauci AS: An HIV vaccine: evolving concepts, N Engl J Med 356:2073–2080, 2007.

Kesselheim A: Safety, supply, and suits—litigation and the vaccine industry, N Engl J Med 364:1485–1487, 2011.

Koff WC: Berkley SF: The renaissance in HIV vaccine development—future directions, N Engl J Med 363:e7, 2010.

Monath TP, Fowler E, Johnson CT, et al: An inactivated cell-culture vaccine against yellow fever, N Engl J Med 364:1326–1332, 2011.

Ohmit SE, Victor JC, Rotthoff JR, et al: Prevention of antigenically drifted influenza by inactivated and live attenuated vaccines, N Engl J Med 355:2513–2522, 2006.

Pallansch MA, Sandhu HS: The eradication of polio: progress and challenges, N Engl J Med 355:2508–2511, 2006.

Poland GA, Jacobson RM: The age-old struggle against the antivaccinationists, N Engl J Med 364:97–100, 2011.

Pulendran B: Tolls and beyond: many roads to vaccine immunity, N Engl J Med 356:1765–1778, 2007.

Relman DA: Microbila genomics and infectious diseases, N Engl J Med 365:347–357, 2011.

Schraeder TL, Campion EW: Smallpox vaccination: the call to arms, N Engl J Med 348:1–2, 2003.

Sirima SB: Protection against malaria by MSP3 candidate vaccine, N Engl J Med 365:1062–1063, 2011.

Thera MA, Doumbo OK, Coulibaly D et al: A field trial to assess a blood-stage malaria vaccine. N Engl J Med 365: 1004–1013.

U.S. Food and Drug Administration: Anthrax, 2012, http://www.fda.gov/Biologics BloodVaccines/Vaccines/ucm061751.htm.

Wilbur DC: Vaccines for preventing cervical cancer: where we are now, CAP Today 21:48, 2007.

CHAPTER 17

Streptococcal Infections

Learning Objectives

At the conclusion of this chapter, the reader should be able to:
- Describe the etiology, epidemiology, signs and symptoms, and complications of streptococcal infection.
- Discuss the immunologic manifestations and diagnostic evaluation of streptococcal infection.
- Analyze and apply laboratory data to a case study.
- Correctly answer case study related multiple choice questions.

- Be prepared to participate in a discussion of critical thinking questions.
- Explain the principle and applications of the classic anti–streptolysin O (ASO) procedure.
- Briefly explain other methods of detection of group A streptococcus.
- Correctly answer end of chapter review questions.

Key Terms

Anti–DNase B (ADN-B)
antistreptolysin O (ASO)
erythrogenic toxin
exogenous endotoxin
exudate
hemoglobinuria

hemolysins
necrotizing fasciitis
neonatal septicemia
osmotic lysis
poststreptococcal glomerulonephritis
purulent

serogroups
streptokinase
streptolysin O (SLO)
streptolysin S
tumor necrosis factor-α (TNF-α)

ETIOLOGY

Most streptococci that contain cell wall antigens of the Lancefield group A (Table 17-1) are known as *Streptococcus pyogenes.* Members of this species are almost always beta-hemolytic streptococci. *S. pyogenes* is the most common causative agent of pharyngitis and its resultant disorder, scarlet fever, and the skin infection, impetigo. The most common type of bacteria causing necrotizing fasciitis is *S. pyogenes.*

In terms of human morbidity and mortality worldwide, however, the role of *S. pyogenes* in the subsequent development of complications such as acute rheumatic fever and poststreptococcal glomerulonephritis is more important. Other *S. pyogenes*–associated infections include otitis media in children, sinusitis in adults, and osteomyelitis, septic arthritis, **neonatal septicemia**, and rare cases of pneumonia.

Necrotizing fasciitis is a rare infection that can destroy skin and soft tissues, including fat and the tissue-covering muscles (fascia). Because these tissues die rapidly, a person with necrotizing fasciitis is sometimes said to be infected with so-called flesh-eating bacteria. A highly invasive group A streptococcal infection is associated with toxic shock syndrome.

Table 17-1	Lancefield Streptococcus Classifications*	
Lancefield Group	**Examples of Bacterial Species in the Group**	**Comments**
A	*Streptococcus pyogenes*	Strains most pathogenic for human beings can cause strep throat, rheumatic fever, scarlet fever, acute glomerulonephritis, and necrotizing fasciitis.
B	*Streptococcus mastitis*	Strains from mastitis in cows and from normal milk, including strains from the human throat and vagina
	Streptococcus agalactiae	Can cause pneumonia and meningitis in neonates and older adults, with occasional systemic bacteremia
C	*Streptococcus equii*	Strains from various lower animals, including cattle, and from the human throat
	Streptococcus dysgalactiae	Can cause pharyngitis and other pyogenic infections similar to group A streptococci
D	*Streptococcus faecalis* (now *Enterococcus faecalis*) Other nonenterococcal group D strains include *Streptococcus bovis* and *Streptococcus equinus*.	Strains from cheese and humans Many former group D streptococci have been reclassified and placed in the genus *Enterococcus*.
E		Strains from certified milk
F	*Streptococcus anginosus* (Lancefield classification) or *Streptococcus milleri* group (European system)	Strains mainly from the human throat, associated with tonsillitis; minute hemolytic
G	*Streptococcus canis* is an example of a GBS Group B streptococcus (GBS) which is typically found in animals, but does not cause infection except in newborns at birth	Strains can cause infection in human beings (a few strains from monkeys and dogs). NOTE: This is not exclusively beta-hemolytic.
H, K, O		Nonpathogenic strains occasionally from normal human respiratory tracts

*This is a serologic classification of hemolytic streptococci, dividing them into groups based on antigenic serocharacteristics. It is based on precipitation tests depending on group-specific carbohydrate substances.

Morphologic Characteristics

S. pyogenes is a gram-positive coccus and the serotype most frequently associated with human infection. Lancefield divided these beta-hemolytic streptococci into **serogroups** A through O on the basis of the immunologic action of the cell wall carbohydrate (Fig. 17-1).

Structures called fimbriae arise near the plasma membrane and project through the cell wall and capsule. These processes contain important surface components of the streptococcus. Lipoteichoic acid on the fimbriae is important in the organism's adherence to human epithelium and the initiation of infection. The M and R antigens, which are structurally similar but immunologically distinct, are also found on the fimbriae. R antigen has no known biological role.

M protein, a cell protein found in association with the hyaluronic capsule, is a major virulence factor of *S. pyogenes*. Strains of *S. pyogenes* that lack M protein cannot cause infection. M protein inhibits phagocytosis and antibody synthesized against M protein provides type-specific immunity to group A streptococci. In addition, M protein is the basis for a subclassification of group A streptococci into more than 60 M serotypes.

Extracellular Products

Extracellular products are important in the pathogenesis of disease and in the serologic diagnosis of streptococcal disease. Antibodies produced in response to these substances provide evidence of recent streptococcal infection. Two **hemolysins,** with the ability to damage human and animal erythrocytes, polymorphonuclear leukocytes (PMNs), and platelets, are produced by most group A strains, as follows:

- **Streptolysin O (SLO),** an oxygen-labile enzyme, binds to sterols in the red blood cell (RBC) membrane, causing stearic rearrangement. This rearrangement produces submicroscopic holes in the RBC membrane and hemoglobin diffuses from the cells. SLO is antigenic; the antibody response to it is the most frequently used serologic indicator of recent streptococcal infection.
- **Streptolysin S,** an oxygen-stable enzyme, is responsible for the beta (clear-appearing) hemolysis on the surface of a blood agar culture plate. Streptolysin S disrupts the selective permeability of the RBC membrane, causing **osmotic lysis.** It is not antigenic.

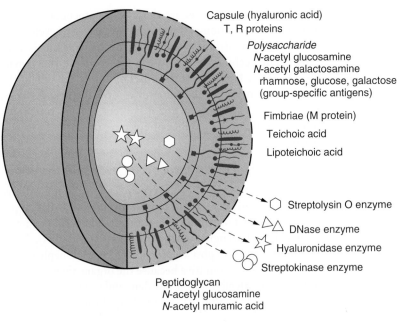

Capsule (hyaluronic acid)
T, R proteins

Polysaccharide
N-acetyl glucosamine
N-acetyl galactosamine
rhamnose, glucose, galactose
(group-specific antigens)

Fimbriae (M protein)

Teichoic acid

Lipoteichoic acid

⬡ Streptolysin O enzyme

△△ DNase enzyme

☆ Hyaluronidase enzyme

◯◯ Streptokinase enzyme

Peptidoglycan
N-acetyl glucosamine
N-acetyl muramic acid

Cytoplasmic membrane

Figure 17-1 *S. pyogenes* contains many antigenic structural components and produces several antigenic enzymes, each of which may elicit a specific antibody response from the infected host. *(Adapted from Forbes BA, Sahm DF, Weissfeld AS: Bailey and Scott's diagnostic microbiology, ed 12, St Louis, 2007, Mosby.)*

- Other substances produced by group A streptococci presumably facilitate rapid spread through subcutaneous or deeper soft tissues and include the following:
  - Hyaluronidase, also called spreading factor, breaks down hyaluronic acid found in the host's connective tissue.
  - Four immunologically distinct deoxyribonucleases (DNases A, B, C, and D) degrade deoxyribonucleic acid (DNA).
  - **Streptokinase,** an enzyme, dissolves clots by converting plasminogen to plasmin.
  - Other extracellular products that can elicit an antibody response include NADase, proteinase, esterase, and amylase.
  - **Erythrogenic toxin** is elaborated by scarlet fever–associated strains and is responsible for the characteristic rash.

EPIDEMIOLOGY

S. pyogenes is one of the most common and ubiquitous of human pathogens. It is found in the human respiratory tract and is always considered a potential pathogen. Upper respiratory infections caused by *S. pyogenes* occur most frequently in school-age children and are uncommon in children younger than 3 years. No gender or race predilection has been described.

Infection is spread by contact with large droplets produced in the upper respiratory tract. Although not as common, food-borne and milkborne epidemics do occur. Crowding enhances the spread of microorganisms.

A number of individuals, particularly school-age children, carry *S. pyogenes* without signs of illness. Carriers have positive cultures without serologic evidence of infection. If a person carries the organisms in the pharynx for prolonged periods after untreated infection, the number of organisms carried and their ability to produce M protein decline during carriage. This results in a progressive decline in the likelihood of spreading infection to others.

The incidence of a major complication of *S. pyogenes,* rheumatic fever, has decreased in the United States. It occurs primarily in the rural South and in areas of crowding and lower socioeconomic status. The incidence of rheumatic fever is 2% to 3% in epidemics and 0.1% to 1% after sporadic cases of streptococcal infection. The probability of developing rheumatic fever is age related, with younger patients more likely to develop carditis than older persons.

Rheumatic fever and resultant valvular heart disease, however, are syndromes of major importance among children in developing nations. Patients with a history of rheumatic heart disease resulting from rheumatic fever are at a significantly increased risk of developing cardiac malfunction and endocarditis later. The risk of recurrent rheumatic fever depends on factors such as the age of the patient at previous recurrences, length of time since the last recurrence, and presence of carditis. In addition, patients who develop streptococcal glomerulonephritis are at risk of later development of renal failure.

SIGNS AND SYMPTOMS

S. pyogenes causes a wide variety of infections, most often acute pharyngitis (strep throat) and upper respiratory infection, as well as impetigo (pyoderma). Other manifestations of infection with *S. pyogenes* include sinusitis, otitis, peritonsillar and retropharyngeal abscess, pneumonia, scarlet fever, erysipelas, cellulitis, puerperal sepsis, and gangrene. A concern still exists that group A streptococcus may be acquiring greater virulence.

Upper Respiratory Infection

The clinical manifestations of *S. pyogenes*–associated upper respiratory infection are age dependent. In an infant or young

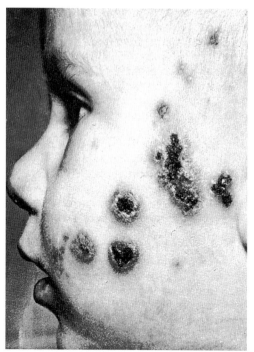

Figure 17-2   Impetigo. Older lesions are dark and encrusted. *(From Wehrle PF, Top FH: Communicable and infectious diseases, ed 9, St Louis, 1981, Mosby.)*

child, the infection is characterized by an insidious onset of rhinorrhea, coughing, fever, vomiting, and anorexia. Cervical adenopathy may also be present. Rhinorrhea is sometimes **purulent.** This syndrome is called streptococcosis.

The classic syndrome of streptococcal pharyngitis is seen in children older than 3 years. It begins with a sudden onset of sore throat and fever, which rapidly progress in severity. Pharyngeal erythema with purulent tonsillar **exudate** and petechiae may be observed on the palate, posterior pharynx, and tonsils. Younger children may have abdominal pain, nausea, and vomiting. Most patients, however, do not manifest the classic syndrome. It is more common for a child with *S. pyogenes* pharyngitis to have a fever, mild sore throat, and pharyngeal erythema without exudate.

Viral pharyngitis can produce many of the same symptoms and cannot be reliably differentiated from streptococcal pharyngitis on the basis of clinical examination alone.

Impetigo and Cellulitis

Impetigo is a skin infection that begins as a papule (Fig. 17-2). The lesion may itch and will eventually crust over and heal. Cellulitis caused by subcutaneous infection with group A streptococci is associated with a warm, red, tender area that may be mildly swollen. Erysipelas, a distinct cellulitis syndrome, usually involves the face and may be associated with pharyngitis. This syndrome is characterized by toxicity and a high fever. If left untreated, erysipelas can be fatal.

Scarlet Fever

Scarlet fever is the result of pharyngeal infection with a strain of group A streptococcus that produces **erythrogenic toxin** and is responsible for the characteristic rash. The signs and

symptoms of scarlet fever are those of streptococcal pharyngitis with the addition of a rash. The rash usually develops on the second day of illness and results in hyperkeratosis with subsequent peeling, similar to the rash of toxic shock syndrome. About 1 week after the onset of illness, the skin of the face begins to peel, which progresses over the next 2 weeks. Exposure to erythrogenic toxin confers specific immunity, limiting to three the number of episodes of scarlet fever in a person.

Complications of *Streptococcus pyogenes* Infection

Not all infections with *S. pyogenes* lead to complications. Acute rheumatic fever, for example, occurs only after upper respiratory tract infection. In contrast, glomerulonephritis occurs after pharyngitis or skin infections (pyoderma). Acute rheumatic fever and poststreptococcal glomerulonephritis are considered nonsuppurative because the organs themselves are not directly infected and a purulent inflammatory response is not present in affected organs (e.g., heart, joints, blood, kidneys).

The pathogenesis of this disease process has not been fully described, but an autoimmune phenomenon may be operational. It is believed that cross-reactive antibodies, originally directed against streptococcal cell membranes, bind to myosin in human heart muscle cells. Other cross-reactive antibodies bind to components of the glomerular basement membrane and form immune complexes at the affected site. These antigen-antibody complexes attract reactive host cells and enzymes that ultimately cause the cellular damage.

All M serotypes that infect the throat appear to be capable of causing rheumatic fever. Researchers have identified a few serotypes, however, that cause a much lower proportion of rheumatic fever cases than would be expected from their frequency as a cause of pharyngitis. The incidence of rheumatic fever is directly proportional to the strength of the antibody response to SLO. The prognosis of rheumatic fever is good when carditis is absent during the initial infection.

Glomerulonephritis may follow an infection of the skin or respiratory tract with one of a limited number of nephritogenic M serotypes. These serotypes are defined by antisera against the M protein, which is also associated with virulence. Why these serotypes cause glomerulonephritis is unknown.

IMMUNOLOGIC MANIFESTATIONS

S. pyogenes is an example of a pathogen that induces the production of several different antibodies. This coccus contains antigenic structural components and produces antigenic enzymes, each of which may elicit a specific antibody response from the infected host. In the course of an infection, the extracellular products act as antigens to which the body responds by producing specific antibodies (indications of infection).

Most infected patients demonstrate increased concentration of antibody against SLO. The concentration of antibody (titer) begins to rise about 7 days after the onset of infection and reaches a maximum after 4 to 6 weeks. A rise in titer of

50 Todd units* in 1 to 2 weeks is of greater diagnostic significance than a single titer.

An elevated titer indicates a relatively recent infection. Peak titers are seen at the time of acute polyarthritis of acute rheumatic fever, but these titers are no longer at their peak during the carditis of acute rheumatic fever. A patient may demonstrate an elevated antibody titer for up to 1 year after infection; therefore, the time of infection is not precisely determined by this technique. Low titers of **antistreptolysin O (ASO)** can be exhibited by apparently healthy persons because of the frequency of subclinical streptococcal infections, but persistently low titers rule out *S. pyogenes* infection.

Of the patients with *S. pyogenes*–related acute glomerulonephritis, 50% display a normal ASO titer but demonstrate an elevated titer to one of the other streptococcal substances (e.g., DNAse and NADase). **Anti–DNase B (ADN-B)** antibody appears to be the most reliable measure of recent *S. pyogenes* skin infection. Titers of ADN-B are elevated in more than two thirds of patients with recent streptococcal impetigo. Anti-NADase antibodies are a particularly good marker in patients who develop nephritis after pharyngitis.

DIAGNOSTIC EVALUATION

In addition to throat cultures in patients with pharyngitis, antibodies to bacterial toxins and other extracellular products that display measurable activity can be tested. ASO and ADN-B are the standard serologic tests. The ability of a patient's serum to neutralize the erythrocyte-lysing capability of SLO (ASO procedure) has been used for many years as a method for detecting previous streptococcal infection. After an infection such as pharyngitis with SLO-producing strains, most patients show a high titer of the antibody ASO. The use of rapid testing (see ASO latex procedure, Chapter 12, and Chapter 14) has replaced the use of the classic ASO procedure archived on the EVOLVE website (and on www.mlturgeon.com).

Streptococci produce the enzyme DNase B. The ADN-B neutralization test prevents the activity of this enzyme and demonstrates recent or previous *S. pyogenes* infection. Antistreptokinase and antihyaluronidase titers (AHTs) have also been used to diagnose streptococcal infection retrospectively.

Serologic testing should compare acute and convalescent sera collected 3 weeks apart. The ASO level becomes elevated in acute or convalescent paired specimens in 80% to 85% of patients with acute rheumatic fever. ADN-B and AHT levels are elevated in the remaining 15% to 20% of patients. In many cases, no acute serum specimen is available; therefore, the antibody titer of the convalescent serum specimen is compared with a reference range value. Reference ranges vary with age, season, and geographic area. False-positive ASO results may be demonstrated because of the presence of beta-lipoprotein, contamination of the serum specimen by bacterial growth products, or

oxidation of ASO. These errors are not encountered with the ADN-B procedure, which is the serologic test of choice for acute rheumatic fever and acute glomerulonephritis after *S. pyogenes* infection.

STREPTOCOCCAL TOXIC SHOCK SYNDROME

Streptococcal toxic shock syndrome (STSS) is caused by a highly invasive group A streptococcal infection and is associated with shock and organ failure.

Etiology

The portal of entry of streptococci in STSS cannot be determined in at least 50% of cases and can only be presumed in many others. The use of tampons has been associated with acquiring the disorder. In other patients, the use of nonsteroidal antiinflammatory drugs (NSAIDs) may have masked the early symptoms or predisposed the patient to more severe streptococcal infection and shock. Usually, STSS appears after streptococci have invaded areas of injured skin (e.g., cuts, scrapes, surgical wounds).

Immunologic Mechanisms

Pyrogenic exotoxins cause fever in human beings and animals and also help induce shock by lowering the threshold to **exogenous endotoxin.** Streptococcal pyrogenic exotoxins A and B induce human mononuclear cells to synthesize not only **tumor necrosis factor-α (TNF-α)** but also interleukin-1 beta (IL-1β) and interleukin-6 (IL-6), suggesting that TNF could mediate the fever, shock, and tissue injury observed in patients with STSS.

M protein contributes to invasiveness through its ability to impede phagocytosis of streptococci by human PMNs.

Superantigens are capable of binding to alpha and beta T cell receptors (TCRs) and major histocompatibility complex (MHC) class II molecules. Superantigens can directly activate 1% to 2% of T cells and create high levels of cytokines in the blood. These high levels can produce shocklike symptoms.

Cytokine production by less exotic mechanisms also likely contributes to the genesis of shock and organ failure. Exotoxins such as SLO are also potent inducers of TNF-α and IL-1β. Pyrogenic exotoxin B, a proteinase precursor, has the ability to cleave pre–IL-1β to release preformed IL-1. Finally, SLO and pyrogenic exotoxin A together have additive effects in the induction of IL-1β by human mononuclear cells. Regardless of the mechanisms, induction of cytokines in vivo is likely the cause of shock and exotoxins, cell wall components, and other substances are potent inducers of TNF and IL-1.

Epidemiology

The rates of STSS are highest in young children and older adults. More than 50% of patients have an underlying chronic illness. STSS is also associated with a substantial risk of transmission in households and health care institutions. Mortality following an outbreak of *S. pyogenes* that progresses to toxic shock can be as high as 70%. The illness is classified as a rare infection because it affects only about 300 people annually. STSS almost never follows a simple streptococcal throat infection.

---

*This is the unit for expressing the results of ASO testing. A Todd unit denotes the reciprocal of the highest dilution of test serum in which there continues to be neutralization of a standard preparation of streptolysin O.

Signs and Symptoms

The symptoms of STSS include shock; fever; blotchy rash; and a red, swollen, and painful area of infected skin. The average incubation period for STSS is 2 to 3 days, usually after minor nonpenetrating trauma.

Pain, the most common initial symptom of STSS, is abrupt in onset and severe and usually precedes tenderness or physical findings. The pain generally involves an extremity but may also mimic peritonitis, pelvic inflammatory disease, pneumonia, acute myocardial infarction, or pericarditis.

About 20% of STSS patients have an influenza-like syndrome characterized by fever, chills, myalgia, nausea, vomiting, and diarrhea. Fever is the most common early sign, although hypothermia may be present in patients with shock.

About 80% of STSS patients have clinical signs of soft tissue infection, such as localized swelling and erythema, which in 70% of one group of patients progressed to necrotizing fasciitis or myositis and required surgical débridement, fasciotomy, or amputation. An ominous sign is the progression of soft tissue swelling to the formation of vesicles and then bullae, which appear violaceous or bluish.

Laboratory Data

The case definition of STSS includes serologic confirmation of group A streptococcal infection by a fourfold rise against SLO and DNAse B. Although initial laboratory studies usually demonstrate only mild leukocytosis, the mean percentage of immature neutrophils can reach 40% to 50%. Blood cultures are positive in 60% of cases.

Renal involvement is indicated by the presence of **hemoglobinuria** and by serum creatinine values that are, on average, more than 2.5 times normal. Renal impairment precedes hypotension in approximately 40% to 50% of patients. Hypoalbuminemia is associated with hypocalcemia on admission and throughout the hospital course.

Treatment

Streptococcal TSS can be deadly and needs immediate treatment. IV fluids and medications to maintain a normal blood pressure are required in acutely ill patients. Penicillin and other beta-lactam antibiotics are most efficacious against rapidly growing bacteria.

After recovery, the skin may peel as the rash heals. Surgery may be necessary to remove areas of dead skin and muscle around an infected wound.

GROUP B STREPTOCOCCAL DISEASE

Group B *Streptococcus agalactiae* infections causes substantial morbidity and mortality in adults and neonates.

Epidemiology

Fatality rate ranges from 26% to 70% among men and non-pregnant women with group B streptococcus (GBS) disease. Despite substantial progress in the prevention of perinatal GBS disease since the 1990s, GBS remains the leading cause of early-onset neonatal sepsis in the United States. Universal screening at 35 to 37 weeks' gestation for maternal GBS colonization and the use of intrapartum antibiotic prophylaxis has resulted in substantial reductions in the burden of early-onset GBS disease in newborns. Although early-onset GBS disease has become relatively uncommon in recent years, the rates of maternal GBS colonization (and therefore the risk for early-onset GBS disease in the absence of intrapartum antibiotic prophylaxis) remain unchanged since the 1970s. GBS disease remains the leading infectious cause of morbidity and mortality in newborns in the United States.

Etiology

GBS, or *S. agalactiae,* is a gram-positive bacterium that causes invasive disease primarily in infants, pregnant or postpartum women, and older adults, with the highest incidence among young infants.

Laboratory Data

Group B streptococci are most frequently isolated from blood, although cerebrospinal fluid (CSF) can also be tested. Serologic identification using latex agglutination with group B streptococcal antisera is available. In addition, more rapid techniques for identifying GBS directly from enrichment broth or after subculture have been developed, including DNA probes and nucleic acid amplification tests (NAATs), such as polymerase chain reaction (PCR) assays.

Signs and Symptoms

The most common clinical finding is skin and soft tissue infection. Early-onset infections are acquired vertically through exposure to GBS from the vagina of a colonized woman. Neonatal infection occurs primarily when GBS ascends from the vagina to the amniotic fluid after the onset of labor or rupture of membranes, although GBS also can invade through intact membranes. Infants also can become infected with GBS during passage through the birth canal; infants who are exposed to the organism through this route can become colonized at mucous membrane sites in the gastrointestinal or respiratory tracts, but these colonized infants usually remain healthy.

Future Directions

Because of the gravity of GBS disease, especially in those who are older and those with chronic diseases, the development of a vaccine is being pursued. Determining the incidence of adult disease and groups at greatest risk helps focus prevention efforts. Intrapartum antibiotics can prevent early-onset neonatal GBS disease but have not been widely used.

CASE STUDY

This 19-year-old woman went to the emergency department (ED) with swelling and redness of her right leg. She had fallen down while rollerblading and had a number of abrasions on the skin of her leg. She also had a body temperature of 37.8° C (100° F). The ED physician ordered

Continued

CASE STUDY—Cont'd

a culture of her leg wound, gave her a prescription for an antibiotic, and discharged her from treatment.

The following evening, the patient collapsed onto the floor of her bedroom. Her roommate found her and called 911. On arrival, the paramedics found an unconscious female with a blood pressure of 80/40 mm Hg and pronounced redness and swelling of her right leg. She was rushed to the ED and admitted to the intensive care unit, where she was immediately placed on IV fluids and medications to raise her blood pressure.

Questions

1. The patient's collapse could be due to:
   a. Dehydration
   b. Streptococcal toxic shock syndrome (STSS)
   c. Lack of sleep
   d. Swollen leg
2. What assay or assays would be a most helpful immunologic/serologic test?
   a. Demonstration of streptolysin O in serum
   b. DNAase B assay
   c. Throat culture for β streptococci
   d. Both a and b

See Appendix A for the answers to these questions.

Critical Thinking Group Discussion Questions

1. Is there any relationship between this patient's problem with her leg and her collapse on the floor?
2. What are the symptoms of streptococcal toxic shock syndrome (STSS)?
3. What is the source of this patient's STSS?
4. Are there any immunologic/serologic manifestations of STSS?

See instructor site ⊜volve for the discussion of the answers to these questions.

Antistreptolysin O (ASO) Latex Test Kit

Principle

In this test (Biotech Laboratories, Suffolk, England), the ASO reagent contains latex particles coated with streptolysin O antigen. When the reagent is mixed with serum containing ASO, the particles will agglutinate, which is interpreted as a positive sample. Detection of ASO in serum may aid in the diagnosis of streptococcal infections.

Infections promoted by acute streptococcal infection result in the production of antistreptolysin O antibodies because of the presence of the SLO antigen liberated by the bacteria.

Reference Intervals

Normal adult levels are less than 200 IU/mL. However, because values may vary with age, gender, diet, or geographic location, it is recommended that each laboratory establish its own reference range.

Limitations

Elevated levels of ASO have also been found in patients suffering from scarlet fever, acute rheumatoid arthritis, tonsillitis, and other streptococcal infections, as well as healthy carriers. Early infections and children aged 6 months to 2 years may cause false-negative results. A single positive ASO result does not provide much information about the state of the disease. Therefore, it is advisable to perform titrations at biweekly intervals over 4 to 6 weeks to follow progression of the disease. The clinical diagnosis should be made in conjunction with clinical and laboratory data, not just on the findings of a single test result.

Clinical Applications

Detection of ASO in serum may aid in the diagnosis of streptococcal infections. Information on the extent and degree of infection can be obtained from the measurement of serum ASO levels. Increased ASO levels are also associated with rheumatic fever and glomerulonephritis.

OSOM Ultra Strep A Test

This is a color immunochromatographic assay (Genzyme, Cambridge, Mass) that uses antibody-labeled color particles. See Chapter 12 and the EVOLVE website for additional information.

Group A Streptococcus Direct Test

This DNA probe assay (Hologic Gen-Probe, San Diego, Calif) uses nucleic acid hybridization for the qualitative detection of group A streptococcal RNA. See Chapter 14 and the EVOLVE website for additional information.

Antistreptolysin O (ASO) Classic Procedure

See the website at www.mlturgeon.com for an archived copy of this traditional procedure.

CHAPTER HIGHLIGHTS

- Most streptococci that contain cell wall antigens of Lancefield group A are known as *Streptococcus pyogenes*. Members of this species are almost always beta-hemolytic streptococci.
- *S. pyogenes* is important in the development of complications such as acute rheumatic fever and poststreptococcal glomerulonephritis.
- Strains of *S. pyogenes* that lack M protein cannot cause infection.
- Extracellular products are important in the pathogenesis and serologic diagnosis of streptococcal disease. Antibodies produced in response to these substances indicate recent streptococcal infection.
- Substances produced by group A streptococci presumably facilitate rapid spread through subcutaneous or deeper soft tissues.

REVIEW QUESTIONS

1. *S. pyogenes* is the most common causative agent of all the following disorders and complications except:
   a. Pharyngitis
   b. Gastroenteritis
   c. Scarlet fever
   d. Impetigo

2. All the following characteristics are descriptive of M protein except:
   a. No known biological role
   b. Found in association with the hyaluronic capsule
   c. Inhibits phagocytosis
   d. Antibody against M protein provides type-specific immunity

3. Substances produced by *S. pyogenes* include all the following except:
   a. Hyaluronidase
   b. DNAses (A, B, C, D)
   c. Erythrogenic toxin
   d. Interferon

4. Laboratory diagnosis of *S. pyogenes* can be made by all the following except:
   a. Culturing of throat or nasal specimens
   b. Febrile agglutinins
   c. ASO procedure
   d. Anti–DNase B

5. False ASO results may be caused by all the following except:
   a. Room temperature reagents and specimens at the time of testing
   b. The presence of beta-lipoprotein
   c. Bacterial contamination of the serum specimen
   d. Oxidation of ASO reagent caused by shaking or aeration of the reagent vial

6. Members of the *S. pyogenes* species are almost always _____ hemolytic.
   a. Alpha-
   b. Beta-
   c. gamma-
   d. Alpha- or beta-

7. Long-term complications of *S. pyogenes* infection can include:
   a. Acute rheumatic fever
   b. Poststreptococcal glomerulonephritis
   c. Rheumatoid arthritis
   d. Both a and b

8. Particularly virulent serotypes of *S. pyogenes* produce proteolytic enzymes that cause _____ in a wound or lesion on an extremity.
   a. Necrotizing fasciitis
   b. Bone degeneration
   c. Burning and itching
   d. Severe inflammation

9-11. Match the substances produced by group A streptococci with the appropriate description.

9. _____ Hyaluronidase

10. _____ Streptokinase

11. _____ Erythrogenic toxin
   a. Degrades DNA
   b. Also called spreading factor
   c. Responsible for characteristic scarlet fever rash
   d. Dissolves clots by converting plasminogen to plasmin

12. All the following characteristics of *S. pyogenes* are correct except:
   a. It is an uncommon pathogen.
   b. It occurs most frequently in school-age children.
   c. It is spread by contact with large droplets produced in the upper respiratory tract.
   d. It has been known to cause foodborne and milkborne epidemics.

13. The clinical manifestations of *S. pyogenes*–associated upper respiratory infection are:
   a. Mild and usually unnoticeable
   b. Age dependent
   c. Associated with cold sores
   d. Difficult to detect

14. The most reliable immunologic test for recent *S. pyogenes* skin infection is:
   a. ASO
   b. Anti–DNAse B
   c. Anti-NADase
   d. Antibody to erythrogenic toxin

15-17. Match each ASO titer situation to the appropriate description. (An answer may be used twice.)

15. _____ Rising titer

16. _____ Declining titer

17. _____ Constant (low) titer
   a. Increase in severity of infection
   b. Not a current infection, but indicates a past infection
   c. Trend toward recovery
   d. No clinical significance

18. If a streptococcal infection is suspected, but the ASO titer does not exceed the reference range, a(n) _____ should be performed.
   a. Repeat titer
   b. Anti–DNAse B test
   c. Anti-NADase test
   d. Throat culture

19. The classic tests to demonstrate the presence of streptococcal infection are:
   a. ASO and anti-NADase
   b. ASO and anti–DNAse B
   c. Anti-NADase and anti-DNAse
   d. Both a and b

20. The highest reported levels of sensitivity testing for group A streptococci are in:
    a. ASO titers
    b. Direct latex agglutination tests
    c. Surface (optical) immunoassay
    d. Both a and b, which are equivalent

BIBLIOGRAPHY

Bisno AL: Group A streptococcal infections and acute rheumatic fever, N Engl J Med 325:783–793, 1991.

Davies HD, McGeer A, Schwartz B, et al: Invasive group A streptococcal infections in Ontario, Canada, N Engl J Med 335:547–554, 1996.

Farley MM, Harvey RC, Stull T, et al: A population-based assessment of invasive disease due to group B streptococcus in nonpregnant adults, N Engl J Med 328:1807–1812, 1993.

Forbes BA, Sahm DF, Weissfeld AS: Bailey & Scott's diagnostic microbiology, ed 12, St Louis, 2007, Mosby.

Hexter DA: Group A streptococcus septicemia in children, JAMA 267:53–54, 1992.

Hoge CW, Schwartz B, Talkington DF, et al: The changing epidemiology of invasive group A streptococcal infections and the emergence of streptococcal toxic-shock-like syndrome, JAMA 269:384–391, 1993.

James E: Testing for strep throat, 2002, http://laboratorian.advanceweb.com/Article/Testing-for-Strep-Throat.aspx.

Mohle-Boetani JC, Schuchat A, Plikaytis BD, et al: Comparison of prevention strategies for neonatal group B streptococcal infection, JAMA 270:1442–1448, 1993.

Schwartz B, Schuchat A, Oxtoby MJ, et al: Invasive group B streptococcal disease in adults, JAMA 266:1112–1114, 1991.

Turner RB, Hendley JO: Streptococcus pyogenes infections. In Stein J, editor: Internal medicine, Boston, 1994, Little, Brown.

Verani JR, McGee L, Schrag SJ: Division of Bacterial Diseases, National Center for Immunization and Respiratory Diseases, Centers for Disease Control and Prevention (CDC): Prevention of perinatal group B streptococcal disease—revised guidelines from CDC, 2010, MMWR Recomm Rep 59(RR-10):1–36, 2010.

Syphilis

Learning Objectives

At the conclusion of this chapter, the reader should be able to:

- Describe the etiology; epidemiology; and signs and symptoms of primary, secondary, latent, and late (tertiary) syphilis.
- Describe the origin and manifestations of congenital syphilis.
- Explain the immunologic manifestations and diagnostic evaluation of syphilis.
- Analyze a case study related to syphilis testing.
- Correctly answer case study related multiple choice questions.

- Be prepared to participate in a discussion of critical thinking questions.
- Discuss the principles and clinical applications of the rapid plasma reagin (RPR) card test and VDRL procedure.
- Discuss the principles and clinical applications of confirmatory syphilis testing, such as the fluorescent treponemal antibody absorption (FTA) test.
- Correctly answer end of chapter review questions.

Key Terms

antitreponemal antibodies
cardiolipin
convalescent sera
darkfield microscopy
granulomatous reactions (gummas)

hutchisonian triad
morbidity
nontreponemal antibodies
rapid plasma reagin (RPR)
reagin antibodies

spirochete
Treponema pallidum antibodies
treponemes
Venereal Disease Research
   Laboratory (VDRL)

The disease syphilis was reported in the medical literature as early as 1495. In 1905, it was discovered that syphilis was caused by a **spirochete** type of bacteria, *Treponema pallidum* (originally called *Spirochaeta pallida*). The first diagnostic blood test for syphilis was the Wassermann test, a complement fixation test developed in 1906. This classic procedure (see www.mlturgeon.com, "Archives of Classic Procedures") has subsequently been replaced by a variety of methods. In the treatment of syphilis, heavy metals, such as arsenic, were replaced by penicillin in the 1940s. Penicillin continues to remain the drug of choice for the treatment of this disease.

ETIOLOGY

T. pallidum is a member of the order Spirochaetales and the family Treponemataceae (Fig. 18-1). The genus *Treponema* includes a number of species that reside in human gastrointestinal and genital tracts. *T. pallidum, Treponema pertenue,* and *Treponema carateum* are human pathogens responsible for significant worldwide **morbidity** (Table 18-1). Yaws, pinta, and bejel are diseases caused by bacteria closely related to *T. pallidum.* Yaws is common in the Caribbean, Latin America, Central Africa, and the Far East. Pinta is found only in Latin America and infection is limited to the skin. Bejel is found in eastern Mediterranean countries, the Balkans, and the cooler areas of North Africa.

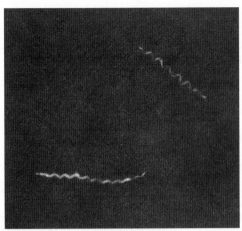

Figure 18-1 *Treponema pallidum. (From Bauer JD: Clinical laboratory methods, ed 9, St Louis, 1982, Mosby.)*

Table 18-1	*Treponema*-Associated Diseases
Bacteria	**Associated Disease**
T. pallidum	Syphilis
T. pallidum (variant)	Bejel
T. pertenue	Yaws
T. carateum	Pinta

Direct examination of the **treponemes** is most often performed with darkfield microscopy. Pathogenic treponemes appear as fine, spiral (8 to 24 coils) organisms approximately 6 to 15 μm long. They have a trilaminar outer membrane similar to that of gram-negative bacteria.

Pathogenic treponemes are not cultivatable with any consistency in artificial laboratory media. Outside of the host, the pathogenic treponemes are extremely susceptible to a variety of physical and chemical agents. Treponemes may remain viable for up to 5 days in tissue specimens removed from diseased animals and from frozen cryoprotected specimens.

EPIDEMIOLOGY

Sexually transmitted diseases (STDs) remain a major public health challenge in the United States. The surveillance report by the Centers for Disease Control and Prevention (CDC) includes data on the three STDs that physicians are required to report to the agency—chlamydia, gonorrhea, and syphilis. Syphilis is considered to be primarily a venereal disease. It is the most common STD in the United States.

The three treponematoses—yaws, pinta, and bejel—are rarely seen in the United States but are prevalent in other countries. These diseases are associated with poverty, overcrowding, and poor hygiene.

In 2009, for the first time in 5 years, the CDC reported that syphilis cases did not increase overall among women. In addition, cases of congenital syphilis (transmitted from mother to infant) did not increase for the first time in 4 years. In 2008, 63% of the reported primary and secondary syphilis cases were among men who have sex with men (MSM). In the surveillance period of 2004 to 2008, rates of P&S syphilis increased the most among 15- to 24-year-old men and women. The incidence of syphilis per capita is higher among blacks and Hispanics than among whites.

Syphilis remains a global problem, with an estimated 12 million people infected each year, despite the existence of effective prevention measures. The last decade has seen a pronounced resurgence of syphilis in countries of the Far East (e.g., China and Africa). Some fundamental social problems (e.g., poverty, inadequate access to health care, lack of education) are associated with disproportionately high levels of syphilis in certain populations.

Pathogenic treponemes are transmitted almost uniformly by direct contact. Treponemal infections of the skin or oral lesions contain many spirochetes that may be transmitted by personal, but not necessarily venereal, contact. These infections are generally acquired during childhood. In each of these diseases, infection elicits antibodies reactive in nontreponemal and treponemal methods.

Syphilis develops in 30% to 50% of the sexual partners of persons with syphilitic lesions. The risk of acquiring syphilis from a single sexual exposure to an infected partner is unknown. A high percentage of partners do seek medical treatment within 90 days of contact.

Syphilis can be acquired by kissing a person with active oral lesions. Very few cases of transfusion-acquired syphilis have been reported in recent years in the United States. During the first half of the twentieth century, however, syphilis was a major bloodborne infectious disease easily transmitted through the prevailing method of direct donor to patient blood transfusion. The danger of syphilis transmission still exists in tropical countries in which the organization of blood banks is deficient and the use of direct blood transfusion prevails in emergency situations. Refrigerated blood storage decreases accidental transmission of the microorganism because *T. pallidum* has a short survival period in stored blood. Spirochetes do not appear to survive in units of citrated blood at 4° C (39° F) for longer than 72 hours.

Cases have been reported of children who acquired syphilis by sharing a bed with an infected parent. In addition, syphilis may be transmitted transplacentally to the fetus. Spirochetes can be transmitted to the fetus during the last trimester of pregnancy, before the mother manifests postpartum evidence of infection.

SIGNS AND SYMPTOMS

Untreated syphilis is a chronic disease with subacute symptomatic periods separated by asymptomatic intervals, during which the diagnosis can be made serologically. The progression of untreated syphilis is generally divided into stages—primary, secondary, latent (hidden), and tertiary (late) (Table 18-2).

Initially, *T. pallidum* penetrates intact mucous membranes or enters the body through tiny defects in the epithelium. On entrance, the microorganism is carried by the circulatory

Table 18-2	Stages of Syphilis	
Phase or Stage	**Features and Comments**	**Test**
Incubating phase	The incubation period usually lasts ≈3 wk but can range from 10-90 days.	Laboratory examination
Primary stage	• During the primary stage, a painless chancre develops at the site where the bacteria entered the body. • A person is highly contagious during the primary stage. • The chancre lasts 28-42 days and heals without treatment.	Darkfield examination
Secondary stage	• This is characterized by a rash that appears from 2-8 wk after the chancre develops. • A person is highly contagious during the secondary stage. • A rash often develops all over the body, including palms of the hands and the soles of the feet. The rash usually heals without scarring in 2-12 wk. • Open sores may be present on mucous membranes and may contain pus (condyloma lata). • Symptoms can include nervous system abnormalities.	• RPR or VDRL • TP-PA used to confirm a syphilis infection after another method tests positive for syphilis. It can be used to detect syphilis in all stages, except during the first 3-4 wk. This test is not done on spinal fluid. • FTA-ABS test detects syphilis except during the first 3-4 wk after exposure to syphilis bacteria. It is more difficult to perform and may be used to confirm a syphilis infection after another method tests positive for the syphilis bacteria. It can be done on a sample of blood or cerebrospinal fluid. CSF
Latent (hidden) stage	• If untreated, an infected person will progress to the latent (hidden) stage of syphilis with no symptoms (latent period). • The latent period may be as brief as 1 yr or range from 5-20 yr. • A person is contagious during the early part of the latent stage and may be contagious during the latent period.	
Relapses of secondary syphilis	• About 20%-30% of people with syphilis have a relapse of the secondary stage of syphilis during the latent stage. • A relapse means that the person had passed through the second stage, was symptom-free, then began to reexperience secondary stage symptoms. Relapses can occur several times. • When relapses no longer occur, a person is not contagious through contact. • A woman in the latent stage of syphilis may still pass the disease to her unborn baby and may have a miscarriage, a stillbirth, or give birth to a baby infected with congenital syphilis.	• Nontreponemal tests measure IgM and IgG antibodies. • It is best for testing for reinfection.
Tertiary (late) stage	• Most destructive stage of syphilis • If untreated, the tertiary stage may begin as early as 1 yr after infection or at any time during a person's lifetime. A person may never experience this stage of the illness. • The symptoms of tertiary (late) syphilis depend on the complications that develop—gummata, large sores inside the body or on the skin, cardiovascular syphilis, or neurosyphilis.	• VDRL on cerebrospinal fluid (CSF) with concurrent RPR serum • If RPR is negative and a high index of suspicion for neurosyphilis remains, perform FTA-Abs on serum. • Some patients have nonreactive nontreponemal tests in late neurosyphilis.

FTA-ABS, Fluorescent treponemal antibody absorption; *RPR,* rapid plasma reagin; *TP-PA, Treponema pallidum* particle agglutination assay; *VDRL,* venereal disease research laboratory.

system to every organ of the body. Spirochetemia occurs very early in infection, even before the first lesions have appeared or blood tests become reactive. Before clinical or serologic manifestations develop, patients are said to be incubating syphilis. The incubation period usually lasts about 3 weeks but can range from 10 to 90 days.

Primary Syphilis

At the end of the incubation period, a patient develops a characteristic, primary inflammatory lesion called a chancre at the point of initial inoculation and multiplication of the spirochetes. The chancre begins as a papule and erodes to form a gradually enlarging ulcer, with a clean base and indurated edge (Fig. 18-2). Generally, it is relatively painless. In most cases, only a single lesion is present, but multiple chancres are not rare.

Chancres are typically located around the genitalia, but in about 10% of cases, lesions may appear almost anywhere else on the body (e.g., throat, lip, hands). In males, spirochetes are present in the lesion on the penis or discharged from deeper sites with semen. In females, infected lesions are usually located in the perineal region or on the labia, vaginal wall, or cervix. If the lesion is located inside the urethra, the only symptom may be a scanty, serous urethral discharge.

Of patients with primary syphilis of the external genitalia, 50% to 70% will subsequently develop inguinal adenopathy. Inguinal adenopathy, however, is less common with chancres involving the cervix or proximal part of the vagina because these sites are drained by the iliac nodes. Regional adenopathy may accompany primary inoculation at other sites; for example, cervical adenopathy may accompany a syphilitic lesion of the oral cavity.

The primary chancre will persist for 1 to 5 weeks and will heal completely in about 4 to 6 weeks, even without treatment. Regional adenopathy will also resolve itself.

Secondary Syphilis

Within 2 to 8 weeks (but occasionally as long as 6 months) after the appearance of the primary chancre, a patient may develop the signs and symptoms of secondary syphilis. In some patients, primary and secondary syphilis overlap and the chancre is still obvious. Other patients never notice the primary chancre and initially have manifestations of secondary syphilis (Fig. 18-3).

The secondary stage is characterized by a generalized illness that usually begins with symptoms suggesting a viral infection—headache, sore throat, low-grade fever, and occasionally a nasal discharge. Blood tests reveal a moderate increase in leukocytes, with a relative increase in lymphocytes.

The disease progresses with the development of lymphadenopathy and lesions of the skin and mucous membranes. Approximately 75% of syphilitic patients develop generalized adenopathy. About 80% have skin lesions, which contain a large number of spirochetes and, when located on exposed surfaces, are highly contagious. Macular lesions are common and a rash invariably involves the genitalia; this rash often is prominent on the palms and soles. Patients may also develop

condylomata lata, flat lesions resembling warts in moist areas of the body (e.g., around the anus or vagina). These lesions do not reflect areas of inoculation but appear to be caused by hematogenous dissemination of spirochetes.

The central nervous system (CNS) is asymptomatically involved in about one third of patients. About 2% of cases manifest as acute syphilitic meningitis. Early CNS involvement may progress to neurosyphilis if untreated. Hepatitis and immune complex glomerulonephritis occasionally accompany secondary syphilis.

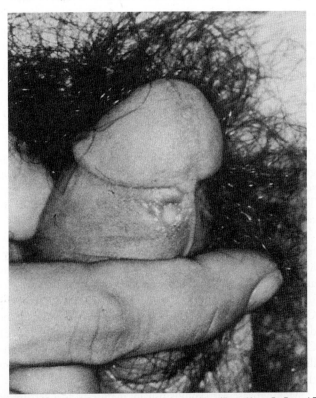

Figure 18-2 A primary chancre of syphilis. *(From Kaye D, Rose LF: Fundamentals of internal medicine, St Louis, 1983, Mosby.)*

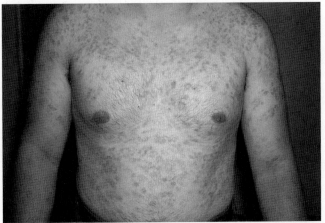

Figure 18-3 Secondary syphilis. *(From James WD, Berger TG, Elston DM: Andrews' diseases of the skin, ed 10, Edinburgh, 2007, Saunders.)*

Secondary syphilis usually resolves within 2 to 6 weeks, even without therapy.

Latent Syphilis

After resolution of untreated secondary syphilis, the patient enters a latent noninfectious state in which diagnosis can be made only by serologic methods. During the first 2 to 4 years of infection, 25% of patients will have one or more mucocutaneous relapses in which the manifestation of secondary syphilis reappears. During these relapses, patients are infectious and the underlying spirochetemia may be passed transplacentally to the fetus. Relapses are extremely rare after 4 years of latency. About one third of patients entering latency are eventually spontaneously cured of the disease, one third will never develop further clinical manifestations of the disease, and the remaining third will eventually develop late syphilis.

Late (Tertiary) Syphilis

The first manifestations of late syphilis are usually seen from 3 to 10 years after primary infection. About 15% of untreated syphilitic individuals eventually develop late benign syphilis, characterized by the presence of destructive granulomas. These granulomas, or gummas, may produce lesions resembling segments of circles that often heal with superficial scarring. The skeletal system is frequently affected, but treponemes are rarely seen.

Of untreated patients, 10% develop cardiovascular manifestations. *T. pallidum* may directly affect the aortic endothelium. Weakening of the blood vessels can occur as a syphilitic aneurysm, usually of the aortic arch.

In about 8% of untreated patients, late syphilis involves the CNS. Initially, CNS disease is asymptomatic and can be detected only by examination of cerebrospinal fluid (CSF). CSF should be examined in all patients being treated for syphilis of unknown duration or who have had syphilis for longer than 1 year.

Meningovascular syphilis usually manifests as a seizure or cerebrovascular accident (stroke). Spirochetes may also involve the brain tissues and cause general paresis, personality changes, dementia, and delusional states. Tabes dorsalis results from involvement of the posterior columns and dorsal roots of the spinal cord and is characterized by a broad-based gait. Impotence and bladder dysfunction are common in this disorder (see later, "Neurosyphilis").

Congenital Syphilis

Congenital syphilis is caused by maternal spirochetemia and transplacental transmission of the microorganism. Untreated syphilis during pregnancy, especially early syphilis, can lead to stillbirth, neonatal death, or infant disorders such as deafness, neurologic impairment, and bone deformities. Congenital syphilis (CS) can be prevented by early detection of maternal infection and treatment at least 30 days before delivery. Changes in the population incidence of P&S syphilis among women usually are followed by similar changes in the incidence of CS. CDC national surveillance data from the period 2003 to 2008 in the United States have indicated that after declining

for 14 years, the CS rate among infants younger than 1 year increased by 23%.

Globally, congenital syphilis is a major health problem in Africa and the Far East. The overarching global goal of the present World Health Organization (WHO) strategy is the elimination of congenital syphilis as a public health problem. This could be achieved through the reduction of prevalence of syphilis in pregnant women and by the prevention of mother to child transmission of syphilis. The strategy rests on four pillars:

1. Ensure sustained political commitment and advocacy.
2. Increase access to, and quality of, maternal and newborn health services.
3. Screen and treat pregnant women and their partners.
4. Establish surveillance, monitoring and evaluation systems.

Classification of congenital syphilis is according to age at diagnosis. The early stage is seen in children younger than 2 years who are untreated. Symptoms of the untreated early stage can include rash, condyloma latum, bone changes, hepatosplenomegaly, jaundice, and/or anemia.

The late stage is seen in children older than 2 years who are untreated. Symptoms of the untreated late stage include eighth nerve deafness, keratitis, and Hutchinson's teeth (Fig. 18-4) **(hutchisonian triad),** as well as arthropathy and neurosyphilis. Residual stigmata can develop. Other characteristics include fissuring around the mouth and anus, skeletal lesions, perforation of the palate, and collapse of nasal bones to produce a saddle-nose deformity.

Neurosyphilis

Although neurosyphilis may be asymptomatic, symptomatic forms include the following:

- Meningeal syphilis, usually less than 1 year after infection
- Meningovascular syphilis, usually 5 to 10 years after infection
- Parenchymatous syphilis

Meningeal neurosyphilis involves the brain or spinal cord. Patients can suffer from headaches and a stiff neck. Meningovascular syphilis involves inflammation of the pia mater and

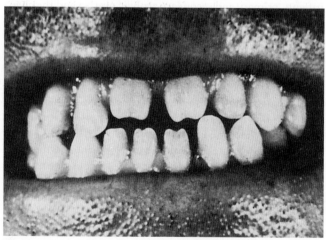

Figure 18-4 Congenital syphilis (Hutchinson's teeth). *(From Kaye D, Rose LF: Fundamentals of internal medicine, St Louis, 1983, Mosby.)*

arachnoid space, with focal arteritis. A stroke syndrome involving middle cerebral artery is common in young adults. Parenchymatous neurosyphilis manifests as general paresis, joint degeneration, and tabes dorsalis (demyelination of posterior columns, dorsal roots, and dorsal root ganglia). Tabes dorsalis is characterized by a gait disturbance and bladder symptoms.

IMMUNOLOGIC MANIFESTATIONS

In the treponemes, two classes of antigen have been recognized:
1. Antigens restricted to one or a few species
2. Antigens shared by many different spirochetes

Specific and nonspecific antibodies are produced in the immunocompetent host. Specific antibodies against *T. pallidum* (**Treponema pallidum antibodies**) and nonspecific antibodies against the protein antigen group common to pathogenic spirochetes are formed. Specific **antitreponemal antibodies** in early or untreated early latent syphilis are predominantly immunoglobulin M (IgM) antibodies. The early immune response to infection is rapidly followed by the appearance of IgG antibodies, which soon become predominant. The greatest elevation in IgG concentration is seen in secondary syphilis.

Nontreponemal antibodies, often called **reagin antibodies,** are produced by infected patients against components of their own or other mammalian cells. Although almost always produced by patients with syphilis, these antibodies are also produced by patients with other infectious diseases. Infectious diseases in which reagin can be demonstrated include measles, chickenpox, hepatitis, infectious mononucleosis, leprosy, tuberculosis, leptospirosis, malaria, rickettsial disease, trypanosomiasis, and lymphogranuloma venereum. Reagin can also be exhibited by patients with noninfectious conditions such as autoimmune disorders, drug addiction, old age, pregnancy, and recent immunization.

Delayed-hypersensitivity immune mechanisms (see Chapter 26) also contribute to the pathophysiology of syphilis. It has been suggested that the **granulomatous reactions (gummas)** result from delayed hypersensitivity in the immune host. In addition, the manifestations of congenital syphilis apparently result in part from an immune inflammatory reaction. Antigen-antibody complexes have been detected in the blood of patients with secondary syphilis and are responsible for the syphilis-associated glomerulonephritis. Suppression of the various aspects of cell-mediated immunity has been noted in syphilis and may contribute to the prolonged survival of *T. pallidum.*

DIAGNOSTIC EVALUATION

The diagnosis of syphilis depends on clinical skills, demonstration of microorganisms in a lesion, and serologic testing. A variety of diagnostic procedures for syphilis are available (Tables 18-3 and 18-4). Classic serologic methods for syphilis measure the presence of two types of antibodies (Table 18-5), nontreponemal methods and treponemal methods.

Testing for syphilis can comply with a logical flow of observations and laboratory testing (Fig. 18-5). Seroconversion between acute and **convalescent sera** is considered strong evidence of recent infection. The best evidence for infection is a significant change in two appropriately timed specimens, in which both tests are performed in the same laboratory at the same time.

Direct Observation of Spirochetes

Two methods of direct observation of spirochetes are available for the examination of a patient specimen from an active syphilitic lesion. These methods are darkfield microscopy and fluorescent antibody microscopy.

Darkfield Microscopy

For symptomatic patients with primary syphilis, **darkfield microscopy** is the test of choice. A darkfield examination is also suggested for immediate results in cases of secondary syphilis, with a titer follow-up test.

Direct and Indirect Fluorescent Antibody

This method of examination uses a fluorescent-labeled antibody conjugate to *T. pallidum.* An alternate indirect method uses antibody specific for *T. pallidum* and a second labeled antiimmunoglobulin antibody. This method offers the advantage of not requiring a live specimen. There is a risk of cross-reactivity with other subspecies of *T. pallidum* when monoclonal antibody is used for the procedure.

Nontreponemal Methods

Nontreponemal methods determine the presence of reagin, an antibody formed against cardiolipin. An antigen composed of **cardiolipin,** a lipid remnant of damaged cells, cholesterol, and lecithin is used to detect the nontreponemal reagin antibodies.

Rapid Plasma Reagin

The **rapid plasma reagin (RPR)** test is the most widely used nontreponemal serologic procedure, although **Venereal Disease Research Laboratory (VDRL)** methods may be used in some clinical and reference laboratories. Both these procedures are flocculation or agglutination tests in which soluble antigen particles coalesce to form larger particles that are visible as clumps when they are aggregated by antibody.

The RPR test, a charcoal agglutination test, can be performed on heated or unheated serum or plasma using a modified VDRL antigen suspension of choline chloride with ethylenediaminetetraacetic acid (EDTA). The RPR card test antigen also contains charcoal particles to which cardiolipin-containing antigen is bound for macroscopic reading. There are three versions of the RPR test. The original RPR method used unmeasured amounts of plasma and was used as a field procedure for screening large numbers of people. The modified RPR test uses the serum reagin test and is performed on measured volumes of unheated serum.

The RPR test measures IgM and IgG antibodies to lipoidal material released from damaged host cells and to

Table 18-3	**Comparison of Tests for Syphilis Diagnosis**				
Test, Methodology	**Antibody**	**Antigen**		**Specimen and Clinical Notes**	**Technical Notes**
Direct Microscopy Observation					
Fluorescent	Antitreponemal antibody with fluorescent tag	T. pallidum		Patient specimen must be swab or discharge from active lesion.	
Darkfield	None	T. pallidum		Patient specimen must be swab or discharge from active lesion.	
Nontreponemal Assay					
RPR	Reagin	Cardiolipin		Use a serum specimen; cannot be used for CSF.	More sensitive than VDRL in primary syphilis
VDRL	Reagin	Cardiolipin		Specimen can be serum or CSF.	Traditional method used less frequently than RPR
Treponemal Test					
DNA probe	None	DNA from patient matched to treponemal DNA			Expensive form of testing
EIA	Anti-IgM or anti-IgG antitreponemal	Enzyme-labeled treponemal antigen		Antibody source is patient serum.	Less sensitive than other methods in later stages of syphilis
FTA-ABS	Antitreponemal	T. pallidum (Nichols strain)			Confirmatory assay; primary stage test results may be negative.
MHA-TP	Antitreponemal	Gel particles or sheep red blood cells; coated carrier particles of T. pallidum cell walls disrupted by high-frequency sound waves.			Less sensitive than FTA-ABS

RPR, Rapid plasma reagin; *VDRL,* venereal disease research laboratory; *FTA-ABS,* fluorescent treponemal antibody absorption; *EIA,* enzyme immunoassay; *MHA-TP,* microhemagglutination assay for antibodies direct against *Treponemal pallidum*; *TP-PA,* Treponemal *pallidum* particle agglutination assay.

Table 18-4	**Select Tests for Syphilis Diagnosis**	
Test	**Methodology**	**Comments**
Darkfield examination	Darkfield microscopy	
RPR	Charcoal agglutination	
T. pallidum (VDRL), serum with reflex to titer	Flocculation	
T. pallidum antibody, serum IgG by IFA	Indirect fluorescent antibody (IFA)	False-positive result in herpes, HIV, malaria, IV drug use, systemic lupus, rheumatoid arthritis, pregnancy, leprosy
T. pallidum antibody, IgM by ELISA	ELISA	If test results are questionable, repeat testing in 10-14 days.
T. pallidum antibody, IgG by ELISA	ELISA	If test results are questionable, repeat testing in 10-14 days.

Adapted from Associated Regional and University Pathologists (ARUP) Laboratories: ARUP's laboratory test directory, 2012 (http://www.aruplab.com/guides/ug/tests/ugs.jsp).
IgG, Immunoglobulin G; *HIV,* human immunodeficiency virus; *IV,* intravenous; *MHA,* microhemagglutination; *VDRL,* Venereal Disease Research Laboratories.
NOTE: VDRL is the preferred test for CSF. Treponemal tests (TP-PA or FTA) are *not* recommended for CSF. FTAs on CSF may be tested, but TP-PA *cannot* be tested on CSF.

Table 18-5	Nontreponemal and Treponemal Assays
Nontreponemal Screening Assays	**Treponemal Confirmatory‡ Assays**
T. pallidum (RPR)*	FTA-ABS
T. pallidum (VDRL)†	*T. pallidum* particle agglutination (antibody to TP-PA)
	T. pallidum antibody IgM by ELISA
	T. pallidum antibody, IgG by Immunoblot
	T. pallidum antibody, IgG by indirect fluorescent antibody (IFA)§

*Serum or CSF with reflex to titer.
†Serum or CSF with reflex to titer.
‡If nontreponemal screening assay is positive.
§CSF.

lipoprotein-like material, and possibly cardiolipin released from the treponemes. If antibodies are present, they combine with the lipid particles of the antigen, causing them to agglutinate. The charcoal particles coagglutinate with the antibodies and show up as black clumps against the white card. If antibodies are not present, the test mixture is uniformly gray.

Antilipoidal antibodies are antibodies that are produced not only as a consequence of syphilis and other treponemal diseases, but also in response to nontreponemal diseases of an acute and chronic nature in which tissue damage occurs. Without some other evidence for the diagnosis of syphilis, a reactive nontreponemal test does not confirm *T. pallidum* infection.

The RPR test is more sensitive than the VDRL test for the detection of primary syphilis.

Venereal Disease Research Laboratory Test

The VDRL test, a flocculation test, is a qualitative and quantitative screening procedure. Flocculation is a specific type of precipitation reaction that takes place over a narrow range of antigen concentration.

Serum for testing must be heated to 56° C (133° F) for 30 minutes to inactivate complement. The test serum should be used promptly after inactivation. The antigen suspension is composed of cardiolipin, cholesterol, and lecithin. The VDRL test measures IgM and IgG antibodies to lipoidal material released from damaged host cells, to lipoprotein-like material, and possibly to cardiolipin released from the treponemes.

Without some other evidence for the diagnosis of syphilis, a reactive nontreponemal test does not confirm *T. pallidum* infection. Antilipoidal antibodies are antibodies that are not only produced as a consequence of syphilis and other treponemal diseases, but also may be produced in response to nontreponemal diseases of an acute and chronic nature in which tissue damage occurs. Without some other evidence for the diagnosis of syphilis, false-positive results may be caused by human immunodeficiency virus (HIV),

herpes simplex virus (HSV), malaria, intravenous drug use (IVDU), systemic lupus erythematosus (SLE), rheumatoid arthritis (RA), pregnancy, leprosy, or endemic treponemal conditions.

VDRL with reflex testing to titer is the preferred test for CSF. A positive VDRL test result on spinal fluid is diagnostic of neurosyphilis.

Treponemal Methods

Treponemal assays can confirm reactive (positive) reagin tests but should not be used as primary screening methods. The most common assays in this category are the following:

- Fluorescent treponemal antibody absorption (FTA-ABS)
- *T. pallidum* particle agglutination (TP-PA)
- *T. pallidum* antibody by enzyme-linked immunosorbent assay (ELISA)
- *T. pallidum* antibody by immunoblot (Western blot) test

Fluorescent Treponemal Antibody Absorption

FTA-ABS can be used to confirm that a positive nontreponemal test result has been caused by syphilis rather than by other biological conditions that can produce a positive serologic result. This test also can determine quantitative titers of antibody, which is useful for following response to therapy.

The FTA-ABS uses a killed suspension of *T. pallidum* spirochetes as the antigen. Most systems use nonviable *T. pallidum* (Nichols strain), extracted from rabbit testicular tissue, as a substrate (antigen). Sorbent, another reagent, is prepared from cultures of nonpathogenic Reiter treponemes. The sorbent that contains an antigen to the Reiter treponeme may or may not specifically absorb the reactivity that occurs in normal sera. Treponema pallidum antigen.

This procedure is performed by overlaying whole treponemes fixed to a slide with serum from patients suspected of having syphilis because of a previously positive syphilis serology. The patient's serum is first absorbed with non–*T. pallidum* treponemal antigens to reduce nonspecific cross-reactivity. Fluorescein-conjugated antihuman antibody reagent is then applied as a marker for specific antitreponemal antibodies in the patient's serum.

FTA-ABS may be helpful in late neurosyphilis when the RPR is negative but there is a high clinical suspicion of syphilis. FTA tests may produce false-positive result in a variety of disorders, such as autoimmune disease, leprosy, febrile illnesses, advanced age, or Lyme disease.

Treponema pallidum Particle Agglutination

This is a semiquantitative particle agglutination assay. It cannot be used to test CSF. This assay cannot differentiate between IgM and IgG antibodies. TP-PA is useful to diagnose infection in patient whose reactive screening test is positive with atypical signs of primary, secondary, or late syphilis. TP-PA compares favorably to the FTA test but is slightly less sensitive in untreated early primary syphilis. This assay is excellent for resolving inconclusive FTA-ABS results.

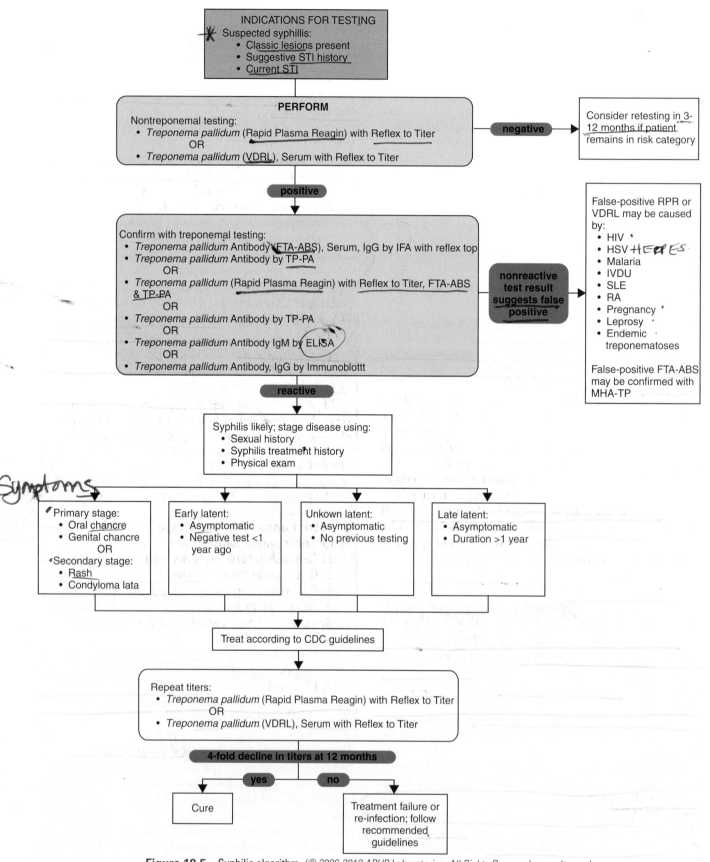

Figure 18-5   Syphilis algorithm. *(© 2006-2012 ARUP Laboratories. All Rights Reserved. consult.com.)*

Treponema pallidum Antibody, Immunoglobulin G, by Enzyme-Linked Immunosorbent Assay

The ELISA assay can discriminate maternally derived IgG antibodies that cross the placenta from IgM antibodies that indicate active infection in a newborn. Congenital syphilis sensitivity is approximately 80%. Hence, congenital syphilis can be confirmed but a negative IgM level does not rule out congenital syphilis. The assay is highly specific (100%) and sensitive (91%).

Treponema pallidum Antibody, Immunoglobulin G, by Immunoblot (Western Blot) Test

A negative result is seen when no specific IgG antibodies against *T. pallidum* are detected. This test should not be used to determine relapse or reinfection of syphilis because of the persistence of reactivity, likely for a lifetime. Repeat testing in 2 to 4 weeks is recommended if results are equivocal. The presence of IgG antibody to *T. pallidum* is suggestive of current or past infection.

Sensitivity of Representative Procedures for Syphilis

Detection of syphilis by serologic methods is related to the stage of the disease and test method (Table 18-6).

In the primary stage, about 30% of cases become serologically active after 1 week and 90% of patients demonstrate reactivity after 3 weeks. Reagin titers increase rapidly during the first 4 weeks of infection and then remain stable for about 6 months. Patients in the secondary stage of syphilis are serologically positive.

During latent syphilis, there is a gradual return of nonreactive serologic manifestations, as seen with nontreponemal methods. About one third of patients in the latent stage will remain seroreactive and presumably infectious. In late syphilis, treponemal tests are generally reactive and nontreponemal methods are nonreactive.

Table 18-6	**Percentage of Positive Tests for Syphilis**			
		Stage		
Test*	Primary	Secondary	Latent	Late
Nontreponemal Assay				
Rapid plasma reagin (RPR)	80-86	99-100		98†
Treponemal Assays				
FTA-ABS	84-85	100		95-100
TP-PA, MHA-TP	85-100	98-100		98-100

Adapted from Tramont E: *Treponema pallidum.* In Mandell GI, Douglas RG Jr, Bennett Jr, editors: Principles and practice of infectious diseases, ed 2, New York, 1985, Wiley & Sons, and LaSalsa L et al: Spirochete infections. In Henry JB, editor: Clinical diagnosis and management by laboratory methods, ed 21, Philadelphia, 2007, WB Saunders, Table 58-1.
MHA-TP, Microhemagglutination assay for antibodies directed against *T. pallidum.*
*Percentage of patients with positive serologic tests in treated or untreated primary or secondary syphilis.
†Treated late syphilis.

Traditional versus Reverse-Screening Algorithm Protocols

The traditional protocol for syphilis screening is to use a nontreponemal test followed by a treponemal antibody test for confirmation of a reactive specimen. The influence of automation presents a reverse protocol. Many automated protocols begin with the detection of IgM and IgG antibodies to treponemal-specific antigen for sensitive detection of primary syphilis infection. A nontreponemal assay is used to detect active disease. Using a reverse protocol, most patient specimen are negative with only a small percentage of specimens requiring a manual nontreponemal test. Proponents of an automated, reverse protocol cite workflow advantages and an increase detection rate of late-stage syphilis.

If discordant results are encountered. The CDC suggests confirmation of discordant results by using the TP-PA which is necessary to rule out a false positive result.

CASE STUDY

History and Physical Examination

A 25-year-old woman comes to an ambulatory center with pain in the right side of her pelvis and a slight temperature. She has a history of two episodes of chlamydial cervicitis and herpes simplex vulvitis.

Physical examination reveals abundant mucopurulent cervical discharge and a painless genital lesion. The patient also has some swelling of her inguinal lymph glands.

Laboratory Data

A stat pregnancy test is ordered. It is positive.

Questions

1. Laboratory assays that would be appropriate for this patient could include:
   a. Cervical culture for gonorrhea and Chlamydia
   b. Gram stain for gonorrhea
   c. Serum testing for HIV and syphilis
   d. All of the above
2. Screening testing for syphilis can include:
   a. Gram stain for *T. pallidum*
   b. RPR test
   c. Treponemal-MHA-TP
   d. FTA-ABS

See Appendix A for the answers to these questions.

Critical Thinking Group Discussion Questions

1. What other laboratory tests would you expect to be ordered?
2. Could this patient have syphilis?
3. If syphilis is suspected, what tests should be ordered?
4. Is there risk of a congenital infection in this woman's unborn child?

See ℮volve for the discussion of the answers to these questions.

See instructor site of ⊖volve for answers to discussion questions.

Classic VDRL Procedure: VDRL Qualitative Slide Test

Principle

During the period of infection with syphilis, reagin, a substance with the properties of an antibody, appears in the serum of infected patients. Reagin has the ability to combine with a colloidal suspension extracted from animal tissue and clump together to form visible masses, a process known as flocculation.

In the VDRL procedure, the patient's heat-inactivated serum is mixed with a buffered saline suspension of cardiolipin-lecithin-cholesterol antigen. This serum-antigen mixture is microscopically examined for flocculation. Positive or reactive sera can be serially diluted and titrated. Syphilis and disorders such as pinta, yaws, bejel, and other treponemal diseases can produce positive reactions.

Procedure

The procedural protocol is posted on the ⊖volve website. The original Wasserman procedure is archived at www.mlturgeon.com for historical reference.

Sources of Error

False-negative reactions can occur in a variety of situations. These include the following:

1. Technical error (e.g., unsatisfactory antigen or technique)
2. Low antibody titers

Patients may have syphilis, but the reagin concentration is too low to produce a reactive test result. A low concentration of reagin may be caused by several factors, such as an infection that is too recent to have produced antibodies, the effects of treatment, latent or inactive disease, and patients who have not produced protective antibodies because of immunologic tolerance. These seronegative patients may demonstrate a positive reaction with more sensitive treponemal tests such as the FTA-ABS.

3. Presence of inhibitors in the patient's serum
4. Reduced ambient temperature (<23° C to 29° C [<73° F to 84° F])
5. Prozone reaction

A prozone reaction is encountered occasionally. This type of reaction is demonstrated when complete or partial inhibition of reactivity occurs with undiluted serum and minimal reactivity is obtained only with diluted serum. The prozone phenomenon may be so pronounced that only a weakly reactive or rough nonreactive result occurs in the qualitative test by a serum that will be strongly reactive when diluted. It is recommended that all sera producing a weak reaction or rough nonreactive results in qualitative testing be retested with a quantitative procedure before a final report of the VDRL slide test is issued.

Weakly reactive results can be caused by the following:

1. Very early infection
2. Lessening of the activity of the disease after treatment
3. Improper technique or questionable reagents

False-positive reactions can also occur. Of all positive serologic tests for syphilis, 10% to 30% may be false-positive biologic reactions. Nonsyphilitic positive VDRL reactions have been reported with the cardiolipin type of antigen in the following:

1. Lupus erythematosus
2. Rheumatic fever
3. Vaccinia and viral pneumonia
4. Pneumococcal pneumonia
5. Infectious mononucleosis
6. Infectious hepatitis
7. Leprosy
8. Malaria
9. Rheumatoid arthritis
10. Pregnancy
11. Older individuals

Contaminated or hemolyzed specimens can also produce false-positive results.

Clinical Applications

The purpose of the VDRL procedure is to demonstrate reagin in cases of syphilis. The procedure may also be positive in treponemal diseases such as yaws and pinta. Reagin, however, is found in some patients who are not infected with treponemes, which can be partially explained by the necrotizing effect of spirochetes on tissues and in other conditions and disorders. It is important that results of the VDRL procedure be correlated with the patient's history and with signs and symptoms.

Limitations

The VDRL procedure is not specific for syphilis but may demonstrate positive reactions in other reagin-producing disorders, autoimmune disorders, infectious diseases, and in pregnancy or aging in normal physiology.

Rapid Plasma Reagin Card Test

Principle

The RPR test is designed to detect reagin, an antibody-like substance present in serum. In this procedure, serum is mixed with an antigen suspension of a carbon particle cardiolipin antigen. If the specimen contains antibody, flocculation occurs with a coagglutination of the carbon particles of antigen. This flocculation appears as black clumps against the white background of a plastic-coated card. The cards are viewed macroscopically.

This is a nontreponemal testing procedure for the serologic detection of syphilis; however, pinta, yaws, bejel, and other treponemal diseases may produce positive results. Positive reactions are occasionally observed with other acute or chronic conditions.

Sources of Error

Error can be introduced into test results because of factors such as contamination of rubber bulbs or an improperly prepared antigen suspension.

False-positive biological reactions have been reported with cardiolipin type of antigens in the following conditions:

- Lupus erythematosus
- Rheumatic fever
- Vaccinia and viral pneumonia
- Pneumococcal pneumonia
- Infectious mononucleosis
- Infectious hepatitis
- Leprosy
- Malaria
- Rheumatoid arthritis
- Pregnancy
- Aging individuals

False-negative reactions can result from the following:

- Poor technique
- Ineffective reagents
- Improper rotation

Again, if mechanical rotation is below or above the 95- to 110–rpm acceptable range, the clumping of the antigen tends to be less intense in procedures with undiluted specimen; thus, some minimal reactions may be missed. In quantitative tests, rotation above 110 rpm tends to produce a decrease in titer, approximately one dilution lower.

Limitations

A diagnosis of syphilis cannot be made based on a single reactive result without clinical signs and symptoms or history. Plasma specimens should not be used to establish a quantitative baseline from which changes in titer can be determined, particularly for evaluating treatment.

The RPR cards should not be used for testing CSF. Little reliance should be placed on cord blood serologic testing for syphilis. The RPR procedure has adequate sensitivity and specificity in relation to the clinical diagnosis.

Clinical Applications

The purpose of the RPR procedure is to demonstrate reagin in cases of syphilis. The test results may also be positive in treponemal diseases such as yaws and pinta. Reagin, however, is found in some patients who are not infected with treponemes, which can be partially explained by the necrotizing effect of spirochetes on tissues and in other conditions and disorders. It is important that results of the procedure be correlated with patient history and with signs and symptoms.

Fluorescent Treponemal Antibody Absorption Test

Principle

The FTA-ABS test is a direct method of observation. Although not recommended for screening, it is the most sensitive serologic procedure in the detection of primary syphilis.

Limitations

The FTA-ABS test is recommended as a confirmatory procedure for syphilis. Its use is discouraged as a screening test. A reagin test such as the RPR is recommended for screening.

Clinical Applications

If a patient has two borderline test results, it is impossible to conclude definitively that the patient has or does not have serologic evidence of syphilitic infection. The attending physician should review the patient's history and physical findings. Diagnosis will rely on the clinical evidence in conjunction with the borderline serologic findings.

The false-positive rate of this test is very low, but it can be associated with autoimmune disorders such as systemic lupus erythematosus. False-positive FTA-ABS results occur in patients with other treponematoses (pinta, yaws, bejel) and in those who have a high titer of antinuclear antibodies or rheumatoid factor. Evidence indicates that pregnant women occasionally have false-positive FTA-ABS test results.

CHAPTER HIGHLIGHTS

- Syphilis is caused by a spirochete, *Treponema pallidum*, usually transmitted in humans by sexual contact.
- Untreated syphilis is a chronic disease with subacute symptomatic periods separated by asymptomatic intervals, during which the diagnosis can be made serologically. The progression of untreated syphilis is generally divided into stages.
- In primary syphilis, the serum in about one third of cases becomes serologically reactive after 1 week and serologically demonstrable in most cases after 3 weeks. The reagin titer increases rapidly during the first 4 weeks and then stabilizes for about 6 months.
- Two to 8 weeks after the appearance of the primary chancre, the patient enters the stage of secondary syphilis, usually characterized by generalized illness suggestive of a viral infection. Skin lesions contain spirochetes and are highly contagious on exposed surfaces. These lesions subside spontaneously after 2 to 6 weeks, even if untreated. In this noninfectious latent stage, serologic tests for syphilis are positive.
- The late (tertiary) stage usually occurs 3 to 10 years after primary infection; gummas can appear in about 15% of untreated syphilitic persons who eventually develop late benign syphilis. Complications include nervous system lesions, causing tabes dorsalis or cardiovascular complications. The tertiary stage is asymptomatic and determined only by serologic testing. Occasionally, the lesions heal so completely that even serologic tests become nonreactive.
- Classic serologic tests for syphilis measure the presence of two types of antibodies, treponemal and nontreponemal.
- Darkfield microscopy is the test of choice for symptomatic patients with primary syphilis.
- The widely used nontreponemal serologic test is the RPR method, a flocculation method.
- Specific treponemal serologic tests include the fluorescent treponemal antibody absorption (FTA-ABS) and *T. pallidum* particle agglutination (TP-PA).

REVIEW QUESTIONS

1-4. Match the *Treponema*-associated diseases (a-d) with the respective causative organism.

1. _____ *T. pallidum*

2. _____ *T. pallidum* (variant)

3. _____ *T. pertenue*

4. _____ *T. carateum*
   a. Yaws
   b. Syphilis
   c. Pinta
   d. Bejel

5-8. Match the following stages of syphilis with the appropriate signs and symptoms.

5. _____ Primary syphilis

6. _____ Secondary syphilis

7. _____ Latent syphilis

8. _____ Late (tertiary) syphilis
   a. Diagnosis only by serologic methods
   b. Presence of gummas
   c. Development of a chancre
   d. Hutchinsonian triad
   e. Generalized illness followed by macular lesions in most patients

9. Which of the following is a term for nontreponemal antibodies produced by an infected patient against components of their own or other mammalian cells?
   a. Autoagglutinins
   b. Reagin antibodies
   c. Alloantibodies
   d. Nonsyphilis antibodies

10-12. Match the following:

10. _____ FTA-ABS test

11. _____ TP-PA test

12. _____ RPR test
   a. Treponemal method
   b. Nontreponemal method

13. In the RPR procedure, a false-positive reaction can result from all the following except:
   a. Infectious mononucleosis
   b. Leprosy
   c. Rheumatoid arthritis
   d. Streptococcal pharyngitis

14. The first diagnostic blood test for syphilis was the:
   a. VDRL
   b. Wassermann
   c. RPR
   d. Colloidal gold

15. Syphilis was initially treated with:
   a. Fuller's earth
   b. Heavy metals (e.g., arsenic)
   c. Sulfonamides (e.g., triple sulfa)
   d. Antibiotics (e.g., penicillin)

16. Direct examination of the treponemes is most often performed by:
   a. Light microscopy
   b. Darkfield microscopy
   c. VDRL testing
   d. RPR testing

17. Pathogenic treponemes _____ cultivatable with consistency in artificial laboratory media.
   a. Are
   b. Are not

18. In infected blood, *T. pallidum* does not appear to survive at 4° C (39 ° F) for longer than:
   a. 1 day
   b. 2 days
   c. 3 days
   d. 5 days

19. The primary incubation period for syphilis *(T. pallidum)* is usually about:
   a. 1 week
   b. 2 weeks
   c. 3 weeks
   d. 4 weeks

20. The stage of syphilis that can be diagnosed only by serologic (laboratory) methods is the:
   a. Incubation phase
   b. Primary phase
   c. Secondary phase
   d. Latent phase

21. Immunocompetent patients infected with *T. pallidum* produce:
   a. Specific antibodies against *T. pallidum*
   b. Nonspecific antibodies against the protein antigen group common to pathogenic spirochetes
   c. Reagin antibodies
   d. All of the above

BIBLIOGRAPHY

Associated Regional and University Pathologists (ARUP) Laboratories: ARUP's laboratory test directory, 2012, http://www.aruplab.com/guides.

Centers for Disease Control and Prevention (CDC): Congenital syphilis—United States, 2003-2008, Morb Mortal Wkly Rep 59:413, 2010.

Centers for Disease Control and Prevention: Sexually transmitted diseases—interactive data: selected STDs by age, race/ethnicity, and gender, 1996-2009, http://wonder.cdc. gov/std-std-race-age.html. 1996-2009.

Cornish N: A new reflex testing algorithm for syphilis screening, MLO Med Lab Obs 43:40, 2011.

Hook EW, Marra CM: Acquired syphilis in adults, N Engl J Med 326:1060-1069, 1992.

Hunter EF, Deacon WE, Meyer PC: An improved test for syphilis—the absorption procedure (FTA-ABS), Public Health Rep 79:5, 1964.

Jaffe HW, Larsen SA, Peters M, et al: Tests for treponemal antibody in CSF, Arch Intern Med 138:252, 1978.

Leclerc G, Giroux M, Birry A, Kasatiya S: Study of fluorescent treponemal antibody test on cerebrospinal fluid using monospecific anti-immunoglobulin conjugates IgG, IgM, and IgA, Br J Vener Dis 54:303, 1978.

Muller F, Moskophidis J: Estimation of the local production of antibodies to *Treponema pallidum* in the central nervous system of patients with neurosyphilis, Br J Vener Dis 59:80, 1983.

Soreng K, Mardis C: Syphilis: evolving screening algorithms and role of automated immunoassays, Med Lab Observer June:30–32, 2012.

World Health Organization: Department of Reproductive Health and Research: the global elimination of congenital syphilis: rationale and strategy for action, 2007, http://whqlibdoc. who.int/publications/2007/9789241595858_eng.pdf.

Yang LG, Tucker JD, Wang C, et al: Syphilis test availability and uptake at medical facilities in southern China, Bull World Health Organ 89:798, 2011.

CHAPTER 19

Vector-Borne Diseases

Learning Objectives

At the conclusion of this chapter, the reader should be able to:
- Describe the etiology, epidemiology, and signs and symptoms of Lyme disease.
- Analyze the immunologic manifestations and diagnostic evaluation of Lyme disease.
- Explain the principle, interpretation, and limitations of an antibody detection assay.
- Describe prevention strategies of Lyme disease.
- Summarize the etiology, epidemiology, and signs and symptoms of ehrlichiosis.
- Analyze the immunologic manifestations and diagnostic evaluation of ehrlichiosis.
- Explain the prevention of ehrlichiosis.
- Summarize the etiology, epidemiology, and signs and symptoms of Rocky Mountain spotted fever.
- Analyze the immunologic manifestations and diagnostic evaluation of Rocky Mountain spotted fever.

- Explain the prevention of Rocky Mountain spotted fever.
- Summarize the etiology, epidemiology, and signs and symptoms of babesiosis.
- Analyze the immunologic manifestations and diagnostic evaluation of babesiosis.
- Explain the prevention of babesiosis.
- Briefly discuss the etiology and laboratory diagnosis of West Nile virus infection.
- Analyze case studies related to the immune response in Lyme disease, Ehrlichiosis, and Babesiosis.
- Correctly answer case study related multiple choice questions.
- Be prepared to participate in a discussion of critical thinking questions.
- Describe the principle, limitations, and clinical applications of the rapid *Borrelia burgdorferi* antibody detection assay.
- Correctly answer end of chapter review questions.

Key Terms

anaplasmosis
anticardiolipin
arthralgia
aseptic meningitis
bacteriostatic
Babesiosis

erythema chronicum migrans (ECM)
human ehrlichiosis
intraerythrocytic
intraleukocytic morulae
Lyme borreliosis
Lyme disease

Plasmodium
rickettsial
Rocky Mountain Spotted Fever
vector-borne
West Nile virus

Globalization has made the world a more connected place. Bacterial and viral diseases transmitted by mosquitoes, ticks, and fleas continue to be an ever-present threat worldwide (Table 19-1). Some of these diseases have been present in the United States for a long time but others have emerged recently. These include some of the world's most destructive diseases, many of which are increasing threats to human health as the environment changes and globalization increases.

The discovery and surveillance of many of these **vector-borne** diseases (e.g., Lyme disease) can be accomplished by serologic testing. Travelers and military personnel may be at risk for exposure to vector-borne disease if they engage in activities that bring them into contact with habitats that

Table 19-1	Examples of Vector-Borne Diseases		
Vector	**Disease**	**Pathogen**	**Distribution**
Mosquitoes			
Aedes triseriatus	California encephalitis	Virus	United States: Upper Midwest, Appalachian region
Aedes aegypti	Dengue fever West Nile encephalitis West Nile fever	Virus Virus	Worldwide: tropical regions United States; spreading nationwide Africa, Asia
Culiseta melanura	Eastern equine encephalitis	Virus	Eastern United States Central and South America, Caribbean
Culex spp.	St. Louis encephalitis Western equine encephalitis	Virus Virus	Eastern United States Central and South America Western United States Central and South America
Ticks			
Deer tick, *Ixodes* spp.	Anaplasmosis (formerly human granulocytic ehrlichiosis)	Bacteria	Worldwide; Europe United States—Northeast, Upper Midwest, northern California
I. scapularis	Babesiosis	Protozoan parasite	United States—primarily northeastern states, rarely Pacific states
Lone star tick, *Amblyomma americanum*	Human monocytic ehrlichiosis	Bacteria	United States—Southeast, south central states
Dog tick, *Rhipicephalus sanguineus*	Mediterranean spotted fever	Bacteria	Europe, Africa, Central Asia
Tickborne, airborne vector	Q fever	Rickettsiae	Worldwide
Dog tick, wood tick, *Dermacentor* spp.	Rocky Mountain spotted fever Tick-associated rash, illness	Bacteria Bacteria	North and South America Southern
Ticks, various	Tickborne relapsing fever	Bacteria	Western United States (endemic*); Southern British Columbia; plateau regions of Mexico; Central and South America; Mediterranean, Central Asia, and much of Africa
Lice, Fleas, Mites			
Human body louse; squirrel flea and louse	Epidemic typhus	Rickettsiae	United States, eastern
Rat flea, *Xenopsylla cheopis*	Murine typhus	Bacteria	Worldwide, where rats are abundant
Cat or dog fleas	Murine typhus–like febrile disease	Rickettsiae	Worldwide

Continued

Table 19-1	Examples of Vector-Borne Diseases—cont'd		
Vector	**Disease**	**Pathogen**	**Distribution**
Mites (chiggers)	Scrub typhus	Rickettsiae	South Asia to Australia, East Asia in recently disturbed habitat (e.g., forest clearings or other persisting mite foci infested with rats and other rodents)
Human body louse	Louse-borne relapsing fever	Bacteria	Africa
	Trench fever	Rickettsiae	Industrialized countries

*Most recent cases and outbreaks have occurred in rustic cabins at higher elevations (≥8000 ft) in coniferous forests in the western United States.

support the vectors or the animal reservoir species associated with these diseases.

Some of the newly emerging infectious diseases in the United States include the following:

- Chagas disease
- Chikungunya
- Dengue
- Leishmaniasis

A few prominent examples of the more commonly occurring vector-borne diseases detectable by serologic methods are presented in this chapter.

LYME DISEASE

Etiology

Lyme disease (Lyme borreliosis) is caused by a spirochete bacterium. It is a cutaneous systemic infection generally transmitted by a hard-bodied tick (Fig. 19-1) and caused by *Borrelia burgdorferi* (Fig. 19-2). The causative agent of Lyme borreliosis currently consists of three pathogenic species—*B. burgdorferi*, *Borrelia afzelii*, and *Borrelia garinii*. Only *B. burgdorferi* strains have been found in the United States. In contrast, most of the illness in Europe is caused by *B. afzelii*, which is associated with the chronic skin condition acrodermatitis chronica atrophicans (ACA), and *B. garinii*, which is associated with neurologic symptoms. Only these two species have been found in Asia. The complete genome of *B. burgdorferi* (strain B31) has now been sequenced.

The spirochete is transmitted by certain ixodid ticks that are part of the *Ixodes* ricinus complex. These include *Ixodes scapularis* (formerly classified as *Ixodes dammini*) in the northeastern and Midwestern United States, *Ixodes pacificus* in the western United States, *Ixodes ricinus* in Europe, and *Ixodes persulcatus* in Asia. The vector has not been identified in Australia. Ixodid ticks are also indigenous to Africa and South America. The lone star tick, *Amblyomma americanum*, does not transmit Lyme disease.

In the United States, the preferred host for larval and nymphal stages of *I. scapularis* is the white-footed mouse, *Peromyscus leucopus*. White-tailed deer, which are not involved in the life cycle of the spirochete, are the preferred host for the *I. scapularis* adult stage and they seem to be critical to tick survival. Ixodid ticks have also been found on at least 30 types of

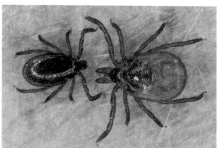
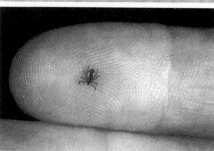

Figure 19-1   Deer tick. *(From Habif TP: Clinical dermatology, ed 2, St Louis, 1990, Mosby.)*

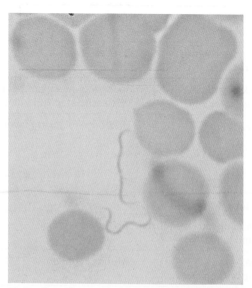

Figure 19-2   *Borrelia* organisms present in the blood of a patient with endemic relapsing fever (Giemsa stain, 1000x magnification). *(From Murray PR et al: Medical microbiology, ed 5, Philadelphia, 2005, Mosby.)*

wild animals and 49 species of birds. Illness is not known to develop in wild animals, but clinical Lyme disease does occur in domestic animals, including dogs, horses, and cattle.

Spirochetes are transmitted from the gut of the tick to human skin at the site of a bite and then migrate outwardly into the skin. This migration causes the unique expanding skin lesion, erythema migrans (EM). Subsequent dissemination of spirochetes to secondary sites may cause major organ system involvement in humans. In dogs, the most common symptom is arthritis.

Epidemiology

Currently, Lyme disease is a global illness. Cases have been reported on all continents except Antarctica. Since its original description more than 25 years ago, Lyme disease has become the most commonly reported (95%) vector-borne illness in the United States. This infection has emerged as a major health hazard for human beings and domestic animals. In 2011, it was the sixth most common nationally notifiable disease. It is endemic in more than 15 states in the United States and in Europe and Asia.

In some patients, Lyme disease may be transitory and of little consequence, but in others it may become chronic and severely disabling. Accurate diagnosis is therefore essential, although better laboratory techniques are still needed.

Retrospectively, the first symptom of Lyme disease apparently was recognized as early as 1908 in Sweden. In the decades that followed, the rash produced by the disease **erythema chronicum migrans (ECM)** was noted elsewhere in Europe, as were other symptoms that seemed to follow ECM's eruption. Secondary symptoms, such as impairment of the nervous system, were described in France, Germany, and again in Sweden.

In the United States the European rash was almost unknown until 1969, when a case of a physician bitten by a tick while hunting in Wisconsin was reported. Although a few ECM cases were seen in Americans who had traveled to Europe, there were no further native American cases until 1975, when physicians at the U.S. Navy base in Groton, Connecticut, reported seeing four patients with a rash similar to that of ECM. At the same time, an epidemiologist at the Connecticut State Department of Health and a rheumatologist at Yale University were notified of an unusual cluster of cases of arthritis occurring in children in Lyme, Connecticut.

It was not until 1982 that Burgdorfer and Barbour isolated a previously unrecognized spirochete, now called *B. burgdorferi*, from *I. scapularis* ticks, and Lyme disease became a recognized vector-borne, infectious disease. Two factors influence the chance that a bitten patient will contract the disease, the likelihood that local ixodid ticks carry the Lyme spirochete and the likelihood of infection after a bite by an infected tick. The probability of infection after an ixodid tick bite in an area of endemic disease is about 3%, but varies in different regions from less than 1% to as high as 5%. It has been suggested that human leukocyte antigen (HLA)–DR4 (HLA-DR4) and, secondarily, HLA-DR2, may increase the risk that Lyme arthritis will become chronic and fail to respond to antibiotics.

Lyme disease does not occur nationwide and is concentrated heavily in the northeast and upper midwest. The highest number of confirmed cases of Lyme disease to date was 29,959 in 2009 (Fig. 19-3). Persons of all ages and both genders are

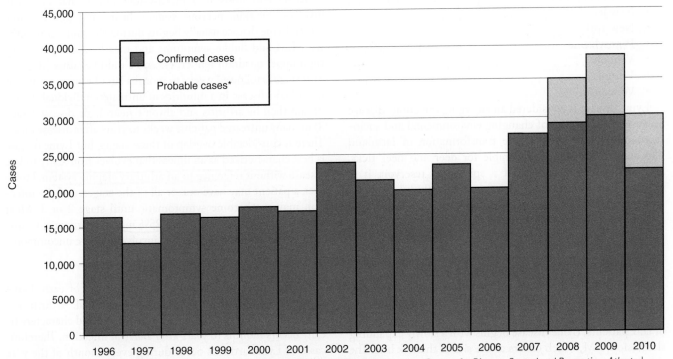

Figure 19-3 **Reported cases of Lyme disease—United States, 1996-2010.** *(Courtesy Centers for Disease Control and Prevention, Atlanta.)*

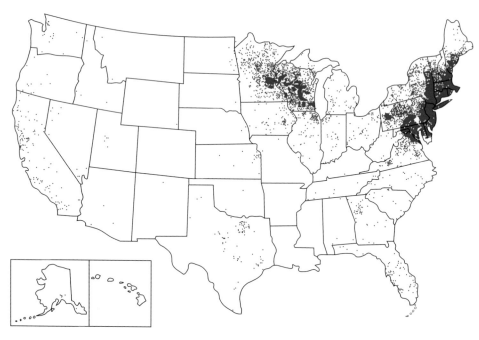

Figure 19-4 Reported cases of Lyme disease—United States, 2011. *(Courtesy Centers for Disease Control and Prevention, Atlanta.)*

One dot is placed randomly within the county of residence for each confirmed case. Though Lyme disease cases have been reported in nearly every state, cases are reported based on the county of residence, not necessarily the county of infection.

equally susceptible. In 2011, 96% of Lyme disease cases were reported from 13 states (Fig. 19-4):

- Connecticut
- Delaware
- Maine
- Maryland
- Massachusetts
- Minnesota
- New Hampshire
- New Jersey
- New York
- Pennsylvania
- Vermont
- Virginia
- Wisconsin

Lyme disease is considered an emerging infectious disease because of the impact of changing environmental and socioeconomic factors, such as the transformation of farmland into suburban woodlots favorable for deer and deer ticks. Although pets may represent a spirochete reservoir, it is unlikely that humans can be infected directly by them. In areas of endemic Lyme disease, however, both adult and nymphal ticks, carried into the household by dogs and cats, may infect humans.

Signs and Symptoms

The basic features of Lyme disease are similar worldwide, but there are regional variations, primarily between the illness in America and that in Europe and Asia. In at least 60% to 80% of U.S. patients, Lyme disease begins with a slowly expanding skin lesion, EM, which occurs at the site of the tick bite. The skin lesion is frequently accompanied by flulike symptoms.

The Centers for Disease Control and Prevention (CDC) clinical case definition for Lyme disease includes the presence of EM or at least one objective, late manifesting sign of musculoskeletal, neurologic, or cardiovascular disease and a positive serologic test for antibodies to *B. burgdorferi*. Many misdiagnosed patients actually have chronic fatigue syndrome or fibromyalgia, both of which can cause similar symptoms, such as joint stiffness or pain, fatigue, and sleep disturbance.

Lyme borreliosis is a multisystem illness that primarily involves the skin, nervous system, heart, and joints (Table 19-2). Lyme disease usually begins during the summer months with EM and flulike symptoms and may be accompanied by right upper quadrant tenderness and a mild hepatitis (stage 1). This stage is followed weeks to months later by acute cardiac or neurologic disease in a minority of untreated individuals (stage 2) and then by arthritis and chronic neurologic disease (stage 3) in many untreated patients weeks to years after disease onset. There is considerable overlap of these stages, but Lyme disease is best characterized as an illness that evolves from early to late disease without reference to an arbitrary staging system. However, a patient may have one or all of the stages, and the infection may not become symptomatic until stage 2 or 3. Most affected patients have EM and 25% manifest arthritis; neurologic manifestations and cardiac involvement are uncommon.

Arthritis

Arthralgia and myalgia are common features of early Lyme disease, but frank arthritis during EM is unusual. Arthritis is a well-described complication of Lyme disease and characteristically occurs months to years after *Borrelia* infection. Therefore, cases of Lyme arthritis occur during every month of the year. Lyme arthritis and parvovirus B19 arthritis can occur in the

Table 19-2		Clinical Features of Lyme Disease
Stage	Duration	Signs and Symptoms
I	4 wk (median) after injection	Cutaneous manifestations (erythema migrans) or other skin eruptions, flulike syndrome, neurologic symptoms
II	Follows a variable latent period	Target organs and systems include nervous system, heart, eyes, and skin, all of which can manifest abnormalities
III	Weeks to years after infection	Arthritis, late neurologic complications, acrodermatitis chronica atrophicans

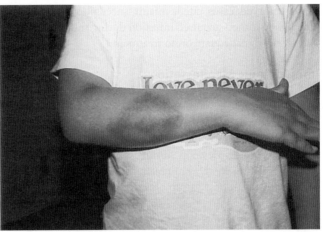

Figure 19-5 **Erythema chronicum migrans.** *(From Forbes BA, Sahm DF, Weissfeld AS: Bailey & Scott's diagnostic microbiology, ed 12, St Louis, 2007, Mosby.)*

absence of other symptoms, such as the characteristic rash. Some suspected cases of Lyme arthritis might be caused by parvovirus B19, particularly those occurring during the parvovirus B19 season.

Arthritis in patients with chronic Lyme disease may be associated with a long-standing infiltration of the joints by *B. burgdorferi* spirochetes, along with a local inflammatory response. It may not be triggered simply by the presence of circulating immunoglobulin G (IgG) antibodies against outer surface proteins.

Cutaneous Manifestations

Cutaneous manifestations can be demonstrated as early ECM (Fig. 19-5), secondary lesions (disseminated lesions and lymphocytoma), and late lesions (ACA). Except for the late lesions, cutaneous manifestations generally resolve spontaneously over weeks to months. The red papule at the site of the tick bite is most often located on the thigh, groin, or axilla. Facial EM is seen more frequently in children.

Several days to weeks after the onset of EM, almost 50% of untreated patients develop secondary skin lesions. A rare early manifestation of Lyme disease is *Borrelia* lymphocytoma, a violaceous, tumor-like swelling or nodule at the base of the earlobe or nipple caused by a dense lymphocytic infiltrate of the dermis. This lesion occurs at the site of a tick bite and in conjunction with other symptoms; it may be confused with lymphoma.

ACA is a late skin manifestation of Lyme disease more prevalent in Europe than in the United States. Lesions display bluish red discoloration, doughy swelling, and fibrotic nodules. Eventually, striking atrophy of the skin and subcutaneous tissues follows. Polyneuropathy coexists in 30% to 45% of patients.

Cardiac Manifestations

Lyme carditis occurs in approximately 8% of untreated patients within 1 to 2 months (range, >1 week to 7 months) after the onset of infection and may be the initial manifestation of Lyme disease. Cardiac features of Lyme disease usually result in a fluctuating degree of atrioventricular conduction defects (first-degree, second-degree, and complete block, as well as

bundle branch and fascicular blocks) or tachyarrhythmias. Myopericarditis can occur, but symptomatic congestive heart failure is uncommon. Patients usually develop signs of light-headedness, syncope, dyspnea, palpitations, and chest pain. Symptoms are more common in patients with more severe degrees of heart block. The carditis usually follows a self-limited and mild course, but temporary pacing may be needed in a small percentage of patients.

Neurologic Manifestations

Neurologic abnormalities occur in approximately 15% of untreated patients. These are usually observed 2 to 8 weeks after disease onset and may include **aseptic meningitis,** cranial nerve palsies, peripheral radiculoneuritis, and peripheral neuropathy. The predominant symptoms of Lyme meningitis are severe headache and mild neck stiffness, which may fluctuate for weeks after a post-EM latent period.

Months to years after the initial infection with *B. burgdorferi,* patients with Lyme disease may have chronic encephalopathy, polyneuropathy or, less often, leukoencephalitis. The appearance of mild encephalopathy has been seen 1 month to 14 years after the onset of disease. Encephalopathy is characterized by memory loss, mood changes, or sleep disturbances. In addition, increased cerebrospinal fluid (CSF) protein levels and evidence of intrathecal production of antibody to *B. burgdorferi* may occur. Chronic neurologic manifestations can also include polyneuropathy with radicular pain or distal paresthesias, fatigue, headache, hearing loss, and verbal memory impairment. These chronic neurologic abnormalities usually improve with antibiotic therapy.

Ocular manifestations may occur in Lyme disease and include cranial nerve palsies, optic neuritis, panophthalmitis with loss of vision, and choroiditis with retinal detachment.

Pregnancy

Transplacental transmission of *B. burgdorferi* with fetal infection has been confirmed. A uniform pattern of congenital malformations has not been identified in maternal-fetal transmission of Lyme disease.

In observed cases cited, infants succumbed shortly after birth. The mothers acquired infection during the first trimester and received inadequate or no treatment.

Immunologic Manifestations

Cellular immune responses to *B. burgdorferi* antigens begin concurrent with early clinical illness. An increase in spontaneous suppressor cell activity and reduction in natural killer (NK) cell activity have been noted. Mononuclear cell, antigen-specific responses develop during spirochetal dissemination and humoral (antibody) immune responses soon follow.

Serodiagnostic tests are insensitive during the first several weeks of infection. In the United States, approximately 20% to 30% of Lyme patients have positive responses, usually of the IgM isotype, during this period, but by convalescence 2 to 4 weeks later, about 70% to 80% have seroreactivity even after antibiotic treatment. After about 1 month, most patients with an active infection have IgG antibody responses. After antibiotic treatment, antibody titers slowly fall, but IgG and even IgM responses may persist for many years after treatment. An IgM response cannot be interpreted as a manifestation of recent infection or reinfection unless the appropriate clinical characteristics are present. Antibodies formed include cryoglobulins, immune complexes, antibodies specific for *B. burgdorferi*, and **anticardiolipin** antibodies. Elevated titers of IgM are noted in early disease. Immunoblot analysis demonstrates that IgM antibodies form initially against the flagellar 41-kilodalton (kDa) polypeptide, but react later to additional cell wall antigens. An overlapping IgG response to these antigens develops in some individuals. These antigen-specific cellular and humoral responses are not known to eradicate infection in early disease or participate in disease pathogenesis.

Specific IgM or IgG antibodies against *B. burgdorferi* are usually not detectable in a patient's serum unless symptoms have been present for at least 2 to 4 weeks. In cases of Lyme arthritis, tests for serum antinuclear antibodies (ANAs) and rheumatoid factor (RF) and Venereal Disease Research Laboratory (VDRL) test results are generally negative. However, anti–*B. burgdorferi* antibodies of the IgG type should be present in the serum of patients with Lyme arthritis.

Outer surface protein A antibodies develop late in the course of human Lyme infection and then only in a subset of patients. A temporal association may exist between the onset of chronic Lyme arthritis in four patients who were HLA-DR4–positive and the development of antibodies to the outer surface protein.

Persistent organisms and spirochetal antigen deposits elicit a vigorous immune reaction, as manifested by a tissue-rich plasma cell and lymphocytic exudate containing abundant T cells, predominantly of the helper subset, plus IgD-bearing B cells. *B. burgdorferi* antigens elicit a strong immune reaction that intensifies with chronicity of arthritis and stimulates macrophages to secrete interleukin-1 (IL-1). IL-1 is capable of stimulating synovial cells and fibroblasts to secrete collagenase and prostaglandin E2; levels of both are elevated in Lyme synovial fluid and can cause erosion of joint cartilage and bone.

Table 19-3	Methods of Lyme Disease Detection
Method	**Comments**
Isolation	Successful cultures have been obtained from ticks, skin biopsies, ear punches, CSF, blood, and synovial fluid; blood is not a reliable sample for culture. Isolation of spirochetes is highly variable.
Histology	Lyme spirochetes are rarely observed in blood smears; examination of tissue is usually performed in addition to an immunologic assay such as fluorescence microscopy. The process is labor-intensive; the test is of limited value.
Serology	FDA-approved IFA and EIA test systems
Molecular	DNA probe with patient DNA matched to *Borrelia* DNA

IFA, Indirect fluorescent antibody; *EIA,* enzyme immunoassay; *FDA,* Food and Drug Administration.

Diagnostic Evaluation

The culture of *B. burgdorferi* from specimens in Barbour-Stoenner-Kelly medium permits a definitive diagnosis. With a few exceptions, positive cultures have only been obtained early in the illness, primarily from biopsy samples of EM lesions, less often from plasma samples, and only occasionally from CSF samples in patients with meningitis. Later in the infection, polymerase chain reaction (PCR) testing is superior to culture for the detection of *B. burgdorferi* in joint fluid.

In the United States, the diagnosis is usually based on the recognition of the characteristic clinical findings, a history of exposure in an area in which the disease is endemic and, except in patients with EM, an antibody response to *B. burgdorferi*. In more than 50% of cases, physicians are comfortable making the diagnosis based on symptoms and patient history. Testing becomes important when the telltale bull's eye rash or other symptoms characteristic of Lyme disease do not appear (Table 19-3).

Antibody Detection

Assays for the detection of antibodies to *B. burgdorferi* are the most practical means for confirming infection. The CDC currently recommends a two-step process when testing blood for evidence of antibodies against the Lyme disease bacteria. Both steps can be done using the same blood sample. The first step uses an enzyme immunoassay (EIA) or, rarely, an indirect immunofluorescence assay (IFA). If the first step is negative, no further testing of the specimen is recommended. If the first step is positive or indeterminate (sometimes called equivocal), the second step should be performed. The second step uses an immunoblot procedure, commonly, a Western blot test. Results are considered positive only if the EIA-IFA and the immunoblot test results are both positive.

The two steps of Lyme disease testing are designed to be done together. CDC does not recommend skipping the first test and just doing the Western blot test. Doing so will increase the frequency of false-positive results and may lead to misdiagnosis and improper treatment.

Enzyme-Linked Immunosorbent Assay

The enzyme-linked immunosorbent assay (ELISA) is the standard test method; it is the most widely available and frequently performed test. The sensitivities of IFA and ELISA methods are usually low during the initial 3 weeks of infection; therefore, negative results are common. The most serious disadvantages of current techniques are low sensitivity and lengthy processing time. In addition, false-positive reactions can result from cross-reactivity in tests for Lyme disease. For example, tick-borne relapsing fever spirochetes, *Borrelia hermsii*, are closely related to *B. burgdorferi*. Antibodies to *B. hermsii*, an agent that coexists with the Lyme disease spirochete in portions of the western United States, strongly cross-react with *B. burgdorferi* in IFA staining and ELISA testing. Common antigens are shared among the *Borrelia* organisms and even with the treponemes. Serum from syphilitic patients reacts positively in assays for Lyme disease. Therefore, serologic test results for antibodies to *B. burgdorferi* should be considered along with clinical data and epidemiologic information when a patient is evaluated for Lyme disease.

Western Blot Analysis

Western blot analysis can verify reactivity of antibody to major surface or flagellar proteins of *B. burgdorferi* (Fig. 19-6). The Western blot test is helpful in determining borderline negative or weakly positive results obtained from other tests, but the values are not always reliable. This procedure is more definitive in later Lyme disease when multiple antibody bands specific for *B. burgdorferi* appear. Reported results from Western blot tests for Lyme disease in its late phase indicates reactive bands for IgM levels. The 41-kDa bands are the earliest to appear, but can cross-react with other spirochetes. The 18-, 23- to 25- (Osp C), 31- (Osp A), 34- (Osp B), 37-, 39-, 83-, and 93-kDa bands are the most specific, but may appear later or not appear at all.

Polymerase Chain Reaction

PCR testing can detect spirochetes in the synovial fluid around the joints or in other clinical samples. The PCR assay looks for DNA of the organism. In the past, positive PCR assay results were taken as definitive evidence that a person had an infection, but it is possible to have antigens in the presence of nonviable organisms. This test amplifies small amounts of DNA that may remain, even when intact organisms are no longer present, an indication that the organism does or did exist. The PCR assay may miss the spirochete in the blood, allowing it to move into other tissues.

The PCR technique directly identifies the pathogen instead of measuring the host's immune response to it. It can detect DNA from as few as one to five organisms, even those that are nonviable. Different specific probes have been developed and the PCR assay has been used to detect *B. burgdorferi* DNA in

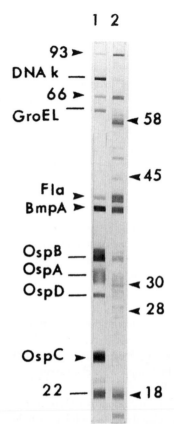

Figure 19-6 Example of immunoblot calibration. *Lane 1,* Monoclonal antibodies defining selected antigens to *B. burgdorferi* B31 separated in a linear SDS-PAGE gel Marblot (MarDx Diagnostics, Carlsbad, Calif). *Lane 2,* Human serum (IgG) reactive with the 10 antigens scored in recommended criteria for blot scoring; lines indicate other calibrating antibodies. Molecular masses are in kilodaltons. *Osp,* Outer surface protein. *(From Detrick B et al, editors: Manual of molecular and clinical laboratory immunology, ed 7, Washington, DC, 2006, American Society for Microbiology Press, p 499.)*

a variety of body fluids. The appeal of the PCR method lies in its rapid turnaround time (2 days versus 6 to 8 weeks for culture) and avoidance of the difficulties associated with culture or immunohistochemistry. It has very high specificity, but the sensitivity may be as low as 70%. The PCR test may be useful in diagnosing early Lyme disease when the patient is still seronegative.

Cerebrospinal Fluid Analysis for Antibody Detection

Spinal taps are not routinely recommended; a negative tap does not rule out Lyme disease. Antibodies to *B. burgdorferi* can be detected in the CSF in only 20% of patients with late disease. Therefore, spinal taps are performed only on patients with pronounced neurologic manifestations. The goal is to rule out other conditions and determine whether *B. burgdorferi* antigens are present. It is especially important to look for elevated protein levels and mononuclear cells, which would dictate the need for more aggressive therapy, and to check the opening CSF pressure, which can be elevated and contribute to headaches, especially in children.

Treatment and Prevention

Treatment decisions after a tick bite are influenced by the following factors:

- Probability that the tick is a carrier of *B. burgdorferi*
- Length of time the tick was attached
- Chance that disease will develop without the telltale rash
- Risk and severity of short- and long-term sequelae
- Accuracy of antibody tests
- Efficacy of antibiotics at various stages of the disease
- Risk of adverse reactions to the antibiotics
- Patient's level of anxiety
- Probability that the patient will comply with follow-up monitoring
- Cost of various strategies; presence of coinfections or immunodeficiencies; prior significant steroid use while infected; age and weight; gastrointestinal (GI) function; blood levels achieved

Antibiotics

It is unclear whether antimicrobial treatment after an *I. scapularis* tick bite will prevent Lyme disease. One study concluded that a single 200-mg dose of doxycycline (MLT) given within 72 hours after an *I. scapularis* tick bite can prevent the development of Lyme disease.

Another study concluded that there is considerable impairment of health-related quality of life in patients with persistent symptoms despite previous antibiotic treatment for acute Lyme disease. In two clinical trials, however, treatment with IV and oral antibiotics for 90 days did not improve symptoms more than placebo.

Various types of antibiotics are in general use for *B. burgdorferi* treatment. The tetracyclines, including doxycycline and minocycline, are **bacteriostatic** unless given in high doses. If high blood levels are not attained, treatment failures in early and late disease are common; however, it is difficult to tolerate high doses.

Penicillins are bactericidal. As would be expected in managing an infection with a gram-negative organism such as *B. burgdorferi*, amoxicillin has been shown to be more effective than oral penicillin V. Because of its short half-life and need for high levels, amoxicillin is usually administered along with probenecid. Because of variability, blood levels are usually measured. Third-generation agents are currently the most effective of the cephalosporins because of their very low blood level counts (0.06×10^9 for ceftriaxone) and they have been shown to be effective in penicillin and tetracycline failures. Cefuroxime axetil (Ceftin), a second-generation agent, is also effective against staphylococci and thus is useful in treating atypical EM, which may represent a mixed infection containing common skin pathogens in addition to *B. burgdorferi*. Because of this agent's GI side effects and high cost, cefuroxime is not used as a first-line drug.

Prevention

When hiking in the woods or mountains, picnicking at local parks, or walking in tall grass in shore areas, individuals should do the following:

- Check daily for ticks.
- Wear light-colored clothing so that tick viewing is easier.
- Tuck pants into socks.

NOTE: On February 26, 2002, GlaxoSmithKline, the maker of the Lyme vaccine LYMErix, pulled the vaccine off the market. Currently, there is no human vaccine for the prevention of Lyme disease, but a veterinary vaccine is available.

HUMAN EHRLICHIOSIS

Human **ehrlichiosis** was first described in the United States in 1986; since then, reports of tickborne illnesses have increased. Unlike Lyme disease, which tends to be indolent, Rocky Mountain spotted fever and ehrlichiosis can be fatal and must be recognized and treated promptly.

Etiology

Tickborne rickettsiae of the genus *Ehrlichia* have been recognized as a cause of human illness in the United States. *Ehrlichia* spp. belong to the same family as the organism that causes Rocky Mountain spotted fever. *Ehrlichia chaffeensis*, the etiologic agent of human monocytic ehrlichiosis in the United States, was demonstrated to cause disease in a patient from Arkansas with tick bites in 1987. Since then, two more *Ehrlichia* spp., *Ehrlichia ewingii* and an *Ehrlichia phagocytophila*–like agent that differs antigenically and genetically from *E. chaffeensis*, have been identified as the cause of anaplasmosis (human granulocytic ehrlichiosis).

Epidemiology

Although the prevalence rates are low, human ehrlichiosis is endemic in the United States. Some fatalities have been reported. Incidence rates increase with age and are higher in men than women. Human ehrlichiosis occurs most frequently in the southern Mid-Atlantic and south central states during spring and summer.

The major vector for *E. chaffeensis* is the lone star tick, *Amblyomma americanum*. The principal reservoir for *E. chaffeensis* is the white-tailed deer, which hosts all stages of *A. americanum*. The primary tick vector for the agent of human granulocytic ehrlichiosis is *I. scapularis* in the eastern United States and *I. pacificus* in California. *Dermacentor variabilis* represents a second tick vector in the United States. The major reservoir for infection may be the white-footed mouse in the eastern United States. The onset of illness in spring and early summer for most cases parallels the time when *A. americanum* and *D. variabilis* ticks are most active.

Signs and Symptoms

Ehrlichiosis is a general term for human granulocytic ehrlichiosis, now called **anaplasmosis,** and human monocytic ehrlichiosis (HME). The syndrome of human ehrlichiosis is not typically recognized by physicians, but should be considered in patients with a history of tick exposure and an acute febrile, flulike illness. Most patients are not suspected of having a **rickettsial** infection. Because ehrlichiosis can cause fatal infections in humans, early detection and treatment with tetracycline or chloramphenicol appear to offer the best chance for complete recovery.

Symptoms are nonspecific and include fever, chills, and headache. Fever and skin rashes are the most common physical findings. In children, fever and headache are universal. Myalgias, nausea, vomiting, and anorexia are also common.

Diagnostic Evaluation

Laboratory studies have indicated that the hematologic, hepatic, and central nervous systems are usually involved in human ehrlichiosis. Definitive diagnosis is based on inclusion in leukocytes (Fig. 19-7). *Ehrlichia* spp. undergo three developmental stages, as follows:

1. Elementary bodies enter a leukocyte by phagocytosis and multiply rapidly.
2. After 3 to 5 days, small numbers of tightly packed elementary bodies (initial bodies) are visible.
3. During the next 7 to 12 days, the initial bodies develop into morular, or mulberry, forms.

For anaplasmosis, direct observation of **intraleukocytic morulae** in Wright-Giemsa–stained peripheral blood or buffy coat smears is a rapid and inexpensive laboratory test. If clinical symptoms and the epidemiologic history are compatible with rickettsial infections, the following diagnostic tests should be used during the acute stage of illness and when antibiotic treatment is initiated:

- PCR test on skin biopsy of rash or eschar, or an ethylenediaminetetraacetic acid (EDTA) whole blood specimen
- Specific immunohistologic detection of rickettsiae in skin biopsy of rash or eschar

In anaplasmosis, the diagnosis is confirmed by seroconversion or by a single serologic titer higher than 1:80 in patients with a supporting history and clinical symptoms. Seroconversion is defined as a fourfold rise in the titer of paired acute and convalescent sera. Detection of IgM class antibody alone should not be interpreted as recent exposure to the rickettsial agents and should be confirmed by detection of IgG or, preferably, IgG seroconversion by parallel evaluation with a convalescent phase serum collected 4 to 6 weeks after onset of the illness.

In HME the diagnosis is confirmed by seroconversion or by a serologic titer higher than 1:128 in patients with a supporting history and clinical symptoms. Serum or CSF can be analyzed for IgM and IgG antibodies to *Ehrlichia* spp.

PCR-based detection of the *E. phagocytophila*–like agent of anaplasmosis represents the most sensitive and direct approach to diagnosis. PCR detection of *E. chaffeensis* includes the amplification of sequences with 16SrDNA.

Treatment and Prevention

HME patients and those with anaplasmosis are treated with doxycycline. No established guidelines have been established for long-term therapy. Prevention consists of reducing the risk of exposure to ticks (see earlier discussion of Lyme disease prevention).

ROCKY MOUNTAIN SPOTTED FEVER

Etiology

Rocky Mountain spotted fever (RMSF) is a tickborne disease caused by the bacterium *Rickettsia rickettsii*. This organism is a cause of potentially fatal human illness in North and South America, and is transmitted to human beings by the bite of infected tick species. In the United States, these include the American dog tick *(Dermacentor variabilis)*, Rocky Mountain wood tick *(Dermacentor andersoni)*, and brown dog tick *(Rhipicephalus sanguineus)*.

Epidemiology

The CDC has noted that the geographic distribution of RMSF correlates with the type of tick found in that area. For example, American dog tick is found in the eastern, central, and Pacific coastal United States; the Rocky Mountain wood tick resides in the western United States. In 2005, the brown dog tick, a vector of RMSF in Mexico was implicated as a vector of this disease in a confined geographic area in Arizona. The cayenne tick *(Amblyomma cajennense)* is a common vector for RMSF in Central and South America and its range extends into the United States in Texas.

During 1997 to 2002, the estimated average annual incidence of RMSF, based on passive surveillance, was 2.2 cases/ million persons. More than half (56%) of reported cases of RMSF were from only five states—North Carolina, South Carolina, Tennessee, Oklahoma, and Arkansas—but cases have been reported from each of the contiguous 48 states, except Vermont and Maine. RMSF is also endemic throughout several countries in Central and South America, including Argentina, Brazil, Columbia, Costa Rica, Mexico, and Panama.

Signs and Symptoms

The first symptoms of RMSF typically begin 2 to 14 days after the bite of an infected tick. A tick bite is usually painless and

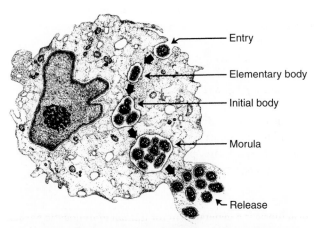

Figure 19-7 Schematic representation of the growth cycle of ehrlichiae in an infected cell. Elementary bodies (EBs; individual ehrlichiae) enter the leukocyte by phagocytosis and multiply. After 3 to 5 days, small numbers of tightly packed EBs are observable and are called initial bodies. During the next 7 to 12 days, additional growth and replication occur, and the initial bodies develop into mature inclusions, which appear by light microscopy as mulberry (morular) forms. This morula is a hallmark of ehrlichial infection. *(From McDade J: Ehrlichiosis—a disease of animals and human beings. J Infect Dis 161:609–617, 1990.)*

Entry

Elementary body

Initial body

Morula

Release

about 50% of those who develop RMSF do not remember being bitten. The disease frequently begins as a sudden onset of fever and headache. Most patients with RMSF (90%) have some type of rash during the course of the illness. The number and combination of symptoms vary greatly from person to person. Symptoms can include fever, rash (occurs 2 to 5 days after fever; may be absent in some cases), headache, nausea, and vomiting.

Diagnostic Evaluation

Blood specimens are not always useful for detection of the organism through PCR assay or culture. If the patient has a rash, PCR testing or immunohistochemical (IHC) staining can be performed on a skin biopsy taken from the rash site or on autopsy specimens. This can yield rapid results with good sensitivity (70%) when applied to tissue specimens collected during the acute phase of illness and before antibiotic treatment has been started, but a negative result should not be used to guide treatment decisions.

During RMSF infection, a patient's immune system develops antibodies to *R. rickettsii,* with detectable antibody titers usually observed within 7-10 days of illness onset. It is important to note that antibodies are not detectable in the first week of illness in 85% of patients; a negative test during this period does not rule out RMSF as a cause of illness.

The gold standard serologic test for diagnosis of RMSF is the IFA with *R. rickettsii* antigen, performed on two paired serum samples to demonstrate a significant (fourfold) rise in antibody titers. The first sample should be taken as early in the disease as possible, preferably in the first week of symptoms, and the second sample should be taken 2 to 4 weeks later.

Typically, in most RMSF cases, the first IgG IFA titer is low or negative and the second shows a significant (fourfold) increase in IgG antibody levels. IgM antibodies usually rise at the same time as IgG near the end of the first week of illness and remain elevated for months or even years. Also, IgM antibodies are less specific than IgG antibodies and more likely to yield a false-positive result. For these reasons, physicians requesting IgM serologic titers should also request a concurrent IgG titer.

Both IgM and IgG levels may remain elevated for months or longer after the disease has resolved or may be detected in persons who were previously exposed to antigenically related organisms. Up to 10% of currently healthy people in some areas may have elevated antibody titers due to past exposure to *R. rickettsii* or similar organisms. If only one sample is tested, it can be difficult to interpret, whereas two paired samples taken weeks apart that demonstrate a significant (fourfold) rise in antibody titer provide the best evidence for the correct diagnosis of RMSF.

Treatment and Prevention

The progression of the disease varies greatly. Patients who are treated early may recover quickly on outpatient medication, whereas those who experience a more severe course may require IV antibiotics, prolonged hospitalization, or intensive care.

Doxycycline is the first-line treatment for adults and children of all ages and is most effective if started before the fifth day of symptoms. Standard duration of treatment is 7 to 14 days.

BABESIOSIS

Starting in January 2011, cases of babesiosis from across the United States will have been formally reported to the CDC. Becoming nationally notifiable is an important step toward monitoring disease occurrence. Babesiosis is a preventable but sometimes life-threatening, tickborne, parasitic disease.

Etiology

Babesiosis is a rare, severe, and sometimes fatal tickborne disease caused by various types of *Babesia,* a microscopic parasite that infects red blood cells (Fig. 19-8). The causative organism of babesiosis was first described by Babes in 1888. In New England and the eastern United States, the disease is caused by *Babesia microti;* in California, it is caused by *Babesia equi.* In Europe, the disease is caused by *Babesia divergens* and *Babesia bovis. Babesia canis* has been found to be responsible for several cases in Mexico and France.

Epidemiology

B. microti is transmitted by tick *I. scapularis* in the northeastern United States. The larvae of the tick feed mainly on the white-footed mouse *(P. leucopus).* When larvae develop into nymphs and adults, they feed on the white-tailed deer *(Odocoileus virginianus),* but may also choose a human host.

Babesiosis is seen most frequently in older individuals, splenectomized patients, or immunocompromised patients. In the 1970s, cases were primarily reported during the spring, summer, and fall in coastal areas in the northeastern United States, especially Nantucket Island off the coast of

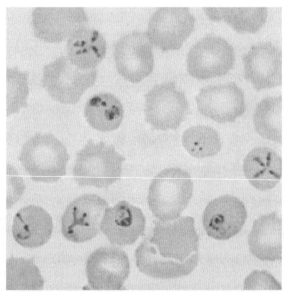

Figure 19-8 *Babesia* in red blood cells (1000x magnification). *(From Forbes BA, Sahm DF, Weissfeld AS: Bailey & Scott's diagnostic microbiology, ed 12, St Louis, 2007, Mosby.)*

Massachusetts and on Long Island in New York. Cases have also been reported in Wisconsin, California, Georgia, and Missouri, as well as in some European countries. The organism has also been transmitted via blood transfusion from asymptomatic donors.

The U.S. blood supply is vulnerable to transfusion-transmitted *Babesia*. Between 1979 and 2009, 159 cases of transfusion-related babesiosis were identified. Most (77%) of the identified cases occurred between 2000 to 2009.

Signs and Symptoms

The incubation period is approximately 7 to 21 days. The clinical presentation is variable, ranging from asymptomatic to rapidly progressive and sometimes fatal. Infections caused by *B. divergens* tend to be more severe (frequently fatal if not appropriately treated) than those caused by *B. microti* (clinical recovery usually occurs).

The disease can cause fever, fatigue, and hemolytic anemia lasting several days to several months. It may take from 1 to 8 weeks, sometimes longer, for symptoms to appear. The disease course is characterized by high fever, massive hemolysis, hemoglobinemia, and hemoglobinuria.

Diagnostic Evaluation

In symptomatic people, babesiosis usually is diagnosed by examining blood specimens under a microscope and observing *Babesia* parasites inside red blood cells. Multiple smears may need to be examined to detect low levels of parasites. Two rapid screening methods are used for the identification of *Babesia* organisms. The gold standard for their identification is the visualization of the **intraerythrocytic** organisms in thick or thin blood films. Sometimes, it is hard to distinguish *Babesia* spp. from *Plasmodium falciparum* (malaria) by blood smear examination. Also, some *Babesia* spp. (e.g., *B. microti*, *B. duncani*) appear identical; they cannot be distinguished from each other by microscopy.

Acute and convalescent antibody titers may be useful for diagnosis. A titer higher than 1:256 is considered diagnostic of acute infection. Only IgG antibody determinations are performed. PCR amplification can be used for diagnosis.

Molecular diagnosis can also be useful. In some infections with intraerythrocytic parasites, the morphologic characteristics observed on microscopic examination of blood smears do not allow an unambiguous differentiation between *Babesia* and *Plasmodium* organisms. In these cases, the diagnosis can be derived from molecular techniques such as PCR testing using the appropriate primers and single-step or the more sensitive nested PCR technique. In addition, molecular approaches are valuable for the investigation of new *Babesia* variants (or species) observed in recent human infections in the United States and Europe.

No *Babesia* test approved by the U.S. Food and Drug Administration (FDA) is currently available for screening prospective blood donors, who may feel healthy despite being infected. Some manufacturers are working with investigators at blood centers to develop FDA-approved tests for *Babesia* for donor screening.

Treatment and Prevention

Standardized treatments for babesiosis have not been developed. However, some drugs used for the treatment of malaria have been found to be effective in some patients with babesiosis.

Antimicrobial therapy is recommended for splenectomized or immunodeficient patients, older patients, and patients with severe infections. The usual regimen consists of a combination of clindamycin and oral quinine. An alternate treatment option is oral azithromycin and oral atovaquone. Exchange transfusion has been effective for patients with a high level of parasites (>10%), severe disease, or massive hemolysis.

Prevention requires vigilance when in tick-infested areas (see earlier discussion of Lyme disease prevention).

WEST NILE VIRUS

Etiology

West Nile virus (WNV) is a member of the Japanese encephalitis virus group of flaviviruses that cause febrile illness and encephalitis in human beings. WNV is a mosquito-borne pathogen.

Epidemiology

The virus has been in the United States since at least the summer of 1999. Figure 19-9 shows the U.S. distribution of WNV in 2011. If WNV infection is reported to the CDC from any area of a state, the entire state is shaded.

Signs and Symptoms

West Nile virus infection is characterized by fever, headache, fatigue, aches, and sometimes a rash. Illness can last from a few days to several weeks.

Diagnostic Evaluation

Historically, flavivirus infections have been diagnosed by serologic tests or virus isolation. IgM antibody is evident in most infected patients 7 to 8 days after the onset of symptoms. IgM antibody has been shown to persist for longer than 500 days in approximately 60% of cases. Most patients demonstrate IgG antibody in 3 to 4 weeks after infection.

Several molecular techniques are available for diagnosis. Molecular detection of WNV is used for prevention of transmission by blood transfusion and transplantation. Laboratory diagnosis of WNV infection is generally accomplished by testing of serum or CSF to detect virus-specific IgM and neutralizing antibodies.

Four FDA-approved WNV IgM ELISA kits from different manufacturers are commercially available in the United States. According to the package inserts, each of these kits is indicated for use on serum to aid in the presumptive laboratory diagnosis of WNV infection in patients with clinical symptoms of meningitis or encephalitis. The package inserts also state that all positive results obtained with any of the commercially available WNV test kits should be confirmed by

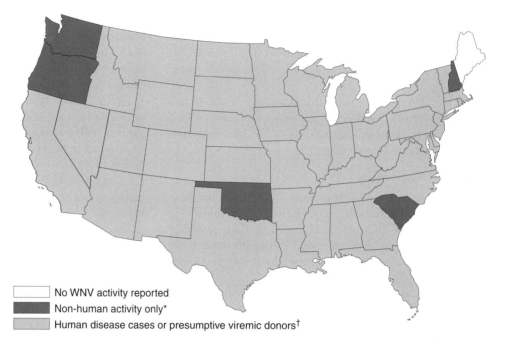

Figure 19-9 Distribution of West Nile virus activity in the United States reported to CDC's ArboNET system, by state, United States, 2011 (as of 11/1/2011). The map shows the distribution of nonhuman activity (light green) and human infections, including PVDs (dark green). If WNV infection is reported from any area of a state, that entire state is shaded. *(From Centers for Disease Control and Prevention, Atlanta [http://www.cdc.gov/ncidod/dvbid/westnile/Mapsactivity/surv&control11MapsAnybyState.htm].)*

☐ No WNV activity reported

■ Non-human activity only*

■ Human disease cases or presumptive viremic donors†

* Includes WNV veterinary disease cases and WNV infections in mosquitoes, birds, and sentinel animals.

† WNV activity in non-human species also might have been reported.

additional testing at a state health department laboratory or by the CDC.

In fatal cases, nucleic acid amplification, histopathology with immunohistochemistry and virus culture of autopsy tissues can also be useful. Only a few state laboratories or other specialized laboratories, including those at the CDC, can carry out this specialized testing.

Treatment and Prevention

There is no specific treatment for WNV infection. In patients with milder disease, symptoms resolve over time, although even healthy people have been sick for several weeks. In patients with more severe disease, hospitalization is usually required for supportive treatment, including IV fluids.

Prevention consists of avoiding mosquito bites.

CASE STUDY 1

A 42-year-old executive lived in New York City. Her company annually sponsored a Memorial Day weekend golf outing at a Long Island club. In early June, she noticed a solid, bright red spot on her left thigh. The spot was about 2 inches wide in the bright red area with an overall diameter of about 6 inches, including the surrounding pale area. The ensuing 11 months passed without further incident.

The following Memorial Day weekend, she was stung several times by bees. Both systemic and local reactions followed. About 1 week later, last year's red ring on the thigh reappeared. During this interval, she experienced fever, malaise, arthromyalgias, headache, and a stiff neck, but recovered completely.

In the fall, the woman noticed insidiously progressive fatigue, malaise, memory deficits, irritability, and inattentiveness to the demands of her job.

She visited a physician, but no abnormalities were noted, and she was referred to a Manhattan neurologist. The patient was eventually diagnosed as having Lyme disease.

Question

1. A major foci of Lyme disease infection is:
   a. Massachusetts to Maryland
   b. Virginia to Florida
   c. Florida to Louisiana
   d. Louisiana to North Dakota

See Appendix A for the answer to this question.

Critical Thinking Group Discussion Questions

1. Did the patient's residence or travel history suggest that she might have been exposed to Lyme disease?
2. Why did it take so long for the patient to develop symptoms of Lyme disease?

See instructor site ⊖**volve** for the discussion of the answers to these questions.

CASE STUDY 2

A 25-year-old graduate student visited his local family physician because of episodic arthromyalgias, sporadic global headaches, fatigue, irritability, and depression. Over the last several months, he had become seriously dysfunctional at work and home.

His residence and travel history revealed a week-long vacation on Cape Cod the previous summer. He could not recall any tick bites or skin lesions fitting the description of EM.

A laboratory test yielded a positive result and a 4-week course of doxycycline was initiated. Two weeks later, he noted significant improvement in symptoms, but 3 months later his previous symptoms recurred. His laboratory test was repeated and again was positive. A 1-month regimen of amoxicillin and probenecid was initiated. This time, there was no improvement. No neurologic findings were apparent. His joints were painful, but no overt synovitis was present. Two months after the second course of antibiotic, his Lyme test result was still positive and the patient was given 2 weeks of infusion therapy with ceftriaxone. His symptoms disappeared after this treatment.

Question

1. The Western Blot procedure is more definitive in the _____ stage of Lyme disease.
   a. Initial
   b. Early
   c. Mid
   d. Late

See Appendix A for the answer to this question.

Critical Thinking Group Discussion Questions

1. Why was the initial treatment regimen unsuccessful?
2. Why did the patient demonstrate a positive laboratory result, even though the usual treatment regimen was unsuccessful?

See instructor site ⊖volve for the discussion of the answers to these questions.

CASE STUDY 3

A 45-year-old man from upstate New York visited his physician because of a worsening headache, myalgia, arthralgia, and generalized weakness. He had been in good health until about 1 week before the appointment. A fever and myalgia began after the patient removed a small tick from his left thigh while on vacation in an area in which *B. burgdorferi* was endemic. In addition, the deer tick found in the area that he visited on vacation is the vector of Lyme disease, babesiosis and, most likely, anaplasmosis.

On physical examination, the patient had a slight fever. His thigh had a rash suggestive of EM. Laboratory results included a complete blood count and liver function tests. A skin scraping was obtained to culture *B. burgdorferi*. Buffy coat smears of peripheral blood were also requested.

The patient had a slight leukopenia, normal white blood cell differential, and normal hemoglobin and hematocrit values. His liver function test results were slightly abnormal. Wright-stained buffy coat smears revealed the presence of morulae of anaplasmosis. The patient was prescribed oral doxycycline twice daily for 14 days. Nine days after initiation of treatment, the patient improved greatly. Repeat laboratory test results were all within the normal reference range. His rash had resolved.

Question

1. *B. burgdorferi* and the agent of anaplasmosis (HE) can be demonstrate by:
   a. Isolation of both organisms from a clinical specimen
   b. Latex agglutination for Lyme disease
   c. ELISA testing
   d. Indirect fluorescent antibody (IFA) testing

See Appendix A for the answer to this question.

Critical Thinking Group Discussion Questions

1. Can the vector of *B. burgdorferi* and the agent of anaplasmosis be the same?
2. Is it important to determine whether one or both infections are present in the same host?
3. How can coinfection with *B. burgdorferi* and the agent of anaplasmosis be demonstrated in the laboratory?

See instructor site ⊖volve for the discussion of the answers to these questions.

CASE STUDY 4

This 73-year-old, previously healthy man had spent the previous summer on Martha's Vineyard. On returning to his home in Boston after Labor Day, he began to feel unusually tired and had difficulty breathing. He also reported that his urine had become dark brown several days after returning home.

On physical examination, the patient was found to be jaundiced and he had an enlarged spleen. A complete blood count, urinalysis, and blood chemistries were ordered. His total white blood cell count was normal but he had an increased percentage of segmented neutrophils. His hemoglobin and hematocrit values and platelet count were all below the normal reference range. He had hematuria and proteinuria. His liver function test results were greatly elevated. His renal function assays were also elevated. A follow-up Wright-stained peripheral blood smear revealed numerous *B. microti* organisms.

The patient was treated with quinine and the antibiotics clindamycin and doxycycline. He also received 2 units of packed red blood cells (RBCs) (MLT). Six days later, the patient was discharged from the hospital.

Question

1. If Babesia cannot be observed by microscopic examination of a peripheral blood smear from a patient who is ill but has no travel history to a malaria-endemic area, an acute infection with Babesia can be diagnosed by:
   a. Repeat blood smear examination in 4 weeks
   b. Testing acute and convalescent patient sera for a rise in the IgG antibody titer
   c. Use of a molecular technique to detect the microorganism
   d. Either b or c

See Appendix A for the answer to this question.

Critical Thinking Group Discussion Questions

1. Would the patient's travel history be suggestive of malaria or another bloodborne infectious disease?
2. What is the definitive diagnosis for babesiosis?
3. What additional laboratory tests are of diagnostic value?

See instructor site ⊖volve for the discussion of the answers to these questions.

CASE STUDY 5

A 35-year-old field biologist from central Missouri was positive for human immunodeficiency virus (HIV). Her work required that she spend a great deal of time in the woods in the surrounding areas. Although she was in good health despite the HIV positivity, she began having back pain, fever, chills, sweats, a productive cough, and extreme tiredness before her visit to the emergency room.

She was admitted to the hospital because her laboratory results demonstrated severe leukopenia and thrombocytopenia. Her liver function tests were also extremely abnormal. Later on the day of admission, renal failure developed. The patient died the next day.

Question

1. In suspected human monocytic ehrlichiosis (HME), if a patient has a supporting history and clinical symptoms, the diagnosis can be confirmed by a serologic titer greater than:
   a. 1:32
   b. 1:64
   c. 1:128
   d. 1:256

See Appendix A for the answer to this question.

Critical Thinking Group Discussion Questions

1. What was the cause of death?
2. What immunologic studies could be performed?
3. Is human monocytic ehrlichiosis a risk in the United States?

See instructor site ⊖volve for the discussion of the answers to these questions.

Rapid *Borrelia burgdorferi* Antibody Detection Assay

The PreVue *Borrelia burgdorferi* assay (Wampole Laboratories, Princeton, NJ) is a Clinical Laboratory Improvement Amendments (CLIA)–waived, single-use, rapid immunographic membrane assay for the qualitative presumptive (first step) detection of IgG and IgM antibodies to *B. burgdorferi* in human serum or whole blood. Positive results must be confirmed with a Western blot test. This procedure uses antigenic proteins developed by recombinant DNA techniques rather than a whole cell *B. burgdorferi* preparation. Antigenic proteins developed by recombinant DNA techniques allow for more accuracy. The false-positive rate is similar to that of other laboratory tests for Lyme disease.

The procedural protocol is posted on the ⊖volve website.

Limitations

The positive predictive value of the test depends on the likelihood of Lyme disease being present. Testing should only be performed when clinical symptoms are present or exposure is suspected.

Clinical Applications

A positive result should only be interpreted as initial evidence for detection of antibodies to *B. burgdorferi* with the recommendation for second-step testing before reporting results to a clinician. A negative result may have a low predictive value early in the infection.

CHAPTER HIGHLIGHTS

- Lyme disease (borreliosis) is caused by the tick-borne spirochete *Borrelia burgdorferi* and is a major health hazard for human beings and domestic animals.
- Lyme disease has been considered an emerging infectious disease because of the impact of changing environmental and socioeconomic factors (e.g., transformation of farmland into suburban woodlots favorable for deer and deer ticks).
- The basic features of Lyme disease are similar worldwide. In at least 60% to 80% of U.S. patients, it begins with a slowly expanding skin lesion, EM, at the site of the tick bite.

- Lyme borreliosis is a multisystem illness that primarily involves the skin, nervous system, heart, and joints. It usually begins during the summer months with EM and flulike symptoms.
- Cellular immune responses to *B. burgdorferi* antigens begin concurrently with early clinical illness, with increased spontaneous suppressor cell and reduced NK cell activity. Mononuclear cell, antigen-specific responses develop during spirochetal dissemination, and humoral (antibody) immune responses soon follow.
- Serodiagnostic tests are insensitive during the first several weeks of *Borrelia* infection. About 20% to 30% of U.S. patients have positive responses, usually of the IgM isotype, during this period, but by convalescence 2 to 4 weeks later, about 70% to 80% have seroreactivity even after antibiotic treatment. After about 1 month, most patients with active infection have IgG antibody responses. After antibiotic treatment, antibody titers fall slowly, but IgG and IgM responses may persist for years.
- Specific IgM or IgG antibodies against *B. burgdorferi* are usually not detectable in a patient's serum unless symptoms have been present for at least 2 to 4 weeks. In Lyme arthritis, test results (ANAs, RF, VDRL) are generally negative, and anti–*B. burgdorferi* antibodies (IgG) should be present.
- The most common laboratory assays for *B. burgdorferi* antibody detection include IFA, ELISA, and PreVue. Immunoblotting techniques can be used with ELISA. PreVue is the first presumptive step in testing individuals with suspected Lyme disease. Positive results must be confirmed by Western blot testing.
- Described first in the United States in 1986, tickborne rickettsiae of the genus *Ehrlichia* cause human illness. Ehrlichiosis is a general term for anaplasmosis and HME.
- Anaplasmosis diagnosis is confirmed by seroconversion (fourfold rise in acute/convalescent sera titer) or single serologic titer greater than 1:80 in patients with a history and symptoms. HME diagnosis is confirmed by seroconversion or serologic titer greater than 1:128.
- Babesiosis is a rare, severe, possibly fatal tickborne disease caused by *Babesia,* which infects RBCs.
- *Babesia* spp. are visualized as intraerythrocytic organisms in thick peripheral (rapid Field's test) or thin blood films. Acute and convalescent antibody titers may be useful; a titer higher than 1:256 is diagnostic of acute infection. Only IgG antibody determinations are performed. PCR amplification can be used for diagnosis.
- West Nile virus, a mosquito-borne virus present in the United States since at least 1999, causes febrile illness and encephalitis in human beings.
- In WNV, IgM antibody is evident in most infected patients 7 to 8 days after the onset of symptoms, persisting for more than 500 days in 60% of cases. Most patients demonstrate IgG antibody in 3 to 4 weeks after infection.

REVIEW QUESTIONS

1. Common vectors of Lyme disease include all the following except:
   a. *I. pacificus*
   b. *I. scapularis*
   c. *I. ricinus*
   d. *D. variabilis*

2. The only continent without Lyme disease is:
   a. Asia
   b. Europe
   c. Africa
   d. Antarctica

3. The primary reservoir in nature for *B. burgdorferi* is the:
   a. White-tailed deer
   b. White-footed mouse
   c. Lizard
   d. Meadowlark

4. The first *B. burgdorferi* antigen to elicit an antibody response is:
   a. Outer surface protein A
   b. Outer surface protein B
   c. Flagellar 41-kDa polypeptide
   d. 60-kDa polypeptide

5. On average, the incidence of infection following an *I. scapularis* tick bite in an endemic area is:
   a. 1%
   b. 3%
   c. 5%
   d. 10%

6. Erythema migrans:
   a. Occurs in all patients
   b. Harbors *B. burgdorferi* in the advancing edge
   c. Is easily distinguished from other erythemas
   d. Is more common in the winter months

7. The predominant symptoms of Lyme meningitis are:
   a. Severe headache and mild neck stiffness
   b. Aseptic meningitis and double vision
   c. Cranial nerve palsies and blurred vision
   d. Peripheral radiculoneuritis and peripheral neuropathy

8. Cardiac involvement in Lyme disease may include:
   a. Murmurs
   b. Conduction abnormalities
   c. Congestive heart failure
   d. Vasculitis

9. Ocular involvement in Lyme disease includes all the following except:
   a. Cranial nerve palsies
   b. Conjunctivitis
   c. Panophthalmitis with loss of vision
   d. Choroiditis with retinal detachment

10. Pregnancy in Lyme disease:
    a. Does not result in high fetal mortality
    b. Has been associated with transplacental infection
    c. Should be terminated because of maternal risk
    d. Is not associated with congenital abnormalities

11. The most useful test for distinguishing between true-positive and false-positive serologic test results is:
    a. Enzyme-linked immunosorbent assay
    b. Immunofluorescence assay
    c. Polymerase chain reaction
    d. T cell assay

12. Preventive methods include all the following except:
    a. Wearing light-colored clothes
    b. Tucking pants into socks
    c. Applying insect repellent to skin and clothes
    d. All of the above

13. Lyme disease, the most common tickborne disease in the United States, is a major health hazard for:
    a. Dogs
    b. Horses and cattle
    c. Humans
    d. All of the above

14. Lyme disease is a _____ type of infection.
    a. Bacterial
    b. Parasitic
    c. Viral
    d. Fungal

15. The first Native American case of what would later be called Lyme disease occurred in:
    a. Connecticut
    b. Wisconsin
    c. Florida
    d. New York

16-19. Fill in the blanks in the chart below, choosing from the following answers.

Possible answers for question 16:

a. 3 days
b. 1 week
c. 4 weeks
d. 3 months

Possible answers for question 17:

a. Neurologic
b. Rheumatoid
c. Cutaneous
   (e.g., erythema migrans)
d. Cardiac

Possible answers for question 18:

a. Hours to weeks
b. Days to weeks
c. Weeks to months
d. Weeks to years

Possible answers for question 19:

a. Arthritis
b. Lyme carditis
c. Transplacental transmission
d. Lymphocytoma

16-19. Fill in the blanks: Clinical features of Lyme disease

Stage	Length of Time	Common Signs and Symptoms
I	16. _____ (median)	17. _____ manifestation after infection
II	Follows a variable latent period	Target organs and systems can manifest abnormalities.
III	18. _____ after infection	19. _____, late neurologic complications

20. Unlike some procedures, the polymerase chain reaction (PCR) assay can be used to detect Lyme disease–causing organisms in:
    a. Urine
    b. Cerebrospinal fluid
    c. Synovial fluid
    d. Blood

21 and 22. Fill in the blanks, choosing from the possible answers (a-d).

Antigen detection systems in Lyme disease testing screen for _____ (21) rather than for _____ (22) associated with the infection.
    a. Antibody
    b. Microorganisms
    c. Antigenic products
    d. An infected tick

23. A patient who has a specific Lyme disease–associated manifestation may be treated with:
    a. Vaccination
    b. Interferon
    c. Antibiotic
    d. Analgesic

24. *Ehrlichia* spp. belong to the same family as the organism that causes:
    a. Lyme disease
    b. Rocky Mountain spotted fever
    c. Toxoplasmosis
    d. Infectious mononucleosis

25. One of the most common physical findings in adults with ehrlichiosis is:
    a. Hives
    b. Fever
    c. Erythema migrans
    d. Nausea

26. Definitive diagnosis of ehrlichiosis requires:
    a. A complete blood count
    b. Detection of the presence of lymphocytopenia
    c. Acute and convalescent serum antibody titers
    d. Direct microscopic observation of inclusions in leukocytes

27. In human granulocytic ehrlichiosis (anaplasmosis), the diagnosis is confirmed by seroconversion or by a single serologic titer of _____ in patients with a supporting history and clinical symptoms.
    a. 1:2
    b. 1:16
    c. 1:80
    d. 1:160

28. In the eastern United States, babesiosis is caused by:
    a. *B. microti*
    b. *B. canis*
    c. *B. bovis*
    d. *B. equi*

29. Babesiosis is characterized by:
    a. Fever
    b. Fatigue
    c. Hemolytic anemia
    d. All of the above

30. *Babesia* organisms can be found in:
    a. Peripheral blood
    b. Sputum
    c. Synovial fluid
    d. Various exudates

31. West Nile virus causes:
    a. Encephalitis
    b. Polio
    c. Measles
    d. Arthritis

32. West Nile virus is transmitted by:
    a. Dogs
    b. Cats
    c. Rats
    d. Mosquitoes

BIBLIOGRAPHY

Centers for Disease Control and Prevention: Lyme disease, 2011, http://www.cdc.gov/lyme.

Centers for Disease Control and Prevention: Tick-borne relapsing fever (TBRF), 2011, http://www.cdc.gov/relapsing-fever.

Centers for Disease Control and Prevention: Ticks, 2011, http://www.cdc.gov/ticks.

Coon D, Versalovic J: Three tick-borne diseases in the northeastern United States: Lyme disease, babesiosis, and ehrlichiosis, TurnAround Times Clin Lab Rev 9:5–10, 2001.

LYMEVAX https://animalhealth.pfizer.com/sites/pahweb/pages/global.aspx: retrieved August 12, 2012.

Niedrig M, Linke S, Zeller H, Drosten C: First international proficiency study on West Nile virus molecular detection, Clin Chem 52:1851–1854, 2006.

Pantanowitz L, Ballesteros E, DeGirolami P: Laboratory diagnosis of babesiosis, Lab Med 32:184–186, 2001.

Steere AC: Lyme disease, N Engl J Med 345:115–123, 2001.

Sullivan E: Food and Drug Administration extends deferral period for blood donors with West Nile virus, Lab Med 36:692–693, 2005.

Vannier E, Krause PJ: Human Babesiosis, NEJM 366(25):2397–2407, June, 2012.

Wampole Laboratories: Wampole PreVue package insert, 2011, http://www.CLIAwaived.comhttp://www.cliawaived.com/web/items/pdf/INV-63220_PreVue_B-Burgdorferi_Testing~1098file1.pdf.

Wormser GP: Early Lyme disease, N Engl J Med 354:2794–2801, 2006.

CHAPTER 20

Toxoplasmosis

Learning Objectives

At the conclusion of this chapter, the reader should be able to:

- Describe the etiology and epidemiology of toxoplasmosis.
- Explain the signs and symptoms of acquired and congenital toxoplasmosis infection.
- Discuss the immunologic manifestations and diagnostic evaluation of toxoplasmosis, including the quantitative determination of IgM antibodies to *Toxoplasma gondii.*

- Analyze a case study related to toxoplasmosis.
- Correctly answer case study related multiple choice questions.
- Be prepared to participate in a discussion of critical thinking questions.
- Describe the principle, interpretation, and limitations of the TORCH procedure.
- Correctly answer end of chapter review questions.

Key Terms

congenital	seroprevalence	transplacental
definitive host	titer	

ETIOLOGY

Toxoplasmosis is a widespread disease in human beings and animals. This infection is caused by *Toxoplasma gondii*, recognized as a tissue coccidian.

EPIDEMIOLOGY

T. gondii was first discovered in a North African rodent and has been observed in numerous birds and mammals worldwide, including human beings. It is a parasite of cosmopolitan distribution able to develop in a wide variety of vertebrate hosts.

Human infections are common in many parts of the world. The prevalence of infection in adults ranges from less than 10% to more than 90%; higher prevalences tend to occur at lower elevations and in latitudes closer to the equator. The highest recorded rate (93%) was in Parisian women who preferred undercooked or raw meat; a 50% rate of occurrence was documented in the children of these women. Toxoplasma infection rates vary around the world. In the United States, it's about 10% to 15%, while rates in Europe and Brazil are much higher, around 50% to 80%. These are only estimates. Calculating exact rates is difficult because most infected people don't have any symptoms.

Toxoplasmosis is not passed from person-to-person, except in cases of mother to child (**congenital**) transmission and blood transfusion or organ transplantation. People typically become infected by three principal routes of transmission:

- Foodborne
- Animal to human (zoonotic)
- Mother to child (congenital)

The **definitive host** is the house cat and other members of the Felidae family (Fig. 20-1). Domestic cats are a source of the disease because oocysts are often present in their feces. Accidental ingestion of oocysts by human beings and animals, including the cat, produces a proliferative infection in the body tissues. Fecal contamination of food or water, soiled hands, inadequately cooked or infected meat, and raw milk can be major sources of human infection. The risk for infection is higher in many developing and tropical countries, especially when people eat undercooked meat, drink untreated water, or are extensively exposed to soil.

Organ transplant recipients can become infected by receiving an organ from a *Toxoplasma*-positive donor. Transfusion-transmitted toxoplasmosis has been associated with the use of leukocyte concentrates. Patients at risk are those receiving immunosuppressive agents or corticosteroids. Laboratory

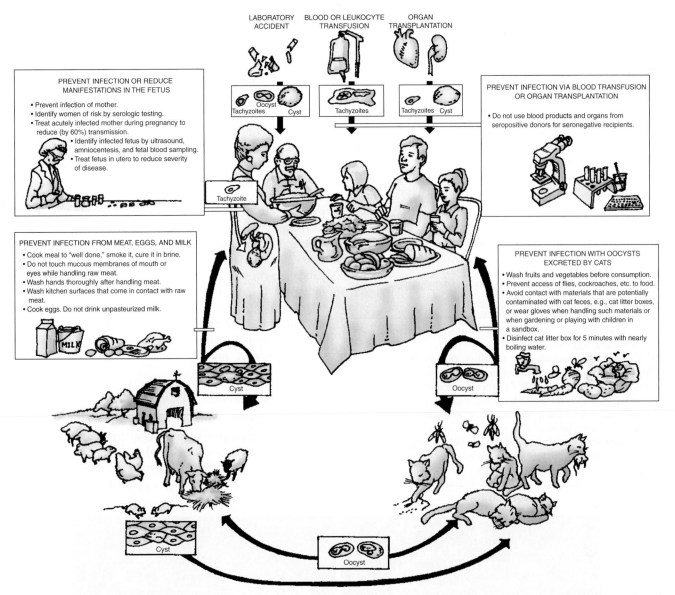

Figure 20-1 Life cycle of *Toxoplasma gondii*. *(Adapted from Katz SL, Gershon AA, Wilfert CM, Krugman S editors: Infectious diseases of children, ed 9, St Louis, 1992, Mosby.)*

workers who handle infected blood can also acquire infection through accidental inoculation.

Transplacental Transmission

All mammals, including human beings, can transmit the infection transplacentally. **Transplacental** transmission usually takes place in the course of an acute but inapparent or undiagnosed maternal infection. Evidence has shown that the number of infants born in the United States each year with congenital *T. gondii* infection is considerably higher than the 3000 previously estimated. It is estimated that 6 of 1000 pregnant women in the United States will acquire primary infection with *Toxoplasma* during a 9-month gestation. Approximately 45% of women who acquire the infection for the first time and who are not treated will give birth to congenitally infected infants. Consequently, the expected incidence of congenital toxoplasmosis is 2.7/1000 live births.

It is recommended that all pregnant women be tested for toxoplasmosis immunity. If a patient is susceptible, screening should be repeated during pregnancy and at delivery. Prevention of infection in pregnant women should be practiced to avert congenital toxoplasmosis (Box 20-1). To further prevent infection of the fetus, women at risk should be identified by serologic testing and pregnant women with primary infection should receive drug therapy.

Seroprevalence

Seroprevalence (antibody to *T. gondii*) varies considerably in the general population. It ranges from 96% in Western Europe to 10% to 40% in the United States. Of patients with acquired immunodeficiency syndrome (AIDS) who are seropositive for *T. gondii*, approximately 25% to 50% will develop toxoplasmic encephalitis (meningoencephalitis). In areas with a lower seroprevalence, such as the United States, the percentage of AIDS patients who develop toxoplasmic encephalitis is lower (5% to 10%).

SIGNS AND SYMPTOMS

In adults and children other than newborns, toxoplasmosis is usually asymptomatic. A generalized infection probably occurs. Although spontaneous recovery follows acute febrile disease, the organism can localize and multiply in any organ of the body or the circulatory system.

Toxoplasma can be harmful to individuals with suppressed immune systems. Toxoplasmic encephalitis in AIDS patients may result in death, even when treated (Fig. 20-2). Persons at risk can be identified by screening patients positive for human immunodeficiency virus (HIV) for antibody to *T. gondii.*

Box 20-1	Methods for Prevention of Congenital Toxoplasmosis

Avoid touching mucous membranes of the mouth and eye while handling raw meat.
Wash hands thoroughly after handling raw meat.
Wash kitchen surfaces that come in contact with raw meat.
Cook meat to >18.8° C (65.8° F); smoke it or cure it in brine.
Wash fruits and vegetables before consumption.
Prevent access of flies, cockroaches, and other insects to fruits and vegetables.
Avoid contact with or wear gloves when handling materials that are potentially contaminated with cat feces (e.g., cat litter boxes) and when gardening.

Acquired Infection

When seen, symptoms are frequently mild. Toxoplasmosis can simulate infectious mononucleosis, with chills, fever, headache, lymphadenopathy, and extreme fatigue. Primary infection may be promoted by immunosuppression. A chronic form of toxoplasmic lymphadenopathy exists. *T. gondii* presents a special problem in immunosuppressed or otherwise compromised hosts. Some of these patients have experienced reactivation of a latent toxoplasmosis. These patients have included those with Hodgkin's and non-Hodgkin's lymphoma, as well as recipients of organ transplants.

Reactivation of cerebral toxoplasmosis is not uncommon in patients with AIDS, in whom toxoplasmic meningoencephalitis is almost always a reactivation of a preexisting latent infection, most often occurring when the total CD4 count falls below 100×10^9/L. *T. gondii*–seropositive, HIV-infected patients may develop toxoplasmic encephalitis because of the following: (1) genetic susceptibility in the human immune response to *T. gondii;* (2) subtle differences in patients' immunocompromised status; (3) differences in the virulence of individual strains of *T. gondii;* (4) possible recurrent infections with different strains; and (5) variable coinfections with other opportunistic pathogens.

Congenital Infection

Toxoplasma can be harmful to fetuses whose mothers become infected during pregnancy. Congenital toxoplasmosis can result in central nervous system (CNS) malformation or prenatal mortality. In infants who are serologically positive at birth, many fail to display neurologic, ophthalmic, or generalized

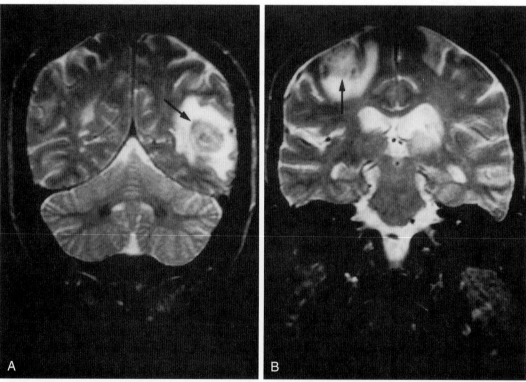

Figure 20-2   Toxoplasmic meningoencephalitis. Shown are magnetic resonance imaging (MRI) brain scans of patients with AIDS. *Arrows* indicate areas infected with toxoplasmosis.

illness at birth. Toxoplasmosis acquired in utero can result in blindness, encephalomyelitis, mental retardation, convulsions, and death in infected neonates.

In as many as 75% of congenitally infected newborns not serologically diagnosed at birth, the disease remains dormant, only to be discovered when other symptoms become apparent, such as chorioretinitis, unilateral blindness, and severe neurologic sequelae.

IMMUNOLOGIC MANIFESTATIONS

Both clinical and laboratory findings in toxoplasmosis resemble those of infectious mononucleosis. An increased number of variant lymphocytes can be seen on a peripheral blood smear.

The diagnosis can be established serologically by detecting a marked elevation of *Toxoplasma* antibodies. Antibodies are demonstrable within the first 2 weeks after infection, rising to high levels early in the infection and then falling slightly, but persisting at an elevated level for many months before declining to low levels after many years. The best evidence for current infection is a significant change on two appropriately timed specimens (paired acute and convalescent specimens), in which both tests are done in the same laboratory at the same time.

If a significant level of *T. gondii* immunoglobulin M (IgM) antibody is detected, it may indicate a current or recent infection. The presence of IgM to *T. gondii* in an adult indicates an infection, but low levels of IgM antibodies occasionally may persist for more than 12 months after infection. The Centers for Disease Control and Prevention (CDC) recommends that any equivocal or positive result should be retested using a different assay from another reference laboratory specializing in toxoplasmosis testing.

DIAGNOSTIC EVALUATION

The diagnosis of toxoplasmosis is typically made by serologic testing. A test that measures immunoglobulin G (IgG) is used to determine whether a person has been infected. If it is necessary to try to estimate the time of infection, which is of particular importance for pregnant women, a test that measures IgM is also used along with other tests, such as an avidity test.

Diagnosis can be made by direct observation of the parasite in stained tissue sections, cerebrospinal fluid (CSF), or other biopsy material. These techniques are used less frequently because of the difficulty of obtaining these specimens.

Parasites can also be isolated from blood or other body fluids (e.g., CSF) but this process can be difficult and requires considerable time. Molecular techniques that can detect the parasite's DNA in the amniotic fluid can be useful in cases of possible mother to child (congenital) transmission.

The diagnosis of toxoplasmosis can be established by the following:

- Serologic tests (Table 20-1)
- Polymerase chain reaction (PCR)
- Indirect fluorescent antibody (IFA)
- Isolation of the organism

Serologic Tests

The mainstay of diagnosis of *T. gondii* infection is serologic testing. A relatively high proportion of people have antibodies to *T. gondii*, which makes interpretation of serologic test results difficult. Assays for different isotypes of antibodies have been developed to support the diagnosis of an acute or chronic *T. gondii* infection.

For the detection of IgM antibodies to *T. gondii*, a variety of procedures are available—IFA, automated enzyme-linked immunosorbent assay (ELISA), and chemiluminescent immunoassay for IgM and IgG antibodies.

IgM Antibodies

The IgM assay was widely used in the past, but this is not recommended for routine use in adults because it may yield frequent false-positive or false-negative results, particularly in pregnant women, immunocompromised patients, and patients from areas in which *Toxoplasma* infection is highly endemic. IgM antibodies tend to appear earlier and decline more rapidly than IgG antibodies. Persistently elevated IgM-specific antibody **titers** after the initial infection can lead to false-positive results and difficulty in interpreting these tests.

In patients with recently acquired infection, IgM *T. gondii* antibodies are detected initially and, in most cases, these titers become negative within a few months. In some patients, however, positive IgM *T. gondii*–specific titers can be observed during the chronic stage of the infection. IgM antibodies have been reported to persist as long as 12 years after the acute infection. However, their persistence does not seem to be clinically relevant and these patients should be considered chronically infected.

Clinicians should be cautious when using IgM antibody levels in prenatal screening. Any positive result in a pregnant patient confirmed positive by a second reference laboratory

Table 20-1	Serologic Evaluation of Toxoplasmosis	
Test	**Method**	**Recommended Use**
T. gondii antibodies, IgG and IgM	Chemiluminescent immunoassay*	First-line test in endemic areas for identifying *T. gondii* infection in pregnant women; diagnosis of opportunistic infections in immunocompromised hosts
T. gondii by PCR		Confirmation of toxoplasmosis infection in immunocompromised hosts

Adapted from Associated Regional and University Pathologists (ARUP): Reference test guide, 2012 (http://www. aruplab.com).
*Note: The CDC suggests that equivocal or positive results be retested using a different assay from another reference laboratory specializing in toxoplasmosis testing (IgG Sabin dye test, IgM ELISA, reflex to avidity and/or other tests).

should be evaluated by amniocentesis and PCR testing for *T. gondii*. A negative result does not rule out the presence of PCR inhibitors in the patient specimen or *T. gondii* DNA concentrations below the level of detection of the assay.

The U.S. Food and Drug Administration (FDA) has recommended that sera with positive IgM test results obtained at nonreference laboratories should be sent to a *Toxoplasma* reference laboratory. After IgM-positive sera undergo confirmatory testing, the results are interpreted as the following: (1) a recently acquired infection; (2) an infection acquired in the past; or (3) a false-positive result.

IgG Antibodies

IgG antibodies appear 1 to 2 weeks after the initial infection, peak after about 6 to 8 weeks, decline gradually over the next 1 to 2 years and, in some cases, persist for life.

Sabin-Feldman Dye Test. IgG antibodies are primarily measured by the Sabin-Feldman dye test (DT), considered the gold standard. The DT is a sensitive and specific neutralization test in which live organisms are lysed in the presence of complement and the patient's IgG *T. gondii*–specific antibody. IgG antibodies usually appear within 1 to 2 weeks of the infection, peak within 1 to 2 months, fall at variable rates, and usually persist for life. The titer does not correlate with the severity of illness. This test is available mainly in reference laboratories.

A negative test result practically rules out prior *T. gondii* exposure—unless the patient is hypogammaglobulinemic. In a small number of patients, IgG antibodies might not be detected within 2 to 3 weeks after initial exposure to the parasite. Rare cases of toxoplasmic chorioretinitis and toxoplasmic encephalitis have been documented in immunocompromised patients negative for *T. gondii*–specific IgG antibodies.

IFA Test. This test uses killed organisms as a substrate, with patient serum assayed for activity against them. IFA is used widely because it measures the same antibodies as the Sabin-Feldman DT and results parallel DT results. False-positive results may occur with sera that contain antinuclear antibodies; false-negative results may occur when using sera from patients with low titers of IgG antibody.

Avidity Test. The functional affinity of specific IgG antibodies is initially low after primary antigenic challenge and increases during subsequent weeks and months. Protein-denaturing reagents are used to dissociate the antibody-antigen complex. The avidity result is determined using the ratios of antibody titration curves of urea-treated and untreated serum.

The avidity test can be used as an additional confirmatory diagnostic tool in patients with a positive or equivocal IgM test or with an acute or equivocal pattern in the differential agglutination test (AC/HS test). Its highest value is observed when laboratory test results reveal high–IgG avidity antibodies and the serum is obtained during the time window of exclusion of acute infection for a particular method (range, 12 to 16 weeks). Low– or equivocal–IgG avidity antibody results should not be interpreted as diagnostic of recently acquired infection. These low- or equivocal-avidity antibodies can persist for months to 1 year or longer.

Studies of the avidity of IgG in pregnant women who have seroconverted during gestation have shown that women with high-avidity test results are infected with *T. gondii* at least 3 to 5 months earlier (time to conversion from low- to high-avidity antibodies varies with the method used). Because low-avidity antibodies may persist for many months, their presence does not necessarily indicate recently acquired infection.

Polymerase Chain Reaction

PCR amplification is used to detect *T. gondii* DNA in body fluids and tissues. The PCR assay can be used to detect the presence or absence of *T. gondii* DNA in fresh or frozen biopsy tissue, CSF, amniotic fluid, serum, or plasma. A negative result does not rule out the presence of PCR inhibitors in the specimen or *T. gondii* DNA concentrations below the level of detection by the assay.

A PCR test performed on amniotic fluid has revolutionized the diagnosis of fetal *T. gondii* infection by enabling an early diagnosis to be made, which avoids the use of more invasive procedures on the fetus.

Histologic Diagnosis

Demonstration of tachyzoites in tissue sections or smears of body fluid (e.g., CSF, amniotic fluid, bronchoalveolar lavage fluid) establishes the diagnosis of the acute infection. The immunoperoxidase method is applicable to unfixed or formalin-fixed paraffin-embedded tissue sections.

A rapid and technically simple method is the detection of *T. gondii* in air-dried, Wright-Giemsa–stained slides of centrifuged (e.g., cytocentrifuged) sediment of CSF or of brain aspirate, or in impression smears of biopsy tissue. Multiple tissue cysts near an inflammatory necrotic lesion indicate acute infection or reactivation of latent infection.

Cell Culture

Detection of *T. gondii* in the blood may represent a major advance in the diagnosis of toxoplasmosis in patients with AIDS. A cell culture method for the growth of *T. gondii* has been developed using monocytes. After 4 days, parasites in the culture are revealed by immunofluorescence with an anti-P30 monoclonal antibody. A quantitative and qualitative analysis by cytofluorometry can then be performed on the cultured cells.

CASE STUDY

History and Physical Examination

A 24-year-old woman with a history of AIDS presents for evaluation of left-sided weakness. She has also been experiencing headaches and seizures and others have observed an alteration in her mental status.

The patient's medical history is notable for an episode of *Pneumocystis jiroveci (previously called Pneumocystis carinii)* pneumonia, primary syphilis treated with penicillin 5 years ago, and occasional thrush. She takes zidovudine and monthly aerosolized pentamidine for *Pneumocystis*

CASE STUDY—Cont'd

prophylaxis. An urgent computed tomography (CT) scan of the head shows two 1-cm lesions in the right basal ganglia, enhanced with IV contrast media.

Laboratory Data

CD4 cell count: 50×10^9/L
Rapid plasma reagin (RPR): Positive at 1:2
Toxoplasmosis IgG: Positive
Toxoplasmosis IgM: Negative

Questions

1. In cases of Toxoplasmosis, diagnosis can be established by:
   a. Isolation of the organism
   b. PCR
   c. IFA
   d. All of the above
2. In cases of current Toxoplasmosis infection, the earliest that Toxoplasma antibodies can be detected is _____ after infection.
   a. 48 hours
   b. 72 hours
   c. Within the first 2 weeks
   d. Within the first 6 months

See Appendix A for the answers to these questions.

Critical Thinking Group Discussion Questions

1. What is the most common cause of lesions in the brain?
2. What is the source of this infection?
3. Is this a newly acquired infection?
4. How can the patient be treated?
5. Should pregnant women be tested for this microorganism?

See instructor site ⊝volve for the discussion of the answers to these questions.

Rapid TORCH Procedure

Principle

The ImmunoDOT TORCH test (GenBio, San Diego, Calif) uses an enzyme immunoassay (EIA) dot technique for the detection of antibodies. The antigens are dispensed as discrete dots onto a solid membrane. After adding specimen to a reaction vessel, an assay strip is inserted, allowing patient antibodies reactive with the test antigen to bind to the strip's solid support membrane. In the second stage, the reaction is enhanced by the removal of nonspecifically bound materials. During the third stage, alkaline phosphatase–conjugated antihuman antibodies are allowed to react with bound patient antibodies. Finally, the strip is transferred to an enzyme substrate reagent that reacts with bound alkaline phosphatase to produce an easily seen distinct dot.

Refer to the ⊝volve website for the procedural protocol.

Interpretation

Negative Results

If no dot is seen or a dot is difficult to see, interpret the results as negative. A negative result for each antigen demonstrates little or no antibody presence, indicating that the patient may be susceptible to primary infection.

Positive Results

This is a dot with an easily seen distinct border that is visible in the center of the window. The outer perimeter of the window must be white to pale gray. A positive result for each antigen demonstrates the presence of that antibody. The presence of *T. gondii* indicates previous or current infection and immunity to future primary infection.

Limitations

If testing of a sample occurs less than 5 days following primary infection, detectable specific antibody may not yet be present.

This test is a qualitative screening procedure and cannot be used to detect increases in antibody titer or to diagnose active infection. The assay is not intended for final selection of cytomegalovirus (CMV)–negative donors for blood transfusion or organ transplantation. The test may be used to screen potential recipients. Antibody screening in the compromised host must be interpreted with caution. The antibody response of an immunosuppressed individual may differ from that of the immunocompetent host. Because maternal antibody will be detected in infants younger than 1 year, the assessment of previous infections or of the immune status of infants is inappropriate using this test alone.

CHAPTER HIGHLIGHTS

- Toxoplasmosis is a widespread disease in human beings and animals caused by *Toxoplasma gondii*, often found in cat feces.
- Fecal contamination of food or water, soiled hands, inadequately cooked or infected meat, and raw milk are sources of human infection. All mammals, including human beings, can transmit the infection transplacentally.
- In adults and children other than newborns, the disease is usually asymptomatic. A generalized infection probably occurs.
- Although spontaneous recovery follows acute febrile disease, the organism can multiply in any organ of the body or circulatory system.
- Congenital toxoplasmosis can result in CNS malformation or prenatal mortality.
- *T. gondii* is difficult to culture and diagnosis must be supported by serologic methods to determine levels of IgM and IgG antibodies to *T. gondii*. The presence of IgM antibodies to *T. gondii* in an adult indicates active infection. Detection of IgM also suggests active infection in the newborn.
- Serologic tests include IFA, chemiluminescent immunoassay, and PCR.

REVIEW QUESTIONS

1. Toxoplasmosis is a _____ infection.
   a. Bacterial
   b. Mycotic
   c. Parasitic
   d. Viral

2. The definitive host of *T. gondii* is the:
   a. Horse
   b. Pig
   c. Dog
   d. Domestic cat

3. All the following are specific methods for preventing congenital toxoplasmosis except:
   a. Avoid touching mucous membranes while handling raw meat.
   b. Wash hands thoroughly after handling raw meat.
   c. Eliminate food contamination by flies, cockroaches, and other insects.
   d. Dispose of fecally contaminated cat litter into plastic garbage bags.

4. The presence of IgM antibodies to *T. gondii* in an adult is indicative of a(an):
   a. Carrier state
   b. Active infection
   c. Chronic infection
   d. Latent disease

5. All the following characteristics are correct regarding toxoplasmosis except:
   a. It is recognized as a tissue coccidian.
   b. Domestic dogs are a source of the disease.
   c. It can be transmitted by infected blood.
   d. It can be transmitted transplacentally.

6. Toxoplasmosis is a serious health threat to:
   a. AIDS patients
   b. Adults
   c. Children older than 2 years
   d. Older patients

7. Congenital toxoplasmosis can cause:
   a. Congenital heart disease
   b. Central nervous system malformation
   c. Urinary tract infections
   d. Muscular disorders

8. Antibodies to *T. gondii* are demonstrable _____ after infection.
   a. 3 to 5 days
   b. Within 10 days
   c. Within 2 weeks
   d. Within 4 weeks

9. The method of choice for detecting IgM antibodies in toxoplasmosis is:
   a. Enzyme-linked immunosorbent assay (ELISA)
   b. Indirect fluorescent antibody (IFA)
   c. Indirect hemagglutination (IHA)
   d. Complement fixation (CF)

BIBLIOGRAPHY

Associated Regional and University Pathologists (ARUP): Reference test guide, 2012, http://www. aruplab.com.

Beaman MH, Luft BJ, Remington JS: Prophylaxis for toxoplasmosis in AIDS, Ann Intern Med 117:163–164, 1992.

Bruce-Chwatt LJ: Transfusion associated parasitic infections. In Bruce-Chwatt LJ, editor: Infection, immunity, and blood transfusion, New York, 1985, Alan R Liss.

Forbes BA, Sahm DF, Weissfeld AS: Bailey and Scott's diagnostic microbiology, ed 12, St Louis, 2007, Mosby.

Hill DE, Chirukandoth S, Dubey JP: Biology and epidemiology of Toxoplasma gondii in man and animals, Anim Health Res Rev 6:41–61, 2005.

Holmes J: MIT researchers study the danger of toxoplasma parasites, MIT News: January 4, 2011. Retrieved August 13, 2012, www.mit.edu.

Jones JL, Schulkin J, Maguire JH: Therapy for common parasitic diseases in pregnancy in the United States: a review and a survey of obstetrician/gynecologists' level of knowledge about these diseases, Obstet Gynecol Surv 60:386–393, 2005.

Kravetz JD, Federman DG: Toxoplasmosis in pregnancy, Am J Med 118:212–216, 2005.

Lopez A, Dietz VJ, Wilson M, et al: Preventing congenital toxoplasmosis, MMWR Recomm Rep 49(RR-2):59–68, 2000.

Montoya JG: Laboratory diagnosis of Toxoplasma gondii infection and toxoplasmosis, J Infect Dis 185(Suppl 1):S73–S82, 2002.

Montoya JG, Kovacs JA, Remington JS: Toxoplasma gondii. In Mandell GL, Bennett JE, Dolin R, editors: Principles and practice of infectious diseases, ed 6, Philadelphia, 2005, Churchill Livingstone, pp 3170–3198.

Montoya JG, Liesenfeld O: Toxoplasmosis, Lancet 363:1965–1976, 2004.

Montoya JG, Rosso F: Diagnosis and management of toxoplasmosis, Clin Perinatol 32:705–726, 2005.

Tirard V, Niel G, Rosenheim M, et al: Diagnosis of toxoplasmosis in patients with AIDS by isolation of the parasite from the blood, N Engl J Med 324:634, 1991.

Turgeon ML: Clinical hematology, ed 5, Philadelphia, 2012, Lippincott Williams & Wilkins.

Cytomegalovirus

Learning Objectives

At the conclusion of this chapter, the reader should be able to:

- Discuss the etiology and epidemiology of acquired, latent, and congenital cytomegalovirus (CMV) infection.
- Explain the signs and symptoms of acquired and congenital CMV infections.
- Describe the immunologic manifestations of CMV.
- Identify and explain the serologic markers and diagnostic evaluation of CMV.
- Discuss the principles and applications of passive latex agglutination and other quantitative determinations of IgM and IgG antibodies.

- Analyze a CMV case study.
- Correctly answer case study related multiple choice questions.
- Be prepared to participate in a discussion of critical thinking questions.
- Describe the principle, reference range, sources of error, limitations, and clinical applications of Latex Agglutination for Antibodies to CMV.
- Describe the principle and clinical applications of antibody detection to CMV.
- Correctly answer end of chapter review questions.

Key Terms

acquired
early antigens

immediate-early antigens
latent infection

primary infection
reactivated infection

ETIOLOGY

Cytomegalovirus (CMV) is a ubiquitous human viral pathogen. The first descriptive report of histologic changes characteristic of those now associated with CMV infection was originally published in 1904, when protozoan-like cells in the lungs, kidneys, and liver of a syphilitic fetus were seen. It was not until 1956 and 1957 that CMV was isolated in the laboratory. Actual isolation of the virus after transfusion, and observation of elevated antibody titers, occurred in 1966.

Human CMV is classified as a member of the herpes family of viruses (herpesviruses). All the herpesviruses are relatively large, enveloped DNA viruses that undergo a replicative cycle involving DNA expression and nucleocapsid assembly within the nucleus. The viral structure gains an envelope when the virus buds through the nuclear membrane, which in turn is altered to contain specific viral proteins.

Although the herpesviruses produce diverse clinical diseases, they share the basic characteristic of being cell associated.

The requirements for cell association vary, but herpesviruses may spread from cell to cell, presumably via intercellular bridges and in the presence of antibody in the extracellular phase. CMV spreads to the lymphoid tissues and proceeds to circulate to systemic lymph nodes. The virus finally comes to rest in the epithelial cells of many tissues. This common characteristic may play a role in the ability of these viruses to produce subclinical infections that can be reactivated under appropriate stimuli.

EPIDEMIOLOGY

CMV infection is endemic worldwide, with most urban adults demonstrating evidence of infection; 50% to 80% of U.S. adults are infected with CMV by age 40 years. The prevalence of CMV seropositivity increases steadily with age. CMV is found in all geographic and socioeconomic groups, but in general it is more widespread in developing countries and areas of lower socioeconomic conditions.

CMV is a major health risk because a large proportion of women, particularly white women, entering their childbearing years lack antibody to CMV. Those at greatest risk of infection are fetuses and immunocompromised persons. CMV is the most common virus transmitted to the fetus. Approximately 1 in 150 children is born with congenital CMV infection, and about 8000 children each year suffer permanent disabilities caused by CMV.

Transmission

Transmission of CMV may be by the oral, respiratory, or venereal route. The virus has been isolated in urine, saliva, feces, breast milk, blood, cervical secretions, virus-infected grafts from a donor, semen, vaginal fluid, and respiratory droplets. It may also be transmitted by the transfusion of fresh blood. Transmission of CMV appears to require intimate contact with secretions or excretions. CMV can be transmitted from a pregnant woman to her fetus during pregnancy. Low-birth-weight (LBW) neonates are also at high risk for CMV infection through transfusion of CMV-infected blood products.

Peripheral blood leukocytes and transplanted tissues have been strongly incriminated as sources of CMV. Transmission of CMV by transfusion of blood or blood components containing white blood cells (WBCs) has assumed increased importance in patients with severely impaired immunity who require supportive therapy. In the United States, CMV screening is required for all units of blood collected from donors. Preventive methods in these patients include effective donor screening, leukocyte-depleted or irradiated blood products, and immune globulin containing passively acquired CMV antibodies. The use of irradiated blood products has become more popular.

Once in a person's body, CMV stays there for life. Most CMV infections are silent, causing no signs or symptoms. Individuals who are CMV-positive (infected with CMV in the past) usually do not have virus in urine or saliva, so the risk of acquiring a CMV infection from casual contact is negligible.

Women who are pregnant or planning a pregnancy should follow hygienic practices (e.g., careful handwashing) to avoid CMV infection. Because young children are more likely to have CMV in their urine or saliva than older children or adults, pregnant women who have or work with young children should be especially careful.

Health care professionals represent a group that has become increasingly concerned about the risks associated with exposure to CMV. Nosocomial transmission from patients to health care workers has not been documented, but observance of good personal hygiene and handwashing offer the best measures for preventing transmission.

Latent Infection

Persistent infections characterized by periods of reactivation are frequently termed **latent infections**. CMV can persist in a latent state and active infections may develop under a variety of conditions (e.g., pregnancy; immunosuppression; after organ, bone, or stem cell transplantation). Of immunosuppressed patients, only seronegative patients appear to be at a significant risk of developing CMV infection. Patients at the highest risk of mortality from CMV infections are allograft transplant, seronegative

patients who receive tissue from a seropositive donor. The great majority of infections in allograft recipients are transmitted by a donated organ or arise from the reactivation of the recipient's latent virus.

True viral latency is defined by the presence of the genetic information in an unexpressed state in the host cell. An operational definition of latency can include the conditions of a dynamic relationship between the virus and host, along with evidence of latency and reactivation of a latent infection. As with any herpesvirus, CMV reactivation is possible at any time, but rarely manifests in immunocompetent individuals.

Congenital Infection

Primary and recurrent maternal CMV infection can be transmitted in utero. Congenital CMV infection is the most common intrauterine infection, affecting 0.4% to 2.3% of all live births in the United States. The presence of maternal antibody to CMV before conception provides substantial protection against damaging, congenital CMV infection in the newborn.

Primary maternal infection during pregnancy, occurring in 1% to 3% of U.S. women, is associated with more severe sequelae of congenital CMV infection. Infected infants can become severely ill and premature infants may die. Most newborns infected with CMV survive, but they may be mentally impaired or may develop other health problems. Approximately 10% of congenitally infected infants have symptoms at birth and, of the 90% who are asymptomatic, 10% to 15% will develop symptoms over months or even years.

SIGNS AND SYMPTOMS

Acquired Infection

Acquired CMV infection is usually asymptomatic and can persist in the host as a chronic or latent infection. The incubation period is believed to be 3 to 12 weeks.

In most patients, CMV infection is asymptomatic. Occasionally, a self-limited, heterophile-negative, mononucleosis-like syndrome results. CMV hepatitis can also develop.

Symptoms include a sore throat and fever, swollen glands, chills, profound malaise, and myalgia. Lymphadenopathy and splenomegaly may be observed. Infections occurring in healthy immunocompetent individuals usually result in seroconversion. Virus may be excreted in the urine during primary and recurrent CMV infections; it can persist sporadically for months or years. Persons experiencing acquired infection, reinfection with the same or different strains of CMV, or reactivation of a latent infection can excrete the virus in titers as high as 10^6 infective units/mL in the urine or saliva for weeks or months.

Normal adults and children usually experience CMV infection without serious complications. Infrequent complications of CMV infection in previously healthy individuals, however, include interstitial pneumonitis, hepatitis, Guillain-Barré syndrome, meningoencephalitis, myocarditis, thrombocytopenia, and hemolytic anemia.

CMV infection can be life-threatening in immunosuppressed patients. Infections in these patients may result in disseminated multisystem involvement, including pneumonitis, hepatitis, gastrointestinal (GI) ulceration, arthralgias, meningoencephalitis, and retinitis. Retinitis and encephalitis are common manifestations of disseminated CMV. Ulcerative damage of tissues (e.g., esophagus) is another demonstration of the cytopathic effects of CMV. Interstitial pneumonitis, frequently associated with CMV infection, is a major cause of death after allogeneic bone marrow transplantation. In premature infants, acquired CMV infection can result in atypical lymphocytosis, hepatosplenomegaly, pneumonia, or death.

Transfusion-acquired CMV infections may cause not only mononucleosis-like syndrome, but also hepatitis and increased rejection of transplanted organs. The following three types of CMV infections are possible in blood transfusion recipients:

1. **Primary infection** occurs when a previously unexposed (seronegative) recipient is transfused with blood from an actively or latently infected donor. This type of infection is accompanied by the presence of virus in the blood and urine, an immediate antibody response, and eventual seroconversion. Patients with primary infections may be symptomatic, but the great majority are asymptomatic.

2. **Reactivated infection** can occur when a seropositive recipient is transfused with blood from a CMV antibody–positive or –negative donor. Donor leukocytes are thought to trigger an allograft reaction, which in turn reactivates the recipient's latent infection. These infections may be accompanied by significant increases in CMV-specific antibody. Some reactivated infections exhibit viral shedding as their only manifestation. Reactivated infections are largely asymptomatic.

3. Reinfection can occur by a CMV strain in the donor's blood that differs from the strain that originally infected the recipient. A significant antibody response is observed and viral shedding occurs. Although it is difficult to differentiate a reactivated infection if the patient and donor are CMV antibody–positive before transfusion, reinfections can be documented if isolates can be obtained from the donor and recipient.

Congenital Infection

About 1 in 750 children in the United States is born with or develops permanent problems due to congenital CMV infection. In the United States, more than 5000 children/year suffer permanent problems caused by CMV infection.

The classic congenital CMV syndrome is manifested by a high incidence of neurologic symptoms, as well as neuromuscular disorders, jaundice, hepatomegaly, and splenomegaly (Fig. 21-1). Petechia is the most common clinical sign, seen in about 50% of CMV-infected infants.

Congenitally infected newborns, especially those who acquire CMV during a maternal primary infection, are more prone to develop severe cytomegalic inclusion disease (CID). The severe form of CID may be fatal or can cause permanent neurologic sequelae, such as intracranial calcifications (Fig. 21-2), mental retardation, deafness, vision defects, microcephaly, and motor dysfunction. Psychomotor impairment is seen in 51% to 75% of survivors. Hearing loss is observed in 21% to 50% and visual impairment in 20% of patients. Infants without symptoms at birth may develop hearing impairment and neurologic impairment later.

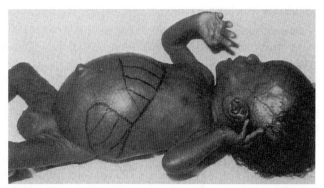

Figure 21-1 Four-month-old child with symptomatic congenital cytomegalovirus (CMV) infection manifesting severe failure to thrive, hepatitis with hepatosplenomegaly, bilateral inguinal hernia, and micropenis. *(From Katz SL, Gershon AA, Wilfert CM, Krugman S, editors: Infectious diseases of children, ed 9, St Louis, 1992, Mosby.)*

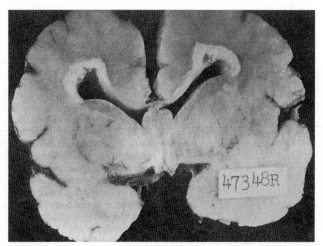

Figure 21-2 **Brain of infant with congenital CMV infection.** Note extensive periventricular necrosis and calcification. *(From Katz SL, Gershon AA, Wilfert CM, Krugman S, editors: Infectious diseases of children, ed 9, St Louis, 1992, Mosby.)*

IMMUNOLOGIC MANIFESTATIONS

Immune System Alterations

CMV infection is known to alter the immune system and to produce overt manifestations of infection. Infection interferes with immune responsiveness in normal and immunocompromised individuals. This diminished responsiveness results in a decreased proliferative response to the CMV antigen, which persists for several months. In patients with CMV mononucleosis-like syndrome, alterations of T lymphocyte subsets result, producing an increase in the absolute number of CD8+ lymphocytes and a decrease in CD4+ lymphocytes. These subset abnormalities persist for months.

Questions have been raised regarding CMV as a potentially oncogenic virus because viral antigens and nucleic acids have been found in human malignancies, including adenocarcinoma of the colon, carcinoma of the cervix, cancer of the prostate, and Kaposi's sarcoma. CMV does have transforming properties in vitro. Although considerable circumstantial evidence exists linking CMV to human malignancies, especially Kaposi's sarcoma, a direct cause and effect relationship has not been established.

Serologic Markers

In cells infected by CMV, several antigens appear at varying times after infection. Before replication of viral DNA takes place, **immediate-early antigens** and **early antigens** are present in the nuclei of infected cells. Immediate-early antigens appear within 1 hour of cellular infection and early antigens are present within 24 hours. At about 72 hours after infection, or the end of the viral replication cycle, late antigens are demonstrable in the nucleus and cytoplasm of infected cells.

The immune antibody response to these various antigens differs in incidence and significance. The presence of antibodies against immediate-early and early antigens is associated with active infection, either primary or reactivated. New CMV infections can be identified by testing for immunoglobulin G (IgG) antibodies on blood samples taken at different times. If the first sample is negative and the second sample is positive, the patient became infected with CMV between the two blood samples.

A newer method, called IgG avidity testing, which measures antibody maturity, has been shown to detect recent primary CMV infection reliably. This test is available on a limited basis in the United States.

Antibody to early antigen undergoes a relatively rapid decline after recovery but can persist for up to 250 days and may identify patients with recent, as well as active, infection. The presence of antibody to early antigen is strongly associated with viral shedding. Antibodies to late antigens persist in high titer long after the recovery from an active infection.

The incidence of viral exposure and subsequent antibody formation (seropositivity) varies greatly, depending on the socioeconomic status and living conditions of the population surveyed. The prevalence of CMV antibody varies with age and geographic location but ranges from 40% to 100%.

The characteristic antibody responses associated with infection are as follows:

- Primary infection, demonstrated by a transient virus-specific IgM antibody response and eventual seroconversion to produce immunoglobulin G (IgG) antibodies to the virus.
- Reactivation of latent infection in seropositive (IgG) individuals, which may be accompanied by significant increases in IgG antibodies to the virus, but elicits no detectable IgM response.
- Reinfection by a strain of CMV different from the original infecting strain. A significant IgG antibody response is demonstrated. It is not known whether an IgM response occurs.

There is no vaccine currently available for preventing congenital CMV disease (present at birth). A few CMV vaccines are being tested in humans, including live attenuated (weakened) virus vaccines and vaccines that contain only pieces of the virus.

In CMV infection, hematologic examination of the blood usually reveals a characteristic leukocytosis. A slight lymphocytosis with more than 20% variant lymphocytes is common. CMV infection is possible in the following situations:

- The patient has mononucleosis-like symptoms but exhibits a negative EBV test result.
- The patient manifests hepatitis symptoms but does not demonstrate any positive results when tested for common hepatitis viruses.

In affected infants, the most common laboratory abnormality is a low platelet count (thrombocytopenia). Clinical chemistry assays may demonstrate abnormal liver function. Presence of infection is also demonstrated by inclusion bodies in leukocytes in urine sediment.

LABORATORY EVALUATION

In immunocompromised patients, CMV serology is not recommended. The preferred method for diagnosis is culture of virus and/or polymerase chain reaction (PCR). A variety of methods can be used for screening purposes (Table 21-1).

A fourfold rise in IgG antibody titer suggests, but does not prove, recent CMV infection. The presence of IgG antibody in

---

CASE STUDY

History and Physical Examination

A 35-year-old man has recently been the recipient of a kidney transplant. He had been feeling well until 2 weeks ago, when he experienced a sore throat, fever, chills, profound malaise, and myalgia. Lymphadenopathy and splenomegaly may be observed. His medications include cyclosporine.

Questions
1. In cytomegalovirus (CMV), the presence of IgM antibodies to CMV can be found in:
   a. Primary CMV
   b. Reactivation of CMV
   c. Reinfection with CMV
   d. All of the above
2. Reactivation of latent CMV may:
   a. Elicit detectable IgM response
   b. Produce significant increase in IgG antibody to CMV
   c. Produce IgM and IgG
   d. Produce neither IgM or IgG

See Appendix A for the answers to these questions.

Critical Thinking Group Discussion Questions
1. Could this patient be suffering from an infectious disease?
2. Why would this patient be susceptible to an opportunistic infection?
3. How could an infection of this type be potentially eliminated?
4. Are health care workers at risk for infections of this type?
5. Can congenital infections of this type occur?
6. How can this disease be diagnosed?

See instructor site ⊖volve for the discussion of the answers to these questions.

Table 21-1	Laboratory Diagnosis of Cytomegalovirus Infection*	
Method	Test Method	Recommended Use
CMV rapid culture	Cell culture, immunofluorescence	Rapid diagnosis of CMV infection Gold standard test for tissue
CMV by Polymerase Chain Reaction (PCR) Blood, bone marrow, amniotic fluid	Qualitative PCR	Rapid test for diagnosing CMV in immunocompromised patients or solid organ donors. Amniotic fluid from a fetus of >21 weeks gestation can be analyzed.
CMV PCR	Quantitative PCR	Diagnose CMV infection. Monitor disease state in solid organ transplant and HIV patients.
CMV antibodies: IgM and IgG	Latex agglutination	Screen pregnant women and infants possibly infected with CMV. Infants may test positive during first 6 months due to maternal antibodies. Discriminate between current (IgM) and prior infections (IgG).
CMV antibodies: total	Solid-phase agglutination	Screen organ donors.
CMV by immunohistochemistry	Immunohistochemistry	Histologic diagnosis of CMV based on tissue from affected site

Adapted from Associated Regional and University Pathologists (ARUP) Laboratories: ARUP's laboratory test directory, 2012 (http://www.aruplab.com/guides).
ELISA, Enzyme-linked immunosorbent assay; *HIV*, human immunodeficiency virus.
*A negative result (<2.6 log copies/mL, or <390 copies/mL) does not rule out the presence of PCR inhibitors in the patient specimen or CMV nucleic acid in concentrations below the assay's level of detection. Inhibition may also lead to underestimation of viral quantitation.

infants complicates the interpretation of serologic results during the first 6 months of life because the antibody may be maternal in origin.

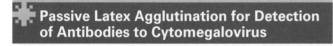

Passive Latex Agglutination for Detection of Antibodies to Cytomegalovirus

Principle

The CMVscan Card Test* is a passive latex agglutination test for the detection of IgM and IgG CMV antibodies. It can be used as a diagnostic tool or to screen donor specimens for antibodies to CMV in human serum and plasma. This assay can be performed qualitatively on undiluted serum to identify antibodies to CMV and quantitatively using serial twofold dilutions to determine the titer of CMV antibody.

In this procedure, latex particles previously sensitized with CMV viral antigen are mixed with serum. If antibody to CMV is present, the agglutinated particles will be macroscopically visible. In the absence of specific antibody or in with low antibody concentration, the latex particles will not agglutinate in the reaction mixture and the particles will appear smooth and evenly dispersed.

The absence of CMV antibodies suggests no viral exposure, whereas the presence of CMV antibodies indicates previous exposure to the virus. Recurrent infection, if it occurs, may not be as severe as primary infection. Because CMV is a blood-borne pathogen, infection is of greatest concern with newborn infants requiring transfusion and immunosuppressed allograft recipients.

The procedural protocol is posted on the ⊖volve website.

Reference Range

- The incidence of CMV infection depends on geographic and socioeconomic factors and patient age.
- Serologic studies indicate that 25% to 50% of the U.S. population demonstrate CMV antibodies by age 15 years.
- In adults, the incidence of antibodies to CMV ranges from 15% to 70%.

Sources of Error

Incorrect test results may be caused by a variety of factors. Specimens that are incorrectly collected or stored can produce errors in the test results. The use of components or procedures other than those previously described may also lead to erroneous results.

Limitations

Several limitations are inherent in CMV antibody detection, as follows:
1. Patients with acute infection may not have detectable antibody.
2. Seroconversion may indicate recent infection, but an increase in antibody titer by this method does not differentiate between a primary and secondary antibody response.
3. The timing of antibody responses during a primary infection may differ slightly. The pattern of antibody response during a primary CMV infection has not been demonstrated.
4. Test results from neonates should be interpreted with caution because the presence of CMV antibody is usually the result of passive transfer from the mother to the fetus.

*Becton Dickinson: Product insert, CMVscan Card Test, Becton Dickinson, revised March 2005, Franklin Lakes, NJ.

5. Although the CMV latex procedure will detect IgM and IgG antibodies, detection of IgA and IgE antibodies has not yet been demonstrated.

A negative CMV test result may be useful in excluding possible infection, but the diagnosis of an actual CMV infection should be documented by demonstrating the presence of the virus directly or by viral culture.

Clinical Applications

The CMVscan Card Test performed as a qualitative test on a single specimen is designed to detect the presence of CMV antibodies. The test will perform satisfactorily with acute-phase or convalescent-phase antibodies. Antibody present in a single specimen is evidence of prior exposure to the virus.

The quantitative test can be used to determine the relative amount of antibody in serum or plasma. When using properly paired specimens, at least 2 weeks apart, demonstration of seroconversion (fourfold or greater rise in antibody titer) may serve as evidence of recent infection. Both specimens should be tested simultaneously. The absence of a fourfold titer rise does not necessarily rule out exposure and infection.

The absence of CMV antibodies suggests that a patient has not been previously exposed to CMV. In the early stages of a primary infection, antibodies may not be detectable. The presence of CMV antibodies in qualitative testing on a single acute or convalescent specimen is an indication of previous exposure to the virus but does not indicate immunity to subsequent reinfection.

When paired specimens are tested simultaneously, the absence of a fourfold rise in titer does not definitively rule out the possibility of exposure and infection. Demonstration of seroconversion in quantitative testing (or a fourfold or greater rise in antibody titer) on paired specimens collected at least 2 weeks apart may suggest recent infection. Conversion from seronegativity to positivity or a change in antibody titer between paired specimens may occasionally be caused by influenza A or *Mycoplasma pneumoniae* infections, suggesting stress reactivation of CMV antibody.

Clinically, the selection of CMV-seronegative blood donors or donor organs by serologic screening for antibody has reportedly been effective in reducing CMV infection in CMV-seronegative recipients. The most suitable candidates for seronegative blood for transfusion are newborn and unborn infants and immunocompromised organ transplant recipients.

Quantitative Determination of IgG Antibodies to Cytomegalovirus*

Principle

Diluted samples are incubated in antigen-coated wells. CMV antibodies, if present, are immobilized in the wells. Residual sample is eliminated by washing and draining, and conjugate (enzyme-labeled antibodies to human IgG) is added and incubated. If IgG antibodies to CMV are present, the conjugate will be immobilized in the wells. Residual conjugate is eliminated by washing and draining and the substrate is added and incubated. In the presence of the enzyme, the substrate is converted to a yellow end product, which is read photometrically for an absorbance maximum at 405 nm. The intensity of the absorbance at 405 nm is proportional to the amount of antibody to CMV present in the sample.

The procedural protocol is posted on the ⊝volve website.

Clinical Applications

The serologic detection of IgM and/or IgG antibodies to CMV is a clinically useful aid in the diagnosis of CMV infection.

The IgG assay is used with serum for diagnostic assessment of prior infections with CMV.

The presence of IgM antibodies to CMV is, in general, indicative of primary CMV infection. Specific IgM antibody, however, has been reported in reactivations and reinfections. IgM antibody may persist for as long as 9 months in immunocompetent individuals and longer in immunosuppressed patients.

IgM responses vary among individuals. Of infants congenitally infected with CMV, 10% to 30% fail to develop IgM antibody responses. Approximately 27% of adults with primary CMV infection may not demonstrate an IgM response. In pregnant women, the presence or absence of CMV IgG or IgM response is of limited value in predicting congenital CMV infection. The presence of CMV-specific IgM antibody in the circulation of the newborn indicates infection.

CHAPTER HIGHLIGHTS

- Cytomegalovirus (CMV) is a herpesvirus. All the herpesviruses are relatively large, enveloped DNA viruses that undergo a replicative cycle involving DNA expression and nucleocapsid assembly within the nucleus. Although the herpesvirus family causes various clinical diseases, herpesviruses share the basic feature of being cell-associated.
- CMV may produce subclinical infections that can be reactivated under appropriate stimuli. Dissemination of the virus may occur by the oral, respiratory, or venereal route, as well as parenterally by organ transplantation or by transfusion of fresh blood.
- The incidence of primary CMV infections during childhood is low. Patients at highest risk of mortality from CMV infections are allograft transplant, seronegative patients who receive tissue from a seropositive donor. Most of these infections are transmitted by the donor organ or from reactivation of the recipient's latent virus.
- Transmission of CMV through transfusion of blood and blood components containing WBCs is increasingly

---

*Information is from the Bio-Rad CMV IgG enzyme immunoassay (EIA) package insert, November 2004 (Bio-Rad, 2012, Hercules, Calif.). NOTE: A CMV IgM EIA is also available from Bio-Rad.

important in immunocompromised patients who require supportive therapy. Low birth weight neonates are also at high risk from CMV infections from infected blood products.

- Persistent infections characterized by periods of reactivation of CMV (latent infections) have not been clearly defined for CMV.
- CMV is a major cause of congenital viral infections in the United States because primary and recurrent maternal CMV infections can be transmitted in utero.
- In CMV-infected cells, antigens appear at various times after infection, before the replication of viral DNA. Immediate-early antigens appear within 1 hour of cellular infection and early antigens within 24 hours. At about 72 hours or the end of the viral replication cycle, late antigens appear.
- The presence of antibodies against immediate-early and early antigens is associated with active infection, primary or reactivated. The following characteristic antibody responses are associated with CMV infection:
- Primary infection is demonstrated by a transient, virus-specific IgM antibody response and eventual seroconversion to produce IgG antibodies to the virus.
- Reactivation of latent CMV infection in seropositive (IgG) individuals may be accompanied by a significant increase in IgG antibodies to the virus, but no detectable IgM response.
- Reinfection by a different CMV strain than the original infecting strain results in a significant IgG antibody response but unknown IgM response.
- Serologic methods (e.g., EIA) to detect CMV-specific IgM can represent primary infection or rare reactivation. Detection of significant increases in CMV-specific IgG antibody suggest, but do not prove, recent infection or reactivation of latent infection.

REVIEW QUESTIONS

1. All the following describe CMV except:
   a. Herpes family virus
   b. DNA virus
   c. Cell-associated virus
   d. Epidemic worldwide

2. Because CMV can persist latently, an active infection may develop as a result of all the following conditions except:
   a. Pregnancy
   b. Immunosuppressive therapy
   c. Organ or bone marrow transplantation
   d. Transfusion of leukocyte-poor blood

3. CMV is recognized as the cause of congenital viral infection in what percentage of all live births?
   a. 0.1% to 0.4%
   b. 0.4 to 2.5%
   c. 2.5% to 4.9%
   d. 4.9% to 9.9%

4. Transfusion-acquired CMV infection can cause:
   a. Mononucleosis-like syndrome
   b. Hepatitis
   c. Rejection of a transplanted organ
   d. All of the above

5-7. Match the three types of CMV infection with their appropriate description.

5. _____ Primary infection

6. _____ Reactivated infection

7. _____ Reinfection
   a. Significant antibody response and viral shedding are caused by different strain of virus.
   b. Seronegative recipient is transfused with blood from actively or latently infected donor.
   c. Seropositive recipient is transfused with blood from a CMV antibody–positive or –negative donor.

8-10. Match the following serologic markers of CMV infection:

8. _____ Early antigens

9. _____ Immediate-early antigens

10. _____ Late antigens
    a. Appear 72 hours after infection or at the end of the viral replication cycle
    b. Appear within 1 hour of cellular infection
    c. Present within 24 hours

11. Antibodies to immediate-early and early antigens are associated with:
    a. Primary active infection
    b. Reactivated active infection
    c. Latent infection
    d. Either a or b

12-14. Match the following:

12. _____ Primary infection

13. _____ Reactivation of latent infection in seropositive IgG patient

14. _____ Reinfection with strain of CMV different from original strain
    a. IgG, but IgM response unknown
    b. Specific IgM antibody response
    c. IgG (no detectable IgM)

15. All the herpesviruses share the feature of being:
    a. RNA viruses
    b. Small viruses
    c. Cell-associated viruses
    d. Nonenveloped viruses

16. A most likely mode of CMV acquisition is:
    a. Irradiated blood products
    b. Non-irradiated blood transfusions containing viable leukocytes

c. Venereal route

d. All of the above

17. Which of the following appears to be the only immuno-suppressed group at significant risk of acquiring CMV infection?

a. Transplant patients

b. Seronegative patients

c. Seropositive patients

d. Health care workers

18. All the following are methods for the prevention of CMV except:

a. Irradiated blood products

b. Leukocyte-depleted blood products

c. Immune globulin with CMV antibodies

d. Transfusion of fresh blood

19-22. Indicate true statements with the letter A and false statements with the letter B.

19. _____ Primary and recurrent maternal CMV infections can be transmitted in utero.

20. _____ CMV is the most common intrauterine infection.

21. _____ Few CMV-infected newborns are asymptomatic.

22. _____ Normal adults and children usually experience CMV infection without serious complications.

BIBLIOGRAPHY

Adler SP: Transfusion-associated cytomegalovirus infections, Rev Infect Dis 5:977–993, 1983.

Bailey TC, Trulock EP, Storch GA, Powderly WG: Ganciclovir for cytomegalovirus after heart transplantation, N Engl J Med 327:891, 1992.

Betts RF: The relationship of epidemiology and treatment factors to infection and allograft survival in renal transplantation. In Platkin SA, et al: CMV pathogenesis and prevention of human infection, New York, 1984, Alan R Liss.

Bowden R, Sayers M, Flournoy N, et al: Cytomegalovirus immune globulin and seronegative blood products to prevent primary cytomegalovirus infection after marrow transplantation, N Engl J Med 314:1006–1010, 1986.

Brady MT: Cytomegalovirus infections: occupational risk for health professionals, Am J Infect Control 14:197–203, 1986.

Brennan D: Dancing partners: cytomegalovirus and allograft injury. Presented at the XVIII International Congress of the Transplantation Society, 2000, Rome.

Burny W, Liesnard C, Donner C, Marchant A: Epidemiology, pathogenesis and prevention of congenital cytomegalovirus infection, Expert Rev Anti Infect Ther 2:881–894, 2004.

Centers for Disease Control and Prevention: Cytomegalovirus (CMV) and congenital CMV infection, 2010, http://www.cdc.gov/cmv/index.html.

Demmler GJ, Six HR, Hurst SM, Yow MD: Enzyme-linked immunosorbent assay for the detection of IgM-class antibodies to cytomegalovirus, J Infect Dis 153:1152–1155, 1986.

Dobbins JG, Stewart JA, Demmler GJ: Surveillance of congenital cytomegalovirus disease, 1990-1991. Collaborating Registry Group, MMWR CDC Surveill Summ 41:35–39, 1992.

Gandhi MK, Khanna R: Human cytomegalovirus: clinical aspects, immune regulation, and emerging treatments, Lancet Infect Dis 4:725–738, 2004.

Griffiths PD, Walter S: Cytomegalovirus, Curr Opin Infect Dis 18:241–245, 2005.

Macé M, Sissoeff L, Rudent A, Grangeot-Keros L: A serological testing algorithm for the diagnosis of primary CMV infection in pregnant women, Prenat Diagn 24:861–863, 2004.

Murph JR, Baron JC, Brown CK, et al: The occupational risk of cytomegalovirus infection among day-care providers, JAMA 265:603–608, 1991.

Preiksaitis JK, Brennan DC, Fishman J, Allen U: Canadian society of transplantation consensus workshop on cytomegalovirus management in solid organ transplantation: final report, Am J Transplant 5:218–227, 2005.

Ross SA, Boppana SB: Congenital cytomegalovirus infection: outcome and diagnosis, Semin Pediatr Infect Dis 16:44–49, 2005.

Rowshani AT, Bemelman FJ, van Leeuwen EM, et al: Clinical and immunologic aspects of cytomegalovirus infection in solid organ transplant recipients, Transplantation 79:381–386, 2005.

Schrier RD, Nelson JA, Nelson MB: Detection of human cytomegalovirus in peripheral blood lymphocytes in a natural infection, Science 230:1048–1051, 1985.

Schuster V, Matz B, Wiegand H, et al: Detection of human cytomegalovirus in urine by DNA-DNA and RNA-DNA hybridization, J Infect Dis 154:309–314, 1986.

Sia IG, Wilson JA, Espy MJ, et al: Evaluation of the COBAS AMPLICOR CMV MONITOR test for detection of viral DNA in specimens taken from patients after liver transplantation, J Clin Microbiol 38:600–606, 2000.

Turgeon ML: Clinical hematology, ed 5, Philadelphia, 2012, Lippincott Williams & Wilkins.

Infectious Mononucleosis

Learning Objectives

At the conclusion of this chapter, the reader should be able to:

- Describe the etiology, epidemiology, and signs and symptoms of infectious mononucleosis.
- Explain the immunologic manifestations of infectious mononucleosis, including heterophile antibodies.
- Discuss the elements of Epstein-Barr virus (EBV) serology and the diagnostic clinical applications of the presence of each component.

- Analyze and apply laboratory data to a case study.
- Correctly answer case study related multiple choice questions.
- Be prepared to participate in a discussion of critical thinking questions.
- Compare the serologic procedures and clinical applications of the Paul-Bunnell, Davidsohn differential, and rapid agglutination techniques.
- Correctly answer end of chapter review questions.

Key Terms

acute
asymptomatic
benign

carcinoma
leukopenia
morphologic

neoplasm
prognostic
splenomegaly

ETIOLOGY

The Epstein-Barr virus (EBV), a human herpesvirus, was discovered in 1964 by Dr. M. Anthony Epstein and his colleague, Yvonne Barr. Subsequently, Drs. Werner and Gertrude Henle screened human serum samples for antibodies to viral capsid antigens of EBV and established the relationship of EBV to several cancers (e.g., Burkitt's lymphoma). EBV became the most intensively studied human cancer virus. The entire genome of one EBV strain was completely sequenced in 1984. The virus parasitizes every cell system—signal transduction, cell cycle control, regulation of gene expression, posttranscriptional RNA processing, protein modification and stability, and DNA replication.

Infectious mononucleosis, caused by EBV, is usually an **acute, benign,** and self-limiting lymphoproliferative condition. EBV is also the cause of Burkitt's lymphoma (a malignant tumor of the lymphoid tissue occurring mainly in African children), nasopharyngeal **carcinoma,** and **neoplasms** of the thymus, parotid gland, and supraglottic larynx. EBV is an important factor in the development of nasopharyngeal carcinoma, an epithelial cancer. Although nasopharyngeal carcinoma is rare in North American and European whites, it is one of the most common cancers in southern China and parts of Southeast Asia. Genetics and environmental factors appear to contribute to the elevated risk of nasopharyngeal carcinoma among the Chinese.

EBV infections can result in complications involving the cardiac, ocular, respiratory, hematologic, digestive, renal, and neurologic systems. EBV-associated neurologic syndromes include Bell's palsy, Guillain-Barré syndrome, meningoencephalitis, Reye's syndrome, myelitis, cranial nerve neuritis, and psychotic disorders. Respiratory paralysis caused by bulbar involvement can be fatal.

EPIDEMIOLOGY

EBV is widely disseminated. It is estimated that 95% of the world's population is exposed to the virus, which makes EBV the most ubiquitous virus known to humans. EBV is a human herpes DNA virus that infects B lymphocytes. The variant lymphocytes produced in response to and seen in microscopic examination of the peripheral blood have T cell characteristics.

The mononucleosis is not from stimulation of B cells by viral infection (EBV will transform cell lines in vitro) but is from a large, effective, CD8 cytotoxic T cell (Tc) response against the EBV-infected circulating B lymphocytes. One of the habitats of the persisting viral genome in hosts with a latent infection is the B lymphocytes of the lymphoreticular system and epithelial cells of the oropharynx.

Although transmitted primarily by close contact with infectious oral pharyngeal secretions, EBV is reportedly transmitted by blood transfusion and transplacental routes. Under normal conditions, EBV transmission through transfusion or transplacental exposure is unlikely. In addition, EBV-associated *posttransplantation lymphoproliferative disorder (PTLD)* develops in 1% to 10% of organ transplant recipients.

The frequency of seronegative patients is almost 100% in early infancy but declines with increasing age, more or less rapidly, depending on socioeconomic conditions, to less than 10% in young adults. After primary exposure, a person is considered to be immune and generally no longer susceptible to overt reinfection. In Western societies, primary exposure to EBV occurs in two waves. Approximately 50% of the population is exposed to the virus before age 5 years; a second wave of seroconversion occurs during late adolescence (age 15 to 24 years). Approximately 90% of adult patients demonstrate antibodies to the virus.

Individuals at risk include those who lack antibodies to the virus. EBV is only a minor problem for immunocompetent persons, but can become a major concern for immunocompromised patients. Blood transfusion from an immune donor to a nonimmune recipient may produce a primary infection in the recipient known as *infectious mononucleosis postperfusion syndrome.* Infectious mononucleosis or an infectious mononucleosis–like illness after blood transfusion often may result from a concomitant cytomegalovirus (CMV) infection rather than EBV. In addition, the association with EBV appears to be a specific finding in malignant lymphoma developing after severe immunosuppression, such as that induced by cyclosporine therapy.

A low percentage of patients experience symptomatic reactivation. Reactivation of latent EBV infection has been implicated in a persistent illness referred to as EBV-associated fatigue syndrome, but this phenomenon is not universally accepted.

Clinically apparent infectious mononucleosis has an estimated frequency of 45/100,000 in adolescents. In immunosuppressed patients, the incidence of EBV infection ranges from 35% to 47%. As with other herpesviruses, there is a carrier state after primary infection.

SIGNS AND SYMPTOMS

Although EBV infects more than 95% of the world's population, most individuals experience no adverse effects. Infants typically have **asymptomatic** infection. The timing of initial infection is a key indicator of the ensuing symptoms. Infectious mononucleosis is the typical illness experienced by adolescents newly infected with EBV.

Most individuals experience seroconversion without any significant clinical signs or symptoms of disease. Immunocompetent

persons maintain EBV as a chronic latent infection. In children younger than 5 years, infection is asymptomatic or frequently characterized by mild, poorly defined signs and symptoms. Although anyone can suffer from this viral disorder, it is typically manifested in young adults.

The incubation period of infectious mononucleosis is from 10 to 50 days; once fully developed, it lasts for 1 to 4 weeks. Clinical manifestations include extreme fatigue, malaise, sore throat, fever, and cervical lymphadenopathy. **Splenomegaly** occurs in about 50% of cases. Jaundice is infrequent, although the most common complication is hepatitis. A smaller percentage of patients develop hepatomegaly or splenomegaly and hepatomegaly. Because abnormal liver function is more marked with EBV-induced than CMV-associated infectious mononucleosis, EBV must be considered in the differential diagnosis of hepatitis.

A significant number of patients with infectious mononucleosis do not manifest classic signs and symptoms.

LABORATORY DIAGNOSTIC EVALUATION

In addition to clinical signs and symptoms, laboratory testing is necessary to establish or confirm the diagnosis of infectious mononucleosis (Table 22-1).

Hematologic studies reveal a leukocyte count ranging from 10 to 20×10^9/L in about two thirds of patients; about 10% of the patients demonstrate **leukopenia.** A differential leukocyte count may initially disclose a neutrophilia, although mononuclear cells usually predominate as the disorder develops. Typical relative lymphocyte counts range from 60% to 90%, with 5% to 30% variant lymphocytes. These variant lymphocytes exhibit diverse **morphologic** features and persist for 1 to 2 months and as long as 4 to 6 months (Fig. 22-1).

If the classic signs and symptoms are absent, a diagnosis of infectious mononucleosis is more difficult to make. A definitive diagnosis can be established by serologic antibody testing. The antibodies present in infectious mononucleosis are heterophile and EBV antibodies.

IMMUNOLOGIC MANIFESTATIONS

Heterophile Antibodies

Heterophile antibodies are composed of a broad class of antibodies. These antibodies are stimulated by one antigen and react

Table 22-1	**Classic Laboratory Findings in Acute Infectious Mononucleosis**
Assay	**Result**
Heterophile antibody test	Positive
Anti-VCA IgM	Elevated titer
Liver enzymes	Elevated
Leukocyte differential	Increased number of variant (atypical) lymphocytes

VCA, Viral capsid antigen; *IgM*, immunoglobulin M.

with an entirely unrelated surface antigen present on cells from different mammalian species. Heterophile antibodies may be present in normal individuals in low concentrations (titers), but a titer of 1:56 or greater is clinically significant in patients with suspected infectious mononucleosis.

The immunoglobulin M (IgM) type of heterophile antibody usually appears during the acute phase of infectious mononucleosis, but the antigen that stimulates its production remains unknown. IgM heterophile antibody is characterized by the following features:

- Reacts with horse, ox, and sheep erythrocytes
- Absorbed by beef erythrocytes

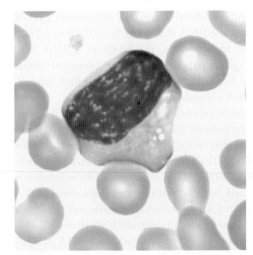

Figure 22-1 Variant lymphocytes seen in Epstein-Barr virus infection (mononucleosis). *(From Rodak BF, Carr JH: Clinical hematology atlas, ed 4, St Louis, 2013, Saunders.)*

- Not absorbed by guinea pig kidney cells
- Does not react with EBV-specific antigens

Paul and Bunnell first associated infectious mononucleosis with sheep cell agglutination and developed a test for the infectious mononucleosis heterophile. Davidsohn modified the original Paul-Bunnell test, introducing a differential adsorption aspect to remove the cross-reacting Forssman and serum sickness heterophile antibodies. Rapid agglutination slide tests are now available.

Epstein-Barr Virus Serology

Within the adult population, 10% to 20% of individuals with acute infectious mononucleosis do not produce infectious mononucleosis heterophile antibody. The pediatric population is of particular concern because more than 50% of children younger than 4 years with infectious mononucleosis are heterophile negative. In diagnostically inconclusive cases of infectious mononucleosis, a more definitive assessment of immune status may be obtained through an EBV serologic panel. Candidates for EBV serology include those who do not exhibit classic symptoms of infectious mononucleosis, who are heterophile negative, or who are immunosuppressed.

Epstein-Barr–infected B lymphocytes express a variety of new antigens encoded by the virus. Infection with EBV results in the expression of viral capsid antigen (VCA), early antigen (EA), and nuclear antigen (NA), with corresponding antibody responses. Assays for IgM and IgG antibodies to these EBV antigens are available. EBV-specific serologic studies are beneficial in defining immune status, and their time of appearance may indicate the stage of disease (Fig. 22-2; Table 22-2). This can provide important information for the diagnosis and management of EBV-associated disease.

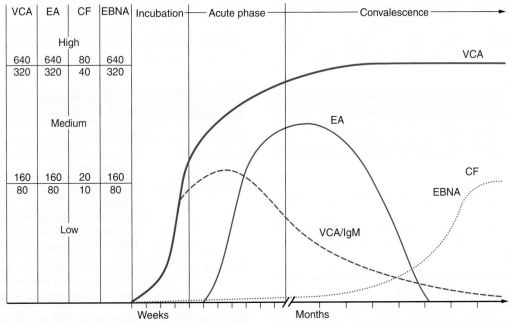

Figure 22-2 Epstein-Barr virus (EBV) antibody response during the course of infectious mononucleosis. *EA,* Early antigen; *VCA,* viral capsid antigen; *EBNA,* Epstein-Barr nuclear antigen; *CF,* complement fixation test. *(Redrawn from Krugman S, et al: Infectious diseases of children, ed 9, St Louis, 1992, Mosby.)*

Patients with nasopharyngeal carcinoma have elevated titers of IgA antibodies to EBV replicative antigens, including VCA. These antibodies, which frequently precede the appearance of the tumor, serve as a **prognostic** indicator of remission and relapse.

Viral Capsid Antigen (VCA)

VCA is produced by infected B cells and can be found in the cytoplasm. Anti-VCA IgM is usually detectable early in the course of infection, but is low in concentration and disappears within 2 to 4 months. Anti-VCA IgG is usually detectable within 4 to 7 days after the onset of signs and symptoms and persists for an extended period, perhaps lifelong.

Early Antigen (EA)

EA is a complex of two components, early antigen–*diffuse* (EA-D), which is found in the nucleus and cytoplasm of the B cells, and early antigen–*restricted* (EA-R), usually found as a mass only in the cytoplasm.

Anti–EA-D of the IgG type is highly indicative of acute infection, but it is not detectable in 10% to 20% of patients with infectious mononucleosis. EA-D disappears in about 3 months; however, a rise in titer is demonstrated during reactivation of a latent EBV infection.

Anti–EA-R IgG is not usually found in young adults during the acute phase but may be seen in the serum of very young children during the acute phase. Anti–EA-R IgG appears transiently in the later, convalescent phase. In general, anti–EA-D and anti–EA-R IgG are not consistent indicators of the disease stage.

Epstein-Barr Nuclear Antigen (EBNA)

EBNA is found in the nucleus of all EBV-infected cells. Although the synthesis of NA precedes EA synthesis during the infection of B cells, EBNA does not become available for antibody stimulation until after the incubation period of infectious mononucleosis, when activated T lymphocytes destroy the EBV genome–carrying B cells. As a result, antibodies to NA are absent or barely detectable during acute infectious mononucleosis.

Anti-EBNA IgG does not appear until a patient has entered the convalescent period. EBNA antibodies are almost always present in sera containing IgG antibodies to VCA of EBV unless the patient is in the early acute phase of infectious mononucleosis. Patients with severe immunologic defects or immunosuppressive disease may not have EBNA antibodies, even if antibodies to VCA are present.

Under normal conditions, antibody titers to NA gradually increase through convalescence and reach a plateau 3 to 12 months after infection. The antibody titer remains at a moderate, measurable level indefinitely because of the persistent viral carrier state established after primary EBV infection. Most healthy individuals with previous exposure to EBV have antibody titers to EBNA that range from 1:10 to 1:160. In EBV-associated malignancies, the levels of EBNA antibody are usually high in patients with nasopharyngeal carcinoma and can range from barely detectable to very high levels in patients with Burkitt's lymphoma.

Test results of antibodies to EBNA should be evaluated in relation to patient symptoms, clinical history, and antibody response patterns to VCA and EA to establish a diagnosis (Table 22-3). The antibody profile can be especially useful. For example, a patient with an infectious mononucleosis–like illness caused by reactivation of a persistent EBV infection resulting from an immunosuppressive malignancy or nonmalignant disease can demonstrate high titers of IgM and IgG VCA antibodies. If the antibody to EBNA is also elevated, however, a diagnosis of primary EBV infection can be excluded.

Additional Testing

Immunofluorescence is a common methology in EBV serology testing. Antigen substrate slides containing EBV-infected B cells are incubated with the patient's serum. The presence of specific antibody is detected by the addition of fluorescein-conjugated antihuman IgG or IgM. The disadvantages of this type of testing are that it is time-consuming, difficult to

Table 22-2	**Characteristic Antibody Formation in Infectious Mononucleosis**					
Parameter	VCA IgM	VCA IgG	EA-D	EA-R	EBNA IgG	Heterophile
No previous exposure	−	−	−	−	−	−
Recent (acute) infection	+	+	±	−	−	+
Past infection (convalescent) period	−	+	−	−	+	−
Reactivation of latent infection	±	+	±	±	+	±

VCA, Viral capsid antigen; *EA-D,* early antigen–diffuse; *EA-R,* early antigen–restricted; *EBNA,* Epstein-Barr nuclear antigen; *IgG,* immunoglobulin G.

Table 22-3	**Characteristic Diagnostic Profile of Epstein-Barr Virus**
Stage	**Description**
Susceptibility	If the patient is seronegative (lacks antibody to VCA)
Primary infection	Antibody (IgM) to VCA is present; EBNA is absent. High or rising titer of antibody (IgG) to VCA and no evidence of antibody to EBNA after at least 4 wk of symptoms
Reactivation	If antibody to EBNA and increased antibodies to EA are present, patient may be experiencing reactivation.
Past infection	Antibodies to VCA and EBNA are present.

VCA, Viral capsid antigen; *EBNA,* Epstein-Barr nuclear antigen; *EA,* early antigen.

interpret, and prone to interference from other serum components (e.g., rheumatoid factor).

The enzyme-linked immunosorbent assay (ELISA) may be used to detect antibodies to EBNA. This ELISA uses a synthetic peptide antigen to determine the relative amounts of IgM and IgG antibodies in patient serum or plasma. Its sensitivity is reportedly 98.9%, with a specificity of 99.0%.

CASE STUDY

History and Physical Examination

A female college freshman reports to the infirmary, complaining of extreme fatigue, frequent headaches, and a sore throat. A routine physical examination by the college physician shows that the patient has swollen lymph nodes (lymphadenopathy), redness of the throat, and a slightly enlarged spleen. A complete blood count (CBC), urinalysis (UA), and mononucleosis screening test are ordered.

Laboratory Data
CBC
- Hemoglobin and microhematocrit—within normal range
- Total leukocyte count—elevated (13.5 × 10⁹/L)
- Leukocyte differential—elevated lymphocytes (56%)
- Many variant forms of lymphocytes (25%)

Urinalysis—normal
Mononucleosis screening test—negative

Therapy and Follow-Up
The physician prescribes bed rest and medication for the patient's headache. A follow-up appointment was scheduled for 10 days later.

Questions
1. Heterophil antibodies can be characterized as:
   a. Reacts with horse and sheep RBCs
   b. Absorbed by beef RBCs
   c. Not absorbed by guinea pig kidney cells
   d. All of the above
2. The antigens expressed by Epstein-Barr (E-B) virus infected lymphocytes encoded by the virus include:
   a. Early antigen (EA)
   b. Viral capsid antigen (VCA)
   c. E-B nuclear antigen (EBNA)
   d. All of the above

See Appendix A for the answers to these questions.

Critical Thinking Group Discussion Questions
1. What is this patient's absolute lymphocyte count? Is this considered normal?
2. What is the most probable diagnosis of this disorder?

3. If repeat testing is performed on the patient after 10 days, could any of the results vary?
4. Discuss the antibodies that could occur in this patient's condition.
5. What type of antigens could be tested for in the blood?

See instructor site ⊖volve for the discussion of the answers to these questions.

Paul-Bunnell Screening Test

Principle
The classic Paul-Bunnell test is a hemagglutination test designed to detect heterophile antibodies in patient serum when mixed with antigen-bearing sheep erythrocytes. Dilutions of inactivated patient serum are mixed with sheep erythrocytes, incubated, centrifuged, and macroscopically examined for agglutination. Positive reactions are preliminary.

See ⊖volve for the procedural protocol on the Evolve website.

Sources of Error
False-positive reactions have been observed in conditions such as hepatitis infection and Hodgkin's disease. An improperly inactivated serum will produce hemolysis.

Clinical Applications
The Paul-Bunnell test is a useful test to screen for the presence of heterophile antibodies because it is simple and inexpensive. Although the specificity of the heterophile assay is rated as good, negative results are demonstrated in individuals who do not produce infectious mononucleosis heterophile antibody. If negative results are displayed, however, EBV serology may be indicated.

Limitations
The test is only indicative of the presence or absence of heterophile antibodies. Demonstrating agglutination by using sheep erythrocytes does **NOT** distinguish between antibodies associated with infectious mononucleosis or serum sickness, or the Forssman antigen.

The heterophile antibody assay lacks sensitivity as a diagnostic criterion for infectious mononucleosis. Sheep erythrocytes are less sensitive than erythrocytes from other species. A patient may take as long as 3 months to develop a detectable heterophile titer.

Davidsohn Differential Test

Principle
This classic procedure distinguishes between the heterophile antibodies that agglutinate the antigen-bearing erythrocytes of sheep. The differential nature of the test is predicated on the

Table 22-4   Agglutinins for Sheep Erythrocytes in Human Serum

Type of Serum	Absorbed by Guinea Pig Kidney	Absorbed by Beef Erythrocytes
Normal	Positive (+)	Negative (−)
Infectious mononucleosis	Negative (−)	Positive (+)
Serum sickness	Positive (+)	Positive (+)

fact that sheep and beef (ox) erythrocytes bear some common antigens not present on the kidney cells of the guinea pig. Exposure of patient serum to guinea pig cells, which are rich in Forssman antigen, and to beef erythrocytes, which are poor in Forssman antigen, produces differential absorption. Any absorbed antibodies are removed by centrifugation and the supernatant fluid is tested with sheep erythrocytes. This classical test differentiates the heterophile types of antibody associated with infectious mononucleosis or serum sickness (Table 22-4).

The Davidsohn differential procedure is performed only if the preliminary Paul-Bunnell test is positive in a titer of 1:56 or greater. Serum sickness occurs as the result of sensitization to animal serum, usually horse serum.

See ⊖volve for the procedural protocol on the Evolve website.

Reporting Results

If the pattern of reactivity demonstrates reduced titers with either beef or guinea pig cells, the antibody source can be attributed to one of the heterophile antibody types. Normal serum is considered to express a titer of 1:28 with an occasional 1:56 result. In infectious mononucleosis, a titer of 1:56 is suspicious and a titer of 1:224 is considered to be a positive result.

Sources of Error

Incorrect pipetting or the use of noninactivated serum can contribute to errors.

Clinical Applications

The Davidsohn differential can distinguish between three types of heterophile antibodies.

Limitations

This test is time-consuming.

🧩 MonoSlide Test

Principle

The BBLMonoSlide procedure (BD BBLMonoSlide, Becton, Dickinson, Franklin Lakes, NJ) is based on the agglutination of horse erythrocytes by heterophile antibody present in infectious mononucleosis. Because horse red blood cells (RBCs) exhibit antigens directed against both Forssman and infectious mononucleosis antibodies, a differential absorption of the

patient's serum is necessary to distinguish the specific heterophile antibody from those of the Forssman type.

The basic principle of the absorption steps in this procedure is comparable to that originally described by Davidsohn in the sheep agglutinin test. Serum or plasma is absorbed with both guinea pig kidney and beef erythrocyte stroma. Guinea pig kidney contains only the Forssman antigen, and beef erythrocytes contain only the antigen associated with infectious mononucleosis. Guinea pig kidney will absorb only heterophile antibodies of the Forssman type and beef erythrocytes will absorb only the heterophile antibody of infectious mononucleosis. Agglutination of horse RBCs by the absorbed patient specimen indicates a positive reaction for heterophile antibody.

The BBLMonoSlide Test uses a disposable card, guinea pig kidney antigen for absorption, and specially treated horse erythrocytes (color-enhanced) to increase specificity and sensitivity and to enhance readability. No special equipment is required to read the BBLMonoSlide Test results.

Reporting Results: Qualitative Method

Positive

A positive infectious mononucleosis reaction will have dark clumps against a blue-green background, distributed uniformly throughout the test circle.

Negative

A negative reaction will have no agglutination but may have fine granularity against a brown-tan background. Peripheral color development associated with fine granularity should be interpreted as negative (e.g., giant blue-green halo on the periphery of the test circle should not be interpreted as a positive result).

Procedure Notes

If a positive qualitative result is demonstrated, a titration procedure may be performed to provide a quantitative indication of the level of heterophile antibody.

Sources of Error

For accurate results, only clear, particle-free serum or plasma specimens should be used.

False-positive results can be caused by the following:
1. Observing agglutination after the observation time
2. Misinterpreting agglutination
3. Simultaneous occurrence of infectious mononucleosis and hepatitis has been reported.

A result interpreted as a false-positive may be caused by residual heterophile antibody present after clinical symptoms have subsided.

Clinical Applications

Infectious diseases such as influenza, rubella, and hepatitis may cause clinical symptoms that mimic those of infectious mononucleosis and present problems in diagnosis. Although the final diagnosis of infectious mononucleosis depends on clinical, hematologic, and serologic findings, a positive test result indicates the presence of the heterophile antibody specific for infectious mononucleosis.

Limitations

The diagnosis of infectious mononucleosis should be based on the results of all clinical and laboratory findings. Some segments of the population do not produce detectable heterophile antibody (e.g., ≈50% of children <4 years old; 10% of adolescents). Detectable levels of heterophile antibody may persist for months and, more rarely, for years, in some individuals.

NOTE: Other forms of rapid testing include Wampole Laboratories Colorcard Mono and Mono-plus.

CHAPTER HIGHLIGHTS

- Epstein-Barr virus (EBV), a DNA virus, is the cause of infectious mononucleosis.
- An estimated 95% of the world's population is exposed to EBV, making it the most ubiquitous virus known. The virus infects B lymphocytes. Although transmitted primarily by infectious oral-pharyngeal secretions, EBV may also be transmitted by blood transfusion and transplacentally.
- The frequency of seronegative patients is almost 100% in early infancy but declines with increasing age to less than 10% in young adults. After primary exposure, a person is considered immune and generally no longer susceptible to overt reinfection.
- In Western societies, primary exposure to EBV occurs in two waves among children and adolescents. EBV is only a minor problem for immunocompetent persons but can become a major concern for immunocompromised individuals.
- The antibodies present in infectious mononucleosis are heterophile and EBV antibodies.
- EBV-infected B lymphocytes express a variety of new antigens encoded by the virus. Infection with EBV results in the expression of viral capsid antigen VCA, early antigen EA, and nuclear antigen NA, with corresponding antibody responses. Assays for IgM and IgG antibodies to these EBV antigens are available.
- EBV-specific serologic studies are beneficial for defining immune status. The time of antibody appearance may indicate the stage of the disease.

REVIEW QUESTIONS

1. The Epstein-Barr virus can cause all the following except:
   a. Infectious mononucleosis
   b. Burkitt's lymphoma
   c. Nasopharyngeal carcinoma
   d. Neoplasms of the bone marrow

2. The primary mode of EBV transmission is:
   a. Exposure to blood
   b. Exposure to oral-pharyngeal secretions
   c. Congenital transmission
   d. Fecal contamination of drinking water

3. Infants infected with EBV are more likely to experience symptomatic infection than EBV-infected adolescents.
   a. True
   b. False

4. IgM heterophile antibody is characterized by all the following features except:
   a. Reacts with horse, ox, and sheep RBCs
   b. Absorbed by beef erythrocytes
   c. Absorbed by guinea pig kidney cells
   d. Does not react with EBV-specific antigens

5. Characteristics of EBV-infected lymphocytes include all the following except:
   a. B type
   b. Expression of viral capsid antigen
   c. Expression of early antigen
   d. Expression of EBV genome

6. Which of the following stages of infectious mononucleosis infection is characterized by antibody to Epstein-Barr nuclear antigen (EBNA)?
   a. Recent (acute) infection
   b. Past infection (convalescent) period
   c. Reactivation of latent infection
   d. Both b and c

7. Which of the following stages of infectious mononucleosis infection is (are) characterized by heterophile antibody?
   a. Recent (acute) infection
   b. Past infection (convalescent) period
   c. Reactivation of latent infection
   d. Both a and c

8. What percentage of the world's population is exposed to EBV?
   a. 25%
   b. 50%
   c. 75%
   d. 95%

9. Infectious mononucleosis postperfusion syndrome is a primary infection resulting from a blood transfusion from a(n) _____ to a(n) _____ recipient.
   a. Immune; nonimmune
   b. Nonimmune; immune
   c. Infected; nonimmune
   d. Infected; immune

10. In infectious mononucleosis, there is no:
    a. Acute state
    b. Latent state
    c. Carrier state
    d. Reactivation

11. The incubation period of infectious mononucleosis is:
    a. 2 to 4 days
    b. 10 to 15 days
    c. 10 to 50 days
    d. 51 to 90 days

12. The use of horse erythrocytes in rapid slide tests for infectious mononucleosis increases their:
    a. Cost
    b. Sensitivity
    c. Specificity
    d. Both b and c

13. EBV-infected B lymphocytes express all the following new antigens except:
    a. Viral capsid antigen VCA
    b. Early antigen EA
    c. Cytoplasmic antigen (CA)
    d. Nuclear antigen NA

14. Anti-EBNA IgG does not appear until a patient has entered the:
    a. Initial phase of infection
    b. Primary infection phase
    c. Convalescent period
    d. Reactivation of infectious stage

15-17. Match each procedure to the appropriate description.

15. _____ Paul-Bunnell screening test

16. _____ Davidsohn differential test

17. _____ MonoSlide agglutination test
    a. Distinguishes between heterophile antibodies; uses beef erythrocytes, guinea pig kidney cells, and sheep erythrocytes
    b. Detects heterophile antibodies and uses horse erythrocytes
    c. Detects heterophile antibodies and uses sheep erythrocytes

BIBLIOGRAPHY

Akashi K, Eizuru Y, Sumiyoshi Y, et al: Severe infectious mononucleosis-like syndrome and primary human herpesvirus 6 infection in an adult, N Engl J Med 329:168–172, 1993.

Andiman W: Use of cloned probes to detect Epstein-Barr viral DNA in tissues of patients with neoplastic and lymphoproliferative diseases, J Infect Dis 148:967, 1983.

Bennett N: Laboratory-based investigations of IM and Epstein-Barr virus, MLO 39:10, 2007.

Horwitz CA, Henle W, Henle G, et al: Long-term serological follow-up of patients for Epstein-Barr virus after recovery from infectious mononucleosis, J Infect Dis 151:1150, 1985.

Lennette ET, Henle W: Epstein-Barr virus infections: clinical and serologic features, Lab Manage 25:23, 1987.

Mori JA, Kurozumi H, Akagi K, et al: Monoclonal proliferation of T cells containing Epstein-Barr virus in fatal mononucleosis, N Engl J Med 327:58, 1992.

Ortho Diagnostics: Monospot product brochures, Raritan, NJ, 1984, Ortho Diagnostics.

Papadopoulos EB, Ladanyi M, Emanuel D, et al: Infusion of donor leukocytes to treat Epstein-Barr virus-associated lymphoproliferative disorders after allogeneic bone marrow transplantation, N Engl J Med 330:1185, 1994.

Pathmanathan R, Prasad U, Sadler R, et al: Clonal proliferations of cells infected with Epstein-Barr virus in preinvasive lesions related to nasopharyngeal carcinoma, N Engl J Med 333:693, 1995.

Randhawa PS, Jaffe R, Demetris AJ, et al: Expression of Epstein-Barr virus-encoded small RNA (by the EBER-1 gene) in liver specimens from transplant recipients with post-transplantation lymphoproliferative disease, N Engl J Med 327:1710, 1992.

Robertson ES: Epstein-Barr virus, N Engl J Med 355:2708, 2006.

Sumaya CV: Serological testing for Epstein-Barr virus: development in interpretation, J Infect Dis 151:984, 1985.

Sumaya CV: Epstein-Barr virus serologic testing: diagnostic indications and interpretations, Pediatr Infect Dis 5:337, 1986.

Sumaya CV: Infectious mononucleosis and other EBV infections: diagnostic factors, Lab Manage 24:37, 1986.

Sumaya CV, Ench Y: Epstein-Barr virus infectious mononucleosis in children. I. Clinical and general laboratory findings, Pediatrics 75:1003, 1985.

Turgeon ML: Leukocytes: clinical hematology, ed 3, Philadelphia, 1999, Lippincott–Williams & Wilkins.

Zijlmans JM, van Rijthoven AW, Kluin PM, et al: Epstein-Barr virus--associated lymphoma in a patient treated with cyclosporine, N Engl J Med 326:1362, 1992.

Viral Hepatitis

Learning Objectives

At the conclusion of this chapter, the reader should be able to:

- Identify and describe the characteristics of the various forms of primary infectious hepatitis, including laboratory assays.
- Compare the etiology, epidemiology, signs and symptoms, laboratory evaluation, and prevention of the various types of hepatitis.
- Analyze case studies related to the immune response various forms of hepatitis.

- Correctly answer case study related multiple choice questions.
- Be prepared to participate in a discussion of critical thinking questions.
- Describe the principle, results, and limitations of the rapid HCV test.
- Correctly answer end of chapter review questions.

Key Terms

anicteric
capsid
chronicity
coinfection
Dane particle

fulminant disease
hepadnavirus
hepatitis B core antigen (HBcAg)
hepatoma
necrosis

nucleocapsid protein
prodromal
sequelae
viremia
virions

GENERAL CHARACTERISTICS OF HEPATITIS

The term *hepatitis* refers to inflammation of the liver. This chapter discusses infectious hepatitis caused by various viruses.

According to the World Health Organization (WHO), 2 billion people are infected with hepatitis. Almost one third of the world's population has been infected with one of the known hepatitis viruses. In the United States, acute viral hepatitis most frequently is caused by infection with hepatitis A virus (HAV), hepatitis B virus (HBV), or hepatitis C virus (HCV). These unrelated viruses are transmitted via different routes and have different epidemiologic profiles. Safe and effective vaccines have been available for hepatitis B since 1981 and for hepatitis A since 1995.

Etiology

Viral hepatitis is the most common liver disease worldwide. The viral agents of acute hepatitis can be divided into two major groups, as follows:
* Primary hepatitis viruses: A, B, C, D, E, and GB virus C
* Secondary hepatitis viruses: Epstein-Barr virus (EBV), cytomegalovirus (CMV), herpesvirus, and others

Incidence

Primary hepatitis viruses account for approximately 95% of the cases of hepatitis. These viruses are classified as primary hepatitis viruses because they attack primarily the liver and have little direct effect on other organ systems. The secondary viruses involve the liver secondarily in the course of systemic infection of another body system. The viruses for hepatitis types A, B, C, D, E, and GB virus C, as well as secondary viruses (e.g., EBV, CMV), have been isolated and identified (Table 23-1).

Signs and Symptoms

As a clinical disease, hepatitis can occur in acute or chronic forms. The signs and symptoms of hepatitis are extremely variable. It can be mild, transient, and completely asymptomatic or it can be severe, prolonged, and ultimately fatal. Many fatalities are attributed to hepatocellular carcinoma in which hepatitis

viruses B and C are the primary causes. The course of viral hepatitis can take one of four forms—acute, fulminant acute, subclinical without jaundice, and chronic (Table 23-2).

HEPATITIS A

Etiology

HAV is a small, RNA-containing picornavirus and the only hepatitis virus that has been successfully grown in culture (Fig. 23-1, *A*). The structure is a simple nonenveloped virus with a nucleocapsid designated as the hepatitis A (HA) antigen (HA Ag). Inside the **capsid** is a single molecule of single-stranded ribonucleic acid (RNA). The RNA has a positive polarity and proteins are translated directly from the RNA. Replication of HAV appears to be limited to the cytoplasm of the hepatocyte.

The highest titers of HAV are detected in acute-phase stool samples. Human infectivity of saliva and urine from patients with acute hepatitis A does not pose a significant risk. Sexual contact has been suggested as a possible mode of transmission.

Epidemiology

Hepatitis A virus was formerly called infectious hepatitis or short-incubation hepatitis. In developing countries, hepatitis A is primarily a disease of young children; the prevalence of infection, as measured by the presence of antibody (immunoglobulin G [IgG] anti-HAV), approaches 100% at or shortly after 5 years of age. The national rate of hepatitis A has declined steadily since the last peak in 1995 (Fig. 23-2). After asymptomatic infection and underreporting were taken into account, an estimated 21,000 new infections occurred in 2009 (the last year for which statistics were available at the time of publication).

The incidence of hepatitis A varies by age. Historically, the highest rates were observed among children and young adults. Effective vaccines have been available since 1995. Since the issuance in 1999 of recommendations for routine childhood vaccination, rates of hepatitis A have declined. In 2005, the

Table 23-1	Characteristics of Viral Hepatitis					
Parameter	Type A: Travelers	Type B: Hospital Personnel	Type D: Delta	Type C: Posttransfusion	Type E	GB Virus C
Agent	Hepatitis A	Hepatitis B	Hepatitis D (delta agent)	Hepatitis C	Hepatitis E	Hepatitis G
	RNA	DNA	RNA	RNA	RNA	RNA
Antigens	HA Ag	HBsAg, HBcAg, HBeAg	Delta	HCV	HEV	GB-C
Antibodies	Anti-HAV	Anti-HBs, anti-HBc, anti-HBe	Antidelta	Anti-HCV	IgM anti-HEV IgG anti-HEV	Anti-HGV
Epidemiology	Fecal-oral	Parenteral, other	Parenteral, other	Parenteral and nonparenteral	Fecal-oral	Parenteral
Incubation period	15-45 days	40-180 days	30-50 days	15-150 days	2-9 wk	?

licensing of hepatitis A vaccines was revised to allow vaccination of children aged 12 to 23 months. Nationwide, hepatitis A vaccination of children is likely to result in lower overall rates of infection.

Susceptibility to infection is independent of gender and race. Crowded unsanitary conditions are a definite risk factor. HAV is transmitted almost exclusively by a fecal-oral route during the early phase of acute illness; the virus is shed in feces for up to 4 weeks after infection. Large outbreaks are usually traceable to a common source, such as an infected food handler, contaminated water supply, or consumption of raw shellfish. Institutions and day care centers are known to be favorable sources for transmission as well.

Hepatitis A infection is noted for occurring in isolated outbreaks or as an epidemic, but it also may occur sporadically. Although rarely a transfusion-acquired hepatitis because of its transient nature, an outbreak of HAV infection that occurred in 52 patients with hemophilia in Italy was documented to have been acquired through infusion of contaminated factor VIII concentrate. This concentrate had been treated by a virucidal method (solvent detergent) that ineffectively inactivates nonenveloped viruses.

Improvements in socioeconomic and sanitary conditions and declining family size may be responsible for a decreasing frequency of infection. The incidence of HAV infection is not increasing among health care workers or in dialysis patients. Maternal-neonatal transmission of HAV is not recognized as an epidemiologic entity. Person to person contact, usually among children and young adults, remains the major route of HAV infection.

The most frequently identified risk factor for hepatitis A has been international travel, reported at 15% of patients overall. Most travel-related cases have been associated with travel to Mexico and Central or South America (70%). As HAV transmission in the United States has decreased, cases among travelers to countries where hepatitis is endemic have accounted for an increased proportion of all cases.

Table 23-2	Forms of Hepatitis
Form	**Characteristics**
Acute hepatitis	Typical form with associated jaundice. Four phases—incubation, preicteric, icteric, and convalescence
	Incubation period, from time of exposure and first day of symptoms, ranges from few days to many months
	Average length of time is 75 days (range, 40-180) in hepatitis B virus (HBV) infection
Fulminant acute hepatitis	Rare form of hepatitis associated with hepatic failure
Subclinical hepatitis without jaundice	Probably accounts for persons with demonstrable antibodies in their serum but no reported history of hepatitis
Chronic hepatitis	Accompanied by hepatic inflammation and necrosis that lasts for at least 6 mo
	Occurs in about 10% of patients with HBV infection

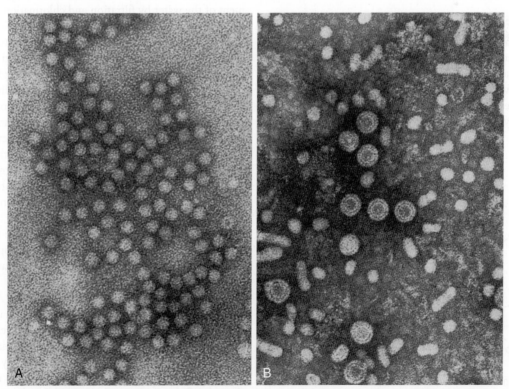

Figure 23-1 **Electron micrographs of hepatitis viruses. A,** Hepatitis A virus (HAV). **B,** Hepatitis B virus (HBV). Note Dane particles. *(From Katz SL, Gershon AA, Wilfert CM, Krugman S, editors: Infectious diseases of children, ed 9, St Louis, 1992, Mosby.)*

Sexual and household contact with another person with hepatitis A have been among the most frequently identified risk factors, reported for 10% of cases in 2006. In 2006, the proportion of HAV-infected persons who reported injection of street drugs was 2.1%.

Signs and Symptoms

Nonimmune adult patients infected with HAV can develop clinical symptoms within 2 to 6 weeks after exposure (average, ≈4 weeks). However, hepatitis A is often a subclinical disease, with many patients being **anicteric.** Clinically apparent cases show elevated serum liver function enzyme and bilirubin levels, with jaundice developing several days later. **Viremia** and fecal shedding of virus disappear at the onset of jaundice. Atypical presentations include prolonged intrahepatic cholestasis, relapsing course, and extrahepatic immune complex deposition, all of which resolve spontaneously.

Complete clinical recovery is anticipated in almost all patients. Hepatitis A rarely causes fulminant hepatitis and does not progress to chronic liver disease. Unusual clinical variants of hepatitis A include cholestatic, relapsing, and protracted hepatitis. In cholestatic hepatitis, serum bilirubin levels may be dramatically elevated (>20 mg/dL) and jaundice persists for weeks to months before resolution. In relapsing hepatitis and protracted hepatitis, complete resolution is anticipated.

A chronic carrier state (persistent infection) and chronic hepatitis (chronic liver disease) do not occur as long-term **sequelae** of hepatitis A. Rarely, injection with HAV may cause fulminant hepatitis, with about 0.1% mortality. Fulminant hepatitis is the most likely complication of coinfection with other hepatitis viruses.

Immunologic Manifestations

Shortly after the onset of fecal shedding, an IgM antibody is detectable in serum, followed within a few days by the appearance of an IgG antibody. IgM anti-HA is almost always detectable in patients with acute HAV. IgG anti-HAV, a manifestation of immunity, peaks after the acute illness and remains detectable indefinitely, perhaps lifelong.

The finding of IgM anti-HAV in a patient with acute viral hepatitis is highly diagnostic of acute HAV. Demonstration of IgG anti-HAV indicates previous infection. The presence of IgG anti-HAV protects against subsequent infection with HAV but is not protective against hepatitis B or other viruses.

Diagnostic Evaluation

Testing methods for HAV include the following:
- Hepatitis A antibodies (total)—enzyme immunoassay (EIA)
- Hepatitis A antibody, IgM antibody

The short period of viremia makes detection difficult. Specific IgM antibody usually appears about 4 weeks after infection and may persist for up to 4 months after onset of clinical symptoms. The presence of IgG or total (IgM and IgG) antibody indicates past infection or immunization and associated immunity. The total assay detects IgM and IgG antibodies but does not differentiate between them. The hepatitis A antibody IgM assay is appropriate when acute HAV infection is suspected. Specific IgG antibody apparently protects an individual from symptomatic infection, but specific IgM may increase with reinfection. In the acute phase of HAV, liver function levels (e.g., serum liver enzyme levels) will be elevated and may aid in establishing the diagnosis.

Prevention and Treatment

The first effective control measures to prevent enterically transmitted viral hepatitis resulted from World War II research. In 1945, the following were demonstrated: (1) infectious virus could be transmitted by contaminated drinking water; (2) treatment of the water by filtration and chlorination made it safe to drink; and (3) gamma globulin derived from convalescent-phase serum from patients with hepatitis could protect adults from clinical hepatitis. For 50 years, refining food and water preparation and establishing standards for immune globulin constituted the methods of HAV prevention. An individual who has had close contact with an HAV-infected person should receive passive immunization with immune globulin intramuscularly.

A safe, highly immunogenic, formalin-inactivated, single-dose vaccine is available to prevent HAV infection (Box 23-1). HAV vaccine should be targeted at high-risk groups (e.g., staff in child care centers; food handlers; international travelers, including military personnel; homosexual men; institutionalized patients).

Universal childhood vaccination may prove to be the most cost-effective method of protecting large populations, both nationally and globally. Routine childhood hepatitis A vaccination is recommended.

In May 2001, the U.S. Food and Drug Administration (FDA) approved a new combination vaccine that protects individuals 18 years of age and older against diseases caused by HAV and HBV. The vaccine, called Twinrix (GlaxoSmithKline Beecham, Philadelphia), combines two already approved vaccines, Havrix (hepatitis A vaccine, inactivated) and Engerix-B (hepatitis B vaccine, recombinant) so that those at high risk for exposure to both viruses can be immunized against both at the

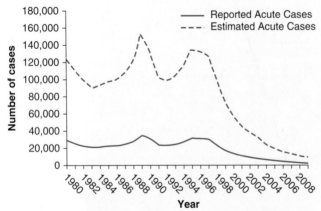

Figure 23-2 Incidence of hepatitis A, by year, 1980-2009. *(Courtesy National Center for HIV/AIDS, Viral Hepatitis, STD, and TB Prevention, Centers for Disease Control and Prevention, Atlanta.)*

Box 23-1	Hepatitis Vaccine: Questions and Answers

Hepatitis A

Who should receive hepatitis A vaccine?

Some people should be routinely vaccinated with hepatitis A vaccine:

- All children ≈1 year (12-23 months) of age
- Persons 1 year of age and older traveling to or working in countries with high or intermediate prevalence of hepatitis A (e.g., those located in Central or South America, Mexico, Asia [except Japan], Africa, and eastern Europe). For more information, see www.cdc.gov/travel.
- Children and adolescents through 18 years of age who live in states or communities in which routine vaccination has been implemented because of high disease incidence
- Men who have sex with men
- Persons who use street drugs
- Persons with chronic liver disease
- Persons who are treated with clotting factor concentrates
- Persons who work with HAV-infected primates or who work with HAV in research laboratories
  Other people might receive hepatitis A vaccine in special situations:
- Hepatitis A vaccine might be recommended for children or adolescents in communities in which outbreaks of hepatitis A are occurring.

At what time before anticipated exposure should the vaccine be administered?

Hepatitis A vaccine must be given at least 1 month before exposure is expected. Travelers with less than 1 month before a trip to an endemic area can receive vaccine and immune globulin (injected at separate anatomic sites).

How long does a vaccination last?

It appears that healthy individuals who receive at least two doses of vaccine are protected for at least 5 years and probably much longer (20 years).

If you are unvaccinated and experience an unusual exposure, what can be done to prevent transmission?

Immune globulin should be given to all close personal contacts including sexual partners and members of the household. Health care workers without unusual exposure to feces or blood do not generally need immune globulin.

Hepatitis B

Who should be vaccinated?

- All babies, at birth
- All children 0-18 years of age who have not been vaccinated
- People of any age whose behavior or job puts them at high risk for HBV infection (see risk factors under general information)

What are the dosages and schedules for hepatitis B vaccines?

The vaccination schedule generally used for adults and children has been three intramuscular injections, the second and third administered 1 and 6 months after the first. Recombivax HB has been approved as a two-dose schedule for ages 11-15 years. Engerix-B has also been approved as a four-dose accelerated schedule.

Can you receive one dose of hepatitis B vaccine from one manufacturer and the other doses from another manufacturer?

Yes. The immune response when one or two doses of a vaccine produced by one manufacturer are followed by subsequent doses from a different manufacturer has been shown to be comparable with that resulting from a full course of vaccination from one manufacturer.

What should be done if there is an interruption between doses of hepatitis B vaccine?

If the vaccination series is interrupted after the first dose, the second dose should be administered as soon as possible. The second and third doses should be separated by an interval of at least 2 months. If only the third dose is delayed, it should be administered when convenient.

Can other vaccines be given at the same time that hepatitis B vaccine is given?

Yes. When hepatitis B vaccine has been administered at the same time as other vaccines, no interference with the antibody response of the other vaccines has been demonstrated.

Are hepatitis B vaccines safe?

Yes. Hepatitis B vaccines have been shown to be safe when administered to both adults and children. Over 4 million adults have been vaccinated in the United States, and at least that many children have received hepatitis B vaccine worldwide.

How long does hepatitis B vaccine protect you?

Recent studies have indicated that immunologic memory remains intact for at least 23 years and confers protection against clinical illness and chronic HBV infection, even though anti-HBs levels might become low or decline below detectable levels.

Can hepatitis B vaccine be given after exposure to HBV?

Yes. After a person has been exposed to HBV, appropriate treatment, given in an appropriate time frame, can effectively prevent infection. The mainstay of postexposure prophylaxis is hepatitis B vaccine, but in some settings the addition of HBIG will provide some increase in protection.

Who should receive postvaccination testing?

Testing for immunity is advised only for persons whose subsequent clinical management depends on knowledge of their immune status (e.g., infants born to HBsAg-positive mothers, immunocompromised persons, health care workers, sex partners of persons with chronic HBV infection).

When should postvaccination testing be done?

When necessary, postvaccination testing, using the anti-HBs test, should be performed 1 to 2 months after completion of the vaccine series—except for postvaccination testing of infants born to HBsAg-positive mothers. Testing of these infants should be performed 3 to 9 months after the completion of the vaccination series.

Who should not receive the vaccine?

A serious allergic reaction to a prior dose of hepatitis B vaccine or a vaccine component is a contraindication to further doses of hepatitis B vaccine. The recombinant vaccines licensed for use in the United States are synthesized by *Saccharomyces cerevisiae* (common baker's yeast), into which a plasmid containing the gene for HBsAg has been inserted. Purified HBsAg is obtained by lysing the yeast cells and separating HBsAg from the yeast components by biochemical.

Adapted from Centers for Disease Control and Prevention: Viral hepatitis, 2012 (http://www.cdc.gov/ hepatitis/index.htm).

same time. Areas with a high rate of both HAV and HBV include Africa, parts of South America, most of the Middle East, and South and Southeast Asia. Clinical trials of Twinrix, given in a three-dose series at ages 0, 1, and 6 months, have shown that the combination vaccine is as safe and effective as the already licensed, separate HAV and HBV vaccines.

HEPATITIS B

Etiology

HBV is the classic example of a virus acquired through blood transfusion. It serves as a model when transfusion-transmitted viral infections are considered (see Fig. 23-1, *B*).

The Australia antigen, now called hepatitis B surface antigen (HBsAg), was discovered in 1966. This discovery, and its subsequent association with HBV, led to the biochemical and epidemiologic characterization of HBV infection.

Hepatitis B is a complex DNA virus that belongs to the family Hepadnaviridae; a member of this family is known as a **hepadnavirus.** Eight different HBV genotypes with differences in clinical outcomes have been identified. Viral proteins of importance include the following:

1. The envelope protein—HBsAg
2. A structural nucleocapsid core protein—**hepatitis B core antigen (HBcAg)**

3. A soluble **nucleocapsid protein**—hepatitis B e antigen (HBeAg)

The unique structure of the DNA of HBV is one of the distinguishing characteristics of a hepadnavirus. The DNA is circular and double stranded, but one of the strands is incomplete, leaving a single-stranded or gap region that accounts for 10% to 50% of the total length of the molecule. The other DNA strand is nicked (3′ and 5′ ends are not joined). The entire DNA molecule is small and all the genetic information for producing both HBsAg and HBcAg is on the complete strand. During the disease process, viral DNA of HBV is actually incorporated into the host's DNA.

HBV relies on a retroviral replication strategy (reverse transcription from RNA to DNA). Eradication of HBV infection is rendered difficult because stable, long-enduring, covalently closed circular DNA (cccDNA) becomes established in hepatocyte nuclei and HBV DNA become integrated into the host genome (Fig. 23-3).

Epidemiology

Hepatitis B infection has been referred to as long-incubation hepatitis. In 2009 (the last year for which statistics were available at the time of publication), a total of 3371 acute symptomatic cases and 38,000 estimated total new infections of hepatitis B were reported in the United States. The overall incidence was

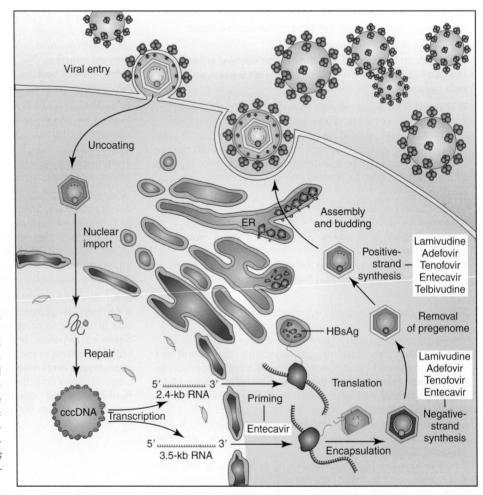

Figure 23-3 Steps of HBV replication. The hepatitis B virus (HBV) establishes covalently closed circular DNA (cccDNA) as a durable miniature chromosome in the host nucleus and relies on a retroviral strategy of reverse transcription from RNA to negative-strand DNA. The steps of HBV replication targeted by nucleoside and nucleotide analogues that are used to treat chronic HBV infection are shown. *ER,* Endoplasmic reticulum; *HBsAg,* hepatitis B surface antigen. *(From Dienstag JL: Hepatitis B virus infection, N Engl J Med 359:1486–1500, 2008.)*

the lowest ever recorded and represents a decline of 81% since 1990 (Fig. 23-4).

About 1.25 million people in the United States have chronic HBV infection, 20% to 30% of whom acquired the infection in childhood. Each year, about 3000 to 5000 people die from cirrhosis or liver cancer caused by HBV. The highest rate of disease occurs in those ages 20 to 49 years. The greatest decline has occurred in children and adolescents as a result of routine hepatitis B vaccination.

The incidence of HBV infection caused by blood transfusion is increasingly rare in developed countries. Transfusion-acquired HBV has been severely reduced because high-risk donor groups (e.g., paid donors, prison inmates, military recruits) have been eliminated as major sources of donated blood and because specific serologic screening procedures have been instituted. This shift to an all-volunteer donor supply probably accounts for a 50% to 60% reduction of transfusion-related hepatitis. The overall incidence of HBV is high among patients who have received multiple transfusions or blood components prepared from multiple-donor plasma pools, hemodialysis patients, drug addicts, and medical personnel (see Table 23-1).

Persons at risk of exposure to HBV, including those mentioned earlier, include members of the following groups:

- Heterosexual men and women
- Homosexual men with multiple partners
- Household contacts and sexual partners of HBV carriers
- Infants born to HBV-infected mothers
- Patients and staff in custodial institutions for developmentally disabled persons
- Recipients of certain plasma-derived products, including patients with congenital coagulation defects
- Health care and public safety workers who may be in contact with infected blood
- Persons born in HBV-endemic areas and their children

Hepatitis B virus does not seem capable of penetrating the skin or mucous membranes; therefore, some break in these barriers is required for disease transmission. Transmission of HBV occurs via percutaneous or permucosal routes and infective blood or body fluids can be introduced at birth, through sexual contact, or by contaminated needles. Infection can also occur in settings of continuous close personal contact. About 50% of patients with acute type B hepatitis have a history of parenteral exposure. Inapparent parenteral exposure involves intimate or sexual contact with an infectious individual. Transmission between siblings and other household contacts readily occurs via transmission from skin lesions such as eczema or impetigo, sharing of potentially blood-contaminated objects such as toothbrushes and razor blades, and occasionally through bites. HBV has been found in saliva, semen, breast milk, tears, sweat, and other biological fluids of HBV carriers. Urine and wound exudate are capable of harboring HBV. Stool is not considered to be infectious.

Signs and Symptoms

Infection with HBV causes a broad spectrum of liver disease, ranging from subclinical infection to acute, self-limited hepatitis and fatal fulminant hepatitis. Exposure to HBV, particularly when it occurs early in life, may also cause an asymptomatic carrier state that can progress to chronic active hepatitis, cirrhosis of the liver, and eventually hepatocellular carcinoma.

A number of factors, including the dose of the agent and an individual's immunologic host response ability, influence the clinical course of HBV infection. Extrahepatic manifestations, reflecting an immune complex–mediated, serum sickness–like syndrome, are seen in fewer than 10% of patients with acute hepatitis B and include rash, glomerulonephritis, vasculitis, arthritis, and angioneurotic edema. Manifestations such as vasculitis, glomerulonephritis, arthritis, and dermatitis are mediated by circulating immune complex deposition (HBV antigen-antibody) in blood vessels.

The progression of liver disease in HBV infection is fostered by active virus replication, manifested by the presence of an HBV DNA level above a threshold of approximately 1000 to 10,000 IU/mL. Patients with lower levels and normal liver enzyme levels are considered to be inactive carriers, with a low risk of clinical progression. Rarely, reactivation in these patients can occur spontaneously or with immunosuppression. Perinatal infection can result in high HBV level replication without substantial liver injury in the early decades of life; however, the risk of progression to cirrhosis and hepatocellular carcinoma is proportional to the level of HBV DNA maintained persistently over time.

Persistent infection is the usual consequence of HBV infection acquired at an early age, signaled by the prolonged presence of HBsAg. Some individuals with chronic HBV infection are asymptomatic carriers, whereas others have clinical, laboratory, and histologic evidence of chronic hepatitis that may be associated with the development of postnecrotic cirrhosis. Persistent HBV infection is believed to be a precursor of primary hepatocellular carcinoma. In about 5% to 10% of individuals with HBV, especially patients with immunodeficiencies (e.g., AIDS), the disease will progress to a chronic state.

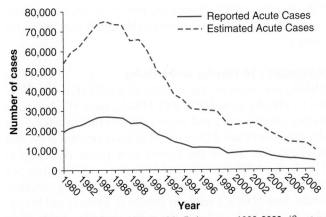

Figure 23-4 Incidence of hepatitis B, by year, 1982-2009. *(Courtesy National Center for HIV/AIDS, Viral Hepatitis, STD, and TB Prevention, Centers for Disease Control and Prevention, Atlanta.)*

Asymptomatic Infection

The most frequent clinical response to HBV is an asymptomatic or subclinical infection. In patients developing clinical symptoms of transfusion-associated hepatitis B, jaundice, and abnormal liver serum enzyme can be manifested from a few weeks to up to 6 months after a single transfusion episode. However, in patients with a classic serologic response associated with HBV, the diagnosis is rarely in doubt, even in the absence of significant symptoms. Diagnosis is more difficult in asymptomatic patients with negative HBV serology who develop a mild elevation of ALT levels a few weeks after a transfusion. Elevated enzyme levels may persist for 1 or 2 weeks.

Laboratory Assays

Laboratory diagnosis (Fig. 23-5) and monitoring of acute and chronic HBV infections involve the use of several of the following tests (Tables 23-3 and 23-4):
1. Hepatitis B surface antigen (HBsAg)
2. Hepatitis B e antigen (HBeAg)
3. Hepatitis B core antibody, total or IgM (anti-HBc)
4. Hepatitis B e antibody (anti-HBe)
5. Hepatitis B surface antibody (anti-HBs)
6. Hepatitis B viral DNA by polymerase chain reaction (PCR, qualitative and quantitative)

Serum testing procedures may be performed by qualitative chemiluminescent immunoassay, qualitative EIA, quantitative real-time PCR, quantitative real-time PCR–nucleic acid sequencing, or real-time PCR with reflex to genotype. Immunohistochemistry may be used to detect HBsAg in liver tissue samples.

Hepatitis B Surface Antigen

Serum HBsAg is a marker of HBV infection. Antibodies against HBsAg signify recovery. The initial detectable marker found in serum during the incubation period of HBV infection is HBsAg. HBsAg usually becomes detectable 2 weeks to 2 months before clinical symptoms and as soon as 2 weeks after infection. This marker is usually present for 2 to 3 months. This procedure screens for the presence of the major coat-protein of the virus (HBsAg) in serum and is considered to be the most reliable method of choice for preventing the transmission of HBV via blood. The presence of HBsAg indicates active HBV infection, acute or chronic.

The titer of HBsAg rises and generally peaks at or shortly after the onset of elevated liver serum enzyme levels (e.g., ALT, SGPT). Clinical improvement of the patient's condition and a decrease in serum enzyme concentrations are paralleled by a fall in the titer of HBsAg, which subsequently disappears. There is variability in the duration of HBsAg positivity and in the relationship between clinical recovery and the disappearance of HBsAg (Fig. 23-6). About 5% of positive HBsAg values are false-positive results.

Among persons infected with HBV with detectable HBsAg in their serum, not all the HBsAg represents complete **Dane particles.** HBsAg-positive serum also contains two other virus-like structures, which are incomplete spherical and tubular forms consisting entirely of HBsAg and devoid of HBcAg, DNA, or DNA polymerase. The incomplete HBsAg particles can be present in serum in extremely high concentrations and form the bulk of the circulating HBsAg.

Hepatitis B–Related Antigen

A hepatitis B–related antigen, HBeAg, is found in the serum of some HBsAg-positive patients. HBV DNA and DNA polymerase will appear along with HBeAg. These are all indicative of active viral replication. HBeAg is rarely found in the absence of HBsAg. HBeAg appears to be associated with the HBV core; however, the relationship between HBeAg and the structure of HBV is unclear. HBeAg appears to be a reliable marker for the presence of high levels of virus and a high degree of infectivity.

Hepatitis B Core Antibody

During the course of most HBV infections, HBsAg forms immune complexes with the antibodies produced as part of the recovery process. Because the HBsAg contained in these complexes is usually undetectable, HBsAg disappears from the serum of up to 50% of symptomatic patients. During this phase, an indicator of a recent hepatitis B infection is anti-HBc, the antibody to the core antigen. The time between the disappearance of detectable HBsAg and the appearance of detectable antibody to HBsAg (anti-HBs) is called the anti-core window or hidden antigen phase of HBV infection. This window phase may last for a few weeks, several months, or 1 year, during which anti-HBc may be the only serologic marker. Anti-HBc is found in 3% to 5% of individuals. Of 100 anti-HBc–positive persons, 97 will have anti-HBs, 2 will have HBsAg, and 1 may have only anti-HBc.

Testing for antibody to the core of the virus (anti-HBc) may provide an additional advantage and lead to the identification of a person recently recovered from an HBV infection who may still be infectious. EIA or microparticle EIA is the method of choice.

An anti-HBc test is the Corzyme test (Abbott Laboratories, Abbott Park, Ill) EIA. The most recent assay to be developed is the test for anti-HBc IgM. This is considered a reliable marker during the window period, diagnostic of acute infection, when most other markers may be absent. The IgM anti-HBc titer rises rapidly in the acute phase and becomes negative in most patients in 3 to 9 months, although it may persist for many years.

Antibodies to HBeAg and HBsAG

HBeAg is a serum marker of active viral replication. Antibodies to HBeAg (anti-HBe) and HBsAg (anti-HBs) develop during convalescence and recovery from HBV infection. The development of anti-HBe in a case of acute hepatitis is the first serologic evidence of the convalescent phase. Antibody to HBsAg (anti-HBs), unlike anti-HBc and anti-HBe, does not arise during the acute disease; it is manifested during convalescence. Anti-HBs is a serologic marker of recovery and immunity. Anti-HBs is probably the major protective antibody in this disease. Thus, hepatitis B immune globulin is so named because it contains high levels of anti-HBs.

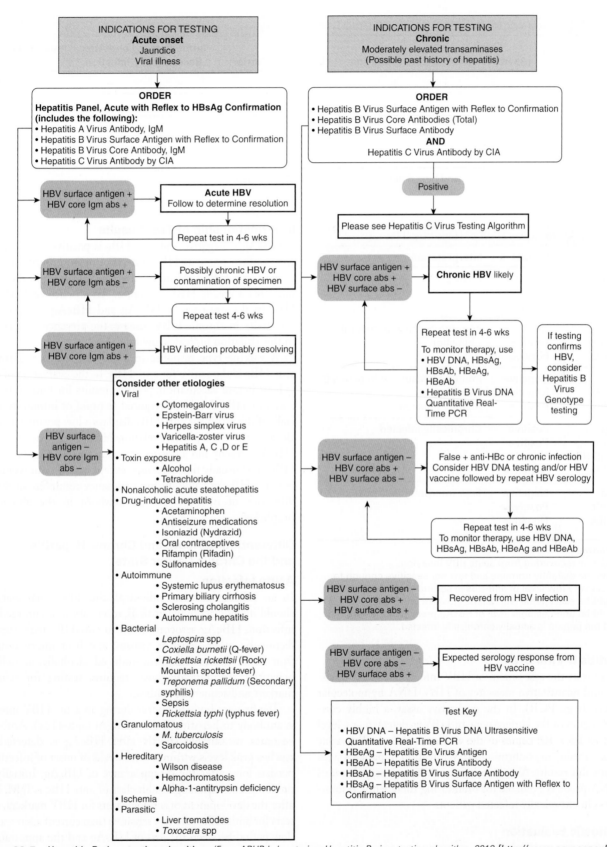

Figure 23-5 Hepatitis B virus testing algorithm. *(From ARUP Laboratories: Hepatitis B virus testing algorithm, 2012 [http://www.arupconsult.com/Algorithms/HBV.pdf].)*

Table 23-3	Serologic Markers for Hepatitis B Virus (HBV) Infection					
Marker	Early (Asymptomatic)	Acute or Chronic	Low-Level Carrier	Immediate Recovery	Long After Infection	Immunized With HBsAg
HBsAg	+	+	−	−	−	−
Anti-HBs	−	±	−	−	±	+
Anti-HBc	−	+	+	+	±	−
Anti-HBc (IgM)	−	+	−	+	−	−

Adapted from Hoofnagle JH: Type A and type B hepatitis, Lab Med 14(11):713 1983.
−, Negative; +, positive; ±, questionable.

Table 23-4	Interpretation of Hepatitis B Panel	
Tests	Results	Interpretation
HBsAg	Negative	Susceptible
Anti-HBc	Negative	
Anti-HBs	Negative	
HBsAg	Negative	Immune because of natural infection
Anti-HBc	Positive	
Anti-HBs	Positive	
HBsAg	Negative	Immune because of hepatitis B vaccination
Anti-HBc	Negative	
Anti-HBs	Positive	Acutely infected
HBsAg	Positive	Chronically infected
Anti-HBc	Positive	
IgM anti-HBc	Negative	
Anti-HBs	Negative	
HBsAg	Negative	Four interpretations possible*
Anti-HBc	Positive	
Anti-HBs	Negative	

*As follows:
1. Might be recovering from acute HBV infection.
2. Might be distantly immune and test not sensitive enough to detect very low level of anti-HBs in serum.
3. Might be susceptible with a false-positive anti-HBc.
4. Might be undetectable level of HBsAg present in the serum and the person is actually chronically infected.

Hepatitis B Viral DNA

Current tests the assessment of HBV infections are the qualitative and quantitative measures of HBV DNA by molecular methods (e.g., PCR). In the qualitative assay, a highly conserved region of the surface gene of HBV is detected at a level as low as 1.5×10^4 copies of the viral genome/mL. This assay may be of value in confirming HBV infection in patients with questionable results. A less sensitive quantitative assay that uses an RNA probe is available for monitoring therapeutic responsiveness in chronically infected patients.

Diagnostic Evaluation

Appropriate diagnostic procedures should be ordered, depending on clinical factors such as patient history, signs and symptoms being evaluated, and cases involving donated blood. The various components of HBV infection can be measured by a laboratory assay.

Interrelationship of Test Results

If HBsAg is negative and anti-HBc is positive, the anti-HBs will confirm previous HBV infection or immunity. The presence of anti-HBc IgM in the absence of HBsAg in the serum indicates a recent HBV infection. An absence of IgM anti-HBc in the presence of HBsAg and HBeAg suggests high infectivity in chronic HBV disease; the presence of anti-HBe in this situation indicates low infectivity.

A vaccine-type response includes test results negative for anti-HBc and positive for anti-HBs. In the evaluation of individuals before vaccination, positive results for both anti-HBc and anti-HBs should be required as proof of immunity, especially if the result for anti-HBs displays a low positive reaction. Because there is a positive relationship between the amount of HBsAg present and a positive reaction for HBeAg, testing for HBeAg is usually not necessary, except in pregnant women. A positive HBsAg value during pregnancy results in an 80% to 90% risk of infection in the newborn in the absence of prophylaxis.

Differentiating Acute and Chronic Hepatitis and the Chronic Carrier State

Acute Infection

In an HBsAg-positive individual, the differential diagnosis should include acute hepatitis B, reactivation of chronic HBV infection, HBeAg seroconversion to anti-HBe flare, superinfection by other hepatitis viruses, and liver injury resulting from other causes (e.g., drug-induced, alcoholic, or ischemic hepatitis). Accurate diagnosis requires testing for serologic markers and sequential studies.

The first antibody to appear during an acute HBV infection is antibody to hepatitis B core antigen (anti-HBc). Anti-HBc becomes measurable shortly after HBsAg is detected and reaches peak levels within several weeks of onset of infection. It persists long after the disappearance of HBsAg. Initially, the predominant immunoglobulin class of anti-HBc is IgM. Early after the development of serologic tests for HBV markers, when tests for anti-HBs were less sensitive than current assays, a window period between the loss of HBsAg and the appearance of anti-HBs was recognized. During this infrequently encountered window, or when levels of HBsAg do not reach detection thresholds, the detection of IgM anti-HBc is the sole marker of acute HBV infection. Over several weeks to months, the titer of IgM anti-HBc falls, tending to become undetectable after

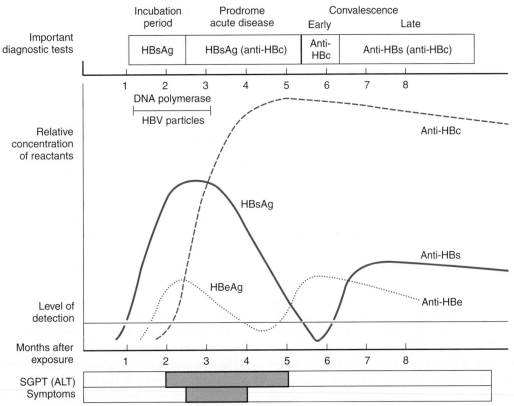

Figure 23-6 Serologic and clinical patterns observed during acute hepatitis B viral infection. *(Adapted from Hollinger FB, Dreesman GR Rose RN, Friedman H, editors: Manual of clinical immunology, ed 2, Washington, DC, 1980, American Society for Microbiology.)*

6 months. Total anti-HBc reactivity declines at a considerably slower rate; the predominant immunoglobulin form of anti-HBc during the late recovery phase is IgG. This IgG anti-HBc persists in slowly declining titers for many years to decades after acute infection.

Within a few days to 1 or 2 weeks of the appearance of HBsAg, hepatitis Be antigen (HBeAg) also becomes detectable in the circulation of acutely infected individuals. HBeAg, a nonstructural nucleocapsid protein, is a marker of HBV replication; its presence is correlated with the presence of complete HBV particles and HBV DNA in the circulation. In acute HBV infection, patients are most infectious during the period in which HBeAg can be detected. In self-limited HBV infection, HBeAg disappears before HBsAg disappears. With the disappearance of HBeAg, its corresponding antibody, anti-HBe, becomes detectable and persists for a prolonged period.

HBV DNA, and possibly HBV **virions,** may persist in circulating immune complexes. The viral genome can remain in an active form in peripheral blood mononuclear cells for more than 5 years after complete clinical and serologic recovery from acute viral hepatitis B.

Chronic Infection

Recent statistics have indicated that 800,000 to 1.4 million persons are living with chronic hepatitis B infection; 3000 patients die annually as the result of chronic liver disease associated with hepatitis B.

Progression from acute to chronic HBV is influenced by a patient's age at acquisition of the virus. Clinical expression of HBV infection is high in Asian but low in Western countries. In the Far East, where HBV infection is acquired perinatally, the immune system does not recognize the difference between the virus and the host. Consequently, a high level of immunologic tolerance emerges. The cellular immune responses to hepatocyte membrane HBV protein associated with acute hepatitis do not occur and chronic, usually lifelong, infection is established in more than 90% of infected patients. In Western countries, most acute HBV infections occur during adolescence and early adulthood. These segments of immunocompetent, HBV-infected patients produce a strong cellular immune response to foreign HBV proteins expressed by hepatocytes, with resulting, clinically apparent acute hepatitis. All but about 1% of infected patients clear the HBV infection.

Hepatitis B virus can lead to chronic infection and HBV patients have been shown to have the viral DNA actually incorporated into the DNA of their liver cells. This integration may be an important factor in the eventual development of liver cell cancer, hepatocellular carcinoma, a well-known long-term outcome of chronic HBV infection.

The hepatitis B virus is not directly cytopathic and the hepatocellular **necrosis** results from the host's immune response to the viral antigens of the replicating virus present in infected hepatocytes. Cytotoxic T cells recognize histocompatibility and HBcAg receptors on the liver cell membrane surface. Attachment of T cells to the receptors, together with natural killer (NK) cells, results in hepatocellular necrosis; in the setting of an effective immune response, HBV replication ceases.

Studies of peripheral blood mononuclear cells have revealed that patients with acute HBV produce vigorous T cell responses against multiple HBV antigenic determinants located on the viral core, envelope, and polymerase proteins, whereas patients with chronic infection have a very weak or undetectable cellular immune response. These findings suggest that a prompt, vigorous, and broad-based cellular immune response results in clearance of the virus from the liver, whereas a qualitatively or quantitatively less efficient or restricted immune response may permit the persistence of virus and the development of ongoing, immunologically mediated liver cell injury. In addition to a patient's immune response, viral factors (HBV genome) may also be important in determining the course of HBV infection.

Chronic HBV occurs in two phases, a more infectious replicative phase (high levels of circulating virions, HBV DNA, HBeAg) and a minimally infectious nonreplicative phase (few virions, circulating spherical and tubular forms of HBsAg, undetectable HBV DNA and HBeAg, but circulating anti-HBe and integrated HBV DNA in hepatocytes). In patients with chronic HBV infection, HBsAg remains detectable for more than 6 months and, in rare cases, HBsAg persists for decades. Spontaneous HBsAg clearance in chronic infection is unusual. Clearance of the virus results in complete clinical and histologic recovery, ultimately leaving the patient with a serologic pattern characterized by hepatitis B core antibody (IgG anti-HBc) and anti-HBs, with the latter conferring immunity.

Asymptomatic individuals in whom test results for HBsAg remain positive are labeled HBsAg carriers. Other chronically infected HBsAg-positive individuals may have clinical or laboratory evidence of chronic liver disease. Anti-HBc is present in all chronic HBV infections. In most chronically infected patients, IgM anti-HBc is a minor fraction of total anti-HBc reactivity. In all patients with HBV infection, HBeAg can be detected during the early phase of infection, but in contrast to the situation with acute self-limited HBV infection, HBeAg may remain detectable in chronically infected individuals for many months to years. In these patients, HBV DNA is also readily detected in the circulation. The presence of circulating HBV DNA is highly correlated with the presence of whole-virus replication, and thus with the potential infectivity of the patient. HBV DNA is also detectable in the hepatocytes of individuals with chronic HBV infection. For a variable but generally prolonged period, this hepatic HBV DNA is present in a free, episomal replicating form. In some patients, HBV DNA becomes integrated into the genome of the host hepatocyte. Viral replication may diminish spontaneously over time or after treatment, signaled by the decline or disappearance of serum HBV DNA, loss of HBeAg, and appearance of anti-HBe in the circulation, as detected by commercial assays. Research has suggested that both anti-HBe and anti-HBs may be present early in chronic hepatitis B complexed to HBeAg and HBsAg.

In 10% to 40% of patients with chronic HBV infection, anti-HBs is detected concurrently with HBsAg. The presence of anti-HBs does not signal reduced infectivity or imminent clearance of HBsAg.

Carrier State

There are an estimated 400 to 500 million HBV carriers worldwide. In the United States, 50,000 to 100,000 people acquire HBV infection each year, even though a highly effective vaccine is available. Immunocompromised patients, including those with human immunodeficiency virus (HIV) infection, are at increased risk for chronic HBV infection. Age at the time of acquisition of HBV infection is a major determinant of **chronicity,** as reflected by the development of the HBsAg carrier state. As many as 90% of infected neonates become carriers. The rate falls progressively with increasing age at the time of infection, so that only 1% to 10% of newly infected adults fail to clear HBsAg. Another important risk factor for chronicity is the presence of intrinsic or iatrogenic immunosuppression. Immunosuppressed individuals are at increased risk of becoming carriers after HBV infection. Gender is a determinant of chronicity. Women are more likely than men to clear HBsAg; therefore, men predominate in all populations of HBsAg carriers.

The worldwide prevalence of the HBsAg carrier state varies widely. In the United States, as in many Western nations, carriers account for approximately 0.2% of the general population. However, among certain groups (e.g., homosexual men, intravenous drug abusers) in the general population, carrier rates 4 to 10 times greater have been identified. Carrier rates as high as 25% have been recognized among Alaskan natives in some Alaskan villages.

Perinatal transmission continues to occur. This rate should be reduced significantly by the implementation of routine screening of all pregnant women for HBsAg, followed by vaccination of their newborns. Hepatitis B vaccination is gradually being incorporated into routine infant immunization programs. A newer multivalent, triple-antigen HBV vaccine should have wide practical application.

Carriers can be divided into two categories based on differing infectivity, depending on the presence in their serum of another antigen, HBeAg, or its antibody (anti-HBe). The types of carrier states include the following:

- The more frequently identified carriers have anti-HBe in their serum and are at a later stage of infection.
- Anti-HBe carriers are less infectious but may transmit infection through blood transfusion.
- HBsAg-positive carriers will become anti-HBe–positive carriers at a rate of about 5% to 10%/year.
- All HBsAg-positive individuals must be excluded from giving blood for transfusion.
- About one in four carriers has HBeAg in their serum. It is likely that these individuals have recently become carriers and that their blood is highly infectious.
- Patients with HBeAg-negative chronic HBV infection, in which precore or core promoter gene mutations preclude or reduce the synthesis of HBeAg, accounts for an increasing proportion of cases. These patients tend to have progressive liver injury, fluctuating liver enzyme activity, and lower levels of HBV DNA than patients with HBeAg-reactive HBV infection.

Prevention and Treatment

Routine hepatitis B vaccination of U.S. children began in 1991. Since then, the reported incidence of acute hepatitis B among children and adolescents (<15 years) has decreased by more than 98% and by 93% in those aged 15 to 24 years. Although not as large as the declines in younger age groups, substantial decreases also have occurred among older persons. The rates are a decrease of 78% in adults aged 25 to 44 years and 61% in adults 45 years of age or older.

The most important factors in preventing transfusion-acquired HBV are donor interviewing, screening of donor blood, use of hepatitis-free products when possible, and appropriate use of blood and blood components. In addition, the avoidance of high-risk blood components such as untreated factor VIII prepared from multiple-donor pools reduces the incidence of HBV.

Elimination of high-risk donors has accounted for at least a 50% reduction in the incidence of hepatitis; routine testing of donated blood for HBsAg has further reduced the incidence by another 20% to 30%. Testing for anti-HBc will detect almost 100% of HBsAg-positive persons, the rare asymptomatic donor in the core window, and the large number of donors who have had subclinical hepatitis B infections and are now immune.

The use of recombinant vaccine against hepatitis B, licensed in 1982, is warranted for high-risk persons, including medical personnel (Box 23-1). HBV vaccine is administered in three doses over 7 months and is about 80% to 95% effective. The vaccine is now included in the childhood vaccination schedule. Hepatitis B vaccine is also a vaccine against cancer (hepatocellular carcinoma). Vaccination offers a new approach to preventing transfusion-acquired HBV and the dependent hepatitis D virus (HDV) in patients who are likely to need ongoing transfusion therapy, such as nonimmune patients with hemophilia, sickle cell anemia, or aplastic anemia.

In cases of accidental needlestick exposure or exposure of mucous membranes or open cuts to HBsAg-positive blood, hepatitis B immune globulin (HBIG) should be administered within 24 hours of exposure and again 25 to 30 days later to nonimmunized patients. Infants born to mothers with acute hepatitis B in the third trimester, or with HBsAg at delivery, should be given HBIG as soon as possible and no later than 24 hours after birth. Persons who are HBsAg-positive or who have anti-HBs need not be given HBIG unless the HBV titer is shown to be low or unknown.

Seven drugs have been licensed in the United States for the treatment of HBV infection. Treatment for about 1 year usually results in the reduction of serum HBV DNA levels and a serum level of HBV DNA that is undetectable by PCR assay.

Liver transplantation is also used for some severe cases of liver disease caused by HBV, although the new organ usually becomes infected with HBV.

HEPATITIS D

Etiology

The hepatitis D virus (HDV), initially called the delta agent and then the hepatitis delta virus, was first described in 1977 as a pathogen that superinfects some patients already infected with HBV (see Table 23-1). Persons with acute or chronic HBV infection, as demonstrated by serum HBsAg, can be infected with HDV. HBV is required as a so-called helper to initiate infection.

The HDV is a replication defective or incomplete RNA virus that by itself, is unable to cause infection. HDV consists of a single-stranded, circular RNA coated in HBsAg. HDV is interesting because it can force the host's RNA polymerase to transcribe the HDV RNA genome.

Epidemiology

Hepatitis D was originally described in Italy and appears to be most common in southern European countries. It also appears to be endemic among Indian tribes living in the Amazon basin. In the United States, Northern Europe, and Asia, infection is uncommon. In the United States, hepatitis D is seen predominantly in intravenous (IV) drug users and their sexual partners, but it has been reported in homosexual men and men with hemophilia. According to the Centers for Disease Control and Prevention (CDC), there are approximately 70,000 people with chronic HDV infection in the United States.

Hepatitis D is a severe and rapidly progressive liver disease for which no therapy has proven effective. Patients with this form of hepatitis are significantly more likely to have cirrhosis and liver failure and to require liver transplantation than patients with HBV infection alone. Chronic HDV infection is responsible for more than 1000 deaths/year in the United States. The mortality rate can be up to 20% of infected patients.

Hepatitis D virus is spread chiefly by direct contact of HBsAg carriers with HDV- or HBV-infected individuals. Family members and intimate contacts of infected individuals are at greatest risk. IV drug users and individuals with multiple sex partners are two other high-risk groups. Maternal-neonatal transmission is uncommon.

Hepatitis D can be acquired either as a co–primary infection (**coinfection**) with HBV (e.g., after inoculation with blood or secretions containing both agents) or as a superinfection in patients with established HBV infection (HBsAg carriers or patients with chronic hepatitis B). A superinfection can make an HBV infection worse by transforming a mild infection into a persistent infection in 80% of patients. In contrast, coinfection rarely leads to a chronic condition. Although HDV is dependent on HBV for its expression and pathogenicity, replication of HDV appears to be independent of the presence of its associated hepadnavirus.

Signs and Symptoms

Hepatitis D infection may be benign and brief, but fulminant hepatitis and chronic hepatitis have been attributed with increasing frequency to HDV. Chronic HDV infection is associated with increased hepatic damage and a more severe clinical course than is expected from chronic HBV infection alone. The occurrence of sequential attacks of HBV in the same patient is probably attributable in most cases to HDV infection superimposed on a previous acute HBV infection.

Infection with HDV agent can occur in several conditions; the symptoms would be typical of acute or chronic hepatitis, as follows:

- Acute hepatitis D with concurrent acute hepatitis B (coinfection)
- Acute hepatitis D in a chronic HBsAg carrier
- Chronic hepatitis D in a chronic HBsAg carrier

Immunologic Manifestations

The HDV probably partially suppresses HBV replication. Hepatitis D infection is diagnosed by the appearance of HDV antigen in serum or the development of IgM or IgG HDV antibodies that appear sequentially in a time frame similar to that described for hepatitis A or B antibodies. HBsAg will also be present.

Coinfection With Hepatitis B Virus

In patients with acute, self-limited HDV coinfection with HBV, various serologic responses indicative of HDV infection have been identified. Serum HDV RNA and HDV antigen (HDAg) may be detected early, concurrently with the detection of HBsAg. HDAg disappears as HBsAg disappears and seroconversion to anti–hepatitis D (anti-HD; initially, IgM and later IgG) follows. The IgM reactivity usually appears several days to a few weeks after the onset of illness, whereas IgG anti-HD appears in the convalescent phase. In about 60% of coinfections, HDAg is not detected by anti-HD, but patients can manifest both IgM and IgG antibodies. IgM anti-HD in self-limited coinfections is usually transient. IgG anti-HD often disappears as well, but occasionally persists in declining titer for many months and may remain detectable as long as 1 to 2 years after the disappearance of HBsAg. In a small number of patients, the early appearance of isolated IgM anti-HD, or its appearance during convalescence of isolated IgG anti-HD, may be the only detectable marker of HDV infection.

Superinfection of Hepatitis B Carrier

Hepatitis D superinfection of HBV (HBsAg) carriers causes the appearance of HDAg and HDV RNA, a simultaneous reduction in HBV replication, and a consequent diminution in the titer of circulating HBsAg. Termination of the HBsAg carrier state appears to occur infrequently after HDV inhibition of HBV replication. Often, HDV infection becomes chronic and HDAg and HDV RNA may remain detectable at low levels in the serum; in persistent HDV infection, large quantities of HDAg can be detected in hepatocytes. High titers of IgM and IgG anti-HD are maintained in persistent infection, reflecting progressive, HDV-induced, chronic liver disease.

Diagnostic Evaluation

The HDV appears in the circulating blood as a particle with a core of delta antigen and a surface component of HBsAg. A person with hepatitis D will have detectable antigen in the liver and antibody in the serum. Test methodologies for HDV use the qualitative EIA (Fig. 23-7)

In addition, HDV antigen can be demonstrated in liver biopsies by double immunodiffusion (DIF) and immunoperoxidase

and in serum by cloned DNA (cDNA). The importance of the detection of antibodies to HDV is largely prognostic. Detection of IgG anti-HDV in the presence of IgM anti-HBc antibody strongly suggests simultaneous infection (coinfection). Detection of IgM anti-HDV in a patient with chronic HBV infection is evidence of HDV superinfection.

Screening for total HDV antibodies in serum is important in the identification of a subpopulation of apparently healthy HBsAg carriers whose risk of serious liver damage is fourfold higher than that of anti-HDV–negative carriers. The combined presence of total anti-HDV antibody and abnormal liver function test results in a symptom-free carrier suggests parenchymal damage and is considered an indication for liver biopsy. Hepatic lesions in anti-HDV–positive carriers often consist of chronic active hepatitis or advanced cirrhosis. A positive test result for IgM anti-HDV increases the likelihood of occult active HBV infection.

HEPATITIS C

Etiology

Hepatitis C, previously called non-A, non-B (NANB) hepatitis, was regarded as a diagnosis of exclusion because of the absence of specific serologic markers and unknown viral origin. HCV has now been identified, with immunologic assays developed for its detection. No homology exists among HAV, HBV, or HDV and HCV.

Viral Characteristics

Hepatitis C virus is an enveloped flavivirus. It is a small, enveloped, single-stranded RNA virus. After binding to the cell surface, HCV particles enter the cell by receptor-mediated endocytosis. Because the virus mutates rapidly, changes in the envelope protein may help it evade the immune system.

There are at least six major HCV genotypes and more than 50 subtypes of HCV. The different genotypes have different geographic distributions. Genotype 1 represents most infection in North and South America, and Europe. Genotypes 1a and 1b are the most common genotypes in the United States. The HCV genotype does not appear to play a role in the severity of disease. Knowing the genotype-specific antibodies of HCV is useful to physicians when making recommendations and counseling patients regarding therapy. Patients with genotypes 2 and 3 have a more favorable prognosis and are more likely to respond to treatment.

Epidemiology

Worldwide, an estimated 180 million people are infected with HCV. In the period 2004 to 2009 (the last year for which statistics were available at the time of publication), 2.7 to 3.9 million persons in the United States were living with chronic infection caused by hepatitis C. Annually, 12,000 patients die in the United States as the result of chronic liver disease associated with HCV. HCV infection is a leading cause of chronic hepatitis, cirrhosis, and liver cancer and is a primary indication for liver transplantation in Western countries.

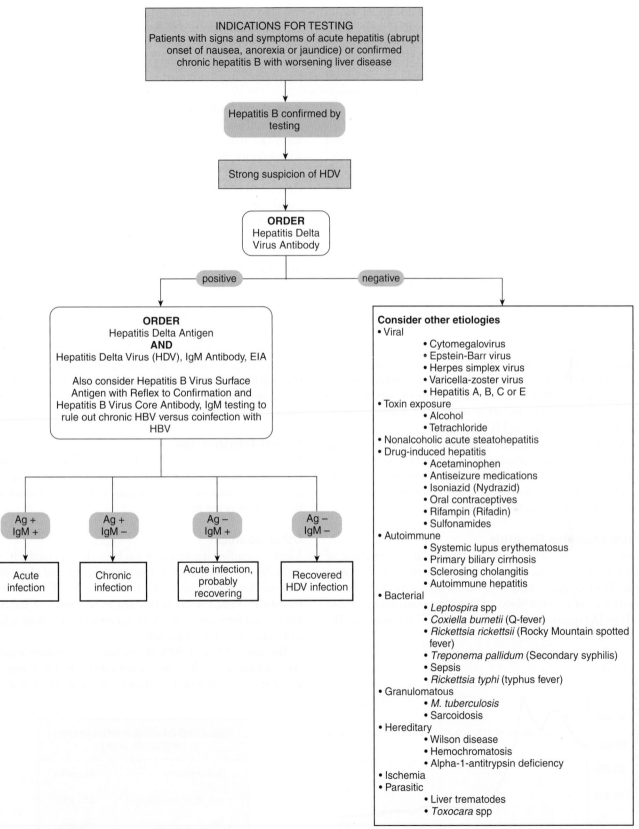

Figure 23-7 Hepatitis delta virus (HDV) testing algorithm. *(From ARUP Laboratories: Hepatitis delta virus [HDV] testing algorithm, 2012 [http://www. arupconsult.com/Algorithms/HDV.pdf].)*

In the past, hepatitis C was considered a disease limited to transfusion recipients. HCV is now recognized in many other epidemiologic settings (see Table 23-1) and as a major cause of chronic hepatitis worldwide. The number of cases reported to the National Notifiable Disease Surveillance System are considered unreliable because of the following: (1) the lack of a serologic marker for acute infection; and (2) the inability of most health departments to determine whether a positive laboratory result for HCV represents acute infection, chronic infection, repeated testing of a person previously reported, or a false-positive result.

In 2009, the total number of reported cases of acute hepatitis was 2600. The estimated total number of new cases of hepatitis C in the United States was 16,000 in 2009 (the last year for which statistics were available at the time of publication). Since the mid-1990s, hepatitis C rates have declined in all age groups, almost reaching a plateau since 2003 (Fig. 23-8). The greatest decline has occurred among persons 25 to 39 years old, the age group traditionally with the highest rates of disease, in whom incidence has declined by 58% since 2000.

Viral Transmission

HCV is spread primarily by percutaneous contact with infected blood or blood products. Currently, injectable drug abuse is the most common risk factor. Workers with needlestick injuries, infants born to HCV-infected mothers, those with multiple sexual partners, and recipients of unscreened donor blood are also at risk for contracting HCV.

Although most hepatitis C patients are injectable drug abusers, many patients acquire HCV without any known exposure to blood or drug use. Sporadic or community-acquired infections without a known source occur in about 10% of acute hepatitis C cases and 30% of chronic cases.

Posttransfusion Hepatitis

After the introduction of serologic testing in the screening of blood donors, the rate of posttransfusion hepatitis C decreased from 33% to approximately 15%. Before laboratory screening, the transfusion of infected blood or blood components (e.g., factor VIII or IX) constituted a clear route of HCV transmission. The incidence of posttransfusion hepatitis C declined in the 1980s because of the effort to replace the pool of high-risk, paid donors. Also, dialysis patients now require fewer blood transfusions because recombinant erythropoietin (EPO) is used to stimulate the patient's own bone marrow to produce red blood cells.

Parenteral and Occupational Exposure

In 2006, illegal IV drug use continued to be the most frequently identified risk factor for HCV infection. Accidental needlestick injuries also are a clearly documented route of hepatitis transmission (Fig. 23-9). The Occupational Safety and Health Administration (OSHA) has estimated that the general risk to health care workers of occupational transmission of HCV is 20 to 40 times higher than the risk of contracting HIV. The CDC has more conservatively estimated that the average risk of HCV transmission after a needlestick injury is six times greater than the risk of HIV transmission. Because of these grim statistics, occupationally acquired HCV infection is a growing concern for health care providers.

A person with a high level of circulating HCV may be capable of transmitting the virus by exposing others percutaneously or mucosally to small amounts of blood or other body fluids. A person with a low level of circulating HCV may be capable of transmitting the virus only by exposing others percutaneously to a large volume of blood. The threshold concentration of virus needed to transmit or cause infection is uncertain.

Sexual Transmission

Sexual transmission is believed to occur, but is infrequent. Spouses of patients with HCV viremia and chronic liver disease have an increased risk of acquiring HCV proportional to the duration of the marriage.

Other Sources

Mother to infant transmission has been documented. HCV is vertically transmitted from mother to infant and the risk of transmission is correlated with the level of HCV RNA in the mother. Personal contact is thought to be a route of infection but has not been conclusively demonstrated; the actual risk for such transmission is unknown.

Between 25% and 50% of sporadic community-acquired cases of hepatitis in the United States are of the HCV type and are unrelated to parenteral exposure. Some of these cases are

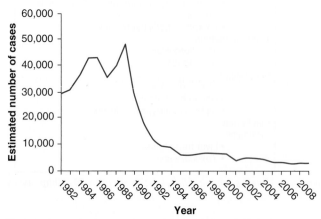

Figure 23-8   Incidence of hepatitis C, by year, 1982-2009. *(Courtesy National Center for HIV/AIDS, Viral Hepatitis, STD, and TB Prevention, Centers for Disease Control and Prevention, Atlanta, GA.)*

Hepatitis C infection after accidental needlestick injury	
Donor source	Hepatitis
• Anti-HCV positive	0%-10%
• HBsAg positive	7%-30%

Figure 23-9   Hepatitis C infection after accidental needlestick injury. *(Adapted from Hernandez ME et al: Risk of needlestick injuries in the transmission of hepatitis C in hospital personnel, J Hepatol 16:56–58, 1992; and Mitsui T et al: Hepatitis C infection in medical personnel after needlestick accident, J Hepatol 16:1109–1114, 1992.)*

believed to result from heterosexual transmission, but in approximately 40% the route of infection cannot be identified. Therefore, transmission can occur by inapparent and apparent parenteral routes; this form of hepatitis cannot be distinguished from other types of viral hepatitis solely by its epidemiologic characteristics.

In addition, liver disease can occur in the recipients of organs from donors with antibodies to HCV. Almost all the recipients of organs from anti-HCV–positive donors become infected with HCV. The current tests for anti-HCV antibodies may underestimate the incidence of transmission and the prevalence of HCV infection in immunosuppressed organ recipients. If the medical condition of the potential recipient is so serious that other options no longer exist, however, the use of an organ from an anti-HCV–seropositive donor should be considered.

Prognosis

Several strains of HCV exist. The genotype of HCV may influence the clinical course of HCV, as well as the response to IFN and newer treatments.

It is believed that about 50% of patients with acute hepatitis C will continue to have elevated serum liver enzyme levels more than 6 months after the onset of illness. These patients usually have persistent HCV RNA detected in their serum and evidence of chronic hepatitis on liver biopsy. Viremia, as detected by HCV RNA assay, may persist for months to years in patients in whom serum liver enzyme levels return to normal, and liver biopsy may reveal chronic hepatitis.

Chronic hepatitis C appears to be a slowly progressive, often silent disease. In addition, HCV may be associated with hepatocellular carcinoma predominantly, if not exclusively, in the setting of cirrhosis.

Signs and Symptoms

Although the clinical characteristics of the acute disease of both types of hepatitis C are basically indistinguishable, the chronic consequences are very different. The signs and symptoms of hepatitis C are extremely variable. It can be mild, transient, and completely asymptomatic, or it can be severe, prolonged, and ultimately fatal.

Hepatitis C more closely resembles HBV than HAV in regard to its transmission and clinical features. Hepatitis C, as with HBV, can be acute and ranges from mild anicteric illness to **fulminant disease.** A fulminant course with a rapidly fatal outcome is rare. Usually, the patient is only mildly symptomatic and nonicteric; less than 25% of patients develop jaundice. Transfusion-associated hepatitis C can be divided into short- and long-incubation types. Incubation periods for the short-duration type range from 1 or 2 to 5 weeks; the longer duration type ranges from 7 to 12 weeks to 6 months or longer.

Hepatitis C is characterized by serum liver enzyme levels in the range of 200 to 800 U/L and marked fluctuations, with intervening periods of normalcy. Mean serum liver enzyme and bilirubin levels of patients with hepatitis C, however, are significantly lower than those of patients with HBV; the extensive overlap of the ranges of elevation precludes the identification of the type of viral hepatitis by the use of these assays.

The diagnosis of hepatitis C has a guarded prognosis. Although hepatitis C was initially thought to be a relatively benign disease, there is increasing evidence of progression to cirrhosis in about 20% of patients, liver failure, and even **hepatoma.** The hepatic damage is caused by the cytopathic effect of the virus and the inflammatory changes secondary to immune activation. Up to 60% of patients with posttransfusion hepatitis C develop chronic liver disease, based on biopsy analysis, and up to 20% of these patients develop cirrhosis.

Posttransfusion hepatitis C affects men and women equally, but a reported 75% of patients developing chronic hepatitis were men. Patients with parenterally acquired (nontransfusion) hepatitis C, including those who have no identifiable source, have the same clinical characteristics and develop chronic liver disease with the same frequency.

Extrahepatic immunologic abnormalities have been shown to occur frequently in patients with chronic HCV infection. HCV infection has been linked to a number of extrahepatic conditions, including Sjögren's syndrome, cryoglobulinemia, urticaria, erythema nodosum, vasculitis, glomerulonephritis, and peripheral neuropathy. HCV apparently causes the cases of mixed cryoglobulinemia previously mentioned.

Laboratory Assays

HCV infection is characterized by two major immunologic fingerprints:

1. Escape of immune response in more than 80% of infected patients
2. Production of monoclonal or polyclonal rheumatoid factor (RF) in 20% to 40% of infected patients

Immunologic failure results in chronic infection, persistent stimulation of the immune system, and subsequent production of circulating immune complexes, of which almost one third become insoluble when exposed to low temperatures and are associated with the clinical picture of cryoglobulinemia. Many epidemiologic studies have demonstrated an association between HCV infection and an increased incidence of B cell, non-Hodgkin's lymphoma (NHL), ranging from 20% to 30% to almost twice that of HCV-negative control subjects.

Traditional Hepatitis C Virus Testing

Traditional testing methods (Fig. 23-10) include a qualitative chemiluminescent immunoassay and qualitative EIA, qualitative recombinant immunoblot assay, quantitative real-time PCR assay, qualitative PCR assay, quantitative branched chain DNA test, polymerase chain reaction–nucleic acid sequencing. interleukin 28 B (IL-28B)–associated variants test, and two single-nucleotide polymorphisms (SNPs) method—qualitative PCR–qualitative fluorescence monitoring.

Western Blot

The Western blot or recombinant immunoblot assay (RIBA) can be used to confirm anti-HCV reactivity. Three successive generations of RIBAs have evolved since 1990, with each providing incrementally improved specificity. In this procedure, serum is incubated on nitrocellulose strips on which four recombinant viral proteins are blotted. Color changes indicate

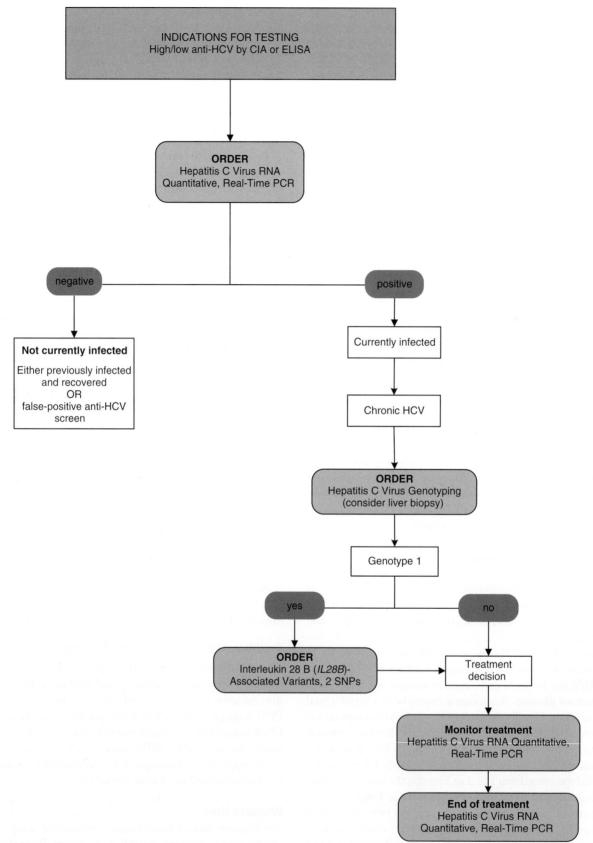

Figure 23-10   Hepatitis C virus testing algorithm. *(From ARUP Laboratories: Hepatitis C virus testing algorithm, 2012 [http://www.arupconsult.com/Algorithms/HCV.pdf].)*

that antibodies are adhering to the proteins. An immunoblot test result is considered positive if two or more proteins react. The assay is considered indeterminate if only one positive band is detected.

Confirmatory testing by immunoblotting is helpful in some clinical situations (e.g., positive anti-HCV detected by EIA but negative for HCV RNA). The positive EIA anti-HCV reactivity could represent the following:

- False-positive reaction
- Recovery from hepatitis C
- Viral infection with levels of virus too low to be detected

If the immunoblot test for anti-HCV is positive, the patient has most likely recovered from hepatitis C and has persistent antibody without virus. If the immunoblot test is negative, the EIA result was probably a false-positive.

Immunoblot tests are used routinely in blood banks when an anti-HCV–positive sample is found by EIA. Immunoblot assays are highly specific and valuable in verifying anti-HCV reactivity. Indeterminate tests require follow-up testing, including attempts to confirm the specificity by repeat testing for HCV RNA.

The current third-generation RIBA uses three recombinant antigens (c33c, c100-3, and NS5) and one synthetic peptide from the core region. Because the RIBA is based on the same recombinant antigens and synthetic peptides as the enzyme-linked immunosorbent assay (ELISA), it is licensed as an additional, more specific test.

Polymerase Chain Reaction

The PCR amplification technique can detect low levels of HCV RNA in serum. Testing for HCV RNA is a reliable way of demonstrating that hepatitis C infection is present and is the most specific test for infection.

Testing for HCV RNA by a PCR assay is particularly useful in the following situations:

- Transaminase levels are normal or only slightly elevated.
- Anti-HCV is not present.
- Several causes of liver disease are possible.

The best confirmatory assay to confirm a diagnosis of hepatitis C is to test for HCV RNA using a PCR assay. In addition, HCV RNA testing is of value when EIA tests for anti-HCV are unreliable (e.g., immunocompromised patients may not produce sufficiently high antibody titer for detection with EIA). Immunosuppressed or immunocompetent patients pose diagnostic problems because of their inability to produce anti-HCV. HCV RNA testing may be required for the following:

- Immunosuppressed patients (e.g., recipients of a solid-organ transplant)
- Patients undergoing dialysis because of chronic renal failure
- Patients taking corticosteroids
- Patients experiencing agammaglobulinemia

Patients exhibiting anti-HCV who have another form of liver disease (e.g., alcoholism, autoimmune disorder) can be difficult to diagnose. In these situations, the anti-HCV may represent a false-positive reaction, previous HCV infection, or mild hepatitis C occurring concurrently with another hepatic abnormality. In these cases, HCV RNA testing can help confirm that hepatitis C is contributing to the liver problem.

Hepatitis C RNA Titers in Serum

Several methods are available for measuring the titer or level of virus in serum, which is an indirect assessment of viral load. These methods include a quantitative PCR and a branched DNA test. Because these assays are not standardized, different laboratories may provide different results on the same specimen. In addition, serum levels of HCV RNA may vary spontaneously by threefold to tenfold over time. With these limitations in mind, however, carefully performed quantitative assays provide important insights into the nature of hepatitis C.

The usefulness of determining the viral load does not correlate with the severity of the hepatitis or with a poor prognosis, but viral load does correlate with the likelihood of a response to antiviral therapy. Monitoring viral load during the early phases of treatment may provide early information on the likelihood of a response. Rates of response to a course of interferon-α (IFN-α) and ribavirin are higher in patients with low levels of HCV RNA. The usual definition of a low level of HCV RNA is less than 2 million copies/mL.

The Heptimax assay (Quest Diagnostics, Madison, NJ) is an ultrasensitive quantitative test that detects levels of HCV based on transcription-mediated amplification technology. Because this technology can detect minute quantities of HCV, physicians can monitor HCV infection better, demonstrate posttreatment resolution, and detect relapses with greater sensitivity.

Acute and Chronic Hepatitis C

Acute Hepatitis C

The coordinated activities of CD4+ T cells and cytotoxic CD8+ T cells, primed in the context of human leukocyte antigen (HLA) class II and I alleles, respectively, on antigen-present cells are critically important for the control of acute HCV infections. The signs and symptoms of acute hepatitis C infection usually include jaundice, fatigue, and nausea. Laboratory manifestations include a significant increase in serum liver enzyme levels (usually >10-fold) and the presence or de novo development of anti-HCV.

Demonstration of HCV antibodies can be problematic because anti-HCV is not always present in the patient with symptoms. In 30% to 40% of patients, anti-HCV is not detected until 2 to 8 weeks after the onset of symptoms. Acute hepatitis C can also be diagnosed by testing for HCV RNA, apparently the earliest detectable marker of acute HCV infection, preceding the appearance of anti-HCV by several weeks. The current ELISA for antibodies to recombinant HCV antigens becomes positive earlier and is more sensitive than preceding ELISAs. Another approach is to repeat the anti-HCV testing 1 month after the onset of illness.

Hepatitis C viremia may persist despite the normalization of serum ALT levels. Intracytoplasmic HCV antigen has been found in the hepatocytes of acutely infected chimpanzees and, by analogy, is presumed to be present in acute hepatitis C in human beings. HCV antigens were not detected in hepatocyte nuclei, Kupffer or sinusoidal lining cells, bile duct epithelium, or blood vessels.

Chronic Hepatitis C

Chronic hepatitis C varies greatly in its course and outcome. At one end of the spectrum are asymptomatic patients who generally have a favorable prognosis; at the other end are patients with severe hepatitis C who have symptoms, HCV RNA in their serum, and elevated serum liver enzyme levels. These patients typically develop cirrhosis and end-stage liver disease.

Episodic fluctuations in serum liver enzyme levels appear to be a feature of chronic hepatitis C. This pattern, presumably reflecting waves of hepatocellular inflammation and necrosis, may last for months to years. Such episodes of disease activity may be related to the emergence of so-called HCV neutralization escape mutants, but other poorly defined mechanisms also may play a role. HCV RNA is detected in the serum by PCR in almost all patients with chronic hepatitis C. HCV replication may be increased in advanced liver disease and may contribute to the progression of disease.

At least 20% of patients with chronic hepatitis C develop cirrhosis, a process that takes 10 to 20 years. After 20 to 40 years, a smaller percentage of patients with chronic disease develop liver cancer. Liver failure from chronic hepatitis C is one of the most common reasons for liver transplantation in the United States.

Chronic hepatitis C is diagnosed when anti-HCV is present and serum liver enzyme levels remain elevated for more than 6 months. Testing for HCV RNA by PCR assay confirms the diagnosis and documents that viremia is present. Most patients with chronic infection will have the viral genome detectable in serum by PCR.

Approximately one third of those infected with HCV manifest anti-HCV antibodies within several weeks; others may take months or, less often, as long as 1 year to express antibodies. The current test antigen represents only 12% of the encoding capacity of the virus.

A reactive test implies infection with HCV, but not infectivity or immunity.

Treatment

The standard of care for HCV treatment since the early 1990s has been interferon, which aimed to boost the immune system rather than attacking the HCV directly. Two new protease inhibitors, boceprevir and telaprevir, approved by the FDA in May 2011, have the potential to transform the management of HCV. The main goal of treatment of chronic hepatitis C is to eliminate detectable viral RNA from the blood. Lack of detectable HCV RNA from blood 6 months after completing therapy is known as a sustained response and has a very favorable prognosis that may be equivalent to a cure. Other, more subtle benefits of treatment may include slowing the progression of fibrosis in patients who do not achieve a sustained response.

All current treatment protocols for hepatitis C are based on the use of various preparations of IFN-α, a naturally occurring glycoprotein secreted by cells in response to viral infections. It exerts its effects by binding to a membrane receptor, which initiates a series of intracellular signaling events that ultimately lead to enhanced expression of certain genes. This leads to enhancement and induction of certain cellular activities, including augmentation of target cell killing by lymphocytes and inhibition of virus replication in infected cells.

Interferon alfa-2a (Roferon-A; Hoffmann-La Roche, Basel, Switzerland), IFN-alfa-2b (Intron-A; Merck/Schering-Plough Pharmaceuticals, North Wales, Pa), and IFN-alfacon-1 (Infergen; Intermune, Kadmon, New York, NY) are all approved in the United States as single agents for the treatment of adults with chronic hepatitis C. Treatment is administered for 6 months to 2 years. Treatment with IFN alone leads to a sustained response in less than 15% of subjects. Because of this low response rate, these IFNs alone are rarely used for the treatment of patients with chronic hepatitis C.

More recently, peginterferon alpha, sometimes called pegylated IFN, has become available for the treatment of chronic hepatitis C. There are two preparations—peginterferon alfa-2b (Peg-Intron; Schering-Plough) and peginterferon alfa-2a (Pegasys; Hoffmann-La Roche). With peginterferon alfa-2a alone, approximately 30% to 40% of patients achieve a sustained response to treatment for 24 to 48 weeks. The addition of ribavirin to IFN-α is superior to IFN-α alone in the treatment of chronic hepatitis C.

Ribavirin is a synthetic nucleoside that has activity against a broad spectrum of viruses. The FDA did not approve ribavirin alone for hepatitis C, but the FDA did approve IFN-alfa-2b plus ribavirin (1998) for the treatment of individuals with chronic hepatitis C who relapsed after previous IFN-α therapy. Relapsers were defined as patients who had normal liver serum enzymes ALT activity at the end of up to 18 months of IFN-α therapy, with abnormal liver serum enzyme activity within 1 year after the end of the most recent course of therapy. The FDA has approved the combination of peginterferon alpha plus ribavirin for the treatment of chronic hepatitis C. For eligible patients with chronic hepatitis C, peginterferon alpha plus ribavirin is likely to be the best treatment option. Clinical trials have shown that a sustained response rate is seen in approximately 50% of patients given this combination for 24 to 48 weeks.

Most studies have indicated that genotypes 1a and 1b are more resistant to treatment with any IFN-α–based therapy than non–type 1 genotypes. Thus, some physicians may prescribe longer a duration of treatment for patients infected with viral genotype 1a or 1b. The best available current treatment for chronic hepatitis C, peginterferon alpha plus ribavirin, leads to an overall sustained response rate in more than 50% of all patients. The sustained response rates are even better for individuals infected with non–type 1 genotypes of the hepatitis C virus.

Several drugs, known as immune modifiers or immunomodulators, that alter the immune response have been tested (some with IFN-α) in clinical trials for chronic hepatitis C. These drugs alter the inflammatory response against liver cells infected with the virus; however, their mechanisms of action are poorly understood. Compounds tested in human beings include thymosin alpha-1 (Zadaxin; SciClone Pharmaceuticals, San Mateo, Calif) and histamine dihydrochloride (Ceplene; EpiCept Tarrytown, NY).

New medications and approaches to treatment are needed for HCV infection. Most promising for the immediate future are newer forms of long-acting IFNs. In addition, promising molecular therapies consist of using ribozymes, enzymes that break down specific viral RNA molecules, and antisense oligonucleotides, small complementary segments of DNA that bind to viral RNA and inhibit viral replication.

Therapeutic vaccines are also being developed to enhance the immune response against the HCV. In contrast to a preventive vaccine (likely a distant development for hepatitis C), a therapeutic vaccine is administered to already infected individuals to stimulate the immune system to fight the infection. Several therapeutic vaccines are in preclinical development for hepatitis C. The most promising of these are DNA vaccines involving the injection of DNA copies of the HCV RNA genome, which are taken up by certain immune system cells. Theoretically, these cells then express viral proteins, stimulating an immune response against the virus.

Who Should and Who Should Not Be Treated?

Patients with anti-HCV, HCV RNA, elevated liver serum enzyme ALT levels, and evidence of chronic hepatitis on liver biopsy, and with no contraindications, should be offered therapy with a combination of IFN-α and ribavirin. The National Institutes of Health Consensus Development Conference Panel has recommended that therapy for hepatitis C be limited to patients who have histologic evidence of progressive disease without signs of decompensation. According to current recommendations, all patients with fibrosis or moderate to severe degrees of inflammation and necrosis on liver biopsy should be treated and patients with less severe histologic disease should be managed on an individual basis. Patient selection should not be based on the presence or absence of symptoms, mode of acquisition, genotype of HCV RNA, or serum HCV RNA levels.

Interferon and combination therapy have not been shown to improve survival or the ultimate outcome in patients with preexisting cirrhosis. The benefit of treatment in patients older than 60 years has not been well documented. The role of IFN therapy in children with hepatitis C remains uncertain.

Prevention

Preventive practices among health care workers to avoid needlestick injuries should be promoted. Investigations have shown that removal of blood from donors with anti-HBcAg from the blood supply and use of third-generation anti-HCV testing can reduce the incidence of posttransfusion hepatitis C.

Vaccines and immunoglobulin products do not exist for the prevention or treatment of hepatitis C. Development of preventive strategies appears unlikely in the near future because these products would require antibodies to all the genotypes and variants of hepatitis C; however, some type of vaccine may eventually be developed.

HEPATITIS E

Etiology

The agent that causes hepatitis E is hepatitis E virus (HEV).

Epidemiology

Only a few cases of hepatitis E have been reported, with none originating in the United States. All have been seen in travelers returning from the Indian subcontinent, northern Africa, the Far East, portions of Russia (the former Soviet Union), and Mexico.

Hepatitis E virus (HEV) is transmitted by the fecal-oral route. Infection is usually the result of poor sanitation conditions. HEV is responsible for large, water-borne outbreaks of hepatitis in the developing world and is the most common cause of sporadic hepatitis in young adults in developing nations. Clinically apparent disease frequently is found in patients 15 to 40 years old.

The HEV infection rate among household contacts of infected patients appears to be low. The seroprevalence of HEV in blood donors is approximately 2%.

Virus-like particles have been observed in the stool from patients with HEV infection. In addition, serologic tests (IgM and IgG anti-HEV) have been developed now that the HEV genome has been cloned and sequenced.

Signs and Symptoms

The incubation period of HEV ranges from 2 to 9 weeks, with an average of 6 weeks. The symptoms of HEV infection are similar to those of other forms of viral hepatitis. HEV particles may appear in feces, inconstantly, during **prodromal** symptoms of hepatitis E. Fecal HEV shedding occurs predominantly during the first week after the onset of jaundice and has not been identified in stool samples obtained at 8 to 15 days. Viremia may occur during the period of fecal HEV shedding.

No form of chronic liver disease has been attributable to infection by HEV. Although most acute infections are self-limited and mild, 10% to 20% of HEV infections in pregnant women about result in fulminant hepatitis, especially in the third trimester of pregnancy.

Immunologic Manifestations

A short-lived, IgM anti-HEV has been found in acute-phase sera. IgG anti-HEV appears and replaces IgM anti-HEV about 2 to 4 weeks after symptoms subside. The duration of detectable IgG anti-HEV remains uncertain.

Diagnostic Evaluation

Specific serologic tests for IgM and IgG anti-HEV are available. HEV can be diagnosed by performing immunoelectron microscopy on a stool specimen. Liver serum enzyme levels, if elevated, are indicative of the acute phase of the infection.

Prevention and Treatment

Standard gamma globulin preparations have not been shown to be effective in the prevention of viral E hepatitis. No effective vaccine has been developed. Treatment of HEV is usually supportive care.

HEPATITIS G

Etiology

The cause of hepatitis G is the hepatitis G virus (HGV), an RNA virus. HGV is almost identical to a viral agent called GB virus type C (GBV-C). In 1995 and 1996, two independent groups discovered and sequenced an agent with limited homology to HCV, named GBV-C/HGV. The viral agents have 96% amino acid identity and represent variants of HGV. It's very common to find people with hepatitis C that are co-infected with GBV-C.

Epidemiology

Hepatitis G virus is a bloodborne agent (Table 23-5). Transfusion recipients and IV drug abusers are at risk of infection. HGV infection frequently occurs as a coinfection with HCV. Prevalence patterns of GBV-C/HGV suggest that the virus is transmitted sexually.

GB virus C infection is common; 1% to 2% of U.S. blood donors have HGV RNA detectable in their serum. HGV is estimated to produce 900 to 2000 infections/year, most of which may be asymptomatic. Chronic infection develops in 90% to 100% of infected persons. Chronic disease is rare or may not occur at all.

Signs and Symptoms

Chronic HGV infection does not appear to be a common cause of important liver disease and does not alter the course of chronic HCV infection. The vast majority of patients with acute, non–A-E hepatitis have no evidence of HGV infection. The role of HGV (GBV-C) in human hepatitis remains unclear.

GB virus C may not be a significant cause of acute or chronic liver disease. In all, 15% of children with chronic hepatitis C or hepatitis B are infected with HGV. In these cases, HGV coinfection does not appear to cause more severe liver disease.

The HGV has not been proven to cause fulminant hepatitis. Studies have suggested that the virus may not even replicate in the liver. The role of HGV in acute and chronic hepatitis remains to be defined fully.

Diagnostic Evaluation

A cDNA expression library was constructed from the plasma of a patient with chronic hepatitis C. Immunoscreening of the expression library with the patient's serum identified several unique HCV and other sequences, from which an anchored PCR method (Table 23-6) was used to amplify overlapping clones for the entire viral genome. The virus was termed the *GB virus C virus*.

Prevention

Confirmation of disease association, establishment of routes of transmission, and development of serologic screening assays are necessary before preventive measures can be considered.

Table 23-5	Summary of Hepatitis Characteristics		
Type of Hepatitis	Molecular Composition	Route of Transmission	Chronicity Possible*
A	RNA	Fecal-oral	No
B	DNA	Parenteral, sexual, perinatal	Yes
C	RNA	Parenteral, sexual, perinatal	Yes
D	RNA	Parenteral, sexual, perinatal Hepatitis B coinfection required	Yes
E	RNA	Fecal, oral	No
G†	RNA	Parenteral, sexual	?

*Progression of virus to an embedded chronic state.
†Can exist as a coinfection with HCV.

Table 23-6	Summary of Hepatitis Markers and Clinical Relationships	
Type of Hepatitis	Serum Expression or Molecular Marker	Clinical Relationship
Hepatitis A (HAV)	HAV RNA	Direct detection of HAV in food or water samples
	IgM anti-HAV	Acute HAV
	IgG anti-HAV	Evidence of previous HAV infection
Hepatitis B	HBsAg	Active hepatitis B infection
	HBeAg	Active hepatitis B infection
	Anti-HBc (Total)	Current or past HBV infection
	Anti-HBe	Recovery phase of hepatitis B
	Anti-HBs	Past infection—evidence of immunity
	HBV DNA	Various manifestations of HBV
Hepatitis C	Anti-HCV	Current or past HCV infections
	HCV RNA	Current HCV infection
Hepatitis D	IgM anti-HDV	Active or chronic hepatitis D infection
	IgG anti-HDV	Chronic hepatitis D, Convalescent hepatitis D status
	HDV RNA	Active HDV infection
Hepatitis E	IgM anti-HEV	Current/new hepatitis E infection
	IgG anti-HEV	Current/former hepatitis E infection
	HEV RNA	Current hepatitis E infection
GB virus C	GB virus C RNA	Chronic GB virus C

TRANFUSION-TRANSMITTED VIRUS

Etiology

A more recent addition to the infectious hepatitis family is the transfusion-transmitted virus (TTV). TTV is a nonenveloped, single-stranded DNA virus with 3739 nucleotides. Two genetic groups have been identified, differing by 30% in nucleotide sequences. It was discovered in 1997 through cloning and DNA sequence analysis by Japanese scientists. This novel, single-stranded linear DNA virus has been designated the TT virus, or TTV, after the initials of the first patient (TT) from whom the virus was isolated.

The most remarkable feature of TTV is the extraordinarily high prevalence of chronic viremia in apparently healthy people, up to almost 100% in some countries.

Epidemiology

The TTV has been associated with posttransfusion hepatitis of unknown etiology (non–A-G). The prevalence in the global population, particularly the United States, United Kingdom, Japan, Germany, and Thailand, can reach 100% in healthy people.

There is evidence that TTV may be transmitted not only by parenteral exposure to blood, but also by the fecal-oral route and from mother to child.

Signs and Symptoms

Although similar to HGV, TTV may be an example of a human virus with no clear disease association. This hypothesis is supported by the fact that the high prevalence of active TTV infection in the general population, both in the United Kingdom and Japan, is not comparable to the rate of significant liver damage.

As with HGV, the pathogenicity of TTV has not been proven.

CASE STUDY 1

History and Physical Examination

Several workers at a local fast food restaurant call in sick and report to the local ambulatory clinic for treatment. All of them complain of extreme fatigue. In addition, another 26-year-old food handler, who returned from visiting his relatives in Costa Rica a month ago, is sick. Within the last 1 or 2 weeks, he has had no energy and "just doesn't feel well." When he recently visited a physician at a local ambulatory clinic, he was slightly jaundiced.

Laboratory Data

Food handler's test results—complete blood count, normal
Serum bilirubin level—slightly elevated

Questions

1. What is the most likely source route of hepatitis infection in this patient?
   a. Fecal-oral
   b. Parenteral
   c. Maternal-neonatal transmission
   d. Blood transfusion
2. Prevention and prophylaxis of hepatitis A consists of:
   a. Handwashing
   b. Vaccination for hepatitis A virus
   c. Immunoglobulin injection if travel to or residence in an endemic area for more than 3 months
   d. All of the above

Answers to these questions can be found in Appendix A.

Critical Thinking Group Discussion Questions

1. What types of additional laboratory tests could be of value in determining the food handler's source of illness?
2. What are the immunologic manifestations?
3. What is the prognosis in this disease?
4. What are the methods of prevention and prophylaxis?
5. Because of this patient's occupation, could particular infectious diseases be of concern?

See instructor site ⊖volve for the discussion of the answers to these questions.

CASE STUDY 2

History and Physical Examination

A 30-year-old phlebotomist presents with fever, persistent fatigue, and joint pain. She reports that a needle in a plastic garbage bag nicked her finger about 2 months ago. Her physical examination was within normal limits.

Laboratory Data

Her laboratory data, however, revealed elevated liver serum enzyme levels and total bilirubin levels. Additional laboratory data included positive HBsAg and positive IgM anti-HBc. Her IgM anti-HAV and anti-HCV tests were negative.

Questions

1. The serologic marker of a low-level hepatitis B (HBV) carrier is:
   a. HbsAg
   b. Anti-HBs
   c. Anti-HBe
   d. Anti-HBc (IgM)
2. During the "window phase" of HBV infection only _____ may be detectable as a marker.
   a. Anti-HBc
   b. Anti-HBe
   c. Anti-HBs
   d. HBsAg

Answers to these questions can be found in Appendix A.

Critical Thinking Group Discussion Questions
1. Does this patient have a form of infectious hepatitis? If so, what type?
2. Can any further tests be done to confirm the diagnosis?
3. What is the patient's prognosis?

See instructor site ⊜volve for the discussion of the answers to these questions.

CASE STUDY 3

History and Physical Examination

A 75-year-old woman had an 18-month history of right-sided abdominal pain and progressive fatigue. Her other medical problems include insulin-dependent diabetes mellitus and hypertension.

She reported no history of blood transfusion, IV drug use, or excessive alcohol use. She had no family history of liver disease. Her physical examination showed no cutaneous stigmata of chronic liver disease, hepatosplenomegaly, or ascites. Her daily medications include Humulin U-100 insulin and a drug for her high blood pressure.

Laboratory Data

Her abnormal laboratory values included elevated liver serum enzyme levels (ALT) and total bilirubin. She also exhibited hypergammaglobulinemia. Other relevant findings included negative HBsAg, positive anti-HCV antibody (by RIBA), and positive HCV RNA (by PCR).

Questions
1. Risk factors for hepatitis C virus (HCV) include:
   a. Illegal IV drug use
   b. Occupational exposure
   c. Multiple sexual partners
   d. All of the above
2. The most specific assay for detection of HCV infection is:
   a. enzyme immunoassay (EIA)
   b. Western Blot
   c. HCV RNA
   d. Recombinant immunoblot assay (RIBA)

Answers to these questions can be found in Appendix A.

Critical Thinking Group Discussion Questions
1. Does this patient have a form of infectious hepatitis? If so, what type?

2. Can any further tests be done to confirm the diagnosis?
3. What is the patient's prognosis?

See instructor site ⊜volve for the discussion of the answers to these questions.

CASE STUDY 4

History and Physical Examination

A 45-year-old, previously healthy medical technologist visited her primary care physician because of increasing fatigue and loss of appetite. She has had a monogamous sexual relationship with her husband for 25 years.

Laboratory Data

After an initial workup for chronic fatigue, including a risk factor history that revealed several needlesticks on the job, she was found to be anti-HCV positive by EIA and RIBA and to have an abnormal liver function profile.

Questions
1. What risk factor for HCV does this patient have?
   a. Recent vaccination
   b. Monogamous sexual relationship
   c. Accidental needlestick (occupational)
   d. Advancing age
2. What percentage of HCV infected individuals do not have the virus circulating in their blood?
   a. 5%
   b. 10%
   c. 15%
   d. 25%

Answers to these questions can be found in Appendix A.

Critical Thinking Group Discussion Questions
1. What is the probable source of the HCV infection?
2. What steps should be taken after exposure?
3. What behavioral changes are necessary now that the patient knows that she has HCV infection?

See instructor site ⊜volve for the discussion of the answers to these questions.

Rapid Hepatitis C Virus Testing

The first FDA-approved, Clinical Laboratory Improvement Amendments (CLIA)–waived rapid HCV test has been approved. The OraQuick HCV Rapid Antibody Test

(OraSure, Bethlehem, Pa) is a single-use immunoassay for the qualitative detection of antibodies to hepatitis C virus in capillary and venipuncture whole blood.

Principle

This test uses an indirect lateral flow immunoassay method to detect antibodies to structural and nonstructural HCV proteins. The device uses synthetic peptides and recombinant antigens from the core, NS3, and NS4 regions of the HCV genome that are immobilized as a single test line on the assay strip.

See the ⊜volve website for the procedural protocol.

Results

Antibodies reacting with these peptides and antigens are visualized by colloidal gold labeled with protein A, generating a visible line in the test zone for a reactive sample. The presence of antibodies to HCV indicates that the individual may be currently infected and capable of transmitting the virus.

In conjunction with other laboratory results and clinical information, the OraQuick HCV Rapid Antibody Test results may be used to provide presumptive evidence of infection with HCV (state of infection or associated disease not determined) in persons with signs or symptoms of hepatitis and in persons at risk for hepatitis C infection.

Limitations

The test is for individuals 15 years or older who are symptomatic or at high risk for hepatitis C infection. The assay is not for use in screening whole blood, plasma, or tissue donors. Performance characteristics have not been established for testing a pediatric population younger than 15 years or for pregnant women.

CHAPTER HIGHLIGHTS

- Viral agents of acute hepatitis can be divided into primary hepatitis viruses—A, B, C, D, E, and G—as well as secondary hepatitis viruses, including Epstein-Barr virus, cytomegalovirus, herpesvirus, and others. Primary hepatitis viruses account for approximately 95% of the cases of hepatitis.
- As a clinical disease, hepatitis can occur in an acute or chronic form.
- Hepatitis A virus (HAV; formerly infectious or short-incubation hepatitis) is common in underdeveloped or developing countries.
- HAV is transmitted almost exclusively by a fecal-oral route during the early phase of acute illness because the virus is shed in feces for up to 4 weeks after infection occurs.
- The incidence of HAV is not increased in health care workers or dialysis patients.
- Hepatitis B virus (HBV) is the classic example of a virus acquired through blood transfusion. Reported cases of

acute hepatitis B have decreased dramatically in the United States in the last 15 years.
- HBV is largely spread parenterally through blood transfusion, needlestick accidents, and contaminated needles, although the virus can be transmitted in the absence of obvious parenteral exposure.
- Serologic markers for HBV infection include HBsAg, HBeAg, anti-HBc, anti-HBe, anti-HBs, and DNA analysis.
- Hepatitis D virus (HDV; initially, the delta agent) superinfects some patients already infected with HBV.
- Hepatitis C virus (HCV) is prevalent in the United States and Western Europe and resembles HBV in terms of transmission characteristics. Health care workers should avoid needlestick injuries.
- Hepatitis E virus (HEV) is transmitted by the fecal-oral route and usually is caused by poor sanitation. No form of chronic liver disease has been attributable to HEV infection. Although most acute infections are self-limited and mild, about 10% to 20% of HEV infections in pregnant women result in fulminant hepatitis, especially in the third trimester of pregnancy.
- GB virus C virus (HGV) is a bloodborne agent. Transfusion recipients and IV drug abusers are at risk of infection. HGV frequently occurs as a coinfection with HCV. HGV is estimated to produce 900 to 2000 infections/year; most are asymptomatic. Chronic disease is rare or may not occur at all.
- Transfusion-transmitted virus (TTV), a recent addition to the infectious hepatitis family. The most remarkable feature of TTV is the extraordinarily high prevalence of chronic viremia in apparently healthy people, almost 100% in some countries. As with HGV, the pathogenicity of TTV has not been proven.

REVIEW QUESTIONS

1-4. Match the following forms of hepatitis with the appropriate description (a-d), using each answer only once.

1. _____ Acute hepatitis

2. _____ Fulminant acute hepatitis

3. _____ Subclinical hepatitis without jaundice

4. _____ Chronic hepatitis
   a. This rare form is associated with hepatic failure.
   b. Typical form of hepatitis with associated jaundice
   c. Probably accounts for persons with serum antibodies but no history of hepatitis
   d. Accompanied by hepatic inflammation and necrosis

5-8. Match the following (use an answer only once).

5. _____ Hepatitis A

6. _____ Hepatitis B

7. _____ Hepatitis D

8. _____ Hepatitis C
   a. Intact virus is the Dane particle
   b. Transmission by both parenteral and nonparenteral routes
   c. Requires HBV as a helper
   d. Most common form of hepatitis

9-12. Match the following (use an answer only once).

9. _____ Hepatitis A

10. _____ Hepatitis B

11. _____ Delta agent

12. _____ Hepatitis C
   a. Should receive immune globulin intramuscularly after exposure
   b. Defective or incomplete RNA virus
   c. Has an epidemiology similar to that of HAV
   d. Previously called Australia antigen

13-17. Match the following serologic markers with the appropriate description.

13. _____ HBsAg

14. _____ HBeAg

15. _____ Anti-HBc

16. _____ Anti-HBe

17. _____ Anti-HBs
   a. Indicator of recent HBV infection may be only serologic marker during the window phase
   b. Found in the serum of some patients who are HBsAg positive; marker for level of virus, infectivity
   c. A serologic marker of recovery and immunity
   d. Initial detectable marker found in serum during incubation period of HBV infection
   e. In the case of acute hepatitis, the first serologic evidence of the convalescent phase

18. Of patients in the United States with chronic hepatitis B, _____ of them acquired the virus in childhood.
   a. Less than 20%
   b. 20% to 30%
   c. 30% to 40%
   d. More than 40%

19. The rate of posttransfusion hepatitis C decreased to _____ after the introduction of serologic testing in the screening of blood donors.
   a. Less than 1%
   b. 5%
   c. 10%
   d. 15%

20-22. Match the following forms of hepatitis with the correct average incubation time.

20. _____ Hepatitis A

21. _____ Hepatitis B

22. _____ Hepatitis C
   a. 5 days
   b. 25 days
   c. 50 days
   d. 75 days
   e. 150 days

23. Which form of hepatitis does not have a chronic form of the disease?
   a. Hepatitis A
   b. Hepatitis B
   c. Hepatitis C

24. Another name for hepatitis B infection is:
   a. Infectious hepatitis
   b. Long incubation hepatitis
   c. Australia antigen
   d. Dane particle

25. The most frequent clinical response to hepatitis B virus is:
   a. Jaundice within 75 days
   b. Asymptomatic infection
   c. Subclinical infection
   d. Both b and c

26. The first laboratory screening test of donor blood was for the detection of:
   a. HBc
   b. HBsAg
   c. HBe
   d. Anti-HBe

27. Which surface marker is a reliable marker for the presence of high levels of hepatitis B virus (HBV) and a high degree of infectivity?
   a. HBeAg
   b. HBsAg
   c. HBcAg
   d. Anti-HBsAg

28. The only serologic marker during the anti-core window period of hepatitis B (the time between disappearance of detectable HBsAg and appearance of detectable anti-HBs) may be:
   a. Anti-HBs
   b. Anti-HBc
   c. Anti-HBe
   d. HBsAg

29. Which of the following is a characteristic of the delta agent?
   a. Is a DNA virus
   b. Usually replicates only in HBV-infected hosts
   c. Infects patients who are HBcAg positive
   d. Is frequently found in the United States

30. Which of the following viruses is rarely implicated in transfusion-associated hepatitis?
   a. Hepatitis A
   b. Hepatitis B
   c. Hepatitis C
   d. Cytomegalovirus

31. In health care workers, the risk of contracting hepatitis C is _____the risk of contracting AIDS.
    a. Lower than
    b. Higher than
    c. The same as
    d. Not something to worry about compared to

32. The specific diagnostic test for hepatitis C is:
    a. Absence of anti-HAV and anti-HBsAg
    b. Increase in liver serum enzyme levels
    c. Detection of non-A, non-B antibodies
    d. Anti-HCV

33. The earliest detectable serologic marker of acute hepatitis C is:
    a. Anti-HCV
    b. Anti-HBc and liver serum enzyme abnormalities
    c. HCV-RNA
    d. Anti-HBs and anti-HBc

34. Primary hepatitis viruses are given this name because they primarily attack:
    a. A variety of body systems
    b. The liver

    c. The skin
    d. The nervous system

35. Hepatitis A has all the following characteristics except:
    a. DNA virus
    b. Short-incubation hepatitis
    c. Crowded, unsanitary conditions as a risk factor
    d. Rare occurrence of transfusion acquisition

36. The Australia antigen is now called:
    a. Dane particle
    b. Long-incubation hepatitis
    c. Hepatitis B surface antigen (HBsAg)
    d. Hepatitis B core antigen (HBcAg)

37-42. Fill in the following table, using a, b, or c, as indicated.
    a. Positive (+)
    b. Negative (–)
    c. Questionable (±)

Serologic Markers for Hepatitis B Virus Infection

	Early (Asymptomatic)	Acute or Chronic	Low-Level Carrier	Immunity With HBsAg
HbsAg	37. _____	38. _____	Negative (–)	Negative (–)
Anti-HBs	Negative (–)	Questionable (±)	Negative (–)	Positive (+)
Anti-HBc	Negative (–)	39. _____	40. _____	41. _____
Anti-HBc (IgM)	Negative (–)	Positive (+)	Negative (–)	42. _____

43. Which category has the highest incidence of acute hepatitis C?
    a. Low socioeconomic status
    b. Dialysis
    c. Transfusion
    d. Illegal drug use

44. Which category has the lowest incidence of acute hepatitis C?
    a. Sexual, household
    b. Dialysis
    c. Drug abuse
    d. Transfusion

45-48. Match each form of hepatitis to the appropriate mode of transmission. (You may use an answer more than once.)

45. _____ Hepatitis A

46. _____ Hepatitis B

47. _____ Hepatitis C

48. _____ Hepatitis E
    a. Fecal-oral
    b. Parenteral
    c. Parenteral and nonparenteral

BIBLIOGRAPHY

Alter MJ, Kuhnert WL, Finelli L, Centers for Disease Control and Prevention: Guidelines for laboratory testing and result reporting of antibody to hepatitis C virus, MMWR Recomm Rep 52(RR-3):1–13, 2003.

Dammacco F, et al: Pegylated interferon-α, ribavirin, and rituximab combined therapy of hepatitis C virus-related mixed cryoglobulinemia: a long-term study, Blood 116:343–353, 2010.

DiBisceglie AM: Interferon therapy for chronic viral hepatitis, N Engl J Med 330:137–138, 1994.

Dienstag JL: Hepatitis B virus infection, N Engl J Med 359:1486–1500, 2008.

Ennishi D, et al: Hepatic toxicity and prognosis in hepatitis C virus-infected patients with diffuse large B-cell lymphoma treated with rituximab-containing chemotherapy regimens: a Japanese multicenter analysis, Blood 116:5119–5125, 2010.

Foran JM: Hepatitis C in the rituximab era, Blood 116:5081–5082, 2010.

Gibb DM, et al: Mother-to-child transmission of hepatitis C virus, Hosp Physician 36:16, 2000.

Gudima S, et al: Origin of hepatitis delta virus mRNA, J Virol 74:7204–7210, 2000.

Hoofnagle JH: Hepatitis B: preventable and now treatable, N Engl J Med 354:1074–1078, 2006.

Jensen DM: A new era of hepatitis C therapy begins, N Engl J Med 364:1272–1273, 2011.

Kangxian J, et al: Epidemiological survey and follow-up of transfusion-transmitted virus after an outbreak of enterically transmitted infection, J Viral Hepat 7:309–312, 2000.

National Institutes of Health: Hepatitis, 2012, http://vsearch.nlm.nih.gov.

Ngo Y, et al: A prospective analysis of the prognostic value of biomarkers (Fibro test) in patients with chronic hepatitis C, Clin Chem 52:1887–1896, 2006.

Petarca A, et al: Safety and efficacy of rituximab in patients with hepatitis C virus–related mixed cryoglobulinemia and severe liver disease, Blood 116:335–342, 2010.

Rollins G: New paradigms for hepatitis C virus treatment, Clin Lab News 38:1–5, 2012.

Rosen HR: Chronic hepatitis C infection, N Engl J Med 364:2429–2438, 2011.

Turgeon ML: Hepatitis C: what's new? Adv Med Lab Prof 12(23):24, 2001.

Wang JT, et al: Incidence and clinical presentation of posttransfusion TT virus infection in prospectively followed transfusion recipients: emphasis on its relevance to hepatitis, Transfusion 40:596–599, 2000.

CHAPTER 24

Rubella and Rubeola Infections

Learning Objectives

At the conclusion of this chapter, the reader should be able to:

- Describe the etiology and epidemiology of rubella (German measles) infection.
- Explain the signs and symptoms of acquired and congenital rubella infection.
- Compare the immunologic manifestations of acquired and congenital rubella infection.
- Explain the laboratory diagnostic evaluation of rubella infection.

- Summarize the epidemiology and laboratory diagnosis of rubeola (measles).
- Analyze a representative case study.
- Correctly answer case study related multiple choice questions.
- Be prepared to participate in a discussion of critical thinking questions.
- Describe the principle, results, limitations, and clinical applications of the passive latex agglutination test for Rubella.
- Correctly answer end of chapter review questions.

Key Terms

clinical manifestations
epidemic

immunity
stillbirth

RUBELLA

Etiology of Rubella

The rubella virus was first isolated in 1962. Acquired rubella, also known as German measles or 3-day measles, is caused by an enveloped, single-stranded RNA virus of the Togaviridae family. Because the virus is endemic to human beings, the disease is highly contagious and is transmitted through respiratory secretions. Before widespread rubella immunization, this viral infection usually occurred in childhood, although it also affected adults.

Epidemiology of Rubella

Three strains of live, attenuated rubella vaccine virus were developed and first licensed for use in the United States in 1969. Before widespread rubella immunization in the United States and Canada, rubella infections occurred in **epidemic** proportion at 6- to 9-year intervals. In 1964, more than 20,000 cases of congenital rubella syndrome and an unknown number of **stillbirths** occurred in the United States as the result of an epidemic that year.

The Pan American Health Organization (PAHO) has made historic achievements in the elimination of measles (rubeola) and has announced a new effort to eliminate (rubella) German

Measles. Many countries in the regions of the Americas have already made great progress in reducing the incidence of congenital rubella syndrome (CRS) through accelerated rubella control programs. Costa Rica, Honduras, Brazil, and Chile, as well as the member countries of the Caribbean, have rubella elimination initiatives underway.

In countries where vaccination is uncommon, the incidence of rubella infection is high and epidemics are frequent. Because vaccination programs have prevented the rubella epidemics that once gave people naturally acquired **immunity,** individuals who have not been vaccinated have a higher level of susceptibility to rubella infection. Primarily, two types of outbreaks have occurred in the United States in the fairly recent past, affecting the following groups:

- Unvaccinated preschool-age children
- Highly vaccinated school-age children

The epidemiology of measles reveals two major impediments to measles elimination: (1) unvaccinated preschool-age children, a factor that allows large outbreaks; and (2) vaccine failures, which account for outbreaks in highly vaccinated school-age populations. On U.S. college and university campuses, the susceptibility to rubella infection among students is estimated to be as high as 20%. Many cases of rubella infection have been unrecognized or unreported because these cases are mild or subclinical.

Contracting the infection and vaccinating against rubella are the only routes to developing immunity. Individuals should be immune to rubella if they have a dated record of rubella vaccination on or after their first birthday, or if they have demonstrable rubella antibody. Even when antibody titers fall to relatively low levels, previous infection or successful vaccination appears to confer permanent immunity to rubella, except in cases of congenital rubella. The only proof of immunity is a positive serologic screening test result for rubella antibody. A history of rubella infection, even if verified by a physician, is not acceptable evidence of immunity.

It is critical to continue to determine the rubella immune status of women of childbearing age and to vaccinate those who are not immune. Individuals requiring rubella immune status determination include those in the following groups:

- Preschool- and school-age children
- All females at or just before childbearing age
- Women about to be married
- Married women

If the woman is not rubella immune, she should be vaccinated and advised not to become pregnant for 3 months because of the remote possibility that the vaccination could lead to an infected fetus.

- Pregnant women

A positive test confirms immunity, but to rule out any possibility of unsuspected current infection, an immunoglobulin M (IgM) screening procedure may also be ordered. If the patient is not rubella-immune, she should be cautioned to avoid exposure to rubella infection. Vaccination is contraindicated in pregnant women; however, a woman should be vaccinated immediately after termination of the pregnancy.

- Health care personnel

Men and women should be vaccinated to prevent possible spread of nosocomial infection to pregnant patients.

Adverse reactions to rubella vaccine have been reported. The Institute of Medicine has determined that a causal relationship exists between rubella vaccine and acute arthritis in adult females. There is weak but consistent evidence for a causal relationship between rubella vaccine and chronic arthritis in adult females. Incidence rates are estimated to average 13% to 15% in adult females after vaccination. Much lower levels of arthritic adverse reactions were noted in children, adolescents, and adult males. Reliable estimates of excess risk of chronic arthritis after rubella vaccination are not available.

Signs and Symptoms of Rubella Infection

A diagnosis of acquired rubella is not based solely on **clinical manifestations.** The signs and symptoms of rubella vary widely from person to person and may not be recognized in some cases, especially if the characteristic rash is light or absent, as may occur in a substantial number of cases. Rubella infection also may resemble other disorders, such as infectious mononucleosis and drug-induced rashes.

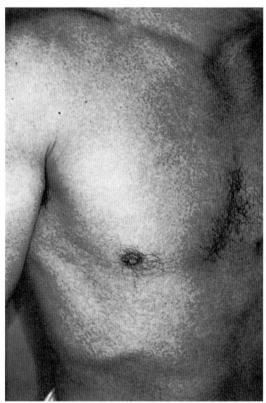

Figure 24-1 Rubella. *(From Odom RB, James WD, Berger TG: Andrews' diseases of the skin: clinical dermatology, ed 9, St Louis, 2000, Saunders.)*

Acquired Rubella Infection

The incubation period of acquired rubella infection varies from 10 to 21 days, and 12 to 14 days is typical. Infected persons are usually contagious for 12 to 15 days, beginning 5 to 7 days before the appearance (if present) of a rash. Acute rubella infection lasts from 3 to 5 days and generally requires minimal treatment. Permanent effects are extremely rare in acquired infections.

The clinical presentation of acquired rubella is usually mild. The clinical manifestations of infection usually begin with a prodromal period of catarrhal symptoms, followed by involvement of the retroauricular, posterior cervical, and postoccipital lymph nodes, and finally by the emergence of a maculopapular rash on the face and then on the neck and trunk (Figs. 24-1 and 24-2). A temperature less than 34.4° C (94° F) is usually present. In older children and adults, self-limiting arthralgia and arthritis are common.

Congenital Rubella Infection

Rubella infection is usually a mild, self-limiting disease with only rare complications in children and adults. In pregnant women, however, especially those infected in the first trimester, rubella can have devastating effects on the fetus (Fig. 24-3). In utero infection can result in fetal death or manifest as rubella syndrome, a spectrum of congenital defects. About 10% to 20% of infants infected in utero fail to survive beyond 18 months.

The point in the gestation cycle at which maternal rubella infection occurs greatly influences the severity of congenital rubella syndrome (Table 24-1); the extent of congenital

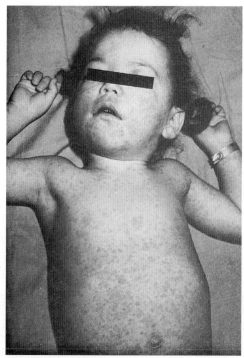

Figure 24-2 Rubella rash. *(From Krugman S et al: Infectious diseases of children, ed 8, St Louis, 1985, Mosby.)*

Table 24-1	Manifestation of Anomalies in Maternal Rubella
Period of Gestation	**Risk of Anomaly**
Prospective Studies	
First trimester	≈25%
Second trimester	
First month	Less than (>)1%
Second month	≥25%
Third month	≥10%
Serologically Confirmed Cases of Maternal Infection	
Before 11 wk	90%
11-12 wk	33%
13-14 wk	11%
15-16 wk	24%
After 16 wk	0%

with maternal rubella infection include encephalitis, hepatomegaly, bone defects, mental retardation, cataracts, thrombocytopenic purpura, cardiovascular defects, splenomegaly, and microcephaly. Severely affected children are likely to have multiple defects in different organ systems. In neonates with congenital rubella syndrome, low birth weight and failure to thrive are common.

Rubella immunity develops in almost all children who have had congenital rubella. In late childhood, however, about one third of these patients lose antibody and become susceptible to acquired rubella. If acquired rubella occurs, it follows a typically benign course. Children with congenital rubella should be screened for rubella immunity in late childhood and vaccinated if necessary.

Immunologic Manifestations

Acquired Rubella Infection

In a patient with primary rubella infection, the appearance of both immunoglobulin G (IgG) and IgM antibodies is associated with the appearance of clinical signs and symptoms, when present.

The IgM antibodies become detectable a few days after the onset of signs and symptoms and reach peak levels at 7 to 10 days. These antibodies persist but rapidly diminish in concentration over the next 4 to 5 weeks, until antibody is no longer clinically detectable. The presence of IgM antibody in a single specimen suggests that the patient has recently experienced a rubella infection. In most cases, the infection probably occurred in the preceding month.

Production of IgG is also associated with the appearance of clinical signs and symptoms. Antibody levels increase rapidly for the next 7 to 21 days and then level off or even decrease in strength. IgG antibodies, however, remain present and protective indefinitely. Detection of IgG antibody is a

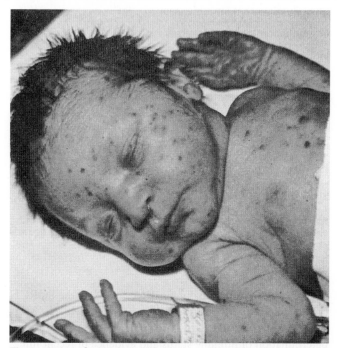

Figure 24-3 Congenital malformations of rubella. *(From Krugman S et al: Infectious diseases of children, ed 8, St Louis, 1985, Mosby.)*

anomalies varies from one infant to another. Some infants manifest almost all the defects associated with rubella, whereas others exhibit few, if any, consequences of infection. Clinical evidence of congenital rubella infection may not be recognized for months or even years after birth.

Rubella syndrome encompasses a number of congenital anomalies. In addition to stillbirth, fetal abnormalities associated

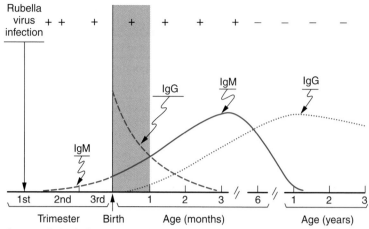

Figure 24-4   Natural history of congenital rubella: pattern of virus excretion and antibody response. *(Adapted from Krugman S et al: Infectious diseases of children, ed 9, St Louis, 1992, Mosby.)*

useful indicator of rubella infection only when the acute and convalescent blood specimens are drawn several weeks apart. Optimum timing for paired testing in the diagnosis of a recent infection is 2 or more weeks apart, with the first (acute) specimen taken before or at the time signs and symptoms appear, or within 2 weeks of exposure.

Paired-specimen testing may demonstrate that the antibody levels are the same. In these cases, either the patient was previously immunized or the acute sample was taken after the antibody had already reached maximum levels. Demonstration of an unequivocal increase in IgG antibody concentration between the acute and convalescent specimens suggests a recent primary infection or a secondary (anamnestic) antibody response to rubella in an immune individual. In cases of an anamnestic response, IgM antibodies are not demonstrable, but IgG production begins quickly. No other signs or symptoms of disease are exhibited.

If both IgM and IgG test results are negative, the patient has never had rubella infection or been vaccinated. Such patients are susceptible to infection. If no IgM is demonstrable but IgG is present in paired specimens, the patient is immune.

When evaluating of the immune status of patients, IgG antibodies present in a dilution of 1:8 or higher indicate past infection with rubella virus and clinical protection against future rubella infection. The clinical significance of lower levels is not currently known. Titers of 1:16, 1:64, 1:512, or higher may be found in acute and past infections; however, the diagnosis of acute infection requires an IgM antibody titer on the same specimen or a paired-specimen comparison. It should be noted that IgM also appears for a transient period after vaccination.

Congenital Rubella Syndrome

Because IgG antibody is capable of crossing the placental barrier, there is no way of distinguishing between IgG antibody of fetal origin and IgG antibody of maternal origin in a neonatal blood specimen (Fig. 24-4).

Testing for IgM antibody is invaluable for the diagnosis of congenital rubella syndrome in the neonate. IgM does not

Table 24-2	**Tests for Rubella Antibodies**
Method	**Antibody Detected**
TORCH antibodies	IgM
TORCH antibodies	IgG
Chemiluminescent immunoassay	IgM
Chemiluminescent Immunoassay	IgG
Immunochromatographic assay	IgG
Indirect immunofluorescence assay (IFA)	Monoclonal antibody (antibodies) to rubella virus virion proteins, E2 and C

cross an intact placental barrier; therefore, demonstration of IgM in a single neonatal specimen is diagnostic of congenital rubella syndrome. In the newborn, serologic confirmation of rubella infection can be made by testing for IgM antibody for at least the first 6 months of life. This is especially useful when clinical evidence of congenital rubella is slow in emerging or is of uncertain origin.

Diagnostic Evaluation

Several screening methods are available, including the TORCH (*Toxoplasma, o*ther [viruses], *r*ubella, *c*ytomegalovirus [CMV], and *h*erpes) procedure (see Chapter 15). The assays for the determination of immune status and evidence of recent infection are presented in Table 24-2.

Persons with infectious mononucleosis sometimes have rubella-specific IgM in low concentrations. Cross-reactions of rubella IgM-positive sera can result from parvovirus IgM. Occasionally, pregnant women will demonstrate IgM antibodies not only to rubella but also to CMV, varicella-zoster virus, and measles virus. In these patients, diagnosis of rubella can be made only by the assessment of rubella-specific IgG antibodies supported by a detailed clinical history.

RUBEOLA (MEASLES)

Rubella and Rubeola are two distinctly different infections. Rubeola is referred to as measles.

Measles is a highly contagious disease caused by the rubeola virus.

Epidemiology

Endemic or sustained measles transmission has not occurred in the United States since the late 1990s. The minimal number of cases yearly in the United States is due to the high rate of vaccination. Occasional small outbreaks from imported cases of measles primarily infects unvaccinated individuals.

Even though the ongoing transmission of endemic (native) measles was declared to be eliminated in the United States in 2000, the disease is still common in many other countries and can be imported into the United States by foreign visitors or returning travelers who are not fully protected against the disease. During 2001 to 2008, a median of 56 cases of measles were reported to the Centers for Disease Control and Prevention (CDC) annually. However, during the first 19 weeks of 2011, 118 cases of measles were reported, the highest number reported for this period since 1996. Of these cases, 87% were imported from the World Health Organization (WHO) European and Southeast Asia regions; 89% of these patients were unvaccinated.

Measles are caused by a single-stranded RNA virus, the only member of the genus *Morbillivirus* (Paramyxoviridae family). Human beings are the only natural reservoirs of this virus, which is spread by respiratory droplets. It is highly contagious, with more than a 90% transmission rate among non-immunized individuals.

Prevention

Prevention includes measles, mumps, and rubella (MMR) vaccine administered to 12- to 15-month-old children, with revaccination between 4 and 12 years of age. A high fever and pulmonary infiltrates can occur in patients exposed to measles that were vaccinated with MMR from 1964 to 1967. Because the vaccine is a live attenuated virus, it should not be used in pregnant women or those with significant immunosuppression.

Laboratory Testing

Laboratory confirmation of measles is made by the detection measles-specific immunoglobulin M antibodies in serum of, isolation of measles virus, or detection of measles virus RNA by nucleic acid amplification in an appropriate clinical specimen (e.g., nasopharyngeal or oropharyngeal swabs, nasal aspirates, throat washes, or urine; Table 24-3).

Serum testing for antibodies is done for the following reasons:

- Can confirm acute infection with measles using IgM and IgG serial testing
- Can confirm seroconversion after vaccination using IgG testing

- IgM and IgG cerebrospinal fluid (CSF) testing to identify subacute sclerosing panencephalitis, which may occur years after the original infection using IgG testing
- Viral culture
- Nasopharyngeal and blood cultures—most sensitive if collected during prodrome up to 1 to 2 days after onset of rash
- Virus can be isolated from urine culture up to 1 week or more after onset of rash
- Difficult to isolate from CSF and brain tissue

The reverse transcription polymerase chain reaction (RT-PCR) assay is not widely available, but is useful for testing CSF.

CASE STUDY

History and Physical Examination

A 20-year-old college junior comes to the student health office because she has been exposed to rubella during a recent outbreak at the college. She had been immunized as a child.

Laboratory Data

- Screening procedure for rubella—negative
- Pregnancy test—positive

Ultrasonography shows that the fetus is in the eighth week of development.

Questions

1. What constitutes proof of immunity to rubella infection?
   a. Physician documented infection
   b. IgG antibody (1:8 dilution or greater)
   c. IgM antibody
   d. Both b and c
2. To confirm congential rubella syndrome _____ antibody must be demonstrated in the newborn's serum.
   a. IgM
   b. IgG
   c. IgA
   d. IgE

See Appendix A for the answers to multiple choice questions.

Critical Thinking Group Discussion Questions

1. Is this woman susceptible to rubella infection?
2. Is the fetus at risk of a congenital defect?
3. Is there any treatment for the infection?
4. What are the immunologic manifestations of infection?

See the instructor site of ⊖volve website for the discussion of the answers to these questions.

Table 24-3	Measles (Rubeola) Antibody Testing	
Test Name	Recommended Use	Comments
Viral culture method—cell culture, immunofluorescence	Gold standard procedure	Nasopharyngeal aspirate, washing, throat swab, lung tissue, CSF or urine samples
Enzyme-linked immunosorbent assay (ELISA)	Measles (rubeola) antibody IgG and IgM; semiquantitative	Low IgM antibody levels occasionally persist >12 mo postinfection or immunization ; residual IgM response may be distinguished from early IgM response by testing patient sera 2-3 wk later for changes in specific IgM antibody levels.
	Measles (rubeola) antibody, IgG; semiquantitative	Screen for vaccination responses.
	Measles (rubeola) antibody, IgM or IgG, CSF; semiquantitative	Diagnose rare but fatal subacute sclerosing panencephalitis (SSPE) in CSF samples; rubeola CSF antibody detection may indicate central nervous system infection; possible contamination by blood or transfer of serum antibodies across blood-brain barrier can affect the results.

Adapted from ARUP Laboratories: Measles virus—rubeola, 2012 (http://www.arupconsult.com/Topics/Rubeola.html).

Passive Latex Rubella Agglutination Test

Principle

Latex particles are sensitized with solubilized rubella virus antigens. When the latex reagent is mixed with serum containing sufficient rubella antibodies, the antigen-antibody complex will form visible clumps. In the absence of antibody, or if the concentration is too low to react, the latex particles will remain smooth and evenly dispersed.

Reporting Results

- A positive reaction demonstrates agglutination.
- A negative reaction demonstrates no agglutination.

Procedure Notes

A single specimen can be used to estimate the immune status of the individual, because any detectable antibody is indicative of immunity and protection against subsequent viral infection. The CLSI has advised that the specimen should not be frozen in a frost-free freezer because the freeze-thaw cycle may be detrimental to serum proteins. These guidelines further suggest that frozen specimens be retained for at least 1 year for later follow-up examination, especially for women of childbearing age who are inadvertently exposed to the rubella virus.

The acute-phase specimen should be collected as closely as possible to the time of exposure, and no later than 3 days after the onset of rash. The convalescent-phase specimen should be taken 7 to 21 days after the onset of the rash or at least 30 days after exposure if no clinical symptoms appear because of a possible inapparent infection. Both specimens should be tested simultaneously.

See the ⊜volve website for the procedural protocol.

Limitations

A single specimen determines immunity; it is not a serodiagnosis of infection or reinfection. At a single dilution, the qualitative protocol will perform satisfactorily with acute-phase and convalescent-phase antibodies; however, when the presence or absence of a fourfold titer rise in paired specimens must be demonstrated, the quantitative protocol is required.

Clinical Applications

The presence of antibodies in a single patient specimen is an indication of previous exposure and immunity to rubella virus. Demonstration of any detectable antibody is indicative of immunity and protection against subsequent viral infection. Demonstration of seroconversion, or a fourfold or higher rise in antibody titer with properly collected paired specimens, is diagnostic of a recent or current infection with rubella virus.

CHAPTER HIGHLIGHTS

- Acquired rubella (German or 3-day measles) is caused by an enveloped, single-stranded RNA virus of the Togaviridae family. It is endemic to human beings, highly contagious, and transmitted through respiratory secretions.
- Contracting rubella infection and vaccinating against rubella are the only ways to develop immunity.
- A diagnosis of acquired rubella is not based solely on clinical manifestations; signs and symptoms vary widely. Although usually mild and self-limiting, with rare complications in children and adults, rubella infections in pregnant women, especially in the first trimester, can result in fetal death or congenital rubella syndrome.
- In primary rubella infection, the appearance of IgG and IgM antibodies is associated with clinical signs and symptoms, when present. IgM antibodies are detectable a few days after onset of symptoms, reach peak levels at 7 to 10 days, and persist but decrease rapidly in concentration over the next 4 to 5 weeks, until no longer clinically detectable.
- IgM antibody in a single specimen suggests a recent rubella infection.
- An unequivocal increase in IgG antibody concentration between the acute and convalescent specimens suggests a

recent primary infection or an anamnestic antibody response to rubella in an immune individual.

- Negative IgM and IgG test results indicate that the patient has never had rubella infection or been vaccinated. These patients are susceptible to infection. If no IgM is demonstrable but IgG is present in paired specimens, the patient is immune.
- IgM does not cross an intact placental barrier, so its demonstration in a single neonatal specimen is diagnostic of congenital rubella syndrome. Rubella infection can be confirmed serologically by IgM antibody testing for at least the first 6 months of life, especially when clinical evidence of congenital rubella is slow in emerging or has an uncertain origin.
- Laboratory confirmation of (rubeola) measles is made by the detection of measles-specific immunoglobulin M antibodies in serum, isolation of measles virus, or detection of measles virus RNA by nucleic acid amplification in an appropriate clinical specimen.

REVIEW QUESTIONS

1. All the following groups of individuals should receive rubella vaccinations except:
   a. School-age children
   b. Women of childbearing age
   c. Pregnant women
   d. Health care personnel

2. The greatest risk of the manifestation of anomalies in maternal rubella is _____ of gestation.
   a. During the first month
   b. During the first trimester
   c. During the third month
   d. During the fourth or fifth month

3. In a patient with primary rubella infection, the appearance of _____ antibodies is associated with the clinical signs and symptoms, when present.
   a. IgG
   b. IgM
   c. IgD
   d. Both a and b

4. Testing for _____ antibody is invaluable for the diagnosis of congenital rubella syndrome.
   a. IgM
   b. IgG
   c. IgD
   d. IgE

5. Before the licensing of rubella vaccine in the United States in 1969, epidemics occurred at _____year intervals.
   a. 2- to 3-
   b. 5- to 7-
   c. 6- to 9-
   d. 10- to 20-

6. Acute rubella infection lasts from _____ days.
   a. 1 to 2
   b. 2 to 4
   c. 3 to 5
   d. 7 to 10

7. IgM antibodies to rubella virus reach peak levels at _____ days.
   a. 2 to 4
   b. 3 to 5
   c. 5 to 7
   d. 7 to 10

8. IgG antibodies to rubella virus increase rapidly for _____ days after the acquisition of infection.
   a. 2 to 8
   b. 3 to 10
   c. 5 to 15
   d. 7 to 21

9. Which percentage of serologically confirmed cases of maternal infection occur before 11 weeks of gestation?
   a. 11%
   b. 24%
   c. 33%
   d. 90%

10. German measles and measles are caused by the same virus.
    a. True
    b. False

11. Laboratory confirmation of rubeola antibody is done by:
    a. Detection of IgM antibodies in serum
    b. Detection of measles virus RNA by nucleic acid amplification in a clinical specimen
    c. Isolation of rubella virus
    d. Either a or b

BIBLIOGRAPHY

ARUP: Laboratories: measles virus—rubeola, 2012, http://www.arupconsult.com/Topics/Rubeola.html.

ARUP: Laboratories: rubella virus, 2012, http://www.arupconsult.com/Topics/RubellaVirus.html.

Centers for Disease Control and Prevention (CDC): Measles—United States, January-May 20, 2011, MMWR Morb Mortal Wkly Rep 60:666–668, 2011.

Centers for Disease Control and Prevention (CDC): Measles outbreak associated with an arriving refugee—Los Angeles county, California, August-September 2011, MMWR Morb Mortal Wkly 61(21):385–389, June 1, 2012.

Centers for Disease Control and Prevention (CDC): Notifiable disease and mortality tables MMWR, Morb Mortal Wkly 61(33):ND452–ND465, August 24, 2012.

Pub Med Health. Rubella. Retrieved August 25, 2012, http://www.ncbi.nlm.nih.gov/pubmedhealth/PMH0002541.

CHAPTER 25

Acquired Immunodeficiency Syndrome

Learning Objectives

At the conclusion of this chapter, the reader should be able to:

- Describe the etiology and viral characteristics of human immunodeficiency virus (HIV-1).
- Explain the epidemiology, including modes of transmission, and prevention of HIV-1.
- Discuss the signs and symptoms of various stages and the classification of HIV infection.
- Describe the immunologic manifestations and cellular abnormalities of HIV-1 infection.
- Explain the serologic markers and diagnostic evaluation of HIV.

- Compare the features of fourth generations HIV testing to other generations of testing.
- Analyze a representative HIV-1 case study.
- Correctly answer case study related multiple choice questions.
- Be prepared to participate in a discussion of critical thinking questions.
- Describe the principles of the Rapid HIV antibody test, GS HIV Combo Antigen/Antibody EIA, and simulation of HIV-1 Detection.
- Correctly answer end of chapter review questions.

Key Terms

acquired immunodeficiency syndrome (AIDS)
antigenemia
antiretroviral therapy
circulating immune (antigen-antibody) complexes
cytochrome P-450
envelope protein

gag region
highly active antiretroviral therapy (HAART)
human immunodeficiency virus (HIV)
long terminal redundancies (LTRs)
protease
proviral genome
retrovirus

reverse transcriptase
single nucleotide polymorphism (SNP)
specific oligomer primers
structural proteins
transcriptase
viral core protein

ETIOLOGY

Human immunodeficiency virus (HIV) is the predominant virus responsible for **acquired immunodeficiency syndrome (AIDS).**

In 1983, researchers at the Pasteur Institute in Paris isolated a retrovirus, termed *lymphadenopathy-associated virus* (LAV), from a homosexual man with lymphadenopathy. Concurrently, an American research team headed by Dr. Robert Gallo isolated the same class of virus, which they labeled *human T-lymphotropic retrovirus* (HTLV) type III. In 1984, the Gallo team was able to demonstrate conclusively through virologic and epidemiologic evidence that HTLV-III was the cause of AIDS. When it was demonstrated that LAV and HTLV-III were the same virus, an international commission changed both names of the virus to HIV to eliminate confusion caused by the two names and to acknowledge that the virus is the cause of AIDS.

Viral Characteristics

Viral Structure

Human immunodeficiency virus is a member of the family Retroviridae, a type D retrovirus that belongs to the lentivirus subfamily. Included in this family are oncoviruses (e.g., HTLV-I, HTLV-II), which primarily induce proliferation of infected cells and formation of tumors. Since the discovery of this virus, much has been learned about the impact of HIV on human cells. Two distinct HIV viruses, types 1 and 2 (HIV-1 and HIV-2), cause AIDS. **HIV-1** is divided into nine subtypes: group M (subtypes A-H), group N, and group O. **HIV-2** is divided into two subtypes, groups A and B.

The HIV-1 virus (Fig. 25-1) is composed of a lipid membrane, **structural proteins,** and glycoproteins that protrude. The viral genome consists of three important structural components—*pol, gag,* and *env.* These gene components code for various products (Table 25-1). **Long terminal redundancies (LTRs)** border these three components. HIV-2 has a different envelope and slightly different core proteins.

Cells infected with HIV can be examined with an electron microscope. The virus may appear as buds of the cell membrane particles. The virion has a double-membrane envelope and an electron-dense laminar crescent or semicircular cores. An intermediate, less electron-dense layer lies between the envelope and core. In a mature, free extracellular virion, the core appears as a bar-shaped nucleoid structure in cross section. This structure appears circular and is frequently located eccentrically. It is composed of structural proteins and glycoproteins that occupy the core and envelope regions of the particle. The virion consists of knoblike structures composed of a protein called glycoprotein (gp) 120, which is anchored to another protein called gp41. Each knob includes three sets of these protein molecules. The core of the virus includes a major structural protein called p25 or p24 encoded for by the gag gene. After human exposure, these and other viral components may induce an antibody response important in serodiagnosis (Table 25-2).

Retroviruses contain a single, positive-stranded ribonucleic acid (RNA) with the genetic information of the virus and a special enzyme called **reverse transcriptase** in their core. Reverse transcriptase enables the virus to convert viral RNA into deoxyribonucleic acid (DNA). This reverses the normal process of transcription in which DNA is converted to RNA—thus, the term *retrovirus.*

The genomes of all known retroviruses are organized in a similar way. In the provirus, which is formed when complementary DNA (cDNA) synthesis is completed from the retroviral RNA template, **viral core protein, envelope protein,** and reverse transcriptase are encoded by the *gag, env,* and *pol* genes, respectively, whereas viral gene expression is regulated by *tat, trs, sor,* and *3'orf* gene products. The *gag* gene encodes a polyprotein found at high levels in infected cells and is subsequently cleaved to form p17 and p24, both of which are associated with viral particles. The *pol* gene encodes for reverse transcriptase, endonuclease, and **protease** activities. The *sor* gene stands for *s*mall *o*pen-*r*eading frame. The *sor* gene product is a protein

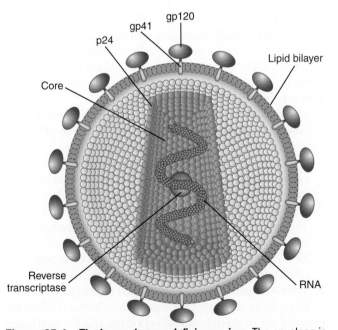

Figure 25-1   The human immunodeficiency virus. The envelope is made up of glycoproteins (gp) of 120 kDa and 41 kDa. The main core protein is p24. As an RNA virus, it relies on reverse transcriptase to produce complementary DNA for transcription and translation. *(From Peakman M, Vergani D: Basic and clinical immunology, ed 2, London, 2009, Churchill Livingstone.)*

Table 25-1	**Viral Genome Components**
Component	**Product**
pol	Produces DNA polymerase Produces endonuclease
gag	Codes for p24 and for proteins such as p17, p9, and p7
env	Codes for two glycoproteins, gp41 and gp120

Table 25-2	**HIV Proteins of Serodiagnostic Importance**		
Virus	**Protein**	**Location**	**Gene**
HIV-1	gp41	Envelope (transmembrane protein)	*env*
	gp160/120	Envelope (external protein)	*env*
	p24	Core (major structural protein)	*gag*
HIV-2	gp34	Envelope (transmembrane protein)	*env*
	gp140	Envelope (external protein)	*env*
	p26	Core (major structural protein)	*gag*

that induces antibody production in the natural course of infection. The *tat* gene also represents a small open-reading frame; the protein product has not been identified to date.

The *env* gene encodes for a polyprotein that contains numerous glycosylation sites. The glycoprotein gp160 is found on infected cells but is deficient on viral particles; however, gp160 gives rise to two glycoproteins, gp120 and gp41, which are associated with the viral envelope. The encoding genes and gene products, or antigens, of the AIDS virus may induce an antibody response after human exposure (Table 25-3).

LTRs, which exist at each end of the proviral genome, play an important role in the control of viral gene expression and the integration of the provirus into the DNA of the hosts. Although a structural similarity exists between the genomes of HIV-1 and HIV-2 (HTLV-IV), the nucleotide sequence homology is limited. There is a nucleotide sequence homology of only 60% between the *gag* genes and 30% to 40% between the remainder of the genes of HIV-1 and HIV-2.

Viral Replication

The replication of HIV is complicated and involves several steps (Fig. 25-2). The HIV life cycle is that of a retrovirus (Box 25-1). Retroviruses are so named because they reverse the normal flow of genetic information. In body cells, the genetic material is DNA. When genes are expressed, DNA is first transcribed into messenger RNA (mRNA), which then serves as the template for the production of proteins. The genes of a retrovirus are encoded in RNA; before they can be expressed, the RNA must be converted into DNA. Only then are the viral genes transcribed and translated into proteins in the usual sequence.

Target Cells. The infectious process begins when the gp120 protein on the viral envelope binds to the protein receptor, called CD4, located on the surface of a target cell. HIV-1 has a marked preference for the CD4+ subset of T lymphocytes (Fig. 25-3). In addition to T lymphocytes, macrophages, peripheral blood monocytes, and cells in the lymph nodes,

skin, and other organs also express measurable amounts of CD4 and can be infected by HIV-1. About 5% of the B lymphocytes may express CD4 and may be susceptible to HIV-1 infection. Macrophages may play an important role in spreading HIV infection in the body, both to other cells and to the target organs of HIV. Monocyte-macrophages enable HIV-1 to enter the immune-protected domain of the central nervous system (CNS), including the brain and spinal cord.

Fusion of the virus to the membrane of a host cell enables the viral RNA and reverse transcriptase to invade the cytoplasm of the cell. However, CD4 receptors are not sufficient for HIV envelope fusion with the T4 cell membrane or for HIV penetration or entry into the interior of the cell. Chemokine coreceptors to CD4, which HIV uses to enter a host cell after binding to it, have been identified. Beta chemokine receptors are cell surface proteins that bind small peptides. They are classified into three groups, depending on the location of the amino acid cysteine (C) in the peptide. These receptors are identified by the individual chemokine(s) that bind(s) to them. In essence, the reference to a specific chemokine also identifies its receptor. The first example of a coreceptor was CXCKR-4 (FUSIN R-4). Other coreceptors include CCKR-2 (R-2), CCKR-3 (R-3), and CC-CKR-5 (R-5). Current research involves exploring ways to block or fill the chemokine receptors with a harmless molecule, thus blocking the binding site of the HIV on the host cell.

Although some cells do not produce detectable amounts of CD4, they contain low levels of mRNA encoding the CD4 protein, which indicates that they do produce some CD4. Because these cells can be infected by HIV in culture, the expression of only minimal CD4 or an alternate receptor molecule may be sufficient for HIV infection to occur. These cell types include certain brain cells, neuroglial cells, a variety of malignant brain tumor cells, and cells derived from bowel cancers. Cells of the gastrointestinal system do not produce appreciable amounts of CD4, although chromaffin cells sometimes appear to be infected by HIV in vivo.

Replication. Retroviruses carry a single, positive-stranded RNA and use reverse transcriptase to convert viral RNA into DNA. The life cycle of the HIV-1 virus consists of five phases (see Box 25-1):

1. The virus attaches and penetrates target cells (e.g., lymphocytes) that express the CD4 receptor. After penetration, the virus loses its protein coat, exposing the RNA core.
2. Reverse transcriptase converts viral RNA into proviral DNA.
3. The proviral DNA is integrated into the genome (genetic complement of the host cell).
4. New virus particles are produced as a result of normal cellular activities of transcription and translation.
5. These new particles bud from the cell membrane.

Once the viral genome is integrated into host cell DNA, the potential for viral production always exists and the viral infection of new cells can continue.

Immunologic activation of CD4+ cells latently infected with HIV induces the production of multiple viral particles, leading to cell death. The extensive destruction of cells leads to the gradual depletion of CD4+ lymphocytes. Progressive defects in

Table 25-3	Encoding Genes and Antigens of AIDS Virus
Encoding Gene	**Antigen**
gag	p55
gag	p24
gag	p17
pol	p66
pol	p51
sor	p24
env	gp160
env	gp120
env	gp41
3′ orf	p27

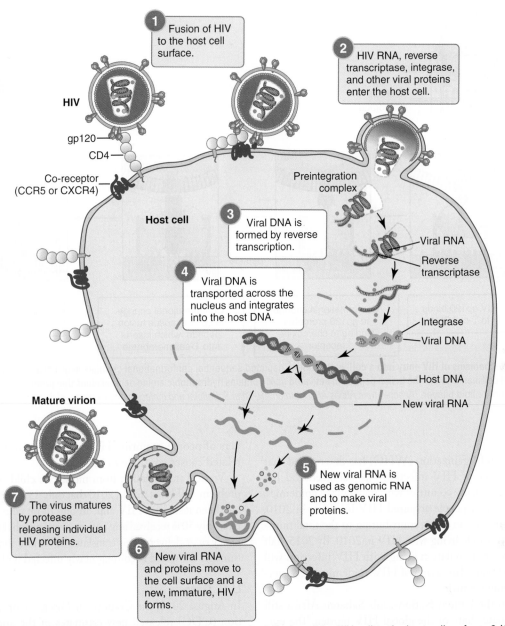

Figure 25-2   HIV replication cycle. Steps in the HIV replication cycle. *1.* Fusion of the HIV cell to the host cell surface; *2.* HIV RNA, reverse transcriptase, integrase, and other viral proteins enter the host cell; *3.* viral DNA is formed by reverse transcription; *4.* viral DNA is transported across the nucleus and integrates into the host DNA; *5.* new viral RNA is used as genomic RNA and to make viral proteins; *6.* new viral RNA and proteins move to the cell surface and a new, immature, HIV virus forms; *7.* the virus matures by protease releasing individual HIV proteins. *(Courtesy National Institute of Allergy and Infectious Diseases, National Institutes of Health, Bethesda, Md.)*

Box 25-1	Summary of HIV-1 Life Cycle

1. The virus attaches to the CD4 membrane receptor and sheds its protein coat, exposing its RNA core.
2. Reverse transcriptase converts viral RNA into proviral DNA.
3. The proviral DNA is integrated into the genome (genetic complement of host cell).
4. New virus particles are produced as the result of normal cellular activities of transcription and translation. Once the viral genome is integrated into host cell DNA, the potential for viral production always exists and the viral infection of new cells can continue.
5. New particles bud from the cell membrane.

the immune system include a severe B cell failure, defects in monocyte function, and defects in granulocyte function.

EPIDEMIOLOGY

HIV causes a chronic infection that leads to a progressive disease. Without treatment, most persons with HIV develop AIDS, which results in substantial morbidity and premature death.

Incidence

More than 25 years after the first clinical evidence of AIDS was reported, it has become the most devastating disease humankind has ever faced.

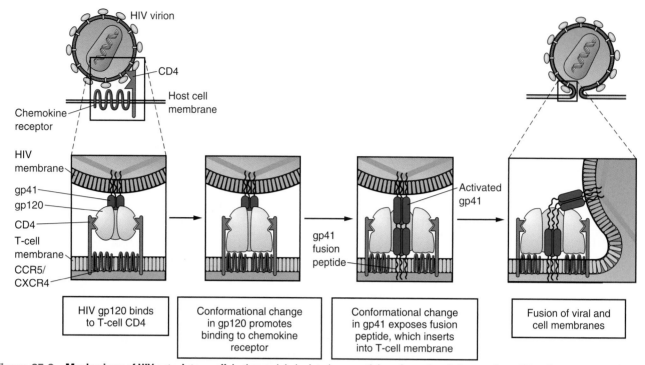

Figure 25-3   **Mechanisms of HIV entry into a cell.** In the model, depicted sequential conformational changes in gp120 and gp41 promote fusion of the HIV-1 and host cell membranes. The fusion peptide of activated gp41 contains hydrophobic amino acid residues that promote insertion into the host cell plasma membrane lipid bilayer. *(Adapted from Abbas AK, Lichtman AH, Pillai S: Cellular and molecular immunology, ed 6, Philadelphia, 2007, Saunders.)*

Global Data

The World Health Organization (WHO) has determined that the global incidence of HIV infection has stabilized and has begun to decline in many countries with generalized epidemics. A total of 2.7 million people acquired HIV infection in 2010, down from 3.1 million in 2001, contributing to the total number of 34 million people living with HIV in 2010. By 2015, half of the United States population living with HIV infection will be older than 50 years. This aging of HIV epidemic will be evident in developing countries.

According to the United Nations, sub-Saharan Africa still bears an inordinate share of the global HIV burden. The epidemics in sub-Saharan Africa vary considerably, with southern Africa still being the most severely affected. An estimated 11.3 million people were living with HIV in southern Africa in 2009, almost one third more than the 8.6 million people living with HIV in the region a decade earlier.

Globally, 34% of people living with HIV in 2009 resided in the 10 countries in southern Africa; 31% of new HIV infections in the same year occurred in these 10 countries, as did 34% of all AIDS-related deaths. About 40% of all women with HIV live in southern Africa.

HIV incidence is falling in 22 countries in sub-Saharan Africa. The HIV incidence appears to have peaked in the mid-1990s and there is evidence of declines in incidence in several countries in sub-Saharan Africa. Between 2001 and 2009, the incidence of HIV infection declined by more than 25% in an estimated 22 African countries. With an estimated 5.6 million people living with HIV in 2009, South Africa's epidemic remains the largest in the world. Emerging concerns are trends affecting Eastern Europe and Central Asia, in which the num-bers of people acquiring HIV infection and dying from HIV-related causes continue to increase.

Vertical transmission from mother to child continues to be a problem. WHO stated in 2010 that only 25% of pregnant women had been tested for HIV and, among those who were HIV positive, only 50% received any antiretroviral prophylaxis during pregnancy or at delivery. This translates into more than 1000 children through the world becoming newly infected with HIV every day.

U.S. Data

In August 2011, the Centers for Disease Control and Prevention (CDC) released new estimates of the annual number of new HIV infections (HIV incidence) in the United States. These estimates suggest that overall HIV incidence in the United States has been relatively stable at approximately 50,000 annual infections between 2006 and 2009.

Each year, the largest number of new HIV infections was in white men who have sex with men (MSM) followed closely by black MSM. Hispanic MSM and black women were also heavily affected. Over the 4-year period, new HIV infections appear to be relatively stable among all populations except young MSM. The overall increase among young MSM was driven by a 48% increase in HIV infections among young black MSM during the 4-year time period.

Classification System

The revised definition of HIV infection, which applies to both HIV-1 and HIV-2, incorporates the reporting criteria for HIV infection and AIDS into a single case definition (Box 25-2). The revised HIV criteria apply to AIDS-defining conditions for adults and children that require laboratory evidence of HIV.

Infectious Patterns

Acquired immunodeficiency syndrome is present worldwide. In some countries and regions (e.g., sub-Saharan Africa, Thailand, India), more than 90% of HIV-1 infections are acquired through heterosexual transmission, in contrast to 10% or less in the United States and Western Europe. HIV-1 and HIV-2 are distinct but related viruses, and both can cause AIDS.

HIV-1

HIV-1 is responsible for the main AIDS epidemic. By analyzing genome sequences of representative strains, HIV-1 has been divided into four groups: group M (for major), including at least nine subtypes, three sub-subtypes of A, and two sub-subtypes of F (A1, A2, A3, B, C, D, F1, F2, G, H, J, and K); group O (for outlier); group N (for non-M, non-O), and group P.

The progression of the natural history and immunopathogenesis of HIV-1 infection can be demonstrated in six discrete stages (Fig. 25-4). These stages are based on the sequential appearance in plasma of HIV-1 viral RNA, the gag p24 protein antigen, antibodies that bind to fixed viral proteins. No matter how HIV-1 was acquired, the timing of the appearance of viral and other markers of infection is generally uniform and follows an orderly pattern.

HIV-2

HIV-2 is endemic in parts of West Africa. HIV-2 strains have been classified into at least five subtypes (A through E). Epidemiologic data have indicated that the prevalence of HIV-2 infections in the U.S. population is extremely low.

The primary mode of transmission of HIV-2 is via heterosexual contact. The period between infection and disease may be longer and milder for persons with HIV-2 than for those with HIV-1. HIV-2 appears to be less harmful (cytopathic) to the cells of the immune system and it reproduces more slowly than HIV-1. Compared with persons infected with HIV-1, those with HIV-2 are less infectious early in the disease course. As the disease advances, HIV-2 infectivity seems to increase compared with HIV-1, but the duration of this increased infectivity is shorter.

Box 25-2   **Revised Surveillance Case Definitions for HIV Infection Among Adults, Adolescents, and Children Aged <18 Months and for HIV Infection and AIDS Among Children Aged 18 Months to <13 Years—United States, 2008**

Summary—For adults and adolescents (i.e., persons aged >13 years), the human immunodeficiency virus (HIV) infection classification system and the surveillance case definitions for HIV infection and acquired immunodeficiency syndrome (AIDS) have been revised and combined into a single case definition for HIV infection (1-3). In addition, the HIV infection case definition for children aged <13 years and the AIDS case definition for children aged 18 months to <13 years have been revised. No changes have been made to the HIV infection classification system, the 24 AIDS-defining conditions for children aged <13 years, or the AIDS case definition for children aged <18 months. These case definitions are intended for public health surveillance only and not as a guide for clinical diagnosis.

Laboratory Criteria for HIV Infection
- Positive result from an HIV antibody screening test (e.g., reactive enzyme immunoassay [EIA*]) confirmed by a positive result from a supplemental HIV antibody test (e.g., Western blot or indirect immunofluorescence assay test).

or
- Positive result or report of a detectable quantity (i.e., within the established limits of the laboratory test) from any of the following HIV virologic (i.e., non-antibody) tests[†]:
  – HIV nucleic acid (DNA or RNA) detection test (e.g., polymerase chain reaction [PCR])
  – HIV p24 antigen test, including neutralization assay
  – HIV isolation (viral culture)

Other Criterion (for Cases that Do Not Meet Laboratory Criteria)
- HIV infection diagnosed by a physician or qualified medical-care provider[‡] based on the laboratory criteria and documented in a medical record.[§] Oral reports of prior laboratory test results are not acceptable.

Case Classification
A confirmed case meets the laboratory criteria for diagnosis of HIV infection and one of the four HIV infection stages (stage 1, stage 2, stage 3, or stage unknown). Although cases with no information on CD4+ T-lymphocyte count or percentage and no information on AIDS-defining conditions can be classified as stage unknown, every effort should be made to report CD4+ T-lymphocyte counts or percentages and the presence of AIDS-defining conditions at the time of diagnosis. Additional CD4+ T-lymphocyte counts or percentages and any identified AIDS-defining conditions can be reported as recommended.

HIV Infection, Stage 1
- No AIDS-defining condition and either CD4+ T-lymphocyte count of >500 cells/µL or CD4+ T-lymphocyte percentage of total lymphocytes of >29.

HIV Infection, Stage 2
- No AIDS-defining condition and either CD4+ T-lymphocyte count of 200-499 cells/µL or CD4+ T-lymphocyte percentage of total lymphocytes of 14-28.

HIV Infection, Stage 3 (AIDS)
- CD4+ T-lymphocyte count of <200 cells/µL or CD4+ T-lymphocyte percentage of total lymphocytes of <14 or documentation of an AIDS-defining condition (see Appendix A). Documentation of an AIDS-defining condition supersedes a CD4+ T-lymphocyte count of >200 cells/µL and a CD4+ T-lymphocyte percentage of total lymphocytes of >14. Definitive diagnostic methods for these conditions are available in Appendix C of the 1993 revised HIV classification system and the expanded AIDS case definition (2) and from the National Notifiable Diseases Surveillance System (available at http://www.cdc.gov/epo/dphsi/casedef/case_definitions.htm).

HIV Infection, Stage Unknown
- No information available on CD4+ T-lymphocyte count or percentage and no information available on AIDS-defining conditions. (Every effort should be made to report CD4+ T-lymphocyte counts or percentages and the presence of AIDS-defining conditions at the time of diagnosis.)

2008 Surveillance Case Definition for HIV Infection Among Children Aged <18 Months

The 2008 case definition of HIV infection among children aged <18 months replaces the definition published in 1999 and applies to all variants of HIV (e.g., HIV-1 or HIV-2). The 2008 definition is intended for public health surveillance only and not as a guide for clinical diagnosis.

Criteria for Definitive or Presumptive HIV Infection

A child aged <18 months is categorized for surveillance purposes as definitively or presumptively HIV infected if born to an HIV-infected mother and if the laboratory criterion or at least one of the other criteria is met.

Laboratory Criterion for Definitive HIV Infection

A child aged <18 months is categorized for surveillance purposes as definitively HIV infected if born to an HIV-infected mother and the following laboratory criterion is met.

- Positive results on two separate specimens (not including cord blood) from one or more of the following HIV virologic (non-antibody) tests:
  - HIV nucleic acid (DNA or RNA) detection[l]
  - HIV p24 antigen test, including neutralization assay, for a child aged >1 month
  - HIV isolation (viral culture)

Laboratory Criterion for Presumptive HIV Infection

A child aged <18 months is categorized for surveillance purposes as presumptively HIV infected if (1) born to an HIV-infected mother, (2) the criterion for definitively HIV infected is not met, and (3) the following laboratory criterion is met.

- Positive results on one specimen (not including cord blood) from the listed HIV virologic tests (HIV nucleic acid detection test; HIV p24 antigen test, including neutralization assay, for a child aged >1 month; or HIV isolation [viral culture] for definitively HIV infected) and no subsequent negative results from HIV virologic or HIV antibody tests.

Other Criteria (for Cases that Do Not Meet Laboratory Criteria for Definitive or Presumptive HIV Infection)

- HIV infection diagnosed by a physician or qualified medical-care provider based on the laboratory criteria and documented in a medical record. Oral reports of prior laboratory test results are not acceptable.

or

- When test results regarding HIV infection status are not available, documentation of a condition that meets the criteria in the 1987 pediatric surveillance case definition for AIDS.

Criteria for Uninfected With HIV, Definitive or Presumptive

A child aged <18 months born to an HIV-infected mother is categorized for surveillance purposes as either definitively or presumptively uninfected with HIV if (1) the criteria for definitive or presumptive HIV infection are not met and (2) at least one of the laboratory criteria or other criteria are met.

Laboratory Criteria for Uninfected With HIV, Definitive

A child aged <18 months born to an HIV-infected mother is categorized for surveillance purposes as definitively uninfected with HIV if (1) the criteria for definitive or presumptive HIV infection are not met and (2) at least one of the laboratory criteria or other criteria are met.[¶]

- At least two negative HIV DNA or RNA virologic tests from separate specimens, both of which were obtained at age ≥1 month and one of which was obtained at age ≥4 months.

or

- At least two negative HIV antibody tests from separate specimens obtained at age >6 months.

and

- No other laboratory or clinical evidence of HIV infection (i.e., no positive results from virologic tests [if tests were performed] and no current or previous AIDS-defining condition)

Laboratory Criteria for Uninfected With HIV, Presumptive

A child aged <18 months born to an HIV-infected mother is categorized for surveillance purposes as presumptively uninfected with HIV if (1) the criteria for definitively uninfected with HIV are not met and (2) at least one of the laboratory criteria are met.

- Two negative RNA or DNA virologic tests, from separate specimens, both of which were obtained at age ≥2 weeks and one of which was obtained at age ≥4 weeks.[#]

or

- One negative RNA or a DNA virologic test from a specimen obtained at age ≥8 weeks.

or

- One negative HIV antibody test from a specimen obtained at age ≥6 months.

or

- One positive HIV virologic test followed by at least two negative tests from separate specimens, one of which is a virologic test from a specimen obtained at age ≥8 weeks or an HIV antibody test from a specimen obtained at age ≥6 months.

and

- No other laboratory or clinical evidence of HIV infection (i.e., no subsequent positive results from virologic tests if tests were performed, and no AIDS-defining condition for which no other underlying condition indicative of immunosuppression exists).

Other Criteria (for Cases that Do Not Meet Laboratory Criteria for Uninfected With HIV, Definitive or Presumptive)

- Determination of uninfected with HIV by a physician or qualified medical-care provider based on the laboratory criteria and who has noted the HIV diagnostic test results in the medical record. Oral reports of prior laboratory test results are not acceptable.

and

- No other laboratory or clinical evidence of HIV infection (i.e., no positive results from virologic tests [if tests were performed] and no AIDS-defining condition for which no other underlying condition indicative of immunosuppression exists).

Criteria for Indeterminate HIV Infection

A child aged <18 months born to an HIV-infected mother is categorized as having perinatal exposure with an indeterminate HIV infection status if the criteria for infected with HIV and uninfected with HIV are not met.

2008 Surveillance Case Definitions for HIV Infection and AIDS Among Children Aged 18 Months to <13 Years

The 2008 laboratory criteria for reportable HIV infection among persons aged 18 months to <13 years exclude confirmation of HIV infection through the diagnosis of AIDS-defining conditions alone. Laboratory-confirmed evidence of

Box 25-2 | **Revised Surveillance Case Definitions for HIV Infection Among Adults, Adolescents, and Children Aged <18 Months and for HIV Infection and AIDS Among Children Aged 18 Months to <13 Years—United States, 2008—cont'd**

HIV infection is now required for all reported cases of HIV infection among children aged 18 months to <13 years.

Criteria for HIV Infection

Children aged 18 months to <13 years are categorized as HIV infected for surveillance purposes if at least one of laboratory criteria or the other criterion is met.**

Laboratory Criteria

- Positive result from a screening test for HIV antibody (e.g., reactive EIA), confirmed by a positive result from a supplemental test for HIV antibody (e.g., Western blot or indirect immunofluorescence assay).

or

- Positive result or a detectable quantity by any of the following HIV virologic (non-antibody) tests[††]:
  - HIV nucleic acid (DNA or RNA) detection (e.g., PCR)
  - HIV p24 antigen test, including neutralization assay
  - HIV isolation (viral culture)

Other Criterion (for Cases that Do Not Meet Laboratory Criteria)

- HIV infection diagnosed by a physician or qualified medical-care provider based on the laboratory criteria and documented in a medical record. Oral reports of prior laboratory test results are not acceptable.

Criteria for AIDS

Children aged 18 months to <13 years are categorized for surveillance purposes as having AIDS if the criteria for HIV infection are met and at least one of the AIDS-defining conditions has been documented.

Adapted from Centers for Disease Control and Prevention: Revised Surveillance Case Definitions for HIV Infection Among Adults, Adolescents, and Children Aged <18 Months and for HIV Infection and AIDS Among Children Aged 18 Months to <13 Years—United States, 2008. MMWR 57(RR10);1-8, December 5, 2008.

*Rapid tests are EIAs that do not have to be repeated but require a confirmatory test if reactive. Most conventional EIAs require a repeatedly reactive EIA that is confirmed by a positive result with a supplemental test for HIV antibody. Standard laboratory testing procedures should always be followed.

†For HIV screening, HIV virologic (non-antibody) tests should not be used in lieu of approved HIV antibody screening tests. A negative result (i.e., undetectable or nonreactive) from an HIV virologic test (e.g., viral RNA nucleic acid test) does not rule out the diagnosis of HIV infection.

‡Qualified medical-care providers might differ by jurisdiction and might include physicians, nurse practitioners, physician assistants, or nurse midwives.

§An original or copy of the laboratory report is preferred; however, in the rare instance the laboratory report is not available, a description of the laboratory report results by a physician or qualified medical-care provider documented in the medical record is acceptable for surveillance purposes. Every effort should be made to obtain a copy of the laboratory report for documentation in the medical record.

‖HIV nucleic acid (DNA or RNA) detection tests are the virologic methods of choice for the diagnosis of exclusion of infection in children aged <18 months. Although HIV culture can be used, culture is less standardized and less sensitive than nucleic acid detection tests. The use of p24 antigen testing to exclude infection in children aged <18 months is not recommended because of poor sensitivity, especially in the presence of HIV antibody. Commercial tests for RNA and DNA detection have become widely available. Quantitative RNA tests have been approved by the Food and Drug Administration (FDA) for monitoring HIV infection, and qualitative RNA tests have been approved to aid diagnosis. The quantitative and qualitative RNA tests meet FDA standards for high analytic and clinical sensitivity and specificity (14-16). All available tests detect the subtypes of group M and strains of group O. HIV-2 can be diagnosed with HIV-2 DNA PCR. HIV RNA tests sometimes do not detect HIV-2 because the viral loads in some HIV-2–infected persons are below detectable levels. Because of the possibility of mutation or recombination involving the sequences detected by a particular test, occasionally, virus might not be detected in a specimen from an HIV-2 infected individual. If HIV-2 infection seems likely but results are negative, testing with a different assay might be advisable.

¶Suspected cases of HIV infection among children aged <18 months who are born to a documented HIV-uninfected mother should be assessed on a case-by-case basis by the appropriate health care and public health specialists.

#If specimens for both negative RNA or DNA virologic tests are obtained at age ≥4 weeks, specimens should be obtained on separate days.

**Children aged 18 months to <13 years with perinatal exposure to HIV are categorized as uninfected with HIV if the criteria for uninfected with HIV among children aged <18 months are met.

††For HIV screening among children aged 18 months to <13 years infected through exposure other than perinatal exposure, HIV virologic (non-antibody) tests should not be used in lieu of approved HIV antibody screening tests. A negative result (i.e., undetectable or nonreactive) by an HIV virologic test (e.g., viral RNA nucleic acid test) does not rule out the diagnosis of HIV infection.

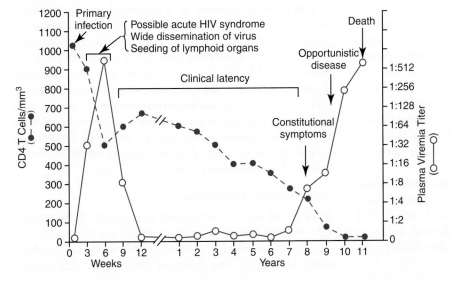

Figure 25-4   Typical course of HIV infection. During the early period after primary infection, there is widespread dissemination of virus and a sharp decrease in the number of CD4 T cells in peripheral blood. An immune response to HIV ensues, with a decrease in detectable viremia followed by a prolonged period of clinical latency. The CD4 T cell count continues to decrease during the following years until it reaches a critical level below which there is a substantial risk of opportunistic diseases. *(From Pantaleo G, Graziosi C, Fauci A: The immunopathogenesis of human immunodeficiency virus infection, N Engl J Med 328:327-335, 1993.)*

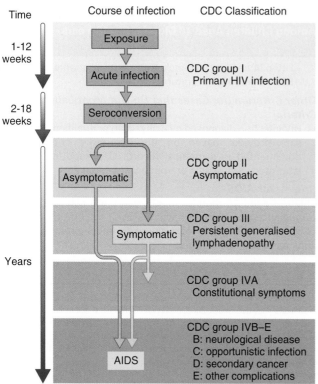

Time

1-12 weeks

2-18 weeks

Years

Course of infection

CDC Classification

Exposure

Acute infection

CDC group I
Primary HIV infection

Seroconversion

Asymptomatic

CDC group II
Asymptomatic

Symptomatic

CDC group III
Persistent generalised
lymphadenopathy

CDC group IVA
Constitutional symptoms

AIDS

CDC group IVB–E
B: neurological disease
C: opportunistic infection
D: secondary cancer
E: other complications

Figure 25-5 CDC classification. The CDC classification is used to define stages of HIV-related illness. *(From Peakman M, Vergani D: Basic and clinical immunology, ed 2, London, 2009, Churchill Livingstone.)*

Modes of Transmission

The HIV virus has been isolated from blood, semen, vaginal secretions, saliva, tears, breast milk, cerebrospinal fluid (CSF), amniotic fluid, and urine. Only blood, semen, vaginal secretions, and breast milk have been implicated in the transmission of HIV to date. HIV has been found in saliva and tears in very low quantities from some AIDS patients. It is important to understand that finding a small amount of HIV in a body fluid does not necessarily mean that HIV can be transmitted by that body fluid. HIV has not been recovered from the sweat of HIV-infected persons. Contact with saliva, tears, or sweat has never been shown to result in transmission of HIV.

HIV can be transmitted as the virus itself or as a cell associated with HIV. The virus is held within leukocytes and carried in fluid (e.g., blood, semen) to the body of another person. Transmission of HIV is believed to be restricted to intimate contact with body fluids from an infected person; casual contact with infected persons has not been documented as a mode of transmission. The risk of HIV infection to children born to women with HIV is 20% to 30%. HIV-2 seems to be less transmissible from an infected woman to her fetus or newborn.

Viral transmission of HIV-1 can be cervicovaginal, penile, rectal, oral, percutaneous, intravenous, in utero or breastfeeding after birth. More than 80% of adults infected with HIV-1 became infected through the exposure of mucosal surface to the virus; most of the remaining 20% were infected by a percutaneous or IV route.

Health care workers have been infected with HIV after being stuck with needles containing HIV-infected blood or, less frequently, after infected blood enters a worker's open cut or a mucous membrane (e.g., eyes, inside of nose). Viral transmission can result from contact with inanimate objects, such as work surfaces or equipment recently contaminated with infected blood or certain body fluids, if the virus is transferred to broken skin or mucous membranes by hand contact.

SIGNS AND SYMPTOMS

The CDC has a classification used to define stages of HIV-related illness (Fig. 25-5). Infection with HIV produces a chronic infection with symptoms that range from asymptomatic to the end-stage complications of AIDS.

Typically, patients in the early stages of HIV infection are completely asymptomatic or show mild chronic lymphadenopathy. The early phase may last from many months to many years after viral exposure. Although the course of HIV-1 infection may vary somewhat in individual patients, a common pattern of development has been recognized. The newly revised HIV classification system provides uniform and simple criteria for categorizing conditions (see Box 25-2).

During the early period after primary infection, widespread dissemination of the virus occurs, with a sharp decrease in the number of CD4+ T cells in peripheral blood. The early burst of virus in the blood, viremia, is often accompanied by flulike symptoms that can be so severe that the affected person may seek help at a hospital emergency department. An immune response to HIV develops, with a concurrent decrease in detectable viremia. It was previously believed that the human immune system could drive the AIDS virus into a latent period that kept it inactive for years. However, this concept has been replaced with the new vision of a virus that is furiously creating copies of itself throughout the disease course, even when the patient appears healthy. Even when HIV cannot be detected in the blood (viremia), it infects lymphatic tissues (in large quantities), including the tonsils and lymph nodes throughout the body. The absence of viremia generally lasts until the end stage of the disease.

This phase is followed by a prolonged period of clinical latency (range, 7 to 11 years; median, 10 years). During the period of clinical latency, the patient is usually asymptomatic. Differences in the infecting virus, host's genetic makeup, and environmental factors (e.g., concomitant infection) have been suggested as causes of the variable duration of clinical latency in persons not receiving **antiretroviral therapy.** Treatment with inhibitors of viral reverse transcriptase (e.g., zidovudine [Retrovir]) and prophylaxis for pneumonia caused by *Pneumocystis jiroveci* (previously called *P. carinii*) have increased AIDS-free time in HIV-1–infected persons.

Opportunistic Infections

Since AIDS was first recognized in the early 1980s, remarkable progress has been made in improving the quality and duration of life for HIV-infected persons in the industrialized world. During the first decade of the epidemic, this progress

Box 25-3	Opportunistic Infections in Immunosuppressed and Immunodeficient Patients

Oral or esophageal candidiasis
Cytomegalovirus
Pneumocystis jiroveci (P. carinii)
Herpes simplex
Entamoeba histolytica
Giardia lamblia
Herpes zoster
Atypical acid-fast bacilli
Shigella
Campylobacter
Cryptococcus neoformans
Adenovirus
Hepatitis
Chlamydia
Salmonella
Syphilis
Anal candidiasis
Dientamoeba fragilis
Blastocystis hominis
Toxoplasma gondii

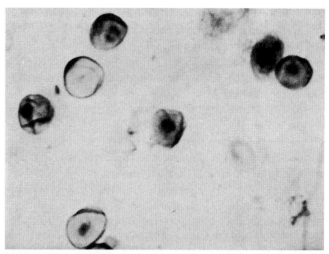

Figure 25-6 *Pneumocystis jiroveci (P. carinii)* from tracheobronchial aspirate (methenamine silver). *(From Markell EK, Voge M: Medical parasitology, ed 5, Philadelphia, 1981, Saunders.)*

resulted from improved recognition of opportunistic disease processes, improved therapy for acute and chronic complications, and introduction of chemoprophylaxis against key opportunistic pathogens. The second decade of the epidemic witnessed extraordinary progress in developing **highly active antiretroviral therapy (HAART),** as well as continuing progress in preventing and treating opportunistic infections. HAART has reduced the incidence of opportunistic infections and extended life. In addition, prophylaxis against specific opportunistic infections continues to provide survival benefits even among patients receiving HAART.

The absolute number of CD4+ T lymphocytes continues to diminish as the disease progresses. When the number of cells reaches a critically low level (<50 to $100 \times 10^9/L$), the risk of opportunistic infection increases. The period of susceptibility to opportunistic processes continues to be accurately indicated by CD4+ T lymphocyte counts for patients receiving HAART.

The end stage of AIDS is characterized by the occurrence of neoplasms and opportunistic infections (Box 25-3). The most common opportunistic infections are *P. jiroveci (P. carinii)* (Fig. 25-6), cytomegalovirus (CMV), *Mycobacterium avium-intracellulare, Cryptococcus, Toxoplasma, Mycobacterium tuberculosis,* herpes simplex, and *Legionella. Histoplasma capsulatum* is being recognized with increasing frequency. The most frequent malignancy observed is an aggressive, invasive variant of Kaposi's sarcoma, discovered in many cases on autopsy. Malignant B cell lymphomas are increasingly recognized in patients with or at high risk for AIDS.

Kaposi's Sarcoma

Kaposi's sarcoma (KS) was first described in 1872 by the dermatologist Moritz Kaposi. Since then, until the AIDS epidemic, KS remained a rare tumor. Classic KS usually occurs in males. The tumor typically presents with one or more asymptomatic red, purple, or brown patches; plaque; or nodular skin lesions. The disease is often limited to single or multiple lesions, usually localized to one or both lower extremities, especially involving the ankle and soles. Classic KS most often has a relatively benign, indolent course for 10 to 15 years or longer, with slow enlargement of the original tumors and gradual development of additional lesions. Up to one third of patients with classic KS develop a second primary malignancy, usually non-Hodgkin's lymphoma. An increased incidence of Hodgkin's disease occurs in HIV-infected homosexual men.

Cryptosporidiosis

Cryptosporidiosis is a disease caused by the parasite *Cryptosporidium parvum.* As late as 1976, this parasite was not thought to cause disease in human beings. In 1993, more than 400,000 people in Milwaukee, Wisconsin, became ill after drinking water contaminated with the parasite. Cryptosporidiosis can be chronic and severe in immunocompromised persons. The watery diarrhea can be prolonged and debilitating, and may be fatal.

Persons at risk of severe cryptosporidiosis include AIDS patients, cancer or organ marrow transplant patients taking drugs that weaken the immune system, and persons born with genetically weakened immune systems.

Disease Progression

Although a large enough dose of the right strain of HIV-1 can cause AIDS on its own, cofactors can influence the progression of disease development. Debilitated patients, weakened by a preexisting medical condition before HIV-1 infection, may progress toward AIDS more quickly than others. Stimulation of the immune system in response to later infections can also hasten disease progression. Other pathogenic microorganisms, such as a herpesvirus called human B lymphotropic virus (human herpesvirus 6 [HHV-6]), can interact with HIV in a way that may increase the severity of HIV infection. HHV-6 is usually easily controlled by the immune system. If HIV compromises the immune system, however, HHV-6 may replicate more freely and become a health threat. The main host of HHV-6 is the B cell, but this virus can also infect CD4+ cells. If these T cells are simultaneously infected by HIV, HHV-6 can stimulate the virus, which further impairs the immune system and promotes disease progression.

The progressive decline of CD4+ cells leads to a general decline in immune function and is the primary factor in determining the clinical progression of AIDS. Plasma HIV-1 RNA is a strong, CD4+ T cell–independent predictor of a rapid progression to AIDS after HIV-1 seroconversion.

Infection with HIV is presently considered to lead to death. When the clinically apparent disease develops, untreated patients usually die within 2 years, some exposed or HIV-1–infected patients never develop AIDS. The current hope is that an AIDS-free generation is on the horizon because of prevention strategies, e.g., safe sex, and pre-exposure prophylaxis.

Although scientists have known since 1986 that CD8 T cells, when stimulated, could release molecules capable of suppressing HIV, the identity of these substances eluded researchers for more than a decade. Studies have suggested that three large proteins, identified as alpha-defensins 1, 2, and 3, could be major contributors to the CD8 antiviral factor that protects some patients against AIDS. In another study, scientists at the National Institutes of Health (NIH) have linked HIV resistance to a different molecule secreted by CD8 T cells, called perforin. More studies related to each category of molecules are needed before either of these theories is confirmed.

Another study at the National Institute of Allergy and Infectious Diseases has examined variations in a gene called *RANTES* (*r*egulated on *a*ctivation, *n*ormal *T* cells *e*xpressed, and presumably *s*ecreted) in HIV-infected and HIV-resistant individuals. This study searched for changes in a **single nucleotide polymorphism (SNP)**. The results showed that one such SNP appears more often in HIV-positive than in HIV-negative persons. In addition, this particular alteration increases the activity of the *RANTES* gene and is associated with up to twice the risk of HIV infection. However, HIV-infected patients with this SNP take about 40% longer to develop AIDS.

IMMUNOLOGIC MANIFESTATIONS

Cellular Abnormalities

The HIV-1 virus has a marked preference for the CD4+ subset of lymphocytes because the CD4 surface marker protein on these cells serves as a receptor site for the virus. Immunologic activation (e.g., participation in an immune response to HIV-1 or viruses in other cells) of CD4+ cells latently infected with HIV-1 induces the production of multiple viral particles, leading to cell death. The extensive destruction of T cells leads to the gradual depletion of the CD4+ lymphocytes. The major phenotypic cell populations affected by AIDS are CD4+ and CD8+ subsets of T lymphocytes. Normally, the CD4+/CD8+ ratio is 2:1 in heterosexuals and 1.5:1 in homosexuals. A reversal of these subsets is evident in, but not diagnostic of, AIDS. In patients with AIDS, the ratio is less than 0.5:1. It is important to note that this results from a marked decrease in the absolute

number of circulating CD4+ cells, rather than from an absolute increase in suppressor or CD8+ cells. This abnormality exists in the lymph nodes and circulating T cells. A diminished CD4+/CD8+ ratio (altered lymphocyte subpopulation) can also be seen in individuals with other disorders, such as cutaneous T cell lymphoma, systemic lupus erythematosus (SLE), and acute viral infections. The ratio, however, reverts back to normal after recovery from a viral infection in non–AIDS patients.

A decreased lymphocyte proliferative response to soluble antigens and mitogens exists in AIDS. Functional testing reveals a diminished response to pokeweed mitogen. This disease also demonstrates defective natural killer (NK) cell activity.

Immune System Alterations

The HIV virus is fragile and, as the virus particle leaves its host cell, a molecule called gp120 frequently breaks off the outer coat of the virus. Glycoprotein 120 can bind to the CD4 molecules of uninfected cells and, when that complex is recognized by the immune system, these cells can be destroyed. The lysis of infected cells and gp120-bound uninfected cells leads to the gradual depletion of the CD4+ lymphocytes. Defects in immunity are related to this T cell depletion. Progressive defects in the immune system also include a severe B cell failure and defects in monocyte and granulocyte function.

Although HIV-1 destroys CD4+ cells directly and hampers the immune system, this process does not cause the severe immunodeficiency seen in AIDS. The severe deficiency can be explained only if the cells are also destroyed by other means. Several indirect mechanisms have been suggested. Infection by HIV can cause infected and uninfected cells to fuse into giant cells called syncytia, which are nonfunctional. Autoimmune responses, in which the immune system attacks the body's own tissues, may also be at work. In addition, HIV-infected cells may send out protein signals that weaken or destroy other cells of the immune system. It is possible that the binding of HIV to a target cell triggers the release of the enzyme protease. Proteases digest proteins; if released in abnormal quantities, they might weaken lymphocytes and other cells and decrease cell survival. The decline in T cells and subsequent alteration of the immune mechanism are the underlying factors in the progression of HIV infection.

Serologic Markers

Detection of Core Antigen

After initial infection, the body mounts a vigorous immune response against the viremia (see Color Plate 10). The first signal of an immune response to HIV-1 infection is the appearance of acute-phase reactants, including α_1-antitrypsin and serum amyloid in plasma 3 to 5 days after transmission. This is followed by a steep rise in the HIV-1 viral load (ramp-up viremia) that coincides with a large burst of inflammatory cytokines led by interferon-α and interleukin-15 (IL 15) and by a burst of plasma microparticles derived from infected and activated CD4 T cells undergoing apoptosis.

Immunologic activities include the production of different types of antibodies against HIV. Some antibodies neutralize the virus, others prevent it from binding to cells, and others stimulate cytotoxic cells to attack HIV-infected cells.

The time and sequence vary for the appearance and disappearance of antibodies specific for the serologically important antigens of HIV-1 during the course of infection. A window period of seronegativity exists from the time of initial infection to 6 or 12 weeks or longer thereafter. Through an enzyme immunofluorescence assay (EIA) based on defined HIV-1 proteins produced by recombinant DNA methods, antibodies specific for gp41 are detectable for weeks or months before assays specific for p24. The appearance of antibodies specific for p24 has been shown to precede that of anti-gp41 in serum specimens undergoing Western blot analysis. This discrepancy in the sequence of antibody appearance is believed to be caused by the greater sensitivity of Western blot compared with viral lysate–based EIAs used for the detection of anti-p24. The gp41 antibodies persist throughout the course of infection. Antibodies specific for p24 not only rise to detectable levels after gp41, but also can disappear unpredictably and abruptly.

Increased production of core antigen is believed to be associated with a burst of viral replication and host cell lysis. The disappearance of antibody directed against p24 occurs concomitantly with an increase in the concentration of core antigen in the serum. This parallel activity may result from the sequestration of antibody in immune complexes; the sudden decrease in anti-p24 is considered to be a grave prognostic sign in HIV-1–infected patients.

Antibodies to HIV-1

Antibodies to HIV-1 appear after a lag period of about 6 weeks between the time of infection and a detectable antibody response. Because of this, some virus-positive, antibody-negative individuals would be missed by initial screening assays.

In addition to a positive HIV antibody test in 85% to 90% of patients, increased antibody titers to other viruses (e.g., cytomegalovirus [CMV], Epstein-Barr virus, hepatitis A or B, *Toxoplasma gondii*) and **circulating immune (antigen-antibody) complexes** can be found. Other ancillary findings include polyclonal hypergammaglobulinemia, elevated levels of interferon-α (IFN-α), α_1-thymosin, and β-microglobulin, and reduced levels of IL-1 or IL-2.

Specific intrathecal synthesis of HIV antibody should be assessed simultaneously with an assay for total CSF immunoglobulin M (IgM) and for the intrathecal synthesis of total immunoglobulin G, as well as IgG specific for an appropriate control organism (e.g., adenovirus). In progressive encephalopathy related to AIDS, an increase in HIV antibody may suggest intrathecal rather than extrathecal synthesis.

DIAGNOSTIC EVALUATION AND MONITORING

Infection with HIV is established by detecting antibodies to the virus, viral antigens, or viral RNA-DNA or by the gold standard, viral culture. The standard test is for antibody detection. Laboratory evaluation of asymptomatic HIV-infected patients consists of the assessment of cellular and humoral components.

Screening of blood donors and patients at risk is usually done by serologic methods. In patients who have developed the

signs and symptoms of AIDS, assessment of T lymphocytes and viral load concentrations are important, along with the diagnosis and treatment of opportunistic infections.

Both leukopenia and lymphocytopenia can exist in the AIDS patient. Total leukocyte and absolute lymphocyte concentrations need to be periodically assessed. The common denominator of AIDS is a deficiency of a specific subset of thymus-derived (CD4+) lymphocytes. Enumeration of lymphocyte subsets is usually performed by flow cytometry (see Plate 11).

Additional testing includes viral load assay and resistance testing, an in vitro method to measure the resistance of HIV to antiretroviral agents. Resistance testing can aid in antiretroviral drug selection but has limitations.

TESTING METHODS

Testing assays for HIV (Table 25-4) are categorized into the following three main types:
1. Detection of HIV antibodies
2. Detection of antigens, particularly p24
3. Detection or quantification of viral nucleic acids

HIV-1 Antibodies

Detection of HIV antibodies by EIA was the first technology developed for HIV diagnosis in 1985. Diagnostic testing is classified as screening or confirmatory testing. Screening tests include traditional EIAs and newer methods. Confirmatory tests include Western blot (WB), indirect immunofluorescent antibody assay (IFA), and HIV RNA detection by nucleic acid amplification testing (NAAT).

Antibodies to HIV can be detected by EIA (specificity 99%, sensitivity 98%; Table 25-5) and confirmed by the immunoblot technique. Antibody testing by EIA remains the standard method for screening potential blood donors. Simultaneous testing for p24 **antigenemia** is considered unnecessary. Third-generation serologic assays have demonstrated that seroconversion typically occurs 3 to 12 weeks after infection, but significant delays can occur in some individuals.

HIV Antigen and Genome Testing

Enzyme Immunoassay: p24 Antigen

The enzyme immunoassay for the HIV-1 antigen detects primarily uncomplexed p24 antigen. This procedure is applicable to blood or CSF testing as evidence of an active infection and can be diagnostic before seroconversion, can predict a patient's prognosis, and is useful for monitoring response to therapy. Disadvantages of the procedure include poor sensitivity, inability to detect in patients with a high titer of p24 antibody, and failure of the method to detect HIV-2 antigen. Antibodies to p24 antigen are a better predictive marker of progression than p24 antigen.

Polymerase Chain Reaction

The polymerase chain reaction (PCR) allows for the direct detection of HIV-1 by DNA amplification. This ultrasensitive PCR technique has revolutionized HIV-1 detection. In addition to confirmatory testing, DNA amplification can be used

Table 25-4	**HIV Assays and Characteristics**		
Assay	**Format**	**Target Molecule**	**Comments**
Lymphocyte CD4 absolute count	Flow cytometry	CD4+	
HIV antigen assay for serum and plasma	EIA	HIV p24 antigen	
HIV types 1 and 2 (HIV-1, HIV-2) antibody detection in serum or plasma	EIA (first- and second-generation tests)	Recombinant HIV-1 *env* and *gag* and HIV-2 env proteins *or* Purified, inactivated HIV-1 virus propagated in T-lymphocyte culture	If reactive, confirm with molecular testing (Western blot).
Detection of HIV-1 groups M and O	EIA (third generation)	Purified, inactivated HIV-1 viral lysate proteins, envelope proteins, and HIV-1 group O transmembrane protein *or* Purified gp160 and p24 recombinant proteins from HIV-1, HIV-2 transmembrane gp36, and synthetic epitope of HIV-1 group O	
Enzyme-linked fluorescence p24 *or* EIA p24	EIA (fourth generation)	HIV-1 gp160, p24 antigen, and peptides representing regions of gp41 from HIV-1 group O and gp36 from HIV-2 *or* HIV-1 antigens p31 and gp41, HIV-2 p36 recombinant protein, HIV-1 group O gp41, and anti-p24 monoclonal antibodies	
HIV antibody detection in serum or plasma	Western blot	Purified and inactivated HIV-1 strain LAV grown in CEM cell line *or* Purified and inactivated HIV-1 propagated in H9/HTLV-IIIB T lymphocyte cell line	
HIV viral load assays	PCR	Reverse-transcriptase PCR *or* Nucleic acid sequence–based amplification *or* Signal amplification, branched-chain DNA	
Rapid testing	Rapid immunoassay	Uses recombinant proteins representing regions of HIV-1 envelope proteins *or* Uses synthetic HIV structural proteins	
Molecular Testing			
HIV-1 RNA	Quantitative real-time PCR		Aids in assessing viral response to antiretroviral treatment
HIV-1 RNA	Quantitative bDNA	Quantitative branched-chain DNA	Aids in assessing viral response to antiretroviral treatment
HIV-1 DNA	Qualitative PCR		Detects HIV-1 proviral DNA in infants <48 hr old; repeat testing at 1-2 mo and 3-6 mo of age
HIV-2 antibody		Qualitative enzyme immunoassay, qualitative immunoblot	Screen for HIV-2 infection in a patient with an epidemiologic link to Africa.
HIV-1 genotyping	Reverse transcription PCR/ nucleic acid sequencing		Detect changes in the viral genome associated with drug resistance. Use in conjunction with CD4 measurement to monitor treatment efficacy.

Table 25-4	HIV Assays and Characteristics—cont'd		
Assay	**Format**	**Target Molecule**	**Comments**
HIV-2 antibody confirmation	Qualitative immunoblot		Confirm positive screening results.
HIV-1 antibody	Qualitative chemiluminescent immunoassay		

Adapted from Zetola N, Klausner JD: HIV testing: an update, MLO Med Lab Obs 38:58–62, 2006.
EIA, Enzyme immunoassay; *PCR,* polymerase chain reaction.

Table 25-5	Causes of False-Positive and False-Negative HIV Enzyme Immunoassay Results	
False-Positive Result	**False-Negative Result**	
Positive RPR (syphilis serology) test	Laboratory glove starch	
Hematologic malignant disorder	Window period before seroconversion	
DNA viral infections	Immunosuppressive therapy	
Autoimmune disorders	Malignancies	
Alcoholic hepatitis	Bone marrow transplantation	
Vaccinations (e.g., hepatitis B, influenza)	Kits that mainly detect antibodies to p24	
Chronic renal failure		
Renal transplantation		

Adapted from Specialty Laboratories, Santa Monica, Calif.
RPR, Rapid plasma reagin.

for the diagnosis of very early, postexposure HIV infection in the window period before production of antibodies.

The goal of direct detection of active virus in patient specimens by an ultrasensitive method is to detect less than 100 molecules of viral nucleic acid in the peripheral blood cells isolated from 1 mL of blood. This number is the assay target because as few as 1 in 10,000 lymphocytes express viral RNA in HIV-1–infected individuals. Therefore, of approximately 10^6 lymphocytes/mL blood, about 100 contain viral nucleic acid, corresponding to 100 to 150 copies of HIV-1 DNA. The presence of HIV-1 DNA in lymphocytes of antibody-positive, asymptomatic patients can be used to confirm exposure to the virus. The presence of viral RNA might be a sensitive indicator of viral replication and possibly of further disease progression.

The basis of PCR is the amplification of minute amounts of viral nucleic acid in lymphocyte DNA. In HIV-1–infected cells, the DNA template is a provirus that exists as integrated or episomal DNA. After amplification, isotope or nonisotope methods can detect the amplified product. The most effective means of target amplification is PCR. A pair of **specific oligomer primers** initiates DNA synthesis in combination with

heat-stable Taq I DNA polymerase. After this first round of primer extension, the material is heated to denature the product from its template and cooled to 37° C (98.6° F) to permit annealing of the primer molecules to the original template DNA and to the newly synthesized DNA fragments. Primer extension is then resumed. By repetition of these cycles of denaturation, annealing, and extension, the original DNA can be increased exponentially.

Viral RNA can also be specifically amplified with some additional steps. The **gag region** is probably the best choice of a sequence for amplification. Detection of viral RNA and DNA in clinical specimens might prove to be a better indicator of biologically active virus than DNA detection alone. The presence of both provirus and viral RNA **transcriptase** would be a strong indication of viral replication. Quantitation of HIV RNA in plasma is useful for determining free viral load, assessing the efficacy of antiviral therapy, and predicting progression and clinical outcome in AIDS patients.

Confirmatory Testing

Western Blot
Before an HIV result is considered positive, the results should be reproducible and confirmable by at least one additional test. Western blot (WB) analysis is currently the standard method for confirming HIV-1 seropositivity (Fig. 25-7).

The WB assay is based on the recognition of the major HIV proteins (p24, gp41, gp120/160) by fractionating them according to their weight by electrophoresis and then visualizing their binding with specific antibodies over nitrocellulose sheets. A positive result is indicated by the presence of any two of the following bands—p24, gp41, and gp120/160. If the test is positive for bands gp41 and/or p24 in conjunction with a positive EIA test result, it is regarded as a confirmatory test. A negative result demonstrates the absence of bands. Indeterminate results can be found in 10% to 20% of EIA-positive tests. In general, the presence of a band at p24, p31, or p55, although still classified as indeterminate, is more indicative of true infection as compared with other band patterns.

The WB appears to work best with samples that contain high levels of antibody. Antibody specificities against known viral components (generally, the core component p24 and envelope component gp41) are considered true-positive results, whereas antibodies specific against nonviral cellular contaminants are nonspecific, false-positive results.

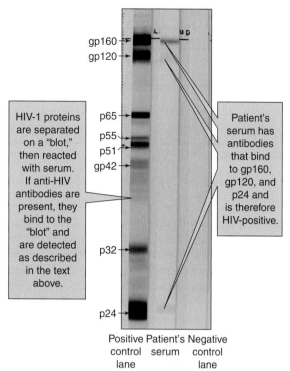

HIV-1 proteins are separated on a "blot," then reacted with serum. If anti-HIV antibodies are present, they bind to the "blot" and are detected as described in the text above.

Patient's serum has antibodies that bind to gp160, gp120, and p24 and is therefore HIV-positive.

gp160
gp120

p65
p55
p51
gp42

p32

p24

Positive Patient's Negative
control serum control
lane   lane

Figure 25-7 Western blot to confirm HIV-positive status. *(From Nairn R, Helbert M: Immunology for medical students, ed 2, Philadelphia, 2007, Mosby.)*

The WB technique is time-consuming and expensive. It is also open to considerable interpretation and has many sources of error. Variables in the test include the following:

- The technical skill and experience of the technologist performing the procedure
- Characteristics of the technical methodology
- General sensitivity of the WB in detecting antibodies specific for various HIV-1 antigens (especially during the window period of seronegativity)
- Frequent lack of specificity because of contamination of the viral reference preparation by histocompatibility and other antigens that electrophoretically migrate with p24 and gp41
- Variation in band reactivity patterns in sera from an individual over the course of HIV-1 infection

Indeterminate test results account for 4% to 20% of WB assays with positive bands for HIV-1 proteins. Indeterminate WB results can be caused by the following:

- Serologic tests in the process of seroconversion; anti-p24 is usually the first antibody to appear.
- End-stage HIV infection, usually with loss of core antibody
- Cross-reacting nonspecific antibodies, as seen with collagen vascular disease, autoimmune diseases, lymphoma, liver disease, injection drug use, multiple sclerosis, parity, or recent immunization
- Infection with O strain or HIV-2
- Recipients of HIV vaccine

- Perinatally exposed infants who are seroconverting (losing maternal antibody)
- Technical or clerical error

In addition, nonspecific reactions producing indeterminate results in uninfected persons have occurred more frequently in pregnant women or mothers than in persons in other groups characterized by low HIV seroprevalence. The incidence of indeterminate WB results is relatively low. The immunofluorescence assay can be used to resolve an EIA-positive, WB-indeterminate sample.

The most important factor in evaluating indeterminate results is risk assessment. Patients in low-risk categories with indeterminate test results are almost never infected with HIV-1 or HIV-2. Repeat testing usually continues to show indeterminate results, and the cause of this pattern is seldom established. Follow-up serology testing at 3 months is recommended to verify the previous results. Patients with indeterminate tests who are in the process of seroconversion usually have positive WB test results within 1 month; repeat tests at 1, 2, and 6 months are generally advocated, with appropriate precautions to prevent viral transmission in the interim.

False-positive WB results, especially those with a majority of bands, are extremely uncommon.

Quantitative RNA Assay

Recently, the U.S. Food and Drug Administration (FDA) approved a quantitative RNA assay for the confirmation of HIV infection.

Immunofluorescence Assay

IFA can provide a definitive diagnosis in samples that test indeterminate with other confirmatory tests. IFA is used to locate the HIV-1 antigen in infected cells. Infected cells are treated with polyclonal or monoclonal antibody against p17 or p24. After being washed, the cells are incubated with fluorescein isothiocyanate or rhodamine conjugate as a secondary antibody and then washed, mounted, and examined using a fluorescence microscope. The limitations of this technique include the need for expensive equipment and the fact that fluorescence fades quickly.

Immunohistochemical Staining

In immunohistochemical (IHC) staining, infected cells are incubated with HIV-1 antibody. After incubation, the cells are treated with an enzyme-labeled secondary antibody (usually alkaline phosphatase or horseradish peroxidase) and an appropriate substrate is added. The cells are washed and examined using simple light microscopy. IHC staining has the advantages of IFA but is simple and inexpensive and does not require extensive expertise. Morphologic changes can also be observed.

Fourth-Generation Testing

Previously, most tests used in the diagnostic setting detected only HIV antibodies. Fourth-generation assays detect HIV-1 p24 antigen up to 20 days earlier than Western blot and 5 to 7 days earlier than third-generation enzyme immunoassays. Levels of p24 antigen increase early after initial infection.

More specific or supplemental tests for HIV-1 and HIV-2 (e.g., NAAT), Western blot, or immunofluorescence, must be performed to verify the presence of HIV-1 p24 antigen or antibodies to HIV-1 or HIV-2.

Fourth-generation assays allow for the differentiation between acute infection (p24 only, no HIV-1 antibody) and established infections (both p24 antigen and HIV-1 antibody). The gold standard for acute infection screening is NAAT. HIV-1 RNA can identify HIV infection as early as 5 days after exposure.

In 2010, the FDA approved the first fourth-generation immunoassay that detects both antigen and antibodies to HIV (ARCHITECT HIV Ag/Ab Combo Assay, Abbott Laboratories, Abbott Park, Ill). This test is a chemiluminescent microparticle immunoassay. The ARCHITECT HIV Ag/Ab Combo Assay was the first diagnostic test approved by the FDA for use in children as young as 2 years of age and pregnant women.

Other fourth-generation assays (e.g., GS HIV Combo Ag/Ab EIA, Bio-Rad Laboratories, Hercules, Calif) use EIA methodology (see later, procedure). These methods simultaneously test for HIV p24 antigen and antibodies to HIV-1 (groups M and O) and HIV-2 in human serum or plasma.

Rapid Testing

Routine HIV testing of whole blood in the emergency department has been shown to find unidentified cases. Currently, six rapid point-of-care testing (POCT) assays have FDA approval, including the OraQuick ADVANCE Rapid HIV-1/2 Antibody Test (OraSure Technologies, Bethlehem, Pa; see later, procedure). OraQuick ADVANCE can screen oral fluid and whole blood. In 2007, Inverness (Waltham, Mass) acquired rights to market the Chembio (Medford, NY) rapid test for the detection of HIV-1 and HIV-2 antibodies in fingertip blood, whole blood, serum, or plasma. Tests use protein A colloidal gold, which allows for the visual detection of HIV antibodies, or second-generation EIA so-called sandwich technology, with HIV-1 gp41 and HIV-2 gp36 synthetic antigen.

A disadvantage of rapid tests includes lower sensitivity than third- and fourth-generation EIA assays. The sensitivity of the currently available rapid tests is similar to that of second-generation EIA assays.

Currently, most protocols recommend confirming any positive rapid tests with WB or EIA. Follow-up with WB or EIA should be done 4 weeks later if confirmatory test results are negative or indeterminate.

Tests for Therapeutic Monitoring

Viral Load Testing

Testing of the viral load should be performed as soon as patient treatment begins. Subsequent viral load testing can be used as a marker for HIV viremia and should be carried out every 3 to 6 months for patients undergoing treatment. New guidelines recommend testing of viral load every 2 to 8 weeks after the initiation of HAART to determine early response to therapy. Fully automated assays have a fast turn-around time. Fully automated assays and real-time PCR are noted to have a lower rate of false-negative results when compared with nucleic acid sequence-based amplification.

CD4 T Lymphocyte Testing

Monitoring of CD4 T lymphocytes measures immune function. This information guides the initiation of antiretroviral therapy (ART) and monitors a patient's response to antiretroviral treatment. CD4 T lymphocyte counts are expressed as absolute counts or as a percentage of the total population of CD4/CD8 as a ratio. Flow cytometry, in conjunction with fluorescence-activated cell sorting (FACS; see Chapter 13) is considered to be the gold standard in CD4 T lymphocyte counting.

PREVENTION

Reducing Viral Transmission

The CDC estimates 1.2 million people in the United States (U.S.) are living with HIV infection. One in five (20%) of those people are unaware of their infection. Despite increases in the total number of people in the U.S. living with HIV infection in recent years. New infections constitute approximately 50,000 Americans becoming infected with HIV each year. The CDC has issued new testing recommendations, making HIV screening a routine part of medical care for all patients 13 to 64 years of age. CDC officials hope that these revised guidelines will increase early HIV diagnosis so that individuals can access treatment, know their health care status, and prevent transmission to others.

Health care personnel should assume that the blood and other body fluids from all patients are potentially infectious (Standard Precautions; see Chapter 6).

Vaccines

Types of potential HIV vaccines include the following:
- Live attenuated vaccines
- Subunit vaccines
- DNA vaccines
- Recombinant vector vaccines

To date, the results of clinical trials have been disappointing (Box 25-4). Live attenuated vaccines are not currently being developed for use in human beings because of safety concerns. The first AIDS vaccine using the subunit concept, AIDSVAX gp120 vaccine, failed to protect against HIV infection in an efficacy trial. Many of the current AIDS vaccines in development are DNA vaccines. DNA vaccines will not cause HIV infection because they do not contain all the genes of the live pathogen. Another common strategy in AIDS vaccine development is recombinant vector vaccines. These will not cause HIV infection because they contain copies of only one or several HIV genes, not all of them. It is hoped that the addition of a vector will allow the vaccine to be more effective in creating an immune response than a DNA vaccine used alone.

Continued testing of vaccines is needed to determine whether they are more immunogenic in different doses, in different populations, and in combination with other candidate HIV vaccines (see Chapter 16).

More than 30 clinical trials have been in progress to develop a vaccine to prevent HIV (see www.iavi.org). The first generation of successful HIV vaccines likely will offer some

Box 25-4	**Clinical Trials for a Candidate HIV-AIDS Vaccine**

Phase I

Phase I trials are the first human tests of a candidate vaccine, generally conducted on small numbers (10 to 30) of healthy adult volunteers who are not at risk for the disease in question. The main goal is evaluation of safety and, to a lesser extent, analysis of the immune responses evoked by the vaccine and of different vaccine doses and immunization schedules. A phase I trial usually takes 8 to 12 months to complete.

Phase II

Phase II testing involves a larger number of volunteers (50 to 500), usually a mixture of low-risk people and higher risk individuals from the population in whom phase III (vaccine efficacy) trials will eventually be conducted. Phase II trials generate additional safety data as well as information for refining the dosage and immunization schedule. Although not set up to determine whether the vaccine actually works, phase II trials are sometimes large enough to yield preliminary indications of efficacy. These trials generally take 18 to 24 months, with the increase over phase I primarily resulting from the additional time required for screening and enrolling larger numbers of trial participants.

Phase III

Phase III trials are the definitive test of whether a vaccine is effective in preventing disease. Using thousands of volunteers from high-risk populations in geographic regions in which HIV is circulating, the incidence of HIV in vaccinated people is compared with that in people who receive a placebo. Successful demonstration of efficacy in a Phase III trial can then lead to an application for licensure of the vaccine.

Phase III trials of AIDS vaccines are generally expected to require a minimum of 3 years for enrollment, immunizations, and assessments of efficacy. Although there has been recent progress in increasing access to treatment and prevention programs, HIV continues to outpace the global response, with at least 80% of those in clinical need of antiretrovirals (ARVs) worldwide not receiving them. Furthermore, although a decline in national HIV prevalence has occurred—for example, in some Sub-Saharan African countries—these trends are not strong or widespread enough to have a major impact on the epidemics.

Adapted from International AIDS Vaccine Initiative: Vaccine science, 2007 (www.iavi.org).

protection but will not be entirely protective—no vaccine is 100% effective. Future generations of a preventive HIV vaccine will become increasingly more effective over time as scientific knowledge improves. However, even partially effective vaccines could make a difference in the following ways:

1. Protect some vaccinated individuals against HIV infection.
2. Reduce the probability that a vaccinated individual who later becomes infected will transmit the infection to others.
3. Slow the rate of progression to AIDS for those who later become infected with HIV.

An HIV vaccine, RV144, is being studied by the U.S Military HIV Research Program at the Walter Reed Army Institute of Research. This clinical trial has involved more than 16,000 adult volunteers in Thailand. In this study, the recipients of the vaccine had a 31% lower chance of becoming infected with HIV than those in the placebo group. Since the study results reported in 2009, more than 100 scientists from 25 institutions have been searching for molecular clues to explain why the vaccine showed a modest protective effect. An antibody formed by vaccinated individuals who made high levels of the antibody resulted in their being significantly less likely to become infected than those who did not. This particular binding antibody attaches to a part of the outer coat of the virus, the first and second variable regions, or V1V2, which may play an important role in HIV infection of human cells. The antibody belongs to the IgG family. Vaccinated study participants who built different antibodies to the vaccine appeared to have less protection from HIV. Further studies of this vaccine will determine whether the V1V2 antibody response is merely a marker of HIV exposure or of decreased susceptibility to HIV infection. The most recent studies of this vaccine have generated the hypothesis that V1V2 antibodies may have contributed to protection against HIV-1 infection, but high levels of Env-specific IgA antibodies may have mitigated the effects of protective antibodies. Vaccines designed to induce higher levels of V1V2 antibodies and lower levels of Env-specific IgA antibodies than are induced by the RV144 vaccine may have improved efficacy against HIV-1 infection.

An HIV vaccine could substantially alter the course of the AIDS pandemic and reduce the number of people newly infected, even if vaccine efficacy and population coverage levels are relatively low.

TREATMENT

Despite declines in morbidity and mortality with combination antiretroviral therapy, its effectiveness is limited by adverse events, problems with patient adherence, and resistance of HIV. Episodic antiretroviral therapy, guided by the CD4+ count, significantly increases the risk of opportunistic disease or death from any cause compared with continuous antiretroviral therapy as a consequence of lowering the CD4+ cell count and increasing the viral load. However, episodic antiretroviral therapy does not reduce the risk of adverse events associated with antiretroviral therapy.

Drug Therapy

Numerous drugs are in use or are in investigational trials for HIV. The FDA has divided drugs into several categories based on their in vivo activity.

Combination Drugs. This category includes drugs that are a non-nucleoside reverse transcriptase inhibitor (NNRTI) combined with a nucleoside reverse transcriptase inhibitor (NRTI), or drugs such as lamivudine-zidovudine, a fixed-dose combination of reverse transcriptase inhibitors (NRTIs).

Entry and Fusion Inhibitors. These drugs block HIV's ability to infect healthy CD4 cells. When used with other anti-HIV agents, these drugs can reduce the amount of HIV in the blood and increase the number of CD4 cells. The first drug in this class, pentafuside (T-20), went into phase III clinical trials in early 2001. The mode of action of the drug is the prevention of HIV entry into the host cell. Zinc finger inhibitors disrupt polyprotein formation essential for HIV replication. An example of a drug in this category is benzamide,

Integrase Inhibitors. This class of drugs blocks the enzyme integrase, which the virus (HIV) needs to make more virus. The drug in this class, zintevir (AR-177), prevents HIV DNA from entering human DNA.

When used with other anti-HIV medicines, a drug in this class may have two functions:

1. Reduces the amount of HIV in the blood (the viral load)
2. Increases the number of white blood cells called CD4 (T) cells

Non-Nucleoside Reverse Transcriptase Inhibitors. NNRTIs work by disrupting one of the early steps in the HIV life cycle, called reverse transcription. During normal reverse transcription, HIV's reverse transcriptase enzyme converts HIV's RNA into DNA. It does this by recoding the RNA building blocks into complementary DNA building blocks. As the HIV life cycle proceeds, the newly formed DNA is used to make more copies of HIV virus.

The first drug in this class, nevirapine, was approved in June 1996. NNRTIs may interact with other cytochrome P-450–processed drugs (e.g., protease inhibitors). NNRTIs have a mixed ability to penetrate the blood-brain barrier.

Nucleoside Reverse Transcriptase Inhibitors. The original NRTI was zidovudine (AZT), approved in March 1987. Zidovudine competes with one of the available DNA building blocks called deoxythymidine 5′-triphosphate. By replacing deoxythymidine 5′-triphosphate in the newly developing HIV DNA, zidovudine is able to stop reverse transcriptase from completing its job. This prevents the HIV DNA strand from being formed and halts the HIV life cycle.

Since zidovudine was approved, additional NRTIs have also been approved. In 2001, the first nucleotide analogue, tenofovir, was approved for HIV treatment. It blocks HIV replication in a manner similar to that of the nucleoside analogues. NRTIs are potent in combination with other drugs. If used alone, resistance to HIV will develop. Some of the drugs in this class (e.g., AZT) can penetrate the blood-brain barrier.

Opportunistic Infection Drug. Acyclovir was approved by the FDA in 1997 for use in the treatment of herpes simplex infections that cause cold sores and genital herpes, as well as herpes zoster infections (shingles) caused by varicella-zoster virus, the virus that causes chickenpox. It does not cure or prevent herpes infection or HIV infection and does not reduce the risk of passing these viruses to other individuals.

Protease Inhibitors. A protease inhibitor (PI) acts by blocking protease, a protein that HIV needs to make more copies of itself. The first drugs in this class for the treatment of HIV were ritonavir and indinavir, approved in 1996. PIs are very potent and may interact with other drugs using **cytochrome P-450**

metabolic pathways. However, poor absorption may affect potency.

Investigational Drugs

New drugs are needed because resistant mutations that protect HIV against existing classes of antiretroviral drugs would be unlikely also to confer resistance to novel agents. Drug discovery and FDA approval currently take an average of 12 to 15 years, and it costs about $400 million for a drug to go from the laboratory to a pharmacy in the United States. Drug approval requires testing in three phases of a clinical trial for safety and efficacy before approval:

- Phase I takes about 1 year and includes 20 to 80 healthy volunteers who are tested for the safety of a new drug.
- Phase II lasts about 2 years and expands the number of volunteers to 100 to 300 persons with the disease to assess the effectiveness of a drug and observe for adverse side reactions.
- Phase III of a clinical trial lasts about 3 years and expands the number of patients with a specific disease to 1000 to 3000 to verify effectiveness further and identify any specific negative side effects of the drug.

Since the FDA Regulatory Modernization Act of 1997, the FDA review process has been streamlined to hasten approval of new therapies to treat severe diseases. Phases I and II have been allowed to be combined to shorten the approval process. It now takes about 18 months for a drug to go through the review process for approval by the FDA. Only about one in five medicines that enters a clinical trial is approved.

Anti-HIV drugs under development include agents that interfere with other steps in the HIV life cycle (e.g., fusion inhibitors, integrase inhibitors) and a second-generation NNRTI.

One rather recent approach involves preventing HIV from invading the human cells in which it replicates, a concept termed *entry inhibition*. To gain entry to host cells, HIV binds to the cell's CD4 receptor in tandem with a coreceptor, usually CXCR5 or CXCR4. This process allows HIV to fuse with the cell membrane and inject its genes inside the cell. Patients with certain mutations in CCR5 are resistant to HIV infection, so drugs that block this receptor might prevent the virus from invading cells.

In addition to new studies of drugs that prevent the virus from binding to host cell receptors, phase III clinical trials have been underway for the T-20 agent, a fusion inhibitor that blocks a different event in viral invasion, the fusion of HIV with the host cell membrane. Another experimental viral entry inhibitor that appears to inhibit activity of gp120, the viral envelope protein that must interact with the host cell's CD4 receptor for HIV invasion to occur, is under development.

Also in early phases of development is an experimental agent intended to block HIV at a later stage, after it has invaded cells. The compound, S-1360, targets integrase, a viral enzyme that enables HIV to splice its DNA into the host cell's DNA. Human trials of the integrase inhibitor AR-177 are now underway.

Also on the horizon are improved versions of NNRTIs. NNRTIs (e.g., efavirenz [EFV], nevirapine) target a key viral enzyme, reverse transcriptase, inhibiting its function by binding to a pocket near the enzyme's catalytic site. However,

NNRTI resistance can develop when HIV acquires one or more mutations that alter the binding pocket. The drug TMC-125, given as a single agent, performed as well as the five-drug regimen containing agents from all three currently licensed classes of anti-HIV medications.

Drug Resistance

Antiviral drug resistance is defined as the reduction in the susceptibility of mutated viruses to specific antiviral drugs. An estimated 50% of U.S. patients receiving antiretroviral therapy are infected with viruses resistant to at least one of the currently available antiretroviral drugs.

The origins of drug resistance are diverse, but drug resistance is associated with the high mutation rate in the HIV genome, which is one of the key biological characteristics of the virus. Genomic mutation is determined by the following:

- The number of mistakes per genome per replication cycle. This is extremely high in HIV because reverse transcriptase has no so-called proofreading ability.
- The number of viral replication cycles per unit of time. This is reflected in an infected patient's viral load.

The relationship between resistance mutations and response to therapy is complex. Each resistance mutation is characterized by the level of associated phenotypic resistance and the specificity of the resistance mutation to one or more drugs.

HIV Antiretroviral Drug Resistance: Genotypes, Phenotypes, Virtual Phenotypes, and Tropism Testing. A patient's response to therapy depends on a number of factors, including patient compliance, percentage of resistant virus population, dosing, and drug pharmacology issues. Genotypic or phenotypic assays can be used to assess HIV drug resistance. The vircoTYPE HIV-1 assay (Janssen Diagnostics, Raritan, NJ) predicts HIV-1 drug resistance based on the nucleic acid sequence of the patient's human immunodeficiency virus. This test analyzes sequences that encompass the entire protease gene and codons 1-335 of the reverse transcriptase gene. An analysis using the Virtual Phenotype Linear Modeling analysis (http://www. janssendiagnostics. com) can be used.

Genotypic Assays. Genotypic assays use sequenced regions of the *pol* gene of the HIV genome, the target site of most antiretroviral drugs. Enzymes coded for in those regions—reverse transcriptase, protease, and integrase—are key to HIV replication. Mutation in these regions can produce enzymes that are not susceptible to antiretroviral drug inhibition. Genotypic tests can be classified using automated rule-based algorithms that label the major species of virus as susceptible, possibly resistant, or resistant. Currently, two FDA-approved testing kits are available.

Phenotypic Assays. Phenotypic assays depend on cell culture–based viral replication assays, with and without drug exposure. Typically, these assays measure the degree to which a specific drug inhibits viral replication in vitro. The intermediate resistance range is the point at which there is a perceptibly diminished clinical response. Full resistance is the point at which there is no drug response. Although testing is expensive, the main advantage is that the procedure may identify resistant strains secondary to novel mutations.

Virtual Phenotypes. Computer algorithms are now able to compare genotypic data from native HIV-1 RNA with a large database of corresponding phenotypes and genotypes to generate a virtual phenotype. A virtual phenotype offers the advantage of producing output that incorporates clinical cutoffs based on viral responses for the 14 most common forms of combination antiretroviral therapy.

Tropism Testing. Resistance testing is necessary to determine the efficacy of drugs that act by blocking HIV entry through coreceptor activation. Tropism or coreceptor testing, like resistance testing, can be done by genotype and phenotype testing. Phenotypic testing requires amplification of the *env* sequence and creation of the viral pseudotypes. After viral material is inoculated onto CD4-, CCR5-, and CXCR4-expressing T cells, gene activity is monitored. The oldest genotypic tropism assay interrogates the coding region of the gp160 HIV-1 envelope protein and is 100% sensitive for detecting certain variants. Charges on amino acids are sought for classification. Currently, phenotype testing is preferred in the United States.

Postexposure Prophylaxis

Among health care workers exposed to HIV occupationally, prompt treatment can decrease the subsequent risk of HIV infection by more than 80%. However, treatment should begin within 1 to 2 hours after exposure. Rapid HIV testing facilitates successful treatment.

The NRTI combinations for postexposure prophylaxis (PEP) include zidovudine (ZDV) and lamivudine (3TC), 3TC and stavudine (d4T), and didanosine (ddI) and d4T. The addition of a third drug for PEP after high-risk exposures is based on demonstrated effectiveness in reducing the viral burden in HIV-infected persons. Previously, indinavir or nelfinavir was recommended as the first-choice agent for inclusion in an expanded PEP regimen. In 1998, the FDA approved EFV, an NNRTI; abacavir (ABC), a potent NRTI; and lopinavir-ritonavir (Kaletra), a PI, for PEP.

Although side effects might be common with NNRTIs, EFV might be considered for expanded PEP regimens, especially when resistance to PIs in the source person's virus is known or suspected. ABC has been associated with dangerous hypersensitivity reactions but, with careful monitoring, may be considered as a third drug for PEP. Kaletra is a potent HIV inhibitor that with expert consultation, may be considered in an expanded PEP regimen. Lopinavir is a newly developed inhibitor that when formulated with ritonavir, has antiviral activity superior to that of a nelfinavir-containing regimen by itself in the initial treatment of HIV-infected adults.

Recommendations for HIV PEP include a basic 4-week regimen of two drugs (ZDV and 3TC, d4T, or ddI and d4T) for most HIV exposures. An expanded regimen includes the addition of a third drug for HIV exposures that pose an increased risk for transmission. When the source person's virus is known or suspected to be resistant to one or more of the drugs considered for the PEP regimen, the recommendation is to select drugs to which the source person's virus is unlikely to be resistant. In addition, consultation with local experts and the

National Clinicians' Postexposure Prophylaxis Hotline (PEP-line; 888-448-4911) is advised under special circumstances (e.g., delayed exposure report, unknown source person, pregnancy in an exposed person, resistance of source virus to antiretroviral agents, toxicity of PEP regimen). Occupational exposures should be considered urgent medical concerns to ensure timely postexposure management.

Failure of PEP to prevent HIV infection in health care personnel (HCP) has been reported in very few cases. Guidelines for the treatment of HIV infection, a condition usually involving a high total-body viral burden, include recommendations for the use of three drugs; however, the applicability of these recommendations to PEP remains unknown. In HIV-infected patients, combination regimens have proved superior to monotherapy regimens in reducing HIV viral load, reducing the incidence of opportunistic infections and death, and delaying onset of drug resistance. A combination of drugs with activity at different stages in the viral replication cycle theoretically could offer an additional preventive effect in PEP, particularly for occupational exposures that pose an increased risk of transmission. Although a three-drug regimen might be justified for exposures that pose an increased risk of transmission, it is uncertain whether the potential added toxicity of a third drug is justified for lower risk exposures.

Information from the National Surveillance System for Health Care Workers and the HIV Postexposure Registry has indicated that almost 50% of HCP experience adverse symptoms (e.g., nausea, malaise, anorexia, headache) while taking PEP and that approximately 33% stop taking PEP because of adverse signs and symptoms. Some studies have shown that side effects and discontinuation of PEP are more common among HCP taking three-drug combination regimens for PEP than HCP taking two-drug regimens. Serious side effects, including nephrolithiasis, hepatitis, and pancytopenia, have been reported with the use of combination drugs for PEP. Known or suspected resistance of the source virus to antiretroviral agents, particularly to agents that might be included in a PEP regimen, is a concern. Resistance to HIV infection occurs with all the available antiretroviral agents and cross-resistance within drug classes is common. Studies have demonstrated the emergence of drug-resistant HIV among source persons for occupational exposures. Despite recent studies and case reports, the relevance of exposure to a resistant virus is still not well understood.

CASE STUDY

History and Physical Examination

A 40-year-old man with a history of IV drug use comes to the emergency room because of a rash and fever. In addition, the patient is complaining of a several day history of malaise, fatigue, fever, headache, and a sore throat.

Physical examination reveals a moderately ill-appearing man with a temperature of 38.8° C (102° F). He has a blanching erythematous, macular-papular rash evident over the trunk, back, and upper and lower extremities. In addition, his throat shows enlarged tonsils and broad-based ulcerations on the buccal mucosa.

He has a history of an episode of endocarditis 2 years ago. At that time, an HIV serology test was performed. It was negative.

Laboratory Data

A complete blood count and liver function tests are ordered. Results show that the patient is anemic (hematocrit, 38%). He also has a severely decreased total leukocyte count and a severely decreased absolute lymphocyte count. Some of his liver function test results are abnormal.

Questions

1. If acute Epstein-Barr Virus (EBV) or human immunodeficiency virus (HIV) are suggested clinically, a difference between the two would be that the HIV patient would have _____.
   a. Atypical lymphocytes present on a peripheral blood film
   b. Atypical lymphocytes absent on a peripheral blood film
   c. Absence of mucosal ulcerations
   d. A positive screening test for infectious mononucleosis
2. The Western Blot assay can recognize ___ major HIV proteins.
   a. p24
   b. gp41
   c. c, gp120/160
   d. All of the above

See Appendix A for the answers to multiple choice questions.

Critical Thinking Group Discussion Questions

1. What is a likely diagnosis of this patient's condition?
2. What is the natural history of this disease?
3. What immunologic laboratory tests might be of value in establishing a diagnosis for this patient?

See instructor site ⊖volve for the discussion of the answers to these questions.

⬛ Rapid HIV Antibody Test

Principle

This point of care test (OraQuick ADVANCE Rapid HIV-1/2 Antibody Test) is a manually performed, visually read, 20-minute qualitative lateral flow immunoassay to detect antibodies to HIV-1 and HIV-2 in oral fluid and blood.

Reporting Results

- Nonreactive: No reddish purple line next to the triangle labeled T; reddish purple line appears next to the triangle labeled C.
  - Interpreted as negative for HIV-1 and HIV-2 antibodies Individuals infected with HIV-1 and/or HIV-2 who are receiving HAART may show false-negative results.
- Reactive: Reddish purple line next to the triangle labeled T; reddish purple line appears next to the triangle labeled C. One line may be darker than the other. A test is reactive if any color appears next to the T triangle and next to the C triangle, regardless of how faint.
  - Interpreted as positive for HIV-1 and/or HIV-2 antibodies

Procedure Notes

After collection of a specimen into the developer solution, the solution facilitates the flow of the specimen into the device and onto the test strip. As the diluted specimen flows through the device, it rehydrates the protein A gold colorimetric reagent in the device. As the specimen continues to migrate up the strip, it encounters the T zone. If the specimen contains antibodies that react with the antigens immobilized on the nitrocellulose membrane, a reddish purple line will appear, indicating qualitatively the presence of antibodies to HIV-1 and/or HIV-2 in the specimen. The intensity of the line color is not directly proportional to the amount of antibody present in the specimen.

- No precision pipetting, predilutions, or special instruments are required to perform the OraQuick ADVANCE Rapid HIV-1/2 Antibody Test.
- Standard Precautions must be practiced throughout the testing procedure.
- The test should be performed at temperatures in the range of 15° C to 37° C (59° F to 98.6° F). All refrigerated reagents must reach room temperature before testing.
- If the test kit is stored at temperatures outside ambient temperatures of 2° C to 27° C (35.6° F to 80.6° F) or used outside the operating temperature of 15° C to 37° C (59° F to 98.6° F), use the kit controls to ensure performance of the test.

GS HIV Combo Ag/Ab EIA

The GS HIV Combo Ag/Ab EIA is an enzyme immunoassay based on the principle of the sandwich technique for the qualitative detection of HIV-1 p24 antigen and detection of envelope antibodies associated with HIV-1 and/or HIV-2 virus in human serum or plasma. The solid phase is coated with the following:
- Monoclonal antibodies against HIV-1 p24 antigen
- HIV antigens: HIV-1 gp160 recombinant protein, a synthetic peptide mimicking a totally artificial (i.e., encoded by no existing virus) HIV-1 group O–specific epitope and a peptide mimicking the immunodominant epitope of the HIV-2 envelope protein. The conjugates are based on the use of biotinylated polyclonal antibodies to HIV p24 Ag (conjugate 1) and peroxidase-conjugated

streptavidin and peroxidase-conjugated HIV-1 antigens (gp41 and gp36 peptides mimicking the immunodominant epitopes of the HIV-1 and HIV-2 envelope glycoproteins, and the same synthetic peptide mimicking a totally artificial HIV-1 group O-specific epitope used for the solid phase; conjugate 2)

During the assay procedure, conjugate 1 (biotinylated polyclonal antibody to HIV p24 Ag) is added to the microplate wells, followed by the addition of samples to be assayed and by controls and a calibrator. If present, HIV p24 antigen binds to the monoclonal antibody on the solid phase and also binds to conjugate 1. HIV-1 and/or HIV-2 antibodies, if present, bind to the antigens immobilized on the solid phase. The addition of conjugate 1 and sample is validated through a color change from yellow-green to blue. After incubation, excess sample is removed by a wash step.

Next, conjugate 2 is added. Peroxidase-labeled streptavidin reacts with biotinylated Ab-Ag-Ab complexes; peroxidase-labeled HIV-1 and HIV-2 antigens bind to the IgG, IgM, or IgA antibodies captured on the solid phase. After incubation, unbound conjugate 2 is removed by washing. A working solution is added to the plate and allowed to incubate. A blue or blue-green color develops in proportion to the amount of HIV antibody and/or antigen present in the sample. Color development is stopped by the addition of acid, which changes the blue-green color to yellow. The optical absorbances of specimens, controls, and the calibrator are determined spectrophotometrically at a wavelength of 450 nm, with a 615- to 630-nm reference.

See the ⊖volve website for the procedural protocol.

Results

This test has been developed to reduce the serologic window significantly for detection of HIV. HIV antigens and antibodies appear and are detectable at different stages of seroconversion and of the infection. Reactive specimens may contain HIV-1 p24 antigen or antibodies to HIV-1 or HIV-2.

Simulation of HIV-1 Detection

Principle

This HIV test (Edvotek, Washington, DC, Kit 271) detects HIV infection indirectly using an enzyme-linked immunosorbent assay (ELISA) against HIV antibodies in the blood. The test detects potential antibodies from a patient's blood by adding it to a microtiter plate coated with HIV antigen. If HIV antibodies are present in the blood, they will bind to the antigens on the plate. This binding is detected with an enzyme-linked secondary antibody that causes a color change on addition of substrate.

This ELISA test uses microtiter plate wells coated with simulated HIV antigen and then tests simulated donor serum for anti-HIV antibodies.

See the ⊖volve website for the procedural protocol.

Results

- One donor should be negative for HIV. The color change should be similar to that of the negative control.
- One donor should be shown positive for HIV. The color change should be similar to that of the positive control.

CHAPTER HIGHLIGHTS

- HIV-1 is the predominant virus responsible for AIDS. In addition to the original HIV-1, a second AIDS-causing virus, HIV-2, was identified in 1985.
- The HIV virus is composed of structural proteins and glycoproteins that occupy the core and envelope regions of the particle.
- Retroviruses contain a single, positive-stranded RNA with the genetic information of the virus and a special enzyme, reverse transcriptase, in their core. Reverse transcriptase enables the virus to convert viral RNA into DNA.
- HIV has a marked preference for the CD4+ subset of lymphocytes. Macrophages, as many as 40% of the peripheral blood monocytes, and cells in the lymph nodes, skin, and other organs also express measurable amounts of CD4 and can be infected by HIV. In addition, about 5% of B lymphocytes may express CD4 and be susceptible to HIV infection.
- Transmission of HIV is believed to be restricted to intimate contact with body fluids from an infected person; casual contact with infected persons has not been documented as a mode of transmission.
- The early phase of HIV-1 infection may last months to years after initial infection. Typically, patients in the early stages of HIV-1 infection are completely asymptomatic or show mild, chronic lymphadenopathy. HIV-1 causes a predictable progressive derangement of immune function; AIDS is one late manifestation of that process.
- Two to 10 years after HIV infection, replication of the virus flares again and the infection enters its final stage. An average of 8 or 9 years may pass before AIDS is fully developed. The virus behaves differently depending on the host cell and its level of mitotic activity. The end stage of AIDS is characterized by neoplasms and opportunistic infections.
- Immunologic activities associated with HIV-1 infection include the production of different types of antibodies against HIV-1. Some antibodies neutralize it, others prevent it from binding to cells, and others stimulate cytotoxic cells to attack HIV-infected cells.
- A window period of seronegativity exists from the time of initial infection to 6 or 12 weeks or longer. Using EIA methods based on defined HIV-1 proteins produced by recombinant DNA methods, antibodies specific for gp41 are detectable for weeks or months before assays specific for p24. The appearance of antibodies specific for p24 precedes that of anti-gp41 in Western blot serum specimens.
- Laboratory evaluation of HIV-infected patients consists of assessment of cellular and humoral components. Screening of blood donors and patients is usually by serologic methods. In patients with signs and symptoms of AIDS, both the assessment of cellular concentrations and function and the diagnosis and treatment of opportunistic infections become important.
- Antibodies to HIV-1 are usually detected by EIA and confirmed by Western blot, currently the standard for confirming HIV-1 seropositivity. If positive for band p41 or p24 with a positive EIA, the test is confirmatory.

REVIEW QUESTIONS

1. The major structural protein (core) of the HIV-1 virus is:
   a. gp41
   b. p24
   c. gp34
   d. gp140

2. The infectious process of AIDS begins when the gp120 protein on the viral envelope bends to the protein receptor, _____, on the surface of a target cell.
   a. CD8
   b. CD4
   c. p24
   d. p26

3. HIV can infect all of the following cells except:
   a. CD4+ subset of lymphocytes
   b. Macrophages
   c. Monocytes
   d. Polymorphonuclear leukocytes

4. The most rapidly growing segment of the HIV-infected population is:
   a. Homosexual males
   b. Lesbians
   c. Health care workers
   d. IV drug users and their sexual partners

5. In HIV infections, a window period of seronegativity extends from the time of initial infection up to:
   a. 2 weeks
   b. 2 to 6 weeks or longer
   c. 6 to 12 weeks or longer
   d. 4 to 8 months or longer

6 and 7. HIV antibodies are usually detected by (6) _____ and confirmed by (7) _____.

Possible answers for question 6:
   a. Latex agglutination
   b. Enzyme immunoassay
   c. Enzyme inhibition
   d. Radioimmunoassay

Possible answers for question 7:
   a. Southern blot
   b. Northern blot
   c. Western blot
   d. DNA hybridization

8. The AIDS-causing virus HIV has also been referred to as:
   a. Human T-lymphotropic virus type III
   b. HTLV-III
   c. Lymphadenopathy-associated virus (LAV)
   d. All of the above

9. HTLV-III was unique when it was isolated because it:
   a. Is a bovine infectious retrovirus
   b. Is a canine infectious retrovirus
   c. Was identified as the cause of AIDS
   d. Is a DNA containing virus

10-12. Fill in the blanks in the following table with the correct letter, choosing from the following answers:
   a. Codes for p24 and for proteins such as p17, p9, and p7
   b. Codes for two glycoproteins, gp41 and gp120
   c. Produces DNA polymerase; produces endonuclease

Viral Genome Structural Components

Component	Product
pol	10. _____
gag	11. _____
env	12. _____

13-17. Arrange the HIV-1 life cycle events in proper order.

13. _____   a. Reverse transcriptase converts viral RNA into proviral DNA.

14. _____   b. New virus particles are produced as the result of normal cellular activities of transcription and translation.

15. _____   c. New particles bud from the cell membrane.

16. _____   d. Virus attaches to CD4 membrane receptor and sheds its protein coat, exposing its RNA core.

17. _____   e. Proviral DNA is integrated into the genome (genetic complement of cell).

18. The criteria for HIV infection for persons 13 years of age or older include:
   a. Repeatedly reactive screening test for HIV antibody
   b. Specific HIV antibody identified by use of supplemental tests
   c. Direct identification of the virus
   d. All of the above

19. After the early period of primary HIV infection, the patient enters a period of clinical latency that lasts a median of _____ years.
   a. 5
   b. 10
   c. 15
   d. 20

20. As AIDS progresses, the quantity of _____ diminishes and the risk of opportunistic infection increases.
   a. HIV antigen
   b. HIV antibody
   c. CD4+ T lymphocytes
   d. CD8+ T lymphocytes

21. The clinical symptoms of the later phase of AIDS are:
   a. Weight loss and decreased polymorphonuclear leukocyte (PMN) cells
   b. Extreme weight loss and fever
   c. Multiple secondary (opportunistic) infections
   d. Both b and c

22. The most frequent malignancy observed in AIDS patients is:
   a. *Pneumocystis jiroveci (P. carinii)*
   b. Kaposi's sarcoma
   c. Toxoplasmosis
   d. Non-Hodgkin's lymphoma

23. Sources of error in the Western blot test include:
   a. Concentration of HIV antigen
   b. Presence of other infectious agents
   c. Technical skill and experience of the technologist performing the test
   d. Age of the blood specimen

24. All the following methods have been developed to detect HIV-1 antigen except:
   a. Transcriptase method
   b. Synthetic peptide approach
   c. Immunofluorescence assay
   d. Immunohistochemical staining

25. All the following methods have been developed to detect the presence of HIV-1 viral gene except:
   a. Radioimmunoassay
   b. In situ hybridization
   c. Southern blot analysis
   d. DNA amplification

BIBLIOGRAPHY

American Association for Clinical Chemistry: Routine HIV testing in the ED catches unidentified cases, 2007, https://www.aacc.org/publications/cln/2007/august/ Pages/newsbrief_0807.aspx#.

Baeten JM, et al: Antiretroviral prophylaxis for HIV prevention in heterosexual men and women, N Eng J Med 367:399–410, 2012.

Bayer R, Oppenheimer GM: Pioneers in AIDS care: reflections on the epidemic's early years, N Engl J Med 355:2273–2278, 2006.

Bio-Rad Laboratories: GS HIV Combo Ab/Ab EIA, product insert, 2011, www.bio-rad.com.

Centers for Disease Control and Prevention: HIV in the United States: at a glance, August 31, 2012, www.cdc.gov/hiv/resources/factsheets/PDF/HIV_at_a_glance.pdf. retrieved.

Cohen JK, Klausner JD: HIV testing update, 2011, http://www.mlo-online.com/ features/201111/clinical-issues/hiv-testing-update.aspx.

Cohen MS, et al: Acute HIV-1 infection, N Engl J Med 364:1943–1954, 2011.

Cohen MS, et al: Prevention of HIV-1, N Engl J Med 365:493–505, 2011.

El-Sadr WM, et al: CD4+ count–guided interruption of antiretroviral treatment, N Engl J Med 355:2283–2294, 2006.

Gallo RC, Montagnier L: AIDS in 1988, Sci Am 259:40–51, 1988.

Haseltine WA, Wong-Stall F: The molecular biology of the AIDS virus, Sci Am 259:52–63, 1988.

Havlir D, Beyer C: The beginning of the end of AIDS? N Eng J Med 367:685–687, 2012.

Haynes BF, et al: Immune-correlates analysis of an HIV-1 vaccine efficacy trial, N Engl J Med 366:1275–1286, 2012.

James E: Clinical clips: FDA approves rapid HIV test, ADVANCE Med Lab Professionals 14:12, 2002.

Janssen Diagnostics: HIV information, 2012, http://www.janssendiagnostics.com.

Kaiser Family Foundation: Fact sheet: the global HIV/AIDS epidemic, 2012, http://www.kff.org/hivaids/. Retrieved August 31, 2012.

Koziel MJ, Peters MG: Viral hepatitis in HIV infection, N Engl J Med 356:1445–1454, 2007.

Lallemant M, Chang S, Cohen R, Pecoul B: Pediatric HIV—a neglected disease? N Engl J Med 365581–365583, 2011.

Malone B: 30 years of HIV/AIDS, Clin Lab News 37(1):3–4, 2011.

McCutchan FE: Understanding the genetic diversity of HIV-1, AIDS 14(Suppl 3):S31–S44, 2000.

McDermott D, et al: Chemokine promoter polymorphism affects risk of both HIV infection and disease progression in multicenter AIDS cohort study, AIDS 14:2671–2678, 2000.

Mills EJ, Bärnighausen, Negrin J: HIV and aging—preparing for the challenges ahead, N Engl J Med 366:1270–1272, 2012.

Moir S, et al: B cells in early and chronic HIV infection: evidence for preservation of immune function associated with early initiation of antiretroviral therapy, Blood 116:5571–5579, 2010.

National Institutes of Health: Possible clues found to why HIV vaccine showed modest protection, 2012, http://www.aidsinfo.nih.gov/news/1228/possible-clues-found-to-why-hiv-vaccine-showed-modest-protection.

Panel on Antiretroviral Guidelines for Adults and Adolescents: U.S. Department of Health and Human Services: Guidelines for the use of antiretroviral agents in HIV-infected adults and adolescents, 2012, http://www.aidsinfo.nih.gov/.

Schim van der Loeff MF, Aaby P: Towards a better understanding of the epidemiology of HIV-2, AIDS 13(Suppl A):S69–S84, 1999.

Scosyrev E: An overview of the human immunodeficiency virus featuring laboratory testing for drug resistance, Clin Lab Sci 19:231–248, 2006.

Sepkowitz KA: One disease, two epidemics: AIDS at 25, N Engl J Med 354:2411–2417, 2006.

Smith T: Employing HIV molecular and rapid testing, ADVANCE Admin Lab 15:44–51, 2006.

Stephenson J: Scientists find some genes a bad omen for anti-HIV drug, JAMA 287:1637, 2002.

Strategies for Management of Antiretroviral Therapy (SMART) Study Group; El-Sadr WM, et al: CD4+ count–guided interruption of antiretroviral treatment, N Engl J Med 355:2283–2296, 2006.

Thigpen M, et al: Antiretroviral preexposure prophylaxis for heterosexual HIV transmission in Botswana, N Eng J Med 367:423–434, 2012.

Turgeon ML: Clinical hematology: theory and procedures, ed 5, Philadelphia, 2012, Lippincott–Williams & Wilkins.

Van Damme L, et al: Preexposure prophylaxis for HIV infection among African women, N Eng J Med 367:411–422, 2012.

Wainberg MA, et al: Development of antiretroviral drug resistance, N Engl J Med 365:637–646, 2011.

Weber JN, Weiss RA: HIV infection: the cellular picture, Sci Am 259:100–109, 1988.

Wong-Stall F, Gallo RC: Human T-lymphotropic retroviruses, Nature 317:395–403, 1985.

World Health Organization: Progress report: Global HIV/AIDS response, 2011, http://www.who.int/hiv/pub/progress_report2011/en. 2011.

CHAPTER 26

Hypersensitivity Reactions

Learning Objectives

At the conclusion of this chapter, the reader should be able to:

- Define the terms hypersensitivity, allergy, sensitization, and immunization.
- Identify and explain the three categories of antigens.
- Compare the basic differences among and give examples of types I, II, III, and IV hypersensitivity reactions.
- Describe the etiology, immunologic activity, signs and symptoms, laboratory evaluation, and treatment of type I hypersensitivity reactions.
- Discuss examples of type II hypersensitivity reactions, including laboratory evaluation.
- Describe the mechanism of tissue injury, clinical manifestations, and laboratory testing for type III hypersensitivity reactions.

- Describe the characteristics and laboratory evaluation of type IV hypersensitivity reactions.
- Discuss the acquisition and consequences of latex sensitivity.
- Analyze case studies related to hypersensitivity reactions.
- Correctly answer case study related multiple choice questions.
- Be prepared to participate in a discussion of critical thinking questions.
- Describe the principle, clinical applications, or sources of error of a food allergy test, and the direct antiglobulin test.
- Correctly answer end of chapter review questions.

Key Terms

allergens
allergy
allergy march
alloimmunization
anaphylactic reactions
Arthus reaction
atopy

autoantibodies
autoantigens
delayed hypersensitivity
desensitization
direct antiglobulin test (DAT)
downregulation
hemolytic reactions

histocompatibility
hypersensitivity
immediate hypersensitivity
immunization
rhinitis
urticaria
vasodilation

WHAT IS HYPERSENSITIVITY?

Hypersensitivity can be defined as a normal but exaggerated or uncontrolled immune response to an antigen that can produce inflammation, cell destruction, or tissue injury. It has traditionally been classified on the basis of time after exposure to an offending antigen. When this criterion is used, the terms immediate hypersensitivity and delayed hypersensitivity are appropriate. Immediate hypersensitivity is antibody mediated; delayed hypersensitivity is cell mediated.

The term **immunization,** or sensitization, describes an immunologic reaction dependent on the host's response to a subsequent exposure of antigen. Small quantities of the antigen may favor sensitization by restricting the quantity of antibody formed. An unusual reaction, such as an allergic or hypersensitive reaction that follows a second exposure to the antigen, reveals the existence of the sensitization.

WHAT IS AN ALLERGY?

Our basic understanding of allergy has evolved from the discovery in 1967 of a previously unknown antibody, immunoglobulin E (IgE). The most significant property of IgE antibodies is that they can be specific for hundreds of different allergens. Common allergens include animal dander, pollens, foods, molds, dust, metals, drugs, and insect stings.

The term **allergy** originally meant any altered reaction to external substances. A related term, **atopy,** refers to immediate hypersensitivity mediated by IgE antibodies. The terms *allergy* and *atopy* are now often used interchangeably. Atopic allergies include hay fever, asthma, food allergies, and latex sensitivity.

Allergies are very common and are increasing in prevalence in the United States, Western Europe, and Australia. Allergies also occur in families, although not necessarily the same allergy.

TYPES OF ANTIGENS AND REACTIONS

Antigens that trigger allergic reactions are called **allergens.** These low-molecular-weight substances can enter the body by being inhaled, eaten, or administered as drugs.

Hypersensitivity reactions can occur in response to different types of antigen, including environmental substances, infectious agents, food, and self antigens.

Environmental Substances

Environmental substances in the form of small molecules can trigger several types of hypersensitivity reactions. Dust can enter the respiratory tract, mimicking parasites, and stimulate an antibody response. An immediate hypersensitivity reaction associated with IgE, such as **rhinitis** or asthma, can result. If dust stimulates immunoglobulin G (IgG) antibody production, it can trigger a different type of hypersensitivity reaction, such as farmer's lung. If small molecules diffuse into the skin and act as haptens, a delayed hypersensitivity reaction, such as contact dermatitis, will result.

Drugs administered orally, by injection, or on the skin can provoke a hypersensitivity reaction mediated by IgE, IgG, or T lymphocytes.

Metals (particularly nickel) and chemicals can also cause type I hypersensitivity reactions. Low-molecular-weight chemicals usually act as a hapten by binding to body proteins or major **histocompatibility** complex (MHC) molecules. The complex of antigen and MHC molecules is then recognized by specific T cells, which initiate the reaction.

Infectious Agents

Not all infectious agents are capable of causing hypersensitivity reactions. The influenza virus can cause hypersensitivity that results in damage to epithelial cells in the respiratory tract. Sometimes, an exaggerated immune response occurs. Influenza virus, for example, can trigger high levels of cytokine secretion or what is called a cytokine storm. In comparison, streptococci can cause a hypersensitivity reaction termed *immune complex disease.*

Self Antigens

Very small immune responses to self antigens is normal and occur in most people. When these become an exaggerated response, however, or when tolerance to other antigens breaks down, hypersensitivity reactions can occur.

Food Allergies

According to the National Institute of Allergy and Infectious Diseases (NIAID), food allergy (FA) is an important public health problem that affects adults and children and may be increasing in prevalence. The prevalence of food allergy in Europe and North America has been reported to range from 6% to 8% in children up to the age of 3 years. A recent U.S. study has estimated that 5% of children under 5 years of age and 4% of teens and adults have food allergies.

Food allergy can cause severe allergic reactions and even death from food-induced anaphylaxis. Despite the risk, there is no current treatment for FA; the disease can only be managed by allergen avoidance or treatment of symptoms. The diagnosis of FA may be problematic because nonallergic food reactions, such as food intolerance, are frequently confused with FAs.

The NIAID guidelines separate diseases defined as FA that include both IgE-mediated reactions to food (food allergies), non–IgE-mediated reactions to certain foods (e.g., celiac disease), and mixed IgE and non-IgE disorders (Table 26-1).

TYPES OF HYPERSENSITIVITY REACTIONS

The four types of hypersensitivity reaction (I to IV) are defined by the principal mechanism responsible for a specific cell or tissue injury that occurs during an immune response (Table 26-2). Types I, II, and III reactions are antibody dependent and type IV is cell mediated. Some overlapping occurs among the various types of hypersensitivity reactions, but there are major differences in how each type is diagnosed and treated.

Type I Reactions

Type I hypersensitivity reactions can range from life-threatening **anaphylactic reactions** to milder manifestations associated with food allergies.

Table 26-1	Classification of Hypersensitivity Reactions			
	Type of Reaction			
Parameter	**I**	**II**	**III**	**IV**
Reaction	Anaphylactic	Cytotoxic	Immune complex	T cell–dependent
Antibody	IgE*	IgG, possibly other immunoglobulins	Antigen-antibody complexes (IgG, IgM)*	None
Complement involved	No	Yes*	Yes*	No
Cells involved	Mast cells, basophils, granules (histamine)*	Effector cells (macrophages, polymorphonuclear leukocytes)*	Macrophages, mast cells	Antigen-specific T cells
Cytokines involved	Yes*	No	Yes*	Yes (T cell cytokines)*
Comparative description	Antibody mediated, immediate	Antibody dependent; complement or cell mediated	Immune complex mediated (immune complex disease)	T cell-mediated, delayed type
Mechanism of tissue injury	Allergic and anaphylactic reactions	Target cell lysis; cell-mediated cytotoxicity	Immune complex deposition, inflammation	Inflammation, cellular infiltration
Examples	Anaphylaxis Hay fever Asthma Food allergy	Transfusion reactions Hemolytic disease of newborn Thrombocytopenia	Arthus reaction Serum sickness Systemic lupus erythematosus	Allergy or infection Contact dermatitis

*Mediator.

Table 26-2	Mediators of Anaphylaxis
Mediator	**Primary Action**
Histamine	Increases vascular permeability; promotes contraction of smooth muscle
Leukotrienes	Alter bronchial smooth muscle and enhance effects of histamine on target organs
Basophil kallikrein	Generates kinins
Serotonin	Contracts smooth muscle
Platelet-activating factor	Enhances the release of histamine and serotonin from platelets that affect smooth muscle tone and vascular permeability
Eosinophil chemotactic factor of anaphylaxis	Attracts eosinophils to area of activity; these cells release secondary mediators that may limit the effects of primary mediators
Prostaglandins	Affect smooth muscle tone and vascular permeability

Etiology

Atopic allergies are mostly naturally occurring, and the source of antigenic exposure is not always known. Atopic illnesses were among the first antibody-associated diseases demonstrating a strong familial or genetic tendency.

Several groups of agents cause anaphylactic reactions. The two most common agents are drugs (e.g., systemic penicillin) and insect stings. Insects of the order Hymenoptera (e.g., common hornet, yellow jacket, yellow hornet, paper wasp) are examples of insects causing the most serious reactions. Immune-mediated IgE adverse food reactions (Box 26-1) can be fatal.

Immunologic Activity

Mast cells (tissue basophils) are the cellular receptors for IgE, which attaches to their outer surface. These cells are common in connective tissues, lungs, and uterus and around blood vessels. They are also abundant in the liver, kidney, spleen, heart, and other organs. The granules contain a complex of heparin, histamine, and zinc ions, with heparin in a ratio of approximately 6:1 with histamine.

Immediate hypersensitivity is the basis of acute allergic reactions caused by molecules released by mast cells when an allergen interacts with membrane-bound IgE (Fig. 26-1). Acute allergic reactions result from the release of preformed granule-associated mediators, membrane-derived lipids, cytokines, and chemokines when an allergen interacts with IgE that is bound to mast cells or basophils by the alpha chain of

| Box 26-1 | **Diagnosis of IgE-Mediated Food Allergy** |

The National Institute of Allergy and Infectious Diseases (NIAID) Expert Panel recommends:

- Considering food allergy in individuals presenting with anaphylaxis or any combination of symptoms that occur within minutes to hours of ingesting food, especially in young children and/or if symptoms have followed the ingestion of a specific food on more than one occasion. In addition, infants, young children, and selected older children diagnosed with certain disorders, such as moderate to severe atopic dermatitis (AD), eosinophilic esophagitis (EoE), enterocolitis, enteropathy, and allergic proctocolitis (AP) should be considered for FA.
- Using medical history and physical examination to aid in the diagnosis of FA.
- Confirming parent and patient reports of FA because multiple studies demonstrate that 50% to 90%of presumed FAs are not allergies.
- Performing an SPT (skin puncture test) to assist in the identification of foods that may be provoking IgE-mediated food-induced allergic reactions, but the SPT alone cannot be considered diagnostic of FA.
- Not using intradermal testing or measuring total serum IgE to make a diagnosis of FA.
- Using allergen-specific serum IgE (sIgE) tests for identifying foods that potentially provoke IgE-mediated food-induced allergic reactions, but not using these tests as diagnostic of FA.
- Not using an atopy patch test (APT) in the routine evaluation of noncontact FA.
- Not using the combination of SPTs, sIgE tests, and APTs for the routine diagnosis of FA.
- Eliminating one or a few specific foods from the diet may be useful in the diagnosis of FA, especially in identifying foods responsible for some non–IgE-mediated food-induced allergic disorders, such as food protein–induced enterocolitis syndrome (FPIES), AP, and Heiner syndrome, and some mixed IgE- and non-IgE–mediated food-induced allergic disorders, such as EoE.
- Using oral food challenges for diagnosing FA. The double-blind, placebo-controlled food challenge is the gold standard. However, a single-blind or open-food challenge may be considered diagnostic under certain circumstances. If either of these challenges elicits no symptoms (i.e., the challenge is negative), then FA can be ruled out, but when either challenge elicits objective symptoms (i.e., the challenge is positive) *and* those objective symptoms correlate with medical history *and* are supported by laboratory tests, then a diagnosis of FA is supported.
- Not using any of the following nonstandardized tests for the routine evaluation of IgE-mediated FA: basophil histamine release or activation, lymphocyte stimulation, facial thermography, gastric juice analysis, endoscopic allergen provocation, hair analysis, applied kinesiology, provocation neutralization allergen-specific IgG4 , cytotoxicity assays, electrodermal test (Vega), mediator release assay (LEAP diet).

Adapted from National Institute of Allergy and Infectious Diseases: Guidelines for the diagnosis and management of food allergy in the United States: summary of the NIAID-sponsored expert panel report, 2011(http://www.niaid.nih.gov/topics/foodAllergy/clinical/Documents/FAguidelinesPatient.pdf).

the high-affinity IgE receptor (FcεRI-α). This antigen receptor also occurs on antigen-presenting cells, where it can facilitate the IgE-dependent trapping and presentation of allergen to T cells.

Histamine, leukotriene C4, interleukin-4 (IL-4), and interleukin-13 (IL-13) are major mediators of allergy and asthma. All are formed by basophils and released in large quantities after stimulation with interleukin-3; IL-3's effect is restricted to basophil granulocytes. Basophil granulocytes should be considered as key effector cells in type 2 helper T (Th2) cell immune responses and allergic inflammation. IL-3 strongly induces messenger ribonucleic acid (mRNA) for granzyme B, a major effector of granule-mediated cytotoxicity.

Anaphylactic Reaction. Anaphylaxis is the clinical response to immunologic formation and fixation between a specific antigen and a tissue-fixing antibody. This reaction is usually mediated by IgE antibody and occurs in the following three stages:

1. The offending antigen attaches to the IgE antibody fixed to the surface membrane of mast cells and basophils. Cross-linking of two IgE molecules is necessary to initiate mediator release from mast cells.
2. Activated mast cells and basophils release various mediators.
3. The effects of mediator release produce vascular changes and activation of platelets, eosinophils, neutrophils, and the coagulation cascade.

It is believed that physical allergies (e.g., to heat, cold, ultraviolet light) cause a physiochemical derangement of proteins or polysaccharides of the skin and transform them into **autoantigens** responsible for the allergic reaction. Most, if not all, of these reactions are caused by the action of a self-directed IgE.

Anaphylactoid Reaction. Anaphylactoid reactions (anaphylaxis-like) are clinically similar to anaphylaxis and can result from immunologically inert materials that activate serum and tissue proteases and the alternate pathway of the complement system. Anaphylactoid reactions are not mediated by antigen-antibody interaction; instead, offending substances act directly on the mast cells, causing release of mediators, or on the tissues, such as anaphylotoxins of the complement cascade (e.g., C3a, C5a). Direct chemical degranulation of mast cells may be the cause of anaphylactoid reactions resulting from the infusion of macromolecules, such as proteins.

Atopic Reaction. In a person with atopy, exposure of the skin, nose, or airway to an allergen produces allergen-specific IgG antibodies. In response to the allergen, the T cells (when tested in vitro) exhibit moderate proliferation and production of interferon-γ (IFN-γ) by type 1 helper T (Th1) cells. In comparison, individuals with atopy have an exaggerated response characterized by the production of allergen-specific IgE antibodies and positive reactions to extracts of common airborne allergens when tested with a skin prick test. T cells from the blood of atopic patients respond to allergens in vitro by inducing cytokines produced by Th2 cells (e.g., IL-4, IL-5, IL-13), rather than cytokines produced by Th1 cells (e.g., IFN-γ, IL-2).

There are always exceptions to the rule, but the immunologic hallmark of allergic disease is the infiltration of affected tissue by Th2 cells.

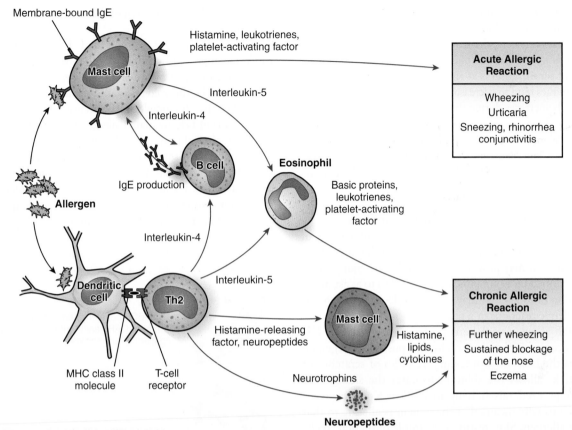

Figure 26-1 **Pathways leading to acute and chronic allergic reactions.** Acute allergic reactions are caused by the antigen-induced release of histamine and lipid mediators from mast cells. In the skin and upper airways, basophils (not shown) may also participate in allergic tissue reactions. Chronic allergic reactions, including the late-phase reaction, may depend on a combination of pathways, including recruitment of eosinophils, liberation of mast cell products by histamine-releasing factors, and neurogenic inflammation involving neurotrophins and neuropeptides. *Th2,* T-helper cell type 2; *MHC,* major histocompatibility complex. *(Adapted from Kay AB: Allergy and allergic disease, N Engl J Med 344:30–38, 2001.)*

Signs and Symptoms

Although everyone inhales airborne allergens derived from pollen, house dust mites, and animal dander, children and adults without atopy produce an asymptomatic, low-grade immunologic response. In a person with atopy, exposure of the skin, nose, or airway to a single dose of allergen produces symptoms (skin redness, sneezing, wheezing) within minutes. Depending on the amount of allergen, immediate hypersensitivity reactions are followed by a late-phase reaction that reaches a peak 6 to 9 hours after exposure to the allergen and then slowly subsides.

Localized Reaction. A localized reaction occurs as an immediate response to mediators released from mast cell degranulation. Local reactions can consist of **urticaria** and angioedema at the site of antigen exposure or angioedema of the bowel after ingestion of certain foods. Localized reactions are severe but rarely fatal. Skin reactions are characterized be the appearance of redness and itching at the site of the introduction of the allergen. This phenomenon is the basic principle of the skin test to diagnose an allergy or confirm sensitivity to a specific antigen.

Generalized Reaction. A generalized (anaphylactic) reaction is produced by mediators such as cytokines and vasoactive amines (e.g., histamine) from mast cells. Anaphylactic reactions are dramatic and rapid in onset. The physiologic effects of the primary and secondary mediators on the target organs, such as the cardiovascular or respiratory system, gastrointestinal (GI) tract, or the skin, define the signs and symptoms of anaphylaxis. Several important pharmacologically active compounds are discharged from mast cells and basophils during anaphylaxis (see Table 26-2).

Histamine release leads to constriction of bronchial smooth muscle, edema of the trachea and larynx, and stimulation of smooth muscle in the GI tract, which causes vomiting and diarrhea. The resulting breakdown of cutaneous vascular integrity results in urticaria and angioedema; **vasodilation** causes a reduction of circulating blood volume and a progressive fall in blood pressure, leading to shock. Kinins also alter vascular permeability and blood pressure.

The body's so-called natural moderators of anaphylaxis are the enzymes that decompose the mediators of anaphylaxis. Antihistamines have no effect on histamine release from mast cells or basophils. In human beings, antihistamines are effective antagonists of edema and pruritus, probably related to their blockage of a histamine-induced increase in capillary permeability but are relatively less effective in preventing bronchoconstriction.

Allergic Disease in Children. Atopic children characteristically experience a progression of allergic disease called **allergy march**

(see later, ImmunoCAP discussion). The formation of IgE antibodies begins early in life, and sensitization can be detected before clinical symptoms. Sensitization to food allergens such as cow's milk is manifested as colic or chronic otitis. The highest incidence of sensitization is at age 2 years. After 3 years of age, food sensitivities tend to decrease; sensitization to inhalant allergens typically increases during the preschool years. In most children with asthma, symptoms begin before age 5 years. Risk factors for allergic asthma include a family history of allergy, sensitization to food allergens, total serum IgE higher than 100 kU/L before age 6 years, living in an allergen-rich environment, and smoking.

Testing for Type I Hypersensitivity Reactions

In addition to a patient history and physical examination, an in vivo testing protocol can be used to assist in the identification of foods that may provoke allergic reactions. Skin testing can be performed by a skin puncture test (SPT) to assist in the identification of foods that may provoke IgE-mediated, food-induced allergic reactions or a patch test.

The SPT alone cannot be considered diagnostic of FA. Placing a drop of a solution containing a possible allergen on the skin is the basis of skin testing. A series of scratches or needle pricks allows the solution to enter the skin. If the skin develops a red, raised, itchy area, this is a positive reaction, which usually means that the person is allergic to that particular allergen. Skin testing is a simple outpatient technique to screen for many potential allergens, but may not be suitable for pediatric patients, pregnant women, or other groups. The procedure carries the risk of triggering a systemic reaction (e.g., anaphylactic reaction) or initiating a new sensitivity.

A patch test may be used for the evaluation of contact food allergies. Skin patch testing involves taping a patch that has been soaked in the allergen solution to the skin for 24 to 72 hours. This type of testing is used to detect contact dermatitis.

Laboratory Evaluation of Allergic Reactions

Advantages of in vitro testing include the lack of risk of a systemic hypersensitivity reaction and the lack of dependence on skin reactivity, which can be influenced by drugs, disease, or the patient's age. Detection of an increased amount of total IgE or allergen-specific IgE in serum indicates an increased probability of an allergic disorder, parasitic infection, or aspergillosis. In vitro laboratory testing can be performed by a variety of methods.

The clinical significance of serum allergen-specific IgE (sIgE) in allergic disorders has long been recognized. The quantitative determination of serum sIgE antibodies is an essential component for differential diagnosis and for identifying the causative allergens for proper medical treatment. The quality and availability of allergens, reagent stability, and degree of automation all influence the method of testing. Based on thousands of test results, a generic curve indicates what an allergen-specific IgE antibody value can mean in relation to symptoms. Although a final diagnosis should always be based on the physicians' overall impression of the patient, a general rule of thumb is that the higher the IgE antibody value, the greater the likelihood of symptoms appearing.

ImmunoCAP. The U.S. Food and Drug Administration (FDA) has approved ImmunoCAP to provide an in vitro quantitative measurement of IgE in human serum (Fig. 26-2). It is considered to be the gold standard for the analysis of allergen-specific IgE. It is intended for in vitro use as an aid in the clinical diagnosis of IgE-mediated allergic disorders in conjunction with other clinical findings (Table 26-3) .

ImmunoCAP assays can be performed for hundreds of allergens, such as weeds, trees, pollens, mold, food, and animal dander. It offers testing for over 650 different allergens and 70 allergen components for sensitive and specific quantitative detection of allergen-specific IgE antibodies.

Test Principle

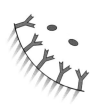

Anti-ECP covalently coupled to ImmunoCAP, reacts with the ECP in the patient serum sample.

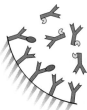

After washing, enzyme-labeled antibodies against ECP are added to form a complex.

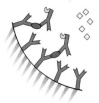

After incubation, unbound enzyme–anti-ECP is washed away, and the bound complex is then incubated with a developing agent.

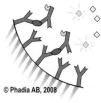

After stopping the reaction, the fluorescence of the eluate is measured. The fluorescence is directly proportional to the concentration of ECP in the serum sample. To evaluate test results, the responses for patient samples are compared directly to the responses for calibrators.

© Phadia AB, 2008

Figure 26-2   ImmunoCAP test—principle, steps, and evaluation. *ECP,* Eosinophilic cationic protein. *(Courtesy Phadia AB, Uppsala, Sweden.)*

Table 26-3	**Comparison of Tests for Specific IgE**		
Parameter	**Skin Prick Testing**	**Intradermal Testing**	**Blood Testing (ImmunoCAP)**
Sensitivity (%)	93.6	60.0	87.2
Specificity (%)	80.1	32.3	90.5

Adapted from Choo-Kang LR: Specific IgE testing: objective laboratory evidence supports allergy diagnosis and treatment, Med Lab Observer MLO 38:10–14, 2006.

The substances to which a patient is exposed will generally dictate the allergens to test. Some allergens are more common as causes of allergy than others. Factors to consider are the following:

- Patient's age
- Symptoms
- Home environment (e.g., pets, hobbies)
- Geographic location of patient's residence

An example of a pediatric allergy, the march (progression) profile, includes testing for allergens to *Alternaria alternata* (*Alternaria tenuis;* mold), cat dander, cockroach (German), *Dermatophagoides pteronyssinus* (*Dermatophagoides farinae;* mites), dog dander, egg white, codfish, whitefish, cow's milk, peanut, soybean, wheat, and total serum IgE. Food profile allergens might include corn, egg white, cow's milk, orange, peanut, shrimp, soybean, and wheat.

Respiratory allergen inhalants can include *A. alternata (A. tenuis)*, cat epithelium and dander, dog dander, elm tree, *Hormodendrum hordei (Cladosporium herbarum;* fungi), house dust, June grass, Kentucky bluegrass, mountain cedar (juniper) tree, and Russian thistle. Respiratory subtropical Florida allergens include *A. alternata (A. tenuis), Aspergillus fumigatus,* pine, Australian pine, Bahia grass, Bermuda grass, cat dander, cockroach (German), common short ragweed, *D. farinae (D. pteronyssinus;* mites), dog dander, *Hormodendrum hordei (Cladosporium herbarum;* fungi), oak tree, pecan (white hickory) tree, *Penicillium notatum,* pigweed, and total serum IgE.

The clinical use of inhaled steroids is becoming increasingly popular because of their antiinflammatory effects, although overtreatment may have serious side effects. To ensure the lowest effective dosage throughout treatment, the laboratory can periodically monitor the occurrence in serum of ECP-2 released from inflammatory cells. Eosinophil cationic protein (ECP) released by eosinophils can be detected in body fluids.

Chemiluminescent Enzyme Immunoassay. A third-generation sIgE method (Immulite 2000; Siemens Healthcare Diagnostics, Tarrytown, NY) is a solid-phase (bead), two-step chemiluminescent enzyme immunoassay (EIA). Allergens are covalently lined to a soluble polymer-ligand matrix, allowing immunochemical reactions to occur in liquid phases for random access automation.

Treatment

Treatment of patients with allergies involves identifying and eliminating or avoiding possible allergens. Drug therapy and desensitization are two treatment strategies.

Drug Therapy. Drug treatments include the following:

- Epinephrine (adrenaline) can be lifesaving in anaphylaxis. Epinephrine stimulates both α-adrenergic and β-adrenergic receptors, decreases vascular permeability, increases blood pressure, and reverses airway obstruction.
- Antihistamines block specific histamine receptors and play an important role in allergies affecting the skin, nose, and mucous membranes. Antihistamines act much slower than epinephrine in treating anaphylaxis and are not very useful in asthma because histamine is not an important allergic mediator released by mast cells in the lung.

- Specific receptor antagonists block the effects of leukotrienes. One drug, montelukast, reduces the amount of airway inflammation in asthma.
- Corticosteroids, often given topically, are widely used in the prevention of symptoms in patients with allergy.
- Other drugs in development aim to block the Th2 cytokine pathway or prevent IgE binding to FcεRI-α.

Desensitization. Desensitization, or immunotherapy, is a well-established technique to improve allergy symptoms caused by specific allergens (e.g., hay fever; Fig. 26-3). If a patient has a history of life-threatening conditions, and if other treatment alternatives are unsatisfactory, desensitization is used to prevent anaphylaxis resulting from insect stings (e.g., yellow jackets). It is best if only one allergen is incriminated.

Specific immunotherapy is associated with **downregulation** of the cytokines produced by Th2 cells, upregulation of cytokines produced by Th1 cells, and induction of regulatory T (Treg) cells. These changes in produce inhibition of allergic inflammation, increases in cytokines that control the production of IgE (IFN-γ and IL-12), production of blocking antibodies (IgG), and release of cytokines involved in allergen-specific hyporesponsiveness (IL-10 and transforming growth factor-β).

Different routes of desensitization induce different T-cell populations—Th1 and Treg cells in the case of subcutaneous administration and Th2 cells in the case of a sting on the skin.

For desensitization to insect venom, venom is injected subcutaneously in increasing doses at fixed intervals. Treatment starts with very small doses of venom because there is a risk of inducing anaphylactic shock. Over time, the patient is injected with increasing quantities of venom, eventually corresponding to the amount of venom in the insect sting. Once desensitization has been carried out, high levels of allergen-specific IgG will bind venom and prevent it from cross-linking IgE on mast cells. After following the prescribed treatment protocol, more than 90% of patients will not develop anaphylaxis if they are stung again.

Type II Reactions

Type II hypersensitivity reactions are a consequence of IgG or IgM binding to the surface of cells. Three different mechanisms of antibody-mediated injury exist in type II hypersensitivity, as follows:

1. Antibody-dependent, complement-mediated cytotoxic reactions. These are characterized by the interaction of IgG or IgM antibody with cell-bound antigen. This binding of an antigen and antibody can result in the activation of complement and destruction of the cell (cytolysis) to which the antigen is bound. Erythrocytes, leukocytes, and platelets can be lysed by this process. Examples of antibody-dependent, complement-mediated cytotoxic reactions include immediate (acute) transfusion reactions and immune hemolytic anemias (e.g., hemolytic disease of the newborn).

2. Antibody-dependent, cell-mediated cytotoxicity. This depends on the initial binding of specific antibodies to target cell surface antigens. The antibody-coated cells are lysed by effector cells, such as natural killer (NK) cells and macrophages, expressing Fc receptors. The Fc receptors of these effector cells attach to the Fc portion of the antibody that is

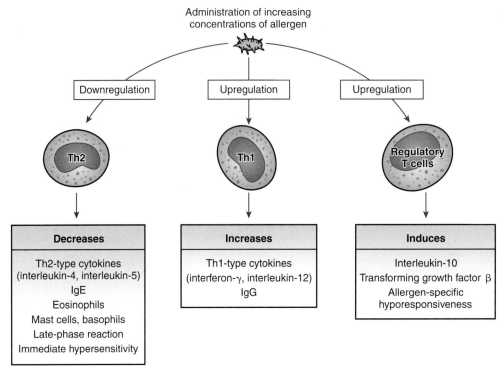

Figure 26-3   Proposed mechanisms of specific immunotherapy (hyposensitization or desensitization).   Specific immunotherapy is associated with downregulation of the cytokines produced by Th2 cells, upregulation of cytokines produced by Th1 cells, and induction of regulatory T cells. These changes in turn lead to inhibition of allergic inflammation, increases in cytokines that control production of IgE (interferon-g and interleukin-12) and blocking antibodies (IgG), and release of cytokines involved in allergen-specific hyporesponsiveness (IL-10 and transforming growth factor-β). *(Adapted from Kay AB: Allergy and allergic disease, N Engl J Med 344:109–113, 2001.)*

coating the target cell. Target cell destruction occurs when cytotoxic substances are released by the effector cells. This is the mechanism of injury in antibody-mediated glomerulonephritis and many other diseases. Antibody binding damages solid tissues, in which the antigen may be cellular or part of the extracellular matrix (e.g., basement membrane).

3. Antireceptor antibodies. These disturb the normal function of receptors. Less often, antibodies may modify the function of cells by binding to receptors for hormones (autoimmune hypersensitivity against solid tissue), as illustrated by autoimmune thyroid disease (see Chapter 28). Hyperacute graft rejection is also an example of type II hypersensitivity (see Chapter 31).

Type II Antibody-Dependent, Complement-Mediated Cytotoxic Reactions

Transfusion Reactions. Transfusion reactions are examples of antibody-dependent, complement-mediated cytotoxic reactions. The term *transfusion reaction* generally refers to the adverse consequences of incompatibility between patient and donor erythrocytes. Transfusion reactions can include hemolytic (red blood cell [RBC]–lysing) reactions occurring during or shortly after a transfusion, shortened posttransfusion survival of RBCs, an allergic response, or disease transmission.

Transfusion reactions can be divided into hemolytic and nonhemolytic types. **Hemolytic reactions** are associated with the infusion of incompatible erythrocytes. These reactions can be further classified into acute (immediate) or delayed in their manifestations

Box 26-2	Types of Transfusion Reactions

Immediate Hemolytic
Intravascular hemolysis of erythrocytes

Delayed Hemolytic
Extravascular hemolysis of erythrocytes

Immediate Nonhemolytic
Febrile reactions
Anaphylaxis
Urticaria
Noncardiac pulmonary edema
Fever and shock
Congestive heart failure
Myocardial failure

Delayed Nonhemolytic
Graft-versus-host disease
Posttransfusion purpura
Iron overload
Alloimmunization to erythrocytes, leukocytes, and platelet antigens or plasma proteins
Infectious disease

(Box 26-2). Several factors influence whether a transfusion reaction will be acute or delayed, including the following:

- Number of incompatible erythrocytes infused
- Antibody class or subclass
- Achievement of the optimal temperature for antibody binding

Immediate Hemolytic Reactions. The most common cause of an acute hemolytic transfusion reaction is the transfusion of ABO group–incompatible blood. In patients with preexisting antibodies resulting from prior transfusion or pregnancy, other blood groups may be responsible.

Epidemiology. Acute hemolytic reactions are the most serious and potentially lethal transfusion reactions. Most fatalities resulting from acute hemolytic transfusion reactions occur in anesthetized or unconscious patients, with the immediate cause of death being uncontrollable hypotension.

Signs and Symptoms. Reactions can occur with the infusion of as little as 10 to 15 mL of incompatible blood. The most common initial symptoms are fever and chills, which mimic a febrile nonhemolytic reaction caused by leukocyte incompatibility. Back pain, shortness of breath, pain at the infusion site, and hypotension are additional symptoms. In addition to shock, the release of thromboplastic substances into the circulation can induce disseminated intravascular coagulation and acute renal failure.

Immunologic Manifestations. Acute hemolytic reactions occur during infusion or immediately after blood has been infused. Infusion of incompatible erythrocytes in the presence of preexisting antibodies initiates an antigen-antibody reaction, with activation of the complement, plasminogen, kinin, and coagulation systems. Other initiators of acute hemolytic reactions include bacterial contamination of blood or infusion of hemolyzed erythrocytes. Many reactions demonstrate extravascular and intravascular hemolysis. If an antibody is capable of activating complement and is sufficiently active in vivo, intravascular hemolysis occurs, producing a rapid increase of free hemoglobin in the circulation. Although uncertain, the cause of the immediate clinical symptoms may be products released by the action of complement on the erythrocytes, which triggers multiple shock mechanisms.

Delayed Hemolytic Reaction. A delayed reaction may not manifest until 7 to 10 days after transfusion. In contrast to an immediate reaction, a delayed reaction occurs in the extravascular spaces. These reactions are associated with decreased RBC survival because of the coating of the RBCs (positive direct antiglobulin test), which promotes phagocytosis and premature removal of RBCs by the mononuclear phagocyte system. If an antibody does not activate complement or activates it very slowly, extravascular hemolysis occurs. Most IgG antibody–coated erythrocytes are destroyed extravascularly, mainly in the spleen.

A delayed hemolytic transfusion reaction may be of two types. It may represent an anamnestic antibody response in a previously immunized recipient on secondary exposure to transfused erythrocyte antigens, or it may result from primary **alloimmunization.** In an anamnestic response, the antibodies are directed against antigens to which the recipient has been previously immunized by transfusion or pregnancy.

Hemolytic Disease of the Fetus and Newborn. Hemolytic disease of the fetus and newborn (HDFN) results from excessive destruction of fetal RBCs by maternal antibodies. HDFN in the fetus or neonate is clinically characterized by anemia and jaundice. If the hemoglobin breakdown product that visibly produces jaundice (bilirubin) reaches excessive levels in the newborn's circulation, it will accumulate in lipid-rich nervous system tissue and can result in mental retardation or death.

Etiology. Antigens possessed by the fetus that are foreign to the mother can provoke an antibody response in the mother. Any blood group antigen that occurs as an IgG antibody is capable of causing HDFN.

Although anti-A and anti-B are present in the absence of their corresponding antigens as environmentally stimulated (IgM) antibodies, infrequent IgG forms may be responsible for HDFN because of ABO incompatibility. High titers of anti-A, anti-B of the IgG type in group O mothers often cause mild HDFN. Anti-A and anti-B antibodies are usually 19S (IgM) in character and, as such, are unable to pass through the placental barrier. In addition, the A and B antigens are not fully expressed on the erythrocytes of the fetus and newborn. In a survey of antibodies that have caused HDFN, more than 70 different antibodies were identified.

Epidemiology. The incidence of HDFN resulting from ABO incompatibility ranges from 1 in 70 to 180, with an estimated average of 1 in 150 births. The most frequent form of ABO incompatibility occurs when the mother is type O and the baby is type A or type B, usually type A.

Until the early 1970s, the Rh antibody anti-D was the most frequent cause of moderate or severe forms of HDFN. Anti-D occurred alone or in combination with another Rh antibody such as anti-C. Anti-D accounted for approximately 93% of cases of non-ABO HDFN. Since the development of modern treatment to prevent primary immunization to the D antigen, the frequency of HDFN caused by anti-D has significantly decreased.

Signs and Symptoms. Hemolytic disease resulting from ABO incompatibility is usually mild because of fewer A and B antigen sites on the fetal or newborn erythrocytes, weaker antigen strength of fetal or newborn A and B antigens, and competition for anti-A and anti-B between tissues and erythrocytes. The number and strength of A and B antigen sites on fetal erythrocytes are less than on adult RBC membranes. In addition, A and B substances are not confined to the RBCs, so only a small fraction of IgG anti-A and anti-B that crosses the placenta combines with the infant's erythrocytes.

Manifestations of HDFN caused by other antibodies can range from mild to severe. In addition to possible death in utero, newborns may demonstrate severe anemia and an increase in RBC breakdown products, such as bilirubin. Accumulation of bilirubin causes jaundice and may result in mental retardation if the bilirubin is not cleared from the infant's body.

Immunologic Mechanisms. For antibody formation to take place, the mother must lack the antigen and the fetus must express the antigen (gene product). The fetus would inherit the gene for antigen expression from the father. HDFN results from the production of maternal antibodies that have been stimulated by the presence of these foreign fetal antigens. The actual production of antibodies depends on a variety of factors: the genetic makeup of the mother, the antigenicity of a specific antigen, and the actual amount of antigen introduced into the maternal circulation.

Transplacental hemorrhage (TPH) can occur at any stage of pregnancy. Immunization resulting from TPH can result from negligible doses during the first 6 months in utero; however, significant immunizing hemorrhage usually occurs during the third trimester or at delivery. Fetal erythrocytes can also enter the maternal circulation as the result of physical trauma from an injury, abortion, ectopic pregnancy, amniocentesis, or normal delivery. Abruptio placentae, cesarean section, and manual removal of the placenta are often associated with a considerable increase in TPH.

An example of the normal pattern of immunization is demonstrated by the case of an Rh(D)-negative mother whose primary immunization (sensitization) was caused by a previously incompatible Rh(D)-positive pregnancy or a blood transfusion, which stimulates the production of low-titered anti-D, predominantly of the IgM class. Subsequent antigenic stimulation, such as fetal-maternal hemorrhage during pregnancy with an Rh(D)-positive fetus, can elicit a secondary (anamnestic) response, characterized by the predominance of increasing titers of anti-D of the IgG class.

Immune antibodies subsequently react with fetal antigens. Erythrocytic antigens, as well as leukocyte and platelet antigens, can induce maternal immunization by the formation of IgG antibodies. In HDFN, the erythrocytes of the fetus become coated with maternal antibodies that correspond to specific fetal antigens. Antibodies to IgG, the only immunoglobulin selectively transported to the fetus, are transferred from the maternal circulation to the fetal circulation through the placenta. The mechanism whereby IgG passes through the placenta has not been definitively established. Most research on transplacental passage supports the hypothesis that all IgG subclasses are capable of crossing the placental barrier between mother and fetus.

When the antigen and its corresponding antibody combine in vivo, increased lysis of RBCs results. Because of this hemolytic process, the normal 45- to 70-day lifespan of the fetal erythrocytes is reduced. To compensate for RBC loss, the fetal liver, spleen, and bone marrow respond by increasing production of erythrocytes. Increased RBC production outside the bone marrow, extramedullary hematopoiesis, can result in enlargement of the liver and spleen and premature release of nucleated erythrocytes from the bone marrow into the fetal circulation. If increased RBC production cannot compensate for the cell being destroyed, a progressively severe anemia develops that can cause the fetus to develop cardiac failure, with generalized edema and death in utero. Less severely affected infants continue to experience erythrocyte destruction after birth, which generates large quantities of unconjugated bilirubin. Bilirubin resulting from excessive hemolysis could result in the accumulation of free bilirubin in lipid-rich tissue of the central nervous system.

Diagnostic Evaluation. The following procedures are generally used for the prenatal or postnatal diagnostic evaluation of HDFN:

- ABO blood grouping
- Rh testing
- Screening for irregular antibodies; identification and titering of any antibodies

- Amniocentesis (prenatal)
- Serum bilirubin of cord or infant blood
- Direct antiglobulin test of cord or infant blood
- Peripheral blood smear
- Kleihauer-Betke test

Prevention. Independent researchers have shown that a passive antibody, Rh IgG, could protect most Rh-negative mothers from becoming immunized after the delivery of Rh(D)-positive infants or similar obstetric conditions. In 1968, Rh IgG was licensed for administration in the United States. Since that time, the incidence of HDFN caused by anti-D has decreased dramatically, although complete elimination may never occur because of the cases in which anti-D is formed before delivery. All pregnant Rh-negative women should receive Rh IgG, even if the Rh status of the fetus is unknown, because fetal D antigen is present on fetal erythrocytes as early as 38 days from conception.

Autoimmune Hemolytic Anemia. Autoimmune hemolytic anemia is an example of a type II hypersensitivity reaction directed against self antigens on RBCs. It can take two forms, cold autoagglutinins and warm autoagglutinins.

Cold Autoimmune Hemolytic Anemia. Cold autoagglutinins, usually IgM, represent about one third of cases of immune hemolytic anemia. Cold agglutinins react best at room temperature or lower.

Warm Autoimmune Hemolytic Anemia. In contrast to the cold form, warm autoagglutinins, usually IgG, represent most cases of autoimmune hemolytic anemia. Although the source of antigen exposure may be unknown, antibodies can be formed to microorganisms or drugs. Warm autoagglutinins react best at 37° C (98.6° F).

Type II Antibody-Dependent, Cell-Mediated Cytotoxicity

Autoantibodies can also attack and damage components of solid tissues, as in Goodpasture's syndrome. In this disorder, IgG autoantibodies bind a glycoprotein in the basement membrane of the kidney's glomeruli and the lungs. Anti–basement membrane antibody activates complement that can trigger an inflammatory response. This group of diseases can be detected by demonstrating the presence of autoantibodies.

Type II Hypersensitivity and Antibodies That Affect Cell Function

In another type II hypersensitivity reaction, antibodies bind to cells and affect their function. These antibodies simply stimulate the target organ function without causing organ damage. In some cases, such as Wegener's granulomatosis, stimulation of cells by autoantibody leads to tissue damage.

Testing for Type II Hypersensitivity

The **direct antiglobulin test (DAT)** is performed to detect transfusion reactions, HDFN, and autoimmune hemolytic anemia (see later procedure). Polyspecific antihuman globulin (AHG), a mixture of antibodies to IgG and complement components (e.g., C3d), is used for preliminary screening. If positive, the DAT can be repeated using monospecific anti-IgG and anti-C3d reagents for a more exact determination. If there is an autoimmune hemolytic anemia caused by IgM, only the C3d assay would be positive.

The indirect AHG assay is used to determine the presence of an unexpected antibody.

Platelet agglutination assays may be of value if idiopathic thrombocytopenic purpura is suspected. If Goodpasture's syndrome is suspected, direct fluorescent examination of a renal tissue biopsy would be helpful.

Type II Autoimmune Hypersensitivity Against Solid Tissue

Autoantibodies can also attack and damage components of solid tissues. These antibodies can simply stimulate the target organ function without causing much target organ damage, as in Graves' disease. In other cases, stimulation of cells by autoantibody leads to tissue damage. As noted, Goodpasture's syndrome involves IgG autoantibodies and a glycoprotein in the basement membrane of the lung and glomeruli. Anti–basement membrane antibody activates complement, which can trigger an inflammatory response. Goodpasture's syndrome can be diagnosed by finding antibodies to glomerular basement membrane in patient serum on indirect immunofluorescence (Fig. 26-4) and autoantibodies in serum.

Prevention and Treatment

Checking the donor and recipient and providing immunization to prevent HDFN are two prevention strategies. Immunosuppressive drugs can reduce B cell autoantibody secretion. Plasmapheresis is a method for reducing the quantity of antibody in a patient's circulating blood.

Type III (Immune Complex) Reactions

Type III hypersensitivity reactions are caused by the deposition of immune complexes in blood vessel walls and tissues. Repeated antigen exposure leads to sensitization with the production of an insoluble antigen-antibody complex. As these complexes are deposited in tissues, the complement system is activated, macrophages and leukocytes are attracted, and immune-mediated damage occurs. Common skin conditions in this category include allergic vasculitis and erythema nodosum. Pulmonary reactions include hypersensitivity pneumonitis, characterized best by farmer's lung, which is a reaction to thermophilic actinomycetes found in moldy hay. Chemicals such as toluene diisocyanate, phthalic anhydride, and trimetallic anhydride can cause bathtub refinisher's lung, epoxy resin lung, and plastic worker's lung, respectively.

Farmer's lung and the **Arthus reaction** (Fig. 26-5) are examples of local immune complex diseases. Poststreptococcal glomerulonephritis is an example of a circulating immune complex disease, as in systemic lupus erythematosus (SLE; see Chapter 29). Immune complexes are lattices of antigen and antibody that may be localized to the site of antigen production or may circulate in the blood. Immune complexes are produced as part of the normal immune response and are usually cleared by mechanisms involving complement. However, they cause disease in various situations. Failure to clear immune complexes can result from the saturation of mechanisms involving excessive ongoing production of immune complexes, as well as antigenemia caused by chronic infection.

The formation of immune complexes under normal conditions protects the host because they facilitate the clearance of various antigens and invading microorganisms by the mononuclear phagocyte system. In immune complex reactions (disease), antigen-antibody complexes form in the soluble or fluid phase of tissues or in the blood and assume unique biological functions, such as interaction with complement and with cellular receptors.

Other type III (immune complex) reactions include serum sickness and certain aspects of autoimmune diseases

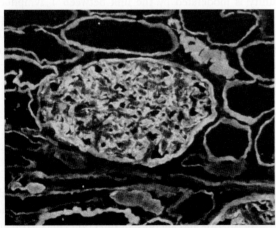

Figure 26-4   Indirect immunofluorescence used to detect autoantibodies in patient with Goodpasture's syndrome. Kidney tissue is used as the target antigen for this test. Linear staining along the glomerular basement membrane appears to be lit up compared with the renal tubules in the background. *(From Nairn R, Helbert M: Immunology for medical students, ed 2, St Louis, 2007, Mosby.)*

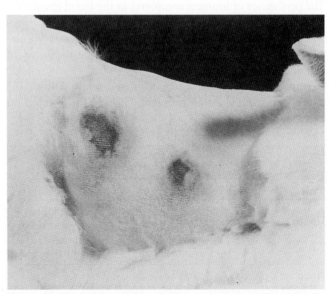

Figure 26-5   Arthus reaction. In these two reactions of the skin of a rabbit, the larger reaction has an extensive zone of erythema and edema surrounding its necrotic center. *(From Markell EK, Voge M: Medical parasitology, ed 5, Philadelphia, 1981, WB Saunders.)*

(e.g., glomerulonephritis in SLE). Circulating soluble immune complexes are responsible for or associated with various human diseases in which exogenous and endogenous antigens can trigger a pathogenic immune response and result in immune complex disease (Table 26-4).

Mechanism of Tissue Injury

Type III reactions are caused by IgG, IgM, and possibly other antibody types. Immune complexes can exhibit a spectrum of biological activities, including suppression or augmentation of the immune response by interacting with B and T cells, inhibition of tumor cell destruction, and deposition in blood vessel walls, glomerular membranes, and other sites. These deposits interrupt normal physiologic processes because of tissue damage secondary to the activation of complement and resulting activities such as mediating immune adherence and attracting leukocytes and macrophages to the sites of immune complex deposition. The release of enzymes and possibly other agents damages the tissues. There are three general anatomic sites of antigen-antibody interactions:

1. Antibody can react with soluble antigens in the circulation and form immune complexes that may disseminate and lodge in any tissue with a large filtration area and cause lesions of immune complex disease.
2. Antibody can react with antigen secreted or injected locally into the interstitial fluid. The classic example is the experimental Arthus reaction, the basic model of local immune complex disease (see Fig. 26-5).
3. Antibody can also react with structural antigens that form part of the cell surface membranes or with fixed intercellular structures such as the basement membranes. Systemic immune complex disease serum sickness is an example of soluble and tissue-fixed antigen involvement.

Clinical Manifestations

The persistence of immune complexes in the blood circulation is not inherently harmful. Immune complex disease develops when these circulating complexes are not cleared from the circulation by phagocytosis and are subsequently deposited in certain tissues.

Serum Sickness. Acute serum sickness develops within 1 to 2 weeks after initial exposure or repeated exposure by injection of heterologous serum protein. There is no preexisting antibody and the disease appears as antibody formation begins. The hallmark of serum sickness is the protracted interaction between antigen and antibody in the circulation, with the formation of antigen-antibody complexes in an environment of antigen excess. Chronic serum sickness can be experimentally induced if small amounts of antigen are given daily and represent just enough antigen to balance antibody production.

Autoimmune Disorders. SLE is an autoimmune disorder characterized by autoantibodies that form immune complexes with autoantigens, which are deposited in the renal glomeruli (see Chapter 29). As a consequence of this type III hypersensitivity reaction, glomerulonephritis (inflammation of capillary vessels in the glomeruli) develops.

Testing for Type III Hypersensitivity Reactions

Specific autoimmune disorders, such as rheumatoid arthritis (see Chapter 30), have specific assays for detecting and monitoring the autoimmune disorder. Common assays use latex agglutination, nephelometry, and chemiluminescence techniques.

Fluorescent staining of tissue biopsy specimens can be used to observe the deposition of immune complexes in tissues. Staining patterns and affected tissues can assist in disease diagnosis and prognosis. Another laboratory assay used in assessment is the quantitation of complement (C3 and C4 components).

Treatment

The most direct treatment is avoidance of the offending antigen. Corticosteroids block some of the damage caused by effector cells. Cyclophosphamide is an alkylating agent that impairs DNA synthesis and prevents rapid proliferation of cells (e.g., lymphocytes reduce B cell proliferation).

Type IV Cell-Mediated Reactions

Type IV cell-mediated immunity consists of immune activities that differ from antibody-mediated immunity. Cell-mediated immunity is moderated by the link between T lymphocytes and phagocytic cells (i.e., monocyte-macrophages). Lymphocytes (T cells) do not recognize the antigens of microorganisms or other living cells but are immunologically active through various types of direct cell to cell contact and by the production of soluble factors.

Characteristics

- Type IV delayed-type hypersensitivity (DTH) involves antigen-sensitized T cells or particles that remain phagocytized in a macrophage and are encountered by previously activated T cells for a second or subsequent time. T cells respond directly, or by the release of lymphokines, to exhibit contact dermatitis and allergies of infection (Figs. 26-6 and 26-7). One of the mechanisms of cell-mediated immunity is delayed hypersensitivity. Delayed hypersensitivity is a major mechanism of defense against various intracellular pathogens, including mycobacteria, fungi, and certain parasites. In

Table 26-4	Diseases Associated With Immune Complexes	
Type	**Examples**
Autoimmune diseases	Rheumatoid arthritis, systemic lupus erythematosus, Sjögren's syndrome, mixed connective tissue disease, systemic sclerosis, glomerulonephritis
Neoplastic disease	Solid and lymphoid tumors
Infectious disease	Bacterial infective endocarditis, streptococcal infection, viral hepatitis, infectious mononucleosis

addition, cell-l-mediated immunity is responsible for the immunologic mechanisms contact sensitivity

- Rejection of foreign tissue grafts, elimination of tumor cells bearing neoantigens and
- Formation of chronic granulomas

Under some of these conditions, the activities of cell-mediated immunity may not be beneficial. Suppression of the normal adaptive immune response (immunosuppression) by drugs or other means is necessary to overcome an unwanted immunologic response in conditions such as organ transplantation, hypersensitivity, and autoimmune disorders.

DTH can be a physiologic reaction to pathogens that are difficult to clear, such as hepatitis B virus and *Mycobacterium tuberculosis*. This triggers the most extreme DTH reactions, characterized by granuloma formation, extensive cell death, and appearance of caseous necrosis. DTH can also occur in response to innocuous environmental antigens (e.g., nickel). Antigens must have a low molecular weight to enter the body. DTH reactions also take place against autoantigens. In insulin-dependent (type 1) diabetes, T cells respond to pancreatic islet cell antigens, damaging the islets and eventually preventing insulin secretion.

DTH reactions are initiated when tissue macrophages recognize the presence of danger signals and initiate the inflammatory response. Dendritic cells loaded with antigen migrate to local lymph nodes, where they present antigen to T cells. Specific T cell clones proliferate in response to antigens and migrate to the site of inflammation. T cells and macrophages stimulate one another through the cytokine network. Tumor necrosis factor-α (TNF-α) is secreted by macrophages and T cells and stimulates much of the damage in DTH reactions. Because of the need for antigen presentation by T cells, DTH reactions are often associated with specific human leukocyte antigen (HLA) alleles.

The hallmark of occupational type IV hypersensitivity is allergic contact dermatitis caused by metals (e.g., nickel, mercury, copper), sunscreen agents, disinfectants, perfumes and fragrances, and pesticides. Pulmonary hypersensitivity can be caused by inorganic dust particles, hard metal, and beryllium. Hard metal exposure involves cobalt from the grinding of steel.

Latex Sensitivity

In the health care setting, natural latex can be an allergen in those who have significant cumulative exposure. Since 1985, policies of Standard Precautions have resulted in an exponential increase in the use of latex gloves. The use of latex condoms has also increased. The increase in total exposure to latex and variations in manufacturing apparently have led to an increase in the number of persons with latex sensitivity.

Once sensitized, an individual may experience allergic symptoms when exposed to any product containing latex. At-risk groups sensitized to natural rubber latex include 8% to 17% of health care workers, as well as children who have repeated surgeries. Less than 1% of the general U.S. population (≈3 million) demonstrate latex sensitivity.

Latex contains low-molecular-weight soluble proteins that cause IgE-mediated allergic reactions. Latex allergy can give rise to a broad range of symptoms. Glove wearers may experience type IV, or delayed hypersensitivity, contact dermatitis that

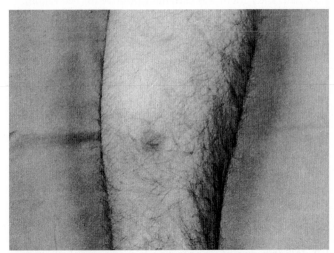

Figure 26-6 Delayed skin reaction. This reaction exhibited an erythematous but nonedematous zone 15 mm in diameter at 48 hours. A control site, inoculated higher on the forearm, showed no reaction at this time. *(From Barrett JT: Textbook of immunology, ed 5, St Louis, 1988, Mosby.)*

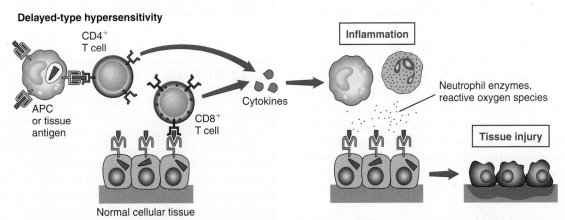

Figure 26-7 Mechanisms of T cell–mediated tissue injury. T cells may cause tissue injury and disease by two mechanisms: (1) delayed-type hypersensitivity reactions (A), which may be triggered by CD4+ and CD8+ T cells, and in which tissue injury is caused by activated macrophages and inflammatory cells; and (2) direct killing of target cells. *(From Abbas AK, Lichtman AH: Basic immunology: functions and disorders of the immune system, ed 3, updated edition, Philadelphia, 2011, Saunders.)*

ranges from nonspecific pruritus to eczematous, red, weepy skin. These symptoms and the irritant contact dermatitis are caused by the accelerators and chemicals used in glove manufacturing, not by the latex itself. Avoidance of latex gloves is often sufficient to prevent these symptoms.

Anaphylactic reactions to latex have been reported in those who had previously experienced only irritant or allergic contact dermatitis. Direct skin contact with latex may cause a type I, or immediate hypersensitivity, IgE-mediated reaction within 30 to 60 minutes of exposure. Urticaria may be local or generalized and the spectrum of progression is notably unpredictable; some persons have experienced anaphylactic reactions after having minimal or no previous symptoms.

Certain fruits, such as bananas, chestnuts, kiwi, avocados, and tomatoes, show cross-reactivity, perhaps because of a similarity to a latex protein component. These foods have been responsible for anaphylactic reactions in latex-sensitive persons. Many other foods, including figs, apples, celery, melons, potatoes, papayas, and pitted fruits (e.g., cherries, peaches), have caused progressive symptoms, beginning with oral itching. Persons with a history of reactions to these foods are at increased risk of developing latex allergy and those who are sensitive to latex should avoid foods to which they have had previous reactions.

Testing for Delayed Hypersensitivity

The skin test for testing of exposure to tuberculosis (TB) is a classic example of a delayed hypersensitivity reaction. The test is based on the principle that soluble antigens from *M. tuberculosis* induce a reaction in individuals who have acquired or been exposed to the tuberculosis microorganism or a related organism at some time. It does not mean that the person has tuberculosis.

A small amount of antigen is injected under the skin (intradermally) with a fine-needle syringe. The site is observed at 48 and 72 hours for the presence of induration (lesion ≥10 mm in diameter).

Other antigens that can be skin-tested include diphtheria toxoid, tetanus toxoid, fungal antigens (e.g., *Trichophyton*, histoplasmin), and *Candida albicans*.

In cases of persistent dermatitis, a patch test may be performed. An adhesive patch containing the suspected allergen is applied to the skin. The skin is checked for redness with papules or tiny blisters, indicating a positive test result, over 48 hours.

Diagnosis of latex allergy is determined by the patient history and immunologic testing. FDA-approved in vitro tests to measure latex-specific IgE are available (Pharmacia CAP, Pharmacia-UpJohn Diagnostics, Kalamazoo, Mich; AlaSTAT, Diagnostic Products, Los Angeles). The low specificity of these tests, which have a false-negative rate of at least 20% and thus unclear positive predictive value, limits their clinical usefulness. Negative serologic testing with a strongly positive history would suggest the value of skin prick testing to confirm the diagnosis.

Treatment

Strategies to avoid a DTH reaction include avoiding antigen exposure. Antiinflammatory drugs or corticosteroids may be useful. In some patients, TNF-α monoclonal antibodies and recombinant interferon-β may be administered.

CASE STUDY 1

Mr. RM, a 60-year-old man, was stung by a bee while gardening. He had been stung once before, earlier in the summer. Within a few seconds, his hand began to itch and he began to experience abdominal cramping. He subsequently had difficulty breathing. Fortunately, he was able to reach a first aid kit in his garage. Inside the kit was an EpiPen (injectable epinephrine) for his wife because she was allergic to bee venom. He used the pen and began to feel somewhat better. He immediately had his wife drive him to the hospital.

He was asymptomatic on arrival at the hospital. RM had no history of adverse reactions to bee venom or antibiotics. Because of the nature of the incident, a diagnosis of anaphylactic shock caused by bee venom sensitivity was made. An IgE level was ordered. The results indicated a level more than twice the (normal) reference range value. In addition, a follow-up skin test was performed. The patient was extremely positive for bee venom.

Question
1. Agents that can produce type I hypersensitivity reactions in susceptible individuals include:
   a. Peanuts
   b. Penicillin
   c. Latex
   d. All of the above

See Appendix A for the answers to multiple choice questions.

Critical Thinking Group Discussion Questions
1. What is the mechanism involved in anaphylaxis?
2. What types of agents can induce anaphylactic shock?

See instructor site ⊜volve website for the discussion of the answers to these questions.

CASE STUDY 2

Mrs. CC, a 35-year-old gravida 4 para 1+ 2, was seen by her gynecologist when she was 8 weeks pregnant. Her first pregnancy 4 years ago was unremarkable. The patient reported that her second and third pregnancies had resulted in a stillbirth at 36 weeks and a spontaneous abortion at 10 weeks of gestation. Her medical history revealed no history of blood transfusions. She remembered being vaccinated for rubella. Her medical records had been destroyed in a fire at the clinic. Repeat blood grouping and Rh testing and an irregular antibody screen were ordered (Box 26-3).

CASE STUDY 2—Cont'd

Mrs. CC returned in 2 weeks for a repeat anti-D titer. The titer had risen to 1:16. At 17 weeks' gestation, an amniocentesis was performed. Severe hemolysis was demonstrated and an intrauterine transfusion of the fetus was carried out using fresh, washed, cytomegalovirus screening test–negative, group O, Rh(D)-negative blood. Because of the continuing risk to the fetus, a cesarean section was performed at 36 weeks' gestation. On delivery, the baby was noted to be jaundiced and pale. The first of three exchange transfusions was performed. Phototherapy was also used to degrade the bilirubin deposited in the skin. The baby made an uneventful recovery with no signs of kernicterus and was discharged from the hospital 5 days after birth.

Question
1. Type II hypersensitivity reactions are related to:
   a. Bee venom
   b. Antibodies (IgM, IgG)
   c. IgE antibodies
   d. Nickel allergy

See Appendix A for the answers to multiple choice questions.

Critical Thinking Group Discussion Questions
1. What is the mechanism of HDFN?
2. What prophylactic measures are used to prevent HDFN caused by the D antigen?

See instructor site ⊖volve website for the discussion of the answers to these questions.

CASE STUDY 3

ZZ's medical history included frequent sore throats as a child. He had been treated with antibiotics, particularly penicillin. Eventually, he developed a rash. He was told that he had developed an allergy to penicillin and that he should not have it again.

A decade later, he developed a urinary tract infection. He was treated with an antibiotic, trimethoprim, for 8 days. A few days after completing the regimen, he developed a headache and some itchy bumps on his skin. The next day he had sore and swollen joints. His physician confirmed that the rash was urticaria. ZZ also had an elevated temperature and swollen glands in his neck. The diagnosis of a drug allergy was made. The patient was given antihistamines. If this medication failed to alleviate the symptoms, more aggressive steroid therapy would be pursued.

ZZ's symptoms did not improve and he was started on an oral corticosteroid, prednisone. When the patient returned to his physician 3 weeks later, he was asymptomatic.

Question
1. Type III diseases associated with immune complexes include:
   a. Autoimme
   b. Neoplastic
   c. Infection
   d. All of the above

See Appendix A for the answers to multiple choice questions.

Critical Thinking Group Discussion Questions
1. What is the likely mechanism of this reaction?
2. What types of agents can lead to drug reactions?

See instructor site ⊖volve website for the discussion of the answers to these questions.

CASE STUDY 4

A 19-year-old college student went to the Student Health Services because she had a slowly developing rash on both earlobes, hands and wrist, and around her neck.

Her medical history revealed that she had eczema in childhood. During her early teens, she had facial acne, for which she was given tetracycline. Physical examination revealed a rash of erythema and small blisters, with marked excoriation because of the itching. Her hands were red, scaly, and dry. The rash on her hands looked different than the eruptions on her neck and ears. A contact hypersensitivity was suspected.

Follow-up patch tests included a standard battery of agents—rubber, cosmetics, plant extracts, perfumes, nickel, and makeup. Strongly positive reactions for rubber and nickel were observed.

The student was advised to eliminate contact with rubber (e.g., rubber gloves) used at home or on the job. Her jewelry probably contained nickel and was believed to be the source of the irritation to her earlobes, neck, and wrists. She was advised to wear only nickel-free jewelry. A mild corticosteroid cream was prescribed for use until her symptoms disappeared.

Question
1. An example of a type IV reaction can be caused by _____.
   a. Nickel
   b. Incompatible blood transfusion
   c. Bacterial contamination of water
   d. An autoimmune disorder

See Appendix A for the answers to multiple choice questions.

Critical Thinking Group Discussion Questions
1. Why did the jewelry cause a rash?
2. What is the mechanism of type IV hypersensitivity involvement in contact eczema?

See instructor site ⊝volve website for the discussion of the answers to these questions.

CASE STUDY 5

A 35-year-old woman reported that she had experienced three bouts of urticaria of unknown origin about 10 years ago. The urticaria affected her mucous membranes and skin. She had experienced similar symptoms after repair of a fractured femur caused by a skiing accident. These symptoms were attributed to an antibiotic reaction.

As an emergency room nurse, she observed occasional localized hives following the use of latex gloves. Even when she used hypoallergenic latex gloves, she continued to have hives every few months. Increased urticaria, at times generalized, continued to occur.

Within 30 minutes of having a routine vaginal examination performed by a health care provider wearing latex gloves, she had an anaphylactic reaction that required resuscitation and hospitalization. A vaginal biopsy 1 week later required a latex-free environment for her safety.

A short time later, she was forced to retire from nursing because of symptoms of asthma. She has also developed food allergies to shellfish.

Question
1. If a person is allergic to latex, a reaction rarely takes place more than _____ after exposure to latex.
   a. 30 minutes
   b. 2 hours
   c. 48 hours
   d. 1 week

See Appendix A for the answers to multiple choice questions.

Critical Thinking Group Discussion Questions
1. What are the most likely type and mechanism of the urticarial hypersensitivity reaction?
2. What are the most likely type and cause of the anaphylactic reaction?

See instructor site ⊝volve website for the discussion of the answers to these questions.

Box 26-3 **Case Study 2: Laboratory Results**

- Mrs. CC: Group A; Rh(D)-negative; irregular antibody screen, positive anti-D (1:8)
- Mr. CC: Group A; Rh(D)-positive; CDe/CDe

⊞ Rapid Test for Food Allergy

Principle

Rapid Test

The RAPID 3-D Casein Test (Tepnel BioSystems, Stamford, Conn) uses a three-line diagnostic dry strip format. When a food extract containing casein is extracted and applied to a collector comb, blue latex particles coated with antibodies to casein are mobilized. These particles bind casein in the sample and flow along the test strip, where they are trapped by a second, immobilized casein antibody, revealing a blue line. RAPID 3-D kits are available for gluten, peanuts, almonds, hazelnuts, and shellfish.

Procedure Notes

See ⊝volve for the procedural protocol.

Limitations

The testing kit is not suitable for the testing of foods consumed at home or in a restaurant by allergic persons.

Clinical Applications

Casein, a protein naturally present in milk, is one of the eight major food allergens, which can initiate reactions ranging from urticaria to anaphylactic shock (types I to IV hypersensitivity reactions).

Identification of casein minimizes the risks posed by food allergens by identifying cross-contamination of ingredient supplies or inadequate cleaning between production batches.

See ⊝volve website for the discussion of the answers to these questions.

⊞ Direct Antiglobulin Test

Principle

The DAT is based on the principle that antiglobulin antibodies induce in vitro agglutination of erythrocytes with immunologically bound antibodies. After erythrocytes (RBCs) are washed to remove free plasma protein from the test mixture, they are tested directly with polyspecific reagents containing anti-IgG and anti-C3d. The DAT procedure is clinically important in the diagnosis of conditions such as hemolytic anemia, including hemolytic disease of the newborn.

Procedure Notes

See ⊝volve website for the procedural protocol.

Reporting Results

- Negative test result: Absence of agglutination in DAT test tube
- Positive test result: Presence of agglutination

Sources of Error

False-positive and false-negative results can occur.

False-positive results in the DAT can be caused by the following:

- Contamination of AHG antisera or supplies
- Overcentrifugation
- Bacterial contamination of specimen or reagents
- Fibrin clot in cell suspension
- Overzealous reading of serum-cell mixture

False-negative results usually occur because of technical error. Common causes of false-negative reactions include the following:

- Failure to add AHG reagent
- Inadequate washing of RBCs
- Weak or inactive AHG

See ⊖volve website for the discussion of the answers to these questions.

CHAPTER HIGHLIGHTS

- The term *immunization*, or *sensitization*, is used to describe an immunologic reaction dependent on the response of the host to a subsequent exposure of antigen.
- Hypersensitivity has traditionally been classified as immediate and delayed based on the time after exposure to an offending antigen.
- Type I hypersensitivity reactions can range from life-threatening anaphylactic reactions to milder manifestations associated with food allergies. This reaction is usually mediated by IgE antibody.
- In vitro evaluation of type I hypersensitivity reactions involves various methods. The advantages of in vitro testing include no risk of a systemic hypersensitivity reaction and no dependence on skin reactivity influenced by drugs, disease, or age.
- Type II cytotoxic reactions are characterized by the interaction of IgG or IgM antibody to cell-bound antigen. This binding of an antigen and antibody can result in activation of complement and destruction of the cell (cytolysis) to which the antigen is bound. Erythrocytes, leukocytes, and platelets can be lysed by this process.
- Examples of type III reactions include the Arthus reaction, serum sickness, and certain aspects of autoimmune disease.

    Type IV cell-mediated immunity consists of immune activities that differ from antibody-mediated immunity. Cell-mediated immunity is moderated by the link between T lymphocytes and phagocytic cells. Delayed hypersensitivity is a major mechanism of defense against various intracellular pathogens, including mycobacteria, fungi, and certain parasites. In addition, cell-mediated immunity is responsible for the immunologic mechanisms of contact sensitivity, rejection of foreign tissue grafts, elimination of tumor cells bearing neoantigens and formation of chronic granulomas.

REVIEW QUESTIONS

Match the following types of hypersensitivity with their respective type of reaction.

1. _____ Type I hypersensitivity
2. _____ Type II hypersensitivity
3. _____ Type III hypersensitivity
4. _____ Type IV hypersensitivity
   a. Cytotoxic reaction
   b. Cell-mediated reaction
   c. Immune complex reaction
   d. Anaphylactic reaction

5. With which cell type are anaphylactic reactions associated?
   a. T lymphocyte
   b. B lymphocyte
   c. Monocyte
   d. Mast

6. Type III reactions are exemplified by all the following except:
   a. Arthus reaction
   b. Serum sickness
   c. Glomerulonephritis
   d. Shingles

7. Type IV reactions are responsible for all the following except:
   a. Contact sensitivity
   b. Delayed hypersensitivity
   c. Elimination of tumor cells bearing neoantigens
   d. Hemolysis of red blood cells

8. Type I hypersensitivity reactions can be associated with:
   a. Food allergies
   b. Hay fever
   c. Asthma
   d. All of the above

9. The most common agents that cause anaphylactic reactions are:
   a. Drugs and food
   b. Drugs and insect stings
   c. Poison ivy and insect stings
   d. Food and insect stings

10-12. Arrange the sequence of events in anaphylaxis in the proper sequence.

10. _____
11. _____
12. _____

   a. The effects of mediator release produce vascular changes, activation of platelets, eosinophils, and neutrophils, and activation of the coagulation cascade.

b. The offending antigen attaches to the IgE antibody fixed to the surface membrane of mast cells and basophils.

c. Activated mast cells and basophils release various mediators.

13-18. Complete the table, choosing from the possible answers provided.

Mediators of Anaphylaxis

Mediator	Primary Action
Histamine	13. _____
Leukotrienes	14. _____
Serotonin	15. _____
Platelet-activating factor	16. _____
Eosinophil chemotactic factors of anaphylaxis	17. _____
Prostaglandins	18. _____

Possible answers to questions 13-15:

a. Enhances the effects of histamine on target organs
b. Increases vascular permeability and promotes contraction of smooth muscle
c. Generates kinins
d. Contracts smooth muscle

Possible answers to questions 16-18:

a. Affects smooth muscle tone and vascular permeability
b. Enhances the release of histamine and serotonin
c. Attracts cells to area of activity; these cells release secondary mediators that may limit the effects of primary mediators.
d. Alters bronchial smooth muscle

19. In vitro evaluation of type I hypersensitivity reactions can include:
    a. RIST
    b. Skin testing
    c. Neither a nor b
    d. Both a and b

20. Cytotoxic reactions are characterized by the interaction of:
    a. IgG to soluble antigen
    b. IgG to cell-bound antigen
    c. IgM to soluble antigen
    d. IgM or IgG to cell-bound antigen

21. An example of a delayed nonhemolytic (type II hypersensitivity) reaction is:
    a. Febrile reaction
    b. Graft-versus-host disease
    c. Urticaria
    d. Congestive heart failure

22. Under normal conditions, immune complexes protect the host because they:
    a. Facilitate the clearance of various antigens
    b. Facilitate the clearance of invading microorganisms
    c. Interact with complement
    d. Both a and b

23. Immune complexes can:
    a. Suppress or augment the immune response by interacting with T and B cells
    b. Inhibit tumor cell destruction
    c. Be deposited in blood vessel walls
    d. All of the above

24. The general anatomic sites of antigen-antibody interaction are:
    a. Tissues with a large filtration area
    b. Interstitial fluids
    c. Cell surface membranes or fixed intercellular structures
    d. All of the above

25. Type IV hypersensitivity reactions are responsible for all the following except:
    a. Contact sensitivity
    b. Elimination of tumor cells
    c. Rejection of foreign tissue grafts
    d. Serum sickness

BIBLIOGRAPHY

American Latex Allergy Association: Patient/public education: fast facts: latex allergy, 2012, http://latexallergyresources.org/.

Bach J: The effect of infections on susceptibility to autoimmune and allergic diseases, N Engl J Med 347:911–920, 2002.

Choo-Kang LR: Specific IgE testing: objective laboratory evidence supports allergy diagnosis and treatment, Med Lab Observer MLO 38:10–14, 2006.

Choo-Kang LR: The progression of allergic disease, Med Lab Observer MLO 38:18, 2006.

Creticos PS, et al: Immunotherapy with a ragweed–toll-like receptor 9 agonist vaccine for allergic rhinitis, N Engl J Med 355:1445–1454, 2006.

Faix JD et al: Multiplexed chemiluminescent immunoassay of specific IgE antibody for in vitro diagnosis of allergic disorders. AACC 2006 Annual Meeting and Clinical Lab Exposition, Chicago, July 2006 (abstract).

Fu P, Zic V: Specific IgE assay on the ImmunoLite 2000 analyzer, AACC 2004 Annual Meeting and Clinical Lab Exposition, Los Angeles, July 2004 (abstract).

Gold DR, Fuhlbrigge AL: Inhaled corticosteroids for young children with wheezing, N Engl J Med 354:2058–2062, 2006.

Kay AB: Allergy and allergic disease, N Engl J Med 344:109–113, 2001. 30-38.

Kay AB: Natural killer T cells and asthma, N Engl J Med 354:1186–1188, 2006.

Kirchner DB: The spectrum of allergic disease in the chemical industry, Int Arch Occup Environ Health 75(Suppl):107–112, 2002.

Lundin P: Evaluation of technical performance of four immunoassay systems for allergy testing: ImmunoCAP 1000, ImmunoCAP 250, Advia Centaur, and Immulite 2000, AACC Annual Meeting, Orlando, Fla, July 2005 (abstract).

Mardis CT, Bal T, Levy R: The masks of allergy undone by IVT, Med Lab Observer MLO 39:12–21, 2007.

Nairn R, Helber M: Immunology for medical students, ed 2, St Louis, 2007, Mosby.

National Institute of Allergy and Infectious Diseases: Guidelines for the diagnosis and management of food allergy in the United States: summary of the NIAID-sponsored expert panel report, 2011, http://www.niaid.nih.gov/topics/foodAllergy/clinical/Documents/ FAguidelinesPatient.pdf.

Nystrand M, et al: A multiplexed immunoassay for rapid detection of specific IgE in allergy diagnosis, 2007, http://www.gesim.de/en/nano-plotter/applications/allergy-diagnosis/allergy-diagnosis.html.

Ollert M, et al: Allergen-specific IgE measured by a continuous random-access immunoanalyzer: interassay comparison and agreement with skin testing, Clin Chem 51:1241–1249, 2005.

Quest Diagnostics: ImmunoCap: specific IgE blood test, 2012, http://www.questdiagnostics. com/home/physicians/testing-services/by-test-name/immunocap.

Roback JD: Technical manual, ed 17, Am Assoc of Blood Banks: Bethesda, MD, 2011.

Sussman GL, Tarlo S, Dolovich J: The spectrum of IgE-mediated responses to latex, JAMA 265:2844–2847, 1991.

Tschopp CM, et al: Granzyme B, a novel mediator of allergic inflammation: its induction and release in blood basophils and human asthma, Blood 108:2290–2298, 2006.

Turgeon ML: Fundamentals of immunohematology, ed 2, Baltimore, 1995, Williams & Wilkins.

CHAPTER 27

Immunoproliferative Disorders

Learning Objectives

At the conclusion of this chapter, the reader should be able to:

• Compare the general characteristics of monoclonal and polyclonal gammopathies.
• Describe and compare the etiology, epidemiology, signs and symptoms, immunologic manifestations, diagnostic evaluation, and treatment of multiple myeloma and Waldenström's primary macroglobulinemia.
• Explain and contrast the characteristics of other monoclonal disorders, such as monoclonal gammopathy of unknown significance.

• Analyze a case study related to immunoproliferation.
• Correctly answer case study related multiple choice questions.
• Be prepared to participate in a discussion of case study related critical thinking questions.
• Describe the principle and application of the Bence Jones Protein Screening Procedure.
• Correctly answer end of chapter review questions.

Key Terms

amyloidosis
Bence Jones (BJ) protein
hypercalcemia
hypergammaglobulinemias
hyperviscosity
indolent

light-chain disease (LCD)
M protein
monoclonal gammopathy
multiple myeloma
osteoclasts
paraprotein

plasma cell dyscrasias
polyclonal gammopathy
rouleaux
smoldering multiple myeloma
Waldenström's primary macroglobulinemia (WM)

A small number of long-lived plasma cells in the bone marrow (<1% of mononuclear cells) produce most of immunoglobulins G and A (IgG and IgA) in normal adult serum. These well-differentiated cells do not divide and have a characteristic phenotype: CD38^{bright}, syndecan-1^{bright}, CD19+, and CD56$^{weak/-}$. Their precursors are slowly proliferating plasmablasts, which migrate to the marrow from lymph nodes after stimulation by antigens and cytokines from helper T (Th) cells in the germinal centers. Events in the germinal centers initiate somatic mutations of the immunoglobulin genes of B cells and a switch from

the production of immunoglobulin M (IgM) to the production of IgG or IgA. After the activated B cells enter the bone marrow, they stop proliferating and differentiate into plasma cells under the influence of adhesion molecules and factors such as interleukin-6. Normal plasma cells die by apoptosis after several weeks or months.

Hypergammaglobulinemias are monoclonal or polyclonal in nature. A monoclonal gammopathy, which can be a benign or malignant condition, results from a single clone of lymphoid plasma cells producing elevated levels of a single class and type of immunoglobulin, referred to as a monoclonal protein, **M protein,** or **paraprotein.** Disorders in this category of **plasma cell dyscrasias** include multiple myeloma (MM), Waldenström's macroglobulinemia (WM), monoclonal gammopathy of undetermined significance (MGUS), light-chain deposition disease, and heavy-chain diseases. In comparison, a polyclonal gammopathy is classified as a secondary disease and characterized by the elevation of two or more immunoglobulins by several clones of plasma cells.

GENERAL CHARACTERISTICS OF GAMMOPATHIES

Monoclonal Gammopathies

Monoclonal gammopathies are characterized by the production of monoclonal immunoglobulin and are associated with suppressed uninvolved immunoglobulins and dysfunctional T cell responses. Although MM is the prototypic **monoclonal gammopathy,** the most common plasma cell disorder is the premalignant precursor of myeloma, MGUS.

Serum and urine electrophoresis and other immunoglobulin assays can demonstrate strikingly abnormal results in disorders such as MM and WM. The gamma region of the electrophoretic pattern can show a dense, highly restricted band from uncontrolled proliferation of one cell clone, whereas the other normal immunoglobulins are deficient. The clinical interpretation of some patterns can be difficult. In contrast, some symptomatic patients do not exhibit the characteristic monoclonal band or spike in their serum protein patterns. This is often the case with **light-chain disease (LCD),** in which only kappa (κ) or lambda (λ) monoclonal light chains are synthesized by the clone. These low-molecular-weight immunoglobulin fragments are filtered through the glomerulus and into the urine, producing a serum electrophoretic pattern that suggests hypogammaglobulinemia, with a very faint monoclonal band or no band at all. These light chains also suggest the presence of a nonsecretory clone, which produces no monoclonal immunoglobulins and frequently demonstrates hypogammaglobulinemia because of the inhibition of normal clones.

Polyclonal Gammopathies

A **polyclonal gammopathy** is a common protein abnormality. It is defined as an increase in more than one immunoglobulin and involves several clones of plasma cells. In contrast to a monoclonal protein, a polyclonal protein consists of one or more heavy-chain classes and both light-chain types. Polyclonal increases are exhibited as secondary manifestations of infection or inflammation. They are often seen in chronic infections, chronic liver disease, especially chronic active hepatitis, rheumatoid connective tissue (autoimmune) diseases, and lymphoproliferative disorders.

A polyclonal protein is characterized by a broad peak or band, usually of gamma mobility, on electrophoresis, by a thickening and elongation of all heavy-chain and light-chain arcs on immunoelectrophoresis, and by the absence of a localized band on immunofixation. A polyclonal gammopathy therefore resembles a normal pattern, with the serum staining more intensely. A selective polyclonal increase is of special interest because only the level of one class of immunoglobulin is significantly elevated; however, the increase is polyclonal because immunoglobulin is produced by several clones of plasma cells and both kappa and lambda types are produced. Immunoglobulin quantitation by specific assay procedures demonstrates which immunoglobulin is increased. Immunofixation is not recommended in cases of polyclonal gammopathy because it presents no additional information.

MULTIPLE MYELOMA

Multiple myeloma is a plasma cell neoplasm characterized by the accumulation of malignant plasma cells within the bone marrow microenvironment, monoclonal protein in the blood or urine, and associated organ dysfunction. Normal bone marrow has about 1% plasma cells, but in MM the plasma cell concentration can rise to 90%. Bone marrow identification of monoclonal plasma cells by histology is an essential part of MM diagnosis and is frequently based on identifying intracellular κ and λ chains using direct immunofluorescent techniques.

Plasma cells produce one of five heavy-chain types together with κ and λ molecules. There is approximately 40% excess production of free light-chain over heavy-chain synthesis to allow proper conformation of the intact immunoglobulin molecules.

Etiology

The cause of MM is unknown. Radiation may be a factor in some cases and a viral cause has been suggested. Other factors may include environmental stimulants, such as exposure to asbestos, benzene, or industrial toxins. The likelihood of a genetic factor in some cases has been supported by well-documented reports of familial clusters with MM.

Pathophysiology

Myelomas arise from an asymptomatic premalignant proliferation of monoclonal plasma cells derived from postgerminal center B cells. In contrast to normal plasma cells, myeloma cells are often immature and may have the appearance of plasmablasts. These cells usually are CD19-CD56[bright], CD38, and syndecan-1, and produce very low amounts of immunoglobulins.

Most patients demonstrate complex karyotype abnormalities with chromosomal gains, deletions, and translocations, some of which are identical to those observed in certain B cell lymphomas. Many numeric and structural abnormalities occur. Primary early chromosomal translocations occur at the immunoglobulin switch region on chromosome 14 (q32.33). This process results in the deregulation of two adjacent genes. Secondary late-onset translocations and gene mutation are implicated in disease progression and include complex karyotypic abnormalities. These genetic abnormalities may prevent the differentiation and apoptosis of myeloma cells, which continue to proliferate and accumulate in the bone marrow. Chromosomal aberrations are of sufficient number to be detected on flow analysis of DNA content, which is aneuploid in about 80% of patients.

Most patients exhibit a slight nuclear DNA excess of 5% to 10%; hypoploidy is observed in only 5% to 10% of patients and is strongly associated with resistance to standard chemotherapy. Deletions of chromosomes 13 and 17 have been observed. The morphologic immaturity, hypodiploidy, and 13q– and 14q+ abnormalities correlate with the resistance to treatment and short survival that are characteristic of aggressive disease.

The somatic mutations of the immunoglobulin genes of myeloma cells indicate that the putative myeloma cell precursors are stimulated by antigens and are memory B cells or migrating plasmablasts.

Myeloma cells proliferate slowly in the marrow (Fig. 27-1; Table 27-1). Less than 1% divide at any one time and myeloma cells do not differentiate. The absolute number of these cells correlates with disease activity and predicts the progression of disease in **smoldering multiple myeloma.** Circulating myeloma cells may disseminate the tumor within the bone marrow and elsewhere.

Interleukin-6 (IL-6) is essential for the survival and growth of myeloma cells, which express specific receptors for this cytokine. Initially identified as a growth factor for myeloma cells, IL-6 has been shown to promote the survival of myeloma cells by preventing spontaneous or dexamethasone-induced apoptosis. An increased level of IL-6 in the serum of patients with MM can be explained by the overproduction of IL-6 in the marrow. The IL-6 system also has a role in the pathogenesis of bone lesions in MM. IL-6, soluble IL-6 receptor alpha (sIL-6Rα), and interleukin-1 beta (IL-1β) activate **osteoclasts** in the vicinity of myeloma cells and thus initiate bone resorption. IL-6 may account for MM-associated anemia

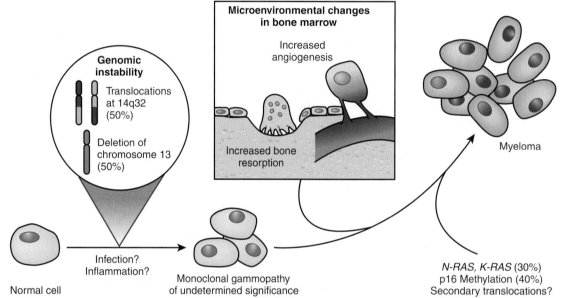

Figure 27-1 **Mechanisms of disease progression in the monoclonal gammopathies.** *(Adapted from Kyle RA, Rajkumar SV: N Engl J Med 351:1860–1871, 2004.)*

Table 27-1	Three Phases of Disease Progression in Multiple Myeloma		
Variable	**Initial Phase**	**Medullary Relapse**	**Extramedullary Relapse**
Site of myeloma-cell accumulation or proliferation	Bone marrow	Bone marrow	Blood, pleural effusion, skin, many other sites
Growth fraction*	<1%	≥1% (1%-95%)	≥1% (1%-95%)
Genetic or oncogenic events	Deregulation of *c-myc* Illegitimate switch recombinations	N-*ras* and K-*ras* point mutations	p53 point mutations
Phenotypic changes	CD19 loss CD56 overexpression	CD28 expression LFA-1 and VLA-5 loss	CD28 expression CD56 loss
Cytologic changes	Detectable plasmablastic compartment in 15% of cases	Plasmablastic compartment growing	Major plasmablastic compartment
Circulating malignant plasma cells	<1%	Increasing	Increasing

From Bataille R, Harousseau JL: Medical progress: multiple myeloma, N Engl J Med 336:1657–1664, 1997.
*Growth fraction is the rate of atypical cells proliferating in the bone marrow.

and for the lack of thrombocytopenia because of its stimulation of megakaryopoiesis.

Epidemiology

Multiple myeloma is the most common form of dysproteinemia. It accounts for 1% of all types of malignant diseases and 10% of hematologic malignancies. The age-adjusted incidence is estimated to be 5.6 cases/100,000 population/year in Western countries. About 10,000 Americans die each year from MM. In Western countries, the frequency of myeloma is likely to increase in the near future as the population ages.

The onset of MM is from 40 to 70 years, with a peak incidence in the seventh decade. It is uncommon (<2% of cases) in patients younger than 40 years. In general, patients with LCD and IgD myeloma are younger than those with IgG or IgA myeloma and have a poorer prognosis because of their high incidence of nephropathy. Males are affected in approximately 62% of cases; the male-to-female ratio is 1.6:1. In addition, blacks are affected twice as often as whites.

IgG myeloma is the most common form of MM (Table 27-2). Four subtypes of IgG heavy chains are known to exist among patients with IgG myeloma. Cases of IgG myeloma are distributed as follows: 65% are gamma G1, 23% gamma G2, 8% gamma G3, and 4% gamma G4 subclass. The only subclass-dependent difference is the greater propensity for patients with IgG3 myeloma to experience **hyperviscosity** syndrome, similar to the manifestation in WM.

Multiple myeloma runs a progressive course, with most patients dying within 1 to 3 years. The β_2-microglobulin level at initial evaluation has been adopted as a predictor of outcome. If the serum β_2-microglobulin level is elevated at the start of therapy, the prognosis is less favorable. The major causes of death are overwhelming infection (sepsis) and renal insufficiency. In patients with sepsis, mortality exceeds 50%, despite antibiotic therapy.

Signs and Symptoms

The signs and symptoms of MM include bone pain, typically in the back or chest, and weakness, fatigue, and pallor associated with anemia or abnormal bleeding. In all, 20% of patients exhibit hepatomegaly and 5% demonstrate splenomegaly. In some cases, the major manifestations of disease result from acute infection, renal insufficiency, **hypercalcemia,** or **amyloidosis.** Weight loss and night sweats are not prominent until the disease is advanced. Bone pain, anemia, and renal insufficiency constitute a triad of signs and symptoms strongly suggestive of MM.

In 1975 a staging system for myeloma was developed. This system defines **indolent** versus severe disease and determines a basis for therapy. Patients are divided into three groups, with classification based on the production of IgG by plasma cells and the total quantity of IgG in the body. The number of abnormal plasma cells is correlated with the hemoglobin value, serum calcium level, serum IgG peak, and presence or absence of lytic bone lesions. Renal function is also considered an important factor, not only because it is essential to survival, but also because IgG light chains can damage the kidneys.

Some physicians use a simpler system of staging based on serum albumin, hemoglobin, and β_2-microglobulin levels.

Skeletal Abnormalities

About 90% of patients with MM have broadly disseminated destruction of the skeleton, which is responsible for the predominance of bone pain. These abnormalities consist of punched-out lytic areas (Fig. 27-2), osteoporosis, and fractures in about 80% of patients. The vertebrae, skull, thoracic cage, pelvis, and proximal humeri and femurs are the most frequent sites of involvement.

Hematologic Features

The diagnosis of MM depends on the demonstration of an increased number of plasma cells in a bone marrow aspirate and/or biopsy and supporting laboratory results (see later, "Diagnostic Evaluation"). Although the bone marrow is typically involved, the disorder may involve other tissues. For example, a positive correlation exists between the production of osteoclast-activating factor by bone marrow cells and the extent of skeletal destruction. Other hematologic factors contributing to the signs and symptoms of pallor and anemia include bleeding, qualitative platelet abnormalities, inhibition of coagulation factors by M protein, and thrombocytopenia. Intravascular coagulation may occur.

Renal Disorders

Acute renal failure (ARF) occurs in about 5% to 10% of patients. Although ARF may occur at any time in the course of myeloma, it can be the initial manifestation of disease. ARF has been observed after infection, hypercalcemia, dehydration, and IV urography. Serum creatinine levels are elevated in about half these patients and approximately one third have hypercalcemia.

Chronic renal failure is a common development in MM patients. As many as two thirds of patients display serum creatinine levels higher than 1.5 mg/dL and 10% to 20% may develop end-stage renal disease (ESRD). Patients with IgD or

Table 27-2	Distribution of Immunoglobulin Types in Patients With Multiple Myeloma
Type of Protein	**Multiple Myeloma (%)**
IgM	12
IgG	52
IgA	22
IgD	2
IgE	Rare
Light chains (kappa or lambda)	11
Heavy chains	Rare
Monoclonal proteins	<1
Nonsecretory myeloma	1

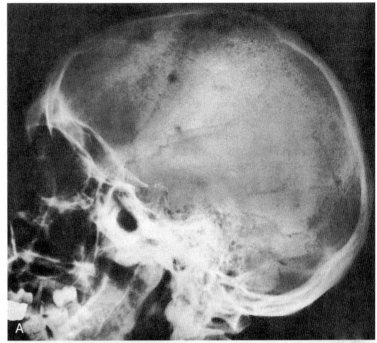

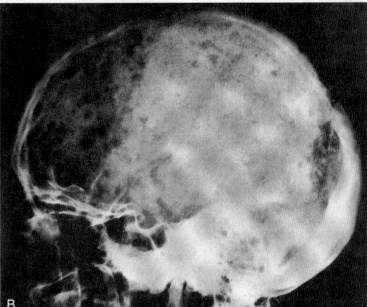

Figure 27-2 **Multiple myeloma.** **A,** Several scattered, small, well-marginated lytic lesions appear in calvarium, located in normally mineralized bone. Multiple lytic lesions can also be seen in the mandible. **B,** Multiple circumscribed lytic lesions crowd bones throughout skull. Lesions are still discrete and margins of most are fairly sharp. *(From Newton TH, Potts DG: Radiology of the skull and brain, St Louis, 1971, Mosby.)*

light-chain myeloma are much more likely to develop renal failure than those with IgG or IgA myeloma. Proteinuria is a common finding, with over half of all MM patients excreting abnormal amounts of **Bence Jones (BJ) protein** (light chains). Patients with BJ proteinuria are much more likely to have renal tubular defects than those without BJ proteinuria.

Studies have suggested that BJ proteins have a deleterious effect on renal function via at least two mechanisms. First, renal failure may result from intratubular precipitation of BJ protein and subsequent intrarenal obstruction. When the distal collecting tubules become obstructed by large casts consisting mainly of BJ protein, the disorder may be referred to as myeloma kidney. The second mechanism of renal failure may be a function of direct tubular cell injury. As a result of these

tubular defects, abnormalities in urine-concentrating ability and renal acidification are observed. Although the presence of a large concentration of BJ proteinuria is usually associated with some degree of renal dysfunction, some patients excrete large amounts of BJ protein for years and maintain renal function.

Lambda light chains have been implicated in nephrotoxicity, but their role has not been firmly established.

Neurologic Features

Pain is a common characteristic of MM, often caused by compression of the spinal cord or nerves. Compression produces back pain, with weakness or paralysis of the lower extremities and bowel or bladder incontinence.

Infectious Diseases

The most frequent cause of death is infection. Patients with MM have increased susceptibility to infectious microorganisms because of an inability to cope with bacterial infections and certain viral diseases. Increased susceptibility principally results from defective antibody synthesis caused by the crowding out and suppression of normal plasma cell precursors.

Repeated bouts of sepsis, often resulting from recurrent infection by microorganisms such as pneumococci or gram-negative bacteria, are common. Pneumonia, pyelonephritis, meningitis, and arthritis are the leading forms of sepsis; when bacteremia ensues, mortality is high.

Immunologic Manifestations

In approximately 20% of patients, multiple myeloma is diagnosed by chance in the absence of symptoms, usually after screening laboratory studies have revealed an increased serum protein concentration. MM cells express not only cytoplasmic immunoglobulins, the hallmark of plasma cells, but early B, T, natural killer (NK), myeloid, erythroid, and megakaryocytic cell markers as well. These phenotypic features are consistent with the hypothesis that MM may originate from a transformed early hematopoietic progenitor cell, which explains the occasional coexistence of MM and acute myelogenous leukemia (AML).

Patients with MM have defects in humoral but not cellular immunity. Humoral immunity is disrupted because plasma cell tumors induce the suppression of antibody synthesis by normal immunoglobulin-secreting cells and the production of antiidiotype antibodies declines proportionately. In addition, selective impairment occurs in the formation of normal antibodies because of increased immunoglobulin catabolism and the release of a protein that incites macrophages to suppress synthesis of normal immunoglobulins by myeloma cells. Depression of normal humoral immunity accounts for the high susceptibility of MM patients to bacterial infection. The normal functioning of cellular immunity is demonstrated by normal resistance to fungal and most viral infections and by normal delayed-type hypersensitivity to skin testing antigens.

Initially, in vivo myeloma clones are subject to control by the immune network via specific idiotype-antiidiotype mechanisms. Each of the million or more potential immunoglobulin variants in every individual carries singular determinants of designated idiotypes. Antiidiotypic antibodies directed against autologous immunoglobulin are elicited during a normal immune response. The presumed mission of antiidiotypic antibodies is to help terminate the immune response by binding complementary idiotypes to form endogenous immune complexes that are removed from the circulation. The antiidiotypic antibodies in turn stimulate production of antibodies to antiidiotype, and so on, to create a modulating network that includes T cells, which recognize idiotype antigens through unique antigen receptors. Antiidiotype- and idiotype-sensitized T cells collaborate most efficiently during highly restricted responses, during which both antibodies and lymphocytes that specifically recognize the dominant idiotype are activated.

These can inhibit or enhance the response of lymphocytes to receptors expressing the idiotype. The overall net direction of the response is determined by the functional influence of T cells linked by antiidiotype receptor interactions to their molecular targets on B cells. In MM, idiotype expression is carried to an extreme. Monoclonal paraproteins secreted by plasma cell tumors induce many immunologic responses capable of acting in concert to contain or modulate tumor growth.

The earliest detectable monoclonal B cell, as identified by idiotypic structures of the myeloma protein, is the transitional form bearing surface IgM, IgD, and IgG. This and the finding that precursor (early) B cells destined to become myeloma cells possess surface IgG (sIgG) indicate that the myeloma tumor clone includes memory B cells that can mature into plasma cells. The use of antiidiotypic antibodies for identifying IgA myeloma clones has revealed clonal expression at the pre–B state, a finding supported by the observation that B cells in the circulation of myeloma patients are clonally frozen at the pre–B stage. As maturing B cell members of the malignant clone differentiate in the marrow, they lose IgD and IgM, in that order, accumulate sIgG, and finally shed sIg to become IgG-producing mature plasma cells, as programmed by the mutant precursor cell. Thus, the mature myeloma cell contains abundant cytoplasmic (secretory) IgG but no sIgG. IgA myeloma cells proceed along the same normal differentiation scheme of B cell maturation. Although MM-associated tumors disseminate widely, the disease is spread through the release of clonal precursors into the blood circulation that show lymphoid rather than plasma cell morphology.

The most consistent immunologic feature of multiple myeloma is the incessant synthesis of a dysfunctional single monoclonal protein or of immunoglobulin chains of fragments, with concurrent suppression of the synthesis of normal functional antibody. In 99% of myeloma patients, an M component is usually found in serum, urine, or both. Different types of M components are associated with various clinical syndromes.

Diagnostic Evaluation

Hematologic Assessment

A normochromic normocytic anemia is present in about two thirds of patients at diagnosis. In part, anemia is related to the hypervolemia caused by the increase in plasma volume because of monoclonal protein production. **Rouleaux** formation is a common finding on peripheral blood smears. The leukocyte count can be normal, although about one third of patients have leukopenia. Relative lymphocytosis is usually present. If lymphocyte subsets are examined, a reduction in CD4+ (helper) and an increase in CD8+ (suppressor-cytotoxic) blood lymphocytes can be noted. Defects in the proliferative responses of lymphocytes to mitogens or antigens are explained by the large portion of B cells in MM that originate from the malignant stem cell clone. Few mature plasma cells are seen in the circulation except at the terminal phase of the disease, but the covert presence of the malignant B cell clone can be unmasked by the laboratory use of monoclonal antibodies (MAbs) or by transforming agents such as phorbol esters. In rare cases, in the terminal stages, plasmablasts and proplasmacytes may amount to 50% of the leukocytes in the peripheral blood.

Bleeding is common. Platelet abnormalities, impaired aggregation of platelets, and interference with platelet function by the abnormal monoclonal protein contribute to bleeding. Inhibitors of coagulation factors and thrombocytopenia from marrow infiltration of plasma cells or chemotherapy may also contribute to bleeding. Some patients have a tendency toward thrombosis, which may manifest as a shortened coagulation time and increased levels of fibrinogen and factor VIII.

Diagnosis of MM, however, depends on the demonstration of an increased number (>10%) of plasma cells in a bone marrow aspirate (Fig. 27-3; see Color Plate 12) and/or biopsy and supporting laboratory results. Cytogenetic analysis or fluorescence in situ hybridization (FISH) of bone marrow aspirate is recommended.

Bence Jones Proteins

Bence Jones proteins have been important diagnostic markers for MM since the mid-19th century (see later, "Bence Jones Protein Screening Procedure"). In about 10% of MM patients, only BJ proteins are produced, with no complete IgM, IgG, or IgA. BJ proteins are single-peptide chains with a molecular weight of 20 to 22 kkDa, but dimerization occurs spontaneously to form molecules of 40 to 44 kDa.

Bence Jones proteins are monoclonal κ or λ immunoglobulin free light chains (FLCs) not attached to the heavy-chain portion of the immunoglobulin molecule. BJ proteins are seen in two types of syndromes:
- With a typical monoclonal gammopathy
- In free LCD

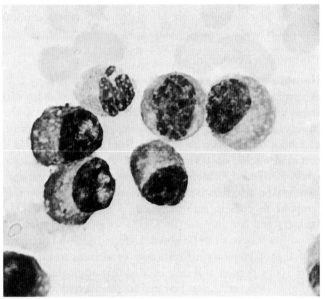

Figure 27-3   Myeloma cells in a bone marrow aspirate. *(From Bauer JD: Clinical laboratory methods, ed 9, St Louis, 1982, Mosby.)*

Serum concentrations of FLCs depend on the balance between production by plasma cells and their precursors and on renal clearance. If there is increased polyclonal immunoglobulin production and/or renal impairment, both κ and λ FLC concentrations can increase by 30% to 40%. Serum FLC tests have been assuming an increasing role in the detection and monitoring of monoclonal gammopathies. Serum FLCs have a short half-life in the blood (κ, 2 to 4 hours; λ, 3 to 6 hours), compared with 21 days for IgG molecules. FLC concentrations allow more rapid assessment of the effects of chemotherapy than monoclonal IgG levels.

Very small amounts of BJ proteins in serum can be associated with significant clinical problems, especially pathologic renal changes. FLCs filter through the glomeruli almost without obstruction because of their small molecular size and accumulate in the tubules. Renal impairment can result from the toxicity of FLCs. Pathologic changes can range from relatively benign tubular proteinuria to ARF or amyloidosis.

BJ proteins can be detected in serum, urine, or both. The level of monoclonal light chains in serum or urine is related to filtration, resorption, or catabolism of the protein by the kidneys. During the early stages of renal disease, when the kidneys are only mildly affected, excretion and reabsorption continue normally, but only partial catabolism occurs. At this point, BJ proteins may be detected in the serum but not in the urine. Progressive renal involvement impairs reabsorption, and diminished reabsorption with decreased catabolism results in FLCs in serum and urine. Later, as resorption is totally blocked, FLCs are present in urine only. In terminal stages of renal disease, uremia occurs, renal clearance is affected, and BJ proteins again appear in the serum.

BJ proteins are unusual in their response to heating. They are soluble at room temperature, become insoluble (forms a precipitate around 60° C to 70° C, and then dissolves at 100° C). This pattern reverses when the temperature is lowered, which is unique to BJ protein.

Serologically, all BJ proteins are not identical, although there are κ and λ types. BJ proteins will react with antisera to the λ chains of IgG and λ chains react with antisera to BJ protein.

Approximately 80% of patients with MM produce intact immunoglobulin monoclonal proteins, of which 46% have excess monoclonal FLCs in the urine by immunofixation electrophoresis. Serum protein electrophoresis is positive less often because of low serum concentrations of FLCs. From 3% to 4% of MM patients have nonsecretory disease. These patients have no detectable monoclonal proteins with serum and urine electrophoretic testing because their tumor cells produce small amounts of monoclonal protein. Their FLC concentrations are below the sensitivity of serum electrophoretic tests and below the threshold for clearance into the urine. These patients can be monitored by serum FLC tests rather than by repeated bone marrow biopsies or whole-body scans.

Free Light Chains

Free light chains are incorporated into immunoglobulin molecules during B lymphocyte development and expressed initially on the surface of immature B cells. Production of FLCs occurs throughout the rest of B cell development and in plasma cells, in which secretion is highest. Tumors associated with the different stages of B cell maturation will secrete monoclonal FLCs into the serum, where they may be detected by FLC immunoassays (Box 27-1; Table 27-3).

Production of FLCs in normal individuals is approximately 500 mg/day from bone marrow and lymph node cells. The molecules enter the blood and are readily partitioned between the intravascular and extravascular compartments. In normal individuals, serum FLCs are rapidly cleared and metabolized by the kidneys, depending on their molecular size.

Immunologic Testing

Traditionally, laboratories have detected the monoclonal immunoglobulins by protein electrophoresis, which began in the 1930s, and have characterized the proteins by immunofixation electrophoresis (IFE), which was developed in the 1980s.

The identification of κ and λ molecules has been accomplished with the use of antibodies specific for each type of protein. Immunodiffusion was initially used, followed by immunoelectrophoresis (in 1953), radial immunodiffusion, and ultimately nephelometry and turbidimetry. An automated nephelometric assay, described in 2001, represented a major breakthrough. This methodology allows for the quantitation of both κ and λ free light chains and can be performed using automated chemistry analyzers (e.g., Dade Behring [now Siemens AG], Beckman Coulter, Roche Hitachi, Olympus) (see Chapter 13).

Box 27-1	Benefits of Serum Free Light-Chain Immunoassays

- Better sensitivity and precision than current electrophoretic assays
- Numeric results for disease monitoring
- Convenience of serum as a test medium
- Identification of AL amyloidosis and NSMM patients who have detectable monoclonal proteins by conventional tests
- More accurate marker of complete disease remission than existing assays
- Short half-life marker for rapid assessment of treatment responses
- Identification of progression risk in individuals with MGUS
- Better screening of symptomatic patients

From Bradwell AR: Serum free light chain analysis, Birmingham, England, 2006, Binding Site, p 4.
FLC, Free light chain; *AL*, immunocyte derived; *NSMM*, nonsecretory multiple myeloma; *MGUS*, monoclonal gammopathy of undetermined significance.

Table 27-3	Assays for Free Light Chains	
Assay	**Advantages**	**Disadvantages**
Total urine protein	Simple, inexpensive, widely used	Inadequate sensitivity for FLC detection
Urine dipstick	Simple, inexpensive, widely used	Inadequate sensitivity for FLC detection
Serum protein electrophoresis	Simple, manual or semiautomated method Well established, inexpensive Monoclonal bands observed Quantitative results with scanning	Insensitive (<500-2000 mg/L) Cannot detect FLCs at low concentration Subjective interpretation of results
Urine protein electrophoresis	Simple, manual, or semiautomated method Well established, inexpensive Monoclonal bands observed Sensitive in concentrated urine (10 mg/L) Quantitative results with scanning	Subjective interpretation of results Urine may require concentration, with possible protein loss False bands from concentrating urine Heavy proteinuria obscures results Cumbersome 24-hour urine collection
Immunofixation electrophoresis (IFE) on serum and urine	Well established Good sensitivity for serum, very sensitive for concentrated urine (5-30 mg/L)	Nonquantitative Serum sensitivity (150-500 mg/L) inadequate for normal serum FLC levels Rather laborious to perform Visual interpretation may be difficult Expensive use of antisera Cannot be used to quantify monoclonal immunoglobulins because of precipitating antibody
Capillary zone electrophoresis	Automated technology Quantitative	Less sensitive (400 mg/L) than IFE for serum FLCs Can fail to detect 5% of positive samples (false-negatives)
Total serum κ and λ assays	Automated immunoassay	Not sensitive enough for routine testing Specificity inadequate for detecting many patients with light-chain multiple myeloma

Adapted from Bradwell AR: Serum free light chain analysis, Birmingham, UK, 2006, Binding Site, pp 23, 47-52.

Box 27-2	**Monoclonal Gammopathies**

1. Malignant monoclonal gammopathies
   a. Multiple myeloma (IgG, IgA, IgD, IgE, and free light chains)
   b. Plasmacytoma
   c. Malignant lymphoproliferative diseases
   d. Heavy-chain diseases
   e. Amyloidosis
2. Monoclonal gammopathies of undetermined significance
   a. Benign (IgG, IgA, IgD, IgM, and rarely, free light chains)
   b. Associated with neoplasms of cell types not known to produce monoclonal proteins
   c. Biclonal gammopathies

Each monoclonal protein (M protein or paraprotein) consists of two heavy-chain polypeptides of the same class and subclass and two light-chain polypeptides of the same type. The different monoclonal proteins are designated by capital letters corresponding to the class of their heavy chains, which are designated by Greek letters: gamma (γ) in IgG, alpha (α) in IgA, mu (μ) in IgM, delta (δ) in IgD, and epsilon (ϵ) in IgE. The subclasses are IgG1, IgG2, IgG, and IgG4, or IgA1 and IgA2, and their light-chain types are κ and λ. A monoclonal protein is characterized by a narrow peak or localized band on electrophoresis, by a thickened bowed arc on immunoelectrophoresis, and by a localized band on immunofixation. Many different entities are associated with M proteins (monoclonal gammopathies; Box 27-2).

Electrophoresis of the serum or urine reveals a tall sharp peak on the densitometer tracing or a dense localized band in most cases of multiple myeloma (Fig. 27-4). A monoclonal protein is demonstrable in the serum and urine in 90% of patients. In all, 60% of patients exhibit IgG, 20% IgA, 10% light chain only (BJ proteinemia), and 1% IgD. Electrophoresis of urine shows a globulin peak in 75% of cases, mainly albumin in 10% of patients, and a normal pattern in 15%. When an M spike is observed on serum protein electrophoresis, the suggested sequence of testing includes testing by immunoelectrophoresis and immunofixation (Table 27-4). Screening for cryoglobulins and viscosity may also be warranted.

Immunoelectrophoresis, also called gamma globulin electrophoresis or immunoglobulin electrophoresis, is a method of determining the blood levels of three major immunoglobulins—IgM, IgG, and IgA—based on their combined electrophoretic and immunologic properties (see Chapter 11). Immunoelectrophoresis is also used frequently to diagnose MM, which affects the bone marrow. Drugs that may cause increased immunoglobulin levels include therapeutic gamma globulin, hydralazine, isoniazid, phenytoin (Dilantin), procainamide, oral contraceptives, methadone, steroids, and tetanus toxoid and antitoxin. The laboratory should be notified if the patient has received any vaccinations or immunizations in the 6 months before the test. Prior immunizations lead to increased immunoglobulin levels, resulting in false-positive results.

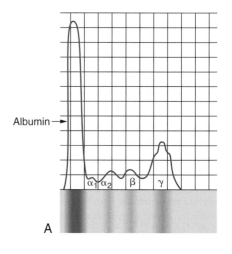

A

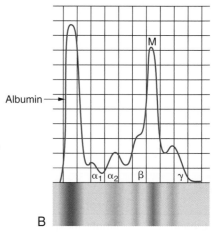

B

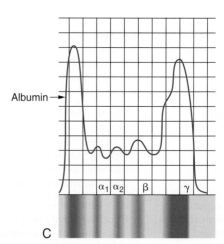

C

Figure 27-4 Serum electrophoretic patterns. A, Normal patient. **B,** Patient with multiple myeloma. **C,** Patient with Waldenström's macroglobulinemia.

Because immunoelectrophoresis is not quantitative, it is being replaced by immunofixation, which is more sensitive and easier to interpret.

Prognosis

In patients diagnosed when they are younger than 60 years, the 10-year survival is approximately 30%. Staging of the disease,

Table 27-4	Suggested Sequence of Immunologic Testing for Monoclonal Proteins	
M Spike on Serum Protein Electrophoresis		
Serum	**Urine**	
Immunoelectrophoresis	Screening of urine for increased protein, (e.g., sulfosalicylic acid)	
Immunofixation	Total protein assay of a 24-hr urine specimen	
Quantitation of immunoglobulins by radial immunodiffusion or nephelometry	Urinary protein electrophoresis	
Screening for cryoglobulins	Urinary immunoelectrophoresis	
Determination of serum viscosity if IgM, IgA, or IgG or signs and symptoms suggestive of hyperviscosity	Immunofixation	

according to the International Staging System, defines three risk groups on the basis of serum β_2-microglobulin and albumin levels. Any chromosomal abnormality detected on standard cytogenetic analysis is associated with a worse outcome than that associated with a normal karyotype. Translocations such as t(4;14), deletion 17p13, and chromosome 1 abnormalities are associated with a poor prognosis.

Standard-risk disease is defined by the presence of hyperdiploidy or t(11;14), normal levels of serum β_2-microglobulin or lactate dehydrogenase, and International Staging System stage I. High-risk disease and a poor prognosis are defined by the presence of one of the following in each category: hypodiploidy, t(4;14), or deletion 17p13; high levels of serum β_2-microglobulin or lactate dehydrogenase, and International Staging System stage III.

The CD200 membrane glycoprotein imparts an immuno-regulatory signal that leads to the suppression of T cell–mediated immune responses. Patients with CD200[absent] MM cells have an increased event-free survival of 24 months; patients with CD200[present] demonstrate an event-free survival of 14 months after high-dose therapy and stem cell transplantation. The presence or absence of CD200 expression in MM cells is considered a predictor of event-free survival for patients who are independent of the stage of disease or β_2M serum levels.

Treatment

Asymptomatic (smoldering) myeloma requires only clinical observation because early treatment with conventional chemotherapy has shown no benefit. Recently, the introduction of autologous stem cell transplantation (see Chapter 32) as a mainstay of myeloma therapy and the availability of agents such as thalidomide, lenalidomide, and bortezomib have changed the medical management of active (symptomatic) myeloma and extended overall survival. New proteasome inhibitors,

immunomodulatory drugs (pomalidomide), targeted therapies, epigenetic agents, and humanized monoclonal antibodies are currently undergoing clinical trial investigations.

When a patient undergoes chemotherapy, the number of myeloma cells in the bone marrow and the amount of monoclonal protein in the blood and urine are closely monitored. A stable monoclonal protein level indicates that the disease is stable, often the result of effective treatment. The monoclonal protein rarely disappears completely from blood and urine.

Vaccination with the myeloma idiotype of a monoclonal immunoglobulin is an investigational means of immunotherapy. DNA hybridization or blotting technology is the newest technology available and can be used to detect abnormal gene arrangements and mutations in cellular oncogenes. Although the gene product of MAbs is the method of detection, DNA probes that can detect the abnormal gene are now available. Blotting techniques may replace the current approach to the laboratory evaluation of monoclonal gammopathies.

Strategies are being investigated to develop risk-adapted approaches to treatment based on knowledge of genetic polymorphisms or mutations that modulate the molecular pathways that underlie the pathogenesis of the disease.

WALDENSTRÖM'S PRIMARY MACROGLOBULINEMIA

Etiology

Waldenström's primary macroglobulinemia (WM), or simply macroglobulinemia, is a B cell disorder characterized by the infiltration of lymphoplasmacytic cells into bone marrow and the presence of an IgM monoclonal gammopathy. WM is considered to be a lymphoplasmacytic lymphoma, as defined by the Revised European American Lymphoma (REAL) and World Health Organization (WHO) classification systems. WM is a malignant lymphocyte–plasma cell proliferative disorder that exhibits abnormally large amounts of immunoglobulin of the 19S IgM type.

The cause of WM is unknown but a possible genetic predisposition may exist. About 20% of WM patients have a familial predisposition to the disease and related B cell malignancies. A greater frequency of IgM monoclonal proteins and quantitative abnormalities have been observed in some relatives of patients with WM. In addition, research has suggested a significantly increased risk of WM after infections—hepatitis B virus, immunodeficiency virus, and rickettsiosis—and found an increased risk of WM in patients with a personal history of autoimmune disease.

Because WM is a malignant offshoot of B cell development before the myelomas, the sole gene product is IgM. Patients with WM have chromosomal rearrangements characteristic of B cell neoplasia, including t(8:14) and trisomy 12.

Epidemiology

Waldenström's macroglobulinemia occurs about 10% as frequently as multiple myeloma. WM has an age-specific incidence; it is most often found in older individuals, with a mean age of onset of 60 to 64 years. No significant gender differences exist in the incidence of WM. Disease onset is usually insidious; the median survival is approximately 3 years after diagnosis.

Signs and Symptoms

The signs and symptoms of WM have an indolent progression over many years. Initially, disease onset is slow and insidious, with the pace of manifestations determined by the rate of proliferation of the IgM-secreting clone. Most clinical signs and symptoms of disease stem from intravascular accumulation of high levels of IgM macroglobulin. When the IgM is precipitable at cold temperatures, as it is in 37% of cases, clinical manifestations of cold sensitivity such as Raynaud's phenomenon, arthralgias, purpura of the extremities, renal insufficiency, and peripheral vascular occlusions may develop. Cold hypersensitivity can occur when serum IgM levels exceed 2 to 3 g/dL and the protein precipitates at temperatures exceeding 20° C (68° F).

Although the patient experiences weakness and fatigue, it is usually the onset of bleeding from the gums or nose that arouses concern. Patients undergo weight loss and the incidence of infection is twice the normal rate. As the disease progresses, about 40% of patients develop hepatomegaly, splenomegaly, and lymphadenopathy. Occasionally, the clinical manifestations may simulate those of diffuse lymphoma. Specific dysfunctions and abnormalities occur in a variety of body systems.

Skeletal Features

In contrast to multiple myeloma, bone pain is almost nonexistent in WM. Diffuse osteoporosis may be seen, but bone lesions are extremely rare.

Hematologic Abnormalities

Patients with WM usually have chronic anemia and bleeding episodes. Bleeding problems in the form of bruising, purpura, and bleeding from the mouth, gums, nose, and gastrointestinal tract are common. The quantities of circulating platelets may be normal or decreased, but the most notable alteration is a disturbance in platelet function. Therefore, thrombocytopenia or hyperviscosity may contribute to the bleeding disorder.

In addition to anemia caused by chronic or recurrent bleeding, the decrease in red blood cells (RBCs) becomes more severe as the disease progresses because of a dilutional effect caused by increased immunoglobulin production. In addition, the presence of macroglobulin also produces an increased erythrocyte sedimentation rate (ESR). Microscopic examination of a peripheral blood smear usually reveals normocytic and frequently hypochromic RBCs with striking rouleaux (rolled coin) formation. The total blood leukocyte count is normal or slightly decreased because of moderate neutropenia. In a terminal patient, the blood may be inundated with malignant lymphoplasmacytic cells.

Renal Dysfunction

Renal function becomes mildly or moderately impaired in about 15% of WM patients. Nephrosis is uncommon. BJ proteinuria, however, is present in about 70% of WM patients, although the quantity of light chains excreted is much less than in multiple myeloma.

Glomerular lesions are the predominant form of renal injury. IgM collects on the endothelial side of the basement membrane of the kidney; sometimes these macroglobulin accumulations obstruct glomerular capillaries.

Ocular Manifestations

Blurred vision is a frequent abnormality of WM. Rouleaux induced by elevations of IgM causes distention of veins and capillaries; retinal oxygenation diminishes as rouleaux-inducing IgM rises. As a result of increased IgM levels, retinal hemorrhage, exudate formation, and varicosities develop, which can lead to more permanent retinal damage unless IgM levels are lowered by therapy.

Neuropsychiatric Problems

The most common serious neurologic consequence of the slowed cerebral perfusion caused by macroglobulinemia is acute cerebral malfunction, beginning with headache, fluctuating confusion, forgetfulness, and slowed mentation. This can progress to somnolence, stupor, and coma–diffuse brain syndrome, sometimes termed *coma paraproteinaemicum*. Neurologic abnormalities can be improved by a reduction of plasma viscosity.

Polyneuropathy affects 5% to 10% of patients with WM. This condition is associated with an increase in spinal fluid protein and deposits of monoclonal IgM on myelin sheaths. Monoclonal IgM found in the plasma and attached to damaged nerves has been shown in some cases to share idiotypic determinants. This suggests that the polyneuropathy of WM may be an autoimmune process caused by monoclonal IgM possessing antibody activity for a component of nerve tissue.

Cardiopulmonary Abnormalities

Congestive heart failure becomes a serious problem in patients with chronic uncontrolled WM. About 90% of IgM remains trapped in the circulating plasma and exerts an unbalanced transendothelial osmotic effect sufficient to cause marked expansion of the plasma volume. This in turn creates a dilutional anemia and augments cardiac filling and cardiac output. As a result, increased cardiac output and blood viscosity overwork the myocardium.

About 10% of patients develop pulmonary lesions. Pulmonary tumors, diffuse infiltrates, and pleural involvement are all about equally represented. The signs and symptoms of pulmonary dysfunction include coughing and dyspnea.

Cutaneous Manifestations

Cold sensitivity is a frequent manifestation of WM; however, skin lesions are uncommon. A small number of patients develop flat, violaceous, macular skin lesions resulting from dense infiltration by lymphoplasmacytoid cells. Pink, pearly-looking papules caused by dense deposits of IgM may be seen.

Immunologic Manifestations

The basic abnormality in this macroglobulinemia is uncontrolled proliferation of B lymphocytes and plasma cells. As a result, there is a heavy accumulation of monoclonal IgM in the circulating plasma and plasmacytoid lymphocytes in the bone marrow.

In many cases, WM is associated with mixed cryoglobulinemia, which reflects the binding of IgG or IgA antiidiotypic antibody to the mutant IgM. In a small number of patients, dysplastic tumor cells secrete 7S IgM monomers, µ chains, or other monoclonal immunoglobulins or fragments. Therefore, the major IgM production indicates that the immunoglobulin (gene) lesion sometimes degenerates and codes for more than one M component.

Diagnostic Evaluation
Hematologic Assessment
Microscopic examination of a bone marrow aspirate reveals that the lymphoplasmacytic cells vary morphologically from small lymphocytes to obvious plasma cells. Frequently, the cellular cytoplasm is ragged and may contain material staining positive with periodic acid–Schiff (PAS) stain, probably identical to the circulating macroglobulin.

The total peripheral blood leukocyte count is usually normal, with an absolute lymphocytosis. Moderate to severe degrees of anemia are frequently observed on peripheral blood smears, as well as rouleaux formation. The patient's plasma volume may be greatly increased and the ESR is also increased.

Platelet counts are usually normal. Faulty platelet aggregation and release of platelet factor 3 are caused by the nonspecific coating of platelets by IgM. The most common coagulation defect is a prolonged thrombin time, resulting from the binding of M component to fibrin monomers and consequent gel clotting of IgM-coated fibrin. Bleeding abnormalities can be demonstrated by the following:

- Faulty platelet adhesiveness
- Defective platelet aggregation
- Abnormal release of platelet factor 3
- Impaired clot retraction
- Prolonged bleeding time
- Positive tourniquet test
- Prolonged thrombin-prothrombin time test
- Decreased levels of factor VIII

Immunologic Assessment
Serum electrophoresis usually demonstrates the overproduction of IgM (19S) antibodies. Diagnosis is made by the demonstration of a homogeneous M component composed of monoclonal IgM. Quantitation of immunoglobulins reveals IgM levels ranging from 1 to 12 g/dL (usually, >3 g/dL), accounting for 20% to 70% of total protein. Characteristically, blood samples are described as having hyperviscosity.

In addition, cryoglobulins can be detected in the patient's serum. Cryoglobulins are proteins that precipitate or gel when cooled to 0° C (32° F) and dissolve when heated. In most cases, monoclonal cryoglobulins are IgM or IgG. Occasionally, the macroglobulin is cryoprecipitable and capable of cold-induced, anti-I–mediated agglutination of RBCs. IgM may also occasionally be a pyroglobulin, which precipitates on heating to 50° C to 60° C (122° F to 140° F) but does not redissolve on cooling or intensified heating, as do typical BJ pyroglobulins. Many cryoglobulins have the ability to fix complement and initiate an inflammatory reaction similar to that of antigen-antibody complexes. Cryoglobulins have been classified into the following three types:

- Type I is composed of a single class. IgM and IgG classes are most common; IgA or light-chain, single cryoglobulins are seen less frequently. Type I constitutes about 25% of cryoglobulins and is generally associated with multiple myeloma, macroglobulinemia, and other, rarer neoplastic proliferations of plasma cells and lymphocytes.
- Type II cryoglobulins consist of two forms. The monoclonal form always has rheumatoid factor activity and usually is an IgM with κ light chains. The second form is polyclonal IgG, which reacts with the monoclonal IgM rheumatoid factor.
- Type III is a mixed cryoglobulin in which both constituent immunoglobulins are polyclonal. More than 90% of type III cryoglobulins contain IgM rheumatoid factor and IgG. Type III cryoglobulins are seen in a variety of autoimmune, systemic rheumatic diseases and persistent infections with immune complexes (e.g., bacterial endocarditis).

Treatment
Current treatment of WM includes single-agent alkylator, nucleoside analogue, or standard-dose rituximab therapy. Newer studies have suggested that extended-dose rituximab and other treatment options are likely to yield as good or even better results than currently recommended therapy. These include therapy with nucleoside analogues or alkylator agents, rituximab in combination with nucleoside analogues, nucleoside analogues plus alkylator agents, and combination chemotherapy (e.g., cyclophosphamide, doxorubicin, vincristine, prednisone [CHOP]) or cyclophosphamide and dexamethasone.

OTHER MONOCLONAL DISORDERS
Monoclonal Gammopathy of Undetermined Significance
MGUS represents the presence of a monoclonal protein in patients with no features of multiple myeloma or related malignant disorders (e.g., WM, B cell lymphoma, chronic lymphocytic leukemia). MGUS was originally considered a benign monoclonal gammopathy, but it is now known that this disorder can evolve into a malignant monoclonal gammopathy.

The International Myeloma Working Group has established the differences between MGUS and plasma cell neoplasms (Table 27-5). Characteristics of MGUS include the following:

- Serum monoclonal protein concentration less than 3 g/dL
- Fewer than 10% plasma cells in the bone marrow
- Absence of lytic bone lesions
- Anemia
- Hypercalcemia

Table 27-5	Diagnostic Criteria for Monoclonal Gammopathy of Undetermined Significance, Multiple Myeloma, and Waldenström's Macroglobulinemia			
	MGUS	**Smoldering Multiple Myeloma**	**Multiple Myeloma**	**Waldenström's Macroglobulinemia**
Bone marrow plasma cells	<10% *and*	≥10% *and/or*	≥10% *and/or*	>10% *and* <10% lymphoplasmacytoid cells
Circulating monoclonal protein	<3 g/dL	≥3 g/dL	≥3 g/dL	>3 g/dL
Clinical signs and symptoms	Absent	Absent	Present	Present

Adapted from International Myeloma Working Group: Criteria for the classification of monoclonal gammopathies, multiple myeloma and related disorders, Br J Haematol 121:749–757, 2003.

- Renal insufficiency
- No clinical signs or symptoms related to the monoclonal gammopathy

In terms of incidence, 50% of patients with a monoclonal gammopathy have MGUS and 15% to 20% have multiple myeloma. The incidence of MGUS increases with age. The median age at diagnosis is about 70 years. MGUS occurs more frequently in men than women and more often in blacks than in whites. IgG is the most common immunoglobulin affected, followed by IgM. The cause is unknown.

The monoclonal gammopathies are characterized by a rearrangement of immunoglobulin genes that result in the production of a monoclonal protein. There are two populations of plasma cells in patients with MGUS: (1) normal and polyclonal (CD38+, CD56+, CD19–); and (2) clonal with an abnormal immunophenotype (CD38+, CD56+, CD19–). The plasma cell clone and associated monoclonal protein concentrations usually remain stable for many years. After a prolonged period, a substantial number of patients with MGUS progress to a malignant plasma cell disorder (e.g., MM, B cell lymphoma, chronic lymphocytic leukemia).

Recommended laboratory testing includes the following:
- Hemoglobin concentration
- Serum calcium concentration
- Creatinine concentration
- Bone marrow aspiration examination
- Total serum protein concentration and serum electrophoresis (serum monoclonal protein concentration)
- 24-hour urine protein excretion concentration and urine electrophoresis (urine monoclonal protein concentration)
- Serum and urine immunofixation (type of monoclonal protein)
- Determination of serum FLC ratio (κ and λ FLCs), particularly for the assessment of prognosis

Light-Chain Disease

Light-chain disease represents about 10% to 15% of monoclonal gammopathies, ranking behind IgG and IgA myelomas, which represent about 60% and 15%, respectively. LCD occurs about as frequently as WM. In LCD, only κ or λ monoclonal light chains or BJ proteins are produced.

Diagnostic evaluation of suspected LCD is similar to the protocol for any lymphoproliferative disorder, but certain changes in approach are necessary because of the low levels of paraprotein that can be involved. Agarose high-resolution protein electrophoresis of serum and urine should be carried out to determine the total protein concentration. A 24-hour urine specimen should be examined electrophoretically because almost all the protein may be BJ protein. Visual examination of the electrophoretic pattern is essential because a small light-chain band frequently does not exhibit a significant peak on densitometric scanning. Serum protein electrophoretic patterns from patients with monoclonal gammopathies may demonstrate the following:
- Typical, well-defined monoclonal band
- Somewhat broad diffuse band caused by polymerization of monoclonal protein
- Normal gamma region
- Hypogammaglobulinemia

Heavy-Chain Disease

As the name implies, heavy-chain disease is characterized by the presence of monoclonal proteins composed of the heavy-chain portion of the immunoglobulin molecule. The term *Franklin's disease* is synonymous with gamma heavy-chain disease. Alpha heavy-chain disease is the most common of the heavy-chain gammopathies and is frequently seen in men of Mediterranean descent. Mu heavy-chain disease is rare.

Heavy chains may be detected in serum, urine, or both (depending on the class of heavy chain involved). When heavy-chain disease is suspected, nonspecific anti-Fab antisera should be used for definitive testing. The serum sample should also be diluted and retested with κ and λ light-chain antisera to rule out prozoning caused by antigen excess.

Gammopathies With More Than One Band

In some cases, more than one monoclonal band is produced. Although gammopathies with two bands may represent a true biclonal condition, routine laboratory techniques cannot distinguish between the various mechanisms that could produce two or more monoclonal bands. Therefore, a serum specimen with an IgG κ and IgA λ band should be appropriately reported as a gammopathy with IgG κ and IgA λ monoclonal bands.

The appearance of more than one band on electrophoresis is often associated with an advanced gammopathy, in which the asynchronous production of the components of the immunoglobulin molecule occurs. In such cases, synthesis of an intact monoclonal immunoglobulin and an excess of monoclonal light chains may be observed. An example of the demonstration of more than one band on electrophoresis can include cases in which the pentameric IgM breaks down into 7S subunits, which appear on electrophoresis as one or more extra monoclonal bands. In addition, monoclonal IgA molecules tend to dimerize and the resulting dimer often has a different mobility than the monomer parent molecule.

CASE STUDY

History and Physical Examination

A 58-year-old nuclear power plant worker sees his family physician because of increasing fatigue and weakness. He also reports pain in his lower back and arms when he walks. Physical examination reveals that the man has pale mucous membranes and hepatosplenomegaly. The physician orders a complete blood count (CBC) and urinalysis (UA). A follow-up appointment is scheduled for the following week.

Laboratory Data

The CBC reveals that the patient has anemia. His leukocyte count and differential count are normal, except for a rouleaux (rolled coin) appearance of the RBCs. The UA is normal. The patient is called and requested to return to the laboratory for additional tests. The physician orders ESR, kidney screening profile, liver blood profile, and radiographic skeletal survey, with the following results:
- ESR—50 mm/hr
- Kidney profile—normal
- Liver profile—normal, except for increased globular protein
- Skeletal survey—bone lesions in various sites

Questions

1. To follow up with the diagnosis of this patient, a _____ would be of value.
   a. Hemoglobin electrophoresis
   b. Serum electrophoresis
   c. Immunoelectrophoresis
   d. Both b and c
2. A risk factor for an immunologic disease is significant in this patient because of:
   a. Age
   b. Occupation
   c. Gender
   d. Recreational lifestyle

See Appendix A for the answers to multiple choice questions.

Critical Thinking Group Discussion Questions

1. What follow-up laboratory tests might be ordered to assist in establishing a definitive diagnosis?
2. What is the nature of the protein found in the urine?
3. What is the most significant laboratory finding in this disorder?
4. What type of immunologic defect exists in this disease process?
5. Does this patient have a risk of occupational exposure?

See instructor site ⊖volve website for the discussion of the answers to these questions.

Bence Jones Protein Screening Procedure

Principle

Heat solubility is used to detect Bence Jones (BJ) protein, the urinary protein characteristic of multiple myeloma (MM). BJ protein is soluble in urine at room and body temperatures. When the urine is heated, BJ protein forms a precipitate around 60° C to 70° C, and then dissolves at 100° C, but reappears on cooling. The minimal detectable concentration of BJ protein is about 30 mg/dL. Excessive amounts of acid or salt will prevent the appearance of the precipitate.

Procedure

Refer to ⊖volve website for the procedural protocol.

Clinical Applications

Bence Jones protein is found in the urine of many patients with MM, osteogenic sarcoma, osteomalacia, and carcinomatosis.

CHAPTER HIGHLIGHTS

- Hypergammaglobulinemias are monoclonal or polyclonal.
- A monoclonal gammopathy can be benign or malignant and results from a single clone of lymphoid plasma cells producing elevated levels of a single class and type of immunoglobulin, referred to as a monoclonal protein, M protein, or paraprotein. These disorders include multiple myeloma (MM) and Waldenström's macroglobulinemia (WM). MM is the most common form of dysproteinemia.
- A polyclonal gammopathy is classified as a secondary disease and is characterized by the elevation of two or more immunoglobulins produced by several clones of plasma cells. Polyclonal protein consists of one or more heavy-chain classes; both light-chain types increase as secondary manifestations of infection or inflammation.
- The cause of MM is unknown, but radiation may be a factor; a viral cause has also been suggested. Other causes may include environmental stimuli or genetic factors.

- Signs and symptoms of MM include bone pain (back or chest), weakness, fatigue, and pallor associated with anemia or abnormal bleeding.
- Proteinuria is a common finding in more than 50% of patients excreting abnormal amounts of Bence Jones (BJ) protein (light chains). Patients have defects in humoral but not cellular immunity.
- Laboratory diagnosis of MM includes electrophoresis of the serum or urine. A monoclonal protein is seen in the serum and urine in 90% of patients. DNA hybridization or blotting technology can be used to detect abnormal genes in B cells. Although the gene product of monoclonal antibodies (MAbs) is the method of detection, DNA probes that detect the abnormal gene are available. Blotting techniques may replace the current laboratory evaluation of monoclonal gammopathies.
- WM is a malignant cell disorder that exhibits abnormally large amounts of 19S IgM. The cause is unknown, but a genetic predisposition may exist.
- WM has an indolent progression over many years. The basic abnormality is uncontrolled proliferation of B lymphocytes and plasma cells.
- Laboratory diagnosis of WM involves serum electrophoresis showing a homogeneous M component composed of monoclonal IgM. Blood samples characteristically display hyperviscosity. In addition, cryoglobulins can be detected.
- Other monoclonal disorders include light-chain disease (LCD), which represents about 10% to 15% of monoclonal gammopathies. In LCD, only κ or λ monoclonal light chains or BJ proteins are produced. A 24-hour urine specimen should be examined electrophoretically because almost all the protein may be BJ.
- Heavy-chain disease is characterized by monoclonal proteins composed of the heavy-chain portion of the immunoglobulin molecule. Alpha heavy-chain disease is most common.

REVIEW QUESTIONS

1. Polyclonal gammopathies can be exhibited as a secondary manifestation of all the following except:
   a.   Chronic infection
   b.   Chronic liver disease
   c.   Multiple myeloma
   d.   Rheumatoid connective disease

2. What is the most frequent cause of death in a patient with multiple myeloma?
   a.   Skeletal destruction
   b.   Chronic renal failure
   c.   Neurologic disorders
   d.   Infectious disease

3. Patients with multiple myeloma have defects in:
   a.   Cellular immunity
   b.   Humoral immunity
   c.   Synthesis of normal immunoglobulins
   d.   Both b and c

4. What is the most consistent immunologic feature of multiple myeloma?
   a.   Synthesis of dysfunctional single monoclonal proteins
   b.   Synthesis of Ig chains or fragments
   c.   Presence of M protein in serum and/or urine
   d.   All of the above

5 and 6.   Fill in the blanks, choosing the correct temperature (a-d).

Bence-Jones proteins are soluble at room temperature, form a precipitate near (5) _____, and then dissolve (resolubilize) at (6) _____.
   a.   37° C
   b.   50° C
   c.   60° C
   d.   100° C

7. M proteins are associated with all the following malignant conditions except:
   a.   Multiple myeloma
   b.   Plasmacytoma
   c.   Malignant lymphoproliferative diseases
   d.   Lymphoma

8. Cryoglobulins are proteins that precipitate or gel at:
   a.   –18° C
   b.   –4° C
   c.   0° C
   d.   4° C

9. Monoclonal gammopathy involves elevated levels of a single class and type of immunoglobulin referred to as:
   a.   Monoclonal protein
   b.   M protein
   c.   Paraprotein
   d.   All of the above

10 and 11.   Fill in the blanks, choosing from the following answers:

In light-chain disease, only (10) _____ or (11) _____ monoclonal light chains are synthesized by a one-cell clone.

Possible answers to question 10:	Possible answers to question 11:
a. beta	a. lambda
b. gamma	b. alpha
c. kappa	c. beta
d. alpha	d. gamma

12. Multiple myeloma is also referred to as:
   a.   Plasma cell myeloma
   b.   Kahler's disease
   c.   Myelomatosis
   d.   All of the above

13. Most patients with multiple myeloma manifest:
    a. Bone pain
    b. Acute renal failure
    c. No symptoms
    d. Hepatomegaly and splenomegaly

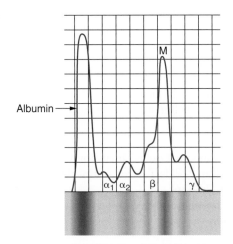

Albumin →

M

α₁ α₂ β γ

14. The figure above represents the serum electrophoresis of a patient with:
    a. Waldenström's macroglobulinemia
    b. Multiple myeloma
    c. No protein abnormality
    d. Polyclonal gammopathy

15. Patients with Waldenström's macroglobulinemia exhibit abnormally large amounts of:
    a. IgM
    b. IgG
    c. IgE
    d. IgA

16. Monoclonal gammopathy of undetermined significance (MGUS) represents a:
    a. Monoclonal protein in patients with no features of multiple myeloma or related malignant disorders
    b. Disorder that can evolve into a malignant monoclonal gammopathy
    c. Serum monoclonal protein concentration less than 3 g/dL
    d. All of the above

17. MGUS is characterized by all the following except:
    a. Fewer than 10% plasma cells in the bone marrow
    b. Presence of lytic bone lesions
    c. Anemia
    d. Hypercalcemia

18. Light-chain disease represents about _____ of monoclonal gammopathies.
    a. 5% to 10%
    b. 10% to 15%
    c. 15% to 25%
    d. 25% to 50%

BIBLIOGRAPHY

Barlogie B, et al: Thalidomide and hematopoietic-cell transplantation for multiple myeloma, N Engl J Med 543:1021–1029, 2006.

Blade J: Monoclonal gammopathy of undetermined significance, N Engl J Med 355: 2765–2670, 2006.

Bradwell AR: Serum free light chain analysis, ed 4, Birmingham, England, 2006, Binding Site.

Cohen AD, Comenzo RL: Systemic light-chain amyloidosis: advances in diagnosis, prognosis, and therapy, Hematology Am Soc Hematol Educ Program 287–294, 2010.

Grass S, et al: Hyperphosphorylated paratarg-7: a new molecularly defined risk factor for monoclonal gammopathy of undetermined significance of the IgM type and Waldenström macroglobulinemia, Blood 117:2918–2923, 2011.

Heher EC, et al: Kidney disease associated with plasma cell dyscrasias, Blood 116:1397–1404, 2010.

Jakubikova J, et al: Lenalidomide targets clonogenic side population in multiple myeloma: pathophysiologic and clinical implications, Blood 117:4409–4419, 2010.

Killingsworth LM, Warren BM: Immunofixation for the identification of monoclonal gammopathies, Beaumont, Tex, 1986, Helena Laboratories.

Kyle A, et al: Prevalence of monclonal gammopathy of undetermined significance, N Engl J Med 354:1362–1369, 2006.

Kyle RA, Rajkumar SV: Multiple myeloma, N Engl J Med 351:1860–1871, 2004.

Martin-Perez D, Piris MA, Sanchez-Beato M: Polycomb proteins in hematologic malignancies, Blood 116:5465–5475, 2010.

Moreaux J, et al: CD200 is a new prognostic factor in multiple myeloma, Blood 108:4194–4197, 2006.

Noonan K, et al: A novel role of IL-17 producing lymphocytes in mediating lytic bone disease in multiple myeloma, Blood 116:3554–3563, 2010.

Palumbo A, Anderson K: Multiple myeloma, N Eng J Med 364:1046–1058, 2011.

Popovic R, Licht JD: MEK and MAF in myeloma therapy, Blood 117:2300–2301, 2011.

Prabhala RH, et al: Dysfunctional T regulatory cells in multiple myeloma, Blood 107:301–304, 2006.

Roccaro AM, et al: MicroRNA-dependent modulation of histone actylation in Waldenström macroglobulinemia, Blood 116:1506–1514, 2010.

Treon SP, et al: Update on treatment recommendations from the Third International Workshop on Waldenström's Macroglobulinemia, Blood 107:3442–3446, 2006.

Treon SP, et al: MYD88 L265P Somatic mutation in Waldenstrom's macroglobulinemia, N Eng J Med 367:1046: 10826-10833, 2012.

Turgeon ML: Clinical hematology: theory and procedures, ed 5, Philadelphia, 2012, Lippincott Williams & Wilkins.

Usmani SZ, et al: Second malignancies in total therapy 2 and 3 for newly diagnosed multiple myeloma: influence of thalidomide and lenalidomide during maintenance, Blood 120:1597–1600, 2012.

Waage A, et al: Melphalan and prednisone plus thalidomide or placebo in elderly patients with multiple myeloma, Blood 116:1405–1412, 2010.

Waxman A, et al: Racial disparities in incidence and outcome in multiple myeloma: a population-based study, Blood 116:5501–5506, 2010.

CHAPTER 28

Autoimmune Disorders

Learning Objectives

At the conclusion of this chapter, the reader should be able to:

- Describe the nature of autoimmune disorders.
- Compare organ-specific and organ-nonspecific characteristics.
- Describe organ-specific and midspectrum disorders.
- Analyze representative case studies.

- Correctly answer case study related multiple choice questions.
- Be prepared to participate in a discussion of case study related critical thinking questions.
- Describe the principle, sources of error, limitations, and application of the antinucleoprotein slide test.
- Correctly answer end of chapter review questions.

Key Terms

antinuclear antibodies (ANAs)
autoantibodies
autoantigens
autoimmune disorder

exogenous factors
IF-blocking antibodies
immune complex
immunocompetent cells

immunoregulation
intrinsic factor (IF)
prealbumin band
vasculitic syndromes

The major autoimmune diseases, e.g., systemic lupus erythematosus (see Chapter 29), rheumatoid arthritis (see Chapter 30), diabetes type 1, and multiple sclerosis share many common features. Chronic and other intermittent inflammation contributes over time to the destruction of target organs that contain inciting antigens or are the sites of immune-complex deposition. Although the adaptive immune system has long been the focus of attention, innate immune mechanisms are now viewed as central to the pathogenesis of these disorders. New genetic findings emphasize the identification of environmental components that interact with host genetic factors are being important to developing a deeper understanding of autoimmunity.

WHAT IS AUTOIMMUNITY?

Autoimmunity represents a breakdown of the immune system's ability to discriminate between self and nonself. The term *autoimmune disorder* refers to a varied group of more than

80 serious, chronic illnesses that involve almost every human organ system. In all these disorders, the underlying problem is similar; the body's immune system becomes misdirected, attacking the organs it was designed to protect.

Autoimmune disorders remain among the most poorly understood and poorly recognized of any category of illnesses. Individually, autoimmune disorders occur infrequently, except for thyroid disease, diabetes, rheumatoid arthritis, and systemic lupus erythematosus. Overall, autoimmune disorders represent the fourth largest cause of disability in Europe and the United States.

The term *autoimmune disorder* is used when demonstrable immunoglobulins (autoantibodies) or cytotoxic T cells display specificity for self antigens, or **autoantigens,** and contribute to the pathogenesis of the disorder (Table 28-1). Autoimmune disorders are characterized by the persistent activation of immunologic effector mechanisms that alter the function and integrity of individual cells and organs. The sites of organ or tissue damage

Table 28-1	Autoimmune Disorders and Associated Abnormalities
Clinical Diagnosis	**Autoantigen**
Addison's disease	P-450 enzymes
Crohn's disease	p-ANCA, pancreatic acinar cells
Ovarian failure/infertility	P-450 enzymes
Pernicious anemia	Parietal cells
Ulcerative colitis	p-ANCA

Box 28-1	Examples of Autoimmune Diseases

Active chronic hepatitis
Addison's disease
Autoimmune atrophic gastritis
Autoimmune hemolytic anemia
Dermatomyositis
Discoid lupus erythematosus
Goodpasture's syndrome
Hashimoto's thyroiditis
Idiopathic thrombocytopenic purpura
Insulin-dependent (juvenile, type 1) diabetes mellitus
Multiple sclerosis
Myasthenia gravis
Pemphigus vulgaris
Pernicious anemia
Primary biliary cirrhosis
Primary myxedema
Rheumatoid arthritis
Scleroderma
Sjögren's syndrome
Systemic lupus erythematosus
Thyrotoxicosis

depend on the location of the immune reaction. The variety of signs and symptoms seen in patients with autoimmune disorders reflects the various forms of the immune response.

It is also important to note that autoantibodies may be formed in patients secondary to tissue damage or when no evidence of clinical disease exists. Unlike autoimmune disorders, autoantibodies can occur as immune correlates of conditions such as blood transfusion reactions. In addition, autoantibodies can be demonstrated in hemolytic disease of the newborn and graft rejection and can result from disorders such as serum sickness, anaphylaxis, and hay fever when the immune response is clearly the cause of the disease.

SPECTRUM OF AUTOIMMUNE DISORDERS

Many disorders are believed to be related to immunologic abnormalities and additional diseases are continually being identified (Box 28-1). Autoimmune disorders exhibit a full spectrum of tissue reactivity (Fig. 28-1). At one extreme are organ-specific disorders such as Hashimoto's disease of the thyroid; at the other extreme are disorders that manifest as organ-nonspecific diseases, such as systemic lupus erythematosus

(SLE; see Chapter 29) and rheumatoid arthritis (RA; see Chapter 30; Table 28-2).

In organ-specific disorders, both the lesions produced by tissue damage and the autoantibodies are directed at a single target organ (e.g., the thyroid). Midspectrum disorders are characterized by localized lesions in a single organ and by organ-nonspecific autoantibodies. For example, in primary biliary cirrhosis, the small bile duct is the main target of inflammatory cell infiltration, but the serum autoantibodies are mainly mitochondrial antibodies and are not liver-specific.

Organ-nonspecific disorders are characterized by the presence of both lesions and autoantibodies not confined to any one organ.

FACTORS INFLUENCING DEVELOPMENT OF AUTOIMMUNITY

Autoimmunity begins with an abnormal interaction of T and B lymphocytes with autoantigens. No single theory or mechanism has been identified as a cause. The potential for autoimmunity, if given appropriate circumstances, is constantly present in every immunocompetent individual because lymphocytes that are potentially reactive with self antigens exist in the body. Antibody expression appears to be regulated by a complex set of interacting factors; these influences include genetic factors, patient age, and **exogenous factors.**

Genetic Factors

Although a direct genetic cause has not been established in autoimmune disease, there is a tendency for familial aggregates to occur. In addition, there is a tendency for more than one autoimmune disorder to occur in the same individual. For example, patients with Hashimoto's disease have a higher incidence of pernicious anemia than would be expected in a random population matched for age and gender.

Another factor related to genetic inheritance is that autoimmune disorders and autoantibodies are found more frequently in women than in men. The presence of certain human leukocyte antigens (HLAs) is also associated with an increased risk of certain autoimmune states.

Patient Age

Autoantibodies are manifested infrequently in the general population. The incidence of autoantibodies, however, increases steadily with age, reaching a peak at around 60 to 70 years.

Exogenous Factors

Ultraviolet radiation, drugs, viruses, and chronic infectious disease may all play a role in the development of autoimmune disorders. These factors may alter antigens, which the body then perceives as nonself antigens.

IMMUNOPATHOGENIC MECHANISMS

Autoimmune disorders are usually prevented by the normal functioning of immunologic regulatory mechanisms. When these controls dysfunction, antibodies to self antigens may be

Organ-Specific Disorders   Organ-Nonspecific Disorders

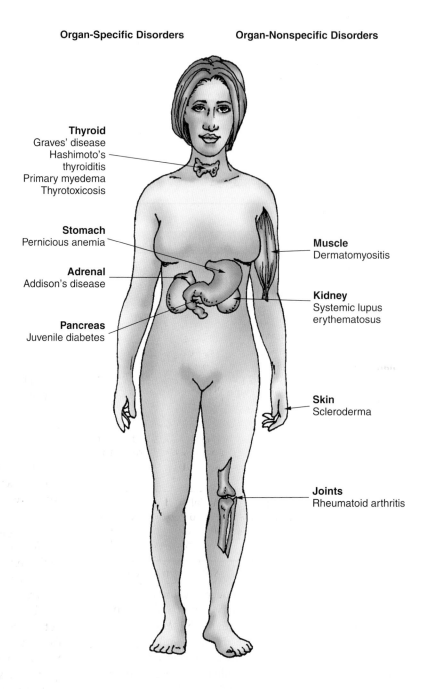

Thyroid
Graves' disease
Hashimoto's
thyroiditis
Primary myedema
Thyrotoxicosis

Stomach
Pernicious anemia

Adrenal
Addison's disease

Pancreas
Juvenile diabetes

Muscle
Dermatomyositis

Kidney
Systemic lupus
erythematosus

Skin
Scleroderma

Joints
Rheumatoid arthritis

Figure 28-1   Autoimmune disorders.

produced and bind to antigens in the circulation to form circulating immune complexes or to antigens deposited in specific tissue sites.

The mechanisms governing the deposition in one organ or another are unknown; however, several mechanisms may be operative in a single disease. Wherever antigen-antibody complexes accumulate, complement can be activated, with the subsequent release of mediators of inflammation. These mediators increase vascular permeability, attract phagocytic cells to the reaction site, and cause local tissue damage. Alternatively, cytotoxic T cells can directly attack body cells bearing the target antigen, which releases mediators that amplify the inflammatory reaction. Autoantibody and complement fragments coat cells bearing the target antigen, which leads to destruction by phagocytes or antibody-seeking K-type lymphocytes.

An individual may develop an autoimmune response to a variety of immunogenic stimuli (Table 28-3). These responses may be caused by the following:

• Antigens that do not normally circulate in the blood

The hidden antigen (sequestered antigen) theory is one of the earliest views of organ-specific antibodies. Antigens are sequestered within the organ and, because of the lack of contact with the mononuclear phagocyte system, they fail to establish immunologic tolerance. Any conditions producing a release of antigen would then provide an opportunity for autoantibody formation. This situation occurs when sperm cells or lens and heart tissues are released directly into the circulation, and autoantibodies are formed. Unmodified extracts of

Table 28-2	**Summary of Organ-Specific and Organ-Nonspecific Disorders**

Similarities

1. Circulating autoantibodies react with normal body constituents.

2. Increased immunoglobulin concentration in serum often found.

3. Antibodies may appear in each of the main immunoglobulin classes.

4. Disease process not always progressive; exacerbations and remissions occur.

5. Autoantibody tests of diagnostic value.

Differences

Organ-Specific	Organ-Nonspecific
Antibodies and lesions are organ-specific.	Antibodies and lesions are organ nonspecific.
Clinical and serologic overlap (e.g., thyroid, stomach, adrenal glands, kidney).	Overlap of SLE, RA, and other connective tissue disorders.
Antigens only available to lymphoid system in low concentrations.	Antigens accessible at higher concentrations.
Antigens evoke organ-specific antibodies in normal animals with complete Freund's adjuvant.	No antibodies produced in animals with comparable stimulation.
Familial tendency to develop organ-specific autoimmunity.	Familial tendency to develop connective tissue disease. Questionable abnormalities in immunoglobulin synthesis in relatives.
Lymphoid invasion, parenchymal destruction by questionable cell-mediated hypersensitivity or antibodies.	Lesions caused by deposition of antigen-antibody (immune) complexes.
Tendency to develop cancer in the organ.	Tendency to develop lymphoreticular neoplasia.

Table 28-3	**Antigens Implicated in Autoimmune Endocrine Diseases**

Disorder	Antigen
Hashimoto's disease	Thyroglobulin Thyroid peroxidase Thyrotropin receptor
Graves' disease	Thyrotropin receptor Thyroid peroxidase Thyroglobulin 64-kDa antigen 70-kDa heat shock protein
Type 1 diabetes	Insulin/proinsulin Insulin receptor Glutamic acid decarboxylase B cell release granule Pancreatic cytokeratin 64-kDa antigen Glucagon 65-kDa heat shock protein
Addison's disease	Adrenal cortical cells 55-kDa microsomal antigen
Idiopathic hypoparathyroidism	130- and 200-kDa antigens Endothelial antigen Mitochondrial antigen

immune response involves interaction of cellular elements such as lymphocytes and macrophages, antigens, antibody, immune complexes, and complement.

SELF-RECOGNITION (TOLERANCE)

In the initial stage of some diseases, infiltration by T lymphocytes may induce inflammation and tissue damage, leading to alterations in self antigens and production of autoantibodies. In other diseases, only the production of autoantibodies is noted with tissue damage. These autoantibodies attack cell surface antigens or membrane receptors or combine with antigen to form immune complexes that are deposited in tissue, subsequently causing complement activation and inflammation.

An immune response requires presentation of a foreign antigen by an antigen-presenting cell (APC) and another signal from the appropriate major histocompatibility complex (MHC) molecule on the host's cells. Both are needed for an immune response. Tolerance is the lack of immune response to self antigens and is initiated during fetal development (central tolerance) by the elimination of cells with the potential to react strongly with self antigens. Peripheral tolerance is a process involving mature lymphocytes and occurs in the circulation. Central tolerance develops in the thymus during fetal life. Self antigens are presented by dendritic cells to self-reactive T cells that are responsible for positive and negative selection of specific lymphocytes. The ultimate goal is to remove T lymphocytes that respond strongly to self antigens. As genes rearrange and code for antigen receptors, the T cell receptors (TCRs) produced may or may not be specific for the MHC expressed on that

tissues involved in organ-specific autoimmune disorders, however, do not readily elicit antibody formation.

- Altered antigens that arise because of chemical, physical, or biological processes (e.g., hapten complexing, physical denaturation, mutation)
- A foreign antigen that is shared or cross-reactive with self antigens or tissue components
- Mutation of **immunocompetent cells** to acquire a response to self antigens
- Loss of the immunoregulatory function by T lymphocyte subsets

Understanding the mechanism of autoimmunity requires an understanding of the regulation of the immune response. The

individual's cells. Positive selection cells that have TCRs capable of responding with self antigens (low-level MHC affinity) are selected for continued growth.

Self-recognition (tolerance) is induced by at least two mechanisms involving contact between antigen and immunocompetent cells:

- Elimination of the small clone of immunocompetent cells programmed to react with the antigen (Burnet's clonal selection theory)
- Induction of unresponsiveness in the immunocompetent cells through excessive antigen binding to them and triggering of a suppressor mechanism

The normal immune response is modulated by antigen-specific and antigen-nonspecific suppressor cell activity.

MAJOR AUTOANTIBODIES

Major autoantibodies can be detected in different disorders. Many diagnostic laboratory tests (Box 28-2) are based on detecting these autoimmune responses. Common autoantibodies include thyroid, gastric, adrenocortical, striated muscle, acetylcholine receptor, smooth muscle, salivary gland, mitochondrial, reticulin, myelin, islet cell, and skin. Antibodies to **antinuclear antibodies (ANAs)** include deoxyribonucleic acid (DNA), histone, and nonhistone protein antibodies.

ORGAN-SPECIFIC AND MIDSPECTRUM DISORDERS

Cardiovascular Disorders

The primary immunologic diseases of the blood vessels are termed *vasculitis;* those of the heart are termed *carditis.*

Vasculitis

Deposition of circulating immune complexes is considered directly or indirectly responsible for many forms of vasculitis. The inflammatory lesions of blood vessels produce variable injury or necrosis of the blood vessel wall. This may result in narrowing, occlusion, or thrombosis of the lumen or aneurysm formation or rupture. Vasculitis occurs as a primary disease process or as a secondary manifestation of another disease (e.g., RA).

Vasculitis is characterized by inflammation within blood vessels, which often results in a compromise of the vessel lumen with ischemia. Ischemia causes the major manifestations of the **vasculitic syndromes** and determines the prognosis. Any size and type of blood vessel may be involved. Therefore, the vasculitic syndromes are a heterogeneous group of diseases (Box 28-3).

Antibodies specific to endothelial cells also contribute to immune vasculopathy. Antiendothelial antibodies are autoantibodies directed against antigens in the cytoplasmic membrane of endothelial cells.

Carditis

The heart shares a susceptibility to immune-mediated injury with other organs. Numerous cardiac diseases are characterized by the presence of inflammatory cells within the myocardium resulting from immune sensitization to endogenous or exogenous cardiac

---

Box 28-2	**Major Autoantibodies**
Acetylcholine receptor (AChR)–binding antibody	Antireticulin antibody
Acetylcholine receptor (AChR)–blocking antibody	Anti–rheumatoid arthritis nuclear antigen (anti-RANA; RA precipitin)
Antiadrenal antibody	Antiribosome antibody
Anticardiolipin antibody	Anti–nuclear ribonucleoprotein (anti-nRNP) antibody
Anticentriole antibody	Anti-Scl antibody or anti–Scl-70 antibody
Anticentromere antibody	Antiskin (dermal-epidermal) antibody
	Antiskin (interepithelial) antibody
Anti-DNA antibody	Anti-Sm antibody
Anti–glomerular basement membrane antibody	Anti–smooth muscle antibody
Anti–intrinsic factor antibody	Antisperm antibody
Anti–islet cell antibody	Anti-SS-A (SS-A precipitin; anti-Ro) antibody
Anti–liver-kidney microsomal (anti-LKM) antibody	Anti-SS-B (SS-B precipitin, anti-La) antibody
Antimitochondrial antibody	Antistriational antibody
Antimyelin antibody	Antithyroglobulin and antithyroid microsome antibody
Antimyocardial antibody	Histone-reactive antinuclear antibody (HR-ANA)
Antineutrophil antibody	Jo-1 antibody
Antinuclear antibody (ANA)	Ku antibody
Anti–parietal cell antibody	Mi-1 antibody
Antiplatelet antibody	PM-1 antibody

BOX 28-3	**Classification of Vasculitic Syndromes**

Systemic necrotizing arteritis
    Polyarteritis nodosa
    Allergic angiitis and granulomatosis
    Overlap syndrome
Hypersensitivity vasculitis
    Henoch-Schönlein purpura
    McDuffie's syndrome
Wegener's granulomatosis
Lymphomatoid granulomatosis
Giant cell arteritis
    Takayasu's arteritis
Mucocutaneous lymph node syndrome
    (Kawasaki's disease)
Behçet's disease
Thromboangiitis obliterans
Central nervous system vasculitis
Miscellaneous
    Cogan's syndrome
    Eales disease
    Hypereosinophilic syndrome with vasculitis

antigens. The consequent reaction of cardiac myocytes to immune injury can range from reversible modulation of their electrical and mechanical capabilities to cell death. Carditis can be caused by a variety of conditions, including acute rheumatic fever, Lyme disease, and cardiac transplant rejection.

Myocardial contractility can be impaired by cell-mediated injury or the local release of cytokines. The study of immune cardiac disease has entered a period of rapid expansion. Primary idiopathic myocarditis is an autoimmune disease characterized by infiltration of the heart by macrophages and lymphocytes. Studies involving the mechanisms whereby immune cells and factors localize in the myocardium, modulate myocyte function, and remodel myocardial architecture are under way.

A diagnosis of acute rheumatic fever requires differentiation from other immunologic and infectious diseases. The immunologic basis for rheumatic heart disease has long been suspected. Patients with rheumatic heart disease exhibit antimyocardial antibodies that bind in vitro to foci in the myocardium and heart valves. These antibodies may be responsible for the deposition of immunoglobulin and complement components found in the same area of rheumatic heart disease tissues at autopsy.

Antimyocardial antibodies appear to be strongly cross-reactive with streptococcal antigens, but they are not toxic to heart tissue unless the latter is damaged previously by some other cause. Because antimyocardial antibodies are often found in patients with a recent myocardial infarction or streptococcal infection without cardiac sequelae, detection of these antibodies has not been a particularly useful differential diagnostic test for cardiac injury. The presence of myocardial antibodies, however, is diagnostic of Dressler's syndrome (cardiac injury) or rheumatic fever.

Collagen Vascular Disorders

Progressive Systemic Sclerosis (Scleroderma)

Scleroderma is a collagen vascular disease of unknown cause that assumes various forms. Eosinophilic fasciitis may be a variant of scleroderma.

The development of scleroderma has been associated with a number of occupations and with drugs such as bleomycin sulfate, tryptophan, and carbidopa. Occupational exposure to vinyl chloride, vibratory stimuli, and silicosis have been associated with the subsequent development of scleroderma.

Epidemiology. Scleroderma occurs in all races and is three times more frequent in women than men.

Signs and Symptoms. Scleroderma is characterized by fibrosis in the skin and internal organs and by arterial occlusions with a distinct proliferative pattern. Initial symptoms usually appear in the third decade of life. Raynaud's phenomenon is the most frequent manifestation. The disease is slowly progressive and chronically disabling, but can be rapidly progressive and fatal.

Immunologic Manifestations. Idiopathic scleroderma is considered an autoimmune disease because of the associated autoantibodies and the overlapping syndromes of scleroderma-polymyositis and scleroderma-SLE.

Antinuclear antibodies are formed in 40% to 90% of patients to the following: (1) extractable nuclear antigens; (2) the

nucleolus; (3) the centromere; and (4) Scl-70. The anticentromere antibody is sensitive and is specific for patients with a subset of scleroderma with CREST syndrome (*c*alcinosis, *R*aynaud's phenomenon, *e*sophageal dysmotility, *s*clerodactyly, and *t*elangiectasia).

In addition, T cell hyperactivity correlates with disease activity. Activated T cells can result in both the vascular changes and increased collagen production in scleroderma. It is now thought that both the vascular disorder and fibrosis result from this cellular immune activation. Vascular injury could be mediated by cytokines or direct cell-cell interaction by activated lymphocytes and endothelial cells.

Signs and Symptoms. Systemic sclerosis is a chronic multisystem disorder that causes thickening of the skin (scleroderma) and involves other organ systems.

In more than 50% of patients, Raynaud's phenomenon occurs before the onset of other manifestations. Skin manifestations can proceed through the stages of pitting edema, a sclerotic hidebound stage, and a final stage of atrophy or softening and a return toward normal. Articular complaints are common. Hypomotility of the gastrointestinal tract is the second most common clinical feature.

Eosinophilia-Myalgia Syndrome

Many people exposed to the agent causing eosinophilia-myalgia syndrome (EMS) may develop illness. Patients develop severe myalgia. More than 50% of patients with EMS develop scleroderma-like manifestations.

The most important predictor of EMS is the ingestion of contaminated L-tryptophan. The association of ingestion of L-tryptophan with a systemic disease now called EMS was first observed in 1989. Some patients have died from the L-tryptophan.

L-Tryptophan was widely used after it was introduced in 1974 as an over-the-counter nostrum for various ailments (e.g., insomnia, premenstrual syndrome, anxiety). Medical professionals also recommended its use for neuropsychiatric or fibromyalgia disorders.

Endocrine Gland Disorders: Thyroid Disease

Numerous endocrine gland disorders are attributable to an autoimmune process. Several of the classic and more common disorders are discussed in this section.

The clinical spectrum of autoimmune thyroid disease is very broad. There are two major forms of autoimmune thyroid disease, chronic autoimmune thyroiditis and Graves' disease.

Lymphoid (Hashimoto's) chronic thyroiditis is a classic example of an organ-specific autoimmune disorder. Other autoimmune disorders affecting the thyroid gland include transient thyroiditis syndrome and idiopathic hypothyroidism.

Lymphoid (Hashimoto's) Chronic Thyroiditis

Etiology. The exact causative mechanism is unknown but is believed to be related to an autoimmune process in which the development of circulating cytotoxic antibodies eventually destroys the thyroid gland, producing hypothyroidism. This disorder is associated with the presence of human

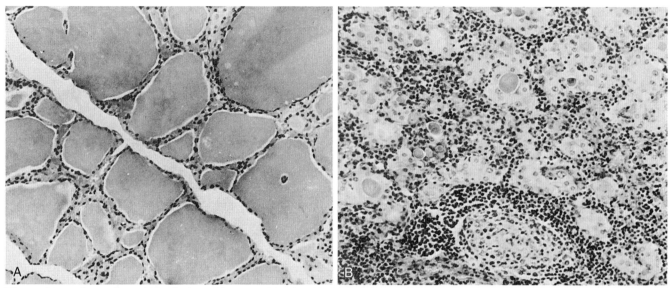

Figure 28-2   Comparison of histologic architecture of the thyroid gland of normal patient, and patient with Hashimoto's disease. A, In the normal thyroid, colloid fills the vesicles, but in a diseased gland **(B)**, only isolated deposits of colloid are seen. The cell infiltrate is lymphoid in nature. Note germinal center in lower middle **(B)**. *(From Anderson JR, Buchanan WW, Goudie RB: Autoimmunity, Springfield, Ill, 1967, Charles C Thomas.)*

leukocyte antigen (HLA)–DR4 and HLA-DR5. However, these associations are not consistent in different races and ethnic groups.

Epidemiology. Lymphoid thyroiditis can occur at any age but is first diagnosed most often in the third to fifth decades of life; it is much more common in women than in men. The fibrous variant of the disease is more often present in middle-aged and older patients.

The mode of inheritance is unknown. However, a genetic tendency to inherit the trait for the development of antibodies against the thyroid gland is highly possible. It is common to have multiple members of a family develop the same disease (e.g., Graves' disease, lymphoid thyroiditis).

Signs and Symptoms. Lymphoid thyroiditis is believed to be the most common cause of sporadic goiter. Characteristically, there is a firm, diffusely enlarged, nontender thyroid gland that may be lobulated. Hypothyroidism, however, is a common late sequela of lymphoid thyroiditis, and patients are usually euthyroid when first seen by a physician. Some individuals have clinical and pathologic evidence of the coexistence of Graves' disease and lymphoid (Hashimoto's) thyroiditis. Histologically, Hashimoto's thyroiditis is characterized by diffuse lymphocytic infiltration (Fig. 28-2).

Immunologic Manifestations

Patients with lymphoid thyroiditis, as well as other autoimmune thyroid disorders, can demonstrate histologic and immunologic manifestations of the disease. Antibodies to thyroid constituents may be observed in these patients. Antibodies to the following constituents may be demonstrated serologically:

- Thyroglobulin
- Thyroid microsome
- Second colloid antigen (CA2 antigen)
- Thyroid membrane receptors
- Thyronine (T_4) and triiodothyronine (T_3)

Thyroglobulin. Antithyroglobulin (TgAb) was the first antibody discovered against a thyroid protein, thyroglobulin. Immunofluorescent laboratory methods using fluorescein-labeled anti–human globulin can demonstrate the binding of antithyroglobulin antibody to thin sections of thyroid tissue in abnormal conditions or in approximately 4% of the normal population. The frequency of positive titers gradually increases in the female population with aging. The absence of antithyroglobulin antibodies, however, does not exclude the diagnosis of Hashimoto's thyroiditis; conversely, the presence of antibodies does not establish the diagnosis because it can be positive in Graves' disease and is occasionally positive in thyroid cancer and subacute thyroiditis. Testing for antibody may also be used to monitor patients with thyroid cancers.

Thyroid Microsomes. Antibodies directed against thyroid microsomes, antithyroid microsomal antibodies, or antithyroperoxidase antibodies (TPO Abs) can be detected in about 7% of the population, with titers ranging from 1:100 to 1:1600. Even a low titer of antithyroid antibodies correlates with a degree of thyroid involvement by an autoimmune process. The absence of antibodies has been documented in diagnosed cases of autoimmune thyroiditis, which may be explained by special characteristics of the antibody, or because it forms complexes with thyroglobulins in the circulation and escapes detection. The presence of these circulating complexes has been documented in patients with thyroid autoimmune disorders.

Second Colloid Antigen. CA2 antigen is directed against a colloid protein and can be detected by immunofluorescent examination. Antibody to CA2 is present in about 50% of patients who have subacute thyroiditis, and it is detectable in some patients with Hashimoto's thyroiditis whose sera show no other evidence of abnormal antibodies.

Thyroid Membrane Receptors. The thyroid membrane receptors are a group of immunoglobulin G (IgG) antibodies that interact with receptors on thyroid membranes. They often produce hyperthyroidism that manifests itself clinically, chemically, and histologically. At present, classification of these IgG antibodies is operational, based on their method of detection. Long-acting thyroid stimulator (LATS) and long-acting thyroid stimulator protector (LATS-P) assays are of importance.

Thyronine and Triiodothyronine. Antibodies to T_4 and T_3 have been found in several patients, most of whom had evidence of a thyroid autoimmune process such as goiter or hypothyroidism. In these cases, the underlying autoimmune process is most likely responsible for the hypothyroidism rather than hormone binding by the circulating antithyronine antibodies.

Diagnostic Evaluation

Fine-needle aspiration biopsy of the thyroid is useful in conjunction with clinical evaluation and serologic studies for the diagnosis of lymphocytic thyroiditis.

Histologic examination of thyroid tissue demonstrates variable infiltration of the entire gland with lymphocytes. Germinal lymphoid centers are characteristic and destruction and distortion of normal thyroid follicles are apparent. The thyroid cells remain intact but are hypertrophied, although the usual heterogeneity of small, enlarged thyroid follicles, some containing flat epithelium, can also be seen. In advanced cases, there is almost complete destruction of normal thyroid tissue, with replacement by lymphocytes or fibrous tissue.

When the disease produces hypothyroidism, a slight increase in plasma thyroid-stimulating hormone (TSH) concentration can usually be demonstrated in the early phase, followed by a decrease in serum T4 and eventually by a decrease in serum T3 levels. Antithyroglobulin and/or antithyroid microsomal antibodies are found in moderate to high titers in more than 50% of patients, but the presence of antimicrosomal antibodies is considered to be more diagnostic.

Antibodies directed against thyroid microsomal antigen (thyroid peroxidase antibody [anti-TPO]) can be detected by various techniques (Table 28-4). Chemiluminescent immunoassay is typically performed to detect anti-TPO autoantibodies. TPO plays a significant role in the biosynthesis of thyroid hormones by catalyzing the iodination of tyrosyl residues in thyroglobulin and the coupling of iodotyrosyl residues to form T_4 and T_3. Autoantibodies produced against TPO are capable of inhibiting enzyme activity. They are also complement-fixing antibodies that can induce cytotoxic changes in cells and consequently cause thyroid dysfunction. More than 90% of patients with autoimmune thyroiditis (Hashimoto's thyroiditis) have anti-TPO. Antibodies to TPO have also been found in most patients with idiopathic hypothyroidism (85%) and Graves' disease (50%).

Graves' Disease

Graves' disease is a form of hyperthyroidism. This disease is most likely if a patient has signs and symptoms of hyperthyroidism. Laboratory chemistry assays usually demonstrate low TSH and elevated free T_4 levels. Of patients with Graves' disease, 50% exhibit thyroid peroxidase antibody (anti-TPO). TSH receptor antibody (TRAb) can discriminate between Graves' disease and toxic nodular goiter. In addition, thyroid-stimulating immunoglobulin can detect thyroid antibodies for diagnosing Graves' disease.

Table 28-4	Antithyroid Antibody Tests
Antigen	**Test to Identify Antibody**
Thyroglobulin	Indirect immunofluorescence on fixed thyroid tissues Tanned RBC hemagglutination Immunometric assays (IMAs) or sandwich methods Radioimmunoassay (RIA)
Microsomal antigen	Enzyme-linked immunosorbent assay (ELISA)
Second colloid antigen (CA2)	Indirect immunofluorescence
Thyroid membrane receptors	LATS LATS-P In vitro assays for thyroid-stimulating immunoglobulin (TSI) or TSH–binding inhibition (TBI)
Triiodothyronine (total T_3)	RIA using different separation methods Electrophoresis with radioactive-labeled thyronines

Pancreatic Disorders

The autoimmune forms of diabetes include type 1 diabetes (T1D), estimated at 5% to 10% of those with diabetes, and latent autoimmune diabetes in adults (LADA), estimated to be 5% to 10% of those diagnosed with type 2 diabetes (T2D). It is now believed that some overlap exists between T1D and T2D. A subset of adult patients diagnosed with T2D actually have LADA.

Insulin-Dependent Diabetes Mellitus

Etiology. Insulin-dependent diabetes mellitus (IDDM), or type 1 diabetes mellitus (T1D), is a disorder of deficient insulin production caused by immune destruction of the B cells of the pancreatic islets. The only definitively identified environmental factor causing T1D is congenital rubella infection. Reports of an association between diabetes and infection with coxsackievirus B and several other viruses have suggested other triggers for the disease.

Genetic susceptibility factors have been identified. T1D is associated with HLA-DR3, DR4, DQ2, and DQ8 antigens. About 90% of white patients with T1D have one or both DR antigens. The presence of both DR3 and DR4 antigens yields an even higher risk of disease development than the additive susceptibility from either antigen, suggesting that other MHC-related genes may be involved in its pathogenesis. Another HLA antigen, DR2, is found less frequently in people with diabetes than in the general population, indicating that this antigen is associated with some type of protective effect. HLA-DQw8 is associated with a twofold to sixfold increased risk for diabetes. Several lines of investigation have implicated the CD4+ T lymphocyte as central in the immune process that leads to the development of diabetes.

Epidemiology. T1D was previously called juvenile-onset diabetes because of when it often presents; 10% of people with diabetes have T1D and approximately 10,000 new cases are diagnosed each year. Most patients develop T1D in childhood or early adolescence, but it may occur at any age. Approximately 95% of patients who develop clinical diabetes before age 30 years have T1D.

Signs and Symptoms. The central clinical feature is the requirement for exogenous insulin to maintain euglycemia.

Immunologic Manifestations. T cells of the CD4+ type are responsible for initiating the immune response to the islets that results in islet cell autoantibodies and B cell destruction. Patients with T1D have the following types of autoantibodies (Box 28-4):

- Insulin autoantibodies (IAAs)
- Glutamic acid decarboxylase (GAD) autoantibodies
- Islet cell antigen-2 (IA-2)

Antibodies reacting with the cells of the pancreatic islets have been found in patients with diabetes accompanying autoimmune endocrine disorders. Autoantibodies to islet-related antigens precede the development of clinical T1D by a prolonged period, often several years. A higher incidence of these anti–islet cell antibodies, however, has been demonstrated in T1D patients.

An immunoglobulin in the sera of patients with insulin-resistant diabetes appears to bind to a tissue receptor for insulin, which prevents some of the biological effects of insulin. In addition, antibodies that bind to and possibly kill pancreatic islet cells have been found in most young patients with T1D.

A small subgroup of patients with T1D has demonstrated antireceptor antibody (InR), an IgG class of antibodies directed against the insulin receptor. Antibodies to InR may be directed to the binding site or to determinants away from the binding site for insulin. This condition is predominant in nonwhite females of all ages.

IA-2 is directed against a phosphatase-type transmembrane 37-kDa islet beta cell antigen (ICA512).

Latent Autoimmune Diabetes in Adults

LADA is now recognized as a slowly developing form of autoimmune diabetes found in patients who are older than 35 years of age. LADA is frequently misdiagnosed as type 2 diabetes. LADA patients progress more rapidly to insulin dependence (T1D) than the typical T2D patient.

Autoimmune Pancreatitis

Autoimmune pancreatitis is a heterogeneous disease. This type of chronic pancreatitis is characterized by an autoimmune inflammatory process in which prominent lymphocyte infiltration with associated fibrosis of the pancreas causes organ dysfunction.

Etiology. Although the cause of the disorder is unknown, it is thought to be a systemic autoimmune disorder. It is frequently associated with other autoimmune disorders (e.g., RA).

Epidemiology. Autoimmune pancreatitis is rare, but an increasing number of cases has been reported since 2000. Although this condition can occur in both genders, it is at least twice as common in men as women. Most patients are older than 50 years at diagnosis.

Signs and Symptoms. Symptoms are variable. Many patients have jaundice; some have abdominal pain. Histologic examination

Box 28-4	**Autoantibody Assays to Differentiate Type 1 Diabetes***
Assay	**Characteristic**
Insulin autoantibodies (IAA)	Autoantibodies specific for beta cells of the pancreas; may aid in proband diagnosis or predict development of type 2 diabetes
Glutamic acid decarboxylase autoantibodies	Aid in the diagnosis and confirmation of type 1 diabetes; may be found in patients who eventually develop type 1 diabetes
Islet antigen-2 autoantibodies	Associated with type 1 diabetes; may be present in patients years before the onset of clinical symptoms

*American Diabetic Association (2008):
- Type 1 diabetes results typically have antibodies and low C-peptide levels.
- Absence of antibodies or normal C-peptide levels does not rule out type 1, but likelihood of type 1 diabetes is low.

United States Preventive Services Task Force (USPSTF; 2008):
- C-peptide testing—use to confirm lack of insulin production, suggesting type 1 diabetes.
- Use of C-peptide levels or insulin levels to diagnose type 1 diabetes is not recommended.

of pancreatic tissue reveals a collar-like periductal infiltrate composed of lymphocytes and plasma cells. Computed tomography (CT) typically reveals a diffuse enlargement of the pancreas, with a halo around its peripheral rim. Various findings on imaging radiography are correlated with serologic and histologic analyses. It is important to diagnose autoimmune pancreatitis correctly on the basis of imaging, histology, and serology because it can mimic pancreatic cancer.

Immunologic Manifestations. In the Japanese population, an association between HLA haplotype DRB1*0405-DQB1*0401 has been observed. Immunologic abnormalities include the following:

- Hypergammaglobulinemia (elevated serum IgG or gamma globulin level) in patients with enhanced peripheral rim halo of the pancreas on CT
- Elevated serum IgG4 concentrations in patients with a diffusely enlarged pancreas
- Autoantibodies against carbonic anhydrase II (ACA II), lactoferrin (antilactoferrin antibody [ALA]), anti–smooth muscle antibody (ASMA), or ANA
- Increased number of CD4+ T lymphocytes in peripheral blood

Adrenal Glands

Idiopathic adrenal atrophy is the primary cause of Addison's disease. It is believed that many of these cases have an autoimmune cause. Women are afflicted twice as often as men. The disease usually presents in the third or fourth decade of life. Although a great potential exists for morbidity, it has a relatively low incidence. The adult form of Addison's disease is associated with HLA class II antigens DR3 and DR4.

Idiopathic Addison's disease is usually diagnosed in patients because of low serum cortisol levels in the presence of elevated levels of corticotropin. Approximately 80% of patients manifest serum antibodies against cortical elements, probably microsomal. Some patients demonstrate antibodies against adrenal cell surfaces. These antibodies generally bind to components in the adrenal cortex but affect only individual zones. Antibodies are generally low in titer and are not a direct reflection of adrenal cell damage. In women with premature ovarian failure, autoimmune destruction of the ovarian stroma has been observed.

Pituitary Gland

Sheehan's syndrome, lymphocytic adenohypophysitis, is a disorder that causes a rapid decline in pituitary function. This disorder is most frequently seen in postpartum women. Antibodies against pituitary cells are observed in some patients. The disorder is distinguished by a mononuclear infiltrate of the pituitary gland and hypophysis.

Parathyroid Gland

Idiopathic hypoparathyroidism occurs as a childhood disorder in type I polyglandular syndrome and, less often, as an isolated disorder in adults. It is associated with complement-mediated cytotoxicity of parathyroid cells, indicating a specific immune response to the parathyroid. Several antigens have been associated with this disorder, including endothelial cell proteins and mitochondria.

Polyglandular Syndromes

Three syndromes of associated endocrinopathies have been defined as the polyglandular syndromes. Type I polyglandular syndrome involves mucocutaneous candidiasis and associated endocrinopathies that begin in early childhood. Patients initially develop candidiasis and hypoparathyroidism, but more than 50% also develop Addison's disease. Gonadal failure, alopecia, and chronic hepatitis are also seen. Patients have organ-specific autoantibodies and poorly defined defects in cell-mediated immunity.

Type II polyglandular syndrome involves the combined occurrence of IDDM or autoimmune thyroid disease with Addison's disease. It is also called Schmidt's syndrome. This type of disorder is seen primarily in women in the second or third decade of life. Most cases are familial, but the mode of inheritance is unknown. There is a strong association with HLA-DR3.

Type III polyglandular syndrome is defined as autoimmune thyroid disease occurring with two other autoimmune disorders, including IDDM, pernicious anemia, and a nonendocrine, organ-specific autoimmune disorder, such as myasthenia gravis. These patients do not have Addison's disease. The HLA-DR3 allele is present in more than 50% of cases. Patients in this category are overwhelmingly female.

Reproductive Disorders

Antibodies against cytoplasmic components of different cells of the ovary have been demonstrated in Addison's disease and in premature ovarian failure, which may be an immune disorder causing reproductive failure and eventually early menopause. A prevalence of smooth muscle antibody, ANA, and antiphospholipid antibodies has been found in women with unexplained infertility. In addition, autoantibodies to the ovary and gonadotropin receptors exist in many women with polyendocrinopathies.

Patients with endometriosis have a defect in natural killer (NK) cell activity. This results in decreased cytotoxicity for autologous endometrial cells. Reduced T lymphocyte–mediated cytotoxicity to endometrial cells has also been found.

A sizable proportion of pregnancy losses may be caused by immunologic factors. The fetus is an immunogenic allograft that evokes a protective immune response from the mother, which is necessary for implantation and growth. The mechanism of pregnancy loss is hypothesized to involve two antiphospholipid antibodies. Lupus anticoagulant and anticardiolipin antibodies are directed against platelets and vascular endothelium. This causes vascular destruction and thrombosis, leading to fetal death and abortion. There is no evidence of a direct immunologic attack on the embryo. A human fetus is capable of survival in utero if it does not share a significant number of maternal MHC antigens, especially HLA-B and HLA-DR and DQ loci.

Antisperm antibodies have been detected in the serum of men and women, in cervical mucus of women, in seminal fluid of men, and attached to sperm cells. In seminal fluid, the immobilizing antibodies to sperm are usually of the IgG class and the agglutinating antibodies are IgA. Elevated levels of antibodies to sperm have been found in more than 40% of men after vasectomy but only occasionally in men with primary testicular agenesis. Allergy-like reactions to seminal fluid have also been observed. These reactions range from local reactions to systemic reactions, including life-threatening anaphylaxis. The allergen is usually one or more prostatic proteins, but it can include IgE to spermatozoa.

Exocrine Gland Disorder

Sjögren's Syndrome

Etiology. Sjögren's syndrome is a chronic inflammatory disease of unknown cause that affects lacrimal, salivary, and other excretory glands. It results in keratoconjunctivitis sicca and xerostomia.

As with RA and SLE, causative factors include infection, abnormalities of immune regulation, and genetic factors. Development of Sjögren's syndrome is strongly associated with HLA-B8 and HLA-DR3. An infectious origin has been suggested. Clear evidence for excessive B cell activity has been demonstrated, but it is not known whether this is caused by B or T cell abnormalities.

Epidemiology. A primary form is not associated with other diseases; a secondary form is associated with RA and other connective tissue diseases. About 90% of patients are women. A 44-fold increased incidence of lymphoma has been noted in patients with Sjögren's syndrome.

Signs and Symptoms. The main clinical manifestations of Sjögren's syndrome are dry eyes, dry mouth, and recurrent salivary gland pain and swelling (Table 28-5). Hoarseness, chronic cough, and increased incidence of infection have been observed. Dryness of the vagina leads to dyspareunia and itching. Dysphagia and atrophic gastritis can also be present. Extraglandular involvement results in interstitial pneumonitis and fibrosis. Renal tubular acidosis and vasculitis involving the peripheral nerves and central nervous system (CNS) can also result from Sjögren's syndrome.

Immunologic Manifestations. The immunologic characteristics of Sjögren's syndrome include hypergammaglobulinemia, ANAs, rheumatoid factor, autoantibodies to salivary duct and other antigens, and lymphocyte and plasma cell infiltration of involved tissue. Antibodies are usually polyclonal and may result in the hyperviscosity syndrome and hypergammaglobulinemic purpura. Speckled or homogeneous ANA patterns are present in 65% of patients and occur more frequently in primary Sjögren's syndrome. Antibodies to Sjögren's syndrome A antigen have been associated with vasculitis in primary Sjögren's syndrome. Antibodies to Sjögren's syndrome B antigen are almost always found in association with Sjögren's syndrome A antigen and only occur in SLE and Sjögren's syndrome. Rheumatoid factor is found in 90% of cases. A rather new autoantibody, anti–α-fodrin, has been found in the sera of most patients with primary Sjögren's syndrome. This antibody may be pathophysiologically associated with some extraglandular manifestations characteristically seen in patients with Sjögren's syndrome.

Autoantibodies to salivary duct antigens are frequently detected in patients with secondary Sjögren's syndrome. They are also common in 25% of patients with RA without Sjögren's syndrome. Mitochondrial antibodies are detected in 10% of patients with primary Sjögren's syndrome and rarely in patients with secondary Sjögren's syndrome and RA. Patients with primary Sjögren's syndrome also have higher levels of antibodies to the thyroid gland, gastric parietal cells, pancreatic epithelial cells, and smooth muscle. Lymphocytic infiltration of the exocrine glands of the eyes, mouth, nose, lower respiratory tract, gastrointestinal (GI) tract, and vagina occurs. The infiltrate is composed of B and T cells. In tissue culture, these cells produce large amounts of IgM and IgG. T cells are predominantly helper cells.

Gastrointestinal Disorders

Atrophic Gastritis and Pernicious Anemia

A malfunctioning immune system can target the stomach lining, resulting in autoimmune gastritis, characterized by chronic inflammation of the gastric mucosa. Persons with autoimmune gastritis may progress to pernicious anemia (PA). Autoimmune gastritis is characterized by the presence of serum autoantibodies against gastric parietal cells, H^+/K^+-ATPase (proton pump), and the cobalamin-absorbing protein, intrinsic factor.

Immunologic Findings. Antibodies against a lipoprotein cytoplasmic component of gastric parietal cells can be detected by immunofluorescence in up to 90% of PA patients and in about 60% of patients with atrophic gastritis without hematologic abnormalities. These antibodies may also be demonstrated in patients with other autoimmune diseases, such as thyroiditis. In addition, antibodies can be found in asymptomatic patients and in those older than 60 years.

Histologic Findings. Atrophic gastritis, which almost always accompanies PA, is characterized by destruction of the gastric mucosa, with lymphocytic infiltration and the absence of parietal and chief cells. The lesions are associated with decreased synthesis of gastric acid and intrinsic factor. Intrinsic factor normally binds ingested vitamin B_{12} at one site and binds to receptors in the distal ileum at another site. Therefore, vitamin B_{12} transport across the ileum is affected.

Vitamin B_{12} (Cobalamin) Transport. Cobalamin transport is mediated by three different binding proteins capable of binding the vitamin at its required physiologic concentrations—intrinsic factor, transcobalamin II, and the R proteins (Table 28-6).

Intrinsic factor (IF), a glycoprotein, is synthesized and secreted by the parietal cells of the mucosa in the fundus region of the stomach in several mammalian species, including human beings. In a healthy state, the amounts of IF secreted by the stomach greatly exceed the quantities required to bind ingested cobalamin in its coenzyme forms. At a very acidic pH, cobalamin splits from dietary protein and combines with IF to form a vitamin-IF complex. Binding by IF is extraordinarily specific and is lost with even slight changes in the cobalamin molecule. This complex is stable and remains unabsorbed until it reaches the ileum. In the ileum, the vitamin-IF complex attaches to specific receptor sites present only on the outer surface of microvillous membranes of ileal enterocytes.

The release of this complex from the mucosal cells, with subsequent transport to the tissues, depends on transcobalamin II (TCII). TCII is a plasma polypeptide synthesized by the liver and probably by several other tissues. TCII, which turns over very rapidly in plasma, acts as the acceptor and principal carrier of the vitamin to the liver and other tissues, as with IF.

Table 28-5	Criteria for Diagnosis Sjögren's Syndrome*
Ocular symptoms	Dry eyes daily for 3 mo, sand or gravel feeling in eyes
Oral symptoms	Dry mouth daily for 3 mo or recurrent or persistent swollen glands
Ocular signs	Post-Schirmer test or rose bengal score >4
Histopathology	Aggregates of ≥50 mononuclear cells/4 mm² of glandular tissue
Autoantibodies	Presence of anti-Ro (SS-A), anti-La (SS-B), ANAs, or rheumatoid factor

*Four or more of these criteria must be present.
From Vitali C, Bombardieri S, Moutsopoulos HM, et al: Preliminary criteria for the classification of Sjögren's syndrome: results of a prospective concerted action supported by the European community, Arthritis Rheum 36:340–347, 1993.

Table 28-6	Vitamin B_{12} (Cobalamin)–Binding Proteins		
Parameter	**Intrinsic Factor**	**Transcobalamin II**	**R Proteins**
Source	Stomach	Liver, other tissues	Leukocytes, ? other tissues
Function	Intestinal absorption	Delivery to cells	Excretion storage
Membrane receptors	Ileal enterocytes	Many cells	Liver cells

Receptors for TCII are observed on the plasma membranes of a wide variety of cells. TCII is also capable of binding a few unusual cobalamin analogues. TCII also stimulates cobalamin uptake by reticulocytes.

The R proteins compose an antigenically cross-reactive group of cobalamin-binding glycoproteins. The R proteins bind cobalamin and various cobalamin analogues. Their function is unknown, but they appear to serve as storage sites and as a means of eliminating excess cobalamin and unwanted analogues from the blood circulation through receptor sites on liver cells. R proteins are produced by leukocytes and perhaps other tissues. They are present in plasma as transcobalamin I and transcobalamin III, as well as in saliva, milk, and other body fluids. Transcobalamin I probably serves only as a backup transport system for endogenous cobalamin. Endogenous vitamin is synthesized in the human GI tract by bacterial action, but none is adsorbed.

Autoimmune Liver Disease

Autoimmune processes are believed to be the possible cause of chronic liver disease. Hypergammaglobulinemia, prominent lymphocyte and plasma cell inflammation of the liver, and the presence of one or more circulating tissue antibodies are typically manifested. These manifestations suggest an organ-localized autoimmune pathogenesis.

Autoimmune hepatitis (AIH), formerly known as *chronic active hepatitis* is an inflammatory condition most common in young women. It is characterized by prominent lymphocyte and plasma cell inflammatory changes, which start in the portal tracts. In some patients, this condition results from a chronic viral infection or inflammation, but in others a number of immunologic abnormalities are present to varying degrees in addition to hypergammaglobulinemia and an elevated erythrocyte sedimentation rate (ESR). A defect in **immunoregulation** is often demonstrated, which may lead to unrestrained immunoglobulin production.

Antinuclear autoantibody using HEp-2 cells will have differing levels of reactivity depending on factors such as the disease activity or multiple ANA specificities. A homogeneous staining pattern (see Color Plate 13) is the most frequent pattern particularly in active AIH. The frequency of positive ANA tests is about 70% in AIH. In remission, the frequency of ANA positivity decreases and the ANA pattern is replaced by a speckled pattern in almost 40% of cases. Other significant antibodies can include an atypical perinuclear ANCA (pANCA) in one type of AIH with a frequency of 65% positivity. In addition, AIH is characterized by autoantibodies to cytoskeletal proteins that support cellular structure, contractility, and locomotion: microfilaments. These autoantibodies to cytoskeleton can be studied by immunofluorescent light (IFL) methodology.

These patients display ANAs and anti–smooth muscle antibodies. A high and persistent titer of antismooth antibodies is suggestive of the autoimmune form of chronic active hepatitis or viral disorders such as infectious mononucleosis.

In some cases this disease is referred to as *lupoid hepatitis*. Patients with aggressive chronic active hepatitis have a poor prognosis, and a significant rate of mortality is reported 5 years after diagnosis.

Idiopathic Biliary Cirrhosis

Idiopathic biliary cirrhosis is a slowly progressive disease that starts as an apparently noninfectious inflammation in the bile ducts of young to middle-aged women. An increased familial incidence has been noted.

Patients exhibit increased serum IgM, depression of cellular immunity, with prominent decreases in suppressor T cells common, and associated autoimmune disorders. It is believed that tissue damage results from an unmodulated attack against host tissue antigens. Antimitochondrial antibodies directed against the cellular ultrastructures, mitochondria, can be displayed. A high titer of antimicrobial antibody strongly suggests primary biliary cirrhosis (PBC); an absence of mitochondrial antibodies is strong evidence against PBC. Other forms of liver disease, however, frequently exhibit low mitochondrial antibody titers.

Inflammatory Bowel Disease

Inflammatory bowel disease (IBD) is the collective name given to Crohn's disease (CD) and ulcerative colitis (UC). A major gene has been identified in these disorders. The Centers for Disease Control and Prevention (CDC) estimates that IBD, which is more common among Ashkenazi Jews than other groups, affects more than 1 million Americans. When researchers examined more than 300,000 single nucleotide polymorphisms (SNPs), the variations that occur when a nucleotide (molecular subunit of DNA) is altered, it was discovered that the frequency of variations in the receptor gene for interleukin-23 (IL-23) is significantly different for those with IBD. A coding variant that apparently protects against IBD is found less frequently in patients with IBD than in healthy patients.

Many factors (e.g., genetic susceptibility, diet) affect the onset and development of IBD. The crux of the disease is an abnormal immune response to harmless bacteria in the gut that benefits the host by providing energy and nutrients. In IBD patients, these microorganisms become a target for attack by the immune system. The inflammation seen in IBD patients has been linked to the following:

- Presence of increased levels of inflammation-promoting cytokines
- Protein molecules used by cells of the immune system to communicate with each other

Studies have suggested that one cytokine, IL-12, is a crucial mediator of this disease. IL-12 causes inflammation by activating a class of different immune cells, type 1 helper T (Th1) cells, which in turn secrete proinflammatory molecules such as interferon-γ (IFN-γ) and tumor necrosis factor-α (TNF-α). These pathways have been suggested as therapeutic targets for human IBD.

The discovery of IL-23 has led some to question the central role of IL-12 and Th1 cells in IBD. Newer studies have indicated that IL-12 and IL-23 are closely related molecules that share a common subunit known as p40. IL-23 has been associated with the activation of a new class of proinflammatory T cells called Th17. These cells secrete the proinflammatory cytokine IL-17, which mediates the inflammatory response in organs such as the brain and joints. Intestinal inflammation is still associated with large increases in IL-17 production in the intestines. Innate immune cells present in inflamed intestines (e.g., granulocytes, monocytes) have been found to contribute to the increased production of IL-17.

Immune Markers. The following serologic markers have been found to be useful in the diagnosis and differentiation of CD and UC:

- Deoxyribonuclease (DNase I)–sensitive perinuclear antineutrophil cytoplasmic autoantibody (p-ANCA). IBD-associated p-ANCA defines an antibody to a nuclear antigen that is sensitive to DNase I.
- Anti–*Saccharomyces cervisiae* antibody (ASCA). This is present in the sera of up to 70% of CD patients.
- Pancreatic antibody. This is observed in approximately 30% of CD patients.
- Anti–outer membrane porin from *Escherichia coli* (anti-OmpC). An IgA response to OmpC is observed in 55% of CD patients.

Celiac Disease

Celiac disease is a lifelong autoimmune intestinal disorder found in individuals who are genetically susceptible. There are also associated clinical disorders of an immune basis (Box 28-5). Damage to the mucosal surface of the small intestine is caused by an immunologically toxic reaction to the ingestion of gluten and interferes with the absorption of nutrients. Celiac disease is unique in that a specific food component, gluten, has been identified as the trigger. Gluten is the common name for the offending proteins in specific cereal grains that are harmful to those with celiac disease. These proteins are found in all forms of wheat (e.g., durum, semolina, spelt, kamut, einkorn, faro) and related grains (rye, barley, triticale) and must be eliminated.

In recent years, key laboratory diagnostic assays comprise testing for autoantibodies against tissue transglutaminase (anti-tTG) or endomysium (EmA) antibodies against deamidated gliadin peptides and the celiac disease (CD)-associated human leukocyte antigens (HLA) DQ2 and DQ8.

New European guidelines have results in two algorithms of testing: symptomatic patients versus asymptomatic patients. For symptomatic patients, the algorithm begins with determination of specific anti-TG antibodies of class IgA in parallel with total IgA or specific IgG measured in parallel testing. If the anti-tTG antibody titer is more than 10 above the upper normal limit, the endomysium (EmA) is positive, and compatible HLA results are found, it is not necessary to perform a small bowel biopsy as was done in the past. Diagnostic tests should be done on individuals on a gluten-containing diet. A biopsy is needed only if serologic and genetic findings are inconclusive. In asymptomatic patients with a high risk factor for CD, e.g., patients with diabetes type 1, Down's syndrome, autoimmune thyroid or liver disease, Turner's syndrome, Williams' syndrome, or selective Ig A deficiency and patients with first-degree relatives of CD patients, HLA-DQ2/DQ8 determination is the first-line of analysis that can be followed up with specific antibody testing. Asymptomatic patients require a duodenal biopsy for a definite diagnosis of CD.

Other Gastrointestinal Tract Immunologic Disorders

Examples of other immunologic disorders related to the GI and hepatobiliary tracts include GI allergy, Whipple's disease, immunoproliferative intestinal disease (alpha heavy-chain disease), and infectious hepatitis (see Chapter 23). Allergy of the GI tract is an IgE-mediated hypersensitivity to food substances that involves the GI tract and, in some cases, the skin and lungs. Examples of systemic autoimmune disease caused by mucosal immune abnormalities are IgA nephropathy (Berger's disease), Henoch-Schönlein purpura, and diseases associated with circulating IgA complexes in the kidney and vasculature. Immunoproliferative intestinal disease is characterized by monoclonal B cells that produce an aberrant alpha heavy chain.

Autoimmune Hematologic Disorders

Various hematologic conditions can be caused by alloantibodies and autoantibodies (Table 28-7).

Box 28-5	Clinical Immune Disorders Associated With Celiac Disease

- Selective IgA deficiency
- Autoimmune thyroid disease
- Chronic autoimmune hepatitis
- Lupus erythematosus
- Sjögren's syndrome
- Type 1 diabetes

Table 28-7	Immunohematologic Diseases
Category	**Examples**
Immune hemolysis	Warm autoimmune hemolytic anemia
	Cold agglutinin disease
	Paroxysmal cold hemoglobinuria
	Drug-induced hemolytic anemias
	Hemolytic disease of the newborn
Immune thrombocytopenia	Idiopathic (autoimmune) thrombocytopenic purpura
	Neonatal alloimmune thrombocytopenia
Immune neutropenia	Autoimmune neutropenia
Immune-mediated transfusion reactions	Acute hemolytic transfusion reaction
	Febrile reactions
	Pulmonary hypersensitivity reaction
	Allergic reactions
	IgA-deficient recipient
	Delayed hemolytic reactions
	Posttransfusion purpura
	Transfusion-associated graft-versus-host disease
Anemias	Pernicious anemia
Deficiency of hemostasis and coagulation	Autoimmune protein S deficiency

Autoimmune Hemolytic Anemia

Autoimmune hemolytic anemia can be classified into the following four groups:

- Warm-reactive autoantibodies (most common)
- Cold-reactive autoantibodies (<20% of cases)
- Paroxysmal cold hemoglobinuria (rare)
- Drug-induced hemolysis (<20% of cases)

Warm Autoimmune Hemolytic Anemia. This anemia is associated with antibodies reactive at warm temperatures (i.e., 37° C [98.6° F]). In more than 75% of cases, the erythrocytes are coated with both IgG and complement, although some may demonstrate coating with IgG alone or, less often, with complement coating. In warm autoimmune hemolytic anemia, negligible serum autoantibody exists because the antibody reacts optimally at 37° C (98.6° F) and is being continuously adsorbed by red blood cells (RBCs) in vivo. Elution of the antibody from the RBCs (mechanical removal of antibodies) can demonstrate an autoantibody, but testing for specificity is not routinely necessary.

Cold Autoimmune Hemolytic Anemia. Cold hemagglutinin disease (CHAD), acute or chronic, is the most common type of hemolytic anemia associated with cold-reactive autoantibodies. The acute form is often secondary to *Mycoplasma pneumoniae* infection or lymphoproliferative disorders such as lymphoma. The chronic form is seen in older patients and produces mild to moderate hemolysis. In addition, Raynaud's phenomenon and hemoglobinuria occur in cold weather.

In CHAD, a cold-reactive IgM autoantibody reacts with RBCs in the peripheral circulation when the body temperature falls to 32° C (89.6° F) or lower and binds complement to the cells. Therefore, complement is the only globulin detected on the erythrocytes. Elutions prepared from RBCs collected at 37° C (98.6° F) will not demonstrate antibody reactivity in the eluate.

Paroxysmal Cold Hemoglobinuria. Previously associated with syphilis, paroxysmal cold hemoglobinuria is now seen more often as an acute transient condition secondary to viral infections, particularly in young children. It may also occur as an idiopathic chronic disease in older people.

The autoantibody is an IgG protein that reacts with RBCs in colder parts of the body; this produces complement components C3 and C4 to bind irreversibly to the erythrocytes. At warmer temperatures, RBCs are hemolyzed and the antibody elutes from the cells. Eluates are also nonreactive. This IgG autoantibody, a biphasic hemolysin, can be demonstrated by performing the classic Donath-Landsteiner test. The autoantibody has anti-p specificity and reacts with all except the rare p or p^k phenotypes. Exceptions that include examples with anti-IH specificity have been described.

Drug-Induced Hemolysis. Coating of RBCs demonstrated by a positive direct anti–human globulin test (DAT) result may be drug induced and accompanied by hemolysis (Table 28-8). The reactivity has been described as being caused by four basic mechanisms: (1) drug adsorption; (2) immune complexing; (3) membrane modification; and (4) autoantibody formation.

Drug Adsorption. Penicillin is a representative example of an agent that displays drug adsorption. In this type of mechanism, the drug strongly binds to any protein, including RBC membrane proteins. This binding produces a drug-RBC-hapten complex that can stimulate antibody formation. The antibody is specific for this complex and no reactions will take place unless the drug is adsorbed on erythrocytes. Massive doses of IV penicillin are needed to coat the erythrocytes sufficiently for antibody attachment to occur.

Approximately 3% of affected patients will demonstrate a positive DAT result and less than 5% will develop hemolytic anemia because of the drug. The hemolysis of RBCs is usually extravascular and occurs slowly. It is not life-threatening and will abate when penicillin is discontinued. There appears to be no connection between this type of antibody production and allergic penicillin sensitivity caused by IgE production.

Other drugs that display drug adsorption are cephalothin derivatives (e.g., cephalothin [Keflin], quinidine).

Immune Complexing. Immune complexing is associated with a variety of drugs, including phenacetin, quinine, rifampin, and stibophen. In this interaction, the drug and antibody form a complex in the serum and attach nonspecifically to the RBCs. Once attached, this complex initiates the complement cascade, which culminates in intravascular hemolysis. The **immune complex** may dissociate from the RBC membrane after complement activation and attach to another erythrocyte. This

Table 28-8	Drug-Induced Positive Direct Antiglobulin Test			
Parameter	**Drug Adsorption**	**Immune Complex**	**Membrane Modification**	**Autoantibody Formation**
Common cause	IgG	Complement	Nonserologic	IgG
Antibody screening	Negative*	Positive†	Negative	Variable‡
Eluate reactivity with reagent RBCs	Nonreactive	Nonreactive	Nonreactive	Reactive§
Penicillin-treated RBCs	Reactive with patient's serum and eluate	Nonreactive	Nonreactive	Nonreactive

*Unless irregular antibodies are present in the sample.
†If the drug and complement are present in the test system.
‡If the autoantibody is high enough in titer, screening tests may be positive with all cells tested.
§Will react with all normal cells tested, occasionally showing Rh-like specificity.

allows a small amount of drug to produce a severe anemia. When the offending drug is discontinued, the hemolytic process disappears quickly.

Membrane Modification. Drugs of the cephalosporin type (e.g., cephalothin) occasionally cause a positive DAT result with polyspecific and monospecific anti–human globulin antisera by membrane modification. In this type of mechanism, the drug alters the membrane so that there is nonspecific absorption of globulins, including IgG, IgM, IgA, and complement. Hemolysis is not a common complication in this type of membrane augmentation.

Autoantibody Formation. Drugs such as methyldopa (Aldomet), levodopa, and mefenamic acid (Ponstel) have been implicated in positive DAT results caused by autoantibody formation. The autoantibody formed recognizes a part of the RBC and therefore reacts with most normal RBCs. Some drug-induced autoantibodies have been shown to have specificities that appear to be of the Rh type, but most have no apparent specificity. Antibody production ceases with withdrawal of the drug.

Idiopathic Thrombocytopenic Purpura

Idiopathic thrombocytopenic purpura is now also known as immunologic thrombocytopenic purpura (ITP). Patients with ITP usually demonstrate petechiae, bruising, menorrhagia, and bleeding after minor trauma. ITP may be acute or chronic. Children are most often affected with the acute type, whereas adults predominantly experience the chronic type. This common disorder may complicate other antibody-associated disorders such as SLE.

Thrombocytopenia, a condition of absent or severely decreased platelets (<10-20×10^9/L), may result from a wide variety of conditions, such as after extracorporeal circulation in cardiac bypass surgery or from alcoholic liver disease. However, most thrombocytopenic conditions can be classified into the following three major categories:

- Decreased production of platelets
- Disorders of platelet distribution
- Increased destruction or use of platelets

Decreased platelet production may result from invasion of the bone marrow by neoplastic cells and is usually not associated with an immunologic cause. Disorders of platelet distribution are associated with a sequestering of platelets in the spleen for various nonimmunologic reasons. Increased destruction or use of platelets, however, is associated with immunologic mechanisms. These mechanisms of destruction are caused by antigens, antibodies, or complement.

Drugs or foreign substances that can cause platelet destruction include quinidine, sulfonamide derivatives, heroin, morphine, and snake venom. Sulfonamide derivative reactions involve the interaction of platelet antigens with drug antibodies. Morphine reactions involve the activation of complement.

Bacterial sepsis causes increased destruction of platelets resulting from the attachment of platelets to bacterial antigen-antibody immune complexes. Certain microbial antigens may initially attach to platelets, followed by specific antibodies to the microorganism. This mechanism has been reported to cause the thrombocytopenia that frequently complicates *Plasmodium falciparum* malaria.

Antibodies of autoimmune or isoimmune origin may cause increased destruction of platelets. Examples of thrombocytopenias of isoimmune origin include posttransfusion purpura and isoimmune neonatal thrombocytopenia. Neonatal autoimmune thrombocytopenia is a condition caused by immunization of a pregnant female by a fetal platelet antigen and by transplacental passage of maternal IgG platelet antibodies. The antigen is inherited by the fetus from the father and is absent on maternal platelets. Posttransfusion purpura is a rare form of isoimmune thrombocytopenia.

Pernicious Anemia

Pernicious anemia is a megaloblastic anemia characterized by a variety of hematologic and chemical manifestations (Table 28-9). PA is caused by a deficiency of vitamin B_{12} that results from the patient's inability to secrete intrinsic factor. In autoimmune cases of PA, anti-IF or antiparietal antibodies have been reported. Demonstration of these antibodies supports the theory that PA is an autoimmune disorder. Nutritional disorders (e.g., vegan diet, gastric bypass surgery, AIDS, small bowel disorders, and competition for vitamin B_{12}) can be nonimmunological causes of PA.

Assays for anti-IF measure antibodies to IF. The presence of **IF–blocking antibodies** is diagnostic of PA. Antibodies can be demonstrated in about 60% of cases. Antiparietal cell assays measure antibodies to parietal cells (large cells on the margins of the peptic glands of the stomach). Most patients with PA (80%) have parietal cell antibodies. In the presence of these antibodies, gastric biopsy almost always demonstrates gastritis. Low antibody titers to parietal cells are often found with no clinical evidence of PA or atrophic gastritis and are sometimes seen in older patients.

Table 28-9	**Hematologic and Chemical Findings in Pernicious Anemia**
Assay	**Finding**
Hematologic Indices	
Hemoglobin (Hb)	Severely decreased
Hematocrit (Hct)	Severely decreased
Erythrocyte (RBC) count	Decreased
Leukocyte (WBC) count	Slightly decreased
Platelet count	Slightly decreased or normal
Mean corpuscular volume (MCV)	Increased
Chemical Indices	
Serum iron	Increased
Total iron-binding capacity (TIBC)	Normal or decreased
Percentage of iron (Fe) saturation	Increased
Serum ferritin	Increased

WBC, White blood cell.

Neuromuscular Disorders

Several important neurologic disorders are related to the immune system. The immune system may play an important role in the pathogenesis and cause of myasthenia gravis and multiple sclerosis. In addition, amyotrophic lateral sclerosis (ALS) has become one of the prime subjects of modern neurologic research.

Amyotrophic Lateral Sclerosis

Along with Alzheimer's disease and Parkinson's disease, ALS is one of the so-called degenerative diseases of the aging nervous system. The immune system has been implicated in ALS. Monoclonal paraproteinemia seems to be disproportionately frequent in patients with ALS. It has also been suggested that ALS patients have a higher incidence of lymphoproliferative disease—lymphoma, Waldenström's macroglobulinemia, and myeloma. There also seems to be an increased frequency of antibodies to a neuronal ganglioside, GM-1.

Inflammatory Polyneuropathies

This group of idiopathic disorders, which includes the acute disorder Guillain-Barré syndrome (GBS), is characterized clinically by the subacute onset of generally symmetric weakness, ranging from modest lower extremity weakness to total, life-threatening involvement of motor and even cranial nerves. Sensory symptoms are less prominent. Unstable blood pressure and potentially fatal arrhythmias have also been observed. Progression of GBS can be rapid; however, most patients do recover.

The cause of GBS is unknown, but it is likely that an abnormal immune response against the peripheral nervous system (PNS) is involved. This may be triggered by an antecedent viral infection. There is infiltration of the PNS with lymphocytes and macrophages and patchy myelin destruction. Some patients display deposition of IgG, IgM, and IgA in PNS tissues. Greatly elevated immunoglobulin levels in the cerebrospinal fluid (CSF), sometimes with oligoclonal bands, suggests locally altered immunoregulation. The antigenic targets of these immunoglobulins remain unknown.

Myasthenia Gravis

Myasthenia gravis is a disorder of the neuromuscular junction characterized by neurophysiologic and immunologic abnormalities (Box 28-6). A postsynaptic defect is caused by a decrease in receptors for acetylcholine and frequently an anatomic defect in the neuromuscular junction plate. Acetylcholine receptor (AChR)–binding antibody is directed against acetylcholine receptors at neuromuscular junctions of skeletal muscle and AChR-blocking antibodies. The ligand bungarotoxin or acetylcholine is important in producing a neuromuscular block. About one third of patients with myasthenia gravis demonstrate AChR-blocking antibodies.

The role of these antibodies in producing disease is unclear. Complement-mediated, antibody-determined damage may be an important mechanism in myasthenia gravis because IgG, C3, and C9 can be demonstrated at the neuromuscular junction and the motor endplate is often abnormal. This suggests that antibody to AChR is capable of increasing the normal rate of degradation, resulting in fewer available receptors.

Multiple Sclerosis

Multiple sclerosis (MS) is the most common demyelinating disorder of the CNS related to abnormalities of the immune system. It is characterized by regions of demyelinization of varying size and age scattered throughout the white matter of the CNS. Demyelinization plaques have a propensity to form in the cerebrum, optic nerves, brainstem, spinal cord, and cerebellum.

Etiology. After more than a century of study, the cause of MS remains unknown. Although research studies support genetic and environmental components of susceptibility, epidemiologic findings are most consistent with an environmental influence against a background of genetic susceptibility as the cause of MS. There is little evidence for a single or unique environmental cause. Viral infection (e.g., human herpesvirus type 6 [HHV-6]) is highly suspected but unconfirmed. In addition, Epstein–Barr virus (EBV), which causes infectious mononucleosis and is associated with other diseases, may increase the risk of MS.

Epidemiology. The incidence, prevalence, and mortality rates of MS vary with latitude. MS is rare in tropical and subtropical areas. The higher risk for MS in Europeans and in relatives of patients with MS and the existence of MS-resistant ethnic groups (e.g., Eskimos, Norwegian Lapps, Australian aborigines) support a genetic predisposition to MS. A low prevalence of MS occurs in Africa, India, China, Japan, and Southeast Asia. In the United States, the incidence is 1/1000 individuals.

MS is the major acquired neurologic disease in young adults. Most patients develop symptoms between the ages of 18 and 50 years. Women are more often affected than men (2:1 ratio). Approximately 1/1000 persons of northern European origin residing in temperate climates will develop prototypical MS in their lifetime. Up to 400,000 people in the United States have MS.

Pathophysiology. MS results from T cell–dependent inflammatory demyelination of the CNS. Inflammatory demyelination caused by T lymphocytes induces B lymphocytes to produce antimyelin antibodies.

The ongoing pathologic process involves the formation of CNS lesions, called plaques, characterized by inflammation and demyelination. Plaques result from a localized inflammatory immune response, initiated by the entry of activated blood T cells into the CNS. These T cells cross the blood-brain barrier by binding to endothelial cells in blood vessels via reciprocal adhesion molecules. The release of enzymes, called matrix

---

Box 28-6	Abnormalities Associated With Myasthenia Gravis

- Thymic hyperplasia with germinal follicles
- Increase in thymic B cells
- Thymoma
- Expression of AChR-binding antibody and AChR-blocking antibody
- Associated with other autoimmune diseases

metalloproteinases (MMPs), allows them to penetrate the basement membrane and extracellular matrix. At the same time, other blood immune system cells penetrate the CNS, causing additional local synthesis and release of damaging inflammatory mediators. The net result is the destruction of myelin sheaths, injury to axons and glial cells, and formation of permanent scar tissue.

Research studies have demonstrated that osteopontin, which is known to play a role in enhancing inflammation, may play a critical role in the immune attack in MS and its progression. Osteopontin has been found to be very active in areas of myelin damage during relapse and remission and in myelin-synthesizing cells and nerve cells. More research is required to determine the exact role of this protein, as well as the therapeutic possibilities it presents.

Signs and Symptoms. MS begins as a relapsing illness with episodes of neurologic dysfunction lasting several weeks, followed by substantial or complete improvement (relapsing-remitting MS). Initial signs of MS are difficulty walking, abnormal sensations (e.g., numbness, possible pain, ineffective vision). Primary symptoms caused by demyelination include fatigue, bladder and bowel dysfunction, loss of balance, loss of memory, slurred speech, difficulty swallowing, and seizures. Depression is a common symptom.

Relapsing MS is the most common form; 85% of patients are symptomatic at onset. The other forms of MS are as follows:

- Primary progressive
- Secondary progressive
- Progressive relapsing

Primary progressive MS advances insidiously from onset, with or without occasional plateaus and minor improvements. Secondary progressive MS develops in about 50% of relapsing MS patients about 10 years into the disease. Progressive relapsing is the rarest form of the disease. Patients begin with primary progression but subsequently experience one or more relapses.

Diagnostic Methods. Magnetic resonance imaging (MRI) is a key imaging modality for establishing a diagnosis of MS. No single laboratory test confirms a diagnosis, but appropriate laboratory test results must be evaluated carefully. Conditions that need to be excluded include collagen vascular disease, vitamin B_{12} deficiency, and endocrine disorders (e.g., thyroid and adrenal gland disease). It is also important to rule out infectious diseases (e.g., Lyme disease, syphilis, human T lymphotropic virus type 1[HTLV-1] infection). CSF analysis may identify the following:

- Oligoclonal IgG band pattern by CSF electrophoresis
- Quantification of CSF IgG and albumin concentrations
- Interpretation of CSF indices (e.g., albumin index, IgG index, IgG synthesis rate, local IgG synthesis)

Immunologic Manifestations. Box 28-7 presents immunologic manifestations of MS suggestive of its autoimmune nature. Antimyelin antibodies directed against components of the myelin sheath of nerves or myelin basic protein can be demonstrated in patients with MS or other neurologic diseases. However, myelin antibodies are not detectable in the CSF of MS patients.

Detection of Oligoclonal Bands. Oligoclonal immunoglobulins may be seen in serum and CSF. An oligoclonal immunoglobulin pattern consists of multiple, homogeneous, narrow, and probably faint bands in the gamma zone on electrophoresis.

Electrophoresis on cellulose acetate will rarely resolve an oligoclonal pattern. Therefore, electrophoretic media with greater resolution, such as agar or agarose gel, are required, and both require the use of concentrated CSF. It is important to perform electrophoresis on a serum specimen concurrently with the CSF specimen to ensure that the demonstrated homogeneous bands are present only in the CSF, which implies endogenous synthesis rather than a serum band that might appear secondarily in the CSF. Infrequently, if a prominent CSF band is present, it may appear in the serum as a homogeneous band. This is most often encountered in subacute sclerosing panencephalitis.

High-resolution electrophoresis attempts to achieve better resolution of proteins beyond the classic five-band pattern. The primary reason for performing high-resolution protein electrophoresis is to detect oligoclonal bands in CSF to increase the diagnostic usefulness of protein patterns. About 80% of CSF proteins originate from the plasma. The electrophoretic pattern of normal CSF is similar to a normal serum protein pattern; however, several differences are detectable, including a prominent **prealbumin band** and two transferrin bands.

Immunofixation has been used in some research studies to show that the oligoclonal bands seen in CSF protein patterns are made up primarily of IgG. Although this may be of academic interest, characterization of the immunoglobulin bands does not significantly improve the diagnostic usefulness of the procedure. Isoelectric focusing, however, is becoming the method of choice for oligoclonal band detection.

Significance of Oligoclonal Bands. If oligoclonal bands are present in CSF but not in the serum, they are the result of increased production of IgG by the CNS. CNS production of IgG occurs in the subarachnoid space of the brain in conjunction with local accumulation of immunocytes. Each has its own specificity that gives rise to oligoclonal bands. Although the immunoglobulin is IgG, it is polyclonal in nature, with several groups of cells producing it. Oligoclonal bands are therefore defined as discrete populations of IgG, with restricted heterogeneity demonstrated by electrophoresis.

One procedure for confirming local CNS production of oligoclonal IgG is to test a matched serum specimen diluted

---

Box 28-7	**Immunologic Manifestations of Multiple Sclerosis**

- Antimyelin antibodies
- Myelinotoxicity and glial toxicity of serum and cerebrospinal fluid in vitro
- In vitro cell-mediated immunity by blood and cerebrospinal fluid cells to myelin components
- Oligoclonal increase in cerebrospinal fluid immunoglobulin
- Increase in certain HLA and Ia antigens (HL-A A3, B7, DW2, and DRW2)

1:100 concurrently with a nonconcentrated CSF sample. Oligoclonal bands present in CSF, but not in the serum, indicate CNS production. This matched sample procedure is especially useful if damage to the blood-brain barrier is suspected because of acute or chronic inflammation, such as meningitis, intracranial tumor, or cerebrovascular disease.

Serum oligoclonal bands may represent immune complexes and are associated with diseases such as Hodgkin's disease or a nonspecific early immune response to other diseases (Box 28-8). **Clinical Findings.** Total CSF protein in patients with MS is usually normal or slightly elevated. In general, patients with no neurologic disease have an IgG concentration of less than 10% of total CSF proteins. Almost 70% of MS patients typically have IgG concentrations of 11% to 35% of total CSF proteins.

Oligoclonal bands in serum are not absolutely indicative of MS; their presence should be used in conjunction with the clinical evaluation and other diagnostic procedures. Although oligoclonal bands can occur in more than 90% of MS patients at some time during the course of their disease, the presence of bands does not correlate with the activity of the disease. The exact number of bands present in MS varies; some studies have demonstrated 7 to 15 bands.

Treatment. Corticosteroid therapy (e.g., methylprednisolone, prednisone) is a common symptomatic treatment for disease relapses. The relapsing form of MS can be treated with immunomodulators such as interferon beta-1b (Betaseron), interferon beta-1a (Avonex), and glatiramer acetate (Copaxone). All these drugs have been approved by the U.S. Food and Drug Administration (FDA). The newest medication for MS is fingolimod (Gilenya), which was approved by the FDA in September 2010. This is the first oral drug available for the long-term treatment of MS. Possible future therapeutic strategies may include combination treatments using existing therapies, standard immunosuppressive drugs, and new immunomodulating agents. Autologous bone marrow transplantation, plasma exchange, TCR peptide vaccine, and gene therapy are other possibilities.

The Myelin Project Cell Culture Units at the University of Wisconsin-Madison and at Sweden's University of Lund have been developing an immortal line of human cells, oligodendrocyte precursors, to repair myelin lesions in MS and the leukodystrophies. Studies have demonstrated that myelin produced as a result of transplantation is capable of restoring nerve conduction. The feasibility of transplanting glial cells derived from human tissue into the CNS is being explored.

French researchers have demonstrated that progesterone promotes remyelination by activating genes that control the synthesis of important myelin proteins.

Neuropathies

A neuropathy is a derangement in the function and structure of peripheral motor, sensory, or autonomic neurons. Autoimmune disorders are one of the disease categories causing neuropathy. In many cases, evidence supports autoimmune pathogenesis. Demonstration of the relationships between specific neuropathic syndromes and antibodies directed against glycolipid and neural antigens are important scientific advances.

In the autoimmune neuropathies, antibodies directed against peripheral nerve components are associated with specific clinical syndromes (Table 28-10). Knowledge of these syndromes and antibody tests can be used to identify a treatable neuropathy. In addition, many autoimmune neuropathic syndromes are associated with malignancies, which they often precede. Recognition of these syndromes can lead to early identification and treatment.

Most antibodies implicated in the development of autoimmune-mediated neuropathies are directed against carbohydrate epitopes of glycoproteins or glycolipids. Glycolipids are concentrated in neural membranes, in which the lipid portion is

Box 28-8	Conditions Associated With Oligoclonal Cerebrospinal Fluid Gamma Globulins

- Multiple sclerosis
- Neurosyphilis-paresthesia
- Paraneoplastic syndrome—subacute sclerosing panencephalitis
- Chronic mycobacterial and fungal meningitis
- Chronic viral meningitis and meningoencephalitis (uncommon)
- Acute viral meningitis (uncommon)
- Primary optic neuritis
- Acute disseminated encephalomyelitis
- Primary optic neuritis
- Peripheral neuropathy
- Guillain-Barré syndrome
- Burkitt's lymphoma
- Psychoneurosis
- Cerebral infarction

Table 28-10	Neuropathy Syndromes Associated With Antibodies Directed Against Peripheral Nerve Components
Clinical Syndrome	**Antibodies**
Chronic sensorimotor demyelinating neuropathy	Antimyelin-associated glycoprotein
Chronic axonal sensory neuropathy	Antisulfatide or anti–chondroitin sulfate
Multifocal motor neuropathy	Anti-GM1 (IgM)
Acute axonal motor neuropathy	Anti-GM1 (IgG)
Fisher syndrome	Anti-GQ1b
Guillain-Barré syndrome	Anti-LM1, GD1b, GD1A, GT1b, sulfatide, B tubulin
Large-fiber sensory neuropathy with ataxia	Anti-GQ1b, GD3, GD1b, GT1b
Subacute sensory neuropathy/encephalomyelitis	Antineuronal nuclear antibody type 1 (anti-Hu)

From Cohen B, Mitsumoto H: Neuropathy syndromes associated with antibodies against the peripheral nerve, Lab Med 26:459–463, 1995.

immersed in the membrane bilayer and the carbohydrate portion is exposed extracellularly. The extracellular domain of the carbohydrate epitopes makes them vulnerable to antibody binding.

Systemic sclerosis (scleroderma) is an autoimmune disease characterized by a wide spectrum of clinical, pathologic, and serologic abnormalities. More than 90% of patients with systemic sclerosis spontaneously produce ANA. The structure and function of the intracellular antigens to which these ANAs are directed have been characterized. These serum autoantibodies are helpful markers because they correlate with certain clinical features of systemic sclerosis (Table 28-11). A more recently developed marker autoantibody, anti–RNA polymerase III antibody, has been identified in many patients who have systemic sclerosis with diffuse or extensive cutaneous involvement.

Renal Disorders

It is generally accepted that most immunologically mediated renal diseases fall into several categories (Box 28-9).

Renal Disease Associated With Circulating Immune Complexes

Renal diseases associated with circulating immune complexes are caused by nonrenal antigens and their corresponding antibodies. These complexes are deposited in one or more of several loci in the glomerulus. Deposition may depend on the size and other characteristics of the complex. Studies have suggested that potentially damaging immune complexes may be formed in situ and involve antigens already present or fixed in the glomerulus. In addition, immune complex activation of complement in the glomerular basement membrane may be augmented by the presence of cells with receptors for C3 located in that area. Activation probably releases biologically active products such as chemotactic substances and causes an inflammatory type of tissue injury. A renal complication of this type can be manifested in SLE.

Membranoproliferative Glomerulonephritis

Another type of glomerular disease, membranoproliferative glomerulonephritis, is believed to be caused by nonimmunologically activated complement. Activation is thought to be analogous to the alternate pathway activation of C3 by certain bacterial products and polysaccharides.

Renal Disease Associated With Anti–Glomerular Basement Membrane Antibody

Anti–glomerular basement membrane (GBM) antibodies are directed against GBM of the glomerulus of the kidney (Fig. 28-3). These antibodies are induced in vivo against the basement membrane of the glomerulus and possibly that of the renal tubule or lung. The factors that stimulate antibody production are not well defined, but it appears likely that binding of drugs (e.g., methicillin), certain infectious agents, or renal damage caused by other immune mechanisms may lead to an immune antibody response. The end result may be direct damage to the bone marrow, with or without complement activation.

Table 28-11	Clinical Types of Systemic Sclerosis (SSc) and Associated Antibody Markers
Clinical Type	**Antibodies**
SSc with diffuse cutaneous involvement (dcSsc)	Anti–RNA polymerase I, anti–topoisomerase I
SSc with limited cutaneous involvement (lcSSc)	Anti–Th ribonucleoprotein anticentromere antibody
SSc-polymyositis overlap syndrome	Anti–PM-Scl

Box 28-9	Categories of Immunologic Renal Disorders

Associated With Circulating Immune Complexes
Systemic lupus erythematosus
Certain vasculitis
Infections
Tumors (possibly)
Immunoglobulins and antiimmunoglobulins

Membranoproliferative Glomerulonephritis
Activation of alternate complement pathway
Possible genetic factors

Associated With Anti–Glomerular Basement Membrane Antibody
Most cases of Goodpasture's syndrome
Some rapidly progressive glomerulonephritides
Membrane altered by virus or drugs (possibly)
Tubulointerstitial Nephritis

Associated With Immune Complex–Mediated Disease
Drugs and possibly infection
Involvement of transplanted kidneys

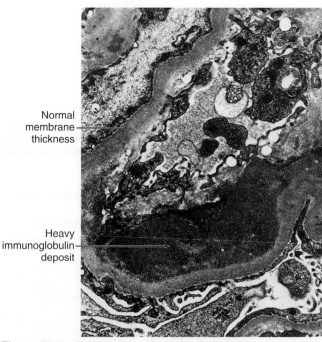

Figure 28-3 Electron photomicrograph demonstrating an immunoglobulin deposit in the basement membrane of a patient with systemic lupus erythematosus (SLE). *(From Barrett JT: Textbook of immunology, ed 5, St Louis, 1988, Mosby.)*

Labels on figure: Normal membrane thickness; Heavy immunoglobulin deposit

Production of anti–bone marrow antibodies, however, appears to be self-limited and lasts for several weeks to months after removal of the inciting agent (i.e., by the kidney).

High antibody titers of anti-GMB are suggestive of Goodpasture's disease, early SLE, or anti-GBM nephritis. The absence of antibodies, however, does not rule out Goodpasture's disease. This type of renal disease represents less than 5% of glomerular disorders.

Tubulointerstitial Nephritis

Tubulointerstitial nephritis involving the renal tubules has been associated with a variety of causes, including immune complex–mediated disease. Precipitating factors can include drugs and possibly infection, as well as the involvement of transplanted kidneys.

Skeletal Muscle Disorders

Inflammatory Myopathy

Polymyositis and dermatomyositis are the most common expressions of a group of chronic inflammatory disorders and can be subclassified into the following six categories:

- Primary idiopathic polymyositis
- Primary idiopathic dermatomyositis
- Polymyositis or dermatomyositis associated with neoplasia
- Childhood polymyositis or dermatomyositis
- Dermatomyositis or polymyositis associated with collagen vascular disease
- Polymyositis or dermatomyositis associated with infections

All these disorders have skeletal muscle damage by a lymphocyte inflammatory process resulting in symmetric weakness, predominantly of proximal muscles.

Polymyositis may be accompanied by inflammation at other sites, especially in the joints, lungs, and heart. The term *dermatomyositis* is used for the disorder when the clinical features of disease are accompanied by characteristic inflammatory manifestations in the skin.

The causes of these disorders remain unknown, but they may develop in genetically susceptible persons after exposure to environmental agents that induce immune activation and inflammation. Infection is the most likely initiating event. As part of the inflammatory response to the infection, susceptible individuals develop a persistent cell-mediated immune attack that continues to destroy muscle after the acute infection is eradicated.

Polymyositis and dermatomyositis are more common in females, with peaks of occurrence in childhood and the fifth decade. Clinically, these disorders present with proximal muscle weakness, sometimes associated with pain, fatigue, and low-grade fever, and lead to atrophy in progressive disease.

Evidence has suggested the polymyositis and dermatomyositis result from immune destruction. Muscle biopsies in patients with dermatomyositis have shown vasculitis, with IgG and complement deposition in the vessel walls in children and infrequently in adults. There is a preponderance of B lymphocytes and an increased CD4+/CD8+ T cell ratio. An increased frequency of activated T cells has been noted in polymyositis and dermatomyositis.

Patients with myositis have many immunologic abnormalities. One unique immunologic feature is the targeting by autoantibodies of certain cytoplasmic proteins and ribonucleic acids (RNAs) involved in the process of protein synthesis. These autoantibodies are found only in patients with myositis and are known as myositis-specific autoantibodies (MSAs; Box 28-10). The MSAs are antigen-driven, arise months before the onset of myositis, correlate in titer with disease activity, disappear after prolonged complete remission, and bind to and inhibit the function of targeted human autoantigenic enzymes on in vitro assays.

Skin Disorders: Bullous Disease and Other Conditions

A wide variety of autoimmune disorders are associated with skin manifestations (Box 28-11).

Two immunologic assays that can be used in conjunction with other clinical information include measurement of antibodies to the basement membrane area of the skin and of antibodies to the intercellular substance of the skin.

Antiskin (dermal-epidermal) antibodies are present in more than 80% of patients with bullous pemphigoid, but the absence of antibodies does not rule out the disorder. Antiskin (interepithelial) antibodies can be detected in 90% of patients with pemphigus. A rising antibody titer may indicate an impending relapse of pemphigus and a decreasing titer suggests effective control of the disease. The absence of demonstrable antibody usually excludes the diagnosis.

Box 28-10	**Myositis-Specific Autoantibodies**

Antisynthetases
Anti–Jo-1
Anti–PL-7
Anti–PL-12 (1)
Anti–PL-12 (II)
Anti-OJ
Anti-EJ
Anti-SRP
Anti–MI-2
Others
Anti-FER
Anti-KJ
Anti-MAS

Box 28-11	**Autoimmune Disorders Associated With Skin Manifestations***

- Discoid lupus
- Bullous pemphigoid
- Pemphigus group
- Dermatitis herpetiformis

*Skin may be involved in the autoimmune reaction in at least three ways:
1. Inflammatory involvement of cutaneous vessels with secondary effects (e.g., some lesions in systemic lupus erythematosus, hypersensitivity angiitis, and syndrome of urticaria and palpable purpura, with or without mixed cryoglobulinemia).
2. Deposition of putative circulating immune complexes in the skin (e.g., SLE).
3. Localized autoreactivity against skin components (e.g., primary skin disorders).

CASE STUDY 1

History and Physical Examination

ZA, a 50-year-old white woman, visited her primary care provider because of extreme fatigue. She also reported experiencing mild pain in her abdominal region.

Physical examination revealed slight hepatomegaly. Her physician ordered a complete blood count and urinalysis. See Table 28-12 for the results of these tests.

Question

1. An immunologic assay of importance in the diagnosis of pernicious anemia is:
   a. Anti-intrinsic factor
   b. Anti-parietal cell antibody
   c. Anti-islet cell antibody
   d. Both a and b

See Appendix A for the answers to multiple choice questions.

Critical Thinking Group Discussion Questions

1. Which chemical and immunologic assays would be helpful in establishing a diagnosis for this patient?
2. What is the prevalence of anti–intrinsic factor in patients with pernicious anemia?
3. What is the prevalence of parietal cell antibodies in patients with pernicious anemia?

See instructor site ⊜volve website for the discussion of the answers to these questions.

CASE STUDY 2

History and Physical Examination

DD is a right-handed 25-year-old woman with no significant medical history. She came to the emergency department because of a sudden onset of slurred speech.

She reported being in excellent health until a month ago, when she began to notice weakness and numbness in her right hand and leg. She felt unsteady when walking and experienced urinary urgency.

Physical examination revealed an overweight young female with a right facial droop. In addition, she staggered on turning around and had difficulty walking in a straight line. A spinal tap and MRI were ordered.

Laboratory and Medical Imaging Data: Laboratory Findings

See Table 28-13 for these findings.

Additional Notes

- CSF agarose electrophoresis: Positive for oligoclonal bands (reference range negative)
- CSF isoelectric focusing: Positive for oligoclonal bands (reference range negative)
- Serum protein electrophoresis interpretation: No apparent monoclonal peak (reference range, no apparent monoclonal peak)
- Serum immunofixation: No paraprotein detected (reference range, no paraprotein detected)

Imaging Studies

MRI revealed a masslike lesion in the region of the corpus callosum, with extensions into the right and left hemispheres of the brain. The location of the lesion was consistent with the patient's presenting symptoms.

A follow-up biopsy of the brain was ordered. Histologically, a biopsy of white matter demonstrated sheets of macrophages, clumps of lymphocytes and plasma cells, and myelin debris.

Question

1. In the diagnosis of multiple sclerosis, the most significant body fluid to analyze is:
   a. Blood
   b. Cerebrospinal fluid
   c. Urine
   d. Biopsy of the brain

See Appendix A for the answers to multiple choice questions.

Critical Thinking Group Discussion Questions

1. What is the cause of the patient's symptoms?
2. Does the patient's age provide a clue to the diagnosis?
3. What is the significance of the laboratory analysis of the CSF?

See instructor site ⊜volve website for the discussion of the answers to these questions.

⊞ Rapid Slide Test for Antinucleoprotein

The SLE latex test provides a suspension of polystyrene latex particles coated with DNP. When the latex reagent is mixed with serum containing the ANAs, binding to the DNP-coated latex particles produces macroscopic agglutination. The procedure is positive in SLE and other autoimmune disorders (e.g., rheumatoid arthritis, scleroderma, Sjögren's syndrome).

See ⊜volve website for the procedural protocol.

Procedure Notes

Sources of Error

Failure to observe the test mixture at the appropriate time can yield false results.

Table 28-12	**Laboratory Data***	
	Patient's Results	Reference Range
Complete Blood Count		
Hemoglobin (Hb)	6.2 g/dL	11.5-16.0 g/dL
Hematocrit (Hct)	0.22 L/L	0.37-0.47 L/L
RBC count	1.7×10^{12}/L	4.2-5.4×10^{12}/L
WBC count	3.8×10^{9}/L	4.5-11.0×10^{9}/L
Red Blood Cell Indices		
Mean corpuscular volume (MCV)	129.4 fL	80-96 fL
Mean corpuscular hemoglobin (MCH)	36.5 pg	27-32 pg
Mean corpuscular hemoglobin concentration (MCHC)	28%	32%-36%

*Blood smear comments: 3 macrocytic RBCs, polychromatophilia, a few nucleated RBCs.

Limitations

No one test has been shown to be completely reliable for the diagnosis of SLE because many of the ANAs accompanying this disease are also demonstrated in other SRDs, such as rheumatoid arthritis.

Clinical Applications

Sera from patients with SLE have been shown to contain several ANAs, as determined by a wide variety of laboratory tests. A specific diagnosis depends on the evaluation of test results and clinical manifestations.

CHAPTER HIGHLIGHTS

- Autoimmunity represents a breakdown of the immune system in its ability to discriminate between self and nonself.
- The term *autoimmune disorder* is used when demonstrable immunoglobulins, autoantibodies, or cytotoxic T cells display a specificity for self antigens and contribute to disease pathogenesis.
- At one extreme are organ-specific disorders; at the other end of the spectrum are disorders that manifest as organ-nonspecific diseases. Midspectrum disorders are characterized by localized lesions in a single organ and organ-nonspecific autoantibodies.
- The potential for autoimmunity is always present in every immunocompetent individual because lymphocytes that are potentially reactive with self antigens exist in the body.
- Antibody expression appears to be regulated by complex interactions that include genetic factors, patient age, and exogenous factors.

Table 28-13	**Cerebrospinal Fluid Examination**	
Assay	Patient Results	Reference Range
Color, clarity	Clear, colorless	Clear, colorless
Total cells	6	0-8
Nucleated cells	2	0-2
Differential, lymphocytes (%)	75	40-60
CSF protein (mg/dL)	125	20-40
CSF glucose (mg/dL)	70	40-80
CSF IgG (mg/dL)	8.5	0-33
Serum albumin (g/dL)	4.2	3.5-5.0
Serum IgG (mg/dL)	941	700-1450
CSF Profile		
CSF—serum IgG index	1.2	0-0.7
CSF IgG-to-albumin ratio	0.28	0-0.23
Albumin index	7.38	0-7.0
CNS IgG synthesis rate (mg/dL)	22.65	0-2.8

- Self-recognition (tolerance) is induced by at least two mechanisms, elimination of a small clone of immunocompetent cells programmed to react with antigen (Burnet's clonal selection theory) or induction of unresponsiveness in immunocompetent cells through excessive antigen binding to them and through triggering of a suppressor mechanism.
- Major autoantibodies can be detected in different disorders. Many diagnostic laboratory tests are based on detecting these autoimmune responses.

REVIEW QUESTIONS

1. All the following characteristics are common to organ-specific and organ-nonspecific disorders except:
   a. Autoantibody tests are of diagnostic value.
   b. Antibodies may appear in each of the main immunoglobulin classes.
   c. Antigens are available to lymphoid system in low concentrations.
   d. Circulatory autoantibodies react with normal body constituents.

2. Antibody expression in the development of autoimmunity is regulated by all the following factors except:
   a. Genetic predisposition
   b. Increasing age
   c. Environmental factors (e.g., ultraviolet [UV] radiation)
   d. Active infectious disease

3. The mechanism responsible for autoimmune disorder is:
   a. Circulating immune complexes
   b. Antigen excess
   c. Antibody excess
   d. Antigen deficiency

4. One of the mechanisms believed to induce self-tolerance is:
   a. Induction of responsiveness in immunocompetent cells
   b. Elimination of clone programmed to react with antigen
   c. Decreased suppressor cell activity
   d. Stimulation of clones of immunocompetent cells

5-8. Match the following (use an answer only once).

5. _____ Acetylcholine receptor–blocking antibodies

6. _____ Anticardiolipin antibody

7. _____ Anti-DNA antibodies

8. _____ Anti–glomerular basement membrane antibodies
   a. Helpful in monitoring Addison's disease
   b. Found in one third of patients with myasthenia gravis
   c. Useful in monitoring the activity and exacerbations of SLE
   d. Suggestive of Goodpasture's disease
   e. Present in SLE and associated with arterial and venous thrombosis

9-12. Match the following:

9. _____ Antinuclear ribonucleoprotein

10. _____ Anti-Scl

11. _____ Anti-Sm

12. _____ Anti–smooth muscle
   a. Antibody to basic nonhistone nuclear protein, diagnostic of systemic sclerosis
   b. Present in bullous pemphigoid
   c. Presence of antibody confirms diagnosis of SLE
   d. Seen in viral disorders
   e. Characteristic of mixed connective tissue disease

13-15. Match the following:

13. _____ Anti SS-A

14. _____ Histone-reactive antinuclear antibody

15. _____ PM-I antibody
   a. Detectable in patients with myasthenia gravis
   b. Demonstrable in Sjögren's syndrome—sicca complex
   c. Highly suggestive of drug-induced lupus erythematosus
   d. Found in one third of patients with uncomplicated polymyositis and some patients with dermatomyositis
   e. Found in most patients with polymyositis

16. The term *autoimmune disorder* is used when:
   a. Demonstrable immunoglobulins display specificity for self antigens.
   b. Cytotoxic T cells display specificity for self antigens.
   c. Cytotoxic T cells contribute to the pathogenesis of the disease.
   d. All of the above

17-21. Indicate true statements (A) and false statements with (B).

17. _____ The presence of autoantibodies are only associated with autoimmune disease.

18. _____ In organ-specific disorders, antigens are only available to the lymphoid system in low concentrations.

19. _____ There is a familial tendency to develop organ-specific disorders.

20. _____ In organ-specific disorders, lesions are caused by deposition of antigen-antibody complexes.

21. _____ In organ-specific disorders, there is a tendency to develop cancer.

22. Self-recognition (tolerance) is induced by:
   a. Burnet's clonal selection theory
   b. Elimination of the small clone of immunocompetent cells programmed to react with the antigen
   c. Induction of unresponsiveness in the immunocompetent cells through excessive antigen binding
   d. All of the above

23-26. Match each term with the correct description.

23. _____ Acetylcholine receptor binding antibody (AChR)

24. _____ Anticentromere antibody

25. _____ Antiintrinsic factor antibody

26. _____ Antimitochondrial antibody
   a. Strongly suggestive, in a high titer, of primary biliary binding antibody cirrhosis
   b. Useful in the diagnosis of myasthenia gravis
   c. Demonstrated in most patients with CREST syndrome
   d. Found in 60% of patients with pernicious anemia

27-30. Match each term below with the correct description.

27. _____ Antimyelin antibody

28. _____ Antimyocardial antibody

29. _____ Cytoplasmic antineutrophil cytoplasmic antibody (c-ANCA)

30. _____ Antinuclear antibody (ANA)
   a. Associated with multiple myeloma
   b. Marker for Wegener's granulomatosis
   c. Characteristic of untreated systemic lupus erythematosus
   d. Diagnostic of Dressler's syndrome or rheumatic fever

31-34. Match each organ in the illustration with the appropriate disease.

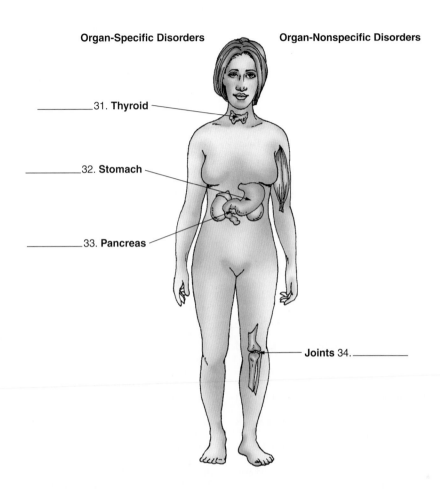

Organ-Specific Disorders   **Organ-Nonspecific Disorders**

_____ 31. **Thyroid**

_____ 32. **Stomach**

_____ 33. **Pancreas**

Joints 34._____

Possible answers to question 31	**Possible answers to question 32**	**Possible answers to question 33**	**Possible answers to question 34**
a. Takayasu arteritis	a. Eosinophilia-myalgia	a. Addison's disease	a. Idiopathic biliary cirrhosis
b. Behçet's disease	b. Hashimoto's thyroiditis	b. Sheehan's syndrome	b. Crohn's disease
c. Graves' disease	c. Raynaud's phenomenon	c. Insulin-dependent diabetes	c. Rheumatoid arthritis
d. Scleroderma	d. Pernicious anemia	d. Sjögren's syndrome	d. Multiple sclerosis

35. The immunologic manifestations of multiple sclerosis include all the following except:
   a.   Antimyelin antibodies
   b.   An oligoclonal increase in CSF immunoglobulin
   c.   In vitro antibody-mediated immunity
   d.   An increase in certain HLA and Ia antigens

36. Most immunologically mediated renal diseases fall into one of the following categories, except for:
   a.   Association with circulating immune complexes
   b.   Association with circulating antigen
   c.   Association with anti–glomerular basement membrane antibody
   d.   Membranoproliferative glomerulonephritis

37. Polymyositis and dermatomyositis are the most common expressions of:
   a.   Rheumatoid heart disease
   b.   Skeletal muscle disorders
   c.   Rheumatoid arthritis
   d.   Either a or b

38-40. Indicate whether each of the following statements is true (A) or false (B) regarding the epidemiology of autoimmune pancreatitis.

38. _____ It is more common in women than men.

39. _____ Most patients are younger than 50 years at diagnosis.

40. _____ The number of reported cases has been decreasing over the last decade.

41. The immunologic abnormality associated with autoimmune pancreatitis in the Japanese population is:
    a. Autoantibodies against carbonic anhydrase
    b. HLA haplotype
    c. Hypogammaglobulinemia
    d. Elevated serum IgE levels

BIBLIOGRAPHY

Ahern P: Gut reactions: study reveals new causes of bowel disease, Dana Foundation Immunol News 6:7–8, 2006.

Ascherio A: Epstein-Barr virus antibodies and risk of multiple sclerosis: a prospective study, JAMA 286:3083–3088, 2001.

Bach J: The effect of infections on susceptibility to autoimmune and allergic diseases, N Engl J Med 347:911–919, 2002.

Bakalar N: Crohn's disease and colitis are linked to mutant gene, Dana Foundation Immunol News 6:1–2, 2006.

Black A: Antiphospholipid syndrome: an overview, Clin Lab Sci 19:144–147, 2006.

Chang A, et al: Research results on myelin repair in long-standing MS brain, N Engl J Med 346:165–173, 2002.

Cho JH, Gregersen PK: Genomics and the multifactorial nature of human autoimmune disease, N Engl J Med 365:1612–1623, 2011.

Davidson A, Diamond B: Autoimmune disease, N Engl J Med 345:340–350, 2001.

Dyment DA, Ebers GC: An array of sunshine in multiple sclerosis, N Engl J Med 347:1445–1447, 2002.

Finkelberg D, Sahani D, Deshpande V, Brugge WR: Autoimmune pancreatitis, N Engl J Med 355:2670–2676, 2006.

Foley KF, Kao P: Biomarkers for inflammatory bowel disease, Clin Lab Sci 20:84–88, 2007.

Frohman EM, Racke MK, Raine CS: Multiple sclerosis—the plaque and its pathogenesis, N Engl J Med 354:942–954, 2006.

Gosink J: Laboratory diagnostics for celiac disease, Med Lab Observer 44(3):30–33, 2012.

Hochberg EP, Gilman MD, Hasserjian RP: Case 17-2006: a 34-year-old man with cavitary lung lesions, N Engl J Med 354:2485–2492, 2006.

Hogancamp WE, Rodriguez M, Weinshenker BG: The epidemiology of multiple sclerosis, Mayo Clin Proc 72:871–878, 1997.

IMMCO Diagnostics: Autoimmune gastritis and pernicious anemia, Buffalo, NY, 2006, IMMCO Diagnostics.

IMMCO Diagnostics: Autoimmunity, Buffalo, NY, 2006, IMMCO Diagnostics.

Kahn AI, Susa J, Ansari Q: Systemic sclerosis (scleroderma), Lab Med 36:723–728, 2005.

Kappos L, et al: Oral fingolimod (FTY 720) for relapsing multiple sclerosis, N Engl J Med 355:1124–1138, 2006.

Keren DF: Anti-ss DNA is not a useful diagnostic test, College of American Pathologists, 2001, http://www.cap.org.

King D: Experts predict advances in autoimmune disease testing, Adv Med Lab Prof 13:8–11, 2001.

Krawitt EL: Autoimmune hepatitis, N Engl J Med 354:54–64, 2006.

Kuhle J, et al: Lack of association between antimyelin antibodies and progression to multiple sclerosis, N Engl J Med 356:371–378, 2007.

Lechner K, Jager U: How I treat autoimmune hemolytic anemias in adults, Blood 116:1831–1838, 2010.

Lyons PA, et al: Genetically distinct subsets within ANCA-associated vasculitis, N Eng J Med 367:214–223, 2012.

Mackay IR: Autoimmune hepatitis: from the clinic to the diagnostic laboratory lab medicine, Lab Medicine vol 42(4):224–232, April 2011.

Mannon PJ, et al: Anti–interleukin-12 antibody for active Crohn's disease, N Engl J Med 351:2069–2078, 2004.

Mooney B: Diagnosing pediatric autoimmune diseases, Adv Med Lab Prof 4:13–14, 26, 2002.

Mueller PW, et al: Type 1 diabetes autoantibodies, Clin Lab News 36:8–10, 2010.

Multiple Sclerosis Foundation: MS information, 2011, www.msfacts.org.

Nakamura RM: Serologic markers in inflammatory bowel disease (IBD), Med Lab Observer MLO 33:8–15, 2001.

National MS: Society: National MS Society Information Resource Center, 2012, http://www.nationalmssociety.org.

Nimmo M: Celiac disease: an update with emphasis on diagnostic considerations, Lab Med 36, 2005.

Noseworthy JH: Multiple sclerosis, N Engl J Med 343:938–952, 2000.

Oksenberk J: Immune protein may play role in MS attacks and progression, Science 294:1613, 2001.

Phelps RG, Rees AJ: The HLA complex in Goodpasture's disease: a model for analyzing susceptibility to autoimmunity, Kidney Int 56:1638–1653, 1999.

Podolsky DK: Inflammatory bowel disease, N Engl J Med 347:417–428, 2002.

Ramsery MK, Owens D: Wegener's granulomatosis: a review of the clinical implications, diagnosis and treatment, Lab Med 37:114–116, 2006.

Robert C, Kupper TS: Inflammatory skin disease, T cells, and immune surveillance, N Engl J Med 341:1817–1827, 1999.

Rosenwasser LJ, Joseph BZ: Immunohematologic diseases, JAMA 268:2940–2945, 1992.

Rutgeerts P, et al: Infliximab for induction and maintenance therapy for ulcerative colitis, N Engl J Med 353:2462–2473, 2005.

Salama AD, et al: Goodpasture's disease, Lancet 358:917, 2001.

Salama AD, et al: Goodpasture's disease, CD4+ T cells escape thymic deletion and are reactive with the autoantigen ∝3(IV)NC1, J Am Soc Nephrol 12:1908–1915, 2001.

Schwartz RS: Autoimmune folate deficiency and the rise and fall of "horror autotoxicus," N Engl J Med 352:1948–1950, 2005.

Sloan EM, et al: Preferential suppression of trisomy 8 compared with normal hematopoietic cell growth by autologous lymphocytes in patients with trisomy 8 myelodysplastic syndrome, Blood 106:841–851, 2005.

Smiroldo J, Coyle PK: Advances in the treatment of multiple sclerosis, Patient Care 33:88–106, 1999.

Smith LA: Autoimmune hemolytic anemias: introduction, Clin Lab Sci 12:109–124, 1999.

Snyder MR, Murray JA: Celiac disease, Clin Lab News 36:8–10, 2010.

Tan FK: Autoantibodies against PDGF receptor in scleroderma, N Engl J Med 354:2709–2711, 2006.

Torassa U: Odd illnesses, strong clues: autoimmune woes target women, San Francisco Chronicle 69, Feb 18, 2001.

Turgeon ML: Fundamentals of immunohematology, ed 2, Baltimore, 1995, Williams & Wilkins.

Turgeon ML: Clinical hematology: theory and procedures, ed 5, Philadelphia, 2012, Lippincott–Williams & Wilkins.

Utiger RD: The pathogenesis of autoimmune thyroid disease, N Engl J Med 325:278–280, 1991.

Voulgarelis M, et al: Malignant lymphoma in primary Sjögren's syndrome, Arthritis Rheum 42:1765–1772, 1999.

Watanabe T, et al: Anti–alpha-Fodrin antibodies in Sjögren syndrome and lupus erythematosus, Arch Dermatol 135:535–539, 1999.

Winter WE: Diabetes disease management, Clin Lab News 31, 2005.

Wright MZ, Dearing LD: The role of HLA testing in autoimmune disease, Adv Med Lab Prof 13:81–84, 2001.

Yorde L: Diagnosing thyroid disorder, Adv Med Lab Prof 12:17, 2000.

Zeher M, et al: Correlation of increased susceptibility to apoptosis of CD4+ T cells with lymphocyte activation and activity of disease in patients with primary Sjögren's syndrome, Arthritis Rheum 42:1673–1681, 1999.

Zinkernagel RM: Maternal antibodies, childhood, infections, and autoimmune diseases, N Engl J Med 345:1331–1335, 2001.

Systemic Lupus Erythematosus

Learning Objectives

At the conclusion of this chapter, the reader should be able to:

- Compare the different forms of lupus, citing manifestations, incidence, and other features.
- Name the two most common drugs that can cause drug-induced lupus.
- Explain the epidemiology and signs and symptoms of SLE.
- Describe the immunologic manifestations of SLE, including diagnostic evaluation.
- Discuss the laboratory evaluation of antinuclear antibodies.

- Analyze selected SLE case studies. Correctly answer case study related multiple choice questions
- Be prepared to participate in a discussion of critical thinking questions.
- Describe the principle, sources of error, limitation, and clinical application of the antinuclear antibody visible method
- Describe the principle and clinical applications of the rapid slide test for antinucleoprotein and autoimmune enzyme immunoassay ANA screening test
- Correctly answer end of chapter review questions.

Key Terms

antineutrophil cytoplasmic antibodies
    (ANCAs)
antinuclear antibody (ANA)
antiphospholipid antibodies
antiphospholipid syndrome

autoimmune
discoid lupus
idiopathic SLE
lupus anticoagulants
lupus erythematosus

neonatal lupus
NETs
nonhistone proteins
Raynaud's phenomenon

Systemic lupus erythematosus (SLE) is the classic model of an **autoimmune** disease. SLE is a systemic rheumatic disorder and the term used most often for the group of disorders that includes SLE and other abnormalities involving multiple systems (e.g., joints, connective tissue, collagen vascular system) in the disease process. Table 29-1 lists the American College of Rheumatology criteria for the classification of SLE.

DIFFERENT FORMS OF LUPUS

There are several forms of lupus, including discoid, systemic, drug-induced, and **neonatal lupus.**

Discoid (cutaneous) lupus is always limited to the skin and is identified by biopsy of the rash that may appear on the face, neck, and scalp. Discoid lupus does not generally involve the

Table 29-1	1997 Update of the 1982 American College of Rheumatology Revised Criteria for Classification of Systemic Lupus Erythematosus
Criterion	**Definition**
1. Malar rash	Fixed erythema, flat or raised, over the malar eminences, tending to spare the nasolabial folds
2. Discoid rash	Erythematous raised patches with adherent keratotic scaling and follicular plugging; atrophic scarring may occur in older lesions
3. Photosensitivity	Skin rash as a result of unusual reaction to sunlight by patient history or physician observation
4. Oral ulcers	Oral or nasopharyngeal ulceration, usually painless, observed by physician
5. Nonerosive arthritis	Involving two or more peripheral joints, characterized by tenderness, swelling, or effusion
6. Pleuritis or pericarditis	1. Pleuritis—convincing history of pleuritic pain or rubbing heard by a physician, or evidence of pleural effusion *OR* 2. Pericarditis—documented by electrocardiogram (ECG) or rub or evidence of pericardial effusion
7. Renal disorder	1. Persistent proteinuria >0.5 g/day, or >3+ if quantitation not performed *OR* 2. Cellular casts—may be red cell, hemoglobin, granular, tubular, or mixed
8. Neurologic disorder	1. Seizures—in the absence of offending drugs or known metabolic derangements (e.g., uremia, ketoacidosis, electrolyte imbalance) *OR* 2. Psychosis—in the absence of offending drugs or known metabolic derangements (e.g., uremia, ketoacidosis, electrolyte imbalance)
9. Hematologic disorder	1. Hemolytic anemia—with reticulocytosis *OR* 2. Leukopenia—<4000/mm^3 total on two or more occasions *OR* 3. Lymphopenia—<1500/mm^3 on two or more occasions *OR* 4. Thrombocytopenia—<100,000/mm^3 in the absence of offending drugs

10. Immunologic disorder	1. Anti-DNA—antibody to native DNA in abnormal titer
	OR
	2. Anti-Sm—presence of antibody to Sm nuclear antigen
	OR
	3. Positive finding of antiphospholipid antibodies on:
	  1. An abnormal serum level of IgG or IgM anticardiolipin antibodies
	  2. A positive test result for lupus anticoagulant using a standard method
	  3. A false-positive test result for at least 6 mo and confirmed by *Treponema pallidum* immobilization or fluorescent treponemal antibody absorption test
	Standard methods should be used in testing for the presence of antiphospholipids.

11. Positive antinuclear antibody	An abnormal titer of antinuclear antibody by immunofluorescence or an equivalent assay at any point in time and in the absence of drugs known to be associated with drug-induced lupus syndrome

From Hochberg MC: Updating the American College of Rheumatology revised criteria for the classification of systemic lupus erythematosus (letter), Arthritis Rheum 40:1725, 1997 and The American College of Rheumatology www.rheumatology.org 2012.

body's internal organs but can evolve into the systemic form of the disease, even if treated. Evolution to systemic lupus cannot be predicted or prevented. The **antinuclear antibody (ANA)** test may be negative or positive at a low titer. Discoid lupus accounts for approximately 10% of all cases of lupus.

Systemic lupus is usually more severe than discoid lupus and can affect the skin, joints, and almost any organ or body system, including the lungs, kidneys, heart, and brain. Systemic lupus may include periods in which few, if any, symptoms are evident (remission) and other times when the disease becomes more active (flare). Most often, when people mention "lupus," they are referring to the systemic form of the disease. Approximately 70% of lupus cases are systemic. In about 50% of these cases, a major organ will be affected.

Drug-induced lupus occurs after the use of certain prescribed drugs (Box 29-1). The most frequently used drugs associated with drug-induced lupus are hydralazine hydrochloride and procainamide hydrochloride. Factors such as the rate of drug metabolism, the drug's influence on immune regulation, and the host's genetic composition are all believed to influence

Box 29-1	**Drugs That Can Produce Clinical and Serologic Features of Systemic Lupus Erythematosus**

- Antiarrhythmics (e.g., procainamide hydrochloride)
- Anticonvulsants (e.g., phenytoin)
- Antihypertensives (e.g., hydralazine hydrochloride)
- Miscellaneous (e.g., chlorpromazine, isoniazid, penicillin, sulfonamides)

pathogenesis. Some drugs (e.g., oral contraceptives, isoniazid) induce serum antinuclear antibodies (ANAs) without symptoms. High antibody titers may exist for months without the development of clinical symptoms.

Procainamide-induced disease does not induce antibodies to double-stranded deoxyribonucleic acid (dsDNA). The ANAs in the drug-induced syndromes are histone-dependent and are never the only ANAs present in the blood. Even with discontinuation of the drug, antibody titers usually remain elevated for months or years.

Only about 4% of patients who take these drugs will develop the antibodies suggestive of lupus. Of those 4%, only an extremely small number will develop overt drug-induced lupus. The symptoms of drug-induced lupus are similar to those of systemic lupus, but milder. Patients with drug-related lupus have a predominance of pulmonary and polyserositic signs and symptoms. Patients with drug-induced lupus have no associated renal or central nervous system (CNS) disease. In addition, lupus-inducing drugs do not appear to exacerbate **idiopathic SLE**. The symptoms usually fade when the medications are discontinued.

Neonatal lupus is a rare condition acquired from the passage of maternal autoantibodies, specifically anti-Ro/SS-A or anti-La/SS-B, that can affect the skin, heart, and blood of the fetus and newborn. Neonatal lupus is associated with a rash that appears within the first several weeks of life and may persist for about 6 months before disappearing. Congenital heart block can occur but is much less common than a rash. Neonatal lupus is not systemic lupus.

ETIOLOGY

The cause of SLE is unknown (idiopathic). Although no single causative agent has been identified, a primary defect in the regulation of the immune system is considered important in the pathogenesis of the disorder. Genetic predisposition can be a factor. Hormones and environmental factors that may trigger the disease include infections, antibiotics (especially sulfonamides and penicillin derivatives), ultraviolet (UV) light, extreme stress, and certain drugs. A combination of these factors may be synergistic.

Antibodies directed against T lymphocytes, including the membrane molecules that mediate their responses, are regularly detected in patients with SLE. Their role in the pathogenesis of autoimmunity is still unclear.

Hormonal Influences

Hormonal factors may explain why lupus occurs more frequently in women than in men. Lupus is often called a woman's

disease because a disproportionate number of women between puberty and menopause suffer from SLE. The increase in disease symptoms may be caused by hormones, particularly estrogen. There is a risk that the disease will worsen during pregnancy and the immediate postpartum period. In addition, postmenopausal therapy is associated with an increased risk for developing SLE. The exact reason for the greater prevalence of lupus in women, and the cyclic increase in symptoms, is unknown.

A condition called the **antiphospholipid syndrome** can be secondary to lupus and may complicate pregnancy. Antibodies against specific autoantigens often present on coagulation factors can cause blood to clot faster than normal or, in some cases, not at all. **Antiphospholipid antibodies** can be found in many patients with lupus and pose a particular risk to pregnant lupus patients because their presence is often associated with miscarriages.

Both the developing fetus and the pregnant mother with lupus are at increased risk of various complications during and after pregnancy. Passive placental transfer of maternal antibodies can produce transient abnormalities such as hepatosplenomegaly, cytopenia, and a photosensitive rash in the newborn. These conditions do resolve themselves in the newborn after the antibody titer declines (see earlier discussion of neonatal lupus).

Genetic Predisposition

Lupus is known to occur within families, but there is no identified gene or genes associated with lupus. Previously, genes on chromosome 6 called immune response genes were associated with the disease. The discovery of a gene on chromosome 1 has been associated with lupus in certain families. Only 10% of lupus patients will have a parent or sibling who already has or may develop lupus. Statistics show that only about 5% of the children born to those with lupus will develop the illness.

Environmental Factors

Various factors, including UV light and bacterial and viral infections, are capable of inducing or exacerbating the signs and symptoms of SLE. These factors may act in different ways. For example, UV light may cause DNA to form thymine dimers, which significantly alters the antigenicity of DNA and could result in the formation of anti-DNA.

EPIDEMIOLOGY

Lupus can occur at any age and in either gender, although it occurs 10 to 15 times more frequently in women than in men after puberty. The Lupus Foundation of America estimates that approximately 1.4 million Americans have a form of lupus. The overall incidence of SLE is estimated to be 50 to 70 new cases/year/1 million population.

Racial groups such as blacks, Native Americans, Puerto Ricans, and Asians (particularly Chinese) demonstrate an increased frequency of SLE. Lupus is two to three times more prevalent among people of color. The incidence of SLE in black women between the 20 and 64 years old is 1 in 245. The reasons for ethnic differences are not clear.

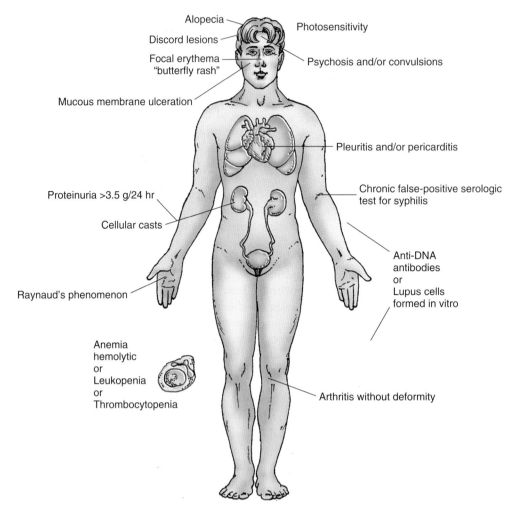

Alopecia
Discord lesions
Focal erythema "butterfly rash"
Mucous membrane ulceration
Photosensitivity
Psychosis and/or convulsions
Pleuritis and/or pericarditis
Chronic false-positive serologic test for syphilis
Proteinuria >3.5 g/24 hr
Cellular casts
Anti-DNA antibodies or Lupus cells formed in vitro
Raynaud's phenomenon
Anemia hemolytic or Leukopenia or Thrombocytopenia
Arthritis without deformity

Figure 29-1   **Signs and symptoms of systemic lupus erythematosus (SLE).**

The prevalence rate, based on a total population, is 1 in 2000, but it is 1 in 700 for women between 20 and 64 years old; 80% of those with systemic lupus develop it between ages 15 and 45 years.

Survival is estimated to be higher than 90% at 10 years after diagnosis. The highest mortality rate is in patients with progressive renal involvement or CNS disease. The two most frequent causes of death are renal failure and infectious complications.

SIGNS AND SYMPTOMS

SLE is a disease of acute and chronic inflammation. Symptoms of SLE often mimic other, less serious illnesses. Fever is one of the most common clinical manifestations of SLE. Disease activity accounts for more than 66% of febrile episodes in patients with SLE. Antibodies with elevated titers that are characteristic of lupus disease activity rather than infection include anti-dsDNA and anti–ribosomal P antibodies, as well as reduced levels of complement and leukopenia.

Many of the clinical manifestations of SLE are a consequence of tissue damage from vasculopathy mediated by immune complexes. Other conditions (e.g., thrombocytopenia, antiphospholipid syndrome) are the direct effects of antibodies to cell surface molecules or serum components.

Manifestations of the disease range from a typical mild illness limited to a photosensitive facial rash and transient diffuse arthritis to life-threatening involvement of the CNS or renal, cardiac, or respiratory system (Fig. 29-1). In the early phases, it is often difficult to distinguish SLE from other systemic rheumatic disorders, such as progressive systemic sclerosis (PSS), polymyositis, primary Sjögren's syndrome, primary Raynaud's phenomenon, and rheumatoid arthritis. Polyarthritis and dermatitis are the most common clinical manifestations.

The course of the disease is highly variable. It usually follows a chronic and irregular course, with periods of exacerbations and remissions. Clinical signs and symptoms can include fever, weight loss, malaise, arthralgia (joint pain) and arthritis (inflammation of the joints), and the characteristic erythematous, maculopapular ("butterfly") rash over the bridge of the nose (Table 29-2). In addition, there is a tendency toward increased susceptibility to common and opportunistic infections. Multiple organ systems may be affected simultaneously.

The onset of lupus can be caused by sun exposure, resulting in sudden development of a rash and then possibly other symptoms. In some patients, an infection, even a cold, does not improve, and complications then arise. These complications may be the first signs of lupus. In some women, the first symptoms develop during pregnancy or soon after delivery.

Table 29-2	Systemic Lupus Erythematosus Symptoms	
Symptom		**Percentage of Cases**
Achy joints (arthralgia)		95
Frequent fevers >37.8° C (100° F)		90
Arthritis (swollen joints)		90
Prolonged or extreme fatigue		81
Skin rashes		74
Anemia		71
Kidney involvement		50
Pain in the chest on deep breathing (pleurisy)		45
Butterfly-shaped rash across the cheek and nose		42
Sun or light sensitivity (photosensitivity)		30
Hair loss		27
Abnormal blood clotting problems		20
Raynaud's phenomenon (fingers turning white and/or blue in the cold)		17
Seizures		15
Mouth or nose ulcers		12

Adapted from Lupus Foundation of America: General Lupus Fact Sheet, 2012 (http://www.lupus.org/webmodules/webarticlesnet/?z=8&a=351org).

Infection

About 20% of episodes of fever are caused by infections in patients with SLE. Infections are the leading cause of death in hospitalized patients. Infections can be caused by bacterial, viral, fungal, or parasitic pathogens. Immunosuppression produced by treatment (e.g., steroids) can interfere with host defense against opportunistic infections (e.g., *Mycobacterium tuberculosis, Histoplasma capsulatum, Listeria monocytogenes*).

Cutaneous Features

Approximately 20% to 25% of patients with SLE develop dermal disorders as the initial manifestation of the disease. As many as 65% of patients will develop a cutaneous abnormality during the course of the disease. The characteristic erythematous, maculopapular butterfly rash across the nose and upper cheeks is the cutaneous feature for which the disease is named—**lupus erythematosus,** the "red wolf" (Fig. 29-2). This rash may also be observed on the arms and trunk. Exposure to UV light will worsen erythematous, as well as other types of, cutaneous lesions.

The spectrum of cutaneous abnormalities includes urticaria, angioedema, nonthrombocytopenic purpura associated with the presence of cryoglobulins, scale formation, and ulcerations of oral and genital mucous membranes. Although neither the collection of immunoglobulins and complement at the dermal-epidermal junction nor the presence of specific antibody

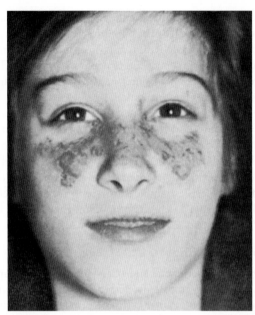

Figure 29-2   Facial rash over bridge of nose in patient with active SLE. *(From Behrman R, Kliegman R, Jenson HB: Nelson's textbook of pediatrics, ed 17, Philadelphia, 2004, Saunders.)*

nuclear ribonucleoprotein (RNP), Sm, native DNA, and single-stranded DNA appears to play a direct role in the pathogenesis of cutaneous lupus lesion, Ro (SS-A) and perhaps La (SS-B) antibodies may be prominent factors.

Diffuse or patchy alopecia is also a common cutaneous manifestation. Hair loss is caused by pustular lesions of the scalp and is usually related to the stress of the disease process. Although the cause of pustular lesions is unknown, these inflammatory infiltrates are characterized by the presence of predominantly Ia-positive (activated) T lymphocytes with both CD4+ and CD8+ phenotypes.

Approximately 2% to 3% of SLE patients demonstrate lupus panniculitis. This condition is characterized by tender or nontender subcutaneous nodules that sometimes ulcerate and discharge a yellowish lipid material. In addition, various nonspecific skin changes are observable secondary to vascular insults. **Raynaud's phenomenon** is demonstrated by approximately one third of patients with SLE and appears to be increased in those who have antibodies to nuclear RNP in their serum.

The presence of lesions does not distinguish between the limited cutaneous (discoid lupus erythematosus) and cutaneous manifestations of SLE. The term **discoid lupus** is used to differentiate the benign dermatitis of cutaneous lupus from the cutaneous involvement of SLE. In discoid lupus, the round lesion is an erythematous inflammatory dermatosis. These lesions are primarily located in light-exposed areas of the skin.

Renal Characteristics

Complement-mediated injury to the renal system is a usual consequence of the high levels of immune complexes in the blood that are deposited in tissues such as the kidneys. Renal disease progression is highly unpredictable. It may be acute, but more typically it progresses slowly. As the kidneys degenerate, the urinary sediment is typical of acute glomerulonephritis and later of chronic glomerulonephritis. Acute glomerulonephritis is characterized by the presence of erythrocytes, leukocytes, and granular and red blood cell (RBC) casts in urinary sediment. The presence of proteinuria may lead to nephrotic syndrome. If end-stage renal disease (renal failure) occurs, it can be managed by dialysis or allograft transplantation.

The systemic necrotizing vasculitis of SLE involves small blood vessels and leads to renal involvement. The most common method of classification of the renal involvement of SLE is the World Health Organization (WHO) system, which is based on histopathologic criteria. The stages of renal disease range from the earliest and least severe form, class II, characterized by mesangial deposits of immunoglobulin and C3, to class V, the most severe form of involvement.

Lymphadenopathy

Enlargement of peripheral and axial lymph nodes and splenomegaly both occur in patients with SLE, but these conditions are usually transient. Patients with SLE may be at greater risk of developing lymphoma than the general population, especially those with secondary Sjögren's syndrome.

Serositis

Serositis is an inflammation of the membrane consisting of mesothelium, a thin layer of connective tissue that lines enclosed body cavities. Mesothelium, a type of epithelium, is originally derived from the mesoderm lining the primitive embryonic body cavity. It becomes the covering of the serous membranes of the body surfaces such as the peritoneum, pleura, and pericardium. Inflammation of these serosal surfaces leads to sterile peritonitis, pleuritis, or pericarditis and is frequently accompanied by severe pain. Serositis is associated with an increased frequency of thrombophlebitis, which may lead to pulmonary embolization.

Cardiopulmonary Characteristics

Inflammation of the myocardium in patients with SLE can produce persistent tachycardia and, occasionally, intractable congestive heart failure. Ischemic disease or, more often, atherosclerotic coronary disease may occur. Patients with severe nephrosis or those treated with corticosteroids for a prolonged period are at an increased risk for developing atherosclerosis.

Pulmonary function studies reveal occult diffusion and obstructive abnormalities in a high proportion of SLE patients, but clinical problems secondary to pulmonary involvement are unusual. Massive hemoptysis may result from acute alveolar hemorrhage. This particular complication occurs in the absence of any detectable bleeding diathesis and is associated with a high rate of mortality.

Gastrointestinal Manifestations

Nonspecific gastrointestinal symptoms are relatively common in patients with SLE, but acute abdominal crises caused by visceral and peritoneal vasculitis are less common. Infarction and perforation of the bowel and viscera are associated with a high rate of mortality. Acute and chronic pancreatitis may also develop as a secondary complication of acute lupus or as a complication during therapy.

Musculoskeletal Features

A characteristic arthritis of SLE is a transient and peripheral polyarthritis with symmetric involvement of small and large joints. Chronic arthritis can result in disability and deformity in SLE patients. Rheumatoid-like hand deformities develop in about 10% of patients. Osteonecrosis develops in 25% of all SLE patients. Arthropathy of osteonecrosis, or avascular necrosis, is often initially detected in weight-bearing joints such as the hips and knees.

Neuropsychiatric Features

In SLE, various neuropsychiatric manifestations develop secondary to involvement of the central and peripheral nervous systems. CNS involvement in SLE includes inflammation of the brain or intracranial blood vessels (vasculitis) and ischemic complications of vasculitis.

The most common abnormalities are disturbances of mental function, ranging from mild confusion, with memory deficiency and impairment of orientation and perception, to psychiatric disturbances such as hypomania, delirium, and schizophrenia. The most common manifestations are cognitive dysfunction, headache, seizures, and psychiatric conditions. Aseptic meningitis, stroke, encephalopathy, movement disorders, and myelopathy can be observed.

Seizures of the grand mal type may be the initial manifestation of SLE and may be present long before the multisystem disease develops. In addition, some patients may have epilepsy and severe headaches.

Antiribosomal P antibodies have been detected in patients with lupus suffer from psychosis or depression.

Late-Onset Lupus

Lupus can occur at any age, in either gender, and in any race. The average age of onset is 59 years; the average age at diagnosis is 62 years. Late-onset lupus affects women eight times more often than men. Late-onset lupus is found primarily in whites, but it occurs in all races.

Symptoms in most cases are relatively mild, but symptoms of lupus in older people can mimic those of other diseases (e.g., rheumatoid arthritis, Sjögren's syndrome, polymyalgia rheumatica). Distinguishing among these disorders can be difficult and may result in a delayed or missed diagnosis. Drug-induced lupus occurs more often in older people because they are more likely to have conditions (e.g., high blood pressure, heart disease) that require treatment that may cause the symptoms of lupus. Symptoms generally fade when the medication is discontinued. Patients with late-onset lupus have a good survival rate and rarely die of the disease or complications of therapy when treated conservatively.

IMMUNOLOGIC MANIFESTATIONS

B lymphocytes, T lymphocytes, and dendritic cells are involved in the pathogenesis of SLE. The pathogenesis of this systemic autoimmune disorder is characterized by the loss of tolerance to nuclear antigens, deposition of immune complexes in tissues, and multiorgan involvement.

Patients with SLE are known to produce multiple autoantibodies. There are two leading hypotheses, not mutually exclusive, as to why so many different antibodies develop. One hypothesis supports the belief that antibody-forming B lymphocytes are stimulated in a relatively nonspecific manner, so-called polyclonal B cell activation. The second hypothesis is that the immune response in SLE is specifically stimulated by antigens. The most compelling evidence in its favor is that the antibody molecules formed over time show evidence of the gene rearrangement and somatic mutation characteristic of an antigen-driven response. Recent studies have suggested that the neutrophilic leukocyte activity is implicated in linked biochemical and cellular events. Findings suggest that in SLE, anti–self antibodies activate neutrophils that consequently release neutrophil extracellular traps (NETs) containing complexes of DNA and antimicrobial peptide. These complexes activate plasmacytoid dendritic cells, which leads to interferon-α release and perpetuation of inflammation and disease. In the future, NETs may serve as a biomarker or predictor of tissue damage in SLE.

Laboratory features of SLE are the presence of ANAs, immune complexes, decreased complement level, tissue deposition of immunoglobulins and complement, circulating anticoagulants, and other autoantibodies. The human **antineutrophil cytoplasmic antibodies (ANCAs),** described for the first time in 1982, are directed against antigenic components mainly present in primary granules of neutrophils. ANCAs are serologic markers of primary necrotizing systemic vasculitis, particularly in Wegener's granulomatosis. In addition, these antibodies have a prognostic interest because, in most cases, their titer is correlated with clinical activity during the disease.

Cellular Aspects

SLE is a disease that results from defects in the regulatory mechanism of the immune system. Studies of the immunopathogenesis of lupus nephritis have demonstrated a variety of aberrations in T cell and B cell function. It is uncertain whether the disease represents a primary dysfunction of T cells or B cells, but alterations in function do occur. Lymphocyte subset abnormalities are a major immunologic feature of SLE. Among the T cell subsets, a lack of or reduced generalized suppressor T cell function and hyperproduction of helper T cells occurs. The formation of lymphocytotoxic antibodies with a predominant specificity for T lymphocytes by patients with SLE at least partially explains the interference with certain functional activities of T lymphocytes associated with SLE. Lymphocytotoxic antibodies are capable of destroying T lymphocytes in the presence of complement and coating peripheral blood T cells.

The regulation of antibody production by B lymphocytes, ordinarily a function of the subpopulation of suppressor T cells, appears to be defective in patients with SLE. Although no single cause can be implicated in the pathogenesis of SLE, patients exhibit a state of spontaneous B lymphocyte hyperactivity, with ensuing uncontrolled production of a wide variety of antibodies to host and exogenous antigens. Host response to some antigens, such as vaccination with influenza, is normal in many cases and the patient manifests a specific, well-controlled humoral immune response.

Humoral Aspects

Circulating immune complexes are the hallmark of SLE. Patients with SLE exhibit multiple serum antibodies that react with native or altered self antigens. Demonstrable antibodies include antibodies to the following:

- Nuclear components
- Cell surface and cytoplasmic antigens of polymorphonuclear and lymphocytic leukocytes, erythrocytes, platelets, and neuronal cells
- Immunoglobulin G (IgG)

SLE is characterized by autoantibodies to almost any organ or tissue in the body. These antibodies may not be specifically diagnostic for SLE. In addition, some may have pathologic significance.

Antibodies to host antigens, particularly nuclear antigens such as DNA, are the principal type of antibody produced in SLE. ANAs are a heterogeneous group of antibodies produced against a variety of antigens within the cell nucleus. ANAs may be found in diseases other than SLE (e.g., other rheumatic or nonrheumatic diseases), as well as in some patients undergoing specific drug therapy and in healthy older individuals. The absence of ANAs almost excludes the diagnosis of SLE unless the patient is being chemically immunosuppressed. ANA titers and specific anti-DNA antibodies fluctuate during the course of the disease. In some cases, a rise in titer may forewarn of an impending disease flare-up.

Antigens to which antibodies are formed are present on nucleic acid molecules (DNA and RNA) or proteins (histones and nonhistones) and on determinants consisting of nucleic acid and protein molecules. Drug-induced cases of lupus have a high incidence of antibodies to histones. Some of these antibodies are directed against the double-stranded helical DNA (native DNA or dsDNA). The presence of anti–native DNA (anti-nDNA) antibodies was reported in 1957. High titers of dsDNA are seen primarily in SLE and closely parallel disease activity. Most SLE patients simultaneously demonstrate antibodies to nucleoprotein and native DNA.

Other nuclear antibodies are directed at the determinants of single-stranded DNA (ssDNA). Antibody titers of 1:32 or higher indicate a substantial concentration of antibody in an autoimmune response. Antibody to the Smith (Sm) antigen, a nuclear acidic protein extractable by aqueous solution, is considered a marker for SLE because anti-Sm has been found almost exclusively in patients with SLE. The presence of anti-Sm is seen in 25% to 30% of patients with SLE, but it rarely occurs in those with other systemic rheumatic (collagen) diseases.

The ANA antideoxyribonucleoprotein (anti-DNP) gives rise to the LE cell, which is found in more than 90% of untreated patients with active SLE. SLE patients with serositis may form LE cells in vivo. The LE cell testing procedure is now an obsolete test. In SLE patients with serositis, LE cells formed in vivo may be observed in aspirate fluid (e.g., pleural fluid). LE cells have been shown to be an expression of the interaction between IgG antibodies and DNP. Anti-DNP is referred to as the LE serum factor.

Antibodies to the Robert (Ro) soluble substance–A (SS-A) nuclear antigens are associated with SLE skin disease and the neonatal SLE syndrome. Antibodies to the Lane soluble substance–B (SS-B) antigens are associated with SLE and with primary and secondary forms of Sjögren's syndrome. Their presence with SS-A antigen in SLE indicates mild disease. When present as the only antibody, SS-B is associated with primary Sjögren's syndrome.

Autoantibodies to RBCs result in hemolytic anemia and can be detected by the anti–human globulin (AHG) test. Membrane-specific autoantibodies to neutrophils and platelets and autoantibodies to lymphocytes (cold-reactive type) are specific for SLE. Antibody titers correlate with disease activity.

Immunologic Consequences

Antibodies combine with their corresponding antigens to form immune complexes. When the mononuclear phagocyte system is unable to eliminate these immune complexes completely, immune complexes accumulate in the blood circulation. These circulating immune complexes are deposited in the subendothelial layers of the vascular basement membranes of multiple target organs, where they mediate inflammation. The sites of deposition are determined in part by the following physiochemical properties of the particular antigens or antibodies involved:

- Size
- Molecular configuration
- Immunoglobulin class
- Complement-fixing ability

After deposition, the immune complexes seem to initiate a localized inflammatory response that stimulates neutrophils to the site of inflammation, activates complement, and results in the release of kinins and prostaglandins. These activities become the basis of antibody-dependent, cell-mediated tissue injury.

DIAGNOSTIC EVALUATION

The manifestations of SLE expressed in laboratory findings are numerous. Histologic, hematologic, and serologic abnormalities reflect the multisystem nature of this disease.

Histologic Changes

The earliest pathologic abnormalities are those of acute vasculitis. Supportive tissue becomes edematous, initially infiltrated with neutrophils and later with plasma cells and lymphocytes. Persistent inflammation results in local deposition of a cellular homogeneous material, histologically similar to fibrin. Nuclear debris from resulting cellular necrosis reacts with ANAs (see later in this section) to form hematoxylin bodies. The presence of immunoglobulins in vascular lesions, predominantly IgM and IgG, can be demonstrated by indirect immunofluorescence.

Renal pathology can also be observed in SLE. The two basic renal abnormalities that manifest are as follows: (1) proliferative glomerulonephritis, which resembles the renal changes in immune complex nephritis; and (2) membranous nephritis.

Hematologic and Hemostatic Findings

In SLE, a moderate anemia (normocytic normochromic anemia) representing chronic disease is a consistent factor. Some patients display coating of erythrocytes, which can be demonstrated by a positive AHG test, but actual hemolysis is infrequent. Lymphocytopenia is common and often reflects disease activity. Thrombocytopenia (50 to 100 × 10^9/L) may also be seen.

Hemostatic Testing

Lupus anticoagulants, antiphospholipid antibodies, are often seen in association with SLE. Antiphospholipid antibodies develop in up to 20% of patients with SLE. These form a group of antibodies detected by tests for lupus anticoagulant and anticardiolipin antibodies.

Circulating anticoagulants are believed to be associated with the presence of false-positive serologic test results for syphilis. Because of the presence of lupus anticoagulant, patients with SLE frequently demonstrate prolonged prothrombin time (PT) and partial thromboplastin time (PTT) results, but lupus anticoagulant rarely causes hemostatic problems. Inhibitors are not necessarily associated with bleeding unless some other defect is present. Because lupus anticoagulant is an inhibitor or prothrombin activator, it is often associated with excessive thrombosis rather than with bleeding. Patients with SLE have a high incidence of thrombotic episodes. Although less common, specific coagulation factor antibodies directed against coagulation factors VIII, IX, XI, and XII have been described. Thrombocytopenia can also occur because of the removal of antiphospholipid antibody–coated platelets.

Serologic Findings

Serologic testing frequently reveals high levels of anti-DNA antibodies, reduced complement levels, and the presence of complement breakdown products of C3 (C3d and C3c). In addition, cryoglobulins, which in some cases represent immune complexes, are frequently present in the serum of patients with SLE. Because monoclonal gammopathies have occasionally been described, a marked increase in gamma globulins may result in a hyperviscosity syndrome or renal tubular acidosis. Serum cryoglobulins of a mixed IgG-IgM type are found in patients with hypocomplementemia. The level of cryoglobulin correlates well with the severity of SLE. The following procedural results are helpful in assessing renal disease:

- Antibody to double-stranded DNA
- Levels of C3 and C4 (with C4 probably being the most sensitive result)
- Cryoglobulin levels

A general correlation exists between abnormal results in each of these procedures and disease activity in many patients, but considerable disagreement surrounds the usefulness of these measurements in predicting renal disease activity. The best laboratory procedures for monitoring the activity of renal disease are the serum creatinine level, urinary protein excretion, and careful examination of urine sediment.

Complement

Inherited deficiencies of several complement components are associated with lupus-like illnesses. Some but not all deficiencies are coded for by autosomal recessive genes of the sixth chromosome, which are in linkage disequilibrium with human leukocyte antigen (HLA)–DRw2. The association of complement deficiencies with SLE may represent the fortuitous association of linked HLA-D region genes, rather than some unusual susceptibility induced by the complement deficiency.

Serum levels of complement typically are reduced, particularly during states of active disease. Deficiencies involving classic and alternative pathway complement components in SLE patients have resulted from consumption of components at the tissue sites of immune complex deposition, impaired synthesis, or both. A depressed level of complement is not specific for the diagnosis of SLE but is a helpful guide in treating patients. Levels of complement (C3, C4) are generally reduced in relationship to disease activity and fluctuation in these levels is often used to monitor disease activity. Patients with decreased levels are at risk for renal and CNS involvement. Deficiencies of C1, C3, and C4 are associated with SLE and other rheumatic diseases.

Antibodies

Nonspecific elevation in immunoglobulin levels, particularly IgM and IgG, frequently occurs in SLE. An actual deficiency of IgA appears to be more common in SLE than in normal individuals.

The ANA procedure (discussed in detail in the next section) is a valuable screening tool for SLE; it has almost replaced the LE cell test because of its wider range of reactivity with nuclear antigens, as well as its greater sensitivity and quality control characteristics.

Antinuclear Antibodies

Characteristics and Implications. ANAs are a heterogeneous group of circulating immunoglobulins that include IgM, IgG, and IgA. These immunoglobulins react with the whole nucleus or nuclear components (e.g., proteins, DNA, histones) in host tissues; therefore, they are true autoantibodies. Generally, ANAs have no organ or species specificity and are capable of cross-reacting with nuclear material from human beings (e.g., human leukocytes) or various animal tissues (e.g., rat liver, mouse kidney). ANAs are found in other diseases (e.g., rheumatoid arthritis), are associated with certain drugs, and are found in older adults without disease (Table 29-3). Thus, assays for ANAs are not specific for SLE. ANAs are present in more than 95% of SLE patients. Because the detection of ANAs is not diagnostic of only SLE, their presence cannot confirm the disease, but the absence of ANAs can be used to help rule out SLE. The significance of the presence of ANAs in a patient's serum must be considered in relation to the patient's age, gender, clinical signs and symptoms, and other laboratory findings.

Systematic Classification. ANAs can be divided into four groups to provide a systematic classification: antibodies to DNA, antibodies to histone, antibodies to nonhistone proteins, and antibodies to nucleolar antigens.

Antibodies to DNA. Antibodies to DNA can be divided into two major groups: (1) antibodies that react with native (double-stranded) DNA; and (2) antibodies that recognize denatured (single-stranded) DNA only.

Table 29-3	**Antibodies in Systemic Rheumatic Diseases**		
Systemic Lupus Erythematosus	**Progressive Systemic Sclerosis**	**Polymyositis**	**Rheumatoid Arthritis**
Antinuclear antibodies	Antinuclear antibodies	Antinuclear antibodies	Antinuclear antibodies
Anti–native DNA	Anti–Scl-1	Anti–Jo-1	Rheumatoid factors
Anti-Sm	—	—	—

Antibodies that react with native DNA appear to interact with antigenic determinants present on the deoxyribose phosphate backbone of the beta helix of DNA. These autoantibodies characteristically stain the kinetoplast of the hemoflagellate *Crithidia luciliae,* a substrate used to detect anti–native DNA antibodies by indirect immunofluorescence. This procedure continues to be the gold standard for testing. Antibodies reactive with denatured DNA probably react with the purine and pyrimidine bases of DNA. These bases are readily accessible on ssDNA; they are buried within the beta helix of dsDNA and are therefore inaccessible. Anti–denatured DNA antibodies are unable to cross-react with native DNA. Conformational changes in the deoxyribose phosphate backbone of denatured DNA appear to be important for antigenicity.

Antibodies to Histones. Antibodies to histones have been shown to react with all major classes of histones—H1, H2A, H2B, H3, and H4. Antihistone antibodies can be induced by drugs such as procainamide and hydralazine. Procainamide-induced lupus erythematosus is characterized by IgG antibodies against the histone complex H2A-H2B in symptomatic patients with SLE. In asymptomatic patients, the antibody may be restricted to the IgM class. Antibodies specific to other nuclear antigens are usually absent in drug-induced lupus in contrast to patients with SLE, who have ANAs of multiple specificity.

Patients with SLE are characterized by the presence of antibodies to multiple antigens, including Sm, RNP, dsDNA, chromatin, and SS-A/Ro (Table 29-4). There are 11 criteria for the diagnosis of SLE and, for a definitive diagnosis, patients must meet at least four of these criteria (see Table 29-1). Two of the criteria are a positive ANA and the detection of antibodies to Sm, dsDNA, or cardiolipin. Antibodies to Sm are detected in 20% to 30% of SLE patients and antibodies to dsDNA may occur in up to 60% of patients. Antibodies to Sm and RNP typically occur together because they react with different proteins that are associated in an RNP particle called a spliceosome. A positive Sm indicates a high probability of SLE.

The presence of antibodies to dsDNA is one of the criteria for the diagnosis of SLE, and these antibodies are associated with active disease. The presence of dsDNA is a major concern in patients with SLE. The formation and deposition of immune complexes can affect various organ systems. Antibodies to dsDNA have also been reported in rheumatoid arthritis

Table 29-4	Immunologic Assays for Detection and Monitoring of SLE	
Name of Assay		**Reference Range**
Antibodies		
Anti–double-stranded (ds) DNA antibody		Negative (1:10)
Anti-La (SS-B) antibody		Negative
Anti–liver cytosol antibody		<15 U/mL
Anti–liver-kidney microsomal (LKM) antibody		<1:40
Antimitochondrial antibody		Negative
Antinuclear antibody		Negative (1:40)
Anti–ribosomal P protein antibody		<20 U/mL
Antiribonucleoprotein (anti-RNP) antibody		Negative
Anti-Ro (SS-A) antibody		Negative
Anti-Smith IgG		Negative
Anti–soluble liver antigen antibody		<5 U/mL
Complement		
Total complement		63-145 U/mL
C3		86-145 mg/dL
C4		20-58 mg/dL

Table 29-5	Antibodies to Nonhistone Proteins (NhPs) and NhP-RNA Complexes in Systemic Rheumatic Diseases	
Antibody	**Disease**	**Incidence (%)**
Centromere-kinetochore	CREST variant of progressive systemic sclerosis (PSS)	70-90
	Diffuse scleroderma	10-20
Jo-1	Polymyositis	31
Ki antigen	Systemic lupus erythematosus (SLE)	20
Ku	Polymyositis/scleroderma overlap	55
Ma antigen	SLE	20
Mi-l	Dermatomyositis	11
NuMa (nuclear mitotic apparatus) antigen	Rheumatoid arthritis (RA) Sjögren's syndrome Carpal tunnel syndrome SLE	3
Proliferating cell nuclear antigen (PCNA)	RA	90
RANA (RA-associated nuclear antigen)	PSS	20
Scl-70	SLE	30
Sm (Smith)	Sjögren's syndrome	70
SS-A/Ro	SLE Other connective tissue diseases	50
	Sjögren's syndrome	40-50
SS-B/La	SLE	15
	Mixed connective tissue disease	>95
Ul-RNP	SLE	35

Adapted from Reimer G, Tan E: Antinuclear antibodies. In Stein J, editor: Internal medicine, Boston, 1987, Little, Brown.

CREST, Calcinosis, Raynaud's phenomenon, esophageal dysmotility, sclerodactyly, and telangiectasia.

patients being treated with the tumor necrosis factor-α (TNF-α) inhibitors. Patients with SLE have antibodies to chromatin more often than antibodies to dsDNA. These chromatin antibodies are also associated with glomerulonephritis and have been identified, along with dsDNA antibodies, in immune complexes eluted from patients' kidneys. Patients with drug-induced lupus develop antibodies to chromatin and, in some cases, to the histone component of chromatin, but not to dsDNA.

The demonstration of only antihistone antibodies may be useful in distinguishing drug-induced lupus from SLE.

Antibodies to Nonhistone Proteins. Another primary class of ANAs in systemic autoimmune disorders is characterized by reactivity with soluble nonhistone nuclear protein and RNA-protein complexes. Clinically important antibodies that react with nuclear **nonhistone proteins** are listed in Table 29-5.

Antibodies to Nucleolar Antigens. The antibodies to nucleolar antigens are as follows:
- U3-RNA-protein complex (enzyme-transcribing ribosomal genes in the nucleolus)
- 7-2-RNP
- RNA polymerase I
- PM-Scl

These antinucleolar antibodies are primarily associated with polymyositis-scleroderma overlap, where they have the highest incidence and titers. However, they are rarely demonstrated in PSS, dermatomyositis, or scleroderma.

Laboratory Evaluation

Demonstrable antibodies include antibodies to nuclear components, cell surface and cytoplasmic antigens of polymorphonuclear and lymphocytic leukocytes, erythrocytes, platelets, and neuronal cells, and IgG. The detection of ANAs is a valuable screening tool for SLE.

Immunofluorescence is extremely sensitive and may show positive results in patients in whom procedures for ANAs (e.g., complement fixation or precipitation) give negative results. At present, immunofluorescence is the most widely used technique for ANA screening. Serologic testing frequently reveals high levels of anti-DNA antibodies, reduced complement levels, and the presence of complement breakdown products of C3 (C3d, C3c).

In addition, cryoglobulins, which may represent immune complexes, are frequently present in the serum of patients with SLE. The level of cryoglobulins correlates well with the severity of SLE. Assays helpful in assessing renal disease associated with SLE are antibodies to dsDNA, levels of C3 andC4, and cryoglobulins.

Indirect Immunofluorescent Tests for Antinuclear Antibody

Indirect immunofluorescent tests for ANA are based on the use of fluorescein-conjugated antiglobulin. These methods are extremely sensitive. In one assay, the serum specimen is delivered into a well on a microscope slide that contains a mouse liver substrate. Substrates of rat or mouse liver or kidney, or cell-cultured fibroblasts, can also be used as the antigen and are fixed to the slides. If antibody is present in the serum of the patient, the unlabeled antibody will attach to the nuclei of the cells in the substrate. After the substrate is washed in buffer, the slide is incubated with fluorescein-labeled goat AHG. If the patient's antibodies have attached themselves to the nuclear antigens in the substrate, the fluorescein-tagged goat AHG will attach to these antibodies. Fluorescence will be seen microscopically using UV light. The slides should be examined as soon as possible. If immediate examination is not possible, the slides can be stored in the dark at 4° C (39° F) for up to 48 hours before being read.

Several different patterns of fluorescence reactivity are seen (see Color Plates #13–#16 and Figure 29-3), depending on whether the ANAs have reacted with the whole nucleus or with nuclear components, such as the nuclear proteins, DNA, or histone (a simple protein). This difference in nuclear fluorescence pattern reflects specificity for various diseases. Patterns are described as being diffused or homogeneous, peripheral, speckled, or nucleolar fluorescence. Nuclear rim (peripheral) patterns correlate with antibody to native DNA and DNP and bear a correlation with SLE, SLE activity, and lupus nephritis. Homogeneous (diffused) patterns suggest SLE or another connective tissue disorder. Speckled patterns are found in many diseases, including SLE. Nucleolar patterns are seen in patients with PSS and Sjögren's syndrome.

After ensuring that the results for positive and negative control specimens are providing the expected reactions, the results for the patient are reported. Results from the screening tests are reported as positive or negative. The normal person is expected to have a negative reaction—no green or gold fluorescence is observed. The degree of positive fluorescence may be semiquantitated on a scale of 1+ to 4+. Positive samples give a green-gold fluorescence of a characteristic pattern (homogeneous, peripheral, speckled, or nucleolar).

Indirect Immunofluorescent Technique

The detection of autoantibodies by immunofluorescence has become an extremely valuable tool. This method is extremely sensitive and may be positive in cases in which procedures for ANAs, such as complement fixation or precipitation, are negative. At present, the indirect immunofluorescent method on a Hep-2 cell substrate is the primary screening test for the diagnosis of systemic rheumatic diseases (SRDs). A negative indirect immunofluorescence result almost rules out a diagnosis of SLE,

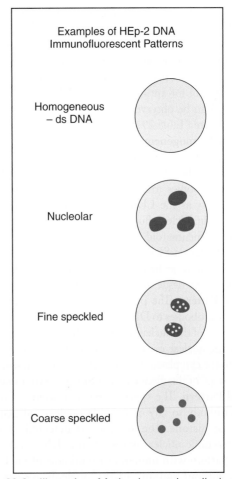

Figure 29-3 Illustration of Antinucleoprotein antibody patterns.

but the patterns observed on Hep-2 slides can provide a key to the diagnosis of other SRDs.

Principles. The antigen in the substrate tissue is fixed to a slide for testing. ANA is not specific for a particular organ; therefore, any tissue containing nuclei may be used as substrate. The tissues most often used are rat or mouse liver or kidney, or cell-cultured fibroblasts grown on slides. If antibody is present in a patient's serum, the unlabeled antibody will attach to the nuclei in the substrate. After the substrate is washed in buffer, it is incubated with fluorescein-tagged goat AHG. If the patient's antibodies have affixed themselves to the nuclear antigens of the substrate, the fluorescein-tagged goat AHG will attach to these antibodies. When the slide is examined microscopically, fluorescence will be visible on UV light.

Interpretation of Staining Patterns of Major Rheumatic Autoantibodies

- Double-stranded DNA (dsDNA)
- Chromatin, Sm
- RNP, SS-A/Ro
- SS-B/La
- Scl-70
- Centromere
- Jo-1, cyclic citrullinated peptide (CCP)

Because ANAs react with the whole nucleus or with nuclear components (e.g., proteins, DNA, histone), reaction patterns reflect the distribution of the various antigens in the nuclei. Major ANAs are detected on all Hep-2 slides, but detection of antibodies to SS-A/Ro varies according to the fixation method. Alcohol diminishes or destroys the SS-A/Ro speckled ANA pattern, leading to a negative ANA. It is always important to include a control for antibodies to SS-A/Ro. Several patterns of reactivity can be observed when a slide is examined in the ANA procedure (Table 29-6).

Diffused or Homogeneous Pattern. The diffused or homogeneous pattern characterizes anti–DNA nucleoprotein antibodies (i.e., antibodies to nDNA, dsDNA, ssDNA, DNP, or histones). Antibodies to DNP have been shown to have the same specificity as the LE factor. Although vacuoles may be seen, the whole nucleus fluoresces evenly. This pattern is typically seen in rheumatoid disorders. High titers of homogeneous ANA suggest SLE, whereas low titers may be found in SLE, rheumatoid arthritis (RA), Sjögren's syndrome, and mixed connective tissue disease (MCTD).

Peripheral Pattern. The peripheral (marginal or rim) pattern results from antibodies to DNA—nDNA, dsDNA, or DNP. The central protein of the nucleus is only lightly stained or not stained at all, but the nuclear margins fluoresce strongly and appear to extend into the cytoplasm. This pattern is associated with SLE in the active stage of the disease and in Sjögren's syndrome.

Speckled Pattern. The speckled pattern occurs in the presence of antibody to any extractable nuclear antigen devoid of DNA or histone. The antibody is detected against the saline extractable nuclear antigens, anti-RNP and anti-Sm. A grainy pattern with numerous round dots of nuclear fluorescence, without staining of the nucleoli, is seen in this pattern type.

Antibodies to Sm antigen have been shown to be highly specific for patients with SLE and appear to be marker antibodies. Anti-RNP has been found in patients with a wide variety of rheumatic diseases, including SLE, RA, Sjögren's syndrome, PSS, MCTD, and dermatomyositis.

Nucleolar Pattern. The nucleolar pattern reflects an antibody to nucleolar RNA (4-6S RNP). A few round smooth nucleoli that vary in size will fluoresce when examined under UV light. The nucleolar pattern is present in about 50% of patients with scleroderma (PSS), Sjögren's syndrome, and SLE. This pattern can also be observed in undiagnosed illnesses manifesting Raynaud's phenomenon.

Centromere. The anticentromere antibody reacts with centromeric chromatin of metaphase and interphase cells. The particular pattern on tissue culture cells is discrete and speckled. This antibody appears to be highly selective for the CREST variant of PSS. The CREST syndrome (*c*alcinosis, *R*aynaud's phenomenon, *e*sophageal dysmotility, *s*clerodactyly, and *t*elangiectasia) is a variant of systemic sclerosis characterized by the presence of calcinosis, Raynaud's phenomenon, esophageal motility abnormalities, sclerodactyly, and telangiectasia. This antibody is found infrequently in the serum of patients with SLE, MCTD, and PSS.

Rapid Slide Test for Antinucleoprotein

The SLE latex test provides a suspension of polystyrene latex particles coated with DNP (see later procedure). When the

Table 29-6	Antinuclear Antibody Patterns and Disorders	
ANA Staining Pattern	**Antibody Specificities**	**Related Disorders**
Homogeneous	nDNA dsDNA ssDNA DNP Histones	Systemic lupus erythematosus (SLE) Rheumatoid arthritis (RA) Sjögren's syndrome Mixed connective tissue disease (MCTD)
Peripheral or rim	nDNA dsDNA DNP	Active SLE Sjögren's syndrome
Speckled	Smith (Sm) RNP	SLE RA Sjögren's syndrome Progressive systemic sclerosis (PSS) MCTD
Nucleolar	4-6S RNP	Scleroderma Sjögren's syndrome Undiagnosed illnesses manifesting Raynaud's phenomenon
Discrete, speckled	Centromere DNA, RNA, ENA	CREST variant of PSS

CREST, Calcinosis, Raynaud's phenomenon, esophageal dysmotility, sclerodactyly, and telangiectasia.

latex reagent is mixed with serum containing the ANAs, binding to the DNP-coated latex particles produces macroscopic agglutination. The procedure is positive in SLE and SRDs (e.g., RA, scleroderma, Sjögren's syndrome).

Autoimmune Enzyme Immunoassay

The autoimmune enzyme immunoassay (EIA) provides a qualitative screening test for the presence of ANAs. In one well, the assay collectively detects total ANAs against dsDNA (nDNA) histones, SS-A/Ro, SS-B/La, Sm, Sm/RNP, Scl-70, Jo-1, and centromeric antigens, along with sera positive for immunofluorescent assay (IFA) Hep-2 ANAs. This assay serves as an alternative to the IFA for screening a patient's serum for ANAs.

TREATMENT

For most patients with lupus, effective treatment and prevention methods can minimize symptoms, reduce inflammation, and maintain normal body functions. For photosensitive patients, avoidance of (excessive) sun exposure and the regular application of sunscreens will usually prevent rashes. Regular exercise helps prevent muscle weakness and fatigue. Immunization protects against specific infections. Support groups and counseling can help alleviate the effects of stress. Lupus patients should avoid smoking, excessive consumption of alcohol, overuse or underuse of prescribed medication, and postponing regular medical checkups.

Medications are often prescribed for patients with lupus, depending on the organ(s) involved and the severity of involvement. Common medications include the following:

- Nonsteroidal antiinflammatory drugs (NSAIDs). NSAIDs are prescribed for a variety of rheumatic diseases, including lupus. Examples include acetylsalicylic acid (aspirin), ibuprofen (Motrin), and naproxen (Naprosyn). These drugs are usually recommended for muscle and joint pain and arthritis. Newer NSAIDs contain a prostaglandin in the same capsule (Arthrotec). The other NSAIDs work in the same way as aspirin, but may be more potent.
- Acetaminophen. Acetaminophen (Tylenol) is a mild analgesic that can often be used for pain. It has the advantage of causing less stomach irritation than aspirin but is not nearly as effective at suppressing inflammation as aspirin.
- Steroids (e.g., prednisone) are used to reduce inflammation and suppress activity of the immune system. Side effects occur more frequently when steroids are taken over long periods at high doses. These side effects include weight gain, a round face, acne, easy bruising, thinning of the bones (osteoporosis), high blood pressure, cataracts, onset of diabetes, increased risk of infection, stomach ulcers, hyperactivity, and increased appetite.
- Antimalarials. Chloroquine (Aralen) or hydroxychloroquine (Plaquenil), typically used to treat malaria, may also be useful for some individuals with lupus. Antimalarials are most often prescribed for the skin and joint symptoms of lupus.
- Immunomodulating drugs. Azathioprine (Imuran) and cyclophosphamide (Cytoxan), cytotoxic drugs, act in a manner similar to that of corticosteroids in that they suppress inflammation and tend to suppress the immune system.

Other agents (e.g., methotrexate, cyclosporin) can be used to control the symptoms of lupus. Some of these are used in conjunction with apheresis, a blood-filtering treatment. Apheresis has been tried by itself in an effort to remove specific antibodies from the blood, but the results have not been promising.

Studies have suggested that immunosuppressive therapy targeted against the calcineurin pathway of T helper (Th) cells, such as tacrolimus, may be effective in the treatment of primary membranous nephropathy.

Newer agents are directed toward specific cells of the immune system. These include agents that block the production of anti-DNA or that suppress the manufacture of antibodies through other mechanisms. Examples are IV immunoglobulin injections, which are given on a regular basis to increase platelet numbers.

- Anticoagulants. Anticoagulants range from aspirin at a very low dose to heparin or coumadin. Generally, such therapy is lifelong in those with lupus and follows an episode of embolus or thrombosis.

Clinical Trials

Drugs are being investigated as therapy for SLE. Currently, 58 clinical trials are being conducted and new research trials are always being initiated. A projection calls for quadruple the number of drugs to treat SLE by 2015.

Belimumab (Benlysta; formerly called LymphoStat-B) is a human monoclonal antibody that specifically recognizes and inhibits the biological activity of B lymphocyte stimulator (BLyS). BLyS is a naturally occurring protein discovered by human genome scientists that is required for B lymphocytes to develop into mature plasma B cells, which produce antibodies, the body's first line of defense against infection. Retrospective and prospective studies have shown elevated levels of BLyS in the blood of many SLE patients and in the blood and joint fluid of RA patients. In lupus, RA, and certain other autoimmune diseases, elevated BLyS levels are believed to contribute to the production of autoantibodies. Preclinical and clinical studies have demonstrated that B cell antagonists can reduce autoantibody levels and help control autoimmune disease activity.

CASE STUDY 1

A 39-year-old black woman with SLE was diagnosed with the illness 20 years ago. Her initial manifestations of illness developed during the postpartum period of her second pregnancy. The pregnancy had been complicated by proteinuria, believed to be caused by toxemia of pregnancy.

The patient had polyarthralgia, alopecia, and erythematous rashes of the face, arms, and legs. A renal biopsy was performed because her urinalysis revealed proteinuria and RBC casts. The renal biopsy revealed diffuse, proliferative glomerulonephritis. In addition to abnormal laboratory results related to renal function, she manifested ANA (titer 1:1280) and antibodies to DNA and the C3 component of complement.

Questions
1. The antibody found in common in systemic rheumatic diseases is
   a. Anti-nuclear antibody (ANA)
   b. Anti-native DNA
   c. Anti-SCI-1
   d. Anti-Jo-1
2. Patients with systemic lupus erythematosus (SLE) are characterized by the presence of antibodies to _____ antigens.
   a. ds DNA
   b. RNA polymerase I
   c. PM-Scl
   d. Anti-centromere

See Appendix A for the answers to multiple choice questions.

Critical Thinking Group Discussion Questions
1. Are the antibodies manifested by the patient typical of SLE?
2. Do patients with SLE have significant morbidity?

See instructor site ⊖volve website for the discussion of the answers to these questions.

CASE STUDY 2

History and Physical Examination

A 27-year-old white woman sought medical attention because of persisting pain in her wrists and ankles and an unexplained skin irritation on her face. On physical examination, swelling of the joints of the hands and ankles was evident, along with erythema of the skin over the bridge of the nose and the upper cheeks. The patient had a slightly elevated temperature.

Laboratory Data

Complete blood count, urinalysis (UA), and rheumatoid arthritis (RA) screening test were ordered, with the following results:

- Hemoglobin and hematocrit—normal
- Total leukocyte count—70×10^9/L
- Differential leukocyte count—normal
- Gross and microscopic UA—normal
- RA screening test—positive

Follow-Up

An ANA screening test was ordered. The results were positive.

Questions

1. Serologic testing frequently reveals _____ in patients with systemic lupus erythematosis (SLE).
   a. Increased titer of anti-DNA
   b. Decreased complement levels in the serum
   c. Presence of C3d and C3c
   d. All of the above
2. A homogeneous anti-nuclear antibody (ANA) (Hep-2) pattern characterizes antibodies to:
   a. n DNA
   b. ds DNA
   c. ss DNA
   d. All of the above

See Appendix A for the answers to multiple choice questions.

Critical Thinking Group Discussion Questions

1. What is the most probable diagnosis in this case?
2. Does this patient fit into the general characteristics of patients with this disease?
3. What is the principle of the ANA test?

See instructor site ⊖volve website for the discussion of the answers to these questions.

⠿ Antinuclear Antibody Visible Method

Principle

This test is an indirect immunoenzyme method that uses tissue culture cells (human epithelial cells) as a substrate for the detection and titration of circulating ANAs in human serum. Patient serum samples are diluted in buffer and added to microscope slide wells with Hep-2 (human epithelial) cells cultured in them. Hep-2 cells are characterized by extremely large nuclei and the presence of mitotic figures to aid in detection. If specific antibodies are present, stable antigen-antibody complexes are formed that bind AHG labeled with horseradish peroxidase (HRP). The presence of HRP is indicated by a reaction with 3,3′-diaminobenzidine stain. The resulting dark-brown to black staining patterns of the nuclei can be seen with a light microscope. The presence of one or more types of circulating autoantibodies is the hallmark of SRDs.

Procedure Note

See ⊖volve website for the procedural protocol.

Reporting Results

- Negative: No cytoplasmic or nuclear-specific stain is observed. The cells may be slightly colored because of some nonspecific reaction of the peroxidase stain reagent.
- Positive: Serum is considered positive if the nuclei of the cells stain more intensely than the negative control well and there is a clearly discernible pattern of colorations.

A grading scale similar to the one shown in Box 29-2 may be helpful in establishing the criteria for each laboratory. Positive specimens should be confirmed by repeating the test with two-fold dilutions of serum. All positive ANA patterns should be titered to end point dilution to detect possible mixed antinuclear reactions that may not be apparent when interpreting a single screening dilution. The end point titer is the last serial dilution in which 1+ coloration with a clearly discernible pattern is detected.

Comments

Indirect immunofluorescence (IIF) and immunoenzyme methods are probably the most practical ways of screening for ANA in the clinical laboratory. The peroxidase enzyme–conjugated antibody method, which is comparable in sensitivity and patterns of reactivity to fluorescent methods, has certain advantages. The HRP technique has the advantages of resulting in a permanent slide and requiring only a conventional light microscope with no special equipment.

Sources of Error

False-negative results can occur if the ANA happens to be specific for an antigen other than the one used in the procedure. False-negative results may also occur if the substrate is fixed in acetone and is inadequately washed. Without fixation, however, some soluble nuclear antigen may be lost. False-negative results may also be related to the binding of antinuclear factor to circulating immune complexes and to a low antibody titer.

Box 29-2	Grading Reactions

Negative

No cytoplasmic or nuclear specific stain observed. The cells may be slightly colored because of some nonspecific reaction of the peroxidase staining reagent.

Borderline

Beige-specific stain

±

Positive

1+: Tan

2+: Light brown

3+: Medium brown

4+: Dark chocolate brown to black

False-positive interpretations may occur because of nonspecific staining, which may resemble a speckled pattern of reactivity. These staining reactions occur whenever the conjugate or serum contains antibodies to other tissue antigens. Careful rinsing and removal of excess fluoresceinated conjugate minimize the risk of some nonspecific staining reactions.

Although IIF is considered to be the gold standard, it suffers from being a nonstandardized manual test, has subjective interpretation of results and has low reproducibility. Recently, manufacturers have automated the preevaluation and evaluation phases of IIF ANA testing, including using automatic fluorescent image analysis to provide a virtual titer, which eliminates the process of staining a series of diluted samples manually. EIAs and solid-phase methods (e.g., microarrays and bead-based assays) are popular. However, IIF currently remains the gold standard of testing.

Limitations

No diagnosis should be based solely on the results of laboratory testing. Clinical data, antibody titers, and other laboratory findings should all be reviewed before a definitive diagnosis is established.

Clinical Applications

In the evaluation of patients with connective tissue disease, the ANA must be interpreted with caution. Under proper testing conditions, a negative ANA generally rules out SLE. A negative ANA result can result from autoimmune disease in remission or nuclear autoantibodies not detectable with indirect immunofluorescent or peroxidase immunoenzyme procedures.

The significance of a positive ANA depends on the titer and to a lesser extent on the observed pattern (see Table 29-6). There is no general agreement on the significance of the various patterns and it should be noted that some patterns may mask other patterns in high concentration. Interpretation of ANA patterns can provide additional information about the type of nuclear component reacting.

Because of the sensitivity of the Hep-2 cell substrate, some apparently normal individuals may show a low degree of staining at the 1:40 screening dilution. ANA titers of 1:10 to 1:80 usually have little significance but may be seen in patients with RA or scleroderma. ANAs are known to be gender- and age-dependent; therefore, a positive low-titer result may be normal for certain individuals in the absence of other clinical signs and symptoms. If a specimen is positive at a 1:10 dilution, it should be retested at dilutions from 1:20 to 1:320. The higher the antibody titer, the more likely is the diagnosis of connective tissue disorder. Changes in the antibody titer can also be used to observe disease activity.

If the ANA test is positive, additional immunologic evaluation is necessary to determine the specificity of the reaction. These evaluations include double immunodiffusion, counterimmunoelectrophoresis, passive hemagglutination, radioimmunoassays, and identification of nuclear antigens by immunoprecipitation or immunoblotting. These evaluations may demonstrate the presence of more than one ANA specificity reaction in the serum. An LE cell preparation is not useful because it is positive in only 75% of patients with confirmed SLE.

Rapid Slide Test for Antinucleoprotein

Principle

The SLE latex test provides a suspension of polystyrene latex particles coated with deoxyribonucleoprotein (DNP). When the latex reagent is mixed with serum containing the ANAs, binding to the DNP-coated latex particles produces macroscopic agglutination. The procedure is positive in SLE and SRDs (e.g., RA, PSS, Sjögren's syndrome, MCTD, drug-induced lupus).

Procedure Notes

See ⊖volve website for the procedural protocol.

Sources of Error

Failure to observe the test mixture at the appropriate time can yield false results.

Limitations

No one test has been shown to be completely reliable for the diagnosis of SLE because many of the ANAs accompanying this disease are also demonstrated in other SRDs (e.g., RA, Sjögren's syndrome, PSS).

Clinical Applications

Sera from patients with SLE have been shown to contain several ANAs, as determined by a wide variety of laboratory tests. A specific diagnosis depends on the evaluation of test results and clinical manifestations.

Autoimmune Enzyme Immunoassay ANA Screening Test

Refer to Chapter 12 for a description of the autoimmune enzyme immunoassay ANA screening test.

Clinical Applications

As with other ANA diagnostic tests, the results are to be used as an aid in diagnosis. Confirmative testing for specific antibodies should be run if a positive assay is obtained. A positive test result suggests certain diseases and should be confirmed by clinical findings.

CHAPTER HIGHLIGHTS

- Systemic lupus erythematosus (SLE) is the classic model of autoimmune disease.
- No single cause of SLE has been identified, but a primary defect in immune system regulation is considered important in its pathogenesis. Other influences include the effect of estrogens, genetic predisposition, and extraneous factors.
- SLE is a disease of acute and chronic inflammation. Lymphocyte subset abnormalities are a major immunologic feature of SLE. The regulation of antibody production of B lymphocytes, ordinarily a function of the subpopulation of T suppressor cells, appears defective in SLE.
- Circulating immune complexes are the hallmark of SLE. Patients exhibit multiple serum antibodies that react with native or altered self antigens. Demonstrable antibodies include antibodies to nuclear components, cell surface and cytoplasmic antigens of polymorphonuclear and lymphocytic leukocytes, erythrocytes, platelets, and neuronal cells, and IgG.
- Antibodies also combine with their corresponding antigens to form immune complexes. When the mononuclear phagocyte system is unable to eliminate them entirely, these immune complexes accumulate in the blood circulation. These circulating immune complexes are deposited in the subendothelial layers of the vascular basement membranes of multiple target organs, where they mediate inflammation.
- The antinuclear antibody (ANA) procedure is a valuable screening tool for SLE. Demonstration of ANAs can indicate various systemic autoimmune connective tissue disorders characterized by antibodies that react with different nuclear components, such as double-stranded DNA, single-stranded DNA, and Sm antigen. ANAs can be found in SLE, MCTD, PSS (or scleroderma), Sjögren's syndrome, polymyositis-dermatomyositis, and RA. A small percentage of patients with neoplastic diseases may also demonstrate the presence of ANAs.
- ANAs are classified into antibodies to DNA, antibodies to histones, antibodies to nonhistone proteins, and antibodies to nuclear antigens. Antibodies to DNA can be divided into two major groups:
  - Antibodies that react with native (double-stranded) DNA
  - Antibodies that recognize denatured (single-stranded) DNA only
- Detection of autoantibodies by immunofluorescence is extremely sensitive and may show positive results when ANA procedures (e.g., complement fixation or precipitation) yield negative results. At present, immunofluorescence is the most widely used technique for ANA screening.

REVIEW QUESTIONS

1. SLE is more common in:
   a. Female infants
   b. Male infants
   c. Adolescent through middle-aged women
   d. Adolescent through middle-aged men

2. One of the most potent inducers of abnormalities and clinical manifestations of SLE is:
   a. Chloramphenicol
   b. Procainamide hydrochloride
   c. Isoniazid
   d. Penicillin

3. The cellular aberrations in SLE include:
   a. B cell depletion
   b. Deficiency of suppressor T cell function
   c. Hyperproduction of helper T cells
   d. Both b and c

4. The principal demonstrable antibody in SLE is antibody to:
   a. Nuclear antigen
   b. Cell surface antigens of hematopoietic cells
   c. Cell surface antigens to neuronal cells
   d. Lymphocytic leukocytes

5. The sites of immune complex deposition in SLE are influenced by all the following factors except:
   a. Molecular size
   b. Molecular configuration
   c. Immune complex specificity
   d. Immunoglobulin class

6. Renal disease secondary to SLE can be assessed by:
   a. Antibody to native dsDNA
   b. Levels of C3 and C4
   c. Levels of ANA
   d. All of the above

7. SLE is a classic model of autoimmune disease and is a(n):
   a. Abnormality of the joints
   b. Systemic rheumatoid disorder
   c. Abnormality of connective tissue
   d. All of the above

8. The overall incidence of SLE has an increased frequency among:
   a. Blacks
   b. Native Americans
   c. Puerto Ricans
   d. All of the above

9. Patients with SLE characteristically manifest:
   a. Butterfly rash over the bridge of the nose
   b. Skin lesions on the arms and legs
   c. Ulcerations on the trunk
   d. Photophobia

10. Laboratory features of SLE include:
    a. The presence of ANAs
    b. Circulating anticoagulant and immune complexes
    c. Decreased levels of complement
    d. All of the above

11. Laboratory procedures that are helpful in assessing renal disease include:
    a. Antibody to double-stranded DNA
    b. Levels of C3 and C4
    c. Cryoglobulin assay
    d. All of the above

12. Antinuclear antibodies (ANAs) are always indicative of SLE.
    a. True
    b. False

13-16. Match the appropriate antibody and disease.

13. _____ Jo-1

14. _____ Mi-I

15. _____ SS-B/La

16. _____ RANA
    a. Systemic lupus erythematosus
    b. Dermatomyositis
    c. Progressive systemic sclerosis
    d. Polymyositis

17 and 18. Match the interpretation of the ANA staining pattern to its respective antibody.

17. _____ Diffused or homogeneous pattern

18. _____ Speckled pattern
    a. Anti–DNA-nucleoprotein antibody
    b. Antibody to nucleolar RNA
    c. Antibody to any extractable nuclear antigen devoid of DNA or histone
    d. Anticentromere antibody

BIBLIOGRAPHY

Bosch X: Systemic lupus erthematosus and the neutrophil, N Engl J Med 365:758–760, 2011.
CenterWatch: Clinical trials, 2011, http://www.centerwatch.com.
Condemi JJ: The autoimmune diseases, JAMA 298:2882–2888, 1992.
Klippel JH: Systemic lupus erythematosus, JAMA 293:1812–1815, 1990.
Lockshin M: Therapy for systemic lupus erythematosus, N Engl J Med 324:189–192, 1991.
Lupus Foundation: Learn About Lupus, 2012, http://www.lupus.org.
Marshall E: Drug market to treat systemic lupus erythematosus will quadruple by 2015, 2006, http://www.decisionresources.com.
Mills JA: Systemic lupus erythematosus, N Engl J Med 330:1871–1879, 1994.
Peebles CL: Antinuclear antibody profiles, Clin Lab News 31:10–12, 2005.
Rollins G: Antinuclear antibody testing dilemmas: does high throughput trump sensitivity? Clin Lab News 37(1):5–7, 2011.
Tsokos GC: Systemic lupus erythematosus, NEJM 365(22):2110–2121, Dec 2011.

CHAPTER 30

Rheumatoid Arthritis

Learning Objectives

At the conclusion of this chapter, the reader should be able to:

- Name significant factors related to the development of arthritis.
- Describe the etiology, epidemiology, and signs and symptoms of rheumatoid arthritis.
- Discuss the immunologic manifestations and diagnostic evaluation of rheumatoid arthritis.
- Briefly describe juvenile rheumatoid arthritis.
- Explain diagnostic procedures used in the identification and evaluation of rheumatoid arthritis.

- Analyze representative rheumatoid arthritis case studies.
- Correctly answer case study related multiple choice questions.
- Be prepared to participate in a discussion of critical thinking questions.
- Describe the principle, sources of error, clinical applications, and limitations of a rapid rheumatoid factor procedure.
- Correctly answer end of chapter review questions.

Key Terms

ankylosing spondylitis
arthrocentesis
articular
cryoglobulins
extra-articular

juvenile idiopathic arthritis
leukotrienes
pathogenesis
polyarthritis
rheumatoid factor (RF)

scleroderma
synovitis
synovium

The word *arthritis* literally means joint inflammation: *arth-* (joint) and *-itis* (inflammation). Arthritis is a large and growing public health problem in the United States. There are more than 100 forms of arthritis and related diseases. With the aging of the U.S. population, even assuming that the prevalence of obesity and other risk factors remain unchanged, the prevalence of physician-diagnosed arthritis and arthritis-attributable activity limitation (AAAL) is expected to increase significantly by 2030. Based on data from the National Health Interview Survey (NHIS; 2007-2009), the estimated distribution of arthritis is:

- 49.9 million (22.2%) of adults aged 18 years or older have self-reported physician-diagnosed arthritis.
- 21.1 million (9.4% of all adults) have AAAL.

The prevalence of arthritis increases significantly with age. Females are more likely than males to suffer from arthritis. Non-Hispanic whites, blacks, Native Americans, and Alaska Natives are more likely to have arthritis than Hispanics, Asians, and Pacific Islanders. Obese and overweight people are diagnosed with arthritis more frequently than underweight or normal weight individuals. Physically inactive people develop arthritis more often than physically active people.

ETIOLOGY

Rheumatic diseases are among the oldest diseases recognized, but the cause of rheumatoid arthritis (RA) remains unknown.

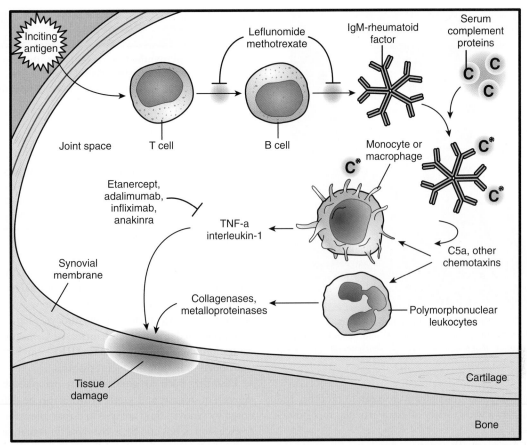

Figure 30-1   Inflammation in the rheumatoid joint. *(Adapted from Olsen NJ, Stein CM: N Engl J Med 350:2167–2179, 2004.)*

Genetic factors are important, as are hormonal and psychosomatic factors. Evidence indicates that immunologic factors are involved in the **articular** and **extra-articular** manifestations of the disease. RA may represent an unusual host response to one or perhaps many causative agents. An infectious cause is possible, although this has not been established.

EPIDEMIOLOGY

Rheumatoid arthritis occurs worldwide, but no definite geographic or climatic variation in incidence has been established. RA affects all races, but the incidence varies across racial and ethnic groups.

Although no specific genetic relationship has been established, a small increase in incidence has been noted in first-degree relatives of patients with RA. Persons with the human leukocyte antigen (HLA)–DR4 haplotype have a significantly higher incidence of RA.

Patients with RA have a shortened lifespan. The most frequent cause of death is cardiovascular disease. The increased prevalence of atherosclerosis in RA patients is suspected to be related to atherogenic side effects of some antirheumatic medications, the effects of chronic systemic inflammation on the vascular endothelium, or shared mechanisms of action between RA and atherosclerosis.

Complications resulting from an increased frequency of local or extra-articular infections in RA patients have been

demonstrated. Mortality may result from conditions such as septicemia, pneumonia, lung abscess, or pyelonephritis. In the past 15 years, the pharmacotherapy of RA has been improved by the development of more effective medications.

SIGNS AND SYMPTOMS

The term *rheumatic disease* does not have a clear boundary; more than 100 different conditions are labeled as rheumatic diseases, including RA, osteoarthritis, autoimmune disorders such as systemic lupus erythematosus (SLE) and **scleroderma,** osteoporosis, back pain, gout, fibromyalgia, and tendinitis.

Rheumatoid arthritis is a chronic, multisystemic, autoimmune disorder and a progressive inflammatory disorder of the joints (Fig. 30-1). It is, however, a highly variable disease that ranges from a mild illness of brief duration to a progressive destructive **polyarthritis** associated with a systemic vasculitis (Fig 30-2). The **pathogenesis** of RA has the following three distinct stages:

1. Initiation of **synovitis** by the primary causative factor
2. Subsequent immunologic events that perpetuate the initial inflammatory reaction
3. Transition of an inflammatory reaction in the **synovium** to a proliferative, destructive tissue process

Rheumatoid arthritis often begins with prodromal symptoms such as fatigue, anorexia, weakness, and generalized aching and stiffness not localized to articular structures. Joint

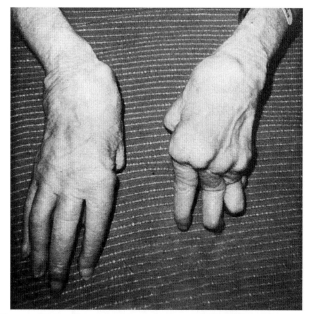

Figure 30-2 *Characteristics of rheumatoid arthritis.* Shown are swan-neck deformity, ulnar deviation, dorsal interosseous atrophy, and swelling of wrist. *(From Kaye D, Rose LF: Fundamentals of internal medicine, St Louis, 1983, Mosby.)*

Box 30-1	**Extra-Articular Manifestations of Rheumatoid Arthritis**

Constitutional manifestations (e.g., weight loss, fatigue)
Subcutaneous rheumatoid nodules
Ocular abnormalities (e.g., inflammatory lesions of episclera and sclera)
Vasculitis
Neuropathy (e.g., mononeuritis multiplex)
Myopathy
Cardiac manifestations (e.g., pericarditis)
Pulmonary manifestations (e.g., pleural effusion)
Osteoporosis
Felty's syndrome—a complex of chronic RA, splenomegaly, anemia, thrombocytopenia, and neutropenia

symptoms usually appear gradually over weeks to months. The patient may display a wide variety of extra-articular manifestations (Box 30-1).

The revised American Rheumatism Association's criteria for diagnosis of RA are presented in Table 30-1. If these conditions are present for at least 6 weeks, the patient is designated as having classic RA. Prognostic markers such as a persistently high number of swollen joints, high serum levels of acute-phase reactants of immunoglobulin M (IgM) rheumatoid factor, early radiographic and functional abnormalities, and the presence of certain HLA class II alleles may help identify patients with more severe RA who are still in the early stages of the disease.

ANATOMY AND PHYSIOLOGY OF JOINTS

Diarthrodial joints are lined at their margins by a synovial membrane (synovium), with synovial cells lining this space. The lining cells synthesize protein and are phagocytic. Synovial (joint) fluid is a transparent viscous fluid. Its function is to lubricate the joint space and transport nutrients to the articular cartilage. Mechanical, chemical, immunologic, or bacteriologic damage may alter the permeability of the membrane and capillaries and may produce varying degrees of an inflammatory response. In addition, inflammatory joint fluids contain lytic enzymes that produce depolymerization of hyaluronic acid, which greatly impairs the lubricating ability of the fluid.

A variety of disorders produce changes in the number and types of cells and chemical composition of the fluid. Analysis of synovial fluid plays a major role in the diagnosis of joint diseases. **Arthrocentesis** constitutes a liquid biopsy of the joint. It is a fundamental part of the clinical database, together with the medical history, physical examination, and plain radiographic films. Analysis of aspirated synovial fluid is essential in the evaluation of any patient with joint disease because it is a better reflection of the events in the articular cavity than abnormal blood test results. For example, abnormal test results—for example, antinuclear antibody (ANA), increased erythrocyte sedimentation rate (ESR), elevated uric acid level, increased C-reactive protein concentration, and **rheumatoid factor (RF)**—can be seen in normal individuals or in unrelated joint diseases.

Disorders such as gout, calcium pyrophosphate dihydrate deposition disease, and septic arthritis can be definitively diagnosed by synovial fluid analysis and may allow for consideration or exclusion of RA and SLE. Synovial fluid analysis can also support a diagnosis of diseases as disparate as amyloidosis, hypothyroidism, ochronosis, hemochromatosis, or even simple edema. In addition, arthrocentesis may alleviate elevated intra-articular pressure. Removal of fluid will relieve symptoms and potentially decrease joint damage. Removal of the products of inflammation is an important component in the treatment of infectious arthritis and may be beneficial for other forms of arthritis.

Routine analysis of synovial fluid should include wet preparation examination for cell count and differential, crystals, Gram stain, and microbiologic culture. Very turbid fluids, or if septic arthritis is considered for other reasons, synovial fluid should be sent for Gram staining and culture. Gram staining is needed if a high likelihood of infection exists. Other observations and procedures can include volume and appearance, viscosity, mucin test, chemical analysis for protein, and glucose.

When examined by the immunofluorescent technique, the rheumatoid synovium can be seen to contain large amounts of immunoglobulin G (IgG) and IgM, alone or together. Immunoglobulins can also be seen in synovial lining cells, blood vessels, and interstitial connective tissues. B cells make immunoglobulin in the synovium of patients with RA. As many as 50% of the plasma cells that can be located in the synovium secrete an IgG RF that combines with similar IgG molecules (self-associating IgG) in the cytoplasm.

IMMUNOLOGIC MANIFESTATIONS

The current model of the pathogenesis of RA proposes that an infective agent or other stimulus binds to receptors on dendritic cells (DCs), which activates the innate immune system

Table 30-1	2010 ACR-EULAR Classification Criteria For Rheumatoid Arthritis*	
Parameter		**Score (Points)**
A. Joint involvement[†,‡]		
• One large joint[§]		0
• Two to ten large joints		1
• One to three small joints (with or without involvement of large joints)[‡]		2
• Four to 10 small joints (with or without involvement of large joints)		3
• >Ten joints (at least one small joint)[‖]		5
B. Serology (at least one test result is needed for classification)[¶]		
• Negative RF *and* negative ACPA		0
• Low-positive RF *or* low-positive ACPA		2
• High-positive RF *or* high-positive ACPA		3
C. Acute-phase reactants (at least one test result is needed for classification)[#]		
• Normal CRP *and* normal ESR		0
• Abnormal CRP *or* abnormal ESR		1
D. Duration of symptoms**		
• <6 wk		0
• ≥6 wk		1

NOTE: These are classification criteria for RA (score-based algorithm). Add scores of categories A to D. A score of 6 to 10 points is needed for classifying a patient as having definite RA. Although patients with a score of 6 to 10 points are not classifiable as having RA, their status can be reassessed and the criteria might be fulfilled cumulatively over time.

Differential diagnoses vary among patients with different presentations, but may include conditions such as SLE, psoriatic arthritis, and gout. If it is unclear about the relevant differential diagnoses to consider, an expert rheumatologist should be consulted.

Adapted from American College of Rheumatology: The 2010 American College of Rheumatology/European League Against Rheumatism classification criteria for rheumatoid arthritis, 2011 (http://www.rheumatology.org/practice/clinical/classification/ra/ra_2010.asp).

ACPA, Anti–citrullinated protein antibody; *CRP,* C-reactive protein; *ESR,* erythrocyte sedimentation rate. *EULAR,* European League Against Rheumatism.

*The criteria are aimed at the classification of newly presenting patients. In addition, patients with erosive disease typical of RA with a history compatible with prior fulfillment of the 2010 criteria should be classified as having RA. Patients with long-standing disease, including those whose disease is inactive (with or without treatment) who, based on retrospectively available data, have previously fulfilled the 2010 criteria should be classified as having RA.

†Joint involvement refers to any swollen or tender joint on examination, which may be confirmed by imaging evidence of synovitis. Distal interphalangeal joints, first carpometacarpal joints, and first metatarsophalangeal joints are excluded from assessment. Categories of joint distribution are classified according to the location and number of involved joints, with placement into the highest category possible based on the pattern of joint involvement.

‡"Small joints" refers to the metacarpophalangeal joints, proximal interphalangeal joints, second through fifth metatarsophalangeal joints, thumb interphalangeal joints, and wrists.

§"Large joints" refers to shoulders, elbows, hips, knees, and ankles.

‖In this category, at least one of the involved joints must be a small joint; the others can include any combination of large and additional small joints, as well as other joints not specifically listed elsewhere (e.g., temporomandibular, acromioclavicular, sternoclavicular).

¶Negative refers to IU values that are ≤ to the upper limit of normal (ULN) for the laboratory and assay; low-positive refers to IU values that are higher than the ULN but ≤3 times the ULN for the laboratory and assay; high-positive refers to IU values that are >3 times the ULN for the laboratory and assay. If RF information is only available as positive or negative, a positive result should be scored as low-positive for RF.

#Normal/abnormal is determined by local laboratory standards.

**Duration of symptoms refers to patient self-report of the duration of signs or symptoms of synovitis (e.g., pain, swelling, tenderness) of joints that are clinically involved at the time of assessment, regardless of treatment status.

(Fig. 30-3). DCs migrate into lymph nodes and present antigen to T lymphocytes, which are activated by two signals—the presentation of antigen and costimulation through CD28. Activated T lymphocytes proliferate and migrate into the joint. Subsequently, T lymphocytes produce interferon-γ (IFN-γ) and other proinflammatory cytokines. This in turn stimulates macrophages and other cells, including B lymphocytes. B cells appear to be pivotal in the pathogenesis of RA because they can be 10,000 times as potent as DCs in presenting antigen.

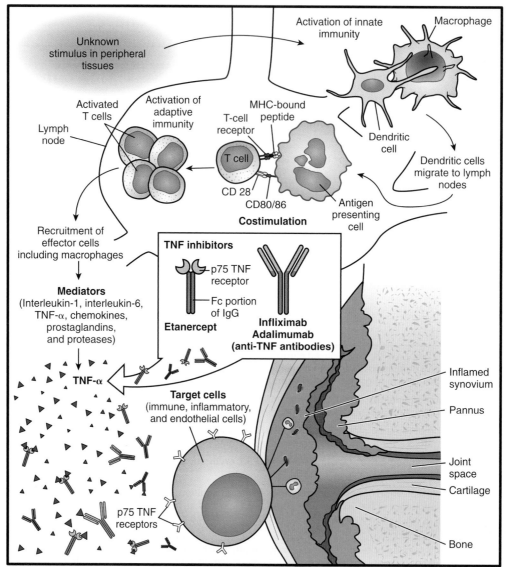

Figure 30-3 **Pathophysiologic role of cytokines and other mediators and their inhibitors in rheumatoid arthritis.** *MHC,* Major histocompatibility complex; *TNF,* tumor necrosis factor. *(Adapted from Scott DL, Kingsley GH: N Engl J Med 355:704–712, 2006.)*

Stimulated macrophages and fibroblasts release cytokines, including tumor necrosis factor-α (TNF-α), a central component in the cascade of cytokines. This results in the production of additional inflammatory mediators and further recruitment of immune and inflammatory cells into a joint. Anti–TNF-α treatment strategies (e.g., monoclonal) prevent interaction with receptors on cell surfaces.

The **leukotrienes** play a major role in the inflammatory response to injury. This class of biologically active molecules has been implicated in the pathogenesis of RA and in other inflammatory diseases (e.g., asthma, psoriasis, inflammatory bowel disease). Leukotrienes are major constituents of a group of oxygenated fatty acids that are synthesized de novo from membrane phospholipid through a cascade of enzymes. Research studies have focused on these molecules because leukotriene inhibitors and antagonists will probably become important agents in the group of antiinflammatory drugs (see later, "Treatment").

DIAGNOSTIC EVALUATION

Low serum iron levels and a normal or low iron-binding capacity are common features in RA. The ESR is elevated to a variable degree in most RA patients and roughly parallels the level of disease activity. Serum protein electrophoresis may demonstrate elevations in the alpha-2 and gamma globulin fractions, with a mild to moderate decrease in serum albumin. The gamma globulin increase is polyclonal.

Immunologic features of RA include RF, anti–cyclic citrullinated peptide (anti-CCP), immune complexes, characteristic complement levels, and ANAs. For example, patients with Felty's syndrome, the association of RA with splenomegaly and leukopenia, almost always develop a high-titer rheumatoid factor assay, a positive ANA assay, and rheumatoid nodules. In addition, these patients have a high titer of immune complex and low total serum complement levels.

Rheumatoid Factor

RFs are immunoglobulins of any isotype with antibody activity directed against antigenic sites on the Fc region of human or animal IgG. RFs have been associated with three major immunoglobulin classes, IgM, IgG, and IgA. IgM and IgG RFs are the most common.

Immunoglobulin M rheumatoid factor is manifested in approximately 70% of adults but is not specific for RA. Being RF-positive correlates with the following:
- Severity of the disease (in general)
- Nodules
- Other organ system involvement (e.g., vasculitis, Felty's syndrome, Sjögren's syndrome)

Agglutination tests for RF, such as the sensitized sheep cell test and latex agglutination, generally detect IgM RFs. Latex agglutination is sensitive but can produce a fairly high number of false-positive results. Because conventional procedures are semiquantitative, they may be insensitive to changes in titer and may detect only those RFs that agglutinate. Immunoturbidimetric assays and enzyme-linked immunosorbent assays (ELISAs) are automated methods of analysis. The presence of abnormal levels of all three RF isotypes—IgM, IgG, and IgA—has a specificity of 99% for RA.

Rheumatoid factor has been associated with some bacterial and viral infections, including hepatitis and infectious mononucleosis, and some chronic infections, such as tuberculosis, parasitic disease, subacute bacterial endocarditis, and cancer. Elevated values may also be observed in the normal older population. The concentration of RF tends to be highest when the disease peaks and tends to decrease during prolonged remission.

Cyclic Citrullinated Peptide Antibodies

CCP antibodies are a highly specific indicator for RA. Antibodies to CCPs (anti-CCP1) were first described in 1998 and, following the introduction of commercial ELISA products using the so-called second-generation peptides (CCP2), there has been increased interest in using this marker in the diagnosis of RA. Anti—CCP IgG antibodies are present in about 69% to 83% of patients with RA and have specificities ranging from 93% to 95%. These autoantibodies may be present in the preclinical phase of disease, are associated with future RA development, and may predict radiographic joint destruction. Antibodies can be detected in sera from individuals up to 14 years before the first clinical symptoms of RA appear.

Compared with other assays for RF, CCP is considered to be more sensitive. This antibody is reported to have high specificity (>95%) and sensitivity (80%) for RA. Early diagnosis and effective treatment provide a window of opportunity for controlling this autoimmune disease. Anti-CCP and rheumatoid factor assays constitute a rheumatoid arthritis panel.

Autoantibodies against mutated and citrullinated vimentin (MCV), a member of the citrullinated protein family, are highly specific markers for RA. A lateral flow immunoassay (LFIA) for the qualitative detection of anti-MCV antibodies, anti-MCV ELISA (ORGENTEC Diagnostics, Mainz, Germany) has been developed as a point of care test.

Other Markers

Antibodies to anti–perinuclear factor (APF) and keratin (anti–keratin antibody [AKA]) are highly specific for RA. Antibodies to APF are reported to be present in the sera of 49% to 91% of RA patients, with specificity greater than 70%.

Immune Complexes

Soluble circulating immune complexes and cryoprecipitable proteins consisting of immunoglobulins, complement components, and RFs are demonstrable in the sera of some patients with RA. Anti–gamma globulin isotypes, IgM, IgG, and IgA classes, are important complexes.

The IgA, IgM, and IgG isotypes of RF are detected years before any symptoms of RA become apparent. The various vascular and parenchymal lesions of RA suggest that the lesions result from injury induced by immune complexes, especially those containing antibodies to IgG. Vasculitis is associated with complexes made up of IgG and 7S IgM RFs. A positive laboratory assay for mixed **cryoglobulins** indicates the presence of a large number of immune complexes and is associated with an increased incidence of extra-articular manifestations, particularly vasculitis.

Complement Levels

Serum complement levels are usually normal in patients with RA, except in those with vasculitis. Hemolytic complement levels are reduced in the serum of less than one third of patients, especially in patients with very high levels of RF and immune complexes. Levels of C4 and C2 are most profoundly depressed in these patients.

Antinuclear Antibodies

Antinuclear antibodies have been found in 14% to 28% of RA patients, who usually have advanced disease. However, disease manifestation is the same in ANA-positive and ANA-negative patients.

JUVENILE IDIOPATHIC ARTHRITIS

Etiology

The term *juvenile rheumatoid arthritis* (JRA) has fallen out of favor worldwide for a number of reasons. JRA is not, as the language implies, simply a pediatric replica of the condition that affects adults. Only about 10% of children have an arthritic disease that closely mirrors rheumatoid arthritis in adults. Researchers have concluded that the JRA category is drawn too narrowly and should include some related diagnoses, such as **ankylosing spondylitis.** Juvenile idiopathic arthritis (JIA) and juvenile rheumatoid arthritis (JRA) can't be used interchangeably because there are differences between the diagnoses they include (Table 30-2).

Juvenile idiopathic arthritis (JIA) is a condition of chronic synovitis beginning during childhood. It is believed that there are a number of causes, including factors such as infection, autoimmunity, and trauma. Research at Tulane University Medical Center have suggested that JIA may be associated with a retroviral particle called human intracisternal A-type particle (HIAP). Antibodies to this particle have been found in

Table 30-2	**Subgroups of Juvenile Idiopathic Arthritis**	
New Classification	**Old Classification**	**Comments**
Systemic arthritis	Systemic-onset JIA	Comprises only ≈10% of JIA cases
Oligoarthritis	Pauciarticular JIA	Accounts for 40% of new JIA patients
Polyarthritis (RF-negative) or polyarthritis (RF-positive)	Polyarticular JIA	
Enthesitis-related arthritis	Excluded in JIA classification, but at onset some patients in this group may be similar to late-onset pauciarticular JIA	
Psoriatic arthritis	Excluded in JIA classification	
Other	Does not fulfill criteria for any categories or fulfills criteria for more than one category	JIA is the most common type of JA but is not the only type. Other forms include juvenile lupus, juvenile scleroderma, and juvenile dermatomyositis. Children can also experience noninflammatory disorders, characterized by chronic pain associated with heredity, injury, or unknown causes.

Adapted from Arthritis Foundation: Juvenile arthritis, 2012 (http://www.arthritis.org/juvenile-arthritis.php).

a very high percentage of patients with JIA. These antibodies have also been found in many patients with three other autoimmune disorders—SLE, Sjögren's syndrome, and Graves' disease. Researchers believe that these four disorders may result from the presence of HIAP, together with genetic factors and some internal or external stimulus, which all combine to dictate the specific symptomatology.

Epidemiology

The incidence of JIA in the U.S. pediatric population is from 0.1 to 1.1/1000.

Signs and Symptoms

Diagnostic criteria include onset before age 16 years, presence of arthritis (i.e., joint swelling for 6 consecutive weeks or longer), and exclusion of other conditions known to cause or mimic childhood arthritis. Several distinct subgroups of JIA have been recognized.

Immunologic Manifestations

Immunologic features of JIA can include the presence of RF, immune complexes, and ANAs.

Rheumatoid Factors

Approximately 20% of children are positive for RF. Most patients who are positive for RF probably represent adult RA occurring in childhood. So-called hidden RF can be detected in 65% of children with negative latex fixation test results. Children in this category do not develop the clinical manifestations of adults with RA.

Immune Complexes

Soluble immune complexes may be detected in patients with active synovitis. Analysis of these complexes is not useful for the diagnosis, prognosis, or monitoring of patients.

Antinuclear Antibodies

ANAs are detectable in few patients with JIA, except that most girls with pauciarthritis and chronic iritis demonstrate a positive ANA test result.

TREATMENT

The major goals of treatment of arthritis are as follows: (1) reduce pain and discomfort; (2) prevent deformities and loss of joint function; and (3) help the patient maintain a productive and active life. Inflammation must be suppressed and mechanical and structural abnormalities corrected or compensated for with assistive devices. Treatment options include reduction of joint stress, physical and occupational therapy, drug therapy, and surgical intervention.

There are several general classes of drugs (Table 30-3) traditionally used in the treatment of RA. A newer class of agents for treatment of RA, recombinant fusion proteins, selectively modulates the CD80 or CD86-CD28 costimulatory signal required for full T cell activation. Other drugs may also be used for treatment.

Nonsteroidal Antiinflammatory Drugs

Traditional treatment of RA consists of nonsteroidal antiinflammatory drugs (NSAIDs; e.g., salicylates, ibuprofen). The major effect of these agents is to reduce acute inflammation. Aspirin is the oldest drug of the nonsteroidal class, but the use of aspirin as the initial choice of drug therapy has largely been replaced by the newer NSAIDs.

Prostaglandins are a group of related compounds that are important mediators of a wide variety of physiologic processes, including immunomodulation. Prostaglandins are derived primarily from arachidonic acid via the cyclooxygenase enzymes (COX) pathway. NSAIDs inhibit prostaglandin synthesis by blocking two isoforms of COX, COX-1, and COX-2. Newer

Table 30-3	**Drugs for Treatment of Rheumatoid Arthritis**	
Drug Type	**Generic Name (Trade Name)**	**Example of Primary Action**
NSAIDs	Over-the-counter NSAIDs include ibuprofen (e.g., Advil, Motrin) and naproxen (Aleve). Stronger NSAIDs are available by prescription.	The effect of NSAIDs is mainly due to their common property of inhibiting cyclooxygenases involved in the formation of prostaglandins, which leads to the normalization of an increased pain threshold.
Disease-modifying antirheumatic drugs (DMARDs)	Methotrexate (Trexall), leflunomide (Arava), hydroxychloroquine (Plaquenil), sulfasalazine (Azulfidine), minocycline (Dynacin, Minocin)	Leflunomide inhibits pyrimidine synthesis and growth factor signal transduction nucleotide synthesis.
Immunosuppressants	Azathioprine (Imuran, Azasan), cyclosporine (Neoral, Sandimmune, Gengraf), cyclophosphamide (Cytoxan)	Azathioprine-inhibits nucleotide synthesis; cyclosporine inhibits transcription.
Steroids	Prednisone	Depress natural immune system activity
TNF-α inhibitors	Etanercept (Enbrel), infliximab (Remicade), adalimumab (Humira), golimumab (Simponi), certolizumab (Cimzia)	Etanercept binds TNF-α and TNF-β; infliximab—chimeric anti–TNF-α antibody; adalimumab—human anti–TNF-α antibody
Other drugs	Anakinra (Kineret), abatacept (Orencia), rituximab (Rituxan), tocilizumab (Actemra)	Anakinra—IL-1 receptor antagonist

Adapted from the Mayo Clinic: Rheumatoid arthritis: Treatments and drugs, 2012.

NSAID agents (e.g., Vioxx, Celebrex) selectively block the COX-2 enzyme that is primarily upregulated in response to tissue damage during inflammation but preserves COX-1 activity and enhances the safety profile.

Corticosteroids and Glucocorticoids

Corticosteroids (e.g., cortisone and prednisolone [prednisone]) have antiinflammatory and immunoregulatory activity. Glucocorticosteroids pass through the cell membrane into the cytoplasm and activate the cytoplasmic glucocorticosteroid receptor, which represses gene expression through the transcriptional interference of activator protein 1 (AP-1) and nuclear factor kappa B (NF-κB). The proteins inhibited by glucocorticosteroids include interleukin-1 (IL-1), IL-2, IL-6, IL-8, TNF-α, and IFN-γ. Glucocorticosteroids were the original selective COX-2 inhibitors. Oral corticosteroids can produce a variety of complications, including high blood pressure, increased susceptibility to infection, and osteoporosis.

Disease-Modifying Antirheumatic Drugs

The disease-modifying antirheumatic drugs (DMARDs) include methotrexate, intramuscular gold salts, hydroxychloroquine, sulfasalazine, D-penicillamine, and immunosuppressive and other cytotoxic drugs (e.g., cyclosporin A, cyclophosphamide, azathioprine). Newer drugs for the treatment of RA include leflunomide, etanercept, adalimumab, infliximab (Remicade), and anakinra Antimalarials may be used as well.

Methotrexate has become the most popular DMARD because of its early onset of action (4 to 6 weeks), good efficacy, ease of administration, and high patient tolerability. Methotrexate is a folic acid antagonist. The immunosuppressive and cytotoxic effects of methotrexate are caused by the inhibition of dihydrofolate reductase.

Immunosuppressive and cytotoxic drugs other than methotrexate are used only for patients who have aggressive disease or extra-articular manifestations such as systemic vasculitis. The most common drugs are azathioprine (Imuran), cyclophosphamide (Cytoxan), and cyclosporin A. Because of the potential for high toxicity, these agents are used for life-threatening extra-articular manifestations or severe articular disease refractory to other therapy.

- Azathioprine is a purine analogue that can cause severe bone marrow suppression, particularly in patients with renal insufficiency or when used concomitantly with allopurinol or angiotensin-converting enzyme (ACE) inhibitors.
- Cyclophosphamide is an alkylating agent associated with serious toxicities, including bone marrow suppression, hemorrhagic cystitis, premature ovarian failure, infection, and secondary malignancy, particularly an increased risk of bladder cancer. Thus, cyclophosphamide is not used in the treatment of uncomplicated RA.
- Cyclosporine (cyclosporin A) is an immunosuppressive agent approved for use for preventing renal and liver allograft rejection. Cyclosporine inhibits T cell function by inhibiting the transcription of IL-2.

Other Drugs

Antimalarial drugs are rapidly absorbed, relatively safe, well tolerated, and often effective remittive agents in the treatment of RA, particularly mild to moderate disease. The mechanism of action of antimalarial drugs in the treatment of patients with RA is unknown.

Recombinant fusion proteins represent a new class of drugs that selectively modulate specific cell surface receptors, CD80 or CD86, on the surface of an antigen-presenting cell that binds to CD28 on the T cell. A recombinant fusion protein, abatacept, has been modified to prevent complement fixation. It competes with CD28 for CD80 and CD86 binding and can be used to modulate T cell activity selectively. This selective costimulation modulator has been proposed to be useful for patients who have an inadequate response to anti–TNF-α therapy.

DIAGNOSTIC PROCEDURES

Diagnostic testing for RA primarily involves RF assays (see rapid agglutination procedure).

CASE STUDY 1

History and Physical Examination

A 62-year-old woman has been experiencing pain in her left knee unrelated to trauma. The pain occurs primarily with weight-bearing. She is currently being treated for hypertension, but is otherwise healthy.

She is obese. An examination of her knee shows tenderness over the medial epicondyle superior to the joint margin. There is a small effusion in her left knee.

Laboratory Data

Her laboratory data are normal, including the RF assay, except for an elevated uric acid level. An x-ray film of her knee was read as normal.

Questions

1. Rhematoid arthritis (RA) has a genetic association with:
   a. HLA-A
   b. HLA-B
   c. HLA-C
   d. HLA-DR4
2. IgM rheumatoid factor (RF) is manifested in approximately _____% of adults but is not specific for rheumatoid arthritis.
   a. 30
   b. 50
   c. 70
   d. 90

See Appendix A for the answers to multiple choice questions.

Critical Thinking Group Discussion Questions

1. What is the cause of her painful knee?
2. What might the effusion in her left knee demonstrate microscopically?
3. Would a restricted diet be of value?

See instructor site ⊝volve website for the discussion of the answers to these questions.

CASE STUDY 2

AD, age 31 years, was referred to a rheumatologist with increasing pain and stiffness in her fingers and wrists. Before her last pregnancy, 3 years earlier, she had experienced similar symptoms, but these had gone away. Since the birth of her last child, she has found it progressively more awkward to carry out a variety of work tasks and hobbies, such as needlepoint. The symptoms are worse in the morning. She has no trouble with her other joints.

Her family history reveals that her mother had RA. On physical examination, the patient was pale. She had bilateral and symmetric tender swelling of her wrists and proximal to the joints of her hands. She had normal range of movement. Her other body systems appeared to be within normal limits.

Laboratory Data

Laboratory assays were ordered (Table 30-4). A diagnosis of early RA was made. The patient was advised to take one aspirin daily. This initially provided some relief of her symptoms.

She returned to her physician 4 months later with worsening symptoms in her hands and pain in both knees. Synovial fluid was removed from her knees. A diagnosis of progressive RA was made.

Questions

1. A highly specific indicator for rheumatoid arthritis is:
   a. Rheumatoid factor
   b. C-reactive protein
   c. Cyclic citrullinated peptide (CCP) antibodies
   d. Depletion of complement
2. An immunoglobulin (Ig) class associated with rheumatoid arthritis is:
   a. IgM
   b. IgG
   c. IgA
   d. All of the above

See Appendix A for the answers to multiple choice questions.

Critical Thinking Group Discussion Questions

1. Do genetic associations exist with RA?
2. Is RA more common in women?
3. What is the immunopathogenesis of RA?
4. What is rheumatoid factor?

See instructor site ⊝volve website for the discussion of the answers to these questions.

Rapid Agglutination

Principle

The principle of serologic testing for rheumatoid arthritis is based on the detection of macroglobulins collectively called RF. RF behaves like antibodies against human gamma globulin (IgG).

In rapid testing, sheep RBCs or latex reagent consists of a stabilized RBC or latex suspension coated with albumin and chemically bonded with denatured human gamma globulin. This reagent serves as an antigen in the procedure. If RFs are present in the serum, macroscopic agglutination will be visible when the reagent is mixed with the serum.

The determination of RFs is important in the prognosis and therapeutic management of rheumatoid arthritis; however, biologically false-positive test results may be observed in a variety of disorders, such as SLE, Sjögren's syndrome, syphilis, and hepatitis.

Procedure Notes

The strength of a positive reaction may be graded as follows:
- 1+: Very small clumping with opaque fluid background
- 2+: Small clumping with slightly opaque fluid background
- 3+: Moderate clumping with fairly clear fluid background
- 4+: Large clumping with clear fluid background

Results

Qualitative Test Results*

- Negative: No agglutination or color change is seen in the reagent. The reagent should have a smooth appearance against a yellow/greenish background.
- Positive: The agglutinated reagent will become visibly blue against a yellow background.
  - If a positive result is obtained with the undiluted specimen, the specimen should be diluted 1:10 to determine the relationship between the level of RF present and a particular disease state.
  - If the 1:10 diluted specimen demonstrates readily visible agglutination, RF is present in the specimen at a level generally associated with RA. If the undiluted specimen demonstrates agglutination and the 1:10 diluted specimen demonstrates the absence of agglutination or a fine granular background, RF is present in the specimen at a low level, which may exist in disease states other than RA.

Semiquantitative Test Results

When positive samples are examined by serial dilution, the titer is the reciprocal of the last dilution that produced a positive result (agglutination).

Sources of Error

False-positive results may be observed if the following occurs:
- Serum specimens are lipemic, hemolyzed, or heavily contaminated with bacteria.

*Wampole ColorCard RF agglutination test (Wampole Laboratories, Cranbury, NJ).

Table 30-4	Case Study: Laboratory Data	
Assay	**Result (Reference Range)**
Erythrocyte sedimentation rate (ESR)	53 mm/hr
C-reactive protein (CRP)	4+
IgM rheumatoid factor (RF)	Positive
Antinuclear antibody (ANA)	Negative
Antibodies to extractable nuclear antigens	Negative
Double-stranded DNA (dsDNA)–binding activity	15%
Serum Complement	
C3	1.1 (0. 75-1.65)
C4	0.4 (0.20-0.65)

- The reaction time is longer than 3 minutes. A false-positive result may also be produced as a result of a drying effect.

Biological false-positive results can be manifested by disorders such as SLE, Sjögren's syndrome, syphilis, and hepatitis. A low rate of positive reactions has been observed in abnormalities such as periarteritis nodosa, rheumatic fever, osteoarthritis, tuberculosis, cancer, some diseases of viral origin, osteoarthrosis, arthritis type undetermined, myositis, and polymyalgia rheumatica. Circulating RF appears to represent a phenomenon of aging, independent of disease.

Clinical Applications

RF is present in the serum of approximately 70% to 80% of patients with clinically diagnosed RA. Almost all patients with variants of RA (e.g., Felty's or Sjögren's syndrome) demonstrate positive results. The highest titers are often found in severe cases of RA. Although the latex agglutination procedure has a 95% correlation with a clinical diagnosis of probable or definite RA, RF is not exclusively limited to patients with RA.

In using latex tests for the detection of RF, a positive result can be expected in less than 5% of healthy individuals. In patients 60 years and older, as many as 30% may be seropositive.

Limitations

As with other diagnostic procedures, the results obtained by an assay yield valuable data that must be evaluated as a component of the total clinical information obtained by the physician. Approximately 25% of patients with definite RA may exhibit negative results for serum RF. Specimens from patients with JIA are usually negative for circulating RF. The strength of the agglutination reaction in the qualitative procedure is not indicative of the actual titer. Weak reactions may occur with slightly elevated or greatly elevated concentrations.

CHAPTER HIGHLIGHTS

- Immunologic factors may be involved in the articular and the extra-articular manifestations of rheumatoid arthritis.
- Rheumatoid arthritis is a chronic, usually progressive, inflammatory disorder of the joints, ranging from mild illness to a progressive, destructive polyarthritis associated with a systemic vasculitis.
- Two pathogenic mechanisms for RA have been hypothesized:
  - The extravascular immune complex hypothesis proposes an interaction of antigens and antibodies in synovial tissues and fluid.
  - An alternative hypothesis is that cell-mediated damage occurs because of accumulation of lymphocytes, primarily T cells, in the rheumatoid synovium, resembling a delayed-type hypersensitivity reaction. The presence of cytokines, which affect articular inflammation and destruction, supports this hypothesis.
- Immunoglobulins can also be observed in synovial lining cells, blood vessels, and interstitial connective tissues. As many as 50% of the plasma cells that can be located in the synovium secrete IgG. The serum of most RA patients has detectable soluble immune complexes. Rheumatoid factors (RFs) have been associated with IgM, IgG, and IgA.
- Cyclic citrullinated peptide (CCP) antibodies are a highly specific and early RA indicator.
- Felty's syndrome is RA with associated splenomegaly and leukopenia. High-titer RF, positive antinuclear antibody (ANA) assay, and rheumatoid nodules are frequently found in patients with Felty's syndrome.
- Juvenile idiopathic arthritis is a condition of chronic synovitis, beginning during childhood.

REVIEW QUESTIONS

1. Rheumatoid arthritis most frequently develops in:
   a. Adolescent females
   b. Adolescent males
   c. Middle-aged women
   d. Middle-aged men

2. Worldwide the incidence of rheumatoid arthritis is:
   a. 1% to 2%
   b. 2% to 4%
   c. 5% to 10%
   d. More than 10%

3. Women are _____ likely than men to develop rheumatoid arthritis.
   a. Less
   b. Equally
   c. Two to three times more
   d. 10 to 20 times more

4. Rheumatoid factor is defined as:
   a. Antigens with specificity for antibody determinants on the Fc fragment of human or certain animal IgG

   b. Antibodies with specificity for antigen determinants on the Fc fragment of human or certain animal IgG
   c. Antigens with specificity for antibody determinants on the Fc fragment of human or certain animal IgD
   d. Antibodies with specificity for antigen determinants on the Fc fragment of human or certain animal IgD

5 and 6. The principle of the rapid agglutination test is based on the reaction of patient (5) _____ and (6)_____ derived from gamma globulin.
   a. Antigen
   b. Antibody
   c. Complement levels
   d. Leukocytes

7-9. Arrange the steps in the pathogenesis of rheumatoid arthritis in the proper order.

   7. _____

   8. _____

   9. _____
   a. Immunologic events perpetuate the initial inflammatory reaction.
   b. The primary etiologic factor initiates synovitis.
   c. An inflammatory reaction in the synovium develops into a proliferative destructive process of tissue.

10. All the following are criteria for rheumatoid arthritis except:
    a. Morning stiffness
    b. Evening stiffness
    c. Rheumatoid nodules
    d. Radiographic changes

11. RF correlates with all the following except:
    a. The severity of the disease in general
    b. The presence of nodules
    c. Other organ system involvement (i.e., vasculitis)
    d. The age of the patient

12. In RA, vascular and parenchymal lesions suggest that lesions result from injury induced by immune complexes, especially those containing antibodies to:
    a. IgM
    b. IgG
    c. IgE
    d. IgD

13. Serum complement levels are usually _____ in patients with rheumatoid arthritis.
    a. Normal
    b. Decreased
    c. Increased
    d. a or b

14. The most common form of juvenile idiopathic arthritis is:
    a. Systemic
    b. Oligoarthritis
    c. Psoriatic
    d. Enthesitis-related

15. In the RF agglutination procedure, a false-positive result may be observed in a serum specimen because of:
    a. Complement interference
    b. High levels of C-reactive protein (CRP)
    c. Antigen excess
    d. Hemolysis

16. In rapid testing for rheumatoid factor, biological false-positive results can be caused by a variety of disorders including:
    a. Infectious mononucleosis
    b. Hepatitis
    c. Systemic lupus erythematosus
    d. Either b or c

BIBLIOGRAPHY

American College of Rheumatology, Ad Hoc Committee on Clinical Guidelines: Guidelines for the management of rheumatoid arthritis, Arthritis Rheum 39:713–722, 1996.

Breedveld FD: New perspectives on treating rheumatoid arthritis, N Engl J Med 333:183–184, 1995.

Centers for Disease Control and Prevention: Prevalence of doctor-diagnosed arthritis and arthritis-attributable activity limitation—United States, 2007-2009, MMWR Morb Mortal Wkly Rep 59:1261–1265, 2010.

Cohen MD: Update: treatment of rheumatoid arthritis, Arthritis Care Res 45:530–532, 2001.

Condemi JJ: The autoimmune diseases, JAMA 268:2885–2888, 1992.

Fantini F: New drugs and treatment strategies for rheumatoid arthritis, Rec Prog Med 94361–94379, 2003.

Genovese M, et al: Abatacept for rheumatoid arthritis refractory to tumor necrosis factor alpha inhibition, N Engl J Med 353:1114–1123, 2005.

Henderson WR: The role of leukotrienes, Ann Intern Med 121:684–696, 1994.

Liang H: Board review: rheumatology, Int Rev Intern Med 41:1467–1473, 1995.

McInnes IB, Schett G: The pathogenesis of rheumatoid arthritis, N Engl J Med 365:2205–2219, 2011.

Olsen NJ, Stein CM: New drugs for rheumatoid arthritis, N Engl J Med 350:2167–2179, 2004.

Renger F, et al: Anti-MCV antibody test for the diagnosis of rheumatoid arthritis using a POCT-immunoassay, 2008, https://acr.confex.com/acr/2008/webprogram/Paper2009.html.

Roose JC, Oster AJ: A new approach to drug development, N Engl J Med 355:2046–2047, 2006.

Sangha O: Epidemiology of rheumatic diseases, Rheumatology 39(Suppl 2):3–12, 2000.

Scott DL, Kingsley GH: Tumor necrosis factor inhibitors for rheumatoid arthritis, N Engl J Med 355:704–712, 2006.

Sullivan, et al: Rheumatoid arthritis: test for anti-CCP antibodies joining RF test as key diagnostic tools, Lab Med 37:17–19, 2006.

Tive L: Celecoxib clinical profile, Rheumatology 39(Suppl 2):21–28, 2000.

Turgeon ML: Synovial fluid. In Turgeon ML: Clinical hematology: theory and procedures, ed 5, Philadelphia, 2012, Lippincott Williams & Wilkins.

Vasishta A: Anti-CCP antibodies: early onset marker in RA, Adv Admin Lab 11:66, 2002.

Wampole ColorCard® package insert, Inverness Medical, 2009.

Wong JB, Ramey DR, Singh G: Long-term morbidity, mortality, and economics of rheumatoid arthritis, Arthritis Rheum 44:2746–2749, 2001.

CHAPTER 31

Solid Organ Transplantation

Mary L. Turgeon and Kyle P. Miller

Learning Objectives

At the conclusion of this chapter, the reader should be able to:

- Identify and describe the histocompatibility antigens.
- Explain the clinical applications of histocompatibility antigens and human leukocyte antigens.
- Identify and describe several laboratory methods for evaluating potential transplant recipients and donors.
- List frequently used terms in transplantation.
- Identify various types of transplants.
- Define graft-versus-host disease.
- Explain the etiology, epidemiology, signs and symptoms, manifestations, diagnosis, and prevention of graft-versus-host disease.

- Describe the types of graft rejection.
- Briefly explain the mechanism of organ or tissue rejection.
- Identify and explain some methods of immunosuppression.
- Analyze a representative transplantation case study.
- Correctly answer case study related multiple choice questions.
- Be prepared to participate in a discussion of critical thinking questions.
- Explain the principle and application of the Longitudinal Assessment of Posttransplant Protocol.
- Correctly answer end of chapter review questions.

Key Terms

accelerated rejection
acute rejection
acute GVHD
alloepitopes
allotype
antibody-dependent, cell-mediated
cytotoxicity (ADCC)

autografts
avascularity
chronic rejection
exons
haplotypes
HLA allele
hyperacute rejection

immunosuppressive agents
major histocompatibility complex
null alleles
proteomics
T cell receptor (TCR)
tolerance
xenotransplantation

The first organ transplantation, using a kidney from an identical twin, was performed in 1954 by Dr. Joseph Murray at Peter Bent Brigham Hospital in Boston. The recipient survived for 9 years. Dr. Murray was ultimately recognized for his work by receiving the Nobel Prize in Medicine in 1990.

At present, a variety of tissues and organs are transplanted in human beings, including bone marrow, peripheral stem cells, bone matrix, skin, kidneys, liver, cardiac valves, heart, pancreas, corneas, and lungs. Transplantation is one of the areas, in addition to hypersensitivity (Chapter 26) and autoimmunity (Chapter 28), in which the immune system functions in a detrimental way.

Early in the history of transplantation, tissue antigens were recognized as important to successful grafting. If significantly different foreign antigens were introduced into an immunocompetent host, the transplanted tissue or organ would undoubtedly fail. Currently, tissue (histocompatibility) matching with concomitant immunosuppression of the host in many cases is used to enhance the probability of success in organ and tissue transplantation.

Transplantation presents the following two basic problems.

- Genetic variation between donor and recipient
- Recognition of genetic differences by a transplant recipient's immune system that causes rejection of a transplanted organ

HISTOCOMPATIBILITY ANTIGENS

The major histocompatibility complex (MHC) is a cluster of genes found on the short arm of chromosome 6 at band 21 (6p21; see Fig 2-1). These genes code for proteins that have a role in immune recognition.

The MHC encodes the human leukocyte antigens (HLAs), which are the molecular basis for T cell discrimination of self from nonself. The HLA complex contains over 200 genes, more than 40 of which encode leukocyte antigens, with the rest an assortment of genes not directly related to the HLA genes. Many genes in this complex have no role in immunity.

Transplanted tissue may trigger a destructive mechanism, rejection, if the recipient's cells recognize the MHC protein products on the surface of the transplanted tissue as foreign, or if immunocompetent cells transplanted on the donor tissue target the foreign cells of the recipient for elimination.

Nomenclature of Human Leukocyte Antigen Alleles

Each **HLA allele** has a unique four-, six-, or eight-letter or digit name (Table 31-1). The length of the allele designation depends on the sequence of the allele and that of its nearest relative. All alleles receive a four-letter or digit name; six- and eight-digit names are only assigned when necessary.

The first two digits describe the type, which often corresponds to the serologic antigen carried by an **allotype**. The third and fourth digits are used to list the subtypes, with numbers assigned in the order in which DNA sequences have been determined.

Alleles whose numbers differ in the first four digits must differ in one or more nucleotide substitutions that change the amino acid sequence of the encoded protein. Alleles that differ

Table 31-1	**HLA Naming System***
Nomenclature	**Indicates**
HLA	Human leukocyte antigen (HLA) region and prefix for an HLA gene
HLA-DRB1	Particular HLA locus (e.g., DRB1)
HLA-DRB1*13	Group of alleles that encode the DR13 antigen
HLA-DRB1*1301	Specific HLA allele
HLA-DRB1*1301N	Null allele
HLA-DRB1*130102	Allele that differs by a synonymous mutation
HLA-DRB1*13010102	Allele that contains a mutation outside the coding region
HLA-A*2409N	Null allele
HLA-A*3014L	Allele encoding a protein with significantly reduced or low cell surface expression
HLA-A*24020102L	Allele encoding a protein with significantly reduced or low cell surface expression, where the mutation is found outside the coding region
HLA-B*44020102S	Allele encoding a protein expressed as a secreted molecule only
HLA-A*3211Q	Allele that has a mutation previously shown to have a significant effect on cell surface expression, but where this has not been confirmed and its expression remains questionable

*As of June 2007, no alleles have been named with the "C" or "A" suffixes.

only by synonymous nucleotide substitutions (also called silent or noncoding substitutions) within the coding sequence are distinguished by the use of fifth and sixth digits. Alleles that only differ by sequence polymorphisms in the introns or in the 5′ or 3′ untranslated regions that flank the **exons** and introns are distinguished by the use of seventh and eighth digits.

In addition to the unique allele designation, optional suffixes may be added to an allele to indicate its expression status. Alleles shown not to be expressed, termed *null alleles,* have been given the suffix N. Alleles shown to be alternatively expressed may have the suffix L, S, C, A, or Q.

The suffix L is used to indicate an allele shown to have *l*ow cell surface expression compared with normal levels. The S suffix is used to denote an allele specifying a protein that is expressed as a soluble *s*ecreted molecule but that is not present on the cell surface. A C suffix indicates an allele product that is present in the *c*ytoplasm but not on the cell surface. An A suffix indicates *a*berrant expression, where there is some doubt as to whether a protein is expressed. A Q suffix is used when the expression of an allele is *q*uestionable, given that the mutation seen in the allele has previously been shown to affect normal expression levels.

Table 31-2	Examples of Nomenclature of HLA Alleles	
Allele (New Nomenclature)	**Frequently Used Shorthand**	
Class I		
HLA-A*0101	HLA-A1	
HLA-B*0801	HLA-B8	
Class II		
HLA-DRB1*0101	HLA-DR1	
HLA-DRB1*0301	HLA-DR3	

Adapted from Peakman M, Vergani D: Basic and clinical immunology, ed 2, New York, 2009, Churchill Livingstone.

Table 31-3	Comparison of Major Histocompatibility Complex Class I and Class II	
Parameter	**Class I**	**Class II**
Loci	HLA-A, B, and C	HLA-DN, DO, DP, DQ, and DR
Distribution	Most nucleated cells	B lymphocytes, macrophages, other antigen-presenting cells, activated T lymphocytes
Function	To present endogenous antigen to cytotoxic T lymphocytes	To present endogenous antigen to helper T lymphocytes

MHC, Major histocompatibility complex.

Major Histocompatibility Complex Regions

The MHC is divided into four major regions (Table 31-2)—D, B, C, and A. The A, B, and C regions are the classic or class Ia genes that code for class I molecules. The D region codes for class II molecules. Class I includes HLA-A, B, and C. The three principal loci (A, B, and C) and their respective antigens are numbered 1, 2, 3, and so on. The class II gene region antigens are encoded in the HLA-D region and can be subdivided into three families, HLA-DR, HLA-DC (DQ), and HLA-SB (DP).

Classes of Human Leukocyte Antigen Molecules

Structurally, there are two classes of HLA molecules, class I and class II (Table 31-3). Both classes are cell surface heterodimeric structures. Class I HLA molecules consist of an alpha chain, a highly polymorphic glycoprotein, encoded within the MHC on chromosome 6. This alpha chain noncovalently associates with beta-2 microglobulin, a nonpolymorphic glycoprotein, encoded by a non-HLA gene on chromosome 15. Class II HLA molecules are composed of alpha chains and beta chains encoded within the MHC. The conformation of class I and class II HLA molecules provides each with a groove in which linear peptides, consisting of 8 to 25 peptides, are displayed for recognition by the cell surface expression on lymphocytes of a transmembrane heterodimeric receptor. All nucleated cells of the body display transmembrane class I HLA molecules in association with the non–transmembrane beta-2 microglobulin molecule.

Class I and class II antigens can be found on body cells and in body fluids. Class I and class II molecules are surface membrane proteins. Class I molecules are transmembrane glycoproteins, but the class II dimer molecule differs from class I in that both dimers span the cell membrane. Class I and class II gene products are biochemically distinct, although they appear to be distantly related through evolution. Class III gene products such as C2, C4A, C4B, and Bf complement components are incomplete but these structures are defined by genes lying between or very near the HLA-B and HLA-DR loci.

Multiple alleles occur at each locus. Genes of class I, II, and III antigens at each locus are inherited as codominant alleles. Inheritance within families closely follows simple mendelian dominant characteristics. Conservation of entire **haplotypes** through generation after generation is the general rule. Very strong linkage disequilibrium is displayed between several HLA loci, creating super or extended haplotypes that may differ from race to race. For example, the most frequent Caucasoid superextended haplotype, AL, Xw7, BB, BfS, C2-1, C4AQOB1, DR3, is almost absent in Asians.

Role of Major Histocompatibility Complex and Human Leukocyte Antigens

The histocompatibility complex that encodes cell surface antigens was first discovered in graft rejection experiments with mice. When the antigens were matched between donor and recipient, the ability of a graft to survive was remarkably improved. A comparable genetic system of alloantigens was subsequently identified in human beings.

The presence of HLA was first recognized when multiply transfused patients experienced transfusion reactions despite proper crossmatching. It was discovered that these reactions were caused by leukocyte antibodies rather than by antibodies directed against erythrocyte antigens. These same antibodies were subsequently discovered in the sera of multiparous women.

The MHC gene products have an important role in clinical immunology. For example, transplants are rejected if performed against MHC barriers; thus, immunosuppressive therapy is required. These antigens are of primary importance and are second only to the ABO antigens in influencing the genetic basis of survival or rejection of transplanted organs.

Although HLA was originally identified by its role in transplant rejection, it is now recognized that the products of HLA genes play a crucial role in our immune system. T cells do not recognize antigens directly but do so when the antigen is presented on the surface of an antigen-presenting cell (APC), the macrophage. In addition to presentation of the antigen, the macrophage must present another molecule for this response to occur. This molecule is a cell surface glycoprotein coded in each species by the MHC. T cells are able to interact with the histocompatibility molecules only if they are genetically identical (MHC restriction).

Both class I and class II antigens function as targets of T lymphocytes that regulate the immune response. Class I molecules regulate interactions between cytolytic T cells and target cells and class II molecules restrict the activity of regulatory T cells (helper, suppressor, and amplifier subsets). Thus, class II molecules regulate the interaction between helper T cells and APCs. Cytotoxic T cells directed against class I antigens are inhibited by CD8 cells; cytotoxic T cells directed against class II antigens are inhibited by CD4 cells. Many genes in both class I and class II gene families have no known functions.

The class I and class II molecules can also bind to self antigens produced in the normal process of cellular protein degradation. Usually, these are not recognized by the **T cell receptor (TCR; tolerance).** In transplant patients, most immune responses are generated not from bacterial antigens, viral antigens, or self antigens, but from the presentation of **alloepitopes** derived from the transplanted tissue to circulating T lymphocytes. Two types of alloepitopes are present on transplanted tissue, private and public. Cross-reactive groups have been defined that categorize the cross-reactive alleles of HLA-A and HLA-B.

Class III molecules bear no clear relationship to class I and II molecules aside from their genetic linkage (presence of the gene in or near the MHC complex). Class III molecules are involved in immunologic phenomenon because they represent components of the complement pathways.

Human Leukocyte Antigen Applications

HLA matching is of value in organ transplantation, as well as in the transplantation of bone marrow. The most important HLA antigens are HLA-A, and HLA-B. Everyone has two types of each of these major HLA antigens; there are many different subtypes of HLA-A and of the others. The best possible match is 6/6; the worst possible match is 0/6.

In kidney allografts, the method of organ preservation, the time elapsed between harvesting and transplanting, the number of pretransplantation blood transfusions, the recipient's age, and the primary cause for kidney failure are all important determinants of early transplantation success or failure. HLA compatibility, however, exerts the strongest influence on long-term kidney survival. The 1-year survival for kidneys transplanted from an HLA-identical sibling approaches 95%. Approximately 50% to 65% of cadaveric kidneys mismatched for all four HLA-A and -B antigens function for 6 months but deteriorate thereafter with time. Only 15% to 25% of these mismatched cadaveric kidneys remain functioning 4 years after transplantation.

It is obligatory to select HLA-identical donors for bone marrow transplantation to reduce the frequency of graft-versus-host disease (GVHD; see later). A method, that depletes donor marrow T cells capable of recognizing foreign host antigens has greatly reduced the incidence of GVHD.

HLA-matched platelets are useful for patients who are refractory to treatment with random donor platelets. In paternity testing, HLA typing is used, along with the determination of ABO, Rh, MNS, Kell, Duffy, and Kidd erythrocyte antigen.

Box 31-1	Relationship of Certain Human Leukocyte Antigens and Diseases
Ankylosing spondylitis	B27
Reiter's syndrome	B27
Psoriasis vulgaris	Cw6
Rheumatoid arthritis	DR4
Behçet's disease	B5 (Bw51)
Type 1 diabetes	DR3
Gold-induced nephropathy	DR5
Congenital adrenal hyperplasia	B47
Chronic lymphatic leukemia	DR5
Kaposi's sarcoma (Mediterranean)	DR5

In the past, most laboratories involved in testing individuals in disputed parentage cases used only the ABO, Rh, and MNS systems. The chances of identifying a falsely accused man with these tests were 58%. Additional testing for Kell, Duffy, and Kidd erythrocyte antigens and for HLA typing has an exclusion rate estimated at 92%.

HLA typing is also useful in forensic medicine, anthropology, and basic research in immunology. In studies of racial ancestry and migration, some antigens are almost excluded or confined to a race (e.g., A1 and B8 are rarely detected in peoples indigenous to central and eastern Asia, and Bw57 is uncommon in whites and African Americans). These distinctions allow for precise conclusions to be drawn regarding origin and ancestry.

HLA testing has increasingly been used as a diagnostic and genetic counseling tool. Knowledge of HLA antigens and their linkage has become important because of the recognized association of certain antigens (Box 31-1) with distinct immunologic-mediated reactions, autoimmune diseases, some neoplasms, and other disorders; these disorders, although nonimmunologic, are influenced by non-HLA genes also located within the major MHC region.

The estimated relative risks or chances of developing a disease if a given antigen is present may be elevated in individuals bearing certain HLA antigens compared to individuals who lack the antigen (Table 31-4). The HLA-B27 antigen is the only HLA antigen with a disease association strong enough to be useful in differential diagnosis. Although the degree of association between HLA antigens and other diseases may be statistically significant, it is not strong enough to be of diagnostic or prognostic value.

Although only 8% of normal whites carry the HLA-B27 antigen, 90% of patients with ankylosing spondylitis (AS) or spondylitis in association with Reiter's syndrome are positive for the antigen. An elevated percentage of HLA-B27–positive patients is also observed in juvenile chronic arthritis with spinal involvement. Therefore, the major indication for screening for HLA-B27 test is to rule out AS when back pain develops in relatives of patients with the disease and to help distinguish incomplete Reiter's syndrome from gonococcal arthritis, or chronic or atypical Reiter's syndrome from rheumatoid arthritis. A negative test for HLA-B27, however, does not exclude the diagnosis of AS or Reiter's syndrome.

Table 31-4	Relationship of Human Leukocyte Antigens to Risk of Disease	
Antigen Present	**Related Disease**	**Risk***
B27	Ankylosing spondylitis	100×[†]
	Reiter's syndrome	40×
	Anterior uveitis	25×
	Arthritic infection with *Yersinia* or *Salmonella*	20×
	Psoriatic arthritis with spinal involvement	11×
	Spondylitis associated with inflammatory bowel disease	9×
	Juvenile chronic arthritis with spinal involvement	5×
B8	Celiac disease	9×
	Addison's disease	6×
	Myasthenia gravis	5×
	Dermatitis herpetiformis	4×
	Chronic active hepatitis	4×
	Sjögren's syndrome	3×
	Diabetes mellitus (insulin dependent)	2×
	Thyrotoxicosis	2×
B5	Behçet's syndrome	6×
BW38	Psoriatic arthritis	7×
BW15	Diabetes mellitus (insulin-dependent)	3×
DR2	Goodpasture's syndrome	16×
	Multiple sclerosis	4×
DR3	Gluten-sensitive enteropathy	21×
	Dermatitis herpetiformis	14×
	Subacute cutaneous lupus erythematosus	12×
	Addison's disease	11×
	Sjögren's syndrome (primary)	10×
DR4	Pemphigus[‡]	32×
	Giant cell arthritis	8×
	Rheumatoid arthritis	6×
	Juvenile (insulin-dependent) diabetes mellitus	5×
DR5	Pauciarticular juvenile arthritis	5×
	Scleroderma	5×
	Hashimoto's thyroiditis	3×

Adapted from Ashman RF: Rheumatic diseases. In Lawlor GJ, Fischer TJ, editors: Manual of allergy and immunology, ed 2, Boston, 1998, Little, Brown.

*Increased risk of developing the disease over a lifetime.

[†]Varies with ethnic group (e.g., 3× for Pima Indians and 300× for Japanese).

[‡]Jewish persons.

Laboratory Evaluation of Potential Transplant Recipients and Donors

Systems developed to ascertain compatibility between donor and recipient include HLA typing and screening of the potential recipient's serum for the presence of antibodies associated with rejection. Graft success is generally correlated with the presence of a compatible crossmatch, although some transplantation teams have proceeded despite a positive (incompatible) crossmatch.

Human Leukocyte Antigen Typing

A potential recipient needs to have HLA typing (Fig. 31-1, *A*). A family search may be conducted for a suitable donor. If a suitable match is not found, the patient is placed on a waiting list (see Fig. 31-1, *B*). When an organ becomes available, the donor is HLA-typed and a computerized search is made for a suitable recipient (see Fig. 31-1, *C*).

A newer method of HLA typing is polymerase chain reaction (PCR) amplification of DNA, followed by probing with sequence-specific oligonucleotide probes (SSOPs) and PCR amplification of alleles at loci using allele-specific primers. A simple computer program has been developed to assign the alleles and genotypes based on the probe hybridization pattern.

The difference between HLA-genotyped and zero mismatches reflects the imperfection of the HLA-typing process. HLA genotype–matched means an HLA-identical sibling when all alleles are truly identical. A zero-mismatched unrelated donor may be mismatched because typing does not distinguish between very closely related alleles. In addition, there may be some effect of non-HLA loci because HLA-identical siblings will share only 50% of their minor histocompatibility loci. The degree of donor-recipient mismatch is somewhat obvious, even in the first year.

Histocompatibility Testing

Because different individuals in a species carry different HLA antigens on their cell surfaces, introduction of foreign antigens can stimulate T cells. These T cells are prominently implicated in graft rejection, and they can also stimulate antibody formation under certain circumstances. Histocompatibility crossmatching is performed to rule out preexisting antibodies capable of causing **hyperacute rejection** (see Fig. 31-1, *D*).

Complement-Mediated Cytotoxicity

Class I antigens are determined by several techniques; the popular classic method is the lymphocyte microcytotoxicity method (complement-mediated cytotoxicity). With this technique, a battery of reagent antisera and isolated target cells are incubated with a source of complement under oil to prevent evaporation. If a specific alloantibody and cell membrane antigen combine, complement-mediated damage to the cell wall allows for penetration of a vital dye and the cells are killed. Cell death is determined by staining. A stain such as trypan blue will penetrate dead cells but not living cells. Unaffected cells remain brilliantly refractile when observed microscopically.

This assay can be insensitive and scoring is subjective. Test sensitivity can be enhanced by the addition of anti–human globulin (AHG) antibody. This assay is used for pretransplantation crossmatching and for antibody specificity analysis. For HLA class I typing or anti–class I antibody identification, a purified T cell population is preferred because human T lymphocytes express class I but not class II molecules. Conversely, B lymphocytes are required for class II typing or antibody identification because human B cells express class I and class II HLA molecules.

Class II HLA-DR and HLA-DQ specificities are also recognized by similar serologic methods, except that isolated B cells are the usual target cells because their surface is rich in these molecules, as well as in class I determinants. At present, HLA-Dw and HLA-DP cannot be serologically defined, and their detection relies on the ability of these molecules to stimulate newly synthesized DNA when added to primary mixed lymphocyte (HLA-Dw) or when re-added to secondary primary lymphocyte (HLA-DP) in vitro cultures.

Class III complement specificities are recognized by the availability of diagnostic reagents, but reagents remain scarce.

Solid-Phase Enzyme-Linked Immunosorbent Assay

The enzyme-linked immunosorbent assay (ELISA) is available for panel-reactive antibody (PRA) determination and antibody-specificity analysis. ELISA-based HLA tests are considered reproducible, sensitive, and objective. Newer assays use pure HLA antigens produced by recombinant technology to improve specificity analysis.

Flow Cytometry

Single-cell analysis by flow cytometry is the most sensitive method for crossmatching and antibody identification (see Chapter 13). Tagged T or B lymphocytes are incubated with the patient's serum to allow the formation of antigen-antibody complexes on the cell surface. Unbound proteins are washed away and the bound antibodies are detected with a second antibody, anti–human immunoglobulin G (IgG) labeled with a chromophore. An alternative flow cytometry format uses microparticles coated with HLA antigens of known specificity (obtained through recombinant techniques) instead of lymphocytes.

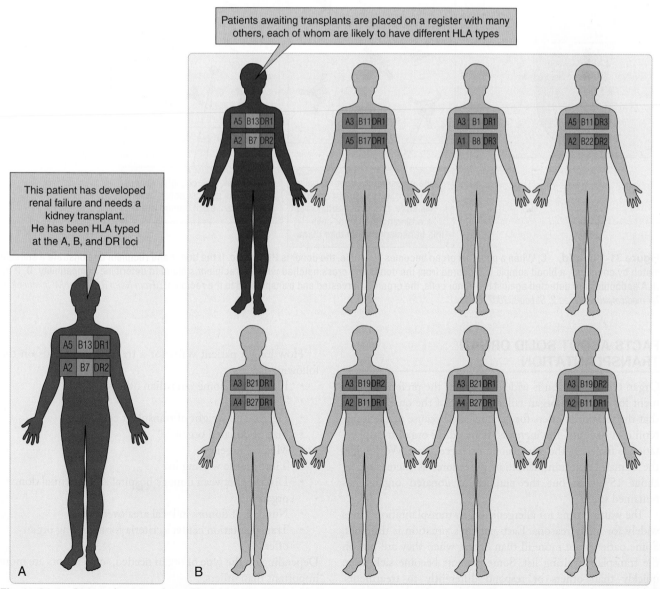

Figure 31-1 Patients (recipients) requiring a solid organ transplant such as a kidney are human leukocyte antigen (HLA)–typed **(A)** and then placed on a transplant registry waiting list **(B)**.

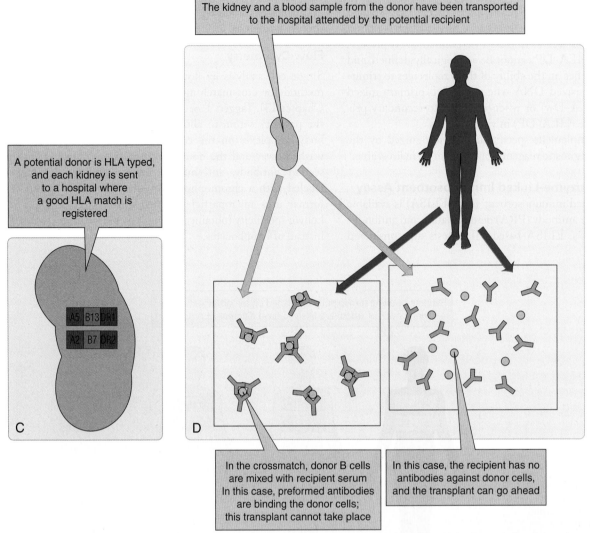

The kidney and a blood sample from the donor have been transported to the hospital attended by the potential recipient

A potential donor is HLA typed, and each kidney is sent to a hospital where a good HLA match is registered

A5 B13 DR1
A2 B7 DR2

C

D

In the crossmatch, donor B cells are mixed with recipient serum
In this case, preformed antibodies are binding the donor cells; this transplant cannot take place

In this case, the recipient has no antibodies against donor cells, and the transplant can go ahead

Figure 31-1 cont'd,   C, When a potential organ becomes available, the donor is HLA-typed. If the donor and recipient demonstrate a suitable match by computer, a blood sample is procured from the donor and crossmatched with the recipient's blood to determine compatibility. **D,** If no HLA antibodies are detected against the donor cells, the organ is harvested and transplanted to the recipient. *(From Nairn R, Helbert M: Immunology for medical students, ed 2, St Louis, 2007, Mosby.)*

FACTS ABOUT SOLID ORGAN TRANSPLANTATION

Organ transplantation is widely viewed as the preferred treatment for end-stage organ failure because of the quality of life that the treatment offers for patients and because of the long-term cost benefits. The increased demand for organ transplantation is fueled by the transplantation success rate. Worldwide, the demand for transplantation procedures is increasing by about 15%/year, but the number of donated organs has remained static.

The waiting time for allergenic organ transplantation varies widely for many reasons. Each patient's situation is different. Some patients are more ill than others when they are put on the transplant waiting list. Some patients become sick more quickly than others or respond differently to treatments. Patients may have medical conditions that make finding a good match more difficult.

How long a patient waits for a transplant depends on the following factors:

- Blood type (some rarer than others)
- Tissue type
- Height and weight of transplant candidate
- Size of donated organ
- Medical urgency
- Time on the waiting list
- Distance between donor's hospital and potential donor organ
- Number of donors in local area over time
- Transplantation center's criteria for accepting organ offers

Depending on the type of organ needed, some factors are more important than others.

In 1984, the U.S. Congress passed the National Organ Transplant Act. The goal of this legislation was to match a low supply of organs with the most critically ill patients, regardless of where they reside. About 79 patients receive an organ transplant every day in the United States. In 2009, more than 28,000 patients received an organ transplant.

On March 22, 2012, the United Network for Organ Sharing patient waiting list contained 113,612 names. The list continues to grow because of the scarcity of organs (Box 31-2). Most of these registrants are waiting for a kidney transplant, followed by those waiting for a liver transplant and heart transplant. Other transplant registrants are waiting for lung, kidney and pancreas, pancreas, pancreatic islet cell, heart and lung, and intestine. Approximately 25% of patients waiting for a liver transplant are children younger than 10 years.

The most common reasons for needing a transplant vary by the type of organ. Kidney recipients usually have diabetes, glomerulonephritis, hypertensive nephrosclerosis, or polycystic

kidneys. Liver recipient patients typically have noncholestatic cirrhosis, cholestatic liver disease, biliary atresia, acute hepatic necrosis, or hepatitis C infection. Patients with cardiomyopathy, congenital heart disease, valvular heart disease, or coronary artery disease are the most frequent heart transplant recipients.

The number of patients living with a function graft has generally increased over the last decade. Graft survival time depends on many factors, including the type of organ transplanted (Fig. 31-2 and Table 31-5).

TRANSPLANTATION TERMINOLOGY

The transplanting or grafting of an organ or tissue ranges from self-transplantation, such as skin grafts from one part of the body to another to correct burn injuries, or hair transplants from one area of the scalp to another to correct pattern baldness, to the grafting of a body component from one species to another, such as transplanting a pig's heart valve to a human. Table 31-6 defines the most recent terms used in transplantation.

TYPES OF TRANSPLANTS

Eleven different organs or human body parts can be transplanted—blood vessels, bone, bone marrow or stem cells (see Chapter 32), cornea, heart, kidneys, liver, lung, middle ear, pancreas, and skin. Successful organ transplants have increased since the advent of the immunosuppressive drug cyclosporine (cyclosporin A).

Box 31-2	**Factors Contributing to the Scarcity of Organs**

Demand for transplantation has increased because more patients are considered eligible.

Age limits for heart and liver transplants eligibility have increased.

Diabetes is no longer an absolute contraindication for transplant eligibility.

The number of donors has shown little growth.

Adapted from Caplan A: Organ procurement and transplantation: ethical and practical issues, 1995 (www.upenn.edu/ldi/issuebrief2_5.html).

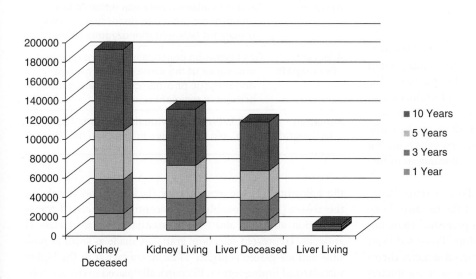

Unadjusted Number of Transplants for Survival Analysis

Figure 31-2 Number of surviving patients after kidney or liver transplants from deceased or living donors. *(From Organ Procurement and Transplantation Network (OPTN) and Scientific Registry of Transplant Recipients (SRTR). OPTN / SRTR 2010 Annual Data Report. Rockville, MD: Department of Health and Human Services, Health Resources and Services Administration, Healthcare Systems Bureau, Division of Transplantation; 2011, www.srtr.org/annual_reports/2010.)*

KEY	Donor	1 Year	3 Years	5 Years	10 Years
Kidney	Kidney Deceased	17760	34901	49989	84554
	Kidney Living	10773	22367	34056	58235
Liver	Liver Deceased	10369	20891	30505	50506
	Liver Living	464	1054	1679	3264

Table 31-5	**Selected Examples of Single Organ Graft Transplant Survival (Unadjusted Graft Survival Expressed in Percentage (%))**				
	Follow–up Period				
	3 Months	**1 Year**	**3 Years**	**5 Years**	**10 Years**
	TX 2007-2008	*TX 2007-2008*	*2005-2008*	*2003-2008*	*1998-2008*
Kidney: Deceased Donor	95.6	91.7	81.8	70.8	44.9
Kidney: Living Donor	98.0	96.5	90.5	82.8	61.2
Pancreas	85.0	74.8	62.6	52.0	35.1
Liver: Deceased Donor	91.7	85.2	75.1	68.5	54.8
Liver: Living Donor	91.3	88.2	80.1	74.6	59.6
Intestine	91.3	81.7	55.2	41.5	24.0
Heart	93.1	88.3	80.7	73.9	54.7
Lung	91.6	81.5	63.3	51.2	26.1

Tx = year or inclusive years of tranplantation.

Source: Organ Procurement and Transplantation Network (OPTN) and Scientific Registry of Transplant Recipients (SRTR). OPTN / SRTR 2010 Annual Data Report. Rockville, MD: Department of Health and Human Services, Health Resources and Services Administration, Healthcare Systems Bureau, Division of Transplantation; 2011. *www.**srtr**.org/annual_reports/**2010***

Living donor transplants have attracted significant media attention. According to the United Network for Organ Sharing and the Health Resources and Services Administration of the U.S. Department of Health and Human Services, a living donor may donate a single kidney, segment of the liver, portion of the pancreas, or the lobe of a lung.

Bone

Bone matrix **autografts** or allografts are common. Transplantation of bone matrix is used after certain limb-sparing tumor resections and to correct congenital bone abnormalities. The major criteria for bone donation are a lack of infection, no history of IV drug use, and no history of prolonged steroid therapy or human growth hormone treatment. Bone can be easily harvested and frozen. Freezing not only preserves the bone but offers the additional benefit of concomitant diminution of histocompatibility antigens.

The major technical requirement for allograft transplantation is maintaining the periosteal sheath of the recipient bone to strip the donor bone completely of all periosteal elements. Transplantation of bone is an easy procedure. Processed bone lacks significant quantities of immunogenic substances; therefore, the need for immunosuppression is almost completely eliminated.

Cornea

Corneal transplants have been a common form of therapy for many years. The first human corneal eye bank was established in New York City in 1944. This type of transplantation has an extremely high success rate because of the ease in obtaining and storing viable corneas.

Corneal grafts are generally performed to replace nonhealing corneal ulcerations. Graft rejection is minimal because of

Table 31-6	**Transplantation Terms**
Term	**Definition**
Autograft	Graft transferred from one position to another in the same individual (e.g., skin, hair, bone)
Syngraft	Graft transplanted between different but identical recipient and donor (e.g., kidney transplant between monozygous twins)
Allograft (homograft)	Graft between genetically different recipient and donor of the same species; grafted donor tissue or organ contains antigens not present in recipient
Xenograft (heterograft)	Graft between individuals of different species (e.g., pig heart valve to a human heart)

the following: (1) the **avascularity** (lack of blood vessels) of this tissue; (2) a reasonably low concentration of class I transplantation antigens; and (3) an essential absence of class II antigens. To prevent rejection, grafts are made as small as possible and are placed centrally to avoid contact with the highly vascularized limbic region. Eccentrically placed grafts are subject to a high rate of immunologic failure because vascularity will allow for lymphocyte contact. Immunosuppressive agents are not routinely administered.

Heart

The first successful allograft cardiac transplantation was performed in 1967 by Dr. Christian Barnard in Cape Town, South Africa. The criteria for selecting the donor and recipient combination for cardiac transplantation are essentially the same as those used for cadaveric renal transplantation. The most significant exclusion for cardiac transplantation, however, is the presence of an active infection. Cardiac transplant donors must have sustained irreversible brain death, but near-normal cardiac function must be maintained. Prophylactic antibiotics and cytotoxic drugs are given to the donor just before harvesting of the heart. Because of the urgency of most situations, most grafts are performed despite multiple HLA incompatibilities. Transplant recipients are maintained on immunosuppressive therapy, anticoagulants, and antithrombotic agents, as well as on a low-lipid diet.

Due to advances in immunosuppression following heart transplantation, there has been an increase in the rate of 1-year survival among recipients to almost 90%, but acute cellular rejection is still observed during the first year after transplantation and at lower rates after the first year. Endomyocardial biopsy remains the primary method for monitoring organ rejection for heart transplants. An alternative method for detecting the rejection of a heart transplant, aside from endomyocardial biopsy, is quantitative assessment of mononuclear cell gene expression in peripheral blood specimens. A study conducted with 602 patients to compare the two methods for monitoring patients for rejection has shown that the overall rate of survival does not differ significantly according to the method of monitoring.

Heart Valves

Xenogenic valve replacement is a standard modality for the treatment of aortic and mitral valve defects. Sources of these xenogenic valves are bovine (cow) or porcine (pig); the valves are chemically or physically modified to reduce antigenicity.

Patients receiving xenoallografts of heart valves are not immunosuppressed after surgery because only minimal or nonexistent graft rejection reactions take place in these modified valves.

Intestine

The first successful intestine transplantation was performed at the University of Toronto in 1986, although the patient only survived for 10 days. The first intestinal transplant recipient to survive for an extended amount of time was a 3½-year-old girl who lived for 192 days in 1987. Intestinal transplantation has improved over the past decade along with the number of intestinal transplantations performed in North America. In 2008, 185 intestinal transplantations were performed. With recent surgical advances, control of acute cellular rejection, and decrease in lethal infections, the rate of patient survival for the first year now exceeds 90%.

When the small intestine is transplanted alone it is referred to as an isolated intestinal transplant, but intestinal transplantations are usually performed with other organs with a composite allograft or with organs implanted separately from the same donor. Suitable intestinal organ donors have stable cardiopulmonary status and liver function. Potential organ transplant recipients with systemic infection and malignancy are excluded.

After a donor is accepted, selective decontamination of the gastrointestinal tract is begun through a nasogastric tube using polyethylene glycol. Generally, the recipient of the transplant is a person suffering from short gut syndrome, in which the intestine had been resected for a variety of reasons.

Kidney

The first successful human kidney transplantation was performed in 1954 between monozygotic twins. Induction of tolerance (see later) was attempted through the use of sublethal total body irradiation and allogeneic bone marrow transplantation, followed by renal transplantation. By 1960, renal transplantation was firmly established as a viable treatment for end-stage renal disease. Because of the continuing problems associated with total-body irradiation, chemical immunosuppression became the mode of treatment. The criteria for recipients of renal allografts generally exclude older patients and patients with a history of malignancy. In addition, patients with active sepsis or patients in whom chronic infection may be reactivated by treatment with steroids or immunosuppressive therapy are also not considered transplantation candidates.

Traditionally, kidney donations are not accepted from individuals older than 65 years because of a decreased likelihood of recipient survival. Donors are excluded if chronic renal disease or sepsis is present. Transplant donations are usually not accepted from those with generalized or systemic diseases such as diabetes mellitus, hypertension, and tuberculosis. Because of the severe shortage of donor kidneys, organs from donors older than 55 years or from donors with a history of hypertension or diabetes mellitus have been used with increasing frequency. Young trauma victims are the most desirable source of cadaveric organ transplants, including the kidneys. Cadaveric organs are not accepted from donors with a history of any malignancy other than that involving the central nervous system.

In addition to tissue compatibility, newer methods of harvesting kidneys have reduced the sensitizing effect related to passenger leukocytes against transplantation antigens borne on these cells. HLA-A and HLA-B loci matches have the best chance for long-term survival of the graft and recipient. The increased survival rate with HLA-A and HLA-B matches is determined not as much by class I compatibility as by the HLA-D region–related antigens associated with these regions. The strongest association between transplantation survival and tissue antigens is with the D region–related antigens (DR, MB, MT). Lewis antigens on the erythrocytes and H-Y antigens associated with X and Y chromosomes are among the other antigen systems that demonstrate a reasonably significant association with graft survival.

Liver

Potential liver transplant recipients must have no extrahepatic disease or infection present. The largest group of transplant recipients has been those with congenital biliary atresia. Patients with cirrhosis may also be good candidates. HLA crossmatching appears to increase the rate of graft survival, but the influence of tissue typing is somewhat unclear. Immunosuppressive regimens such as azathioprine and corticosteroids or cyclosporin A increase survival. Major complications of this procedure have been biliary tract fistulae or leaks, which have occurred in 30% to 50% of patients.

Lung

Successful lung transplantation has been difficult to achieve because of technical, logistic, and immunologic problems. Technically, the lung donor and recipient must have essentially identical bronchial circumferences to obtain a good match. An additional technical problem is that the lungs are extremely sensitive to ischemic damage, and successful preservation after harvesting has been unsuccessful. Occasionally, lung-heart combination transplantation has been attempted. The combined procedure is less difficult than single-organ transplantation.

The lungs are susceptible to infection; sepsis is very common among potential donors. Severe rejection is common because of the high density of Ia-positive cells in the vasculature and the high concentration of passenger leukocytes trapped in the alveoli and blood vessels. Intensive immunosuppressive therapy is needed to maintain the graft. Many lung recipients have died from massive infection and sepsis.

Pancreas

Newer modes of transplantation include full pancreatic or isolated islet cell transplantation. Pancreatic grafts have been successful for only a short period because of a high rate of technical failure or irreversible rejection. Transplantation of small quantities of isolated islet cells into the retroperitoneal space, however, has demonstrated a reasonably good success rate.

Pancreatic islet transplants are risky and experimental, with about 50% of patients achieving insulin dependency after 1 year. From December 16, 1966 to December 31, 2008, more than 30,000 pancreas transplants were reported to the International Pancreas Transplant Registry (IPTR). There are three types of pancreatic transplantations that can be done: pancreas-kidney transplantation (SPK, the most common; 73%); pancreas transplantation after kidney transplantation (PAK; 18%); and pancreas transplantation alone (PTA; 9%).

Skin

The development of nonimmunogenic skin replacement materials has lowered the demand for skin allografts. Skin allografts elicit the rejection phenomenon because skin has an extremely high density of MHC class I antigens. Therefore, sensitization and recognition of antigenic differences are likely, with resultant rejection of the grafted skin. If done, skin allografts are performed and supported with immunosuppressive therapy.

GRAFT-VERSUS-HOST DISEASE

Graft-versus-host disease (GVHD) can be an unintentional consequence of blood transfusion or transplantation in severely immunocompromised or immunosuppressed patients. The degree of immunodeficiency in the host, rather than the number of transfused immunocompetent lymphocytes, determines whether GVHD will occur.

Etiology

When immunocompetent T lymphocytes are transfused from a donor to an immunodeficient or immunosuppressed recipient, the transfused or grafted lymphocytes recognize

Table 31-7	Requirements for Potential Graft-versus-Host Disease
Factor	Comments
1. Source of immunocompetent lymphocytes	Blood products, bone marrow transplant, organ transplant
2. Human leukocyte antigen differences between patient and recipient	The stronger the antigen difference, the more severe the reaction.
3. Inability to reject donor cells	Patients are severely immunocompromised or immunosuppressed.

that the antigens of the host are foreign and react immunologically against them (Table 31-7). Instead of the usual transplantation reaction of host against graft, the reverse graft-versus-host reaction occurs and produces an inflammatory response.

In a normal lymphocyte transfer reaction, the results of a GVHD are usually not serious because the recipient is capable of destroying the foreign lymphocytes. However, engraftment and multiplication of donor lymphocytes in an immunosuppressed recipient are a real possibility because lymphocytes capable of mitosis can be found in stored blood products. If the recipient cannot reject the transfused lymphocytes, the grafted lymphocytes may cause uncontrolled destruction of the host's tissues and eventually death. A patient can develop chronic or **acute GVHD.** The stronger the antigen difference, the more severe is the reaction.

Epidemiology

It is now accepted that GVHD can occur whenever immunologically competent allogeneic lymphocytes are transfused into a severely immunocompromised host. Patients at risk include those who are immunodeficient or immunosuppressed with severe lymphocytopenia and bone marrow suppression. Despite chemotherapy at the time of bone marrow transplantation, patients are highly likely to develop acute GVHD and some of these immunocompromised patients will die of GVHD or associated infections.

Chronic GVHD affects 20% to 40% of patients within 6 months after transplantation. Two factors closely associated with the development of chronic GVHD are increasing age and a preceding episode of acute GVHD.

Cases of transfusion-related GVHD have increased significantly in the past 2 decades. This reaction has been reported subsequent to blood transfusion in bone marrow transplant recipients after total-body irradiation and in adults receiving intensive chemotherapy for hematologic malignancies. GVHD has also occurred in infants with severe congenital immunodeficiency and in those who received intrauterine transfusions followed by exchange transfusion. Almost 90% of patients with posttransfusion GVHD will die of acute complications of the disease. The usual cause of death is generalized infection.

Signs and Symptoms

GVHD causes an inflammatory response. Posttransfusion symptoms begin within 3 to 30 days after transfusion. Because of lymphocytic infiltration of the intestine, skin, and liver, mucosal destruction results, including ulcerative skin and mouth lesions, diarrhea, and liver destruction. Other clinical symptoms include jaundice, fever, anemia, weight loss, skin rash, and splenomegaly.

In bone marrow transplant patients, acute GVHD develops within the first 3 months of transplantation. The initial manifestations are lesions of the skin, liver, and gastrointestinal tract. An erythematous maculopapular skin rash, particularly on the palms and soles, is usually the first sign of GVHD. Disease progression is characterized by diarrhea, often with abdominal pain, and liver disease. Other signs and symptoms of complications related to therapy include fever, granulocytopenia, and bacteremia. Interstitial pneumonia, frequently associated with cytomegalovirus (CMV), can also occur.

Chronic GVHD resembles a collagen vascular disease, with skin changes such as erythema and cutaneous ulcers, and a liver dysfunction characterized by bile duct degeneration and cholestasis. Patients with chronic GVHD are susceptible to bacterial infections. For example, increasing age and preexisting lung disease increase the incidence of interstitial pneumonia.

Immunologic Manifestation

In immunocompromised patients, the transfused or grafted lymphocytes recognize the antigens of the host as foreign and react immunologically against them. Instead of the usual transplantation reaction of host against graft, the reverse GVHD occurs.

Diagnostic Evaluation

Laboratory evidence of immunosuppression or immunodeficiency, such as a decreased total lymphocyte concentration, suggests that a patient may develop GVHD. Evidence of inflammation, such as an increased C-reactive protein (CRP) level, elevated leukocyte count with granulocytosis, and increased erythrocyte sedimentation rate (ESR), may suggest that GVHD has developed in GVHD candidates. Complications of anemia and liver disease, characterized by increased levels of bilirubin and blood enzymes (e.g., transaminases, alkaline phosphatase), and the presence of opportunistic pathogens (e.g., CMV) can further support the diagnosis.

Pathologic features include lymphocytic and monocytic infiltration into perivascular spaces in the dermis and dermoepidermal junction of the skin and into the epithelium of the oropharynx, tongue, and esophagus. Infiltration can also be observed into the base of the intestinal crypts of the small and large bowels and into the periportal area of the liver, with secondary necrosis of cells in infiltrated tissues.

Prevention

The incidence of GVHD can be minimized by depletion of mature lymphocytes from the marrow by using monoclonal antibodies or physical methods. The risk of GVHD can be minimized, if not eliminated, by irradiation of the marrow transplant or blood products. Blood product irradiation is believed to be the most efficient and probably the most economical method available for the prevention of posttransfusion GVHD.

No cases of posttransfusion GVHD have been reported after the administration of irradiated blood products irradiated with an effective and appropriate radiation dose. Several categories of patients possess the clinical indications for the use of irradiated products.

High-Risk Patients

Patients at the highest risk with an absolute need for irradiated blood products include the following:

- Recipients of autologous or allogeneic bone marrow grafts. Recipients of autologous bone marrow may be expected to have the same risk of posttransfusion GVHD as patients receiving allogeneic bone marrow.
- Children with severe congenital immunodeficiency syndromes involving T lymphocytes. The degree of immunodeficiency in the host, rather than the number of transfused immunocompetent cells, determines whether GVHD will occur.

Intermediate-Risk Patients

Patients considered to be at a lower risk of developing GVHD include the following:

- Infants receiving intrauterine transfusions, followed by exchange transfusions, and possibly infants receiving only exchange transfusions. The immune mechanism of the fetus and newborn may not be sufficiently mature to reject foreign lymphocytes and prior transfusions may induce a state of immune tolerance in the newborn. Transfused lymphocytes may continue to circulate for a prolonged period in some immunologically tolerant hosts without the development of GVHD. There is insufficient evidence to recommend irradiation of blood given to all premature infants.
- Patients receiving total-body radiation or immunosuppressive therapy for disorders such as lymphoma and acute leukemia. Although routine irradiation of blood products given to these patients can be justified, it cannot be regarded as absolutely indicated because the risk of developing GVHD is so low. Blood product irradiation, however, is advised for selected patients with hematologic malignancies, especially when transfusions are given during or near the time of sustained and severe therapy-induced immunosuppression.

Low-Risk Patients

Patients also at risk but considered the least susceptible include the following:

- Patients with solid tumors. The incidence of the development of GVHD in these patients is difficult to determine. However, it has developed in nonhematologic malignancies such as neuroblastoma. In one case, GVHD developed after infusion of a single unit of packed red blood cells (RBCs).
- Patients with aplastic anemia receiving antithymocyte globulin theoretically may be at increased risk of posttransfusion GVHD during therapy-induced periods of lymphocytopenia.

- Although a theoretical risk of posttransfusion GVHD may exist in patients with acquired immunodeficiency syndrome (AIDS), the disease has not actually been observed in this disorder. The routine use of irradiated blood is not recommended.

Effects of Radiation on Specific Cellular Components

Lymphocytes. Ionizing radiation is known to inhibit lymphocyte mitotic activity and blast transformation. Irradiation of normal donor lymphocytes with 1500 rad from a cesium-137 source results in a 90% reduction in mitogen-stimulated ^{14}C-thymidine incorporation. An 85% reduction in mitogen-induced blast transformation after exposure to 1500 rad and a 97% to 98.5% reduction in mitogenic response have been noted after an appropriate exposure to radiation.

Granulocytes. Ionizing radiation may impair granulocyte function in a dose-dependent manner. The degree of actual damage to granulocytes is controversial. Chemotactic activity decreased linearly with increasing doses of irradiation from 500 to 120,000 rad, but the reduction only reached statistical significance at 10,000 rad. A linear dose-response curve demonstrates that granulocyte locomotion is affected by very small doses of irradiation. An appropriate dose of radiation is likely to eliminate lymphocytic mitotic activity and prevent GVHD without causing significant damage to granulocytes or altering their chemotactic or bactericidal ability. Irradiation before transfusion has been demonstrated to contribute to defective oxidative metabolism, but this effect is highly variable.

Mature Red Blood Cells. Mature RBCs appear to be highly resistant to radiation damage. After RBCs were exposed to 10,000 rad, ^{52}Cr-labeled in vivo RBC survival was the same as that of untreated controls. Stored erythrocytes can be treated with up to 20,000 rad without changing their viability or in vitro properties, including adenosine triphosphate (ATP) and 2,3-diphosphoglycerate (2,3-DPG) levels, plasma hemoglobin (Hb), and potassium ions (K$^+$).

Platelets. Ionizing radiation may impair platelet function. Although this impairment is dose-dependent, the effects of irradiation on platelets have been difficult to characterize. Several studies have demonstrated unchanged in vivo platelet survival after exposure to 5000 to 75,000 rad. A 33% decrease in the expected platelet count increase was noted after transfusion of platelets exposed to 5000 rad, and similarly irradiated autologous platelets had a diminished ability to correct the bleeding times in a small number of volunteers who had consumed aspirin.

Immunologic Tolerance

The importance of tolerance to self antigens was recognized early in the study of immunology. Immunologic tolerance is the acquisition of nonreactivity toward particular antigens. Self-recognition (tolerance) is a critical process, and the failure to recognize self antigens can result in autoimmune disease (see Chapter 28).

Various pathways to immunologic tolerance have been recognized. It has been suggested that T and B cells are affected independently and differently and may be tolerated under certain circumstances. Several mechanisms may operate simultaneously in a single host. During fetal development of the immune system and during the first few weeks of neonatal life, none of the cells of the immune system has reached maturity. For this reason, the entire immune system is particularly susceptible to tolerance induction at this stage of development.

T Cell Tolerance

T cells do not show a marked difference in tolerance at different stages of maturation. The antigen required to produce tolerance and the circumstance of its presentation are specific for each individual T cell subset. At least three pathways have been recognized for T cell tolerance:

1. Clonal abortion. Immature T cell clones may be aborted in a manner similar to that of B cells.
2. Functional deletion. The subsets of a mature T cell may be individually deleted, leading to the loss of only one of the functions of the T cell group.
3. T cell suppression. T cell suppressors actively suppress the actions of other T cell subsets or B cells.

B Cell Tolerance

As a B cell matures, it becomes less susceptible to tolerization. In addition, during B cell maturation, the forms of antigen presentation that will produce tolerance also vary. Four pathways have been established for the induction of B cell tolerance. Therefore, the mode of tolerance depends on the maturity of the cell, antigen, and manner of antigen presentation to the immune system.

The pathways of B cell tolerance are as follows:

1. Clonal abortion. A low concentration of multivalent antigen may cause the immature clone to abort. Tolerance of immature B cells by this mechanism is high.
2. Clonal exhaustion. Repeated antigen challenge with a T-independent antigen may remove all mature functional B cell clones. Tolerance of mature B cells is moderate.
3. Functional deletion. The combined absence of the helper T subset and presence of T-dependent antigen (or with T suppressor cells), or an excess of T-independent antigen, prevents mature B cells from functioning normally. The ability to tolerize B cells by this mechanism is moderate.
4. Antibody-forming cell blockade. An excess of T-independent antigen interferes with the secretion of antibody by antibody-forming cells. B cell tolerance by this mechanism is low.

Immune Response Gene–Associated Antigens

The specific immune responses to a variety of antigenic substances are now known to be regulated by an immune response (Ir) gene. Ir gene control is considered genetically dominant. The homology of the HLA-D region with the animal I region suggests that the human Ir gene might be linked to the HLA complex. Evidence for the existence of the Ir gene has been obtained from family and population studies. Additional evidence for the presence of Ir genes comes from HLA-linked disease susceptibility genes and HLA-disease associations. It is believed that individuals who lack this gene are unresponsive.

The generally accepted concept is that the Ir gene is responsible for the interaction of T cells with B cells and macrophages, which are necessary for T cell activation. Activation of T cells is required for the following:

- Conversion to active helper function
- Production of lymphokines

Mediation of delayed and contact hypersensitivity, as the proliferative response to antigen, depends on the interaction of a T cell with an APC, usually macrophage-monocytes. Helper function also depends on T cell interaction with precursors of antibody-secreting cells. T cells interact with these cells by recognizing specific antigen bound to macrophages or to B cells and the I region gene products expressed on the surface of these cells. T cells are able to recognize the precise details of antigen structure and distinguish between two closely related Ir gene–associated molecules expressed on the surface of these APCs or on the B cell.

GRAFT REJECTION

Organs vary with respect to their susceptibility to rejection based on inherent immunogenicity (Box 31-3), which is influenced by factors such as vascularity.

The role of sensitized lymphocytes and antibodies in graft rejection differs and is influenced by the type of organ transplanted. Lymphocytes, particularly recirculating small lymphocytes, are effective in shortening graft survival. Cell-mediated immunity is responsible for the rejection of skin and solid tumors. However, humoral antibodies can also be involved in the rejection process. The complexity of the action and interaction of cellular and humoral factors in grafts is considerable. Five possible categories of graft rejection have been demonstrated in human kidney transplant rejection—hyperacute, accelerated, acute, chronic, and immunopathologic (Table 31-8; Color Plate 17).

First-Set and Second-Set Rejections

Skin transplantation is the most common experimental model for transplantation research (Fig. 31-3). Rejection of skin and

solid tumors can be divided into first-set and second-set rejections. Activation of cellular immunity by T cells is the predominant cause of the first-set allograft rejection. Lymphocytes can directly attack cellular antigens to which they are sensitized by previous exposure or by cytotoxic lymphokines. The primary role of lymphocytes in first-set rejection is consistent with the histology of early reaction and shows infiltration by mononuclear cells, with very few polymorphonuclear leukocytes or plasma cells. Sensitization occurs within the first few days of transplantation, and the tissue is lost in 10 to 20 days.

When sensitized lymphocytes are already present because of prior graft rejection, an **accelerated rejection** of tissue results from regrafting, called second-set rejection. Lymphocytes from a sensitized animal transferred to a first-graft recipient will accelerate rejection of the graft. Graft rejection is primarily a T cell function, with some assistance from antibodies.

Hyperacute Rejection

Hyperacute reactions are caused entirely by the presence of preformed humoral antibodies in the host, which react with donor tissue cellular antigens. These antibodies are usually anti-A–related or anti-B–related antibodies to the ABO blood group systems or antibodies to class I MHC antigens (hypersensitivity type II). Potential recipients harboring antibodies to HLA-A, HLA-B, and HLA-C (class I) but not HLA-DR (class II) antigens are at high risk for this process.

Box 31-3	Immunogenicity of Different Transplant Tissues
Most Immunogenic	
Bone marrow	
Skin	
Islets of Langerhans	
Heart	
Kidney	
Liver	
Bone	
Xenogeneic valve replacements	
Least Immunogenic	
Cornea	

Table 31-8	Categories and Characteristics of Graft Rejection Based on Immune Destruction of Kidney Grafts		
Type	Time of Tissue Damage	Predominant Mechanism	Cause
Hyperacute	Within minutes	Humoral	Preformed cytotoxic antibodies to donor antigens
Accelerated	2-5 days	Cell-mediated	Previous sensitization to donor antigens
Acute	7-21 days	Cell-mediated (possibly antibody cell-mediated cytotoxicity)	Development of allogeneic reaction to donor antigens
Chronic	Later than 3 mo	Cell-mediated	Disturbance of host-graft tolerance
Immunopathologic damage to the new organ	Later than 3 mo	1. Immune complex disorder 2. Complex formation with soluble antigens	Immunopathologic mechanisms related to circumstances necessitating transplantation

The interaction of cellular antigens with antibodies activates the complement system and leads to grafted cell lysis and clotting in the grafted tissue. Kidney allografts can be rejected by the hyperacute rejection process within minutes of transplantation. The irreversible kidney damage of hyperacute rejection is characterized by sludging of erythrocytes, development of microthrombi in the small arterioles and glomerular capillaries, and infiltration of phagocytic cells.

Genetically altered pig organs could be available for transplantation into human beings within 2 years, but it is likely to be at least 5 years before full-scale studies can begin. Future xenotransplantation will depend on overcoming problems of hyperacute rejection. In hyperacute rejection, the recipient of the organ produces xenoreactive antibodies, which lodge on the cells lining the blood vessels of the new organ and trigger the release of complement. This release triggers inflammation, swelling, and ultimately blockage of the blood vessels, leading to death of the organ.

Accelerated Rejection

Accelerated rejection is comparable to the second-set rejection phenomenon observed in animal models. In these cases, retransplantation is less severe than hyperacute rejection and is considered to be accelerated rejection. Accelerated rejection is caused by activation of the T cell–mediated response.

Acute Rejection

Acute rejection can result after the first exposure to alloantigens. In this reaction, donor antigens select reactive T cell

Hyperacute rejection

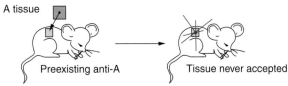
A tissue

Preexisting anti-A → Tissue never accepted

First set rejection

A tissue

Normal B mouse → Tissue rejected 10 to 20 days

Second set rejection

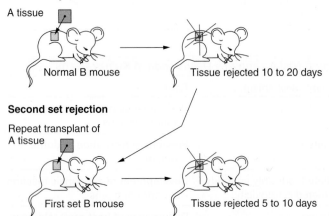
Repeat transplant of A tissue

First set B mouse → Tissue rejected 5 to 10 days

Figure 31-3 Hyperacute rejection results from placement of tissue in an animal already possessing antibodies to antigens of grafted tissue. Second-set rejection is an accelerated first-set reaction and is seen in animals that have already rejected tissue at least once. *(Adapted from Barrett JT: Textbook of immunology, ed 5, St Louis, 1988, Mosby.)*

clones and initiate visible manifestation of rejection within 6 to 14 days. The early processes in acute rejection appear to be T cell–mediated; however, later aspects may involve antibodies and complement.

Acute rejection is equivalent to a first-set allograft rejection in experimental animals and is primarily mediated by cells, as in accelerated rejection. Immunopathologic changes include the presence of immune complex deposition and other hypersensitivity reactions already present in the recipient.

Acute rejection takes place when there is HLA incompatibility. Recipient T cells can respond to donor peptides presented by a recipient MHC or to donor MHC molecules themselves. The better the HLA match, the more successful are the prospects for nonrejection. Because of the shortage of organs and the huge demand for organs, partially mismatched organs (e.g., kidneys) may be used. The survival of the kidney is related to the degree of mismatching, especially at the HLA-DR loci. Despite mismatching, 1-year survival with five mismatches was almost 80% because of the effect of potent immunosuppressive drugs.

A recipient may respond to minor histocompatibility antigens. Minor antigens are encoded by genes outside the HLA. These minor histocompatibility antigen mismatches are not detected by standard tissue typing techniques but may cause rejection despite a good HLA match. Up to one third of transplants can be rejected because of minor antigens.

Acute early rejection, which occurs up to about 10 days after transplantation, is histologically characterized by dense cellular infiltration and rupture of peritubular capillaries. It appears to be a cell-mediated hypersensitivity reaction involving T cells. In comparison, acute late rejection occurs 11 days or more after transplantation in patients suppressed with prednisone and azathioprine. In kidney allografts, acute late rejection is probably caused by the binding of immunoglobulin, presumably antibody and complement, to the arterioles and glomerular capillaries, where they can be visualized by immunofluorescent techniques. These immunoglobulin deposits on the vessel walls include platelet aggregates in glomerular capillaries, which cause acute renal shutdown. The possibility of damage to antibody-coated cells through **antibody-dependent, cell-mediated cytotoxicity (ADCC)** may also take place.

Chronic Rejection

Chronic rejection occurs in most graft recipients. The process results in a slow but continual loss of organ function over months or years. However, chronic rejection is often responsive to various immunosuppressive therapies.

In kidney allografts, this insidious rejection is associated with subendothelial deposits of immunoglobulin and the C3 component of complement on the glomerular basement membranes. This may occasionally be an expression of an underlying immune complex disorder that may have originally necessitated the transplantation, or it may result from complex formation with soluble antigens derived from the grafted kidney.

MECHANISMS OF REJECTION

General Characteristics

Variations in the expression of class II histocompatibility antigens by different tissues and the presence of APCs in some tissues greatly influence the success of a transplant. APCs that enter the graft through the donor's circulation are likely to elicit graft rejection. If these so-called passenger lymphocytes leave the graft after transplantation and enter the draining lymphatic system, they are particularly effective in sensitizing the host.

Rejection of a graft displays the following two key features of adaptive immunity:

* Memory
* Specificity

Only sites accessible to the immune system in the recipient are susceptible to graft rejection. Certain privileged sites in the body allow allogeneic grafts to survive indefinitely.

Role of T Cells

Graft rejection is primarily regulated by the interaction of the host's T cells with the antigens of the graft. Unmodified rejection, however, results from the destructive effects of cytotoxic T (Tc) cells, activated macrophages, and antibody.

In tissue transplants, the graft consists of tissue cells that carry class I antigens (HLA-A, HLA-B, and HLA-C) and of lymphocytes that carry class I and class II antigens (HLA-D and related antigens of an associated Ir gene). Activated T cells specific for class I antigens have the potential to express cytotoxic activity, which damages the endothelium and parenchymal cells of the graft. Binding of these cells to the class I antigens on target cells of the donor organ triggers the release of lymphokines and subsequently activates a nonspecific inflammatory response in the allograft.

T cells specific for class II antigens of the donor tissue cannot react directly with the parenchymal cells of the graft not expressing class II antigens. However, these cells can activate lymphocytes in the transplant through lymphocyte release. Therefore, damage to the graft can result from a cytotoxic reaction directed against cells of the transplanted organ, a severe nonspecific inflammatory response, or both.

Activation of helper T (Th) cells by class II antigens such as HLA-DR probably stimulates the release of interleukin-1 (IL-1). IL-1 subsequently stimulates the release of various lymphokines from Th cells, which in turn activate macrophages, Tc cells, and antibody-releasing B cells, as well as increase the immunogenicity of the graft. In addition, macrophages and other accessory cells are subsequently stimulated by T cell products and release IL-1, which in turn stimulates the formation of IL-2 receptors and the release of IL-2 by Th cells. IL-2 interacts with specific IL-2 receptors expressed on activated Th and Tc cells. This interaction stimulates the initiation of DNA synthesis and the eventual clonal proliferation of IL-2 receptor–bearing cells. IL-2 also causes the release of interferon-γ (IFN-γ), which activates macrophages and stimulates the release of B cell differentiation factors required for the proliferation of antigen-activated B cells. The release of IL-2–dependent IFN-γ by activated T cells may initiate a vicious circle, because IFN-γ induces the expression of class II molecules on endothelial cells, as well as the expression of certain class II–negative macrophages.

Histologic examination of an allogenic skin graft during the process of rejection demonstrates that the dermis becomes infiltrated by mononuclear cells, many of which are small lymphocytes. This accumulation of lymphocytes precedes the destruction of the graft by several days. Although this graft rejection process is caused by Tc cells, in some cases Th cells are also elicited by MHC gene differences. Graft rejection may be a special form of response related to delayed hypersensitivity reactions, in which case the ultimate effectors of graft destruction are the monocyte-macrophages recruited to the site. It is debatable whether the macrophages seen in grafts are effectors of graft destruction or arrive only as a consequence of the inflammatory process and cell damage.

Antibody Effects

Cell-mediated immunity is the major effector mechanism in graft rejection. Antibodies, however, can also be involved in graft rejection. Antibodies can cause rapid (hyperacute) graft rejection, but they are usually less significant than cell-mediated immunity. Exceptions include cases in which the recipient has been previously sensitized to a particular antigen, reactions occur to hematopoietic cells, or the graft is directly connected to the host's blood circulation (e.g., kidney allograft).

In dispersed cellular grafts, such as infusion of erythrocytes, leukocytes, and platelets, antibodies (humoral immunity) may dominate the rejection process because antigens are fully exposed to a preexisting or developing antibody response. Cells are highly susceptible to complement-activated membrane damage. If cytolysis does not occur immediately, antibodies may function as opsonins to encourage phagocytic destruction of transfused cells.

Humoral immunity is suspected of playing a major role in the rejection of xenografts. Xenografts possess a large number of antigens shared between donor and recipient. One species can possess agglutinins for cells of distantly related species, which can attack the xenogenic tissue as soon as it is transplanted.

Immunosuppression

For most patients who receive a donated organ, immunosuppressant drug therapy and monitoring of the concentration of immunosuppressants play a critical role in the success of the transplant. Laboratory methods for measuring immunosuppressant drug concentrations in blood include immunoassay, high-performance liquid chromatography (HPLC), and liquid chromatography with mass spectrometry (LC-MS). Clinical laboratories are increasingly using LC-MS for routine measurement of immunosuppressants.

Immunosuppression is used for the following:

* Induction (intense immunosuppression in the initial days after transplantation)
* Maintenance of transplant
* Reversal of established rejection

Forms of immunosuppression include chemical (Box 31-4), biologic, and irradiation of the lymphoid system or the donated

Box 31-4	Immunosuppression in Human Organ Transplantation
1945-1955	Research on antimetabolites, including 6-mercaptopurine, azathioprine, and corticosteroids, used to improve kidney graft survival.
Late 1960s	Antilymphocyte globulin proved successful.
1976	Cyclosporine developed.
1983	Cyclosporine approved by FDA.
1984	OKT3 (muromonab-CD3) approved by FDA.
1994	Tacrolimus (FK-506) approved by FDA.
1995	Mycophenolic acid approved by FDA (almost 30 years after development).
1996	Cyclosporine microemulsion (Neoral) approved by FDA.
1997	Antithymocyte globulin approved by FDA. Dacliximab (Zenapax) approved by FDA.
1999	Sirolimus (Rapamune) approved by FDA.
2004	Enteric-coated mycophenolic acid approved by FDA, generic formulations of both
2008-2010	tacrolimus and mycophenolate mofetil approved by FDA.
2011	Nulojix (belatacept) approved by FDA.

FDA, U.S. Food and Drug Administration.

Table 31-9	Types of Immunosuppressive Treatment
Drug	**Mechanism of Action**
Corticosteroids	Reduce inflammation by inhibiting macrophage cytokine secretion
Cyclosporine and FK506	Blocks T cell cytokine production by inhibiting the phosphatase calcineurin and then blocking activation of the NFAT transcription factor
Mycophenolate mofetil	Blocks lymphocyte proliferation by inhibiting guanine nucleotide synthesis in lymphocytes
Rapamycin	Blocks lymphocyte proliferation by inhibiting IL-2 signaling
Anti-CD3 monoclonal antibody	Depletes T cells by binding to CD3 and promoting phagocytosis or complement-mediated lysis (used to treat acute rejection)
Anti–IL-2 receptor antibody	Inhibits T cell proliferation by blocking IL-2 binding; may also opsonize and help eliminate activated IL-2R-expressing T cells
CTLA4-Ig	Inhibits T cell activation by blocking B7 costimulator binding to T cell CD28 (clinical trials)
Nulojix (belatacept)	A selective T cell costimulation blocker

Adapted from Abbas AK, Lichtman AH: Basic immunology, ed 3, St Louis, 2011, Saunders.

NFAT, Nuclear factor of activated T cells. *IL*, interleukin, *CTLA4-Ig*, cytotoxic T lymphocyte-associated protein-4-immunoglobulin (fusion protein).

FDA approves Nulojix for kidney transplant patients www.fda.gov/NewsEvents

organ. The immunosuppressive activities of therapeutic agents used in transplantation directly interfere with the allograft rejection response. The problem arising from all immunosuppressive techniques is that the person is more susceptible to infection. If infection occurs, immunosuppression must be suspended, at which time allogeneic reactions frequently develop.

Immunosuppressive measures may be antigen-specific or antigen-nonspecific (Table 31-9). Antigen-nonspecific immunosuppression includes drugs and other methods of specifically altering T cell function. Many cytotoxic drugs are primarily active against dividing cells and therefore have some functional specificity for any cells activated to divide by donor antigens. The use of these drugs is limited by the toxic effects that they may have on other dividing cells or on the physiologic functioning of organs such as the liver.

Antigen-specific immunosuppression is an ideal form of immunosuppression. Antigen-specific tolerance is that induced by the infusion of donor cells. This is generally impractical in transplantation, but may be useful in the phenomenon of immunologic enhancement. Enhancement of tolerance has been attempted in renal allograft patients. In a donor-specific blood transfusion program, the patient is transfused several times before elective transplantation with blood from the prospective kidney donor. The overall effect of these transfusions appears to be a tolerance of the recipient to donor transplantation antigens other than those in the HLA-linked regions, such as minor histocompatibility loci, RBC loci, and leukocyte surface antigens. This treatment has greatly prolonged graft survival in these patients.

Cytotoxic Drugs

Cytotoxic drugs are the most common form of therapy and usually include alkylating agents, purine and pyrimidine analogues (Fig. 31-4), folic acid analogues, or the alkaloids. The drugs of choice, excluding alkylating drugs, are azathioprine, 6-mercaptopurine, 6-thioguanine, 5-fluorouracil, cytosine arabinoside, methotrexate and aminopterin, and vinblastine and vincristine.

Most immunosuppressive drugs administered alone cannot produce antigen-specific tolerance because they act equally on all susceptible clones. Except for certain drugs (e.g., cyclosporin A), most immunosuppressive agents can be rendered antigen-specific only by including an antigen-specific element in the tolerizing regimen. In these cases, the drugs act as cofactors in tolerogenesis. Experimental evidence has suggested that these regimens may act as follows:

- Lowering the threshold for tolerance induction
- Blocking the differentiation sequence in cells triggered by antigen

Azathioprine

Since its introduction in 1961, azathioprine, an oral purine analogue that is an antimetabolite with multiple activities, has been the mainstay of antirejection therapy. Azathioprine requires activation to 6-mercaptopurine, which is further metabolized

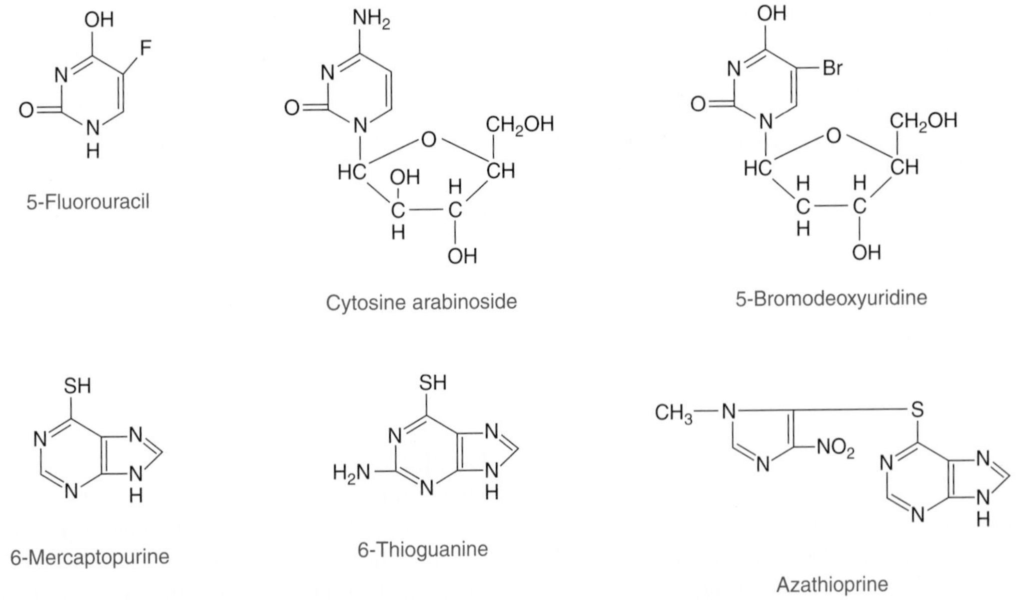

Figure 31-4   Pyrimidine analogues *(upper row)* and purine analogues *(lower row)* with B and T cell–suppressing activity. A large number of similar compounds are available for human use. *(Adapted from Barrett JT: Textbook of immunology, ed 5, St Louis, 1988, Mosby.)*

to active 6-thioguanine nucleotides. Metabolites of azathioprine, such as the in vivo metabolite 6-mercaptopurine, are incorporated into cellular DNA. This inhibits purine nucleotide synthesis and metabolism and alters the synthesis and function of ribonucleic acid (RNA). Therefore, azathioprine acts at an early stage in T cell or B cell activation during the proliferative cycle of effector lymphocyte clones. Azathioprine is useful in preventing acute rejection because it inhibits the primary immune response; however, it has little or no effect on secondary responses. Adverse effects include bone marrow suppression, myopathy, alopecia, pancreatitis, and hepatitis. A drug interaction can occur with allopurinol.

Corticosteroids

Corticosteroids can be used in conjunction with azathioprine or other immunosuppressants such as cyclosporine. Corticosteroids directly inhibit antigen-driven T cell proliferation, but steroids do not act directly on the IL-2–producing T cell. They do, however, inhibit production of lymphokines by preventing monocytes from releasing IL-1, thereby blocking IL-1–dependent release of IL-2 from antigen-activated T cells. Other activities of monocytes, such as inhibition of chemotaxis, are also likely to be important in the immunosuppressive process.

High doses of corticosteroids are used to treat acute rejection. In addition, steroids probably reverse in vivo rejection episodes by preventing the production of IL-2, which would inhibit activated T cells as an essential trophic factor.

Cyclosporine (Cyclosporin A)

Cyclosporine, isolated in 1971 from the fungus *Tolypocladium inflatum*, has become the mainstay of immunosuppressive therapy in transplantation. Cyclosporine affects T cells preferentially by inhibiting the induction of cytotoxic T cells. Unlike corticosteroids, cyclosporine does not inhibit the capacity of all

accessory cells to release IL-1. Cyclosporine blocks calcineurin to the IL-2 gene transcription pathway and the release of certain other lymphokines (e.g., IFN-γ). Cyclosporine binds to cyclophilin and the complex binds to and inhibits calcineurin (a protein phosphatase). This prevents activation of the IL-2 transcription factor.

The secretion of B cell growth and differentiation factors by activated T cells is also inhibited by cyclosporin A. Therefore, under the influence of cyclosporin A, Th cell–dependent B cells are not fully activated because of a lack of necessary Th cell stimulation. In pharmacologic doses, however, cyclosporin A does not grossly interfere with the activation and proliferation of suppressor T cells. Studies have shown prolonged renal allograft survival with cyclosporin A, despite potential mismatches of the HLA system. Adverse effects of corticosteroids include fluid retention, electrolyte abnormalities, hyperglycemia, hypertension, peptic ulcer disease, osteoporosis, and adrenal insufficiency. Hepatotoxicity has been observed in 4% to 7% of patients. Drug interactions can occur with grapefruit juice, erythromycin, oral contraceptives, and a variety of other drugs. Drug monitoring is critical because of the narrow therapeutic range.

A newer cyclosporine microemulsion offers the advantage of improved trough measurement correlation with the actual patient circulating concentration.

Tacrolimus

Tacrolimus (FK-506), a macrolide with mechanisms similar to that of cyclosporine, is derived from a fungus, *Streptomyces tsukubaensis*, found in soil samples in Japan. FK-506 is 50 to 100 times more powerful than cyclosporine. Its primary target appears to be the Th lymphocytes, with little effect on other aspects of the immune response. FK-506 acts early in the process of T cell activation and inhibits the production of IL-2. As a result, T lymphocytes do not proliferate, secretion of

IFN-γ is inhibited, MHC class II antigens are not induced, and further activation of macrophages does not occur.

Because FK-506 is a more potent immunosuppressant than cyclosporine, patient recovery time is faster. FK-506 has higher toxicity compared with cyclosporine. Nephrotoxicity, hyperkalemia, hypokalemia, hypomagnesemia, hypertension, and other side effects may occur, but FK-506 causes no serious side effects (e.g., kidney damage, elevated blood pressure, mood swings). Patients receiving FK-506 have increased susceptibility to infections (e.g., CMV) and an increased risk of developing lymphoma or posttransplantation lymphoproliferative diseases. Inhibitors and inducers of P-450 3A4 may demonstrate an altered rate of metabolism that requires an adjustment in drug dose.

Sirolimus

Sirolimus (Rapamune), previously referred to as rapamycin, was under development for more than 20 years before gaining approval by the U.S. Food and Drug Administration (FDA). Sirolimus is derived from the fungus *Streptomyces hygroscopicus* from the soil of Easter Island. Structurally, sirolimus resembles tacrolimus and has the same intracellular binding protein or immunophilin, known as FKBP-12, but sirolimus has a novel mechanism of action. Sirolimus is a substrate for P-450 3A4 and inhibits the activation and proliferation of T lymphocytes and subsequent production of IL-2, IL-4, and IL-15. Sirolimus also inhibits antibody production. Sirolimus has been approved as an adjunctive agent (in combination with steroids) for the prevention of acute renal allograft rejection. The main side effects include increased risk of infections and lymphoma, hypercholesterolemia, hypertriglyceridemia, interstitial pneumonitis, insomnia and tremor, and thrombocytopenia.

Mycophenolate Mofetil

Mycophenolate mofetil (RS-61443) inhibits de novo guanosine synthesis by inhibiting inosine monophosphate dehydrogenase. This drug inhibits T and B lymphocyte proliferation and antibody formation by B lymphocytes and has been efficacious as prophylactic and rescue therapy in refractory renal allograft rejection in clinical trials.

Mycophenolate mofetil (MMF; CellCept), is a drug that is now being used more frequently in treatment plans as a substitute for azathioprine. MMF prevents the production of cells such as azathioprine but is believed to be more effective for preventing rejection in patients. Studies have suggested that mycophenolate is effective in preventing acute rejection and may also slow the progression to chronic rejection. Adverse side effects include a lowering in blood cell development, which can cause abdominal pain, vomiting, and diarrhea, but generally it is a well-tolerated drug.

Antilymphocyte (Antithymocyte) Globulin

Other immunosuppressive measures directed at T cells include the use of antilymphocyte (antithymocyte) globulin (ATG), an IgG polyclonal antibody, at the time of transplantation and the use of lymphoid irradiation before transplantation. The usefulness of ATG for preventing or reversing rejection in renal allograft recipients has been well established. Adverse side

effects can include complement-mediated lysis of lymphocytes, serum sickness, leukopenia, and thrombocytopenia.

Among patients at high risk for acute rejection or delayed graft function who have received a kidney transplant from a cadaveric donor, induction therapy consisting of a 5-day course of antithymocyte globulin, as compared with basiliximab, reduces the incidence and severity of acute rejection but not the incidence of delayed graft function.

A regimen of total lymphoid irradiation plus antithymocyte globulin decreases the incidence of acute GVHD and allows graft antitumor activity in patients with lymphoid malignant diseases or acute leukemia treated with hematopoietic cell transplantation.

Nulojix

One of the newest drugs is Nulojix (belatacept). This drug was approved by the FDA in 2011 to prevent acute rejection in adult patients who have had a kidney transplant. This drug is approved for use with other immunosuppressants, e.g., basiliximab, mycophenolate mofetil, and corticosteroids. This type of drug is called a selective T cell costimulation blocker.

Monoclonal Antibodies

Monoclonal antibody (muromonab-CD3, OKT2 [Orthoclone, OKT3]) is used because the CD3 surface membrane marker is found on all mature post-thymic T cells. Interaction between OKT3 and the surface of mature T lymphocytes causes T cell depletion. The use of OKT3 reverses almost all acute renal transplant rejection and is indicated for the treatment of steroid-resistant rejection. A side effect of this drug is cytokine-release syndrome, a condition of flulike symptoms, dyspnea, aseptic meningitis, and pulmonary edema.

Dacliximab (Zenapax) is a recently approved humanized monoclonal antibody to the alpha subunit of the IL-2 receptor. A decreased incidence of renal allograft rejection has been observed with triple- and/or double-immunosuppressive regimens.

Immunosuppressive Protocols

Protocols for immunosuppression of transplant recipients vary widely, depending on the transplantation center, type of organ transplanted, after transplantation, underlying cause of organ failure, and preexisting conditions (Box 31-5). Protocols are becoming more complex because of more immunosuppressive drug choices. In general, protocols include the following:
- Lymphokine synthesis inhibitors (e.g., cyclosporine, tacrolimus).
- Nucleoside synthetase inhibitors (e.g., azathioprine, mycophenolate mofetil).
- Steroids (e.g., prednisone).
- Induction or pretransplantation therapy—may include antithymocyte globulin, CD3 or CD25, or dacliximab

New Approaches in Immunosuppression

Survival after solid organ transplantation has increased in the era of tacrolimus and mycophenolate. These drugs have enhanced specificity and potency for T and B lymphocytes compared with their predecessors, cyclosporine and azathioprine. Between

2008 and 2010, the United States Food and Drug Administration approved several generic formulations of both tacrolimus and mycophenolate mofetil. Deciding whether generic products can be safely substituted for the innovator product is a clinical dilemma similar to that which occurred when generic formulations of cyclosporine became available.

Suggested new strategies include the following:
- Cellular transplants
- Transgenic organs
- Development of chimerism
- Localized immunosuppression
- Prevention of chronic rejection

Post–Organ Transplantation Complications

Because complications are associated with transplantation, their early diagnosis and treatment are essential. The primary risks of transplantation are rejection and infection. Five other major complications of organ transplantation are cancer, osteoporosis, diabetes, hypertension, and hypercholesterolemia.

Infectious Diseases

Infections can be viral, such as CMV (80%), Epstein-Barr virus (20% to 30%), hepatitis B, or hepatitis C. Even rabies has been associated with organ transplantation. Other pathogens include *Pneumocystis jiroveci* (formerly known as *P. carinii*). Organisms associated with central nervous system infection in renal transplant recipients, in decreasing order of frequency, are *Listeria, Cryptococcus, Mycobacterium, Nocardia, Aspergillus, Mucor, Toxoplasma,* and *Strongyloides* spp. Published guidelines advise transplant teams to do the following to minimize transplant risk:

1. Screen for infectious disease agents in the donor and recipient before transplantation.
2. Culture and identify known and novel pathogens in recipients after transplantation.
3. Archive serologic samples before transplantation for identification of new infections later.

Cancer

Organ transplant recipients have a 20% greater risk of the development of cancer. The incidence of non-Hodgkin's lymphoma is increased by 40%. The greatest risk for lymphoma is within the first 6 to 12 months after transplantation. Transplant recipients also have a greater risk of skin cancer and a slightly increased risk of cervical cancer. An increased risk of the development of cancer may be the result of chemotherapy and radiation therapy.

Osteoporosis

In the general population, osteoporosis affects one in four women and one in eight men. The general risk factors are age, postmenopausal state, sedentary lifestyle, and inadequate calcium intake. Transplant recipients are at an increased risk of developing osteoporosis because of pretransplantation immobility and long-term effects of steroid therapy. Regular bone density scanning should be a routine component of posttransplantation care.

Diabetes

Diabetes mellitus is a concern in two risk groups, patients with preexisting diabetes (25%) and those who develop diabetes after transplantation (20%). Patients with preexisting diabetes may require increased doses of insulin until stabilized on medications. Posttransplantation steroid-induced hyperglycemia can produce physiologic conditions that negatively affect a graft. Steroid medication might aggravate a familial tendency toward diabetes. The use of steroids results in decreased use of insulin by peripheral tissues, eventual insulin resistance with decreasing receptor sites, reduction in insulin production, and accelerated glycogenolysis by the liver to assist in glucose availability. These metabolic activities perpetuate hyperglycemia. In addition to threatening graft survival, diabetes can have other negative health consequences, such as adult blindness, vasculopathy, neuropathy, retinopathy, bladder infections, and a shortened lifespan.

Hypertension

An abnormal increase in blood pressure is usually a preexisting medical condition in transplant recipients. This condition is often associated with renal failure. Hypertension can negatively affect the patient's general health and graft survival.

Hypercholesterolemia

An increased blood cholesterol is a serious posttransplantation concern because of long-term vascular effects to the patient and engrafted organ. Hypercholesterolemia can result from the return of the patient's appetite and the lifting of dietary restrictions.

Xenotransplantation

Xenotransplantation is any procedure that involves the transplantation, implantation or infusion into a human recipient of either (a) live cells, tissues, or organs from a nonhuman animal source, or (b) human body fluids, cells, tissues or organs that have had *ex vivo* contact with live nonhuman animal cells, tissues or organs. The development of xenotransplantation is, in part, driven by the fact that the demand for human organs for clinical transplantation far exceeds the

Box 31-5	Sample Protocol (Liver)
Intraoperative	Methylprednisolone
Day 0	Methylprednisolone,
Day 1	Prednisolone
Day 2	Taper
Days 0-5	Antilymphocyte globulin (ATG), IV; given until adequate cyclosporin A levels obtained
Days 0-5	Azathioprine IV
Day 6	Azathioprine, PO
Day ?	Cyclosporin A

From Tsunoda S: Update on immunosuppression, Boston, 2000, Tufts University School of Medicine Transplant Teleconference Series.

supply (Box 31-6). There is a global shortage of organs for transplantation. Pig heart valves are already used to repair human hearts, and porcine pancreatic islet cells are used to treat diabetes, so it is not a big leap to envision trans-species, whole-organ transplantation. Pigs are considered the most likely organ transplant donors for human beings because their organs are similar in size to human organs, they are easy to breed, and the extensive biologic differences between pigs and human beings make it unlikely for porcine diseases to infect human beings.

Another application of cross-species organ use was successfully demonstrated in a phase I clinical trial that used transgenic pig livers as an ex vivo (outside the body) support system for patients with acute liver failure. The pig liver was used to bridge the gap between organ failure and obtaining an appropriate human liver for transplantation in these patients. Protocols are being developed for a phase I in vivo (inside the body) clinical trial.

Other procedures, some in clinical trials, use cells or tissues from other species to treat life-threatening illnesses such as cancer, AIDS, diabetes, liver failure, and Parkinson's disease. Even if whole organs are not transplanted, animal cells or tissues will likely be used to treat many diseases. In 1995, physicians in California transplanted bone marrow from a baboon into an AIDS patient in a highly controversial procedure that prompted the creation of strict guidelines for transplantation by the FDA, National Institutes of Health (NIH), and Centers for Disease Control and Prevention (CDC).

Ethical and medical concerns surround xenotransplantation. Ethical concerns relate to selling organs. Donors may be paid as little as $1000 for a donated kidney in countries such as Brazil, India, or Moldova. A serious medical concern is the risk that transplanted tissue may carry unknown latent infections that once introduced into the recipient, could be activated and give rise to infection.

BIOMARKERS FOR REJECTION

Emerging technologies, such as gene expression profiling, **proteomics**, metabolomics, and genomics, are rapidly advancing the pace of discovery of new biomarkers for rejection. These approaches are expected to generate improved diagnostic tests and knowledge that will lead to more effective therapies.

One of the most promising areas of transplant research, especially kidney transplantation, has been the discovery of biomarkers for rejection that are detectable in blood and urine. Biopsy-confirmed rejection, the current gold standard for diagnosis of allograft rejection, is invasive and subject to sampling errors. Development of noninvasive assays that detect molecular biomarkers for rejection could revolutionize the management of transplant recipients by the following:

- Detecting a prerejection profile that will allow therapeutic interventions before rejection causes graft dysfunction
- Improving the sensitivity and specificity of rejection diagnosis
- Developing new classification systems for rejection that will improve prognosis
- Providing information for designing individualized immunosuppressive regimens that could prevent rejection while minimizing drug toxicity
- Performing a Longitudinal Assessment of Posttransplant Immune Status (see Procedural Protocol)

FOXP3 mRNA

By studying concentrations of particular messenger RNAs (mRNAs) or proteins associated with immune activation or tissue stress, several gene products with altered expression in blood, urine, and biopsy tissue during rejection episodes have been identified. Urine concentrations of *FOXP3* mRNA, a member of the forkhead family of cell differentiation genes and a lineage-specific transcript for graft-protecting regulatory T cells, can predict reversal of acute renal allograft rejection with high sensitivity and specificity.

Measurement of the products of individual genes such as *FOXP3* probably will not supplant conventional biopsies for the diagnosis of rejection, but the development of panels of informative gene products in blood and urine, coupled with renal function and immune response markers, ultimately should achieve the sensitivities and specificities required for diagnosis and clinical management of kidney rejection.

Analyses of more than 1300 genes that were differentially expressed in kidney allografts have revealed three distinct molecular signatures of acute rejection that were more predictive of allograft survival than traditional histologic analysis. These data have also generated new hypotheses for the molecular mechanisms of rejection. For example, B cell infiltration is characteristic of aggressive acute rejection.

A new gene expression test, AlloMap (XDx, San Francisco), is being tested to explore its ability to predict acute cardiac allograft rejection. The test appears to detect the absence of moderate to severe cellular rejection, which might reduce the need for frequent biopsies.

Box 31-6	Milestones in Xenotransplantation
1963-1964	Chimpanzee to human renal transplants
1964	Pig heart valve transplant
1968	Sheep heart transplant
1984	"Baby Fae" transplanted with a baboon heart
1992	Baboon to human liver transplant
1994	Pig pancreatic islets transplanted to insulin-dependent patients
1995	Neuronal cells from fetal pig transplanted to patients with Parkinson's disease
1996	Baboon bone marrow transplanted to AIDS patient

Adapted from Wilde M: Rejection, retroviruses: major barriers to xenotransplantation, Adv Med Lab Prof 9:14–19, 1997.

CASE STUDY

Forty-year-old CG was seen by her family physician after several episodes of painless hematuria. On direct questioning, she complained of worsening malaise and swelling of her legs and hands over the previous 2 weeks. She also reported that despite a high fluid intake, she was urinating much less frequently than normal. She had no significant medical history.

On examination, the patient was pale and had generalized swelling of her extremities. Her temperature was 38.5° C (101° F) and her blood pressure was 160/110 mm Hg. She had no palpable masses or hepatosplenomegaly.

A diagnosis of idiopathic and rapidly progressive glomerulonephritis was made. She was given antihypertensive agents, corticosteroids, and azathioprine for 2 weeks, but her renal function deteriorated and end-stage renal failure was diagnosed. Hemodialysis was initiated.

In preparation for a possible renal transplant, she was tissue-typed for MHC antigens using anti-HLA antibodies. She was found to be HLA-A10, A28, B7, Bw52, Cw2, Cw6, DR2, DRw10, and blood group B positive. A suitable cadaveric kidney was found from a donor of HLA-A9, A28, B7, B17, Cw2, Cw6, DR2, DR4, and blood group B positive. A crossmatch of the patient's serum with donor lymphocytes was satisfactory.

She underwent successful kidney transplantation. Her posttransplantation treatment was a combined triple-immunosuppressive regimen of prednisolone, cyclosporin A, and azathioprine. She progressed well immediately after transplantation.

Twelve days after engraftment, the patient developed a fever and was noted to be lethargic. Physical examination revealed generalized edema. Her blood pressure was 165/110 mm Hg. Her urine output had dropped significantly. A renal biopsy was performed. Histologic examination demonstrated significant interstitial mononuclear cell infiltration. This finding was consistent with the diagnosis of acute graft rejection. She was immediately treated with parenteral methylprednisolone. This treatment failed to improve her renal function and an antilymphocyte monoclonal antibody was administered. Her renal function improved and she was eventually discharged receiving cyclosporin A therapy.

Questions
1. Class II major histocompatibility complex (MHC) are encoded for in the ____ region.
   a. A
   b. B
   c. C
   d. D
2. In a kidney transplant, antibody to ABO antigens of donor tissue will produce _____ rejection.
   a. Hyperacute
   b. Acute
   c. Delayed
   d. Chronic

See Appendix A for the answers to multiple choice questions.

Critical Thinking Group Discussion Questions
1. What factors are important in matching donor to recipient in renal transplantation?
2. How does this patient's graft rejection compare with other types of graft rejection?

See instructor site ⊖volve for the discussion of the answers to these questions.

Longitudinal Assessment of Posttransplant Immune Status

Principle
• A noninvasive means of providing a biomarker of patient cellular immune status over time is the ImmuKnow assay (Figure 31-5).

Clinical Application
• This assay assists in identification of transplant patients who are at risk of developing an infection due to over-immunosuppression. Periodic monitoring (Table 31-10) guides clinicians in making therapeutic decisions that avoid overimmunosuppression and underimmunosuppression.

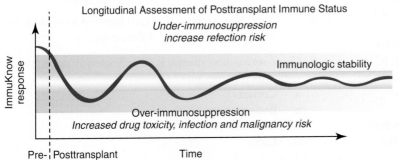

Figure 31-5 Longitudinal assessment of posttransplant immune status. *(With permission from Cylex, Inc., Columbia, Maryland, www.cylex.net.)*

Table 31-10	**Patient Immune System Monitoring***
Time	**Interval**
Pretransplant	Test as needed
Months 1-6	Test every 2 weeks
Months 7-12	Test monthly
After year 1	Perform routine monitoring (at minimum, test quarterly)

From Cylex, Inc (with permission) www.cylex.net. Accessed August 22, 2012.

*Additional assays may be required in the event of changes in clinical status or posttransplant complications. This information is based on therapeutic drug monitoring recommendations described in immunosuppressant agent prescribing information.

CHAPTER HIGHLIGHTS

- All vertebrates capable of acute rejection of foreign skin grafts possess a localized complex involving many genes that exert major control over the organism's immune reactions.
- Some of these antigens are much more potent than others in provoking an immune response and therefore are called the major histocompatibility complex (MHC). In human beings, the MHC is referred to as human leukocyte antigens (HLAs).
- The MHC is divided into four major regions—D, B, C, and A. The A, B, and C regions code for class I molecules, whereas the D region codes for class II molecules.
- Class I and class II antigens can be found on surface membrane proteins of body cells and in body fluids.
- The MHC gene products have an important role in clinical immunology. For example, transplants are rejected if performed against MHC barriers; thus, immunosuppressive therapy is required. These antigens are of primary importance in influencing the genetic basis of survival or rejection of transplanted organs.
- Although HLA was originally identified by its role in transplant rejection, it is now recognized that the products of HLA genes play a crucial role in our immune system. T cells do not recognize antigens directly but do so when the antigen is presented on the surface of an antigen-presenting cell (APC), the macrophage. In addition to presenting the antigen, the macrophage must present another molecule for this response to occur. This molecule is a cell surface glycoprotein coded in each species by the MHC.
- T cells are able to interact with the histocompatibility molecules only if they are genetically identical (MHC restriction). Both class I and class II antigens function as targets of T lymphocytes that regulate the immune response.
- Class I molecules regulate interaction between cytolytic T cells and target cells; class II molecules restrict the activity of regulatory T cells (helper, suppressor, and amplifier subsets).
- Class II molecules regulate the interaction between helper T cells and APCs.
- HLA matching is of value in organ transplantation and in the transplantation of bone marrow.
- Transplantation is one of the areas (in addition to hypersensitivity and autoimmunity) in which the immune system functions in a detrimental way. Tissues and organs transplanted include peripheral stem cells or bone marrow, bone matrix, skin, kidneys, liver, cardiac valves, heart, pancreas, corneas, and lungs.
- Host immunity to the donor can cause graft-versus-host disease (GVHD), believed to result from the patient being sensitized to unshared HLA antigens before transplantation or transfusion. When allogenic T lymphocytes are transfused from donor to recipient with a graft or blood transfusion, the patient can develop acute or chronic GVHD. Patients at risk for GVHD include those who are immunodeficient or immunosuppressed with severe lymphocytopenia and bone marrow suppression.
- Immunologic tolerance is the acquisition of nonreactivity toward particular antigens. Self-recognition (tolerance) is a critical process; the failure to recognize self antigens can result in autoimmune disease.
- Immunosuppressive measures may be antigen-specific or antigen-nonspecific. Antigen-nonspecific immunosuppression includes drugs and other methods of specifically altering T cell function. Immunosuppressive measures directed at T cells include the use of ATG at the time of transplantation and of lymphoid irradiation before transplantation.

REVIEW QUESTIONS

1-4. Match the following items.

1. _____ Autograft

2. _____ Syngraft

3. _____ Allograft (hemograft)

4. _____ Xenograft

a. Graft transplanted between different but identical recipient and donor

b. Graft transferred from one position to another in the same individual

c. Graft between genetically different recipient and donor of the same species

d. Graft between individuals of different species

5. Graft-versus-host disease is most frequently associated with which transplant?
    a. Cornea
    b. Bone marrow
    c. Bone matrix
    d. Lung

6-9. Match the following types of graft rejection.

6. _____ Hyperacute   a. Caused by preformed cytotoxic antibodies

7. _____ Accelerated   b. An immunopathologic mechanism

8. _____ Acute   c. Caused by previous sensitization to donor antigens

9. _____ Chronic   d. Disturbance of host-graft tolerance

10. The immune system functions in a detrimental way in:
    a. Hypersensitivity reactions
    b. Autoimmunity
    c. Transplantation
    d. All of the above

11. The probability of success in organ and tissue transplantation increases as a result of:
    a. Histocompatibility testing
    b. Immunosuppression
    c. Surgical technique
    d. Both a and b

12. The D region of the major histocompatibility complex (MHC) codes for class _____ molecules.
    a. I
    b. II
    c. III
    d. IV

13. Class I includes HLA-_____ antigens.
    a. A, B, and C
    b. B, C, and D
    c. DR, DC(DQ), and A
    d. DR, DC(DQ), and SB

14. Class I molecules:
    a. Regulate interaction between cytolytic T cells and target cells.
    b. Restrict activity of regulatory T cells and target cells.
    c. Regulate interaction between helper T cells and antigen-presenting cells.
    d. Represent components of the complement pathways.

15. The 1-year survival for kidney transplantation from HLA-identical siblings approaches:
    a. 50%.
    b. 75%.
    c. 95%.
    d. 100%.

16-19. Match the following to show the relationship between certain HLA antigens and diseases.

16. _____ Ankylosing spondylitis   a. B8

17. _____ Type I diabetes   b. B27

18. _____ Myasthenia gravis   c. DR2

19. _____ Multiple sclerosis   d. DR3

20. The most common form of bone marrow transplant is:
    a. Allogeneic
    b. Autologous
    c. Xenograft
    d. Syngraft

21. Potential GVHD has all the following characteristics except:
    a. Source of immunocompetent T lymphocytes
    b. Source of immunocompetent B lymphocytes
    c. HLA differences between patient and recipient
    d. Inability to reject donor cells

22. In GVHD posttransfusion, symptoms begin within _____ day(s) after transfusion.
    a. 1
    b. 2 to 4
    c. 3 to 5
    d. 3 to 30

23. GVHD can be prevented by:
    a. Irradiating the patient pretransfusion
    b. Irradiating the blood component pretransfusion
    c. Administering antibiotics pretransfusion
    d. Administering steroids posttransfusion

24. The mainstay of immunosuppression therapy in transplantation is:
    a. Azathioprine
    b. Corticosteroids
    c. Cyclosporine
    d. Antilymphocyte globulin

BIBLIOGRAPHY

Baxter-Lowe LA, Busch MP: DNA microchimerism and organ transplant rejection, Clin Chem 52:559–560, 2006.

Brennan DC, et al: Rabbit antithymocyte globulin versus basiliximab in renal transplantation, N Engl J Med 355:1967–1977, 2006.

Clinical Clips: Cell transplants help brain repair after stroke, Adv Med Lab Prof 13:35, 2001.

Dantal J, Soulillou JP: Immunosuppressive drugs and the risk of cancer after organ transplantation, N Engl J Med 353:1371–1372, 2005.

Delmonico FL, Burdick JF: Maximizing the success of transplantation with kidneys from older donors, N Engl J Med 354:411–412, 2006.

Fishbein TM: Intestinal transplantation, N Engl J Med 361:998–1008, 2009.

Gadi VK, et al: Soluble donor DNA concentrations in recipient serum correlate with pancreas-kidney rejection, Clin Chem 52:379–382, 2006.

Gruessner AC, Sutherland DE: Pancreas transplant outcomes for United States cases as reported to the United Network for Organ Sharing and the International Pancreas Transplant Registry, Clin Transpl 45–56, 2008.

Halloran PF: Immunosuppressive drugs for kidney transplantation, N Engl J Med 351:2715–2726, 2004.

Ingelfinger JR: Risks and benefits to the living donor, N Engl J Med 353:447–449, 2005.

Lowsky R, et al: Protective conditioning for acute graft-versus-host disease, N Engl J Med 353:1321, 2005.

Peters TG: Transplant drugs: medicines that prevent rejection, 2003, (http://www.aakp.org/aakp-library/Transplant-Drugs).

Pham MX, et al: Gene-expression profiling for rejection surveillance after cardiac transplantation, N Engl J Med 362:1890–1900, 2010.

Plath KB, Talmon GA, Stickle DF: Immunosuppressant drugs, Clin Lab News 32:10–12, 2006.

Remuzzi G, et al: Long-term outcome of renal transplantation from older donors, N Engl J Med 354:343–352, 2006.

Sayegh MH, Carpenter CB: Transplantation 50 years later: progress, challenges, and promises, N Engl J Med 351:2761–2766, 2004.

Shelton C: Post–organ transplantation complications, Transplantation Issues for Nurses Toronto, 1999, (workshop handout).

Titus K: Steering the straits of transplant testing, CAP Today 20:68–72, 2006.

Todo Satoru MD, et al: Current status of intestinal transplantation, Adv Surg 27:295–303, 1994.

Todo Satoru MD, et al: Intestinal transplantation in composite visceral grafts or alone, Ann Surg 216:223–234, 1992.

Tsunoda SM: Update on immunosuppression, Boston, 2000, Tufts University School of Medicine Transplant Teleconference Series.

Turgeon ML: Fundamentals of immunohematology, ed 2, Baltimore, 1995, Williams & Wilkins.

United Network for Organ Sharing: Critical data: U.S. facts about transplantation, 2007, (www.unos.org).

Upton H: Origin of drugs in current use: the cyclosporin story, 2001, (http://www.davidmoore.org.uk/Sec04_01.htm).

Venkataramanan R, et al: Clinical utility of monitoring tacrolimus concentrations in liver transplant patient, J Clin Pharmacol 41:542–551, 2001.

Wilde M: Rejection, retroviruses: major barriers to xenotransplantation, Adv Med Lab Prof 9:14–19, 1997.

Learning Objectives

At the conclusion of this chapter, the reader should be able to:
- Identify and discuss various types of cancer treated with progenitor cell transplants.
- Define the term *progenitor cell*.
- Name three types of stem cell transplants.
- Discuss available treatment options for cancer.
- Discuss the evaluation of candidates for transplantation.
- Describe the process of obtaining blood stem cells.
- Discuss the transplantation protocol, related complications, graft manipulation and storage, and cell infusion.

- Compare at least three current directions in bone marrow transplantation.
- Identify and discuss directions in bone marrow transplantation.
- Analyze laboratory and clinical data of the cited case study and apply these concepts to the field of bone marrow transplantation.
- Correctly answer case study related multiple choice questions.
- Be prepared to participate in a discussion of critical thinking questions.
- Correctly answer end of chapter review questions.

Key Terms

alkylating agents	**cytotoxicity**	**immunotherapy**
antimetabolites	**engraftment**	**peripheral blood stem cells (PBSCs)**
CD34+ cells	**graft-versus-host disease (GVHD)**	**vinca alkaloids**
cryopreservation	**hematopoietic stem cells**	

Stem cell transplantation is currently being used to treat patients with malignant and nonmalignant diseases (e.g., chronic myelogenous leukemia, severe combined immunodeficiency disease, non-Hodgkin's lymphoma). The goal of transplanting bone marrow or peripheral blood progenitor cells is to achieve a potential cure or help patients recover from high-dose chemotherapy that has destroyed stem or marrow cells, a condition known as myeloablation.

CANCERS TREATED WITH PROGENITOR CELL TRANSPLANTS

Leukemia

In most types of leukemia, the body produces large numbers of immature white blood cells (WBCs) that do not function properly. Under appropriate conditions, bone marrow transplantation may be useful in treating certain types of leukemia (Box 32-1).

Acute lymphoblastic leukemia is the most common type of leukemia in young children but may also affect adults, especially those age 65 years and older. It is a rapidly progressive malignant disorder involving the production of immature WBCs (blasts), which often results in the replacement of normal bone marrow with blast cells. Acute myeloid leukemia, also referred to as non-lymphoblastic leukemia, occurs in adults and children.

Although chronic lymphocytic leukemia most often affects adults older than 55 years, it sometimes occurs in younger adults, but rarely affects children. Chronic myeloid leukemia occurs mainly in adults and affects a very small number of children.

Box 32-1	Diseases Treatable by Stem Cell Transplantation

Acute Leukemias
Acute lymphoblastic leukemia
Acute myelogenous leukemia

Chronic Leukemias
Chronic myelogenous leukemia
Chronic lymphocytic leukemia

Myelodysplastic Syndromes
Refractory anemias
Chronic myelomonocytic leukemia

Stem Cell Disorders
Aplastic anemia
Fanconi's anemia
Paroxysmal nocturnal hemoglobinuria

Myeloproliferative Disorders
Primary myelofibrosis
Polycythemia vera

Lymphoproliferative Disorders
Non-Hodgkin's lymphoma
Hodgkin's disease

Phagocyte Disorders
Chédiak-Higashi syndrome
Chronic granulomatous disease
Immunodeficiencies
Severe combined immunodeficiency

Inherited Platelet Abnormalities
Congenital thrombocytopenia
Plasma cell disorders
Multiple myeloma
Plasma cell leukemia
Waldenström's macroglobulinemia

Other Malignancies
Breast cancer
Ewing's sarcoma
Neuroblastoma
Renal cell carcinoma

Inherited Erythrocyte Abnormalities
Beta-thalassemia major
Pure red cell aplasia
Sickle cell disease

Liposomal Storage Diseases
Mucopolysaccharidoses
Hurler's syndrome
Gaucher's disease
Niemann-Pick disease

Table 32-1	Estimated 5-Year Survival Rates after Transplantation*	
Disease	**Allogeneic (%)**	**Autologous (%)**
Severe combined immunodeficiency	90	N/A
Aplastic anemia	90	N/A
Thalassemia	90	N/A
Acute myeloid leukemia		
First remission	55-60	50
Second remission	40	30
Acute lymphocytic leukemia		
First remission	50	40
Second remission	40	30
Chronic myeloid leukemia		
Chronic phase	70	ID
Blast crisis	15	ID
Chronic lymphocytic leukemia	50	ID
Myelodysplasia	45	ID
Multiple myeloma	30	35
Non-Hodgkin's lymphoma, first relapse, second remission	40	40
Hodgkin's disease, first relapse, second remission	40	50

ID, Insufficient data; *N/A,* not applicable.

*These estimates are based on data reported by the International Bone Marrow Transplant Registry.

For patients with lymphoma, chances of survival depend on the grade and stage of cancer, overall patient health, and response to treatment. Hodgkin's lymphoma is one of the most curable forms of cancer. Patients diagnosed with stage I disease have more than a 90% chance of living 10 years or longer. Of interest, higher grade aggressive types are more likely to be cured with chemotherapy. Lower-grade lymphoma often can have longer average survival times, with a mean survival of 10 years in some cases. Most children respond well to treatment, even though children tend to have the higher grades of lymphoma. From 70% to 90% of these children survive 5 years or longer (Table 32-1).

WHAT ARE PROGENITOR BLOOD CELLS?

Progenitor cells have the ability to evolve into different types of cells. Bone marrow and peripheral blood progenitor cells are capable of reconstituting a person's immune system because they contain the precursor to the cells that make up the blood: lymphocytes, granulocytes, macrophages, and platelets. Progenitor cells that circulate in the bloodstream are called **peripheral blood stem cells (PBSCs)**. PBSCs are found in much

Non-Hodgkin's and Hodgkin's Lymphoma

In Hodgkin's disease and non-Hodgkin's lymphoma, cells in the lymphatic system become abnormal. They divide too rapidly and grow without any order or control, and old cells do not die as cells normally do. Because lymphatic tissue is present in many parts of the body, Hodgkin's disease and non-Hodgkin's lymphoma can start almost anywhere. These diseases may occur in a single lymph node, in a group of lymph nodes, or sometimes in other parts of the lymphatic system (e.g., bone marrow, spleen).

smaller quantities in the circulating blood than in the bone marrow. **Hematopoietic stem cells** are found in very small numbers in the peripheral blood and greater numbers in the marrow.

The hematopoietic stem cell population is not fully characterized, but the cell marker, CD34+ antigen, identifies a population of stem cells that can repopulate the bone marrow after chemotherapy. The required minimal dose of **CD34+ cells** is difficult to define, but most transplantation centers will infuse a minimal dose of 2×10^6 CD34+ cells/kg patient weight in the autologous and allogeneic PBSC setting.

Historically, the dose of bone marrow has been based on the nucleated cell (NC) count (i.e., 2 to 4×10^8 NC/kg recipient weight). There is no established amount of CD34+ bone marrow stem cells to infuse because there may be more primitive cells, and therefore likely to be CD34– cells, in the marrow that are capable of reconstituting the recipient's marrow.

TYPES OF TRANSPLANTS

There are three major types of transplants:
- Allogeneic
- Syngeneic
- Autologous

In an allogeneic setting, a person receives bone marrow or PBSCs from a related or an unrelated donor, depending on the availability of a good human leukocyte antigen (HLA) match. Because HLA tissue types are inherited, patients are more likely to find a matched donor from within their own family, racial, or ethnic group. In syngeneic transplantation, patients receive stem cells from their identical twin. Patients who undergo an autologous transplantation have donated their own cells after PBSC mobilization with granulocyte colony-stimulating factor (G-CSF) or granulocyte-macrophage colony-stimulating factor (GM-CSF).

TRADITIONAL TREATMENT OPTIONS

To understand why bone marrow and PBSCs are used and how they work, it is helpful to understand how chemotherapy and radiation therapies affect these cells. Chemotherapy and radiation target rapidly dividing cells. These therapies are used to treat cancers because cancer cells divide more rapidly than healthy cells. Bone marrow cells also divide at a rapid rate and can be severely damaged or destroyed by high-dose treatment. Without healthy bone marrow, the patient cannot make the blood cells that are able to fight off infections, carry oxygen, and prevent bleeding.

Treatment for cancer includes chemotherapy, radiation therapy, surgery, hormone therapy, and/or **immunotherapy.** These therapies may be administered alone or in combination to eliminate malignant cells most effectively.

Chemotherapy

Chemotherapy may involve one drug or a combination of two or more drugs, depending on the type of cancer and its rate of progression.

Box 32-2	Cancer Chemotherapy Agents
Direct DNA-Interacting Agents	**Indirect DNA-Interacting Agents**
Alkylators	**Antimetabolites**
Cyclophosphamide	Deoxycoformycin
Chlorambucil	6-Mercaptopurine
Melphalan	2-Chlorodeoxyadenosine
BCNU (carmustine)	Hydroxyurea
CCNU (lomustine)	Methotrexate
Ifosfamide	5-Fluorouracil (5-FU)
Procarbazine	Cytosine arabinoside (ARA-C)
Cisplatin	Gemcitabine
Carboplatin	Fludarabine phosphate
	Asparaginase
Antitumor Antibiotics	**Antimitotic Agents**
Bleomycin	Vincristine
Actinomycin D	Vinblastine
Mithramycin	Paclitaxel
Mitomycin C	Estramustine phosphate
Etoposide (VP-16)	
Topotecan	
Doxorubicin and daunorubicin	
Idarubicin	
Mitoxantrone	

Chemotherapeutic drugs can be divided into the following:
1. Agents that are active against both dividing and nondividing cells
2. Drugs that are active against dividing cells and affect a particular phase of cell division
3. Agents that affect all or most of the phases of the cell cycle (Box 32-2)

Whatever the mode of action of these drugs, they destroy malignant cells in the same proportion of cells that is killed for each dose of chemotherapeutic agent.

Alkylating Agents, Antimetabolites, and Alkaloids

The first chemotherapeutic agents to be used in bone marrow transplantation were **alkylating agents** such as cyclophosphamide and busulfan. Their common mechanism of action is that on entering the cells, the alkyl groups bind to the electrophilic sites in DNA and other biologically active molecules. This bifunctional alkylation of DNA results in efficient cross-linking of the DNA, leading to strand breakage and ultimately cell death.

Antimetabolites such as 5-fluorouracil (5-FU), cytarabine, and fludarabine induce **cytotoxicity** by serving as false substrates in biochemical pathways. Many are nucleoside analogues that are incorporated into DNA and RNA and therefore inhibit nucleic acid synthesis. They are cell cycle active and are specific mainly for cells in the S phase.

The **vinca alkaloids,** vincristine and vinblastine, which were isolated from the periwinkle plant, inhibit microtubule assembly by binding to tubulin. This microtubule stabilization prevents the cells from dividing; thus these alkaloids are cytotoxic predominantly during the M phase of the cell cycle. Bleomycin, an antitumor antibiotic, induces single-strand and double-strand breaks through free radical generation and is cytotoxic mainly during the G2 and M phases of the cell cycle.

Radiotherapy

Radiotherapy uses large doses of high-energy beams or particles to destroy cancer cells in a specifically targeted area. Radiation damages DNA and keeps the cells from dividing.

Radiotherapy is most often used on localized solid tumors and on cancers such as leukemia and lymphoma that affect the bloodstream. More than 50% of patients with cancer undergo radiation therapy; for some, it will be the only cancer treatment that they need. Radiation is often used in combination with other treatments to shrink the tumor or make surgery or chemotherapy more effective. Used after chemotherapy or surgery, radiation destroys any cancer cells that might remain. Normal cells that may be affected by radiotherapy will usually repair themselves.

EVALUATION OF CANDIDATES FOR PERIPHERAL BLOOD STEM CELL AND BONE MARROW TRANSPLANTATION

Factors that influence the eligibility for bone marrow transplantation include age, disease status, performance status for the recipient, organ function (i.e., heart, lung, liver, and kidney function), infectious disease status, compatibility of the donor and recipient, and psychosocial status. Patients who undergo high-dose chemotherapy and hematopoietic stem cell transplantation require a careful evaluation of all body systems to ensure that they are able to tolerate the aggressive therapy and the isolation of their hospital stay, which can last days to months.

Pretransplantation evaluation and testing (Fig. 32-1) may include HLA tissue typing, bone marrow biopsy and aspiration, electrocardiography, echocardiography, complete history and physical examination, chest x-ray study, pulmonary function tests, dental cleaning, blood tests such as complete blood count (CBC) and blood chemistries, and screening for viruses such as hepatitis, human T lymphotropic virus I and II, cytomegalovirus (CMV), herpes, and human immunodeficiency virus (HIV).

At some point before transplantation, a central venous catheter is usually placed in a large vein to help in drawing blood samples, infusing medications during and after the transplantation, and actually infusing bone marrow or PBSCs.

ABO Blood Group and Human Leukocyte Antigen Matching

The donor and recipient may be incompatible. HLA matching is the primary consideration in assessing whether a donor is acceptable for a given patient and overshadows any other non-HLA factors, including ABO incompatibility.

HLA matching is important because a close HLA match does the following:
• Improves the chances for a successful transplantation

• Promotes **engraftment,** the process of donated cells beginning to grow and produce new blood cells in the host
• Reduces the risk of post-transplantation **graft-versus-host disease (GVHD)**

There are a number of HLA markers. Some markers, such as HLA-A, HLA-B, HLA-C, and HLA-DRB1 are most important to the success of transplantation. The HLA-DQ is used for evaluation by some transplant centers but not by others. The impact of DQ is minimal.

Minimum matching levels must be met before a donor or unit of cord blood cells can be transplanted. The National Marrow Donor Program (NMDP) program requires that at least a 6 out of 8 match exist. However, some transplant centers set more stringent requirements for a 7 out of 8 match between patient and donor (Fig. 32-2).

For adult donors, a match of at least six of these eight HLA markers is required. For cord blood units, which require less strict matching criteria, a match of at least four of six markers is required at HLA-A, HLA-B, and HLA-DRB1.

OBTAINING CELLS FOR TRANSPLANTATION

Bone Marrow

In the procedure for harvesting bone marrow, the donor is given general or regional anesthesia and marrow is usually aspirated with large needles from the posterior iliac crest; the anterior crest can also be used in certain cases (Fig. 32-3). The goal of the procedure is to collect 10 to 15 mL of marrow/kg of recipient weight. Approximately 600 to 900 mL of marrow is collected. The aspirated marrow is collected in bags containing a buffered isotonic solution and heparin to prevent coagulation.

After the marrow has been collected, it is filtered to remove any bone chips, fat, and clots that may have been collected or formed during the procedure. The bone marrow is frequently processed to remove undesired volume and cells. If the marrow is matched and no further manipulation is needed, it is transfused within 12 to 24 hours after collection, depending on the location of the recipient. If it is not transfused within 24 hours, it is cryopreserved.

Peripheral Blood Progenitor Cells

Peripheral blood progenitor cells have been increasingly used in place of bone marrow as a source of stem cells for allogeneic transplants. Reasons for this trend are the large amount of hematopoietic stem cells that can be collected, more rapid hematologic recovery, elimination of the surgical procedure and anesthesia risk for the donor, and reduced transplantation costs. However, a patient who receives allogeneic peripheral blood progenitor cells may be at a greater risk for chronic graft-versus-host disease (GVHD; see following discussion and Chapter 31), possibly because of the high amount of lymphocytes in the product. Up to a log increase in lymphocytes is collected in a PBSC collection compared with a bone marrow collection. Conversely, this increase in lymphocytes could aid in the patient's immune reconstitution and also impart a graft-versus-leukemia effect.

**Pre-Transplant Checklist for
Allogeneic Donor**

Name:_____   Medical Record #:_____

Date of Collection:_____   Pre-Test:_____ Where:_____

Contact:_____   Phone:_____ Fax:_____

Protocol:_____

HLA Typing Performed by _____   Date of Repeat HLA at Hospital:_____

Name of Recipient:_____   Medical Record #:_____

Type of Collection (circle):   Marrow/PBSC   Syngeneic/Related/Unrelated

Test	Required (÷)	Date Ordered	Date Report Received	Eligibility Criteria	Meets Eligibility (÷)
History and Physical	÷				
Transfusion History	÷				
Vaccination History	÷				
Chest X-Ray	÷				
EKG	÷				
Laboratory Tests					
ABO group / Rh type	÷				
HLA typing	÷				
Confirmatory HLA	÷				
Toxoplasma antibody	÷				
CMV	÷				
HSV I and II	÷				
Infectious Disease Markers					
HIV consent obtained	÷	Date:			
Anti-HIV 1 / 2	÷			**negative**	
HIV-1-Ag	÷			**negative**	
Anti-HTLV	÷				
HBsAg	÷				
Anti-HBc	÷				
HCV	÷				
RPR	÷				
CBC with differential	÷				
Electrolytes	÷				
BUN	÷				
Creatinine	÷				

Originated: 11/99
Revised: Form 9929

Figure 32-1 Pretransplantation checklist for allogeneic donor.

Continued

**Pre-Transplant Checklist for
Allogeneic Donor**

Test	Required (÷)	Date Performed	Date Report Received	Eligibility Criteria	Meets Eligibility (÷)
Beta HCG - **females only**				negative	
Liver Function Tests					
SGOT	÷				
SGPT	÷				
LDH	÷				
Alkaline phosphatase.					
Total bilirubin	÷				
Chimerism - peripheral blood					
Urinalysis	÷				
PT	÷				
PTT	÷				

High-risk behavior yes no	Comments:

Additional Testing:

ABO compatibility	Donor ABO/Rh _____ Recipient ABO/Rh _____ compatible _____ major incompatibility _____ minor incompatibility _____
CMV Compatible yes no	Donor _____ Recipient _____
OR Date _____	
Autologous blood stored yes no	No. of units _____

PBSC donors	
Sent to blood bank for donor evaluation	Date: _____ Cleared by blood bank yes no If no, comments _____

Request for Hematopoietic Progenitor Cell Product Collection Form #9904 completed	Date:
Informed Consent obtained and donor given opportunity to ask questions.	Date:

The above results have been reviewed, and the donor meets all eligibility criteria for donation of PBSC/Bone Marrow. Any abnormal results have been discussed with the donor.

Attending Physician

_____   _____

Signature   Date

Originated: 11/99   Form 9929
Revised:

Figure 32-1—cont'd

Peripheral blood progenitor cells are obtained for transplant by a procedure called apheresis or leukapheresis. For 4 or 5 days before apheresis, normal donors are given G-CSF, which increases the amount of stem cells released into the bloodstream. Typically, in the autologous setting, the patient is mobilized, with G-CSF given for 7 to 10 days after myelosuppressive chemotherapy. Disease status and prior treatment influence the ability to mobilize autologous PBSCs. The levels of hematopoietic stem cells rise up to 50-fold in the recovery phase after myelosuppressive chemotherapy and the administration of G-CSF.

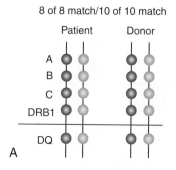

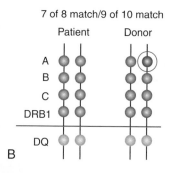

Figure 32-2 **HLA matching of patient and donor. A,** All the patient's markers match the donor's. The 8 of 8 match means that there is a match at A, B, C, and DRB1. A 10 of 10 match means that there is a match at A, B, DRB1, C and DQ. **B,** One of the patient's A markers does not match one of the donor's A markers. Therefore, this is a 7 of 8 match or a 9 of 10 match. *(©National Marrow Donor Program, 2012,* www.marrow.org/pati ent. *Reprinted with permission.)*

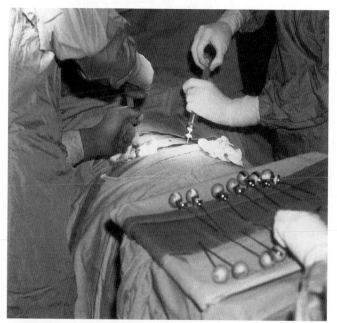

Figure 32-3 Bone marrow harvest from posterior iliac crest. *(Courtesy Bone Marrow Transplant Unit, Massachusetts General Hospital, Boston.)*

In apheresis, the blood is removed through a central venous catheter or vein in the arm. The blood goes through a continuous flow apheresis machine in which mononuclear cells (presumably including the desired stem cells) are separated by centrifugation from the red blood cell (RBC) and plasma fractions, which are returned to the donor during the procedure. The process usually takes one or two sessions of 3 to 5 hours per collection. The collected cells are then cryopreserved (frozen) in liquid nitrogen for later use or transplanted into the recipient.

Similarly, stem cells from a newborn's cord blood, considered adult cells because they are not from embryos, produce only blood cells. In general, adult stem cells are scarcer in the body and more difficult to culture than embryonic cells, yet large numbers are needed for therapy.

TRANSPLANTATION

The high-dose chemotherapy given before transplantation leads to prolonged cytopenias, which account for much of the morbidity and mortality associated with the procedure. After

the bone marrow or PBSCs are transplanted into the recipient via a central catheter, the cells migrate to the bone marrow, where they begin to produce new blood cells in a process known as engraftment. The primary measure of hematopoietic recovery, or engraftment, is when the neutrophil count reaches at least $0.5 \times 10^9/L$ for 3 consecutive days and a platelet count of $20 \times 10^9/L$ is maintained without platelet transfusion. Engraftment usually occurs within 2 to 4 weeks after the infusion of stem cells. The type of transplant, source, and dose of stem cells are factors influencing engraftment times. Complete recovery of immune function takes much longer, up to several months for autologous transplant recipients and 1 to 2 years for allogeneic transplant recipients. Studies have shown that patients receiving allogeneic PBSCs are less likely to have infections after transplantation than bone marrow recipients.

Transplantation-Related Complications

Complications after transplantation of bone marrow or PBSCs can range from infection, GVHD, rejection, and organ damage to infertility and death. Early complications usually occur within the first 100 days after transplantation. After receiving an allogeneic transplant, rejection rates can range between 1% and 2% in HLA-matched recipients and 5% to 10% in the mismatched recipients. GVHD can be attributed to many factors, including HLA mismatch between donor and recipient, conditioning regimen, viral exposure of donor and recipient, and dose of T cells infused into the patient.

Acute GVHD affects at least 40% to 60% of allogeneic hematopoietic stem cell transplant patients after conditioning with myeloablative regimens and is a major cause of early morbidity and nonrelapse mortality in these patients. Acute GVHD occurs within the first weeks after transplantation, is the result of complex interactions among the donor T cells, and involves the recognition of major histocompatibility complex (MHC) antigens on the recipient's organs (liver, gastrointestinal tract, skin, mucosal membranes).

Chronic GVHD occurs later and is defined as the presence or persistence of GVHD beyond 100 days since transplantation.

GVHD can be prevented or controlled by corticosteroids, calcineurin inhibitors (e.g., cyclosporin A, tacrolimus), and T cell depletion of the graft.

Graft Manipulation and Storage

The processing of bone marrow and PBSCs varies from laboratory to laboratory, with different techniques to accomplish the same result. A bone marrow harvest results in the collection of a large volume of marrow that contains progenitor blood cells. Therefore, it is desirable to concentrate the marrow in the autologous and allogeneic settings. The purpose is twofold, to reduce the volume and remove RBCs.

ABO incompatibility between donor and recipient is encountered in 23% to 30% of all hematopoietic cell transplantations. A major incompatibility exists between donor and recipient when the recipient possesses antibodies against the RBC antigens of the donor, which would result in lysis of the transfused donor cells (e.g., group A donor and group O recipient).

Differences between donor and recipient's ABO or Rh blood groups have no effect on marrow engraftment, rejection, or GVHD. As long as the transplant recipient has antibodies against the RBCs of the donor, erythrocytes will be destroyed inside the marrow at an early stage. This could result in a state of chronic hemolysis that can last for 4 to 6 weeks after the marrow infusion, although durations of up to 8 months have been reported.

To prevent acute hemolysis, the main objective of the laboratory is to remove as many RBCs as possible while preserving the hematopoietic progenitor cells to ensure timely engraftment. This is mainly accomplished by automated means, but manual methods are still used. Low-speed centrifugation sediments the cellular elements of the marrow so that the plasma and collection media can be removed and the WBC-rich buffy coat expressed into a separate container while the RBCs are retained in the original container. This manual method has an increased risk of contamination of the graft, depends on the technique of the technologist for good recovery of the cells, and is labor-intensive.

Automated procedures involving apheresis equipment; such as the COBE Spectra (Terumo BCT, Lakewood, Colo) and Fenwall (Americus, Lake Zurich, IL) use a closed sterile system that rapidly recovers the desired mononuclear cells (Fig. 32-4). Minor ABO mismatches are present in 15% to 20% of HLA-matched donor-recipient pairs. Patients who receive hematopoietic progenitor cells from a minor ABO-incompatible donor are at risk of developing immediate immune hemolysis caused by isohemagglutinins infused with the marrow or PBSCs, or delayed hemolysis caused by isohemagglutinins produced by the donor lymphocytes (i.e., B cells). Immediate hemolysis can be avoided by simple removal of plasma from the graft before infusion. However, delayed hemolysis caused by antibody production from donor-derived B lymphocytes requires the ex vivo removal of lymphocytes or suppression of T lymphocyte function by cyclosporine.

Removal of the plasma from the graft is used to minimize the risk of immediate hemolysis. This is accomplished by placing the marrow or PBSCs into standard blood transfer bags, centrifuging, and removing supernatant plasma. Normal saline or other media can be added to the product in a volume equivalent to about 50% of the volume of the discarded plasma to dilute the remaining donor antibody and lower the hematocrit for easier infusion.

With the development of monoclonal antibodies (MAbs), there has been an increase in stem cell selection (e.g., CD34+ cells) and purging of grafts (e.g., CD19+/CD20+ B cells).

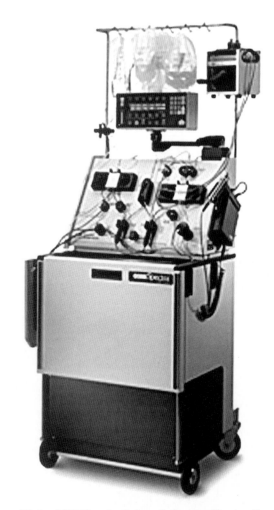

Figure 32-4 COBE Spectra Apheresis System. *(Courtesy Terumo BCT, Lakewood, Colo.)*

These techniques have resulted in decreased tumor reinfusion into autologous recipients and decreases in the amount of T cells infused in allogeneic recipients. **Cryopreservation** of the product is usually accomplished by the addition of 10% dimethyl sulfoxide (DMSO) and autologous plasma or 5% DMSO with 6% pentastarch and 4% human albumin. DMSO and pentastarch are thought to keep the cells from dehydrating during the freezing process, which would cause them to lyse. The product is then frozen in a controlled-rate freezer, which reduces the temperature of the product by 1° to 3° C (34° to 37° F)/minute, or by dump freezing in a –80° C (–112° F) freezer. After the product is frozen, it is kept in a liquid nitrogen freezer, vapor or liquid phase, until the time of transplantation.

Cell Infusion

At transplantation, the product is thawed in a 37° C (98.6° F) water bath in the laboratory or at the patient's bedside and is then infused without a filter through a central line. Toxicities and side effects have been associated with the infusion of cryopreserved products, mainly from the DMSO and volume overload. The most common symptoms are mild nausea, vomiting, and hypertension. Side effects of the infusion are rare and often mild. DMSO can cause patients to experience an immediate garlic-like taste. Sucking on hard candies during and after the infusion may help. Most patients undergoing allogeneic or syngeneic transplantation do not experience this problem, because the cells most likely were not mixed with DMSO or cryopreserved.

TRANSPLANTS FROM UNRELATED DONORS

About 70% of patients who need a transplant do not have a suitable donor in their family. The National Marrow Donor Program (NMDP), which operates Be The Match, is a nonprofit organization that facilitates unrelated marrow and blood stem cell transplants for patients who do not have matching donors in their families. Through a network of national and international affiliates, the program aids in more than 450 transplants each month. More than 18.5 million potential donors and more than 590,000 cord blood units are connected in the affiliated system. Approximately 40% of the transplants facilitated by the NMDP involve a U.S. patient receiving stem cells from an international donor or an international patient receiving stem cells from a U.S. donor.

Cord blood from unrelated donors has become an important source of hematopoietic stem cells (HSCs). Benefits include greater availability of stem cells and possible antileukemia effects in patients with hematologic malignancies when a noninherited maternal antigen of the cord blood donor matches the patient's mismatched antigen.

The donor-recipient HLA mismatch level affects the outcome of unrelated cord blood transplantation. Possible permissive mismatches involve the relationship between direction HLA mismatch vector or direction and transplantation outcomes. In most cord blood transplants, a mismatched HLA antigen is present in recipient and donor. This type of mismatch is bidirectional between the graft and host. The preferred type of mismatch is when the donor is homozygous at an HLA locus but the patient has two antigens identified (one matching the donor) at that locus, only donor cells have an HLA target, and the mismatch is in the graft-versus-host (GVH) direction with a rejection mismatch. If all mismatched loci have this type of mismatch, these are GVH-only mismatches. Engraftment of myeloid cells is significantly faster with grafts having GVH-only mismatches.

A major advantage of cord blood has been the ability to transplant grafts that are partially HLA-mismatched because of a relatively low incidence and severity of GVHD for the level of mismatch, a probable consequence of immunologic tolerance of this neonatal HSC source. Most cord blood transplantations to date (estimated at >30,000 globally) have been performed with grafts having one or two HLA-A, HLA-B, and HLA-DRB1 mismatches.

Immune reconstitution after stem cell transplantation is a complex process involving various components of the innate and adaptive immune systems. Two main pathways of T cell regeneration contribute to post–T lymphocyte recovery, thymopoiesis and peripheral blood expansion of mature T cells. Thymopoiesis provides a new pool of naïve T cells that is essential for sustained long-term immunity. Challenges to thymopoiesis can lead to a higher risk of opportunistic infections and an adverse outcome. Secondary cytopenia is a common complication of stem cell transplantation. Causes of secondary cytopenia include viral infection, septicemia, GVHD, and myelotoxic drugs. Older patients appear to be more prone to cumulative toxicities of post-transplantation drug regimens, but nonmyeloablative conditions, optimized HLA matching, and higher doses of CD34+ cell infusion may reduce the risk of cytopenia after day 28.

CURRENT DIRECTIONS

Genetic engineering of hematopoietic stem cells holds the promise of potentially treating many hereditary and acquired diseases. The promise of this therapy is laudable but it does have limitations. The technologies used to date have occasionally resulted in clonal expansion, myelodysplasia, or leukemogenesis.

At present, technology is challenged by the inability to expand or clone genetically modified HSCs from adult or cord blood specimens. New genetic material must be permanently introduced to correct the underlying disease mutation in the treatment of genetic disorders. Patient-specific induced pluripotent stem (iPS) cells can be generated from various cell types obtained from patients with inherited or acquired disorders. Safer and more effective methods will rely on the therapeutic use of pluripotent stem cells. One recent approach bypasses the need for iPS cells and the obstacles to generating human stem cells from embryonic-type cells. It consists of direct reprogramming of skin cells to a multipotent progenitor stage by the introduction of a single transcription factor, Oct4. Oct4-reprogrammed progenitor cells may possess desirable traits. Another potential game-changing advancement would be the ability to reprogram human adult stem cells to an expandable condition without reducing the long-term self-renewal properties and their safety.

Another aspect of adult stem cell transplantation has been studied in the field of regenerative medicine. The general goal of this field is transplanting donor stem cells to replace or repair defective cells in a patient. In the case of an HLA mismatch between donor and recipient, transplantation is hampered by the risks of immunologic recognition and rejection of the stem cell graft.

There are two critical concerns in the transplantation of umbilical cord blood:

1. Initial time to engraftment
2. Restoration of immune function

Umbilical cord blood transplantation (CBT) has been a successful alternative therapeutic option for transplant patient who have no suitable related allogeneic donors. But the significant delay in recovery of all hematopoietic blood cell lines is a major complication. The initial engraftment of cells that develop into the myeloid cell line (red blood cells, platelets, and granulocyte/monocyte) is 1 month. Development of T- and B-lymphocytes commonly takes 6 months or more after transplantation. Two factors have been found to be of extreme importance: (1) the total dose of progenitor (CD34+) cells in a cord blood unit has been associated with patient survival; and (2) the total dose of clonogenic progenitors with the graft correlates with engraftment of the transplant. Research studies continue to delineate these challenging issues.

A new idea is to transplant stem cells into a fetus early in gestation. The benefit is that in utero transplantation would occur when the immune system of the fetus is immature, which would provide the theoretical opportunity to induce fetal tolerance of foreign cells. This would avoid rejection and the need for immunosuppressive therapy. To date, a major problem has been achieving adequate levels of engraftment.

CASE STUDY

MC is an obese 46-year-old white woman with diabetes. She came to the emergency department with complaints of rectal bleeding and a feeling of significant fatigue.

History and Physical Examination

Medical History

The patient has a long-standing history of infected foot ulcerations that are not secondary to vascular insufficiency or diabetes. She received a prolonged course of chloramphenicol for the foot infections in Brazil. After treatment, she was found to be pancytopenic and required transfusions of packed RBCs and platelets on a regular basis.

Her medical history also includes a history of a positive purified protein derivative (PPD) test, for which she received antituberculosis therapy for 4 months. She sustained facial fractures in a car accident several years ago.

Medications

The patient takes rifampin (daily), INH (daily), pyridoxine (daily), cyclosporine (Sandimmune), insulin morning and evening, and metformin (Glucophage).

Social History

MC is a citizen of Brazil. Her husband died several years ago. She has three children, one living in the United States and two living in Brazil.

Allergies

She has no known allergies.

Family History

The patient's father died of heart disease at age 63; her mother died of cancer at age 48. The patient has nine siblings, six in Brazil and three in the United States. One sister, age 42, lives in the United States and is HLA-matched.

Physical Examination

The patient weighs 233 lb; her blood pressure is 120/70 mm Hg; and her pulse is 66 beats/min and regular.

Her temperature is 37.1° C (98.8 ° F). She has ecchymoses and petechiae of the skin, with mild bruising on her left shoulder. She has multiple scars on her feet and legs. There are no other abnormal physical findings.

Laboratory Data

See Table 32-2.

Immunologic Studies

- Hepatitis A antigen—positive.
- Hepatitis B and hepatitis C screening tests—negative.

Follow-up Evaluation

A bone marrow biopsy was performed. Histologic study of the aspirate and clot revealed a hypocellular marrow with trilineage hematopoiesis and dyserythropoiesis. Cytogenetic studies were normal (karyotype: 46,XX). Flow cytometry revealed polyclonal (kappa+ and lambda+) CD19+ B cells and CD4+ and CD8+ T cells. The iron stain was normal.

HLA Typing

- Patient: A11, 68; B18, 52; DR4, 15; DQ3, 6
- Donor: A11, 28; B18, 52; DR4, 15; DQ3, 6

At 3 Months

The patient is feeling well. The pain and swelling in her right arm have resolved. She has had no fever, nausea, vomiting, diarrhea, rash, chest pain, shortness of breath, dysuria, hematuria, headache, or edema.

Medications

The patient was receiving fluconazole (Diflucan), ursodiol (Actigall), valganciclovir, cyclosporine, sulfamethoxazole, magnesium oxide (norgestimate–ethinyl estradiol).

Physical Examination

The patient now weighs 152.6 lb; her blood pressure is 139/93 mm Hg, temperature 35.9° C (96.6° F), and pulse 69 beats/min and regular. She has no skin rash.

Her eyes and mouth are without scleral icterus or mucositis and the lungs are clear. Her heartbeat has a regular rate and rhythm. Her abdomen is soft and nontender, without masses or organomegaly. Extremities are without edema. Her neurologic examination revealed no tremors.

Laboratory Data

See Table 32-3.

Comments

1. Day +88 after HLA-matched donor stem cell transplantation for severe aplastic anemia: stable trilineage hematopoiesis. Mild leukopenia is probably a result of valganciclovir and/or sulfamethoxazole.
2. Right arm cellulitis, resolved.
3. Renal insufficiency secondary to focal glomerulosclerosis—persistent proteinuria (1.4 g/24 hr)

and elevated BUN and creatinine levels (despite a low therapeutic cyclosporine level).

Treatment Plan

1. Check cyclosporine level today and adjust dose accordingly.
2. Refill norgestimate–ethinyl estradiol.
3. Continue sulfamethoxazole DS for *Pneumocystis jiroveci* (formerly *P. carinii*) prophylaxis and valganciclovir for previous CMV infection.

Questions

1. A risk involved in bone marrow transplant is:
   a. Graft-versus-host disease (GVHD)
   b. Fungal infections
   c. Reactivation of cytomegalovirus (CMV) infection
   d. All of the above
2. The breakthrough drug for preventing bone marrow transplant rejection was:
   a. Prednisone
   b. FK-506
   c. Cyclosporine A
   d. Immunoglobulins

See Appendix A for the answers to multiple choice questions.

Critical Thinking Group Discussion Questions

1. What is the cause of this patient's aplastic anemia?
2. Did the patient have any other treatment options?
3. What are the risks involved in bone marrow transplant?
4. What drug is highly effective in preventing rejection?

See the instructor site ⊖volve for the discussion of the answers to these questions.

Table 32-2	Case Study: Laboratory Results (1)	
Parameter	**Patient Result**	**Reference Range**
White blood cell (WBC) count	2.1 × 10⁹/L	4.5-11 × 10⁹/L
Hematocrit (Hct)	20.4%	36%-46%
Hemoglobin (Hgb, Hb)	6.9 g/dL	12-16 g/dL
Red blood cell (RBC) count	1.83 × 10¹²/L	4-5.20 × 10¹²/L
Platelet count*	49 × 10⁹/L	150-350 × 10⁹/L
Mean corpuscular volume (MCV)	112 fL	80-100 fL
Red cell distribution width (RDW)	20.2%	11.5%-14.5%
Reticulocyte count	1.5%	0.5%-1.9%
Leukocyte differential		
Segmented neutrophils	27%	40%-70%
Lymphocytes	57%	22%-44%
Monocytes	13%	4%-11%
Eosinophils	0%	0%-8%
Basophils	0%	0%-3%
Variant lymphocytes: 3%		
Anisocytosis: 2+		
Hypochromia: 1+		
Macrocytes: 3+		
Blood Chemistry		
Electrolytes: within normal limits		
Liver Function Tests		
Alkaline phosphatase (ALP)	131 IU/L	30-100 IU/L
Alanine transaminase (ALT/SGPT)	167 IU/L	7-30 IU/L
Aspartate transaminase (AST/SGOT)	56 IU/L	9-25 IU/L
Lactic dehydrogenase (LDH)	266 IU/L	110-210 IU/L
Plasma glucose	123 mg/dL	70-110 mg/dL

*Posttransfusion.

CHAPTER HIGHLIGHTS

- The goal of transplanting bone marrow or peripheral blood progenitor cells is to achieve a potential cure or help patients recover from high-dose chemotherapy that has destroyed healthy stem cells or marrow cells.
- Bone marrow and peripheral blood progenitor cells are capable of reconstituting a patient's immune system because they contain the precursor to the cells that make up the blood. Some stem cells circulate in the bloodstream and are called peripheral blood stem cells (PBSCs).
- There are three major types of transplants—allogeneic, syngeneic, and autologous.

- Chemotherapy and radiation target rapidly dividing cells. These therapies are used to treat cancers because cancer cells divide more rapidly than healthy cells. Bone marrow cells also divide at a rapid rate and can be severely damaged or destroyed by high-dose treatment.
- Without healthy bone marrow, a patient cannot make the blood cells that are needed to fight off infections, carry oxygen, and prevent bleeding. Bone marrow and PBSC

Table 32-3	Case Study: Laboratory Results (2)	
Assay	Patient Result	Reference Range
Sodium (Na⁺)	139 mEq/L	135-145 mEq/L
Potassium (K⁺)	4.7 mEq/L	3.5-5 mEq/L
Magnesium (Mg²⁺)	1.6 mEq/L	1.4-2 mEq/L
Blood urea nitrogen (BUN)	28 mg/dL	8-25 mg/dL
Creatinine	1.8 mg/dL	0.6-1.5 mg/dL
Total bilirubin	0.2 mg/dL	0-1 mg/dL
Direct bilirubin	0.1 mg/dL	0-0.4 mg/dL
ALP	99 IU/L	30-100 IU/L
AST/SGOT	16 IU/L	9-25 IU/L
LDH	208 IU/L	100-210 IU/L
WBC count	3.7×10^9/L	$4.5\text{-}11 \times 10^9$/L
Hct	39%	36%-46%
Platelet count	173,000	$200\text{-}400 \times 10^{12}$/L

transplants can replace the normal and abnormal cells that were destroyed during treatment.

- Factors that influence the eligibility for bone marrow transplantation include age, disease status, performance status for the recipient, organ function, infectious disease status, compatibility of the donor and recipient, and psychosocial status.
- The procedure for obtaining or harvesting bone marrow is the same for all types of transplants. The goal of the harvest procedure is to collect 10 to 15 mL of bone marrow/kg recipient weight.
- Complications that develop from transplantation of bone marrow or PBSCs range from infection, GVHD, rejection, and organ damage to infertility and death.

REVIEW QUESTIONS

1. The following diseases are treatable by stem cell transplantation:
   a. Acute lymphoblastic leukemia and acute myelogenous leukemia
   b. Aplastic anemia and non-Hodgkin's lymphoma
   c. Severe combined immunodeficiency disease and chronic myeloid leukemia
   d. All of the above

2. Progenitor blood cells are:
   a. Pluripotent
   b. Found only in bone marrow
   c. Not useful in reconstituting a person's immune system
   d. Determined by the exact number of CD34+ and stem cells

3-5. Match the following transplants:

3. _____ Allogeneic   a. Stem cells from identical twins.

4. _____ Autologous   b. Marrow from a related or unrelated donor.

5. _____ Syngeneic   c. Transplant of own cells.

6. Radiotherapy is most often used for:
   a. Myelodysplastic syndrome
   b. Localized solid tumors
   c. Hodgkin's disease
   d. Both b and c

7. Pretransplantation evaluation includes:
   a. HLA tissue typing and hepatitis screening
   b. Electrocardiography and CBC
   c. Bone marrow biopsy and complete history, including physical examination
   d. All of the above

8. Bone marrow is usually aspirated from:
   a. Sternum
   b. Anterior iliac crest
   c. Posterior iliac crest
   d. Vertebrae

9. Peripheral blood stem cells (PBSCs) are obtained by:
   a. Phlebotomy
   b. Apheresis
   c. Leukapheresis
   d. Both b and c

10. Engraftment of bone marrow or PBSCs is:
    a. Cell production in the bone marrow
    b. Matching the donor and patient
    c. Measured by the number of lymphocytes in circulation
    d. Antibody production

11. Complications of bone marrow or PBSC transplantation include:
    a. Infection and graft-versus-host disease (GVHD)
    b. Acute rejection and organ damage
    c. Chronic rejection and death
    d. All of the above

12. Differences between donor and recipient's ABO or Rh blood groups have _____ effect on marrow engraftment.
    a. No
    b. Some
    c. A major
    d. A total

13. Stem cell selection can be improved using the CD_____ cell surface marker.
    a. 4+
    b. 8+
    c. 34+
    d. 56+

14. Increased cell selection and purging of grafts using cell surface membrane markers has resulted in:
    a. Decreased risk of tumor reinfusion
    b. Lesser GVHD
    c. Transfusing fewer erythrocytes as contaminants
    d. All of the above

15. Toxicity associated with infusion of cryopreserved products is mainly caused by:
    a. Dimethyl sulfoxide (DMSO)
    b. Pentastarch
    c. Human albumin
    d. Glycerol

BIBLIOGRAPHY

Aiutii A, Roncarolo MG: Ten years of gene therapy for primary immune deficiencies, Hematology Am Soc Hematol Educ Program 682–689, 2009.

American Association of Blood Banks: Standards for hematopoietic progenitor cell services, ed 2, Bethesda, Md, 2000, American Association of Blood Banks.

Antin J, et al: Peripheral blood stem cells for allogenic transplantation: a review, Stem Cells 19:108–117, 2001.

Baynes RD, et al: Bone marrow and peripheral blood hematopoietic stem cell transplantation: focus on autografting, Clin Chem 46(Pt 2):1239–1251, 2000.

Bensinger W, et al: Transplantation of bone marrow as compared with peripheral blood cells from HLA-identical relatives in patients with hematologic cancers, N Engl J Med 344:175–181, 2001.

Blaser B, et al: Trans-presentation of donor-derived interleukin-15 is necessary for the rapid onset of acute graft-versus-host disease but not for graft-versus-tumor activity, Blood 108:2463–2469, 2006.

Blume KG, et al: A review of autologous hematopoietic cell transplantation, Biol Blood Marrow Transplant 6:1–12, 2000.

Braziel RM, et al: The Burkitt-like lymphomas: a Southwest Oncology Group study delineating phenotypic, genotypic and clinical features, Blood 97:3713–3720, 2001.

Chabner BA, Longo DL, editors: Cancer chemotherapy and biotherapy: principles and practice, ed 3, Philadelphia, 2001, Lippincott–Williams & Wilkins.

Contassot E, et al: Ganciclovir-sensitive acute graft-versus-host disease in mice receiving herpes simplex virus–thymidine kinase expressing donor T cells in a bone marrow transplantation setting, Transplantation 4:503–508, 2000.

Copelan EA: Hematopoietic stem cell transplantation, N Engl J Med 354:1813–1826, 2006.

Davies SM, et al: Engraftment and survival after unrelated-donor bone marrow transplantation: a report from the National Marrow Donor Program, Blood 96:4096–4103, 2000.

Focosi D, Petrini M: More on donor-derived T-cell leukemia after bone marrow transplantation, N Engl J Med 355:2, 2006.

Franks LM, Teich NM: Introduction to the cellular and molecular biology of cancer, ed 3, New York, 1999, Oxford University Press.

Highfill SL, et al: Bone marrow myeloid-derived suppressor cells (MDSCs) inhibit graft-versus-host disease (GVHD) via an arginase-1-dependent mechanism that is up-regulated by interleukin-13, Blood 116:5738–5747, 2010.

Johnston LJ, Horning SJ: Autologous hematopoietic cell transplantation in Hodgkin's disease, Biol Blood Marrow Transplant 6:289–300, 2000.

Krause D, et al: Isolation and flow cytometric analysis of T-cell-depleted CD34+ PBPCs, Transfusion 40:1475–1481, 2000.

Laughlin MJ, et al: Outcomes after transplantation of cord blood or bone marrow from unrelated donors in adults with leukemia, N Engl J Med 351:2265–2275, 2004.

Leisenrig WM, et al: It's about time: a new prognostic tool for acute graft-versus-host disease, Blood 108:749–755, 2006.

Liu C, et al: Progenitor cell dose determines the pace and completeness of engraftment in a xenograft model for cord blood transplantation, Blood 116:5518–5527, 2010.

Martin-Henao GA, et al: Isolation of CD34+ progenitor cells from peripheral blood by use of an automated immunomagnetic selection system: factors affecting the results, Transfusion 40:35–43, 2000.

Moretta L, et al: Killer Ig-like receptor-mediated control of natural killer cell alloreactivity in haploidentical hematopoietic stem cell transplantation, Blood 117:764–771, 2011.

Nakamae H, et al: Cytopenias after day 28 in allogeneic hematopoietic cell transplantation: impact of recipient/donor factors, transplant conditions and myelotoxic drugs, Haematologica 96:1838–1844, 2011.

National Marrow Donor Program 2012 (http://www.nmdp.org).

Nikolic B, et al: A novel application of cyclosporin A in nonmyeloablative pretransplant host conditioning for allogeneic BMT, Blood 96:1166–1172, 2000.

Parolini O: In utero hematopoietic stem-cell transplantation—a match for mom, N Engl J Med 364:1174–1175, 2011.

Penno K: Combining forces, Adv Med Lab Prof 17:18–20, 27, 2005.

Reya T: Illuminating immune privilege—a role for regulatory T cells in preventing rejection, N Engl J Med 365:956–957, 2011.

Rivière I, Dunbar CE, Sadelain M: Hematopoietic stem cell engineering at a crossroads, Blood 119:1107–1116, 2012.

Ross DW: Introduction to oncogenes and molecular cancer medicine, New York, 1998, Springer.

Sanz MA: Cord-blood transplantation in patients with leukemia: a real alternative for adults, N Engl J Med 351:2328–2338, 2004.

Serody JS, et al: Comparison of granulocyte colony-stimulating factor (G-CSF)–mobilized peripheral blood progenitor cells and G-CSF–stimulated bone marrow as a source of stem cells in HLA-matched sibling transplantation, Biol Blood Marrow Transplant 6:434–440, 2000.

Socié G: Graft-versus-host disease: from the bench to the bedside? N Engl J Med 353:1396–1397, 2005.

Spitzer TR: Nonmyeloablative allogeneic stem cell transplant strategies and the role of mixed chimerism, Oncologist 5:215–223, 2000.

Spitzer TR, et al: Intentional induction of mixed chimerism and achievement of antitumor response after nonmyeloablative conditioning therapy and HLA-matched donor bone marrow transplantation for refractory hematologic malignancies, Biol Blood Marrow Transplant 6:309–320, 2000.

Stevens CE, et al: HLA mismatch direction in cored blood transplantation: impact on outcome and implications for cored blood unit selection, Blood 118:3969–3978, 2011.

Storek J, et al: Immune reconstitution after allogeneic marrow transplantation compared with blood stem cell transplantation, Blood 97:3380–3389, 2001.

Sutherland R, et al: The CD 34 antigen: structure, biology and potential clinical applications, J Hematotherapy 1:115–129, 1992.

Sykes M, et al: Mixed lymphohaemopoietic chimerism and graft-versus-lymphoma effects after non-myeloablative therapy and HLA-mismatched bone marrow transplantation, Lancet 353:1755–1759, 1999.

Ullmann AJ, et al: Posaconazole or fluconazole for prophylaxis in severe graft-versus-host disease, N Engl J Med 356:335–346, 2007.

Vincent K, Denis-Claude R, Perreault C: Next-generation leukemia immunotherapy: Blood 118:2951–2959, 2011.

Visigalli I, et al: Gene therapy augments the efficacy of hematopoietic cell transplantation and fully corrects mucopolysaccharidosis type I phenotype in the mouse model, Blood 116:5130–5139, 2010.

Wils E, et al: Insufficient recovery of thymopoiesis predicts for opportunistic infections in allogeneic hematopoietic stem cell transplant recipients, Haematologica 96:1846–1854, 2011.

Zambelli A, et al: Clinical toxicity of cryopreserved circulating progenitor cells infusion, Anticancer Res 18:4705–4708, 1998.

Zhang C, et al: Donor CD4+ T and B cells in transplants induce chronic graft-versus-host disease with autoimmune manifestations, Blood 107:2993–3000, 2006.

Learning Objectives

At the conclusion of this chapter, the reader should be able to:

- Compare the characteristics of benign and malignant tumors.
- Describe the epidemiology of cancer in adults and children.
- Explain the characteristics of the three major causative factors in human cancer.
- Compare the stages of carcinogenesis.
- Describe the aspects of cancer-related genes.
- Define and give examples of proto-oncogenes.
- Describe the role of oncogenes.
- Describe the characteristics of the major body defenses against cancer.

- Identify and discuss the characteristics of tumor markers.
- Discuss what's new in cancer diagnostic testing.
- Compare various modalities for treating cancer.
- Analyze representative case studies.
- Correctly answer case study related multiple choice questions.
- Be prepared to participate in a discussion of critical thinking questions.
- Describe the principle and clinical applications of the prostate-specific antigen procedure.
- Correctly answer end of chapter review questions.

Key Terms

abl proto-oncogene
adenomas
alpha-fetoprotein (AFP)
antioncogenes
benign
carcinoembryonic antigen (CEA)
carcinoma

carcinoma in situ
cytochrome P-450
DNA microarray technology
immunosurveillance
malignant
neoplasms
oncofetal proteins

oncogenes
p53 gene
proto-oncogenes
purine analogues
spontaneous tumor antigens
tumor necrosis factor
tumor-specific antigens (TSAs)

Oncology is that branch of medicine devoted to the study and treatment of tumors. The term *tumor* is commonly used to describe a proliferation of cells that produces a mass rather than a reaction or inflammatory condition. Tumors are **neoplasms** and are described as **benign** or **malignant.** Most tumors are of epithelial origin (ectoderm, endoderm, or mesoderm); the remaining tumors are of connective tissue origin (Fig. 33-1). The key distinction between benign and malignant tumors is the ability of malignant tumors to invade normal tissue and metastasize to other secondary sites.

CANCER STEM CELLS

Biology research studies have discovered that stem cells are critical for the generation of complex multicellular organisms and the development of tumors. To cure a cancer through stable long-term remission, the stem cell compartment of a tumor needs to be eradicated. Stem cells have three distinctive properties:

- Self-renewal when daughter cells retain the same biologic properties as the parent cell
- Capability to develop into multiple lineages
- Potential to proliferate extensively

If normal self-renewal is subverted, it becomes abnormal self-renewal. If increased self-renewal occurs, combined with the intrinsic growth potential of stem cells, it may yield a malignant phenotype. It is possible that cancer stem cells can arise by mutation from normal stem cells or mutated progenitor cells (Fig. 33-2).

TYPES OF TUMORS

Benign Tumors

Benign tumors are often named by adding the suffix *-oma* to the cell type (e.g., lipoma), but there are exceptions (e.g., lymphomas, melanomas, hepatomas). Benign tumors arising from glands are called **adenomas;** those from epithelial surfaces are termed *polyps* or papillomas.

Benign tumors are characterized by the following:
- Usually are encapsulated
- Grow slowly
- Usually are nonspreading
- Have minimal mitotic activity
- Resemble the parent tissue

Other types of tumors include non-neoplastic lesions associated with an overgrowth of tissue that is normally present in the organ (e.g., hyperplastic tissue) and choristomas, normal tissue in a foreign location (e.g., pancreatic tissue in the stomach).

Malignant Tumors

A malignant neoplasm of epithelial origin is referred to as **carcinoma,** or cancer. Those arising from squamous epithelium (e.g., esophagus, lung) are called squamous cell carcinomas, those arising from glandular epithelium (e.g., stomach, colon, pancreas) are called adenocarcinomas, and those arising from transitional epithelium in the urinary system are called transitional cell carcinomas.

Other types of malignant tumors include amine precursor uptake and decarboxylational tumors. These are neuroendocrine tumors that commonly develop from neural crest and neural ectoderm (e.g., small cell carcinoma of lung). Sarcomas, malignant tumors of connective tissue origin (e.g., fibrosarcoma), and teratomas are derived from all three germ cell layers (e.g., teratoma of the ovary or testis).

Malignant tumors are characterized by the following:
- Increase in the number of cells that accumulate
- Usually, invasion of tissues
- Dissemination by lymphatic spread or by seeding within a body cavity
- Metastasis
- Characteristic nuclear cellular features
- Receptors for integrin molecules (e.g., fibronectin), which help malignant cells adhere to extracellular matrix, type IV collagenases, which dissolve basement membranes, and proteases

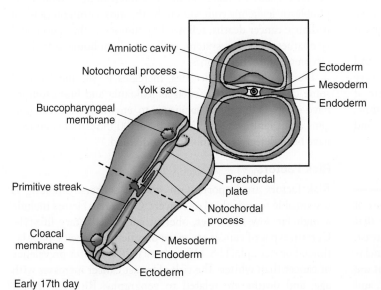

Amniotic cavity
Notochordal process
Yolk sac
Buccopharyngeal membrane
Ectoderm
Mesoderm
Endoderm
Primitive streak
Prechordal plate
Notochordal process
Cloacal membrane
Mesoderm
Endoderm
Ectoderm
Early 17th day

Figure 33-1 Embryonic primary germ layers. *(Adapted from Larsen WJ: Human embryology, ed 3, Philadelphia, 2001, Churchill Livingstone.)*

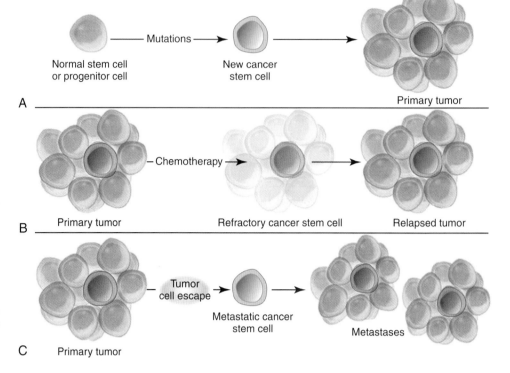

Figure 33-2 **For tumors in which cancer stem cells play a role, at least three scenarios are possible.** **A,** Mutation of a normal stem cell or progenitor cell may create a cancer stem cell, which will then generate a primary tumor (Panel A). **B,** During treatment with chemotherapy, most cells in a primary tumor may be destroyed, but if the cancer stem cells are not eradicated, the tumor may regrow and cause a relapse (Panel B). **C,** Cancer stem cells arising from a primary tumor may emigrate to distal sites and create metastatic lesions (Panel C). *(From Jordan CT, Guzman ML, Noble M: Cancer stem cells, N Engl J Med 355:1253–1260, 2006.)*

- Secretion of transforming growth factor α (TGF-α) and transforming growth factor β (TGF-β) to promote angiogenesis and collagen deposition
- Often, recurrence after attempts to eradicate the tumor by surgery, radiation, or chemotherapy

Biologically distinct and relatively rare populations of tumor-initiating cells have been identified in cancers of the hematopoietic system, brain, and breast. Cells of this type have the capacity for self-renewal, the potential to develop into any cell in the overall tumor population, and the proliferative ability to drive continued expansion of the population of malignant cells. The properties of these tumor-initiating cells closely parallel the three features that define normal stem cells. Malignant cells with these functional properties are termed *cancer stem cells* (Fig. 33-3). Cancer stem cells can be the source of all the malignant cells in a primary tumor.

Despite decreases in the incidence of some cancers and associated mortality, cancer remains highly lethal and very common. About 41% of Americans will develop some form of cancer, including nonmelanoma skin cancer, in their lifetime; 20% of Americans will die from cancer. Cancer is the second leading cause of death in the United States.

EPIDEMIOLOGY

Lung, colorectal, and breast cancers are the leading causes of cancer deaths in the United States. The types of cancer that have been increasing in incidence are cancer of the lung, breast, prostate, and pancreas and multiple myeloma, malignant melanoma, and Hodgkin's lymphoma. The types of cancer that are decreasing in incidence are cancer of the stomach, cervix, and endometrium.

Cancer in Adults

The lifetime probability of developing cancer is higher in men than in women. The three most common cancers in men are prostate, lung and bronchus, and colorectal, accounting for about 54% of all newly diagnosed cancers. The three most common cancers in women are breast, lung and bronchus, and colorectal, accounting for about 52% of cancer cases in women. Breast cancer alone is expected to account for 26% of all new cancer cases among women. Cancer accounts for more deaths than heart disease in persons younger than 85 years.

Cancer in Children

Cancer is the second leading cause of death among children between 1 and 14 years old in the United States. Acute lymphoblastic leukemia continues to be the most common cause of pediatric cancer deaths, followed by tumors of the central and sympathetic nervous system, malignant lymphoma, soft tissue sarcomas, and renal tumors.

During the past 3 decades, increases in the incidence of some childhood cancers, such as leukemia and brain tumors, have suggested prenatal exposure to environmental carcinogens as a causative factor. More than 300 industrial chemicals have been detected in umbilical cord blood.

Risk Factors

Risk factors are important in specific cancers. Smoking is responsible for one third of cancers. Other risk factors include a high-fat, low-fiber diet, obesity, and a sedentary lifestyle. Certain types of cancer are more prevalent in specific populations. For example, U.S. blacks have a 20% greater prevalence of cancer than whites. The risk of breast cancer increases with age, and deaths are related to geography. Risk factors for breast cancer include family history, particularly breast cancer

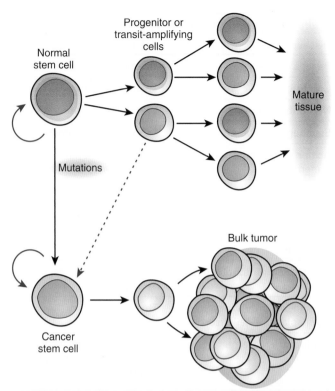

Figure 33-3   Stem cell systems. Normal tissues arise from a central stem cell that grows and differentiates to create progenitor and mature cell populations. Key properties of normal stem cells are the ability to self-renew *(curved arrow),* multilineage potential, and extensive proliferative capacity. Cancer stem cells arise by means of mutation in normal stem cells or progenitor cells and subsequently grow and differentiate to create primary tumors *(broken arrow* indicates that specific types of progenitors involved in the generation of cancer stem cells are unclear). As with normal stem cells, cancer stem cells can self-renew, give rise to heterogeneous populations of daughter cells, and proliferate extensively. *(Adapted from Jordan CT, Guzman ML, Noble M: N Engl J Med 355:1253-1260, 2006.)*

Table 33-1	Selected Environmental Factors Associated With Cancer
Factor	**Type of Cancer**
Aerosol and Industrial Pollutants	
Asbestos (silica)	Mesothelioma
Lead, copper, zinc, arsenic, cyclic aromatics, tobacco	Lung cancer
Vinyl chloride	Liver angiosarcoma
Benzene	Leukemia
Aniline dyes, coal	Skin and bladder carcinoma
Drugs	
Androgenic steroids	Hepatocellular carcinoma
Stilbestrol (prenatal)	Vaginal adenocarcinoma
Estrogen (postmenopausal)	Endometrial carcinoma
Hydantoins	Lymphoma
Chloramphenicol, alkylating agents	Leukemias, lymphomas
Infectious Agents	
Epstein-Barr virus	Burkitt's lymphoma, nasopharyngeal cancer (?) Hodgkin's disease
Human papillomavirus	Cervical cancer
Herpesvirus type 2	Cervical cancer
Human immunodeficiency virus (HTLV-III)	Kaposi's sarcoma, non-Hodgkin's lymphoma, primary lymphoma of the brain, bladder cancer
HTLV-I	Non-Hodgkin's lymphoma
Hepatitis B	Hepatocellular carcinoma

in a first-degree relative, first pregnancy after age 30 years, presence of fibrocystic disease, probably the use of oral contraceptives or hormone replacement therapy, prior breast or chest wall radiation, prior breast cancer, and ethanol consumption.

Survivors of childhood and adolescent cancer constitute one of the higher risk populations. The curative therapy (e.g., chemotherapy, radiation) administered for the cancer also affects growing and developing tissues. These patients are at increased risk for early mortality caused by second cancers and cardiac or pulmonary disease. Two thirds of survivors have at least one chronic or late-occurring health problem.

CAUSATIVE FACTORS IN HUMAN CANCER

Factors that cause most neoplasms are unknown. They can be classified as environmental factors (e.g., chemical and radiation), host factors and disease associations, and viruses.

Environmental Factors

The incidence of cancer has been correlated with certain environmental factors. Table 33-1 lists environmental factors that have been definitively linked with cancer, including aerosol and industrial pollutants, drugs, and infectious agents. Radiation exposure is also known to be associated with specific types of cancer (e.g., acute leukemia, thyroid cancer, sarcomas, breast cancer). Women concerned about organochlorine substances (e.g., polychlorinated biphenyls [PCBs], dioxins, pesticides [DDT, banned in 1972]) can be reassured that available evidence does not suggest an association between exposure to these chemicals and breast cancer.

Most chemical carcinogens are inactive in their native state and must be activated by enzymes in the **cytochrome P-450** or other enzyme systems (e.g., bacterial enzymes or enzymes induced by alcohol).

In radiation carcinogenesis, ionizing particles (e.g., alpha and beta particles, gamma rays, x-rays) hydrolyze water into free radicals, which are mutagenic to DNA by activating proto-oncogenes. Ultraviolet (UV) light, especially UVB, induces the formation of thymidine dimers, which distort the DNA molecule, leading to skin cancers (e.g., basal cell carcinoma, malignant melanoma).

Host Factors and Disease Associations

Various host factors have been linked to a higher than expected incidence of cancer. For example, the presence of certain genetic disorders (e.g., Down syndrome) is associated with an increased incidence of leukemia. The link between certain genetic abnormalities and leukemia is consistent with a germinal or somatic mutation in a stem cell line.

Familial clustering of germ cell tumors, malignant tumors arising in the testis, has been observed, particularly among siblings. Cryptorchidism and Klinefelter's syndrome are predisposing factors in the development of germ cell tumors arising from the testis and mediastinum, respectively.

The incidence of cancer is 10,000 times greater than expected in patients with an immunodeficiency syndrome. The increased incidence of lymphomas in congenital, acquired, and drug-induced immunosuppression is consistent with the failure of normal immune mechanisms or antigen overstimulation with a loss of normal feedback control. Table 33-2 lists other cancer-related conditions.

Viruses

Viral causes of some cancers are known. Viruses associated with specific cancers are listed in Table 33-1. Nonpermissive cells that prevent an oncogenic RNA or DNA virus from completing its replication cycle often produce changes in the genome that result in the activation of proto-oncogenes or inactivation of suppressor genes.

STAGES OF CARCINOGENESIS

Some precancerous conditions progress through a series of growth alterations before becoming cancerous. For example, cervical cancer progresses from squamous metaplasia to squamous dysplasia to **carcinoma in situ,** and finally to invasive cancer. Endometrial cancer progresses from endometrial hyperplasia to atypical endometrial hyperplasia to carcinoma in situ, and finally to invasive cancer.

Cancer (Box 33-1) results from a series of genetic alterations that can include the following:
- Activation of oncogenes that promote cell growth
- Loss of tumor suppressor gene activity, which inhibits cell growth

Mutation or overexpression of oncogenes produces proteins that can stimulate uncontrolled cell growth, whereas mutation or deletion of tumor suppressor genes results in the production of nonfunctional proteins that can no longer control cell proliferation. The mutant cell multiplies and the succeeding generations of cells aggregate to form a malignant tumor.

Interleukin-24 (IL-24), initially called MOB-5, is a protein that is usually secreted by immune system cells in response to injury or infection. Research on colon cancer cells has demonstrated that IL-24, in conjunction with its receptors, appears to give a cancer cell the ability to fuel its own growth. The secreted proteins are released from one cell to transmit a signal to grow, migrate, or survive to another cell. These proteins cannot act alone and must act through a receptor or receptors on the receiving cell.

Table 33-2	Cancer-Related Conditions
Disease	**Related Cancer**
Paget's disease	Osteogenic sarcoma
Cryptorchidism	Testicular cancer
Neurofibromatosis	Brain tumors, sarcoma
Esophageal webbing	Esophageal carcinoma
Achlorhydria and pernicious anemia	Gastric carcinoma
Cirrhosis	Hepatoma
Cholelithiasis	Gallbladder cancer
Chronic inflammatory bowel disease	Colon cancer
Migratory thrombophlebitis	Adenocarcinoma, especially pancreatic
Myasthenia gravis, pure red cell aplasia, T cell disorder	Thymoma
Nephrotic syndrome	Membranous carcinomas; lymphomas, especially Hodgkin's

Box 33-1	The Process of Cancer

Cancer is a multistep process involving the following:
- Initiation (irreversible mutations involving proto-oncogenes)
- Promotion (growth enhancement to pass on the mutation to other cells)
- Progression (e.g., development of tumor heterogeneity for metastasis, drug resistance)

CANCER-PREDISPOSING GENES

Cancer-predisposing genes may act in the following ways:
- Affect the rate at which exogenous precarcinogens are metabolized to actively carcinogenic forms that can damage the cellular genome directly
- Affect a host's ability to repair resulting damage to DNA
- Alter the immune ability of the body to recognize and eradicate incipient tumors
- Affect the function of the apparatus responsible for the regulation of normal cell growth and associated proliferation of tissue

Relatively few cancer-predisposing genes have been described. An absence of functional alleles at specific loci, however, allows the genesis of the malignant process (Table 33-3). For example, individuals with certain mutations in the gene *BRCA2* are at a very high risk (up to 85%) for developing breast cancer and other cancers (e.g., ovarian cancer) because a DNA repair path cannot properly repair ongoing wear and tear to the DNA.

A mutation in a gene thought to be responsible for colon cancer may initially cause it. This gene, APC, normally limits

Table 33-3	Tumors Associated With Homozygous Loss of Specific Chromosomal Loci	
Tumor Type		**Chromosomal Linkage**
Multiple endocrine neoplasia, type 2		1
Renal cell carcinoma		3
Lung carcinoma		3
Colon carcinoma, familial polyposis		5
Multiple endocrine neoplasia, type 2a		10
Wilms' tumor, hepatoblastoma, rhabdomyosarcoma		11
Retinoblastoma		13
Ductal breast carcinoma		13
Colon carcinoma		17
Acoustic neuroma, meningioma		22

the expression of a protein, survivin. When APC is altered, survivin works overtime and, instead of dying, stem cells in the colon overpopulate, resulting in cancer. Survivin is overexpressed in colon cancer. It prevents programmed cell death, or apoptosis, the process whereby cells normally die. Rather than dying on schedule, cancer cells instead grow out of control. The APC gene controls the amount of survivin by shutting down its production.

PROTO-ONCOGENES

Proto-oncogenes act as central regulators of the growth in normal cells that code for proteins involved in growth and repair processes in the body. Proteins such as growth factors or transcription factors are necessary for normal growth.

Genetic mutations in proto-oncogenes produce **oncogenes.** Oncogene activation causes the overexpression of growth-promoting proteins, resulting in hypercellular proliferation and tumorigenesis. Tumor suppressor genes normally counteract proto-oncogenes by encoding proteins that prevent cellular differentiation. When mutations in tumor suppressor genes cause loss of function, the expressed tumor suppressor proteins are no longer able to suppress cellular growth.

For example, the activation of proto-oncogenes (e.g., *ras*) involved in the growth process or inactivation of suppressor genes (e.g., *p53*), which keeps growth in check by binding and activating genes that put the brakes on cell division, is responsible for neoplastic transformation of a cell. Defects in the gene for p53 cause about 50% of all cancers.

p53 Protein

The **p53 gene** (tumor suppressor gene) is located on chromosome 17 and produces a protein that downregulates the cell cycle. A mutation of p53 is associated with an increased incidence of many types of cancer. The p53 tumor suppressor protein is dysfunctional in most human cancers. Even when p53 is

not itself mutant, its regulators (e.g., p14^{ARF}, a p53-stabilizing protein) are often altered. The p53 protein is a key responder to various stresses, including DNA damage, hypoxia, and cell cycle aberrations. Specific molecular pathways that activate p53 depend on the nature of the stress and the cell type. Consequently, these determine the specific downstream effectors and cellular response—apoptosis, growth arrest, or senescence.

It is widely believed that the central role of p53 in tumor suppression is to mediate the response to DNA damage. If p53 is missing when damage occurs, cells do not undergo p53-mediated arrest or apoptosis. Cells that have sustained mutations in oncogenes or tumor suppressor genes because of the damage obtain a growth advantage that fuels the development of cancer.

Apparently, DNA damage itself is not the critical event that leads to cancer, as long as the oncogenic stress pathways that activate p53 are intact. For any given cancer type, p53 dysfunction generally correlates with poor treatment response and poor prognosis; therefore, restoration of p53 function is a potential avenue for therapeutic development. Drugs currently being developed will enhance the function of kinases that activate p53 in response to DNA damage.

ROLE OF ONCOGENES

The genetic targets of carcinogens are oncogenes. Oncogenes have been associated with various tumor types (e.g., HER-2/*neu* with breast, kidney, and ovarian cancers). Oncogenes are considered altered versions of normal genes. Over a lifetime, a variety of mutations can convert a normal gene into a malignant oncogene.

Once an oncogene is activated by mutation, it promotes excessive or inappropriate cell proliferation. Oncogenes have been detected in about 15% to 20% of a variety of human tumors and appear to be responsible for specifying many of the malignant traits of these cells. More than 30 distinct oncogenes, some of which are associated with specific tumor types, have been identified (Table 33-4). Each gene has the ability to evoke many of the phenotypes characteristic of cancer cells.

Major classes of oncogene products involved in the normal growth process of cells include the following:
- Growth factors (e.g., *sis* oncogene)
- Epidermal growth factor receptors (EGFRs)
- Membrane-associated protein kinases (e.g., *src* oncogene)
- Membrane-related guanine triphosphate (GTP)–binding proteins (e.g., *ras* oncogene)
- Cytoplasmic protein kinases (e.g., *ras* oncogene)
- Transcription regulators located in the nucleus (e.g., *c-myc* oncogene)

In addition, tumor suppressor genes (**antioncogenes**) are guardians of unregulated cell growth (e.g., *p53, Rb* oncogenes).

Mechanisms of Activation

Point mutations, translocations (e.g., t8;142 in Burkitt's lymphoma) and gene amplification (multiple copies of the gene

Table 33-4	Some Oncogenes Formed by Somatic Mutation of Normal Genetic Loci
Oncogene	**Disorder**
ab1	Chronic myelogenous leukemia
myc	Burkitt's lymphoma
N-myc	Neuroblastoma
EGFR, HER2	Mammary carcinoma
Ras type	Wide variety of tumors

EGFR, Epidermal growth factor receptor; *HER2,* human EGFR-2.

Box 33-2	Oncogenic Viruses

- Ribonucleic acid (RNA)—leukemia, carcinoma viruses, mammary tumor viruses
- Deoxyribonucleic acid (DNA)—herpesviruses, adenoviruses, papilloma viruses

with overexpression of products) are mechanisms of activation, as follows:

- Overexpression of the c-erbB-2 (HER2/*neu*) oncogene is noted in up to 34% of patients with invasive ductal breast carcinoma and predicts poor survival.
- Activation of the *ras* proto-oncogene (point mutation) is associated with about 30% of all human cancers. About 25% of patients with acute myelogenous leukemia display this point mutation. *Ras* is mutated frequently in colon and pancreatic cancers; it appears that *ras* activation leads to unregulated expression of IL-24 and its receptors.
- Translocation of the **abl proto-oncogene** from chromosome 9 to chromosome 22 with formation of a large *bcr-abl* hybrid gene on chromosome 22 (Philadelphia chromosome) results in chronic myelogenous leukemia.
- Inactivation of suppressor genes (point mutations) leads to unrestricted cell division, inactivation of each of the RB1 suppressor genes on chromosome 13 is associated with malignant retinoblastoma in children, and inactivation of the *p53* suppressor gene on chromosome 17 accounts for 25% to 50% of all malignancies involving the colon, breast, lung, and central nervous system.

Viral Oncogenes

Various RNA and DNA viruses have been associated with human malignancies (Box 33-2). Some viral agents have a clear causative role, such as the Epstein-Barr virus and certain papillomaviruses, which are the causative agents in Burkitt's lymphoma and cervical carcinoma, respectively.

Viruses carry viral oncogenes into target cells, where they become firmly established. Clonal descendants then carry the viral genes, which maintain the malignant phenotype of the cell clones.

Tumor-Suppressing Genes

A very different class of cancer genes has been discovered. These tumor-suppressing genes in normal cells appear to regulate the proliferation of cell growth. When this type of gene is inactivated, a block to proliferation is removed and cells begin a program of deregulated growth, or the genetically depleted cell itself may proliferate uncontrollably. Thus, tumor-suppressing genes are referred to as antioncogenes. In time, their discovery will lead to the reformulation of ideas about how the growth of normal cells is regulated.

Much speculation surrounds the operation of tumor-suppressing genes in normal tissue. It is known that normal cells exert a negative growth influence on each other within a tissue. Normal cells also secrete factors that are negative regulators of their own growth and that of adjacent cells. Diffusible factors may also be released by normal cells to induce the end-stage differentiation of other cells in the immediate environment; these factors include the following:

- Interferon-β (IFN-β)
- Transforming (tumor) growth factor (TGF)
- Tumor necrosis factor (TNF)

Normal gene products appear to prevent malignant transformation in some way. It is speculated that normal cells must have receptors that detect the presence of these growth-inhibiting and differentiation-inducing factors, which allow them to process the signals of negative growth and respond with appropriate modulation of growth. Genes may specify proteins necessary to detect and respond to the negative regulators of growth. If this process becomes dysfunctional as a result of inactivation or the absence of a critical component, such as the loss of chromosomal loci, a cell may continue to respond to mitogenic stimulation but lose its ability to respond to negative feedback to cease proliferation. Animal experiments have suggested that human beings carry a repertoire of genes, each of which is involved in the negative regulation of the growth of specific cell types. Somatic inactivation of these genes may be involved in the initiation of tumor cell growth or the transformation of benign tumors into malignant ones. Therefore, the somatic inactivation of tumor-suppressing genes may be as important to carcinogenesis as the somatic activation of oncogenes.

BODY DEFENSES AGAINST CANCER

Although there is no single satisfactory explanation for the success of tumors in escaping the immune rejection process, it is believed that early clones of neoplastic cells are eliminated by the immune response. The growth of malignant tumors is primarily determined by the proliferative capacity of the tumor cells and by the ability of these cells to invade host tissues and metastasize to distant sites. It is believed that malignant tumors can evade or overcome the mechanisms of host defenses (Color Plate 18).

Tumor immunity has the following general features:

1. Tumors express antigens that are recognized as foreign by the immune system of the tumor-bearing host.
2. The normal immune response frequently fails to prevent the growth of tumors.
3. The immune system can be stimulated to kill tumor cells and rid the host of the tumor.

Host defense mechanisms against tumors are both humoral and cellular. Effector mechanisms include the following:

- T lymphocytes
- Natural killer cells
- Macrophages
- Antibodies

T Lymphocytes

Cytolytic T lymphocytes (CTLs) provide effective antitumor immunity in vivo. CTL-mediated rejection of transplanted tumors is the only established example of completely effective specific antitumor immunity in vivo. Mononuclear cells derived from the inflammatory infiltrate in human solid tumors, called tumor-infiltrating lymphocytes, also include CTLs with the capacity to lyse the tumor from which they were derived. CD4+ T cells may play a role in antitumor responses by providing cytokines for effective CTL development.

Natural Killer Cells

Natural killer (NK) cells can be activated by direct recognition of tumors or as a consequence of cytokines produced by tumor-specific T lymphocytes. These cells use the same lytic mechanisms as CTLs to kill cells but do not express T cell antigen receptors, and they have a broad range of specificities. Research has also focused on the role of IL-2–activated NK cells in tumor killing. These cells, referred to as lymphokine-activated killer cells, are derived in vitro by culture of peripheral blood cells or tumor-infiltrating lymphocytes from tumor patients with high doses of IL-2.

NK cells may play a role in **immunosurveillance** against developing tumors, especially those expressing viral antigens.

Macrophages

Activated macrophages produce the cytokine **tumor necrosis factor.** As the name implies, TNF can kill tumors but not normal cells. TNF kills tumors by direct toxic effects and indirectly by effects on tumor vasculature.

Antibodies

Antibodies are probably less important than T lymphocytes in mediating the effect of antitumor immune responses, but tumor-bearing hosts produce antibodies against various tumor antigens. These serve as tumor markers.

Although malignant tumors may express protein antigens that are recognized as foreign by the tumor host, and despite the fact that immunosurveillance may limit the outgrowth of some tumors, the immune system often does not prevent the occurrence of cancer. The simplest explanation is that the rapid growth and spread of a tumor overwhelm the effector mechanisms of the immune response.

TUMOR MARKERS

In tumor immunology, a fundamental tenet is that when a normal cell is transformed into a malignant cell, it develops unique antigens not normally present on the mature normal cell.

Table 33-5	**Cancer Biomarkers**	
Type of Molecule	**Biomarkers in Blood or Body Fluid**	**Type of Cancer Detected**
Enzyme	Prostate-specific antigen (PSA)	Prostate
Oncofetal proteins	Alpha-fetoprotein (AFP); carcinoembryonic antigen (CEA)	Hepatocellular, germ cell Colorectal
Hormones	β-Human chorionic gonadotropin (β-hCG); calcitonin; adrenocorticotropic hormone (ACTH)	Trophoblastic Medullary thyroid Small cell lung
Mucins	CA 125, CA 19-9, CA 27.29, CA 15-3	Ovarian Breast
Immunoglobulins	Bence-Jones protein (urine)	Multiple myeloma
Genetic alteration	HER2/neu	Breast
Other proteins	HE4 Tg Nuclear matrix protein 22 (NMP-22); bladder tumor–associated antigen (BTA)/ complement factor H–related protein (CFHrp)	Ovarian Thyroid Bladder

Adapted from Snyder J: Genomic, proteomic developments in tumor markers, Adv Med Lab Prof 16:42–48, 2004; and Rhea JM, Molinaro RJ: Cancer biomarkers, MLO Med Lab Observer, 43:10–18, 2011.

Tumors frequently produce **tumor-specific antigens (TSAs)** to which the host may develop antibodies. Virus-induced cancers are the most antigenic; chemical-induced cancers are the least antigenic.

Tumor markers are substances present in or produced by tumors that can be used to detect the presence of cancer based on their measurement in blood, body fluids, cells, or tissue (Table 33-5). A tumor marker may be produced by the host in response to a tumor that can be used to differentiate a tumor from normal tissue or to determine the presence of a tumor. Non-neoplastic conditions can also exhibit tumor marker activity (Table 33-6). Some tumor markers are used to screen for cancer, but markers are more often used to monitor recurrence of cancer or determine the degree of tumor burden in the patient. To be of any practical use, the tumor marker must be able to reveal the presence of the tumor while it is still susceptible to destructive treatment by surgical or other means. Tumor markers can be measured quantitatively in tissues and body fluids using biochemical, immunochemical, or molecular tests (Table 33-7).

The search for tumor markers goes back more than 150 years. The earliest identified tumor marker was Bence-Jones protein, a light-chain immunoglobulin, found in patients with multiple

Table 33-6   Non-neoplastic Conditions With Elevated Serum and Plasma Concentrations of Tumor Markers

Tumor Marker	Concentration in Normal Serum (ng/mL)	Non-neoplastic Conditions
CEA	<2.5	Inflammatory bowel disease, pancreatitis, gastritis, smoker's chronic bronchitis, alcoholic liver disease, hepatitis
AFP	<40	Pregnancy, regenerating liver tissue after viral hepatitis, chemically induced liver necrosis, partial hepatectomy, cystic fibrosis, ataxia-telangiectasia, premature infants, tyrosinemia
β-hCG	Negative	Pregnancy
Serum acid phosphatase	Negative	Pregnancy
Placental alkaline phosphatase	Negative	Pregnancy

Table 33-7   Tumor Markers in Neoplasms

Tumor Markers	Clinical Value
CEA	Monitors response to therapy of patients with various types of cancer
AFP	Diagnosis of germ cell and hepatic tumors
CA 125	Diagnosis of ovarian cancer
β-hCG	Diagnosis of germ cell tumors
Prostate acid phosphatase	Diagnosis of prostate cancer

AFP, Alpha₁-fetoprotein; *β-hCG,* beta subunit of chorionic gonadotropin; *CEA,* carcinoembryonic antigen.

myeloma (see Chapter 27). Over the last 15 years, the use of tumor markers in the United States has risen dramatically. Tumor markers play an especially important role in the diagnosis and monitoring of patients with prostate, breast, and bladder cancers.

Older, well-established markers include alkaline phosphatase and collagen-type markers in bone cancer, immunoglobulins in myeloma, catecholamines and their derivatives in neuroblastoma and pheochromocytoma, and serotonin metabolites in carcinoid. In addition, there are many breast tissue prognostic markers (e.g., hormone receptors, cathepsin-D, HER2/*neu* oncogenes, plasminogen receptors and inhibitors).

The list of tumor markers approved by the U.S. Food and Drug Administration (FDA) continues to grow (Table 33-8).

Nine of these biomarkers are protein biomarkers identifiable in blood. Other recently approved protein biomarkers can be detected in urine, such as nuclear matrix protein 22, fibrin and fibrinogen degradation products, and bladder tumor antigen for monitoring bladder cancer, and by immunohistochemical methods using tumor tissues, such as estrogen receptor for breast cancer. Additional FDA-approved cancer biomarkers are DNA-based, such as human epidermal growth factor receptor 2 and HER2/*neu* for breast cancer, and can be assayed by fluorescent in situ hybridization (FISH). Multiple-marker combinations are useful in the management of some cancers (Table 33-9), but the use of more than two markers is questionable.

An ideal tumor marker would be an assay in which a positive result would only occur in patients with a malignancy, would correlate with stage and response to treatment, and is easily reproducible. No tumor marker to date has met this ideal marker description, nor has any tumor marker has been established as a practical screening test in a general healthy population or in most high-risk populations. The rationale for this poor predictive value of tumor markers is the lack of sensitivity and specificity in the low cancer rates that prevail in population groups. Because of the low prevalence of cancer, in general, even assays that are highly sensitive and specific may have a low predictive value.

Categories of Tumor Antigens

Tumor cells manifest tumor antigens, as well as self HLA antigens. There are four types of tumor antigens identified:
1. Tumor-specific antigens (TSAs) on chemically induced tumors
2. Tumor-associated antigens (TAAs) on virally induced tumors
3. Carcinofetal antigens
4. Spontaneous tumor antigens

Tumor-Specific Antigens

Chemically induced tumors are known to develop TSAs, which are uniquely associated with each tumor. These antigens are not found in normal cells. TSAs demonstrate little or no cross-reactivity between different tumors caused by the same carcinogen, perhaps because every tumor caused by chemical agents has unique surface characteristics.

Tumor-Associated Antigens

TAAs are cell surface molecules coded for by tumorigenic viruses. These antigens are not expressed on the virion but are synthesized by the host cell. In contrast to TSAs, TAAs are virus-specific. Therefore, each specific virus induces the same antigens, regardless of the tissue of origin or the animal species.

Carcinofetal Antigens

Well-differentiated tissue produces and secretes little or no fetal gene products. The abnormal behavior of malignant cells is believed to derepress genes normally expressed only during fetal life. Because the products of these fetally active genes are recognized as self, they do not elicit humoral or cell-mediated responses.

Table 33-8	Some Common Serum Tumour Markers and Their Clinical Utility*					
Tumor Type	Cancer Deaths (USA) (%)	Tumour Markers	Specificity	Sensitivity	Tumour Detection	Clinical Utility
Lung + bronchus	28	Neuron specific enolase	Poor	Poor	Late	Poor
Colon + rectum	9	Carcinoembryonic antigen (CEA)	Poor	Modest	Late	Modest
Breast	7	AA 15-3; CEA	Poor	Modest	Late	Modest
Pancreas	6	CA 19-9: CEA	Poor	Poor	Late	Poor
Prostate	5	Prostate-specific antigen	Modest	Good	Good	Good
Stomach	2	CEA; CA 19-9	Modest	Modest	Late	Poor
Ovary	2.5	CA 125	Modest	Modest	Intermediate	Good
Liver	3	Alpha-feto-protein α-FP	Good	Good	Intermediate	Good
Myeloma	1.9	Monoclonal protein/FLC	Good	Good	Early	Very good
AL amylidosis	0.3	Monoclonal protein/FLC	Good	Good	Early	Very good
Germ cell	0.1	α-FP; human chorionic gonadotrophin (HCG)	Good	Good	Early	Very good
Choriocarcinoma	<0.1	HCG	Good	Good	Early	Very good
Neuroendocrine	<0.1	Chromogranin, A, gastrin	Modest	Good	Early	Very good

From Bradwell AR: Serum free light chain analysis, Birmingham, UK, 2010, Binding Site, p 2.
FLC, Free light chains.
*All of these are measured using highly sensitive immunoassays apart from monoclonal proteins.

Table 33-9	Related Multiple Tumor Markers
Markers	Comments
AFP and β-hCG	Valuable combination in therapy and follow-up in patients with germ cell tumors of the testes.
CEA, AFP, and LDH	Combination seems to help differentiate primary liver cancer from liver metastases related to another organ.
Ratio of free to total PSA	The ratio may distinguish benign prostatic hypertrophy (BPH) from prostate cancer.
CEA and numerous mucin-type markers	May complement each other

AFP, Alpha-fetoprotein; *β-hCG,* beta subunit of chorionic gonadotropin; *CEA,* carcinoembryonic antigen; *LDH,* lactate dehydrogenase; *PSA,* prostate-specific antigen.

During malignant transformation, however, gene derepression is responsible for the production of increased concentrations of these gene products, which are known as **oncofetal proteins.** Carcinoembryonic antigen is an example of a carcinofetal antigen.

Spontaneous Tumor Antigens

Tumors caused by no known mechanism, known as **spontaneous tumor antigens,** are thought to produce antigens. Disagreement exists regarding whether these tumors are similar to those produced experimentally by chemical, viral, or physical agents. Although substantial evidence supports the contention that these tumors do not produce unique antigens, some evidence has refuted this contention. The importance of these findings remains unclear.

Specific Tumor Markers

Ten protein cancer biomarkers have been FDA-approved for clinical use:

1. Alpha-fetoprotein
2. CA 125
3. Human epididymis protein 4
4. Thyroglobulin
5. Prostate-specific antigen (PSA)
6. Carcinoembryonic antigen
7. CA 19-9
8. CA 15-3
9. CA 27.29
10. HER2/*neu*

Other markers include the beta subunit of human chorionic gonadotropin (β-hCG) and miscellaneous enzyme and hormone markers.

Alpha-Fetoprotein

Alpha-fetoprotein (AFP) is normally synthesized by the fetal liver and yolk sac. AFP is secreted in the serum in nanogram to milligram quantities in hepatocarcinoma, endodermal sinus tumors, nonseminomatous germ cell (testicular) cancer, teratocarcinoma of the testis or ovary, and malignant tumors of the mediastinum and sacrococcyx. In addition, a small percentage of patients with gastric and pancreatic cancer with liver metastasis may have elevated AFP levels. Both AFP and β-hCG should be quantitated initially in all patients with teratocarcinoma because one or both markers may be secreted in 85% of patients. The concentration of AFP may be elevated in nonneoplastic conditions such as hepatitis and cystic fibrosis.

AFP is a reliable marker for following a patient's response to chemotherapy and radiation therapy. Levels should be obtained every 2 to 4 weeks (metabolic half-life in vivo, 4 days).

CA 125

CA 125, a mucin-like glycoprotein, is expressed on the surface of coelomic epithelium and human ovarian carcinoma cells. CA 125 is relatively more sensitive in low-stage ovarian cancer. It reacts against an MAb developed against a cell line from one patient's ovarian cystadenocarcinoma. It is elevated in carcinomas and benign disease of various organs (e.g., pelvic inflammatory disease, endometriosis), but is most useful in ovarian and endometrial carcinomas.

Human Epididymis Protein 4

Human epididymis protein 4 (HE4) was approved in 2009. It is recommended for monitoring patients for recurring epithelial ovarian cancer. Disease recurrence or progression can be indicated if HE4 levels are ≥150.1 pM. This marker is not specific for ovarian cancer. Therefore, it is not suitable for use in the screening or diagnosis of ovarian cancer.

Thyroglobulin

Thyroglobulin (Tg) is produced and used exclusively by the thyroid gland. A Tg assay is frequently ordered prior to thyroid surgery to determine whether the tumor is producing Tg. This assay can be performed to monitor cancer recurrence because of rising levels over time following thyroid surgery. Tg levels can be elevated not only in thyroid cancer, but in Graves' disease and thyroiditis.

Prostate-Specific Antigen and Prostatic Acid Phosphatase

Prostate cancer is a leading cause of cancer death in U.S. men. Although there has been controversy in recent years about the application of prostate assays, there are two tumor markers for cancer of the prostate, prostate-specific antigen (PSA) and prostatic acid phosphatase.

Prostate-Specific Antigen. PSA screening has been controversial in recent years. Research on PSA testing offers mixed results on the benefits of PSA screening testing. However, some investigators suggest that PSA-screened men were more likely to be treated for prostate cancer at academic centers, where they got more state-of-the-art treatment.

PSA is a prostate tissue–specific marker, but not a prostate cancer–specific marker. It is a protease enzyme secreted almost exclusively by prostatic epithelial cells. Blood levels of PSA are increased when normal glandular structure is disrupted by benign or malignant tumor inflammation. The serum PSA level is directly proportional to tumor volume, with a greater increase per unit volume of cancer compared with benign hyperplasia. However, elevated PSA levels can be detected in prostate infection, irritation, benign prostatic hypertrophy, and recent ejaculation.

Free PSA assists in distinguishing cancer of the prostate from benign prostatic hypertrophy (BPH). Comparison of free PSA to PSA levels is used to assess the risk of cancer because the ratio of free PSA to PSA in prostate cancer is decreased. PSA levels appear useful for monitoring progression and response to treatment in patients with prostate cancer.

Other techniques that have been used for the detection of prostate cancer include PSA velocity (incremental increase of PSA over time), PSA density (ratio of serum PSA to prostate volume), age-adjusted PSA (PSA increases with age), biostatistically derived algorithms, free and total PSA, complexed PSA and, most recently, human kallikrein II, a molecule similar but not identical to PSA.

Other Prostate Cancer Biomarkers. Prostatic acid phosphatase is another older marker for prostate cancer. It is a serum enzyme exclusively diagnostic of prostatic carcinoma.

Isoforms of PSA represent the next generation of prostate cancer detection. An alternative marker is hK2. Its serum level is also elevated in men with prostate cancer. Another marker, early prostate cancer antigen-2 (EPCA-2), can specifically identify prostate cancer and distinguish aggressive from nonaggressive disease. These newer PSA-based screening assays will also be helpful for diagnosis and monitoring treatment.

Carcinoembryonic Antigen

The cell surface protein **carcinoembryonic antigen (CEA)** is found predominantly on normal fetal endocrine tissues in the second trimester of gestation. If CEA is detected in mature individuals, it is of limited diagnostic value but is helpful in differentiating between benign and malignant pleural and ascites effusions. CEA was first described in 1965 as a tumor marker specifically elevated in patients with colon cancer; it was later found to be elevated in patients with breast, lung, liver, and pancreatic cancers. Plasma levels higher than 12 ng/mL are strongly correlated with malignancy. Elevated neoplastic states frequently associated with an increased CEA level are endodermally derived gastrointestinal neoplasms and neck and breast carcinomas. Also, 20% of smokers and 7% of former smokers have elevated CEA levels.

CEA is used clinically to monitor tumor progress in patients who have diagnosed cancer with a high blood CEA level. If treatment leads to a decline to normal levels (<2.5 ng/mL), a rise in CEA level may indicate cancer recurrence to the clinician. A persistent elevation is indicative of residual disease or poor therapeutic response. In patients who have undergone colon cancer resection surgery, the rate of clearance of CEA levels usually return to normal within 1 month, but may take as long as 4 months. Blood specimens should be obtained 2 to 4 weeks apart to detect a trend.

CA 19-9

CA 19-9 is a glycolipid, Lewis blood group carbohydrate. Elevated levels have been found in patients with pancreatic, hepatobiliary, colorectal, gastric, hepatocellular, pancreatic, and breast cancers. Its main use is as a marker for colorectal and pancreatic carcinoma. This marker has greater specificity for pancreatic cancers than CEA. CA 19-9 is also known as gastrointestinal cancer–associated antigen.

CA 15-3

CA 15-3 is a biomarker used in conjunction with patient history, physical examination, and mammography during active cancer therapy to monitor metastasis. CA 15-3 is a high-molecular-weight (HMW) glycoprotein coded by the MUC-II gene and expressed on the ductal cell surface of most glandular epithelial cells. The main purpose of the assay is to monitor patients after mastectomy. Using a cutoff of 25 U/mL for CA 15-3, the detection rate is only 5% for stage I breast cancer.

The sensitivity is much better in higher stage disease, which makes it a good measure of tumor burden. CA 15-3 is positive in other conditions, including liver disease, some inflammatory conditions, and other carcinomas. A change in the CA 15-3 concentration is more predictive than the absolute concentration. Over time, tumor markers exhibit a steady state in the body, a balance between antigen production by the tumor and degradation and excretion. Changes in tumor burden are reflected by changes in the tumor marker concentration.

A high CA 15-3 level (>32 U/mL) usually indicates advanced breast cancer and a large tumor burden. This biomarker lacks sensitivity and specificity and is approved only for monitoring patient response to treatment and recurrence.

CA 27.29: Breast Carcinoma–Associated Antigen

Carcinoma of the breast often produces mucinous antigens that are HMW glycoproteins with O-linked oligosaccharide chains. Monoclonal antibodies (MAbs) directed against breast carcinoma–associated antigen (CA 27.29) can quantitate the levels of this antigen in serum. The antibodies recognize epitopes of a breast cancer–associated antigen encoded by the human *MUC1* gene, which is also referred to as MAM6, milk mucin antigen, CA 27.29, and CA 15-3. This tumor marker may be useful in conjunction with other clinical methods for predicting early recurrence of breast cancer. It is not recommended as a breast cancer screening assay. Increased levels of CA 27.29 (>38 U/mL) may indicate recurrent disease in a woman with treated breast carcinoma and may indicate the need for additional testing or procedures. Some clinical investigators do not endorse the routine use of this new marker.

HER2/*neu*

HER2/*neu* is encoded by an oncogene and is over expressed in 15% to 20% of invasive breast cancers. It is associated with increased tumor aggressiveness and a reduced survival rate. This biomarker is a predictive assay to assess tumor susceptibility to therapy, such as lapatinib and trastuzumab (Herceptin, a humanized monoclonal antibody that targets HER2/*neu*).

Other Cancer Biomarkers

β-Human Chorionic Gonadotropin (β-Beta Subunit)

β-hCG, an ectopic protein, is a sensitive tumor marker with a metabolic half-life in vivo of 16 hours. A serum level of β-hCG higher than 1 ng/mL is strongly suggestive of pregnancy or a malignant tumor such as an endodermal sinus tumor, teratocarcinoma, choriocarcinoma, molar pregnancy, testicular embryonal carcinoma, or oat cell carcinoma of the lung.

Miscellaneous Enzyme Markers

Lactic dehydrogenase (LDH) is a frequently measured enzyme of the glycolytic pathway. The level of LDH is elevated in a wide variety of malignancies and other medical disorders. Its level has been shown to correlate to tumor mass in solid tumors so it can be used to monitor progression of these tumors.

Neuron-specific enolase is an isoenzyme specific for all tumor cells derived from the neural crest. An enzyme increase has been detected in neuroblastoma, pheochromocytoma, oat cell carcinomas, medullary thyroid and C cell parathyroid carcinomas, and other neural crest–derived cancers. Serum levels are frequently elevated in disseminated disease.

Placental alkaline phosphatase (ALP) can be detected during pregnancy. ALP is also associated with the neoplastic conditions of seminoma and ovarian cancer.

Miscellaneous Hormone Markers

Elevated or inappropriate serum levels of hormones can function as tumor markers. Adrenocorticotropic hormone (ACTH), calcitonin, and catecholamines may be secreted by differentiated tumors of endocrine organs and squamous cell lung tumors. Oat cell carcinomas may produce β-hCG, antidiuretic hormone (ADH), serotonin, calcitonin, parathyroid hormone (PTH), and ACTH. These hormones can be used to follow a patient's response to therapy.

In addition, some breast cancers demonstrate progesterone and estradiol (estrogen) receptors, which are strongly correlated with a positive response to antihormone therapy. Patients with neuroblastoma and pheochromocytoma secrete catecholamine metabolites that can be detected in the urine. Neuroblastomas also release neuron-specific enolase and ferritin; these markers can be used for diagnosis and prognosis.

Breast, Ovarian, and Cervical Cancer Markers

For more than 15 years, circulating breast cancer antigens have been used to monitor therapy and evaluate recurrence of the cancer. Estrogen and progesterone receptors are universally accepted as prognostic markers and therapeutic choice indicators. A relatively new approach has been the use of the oncogene HER2/*neu* as a prognostic indicator and a marker related to the choice of therapy. This has been particularly useful since the introduction of trastuzamab as a chemotherapeutic agent that targets the HER2/*neu* receptor. Breast cancer patients who express HER2/*neu* in their cancers have a poor prognosis with shorter disease-free and overall survival than patients who do not express HER2/*neu*. The evaluation of HER2/*neu* has two clinical functions: (1) predictive marker for response to trastuzumab therapy; and (2) prognostic marker.

A newer and more powerful predictor of the outcome of primary breast cancer in young women has been reported. Microarray analysis of a previously established 70-gene profile has demonstrated that a good prognosis gene expression signature is a strongly independent factor in predicting disease outcome.

Epidermal Growth Factor Receptor

EGFR and human epidermal growth factor receptor-2 (HER-2, HER2/*neu*, or c-erB-2) are both transmembrane tyrosine kinase receptors expressed on normal epithelial cells but overexpressed in some cancer cells. A portion of both receptors is released from the cell surface and circulates in normal people and in abnormally high levels in cancer patients. The shed portions can be measured in serum or plasma using antibody-based immunoassays. These assays allow real-time assessment of the patient's HER2/*neu* or EGFR status and repeat testing for patient monitoring; they can be performed in a standardized and quantitative manner.

HER2 and EGFR have been the targets of considerable pharmaceutical activity to develop therapies that will interfere with the oncogenic potential of these growth factor receptors. These therapies include small-molecule inhibitors designed to target and block the function of HER2 protein overexpression. One drug, trastuzumab, is a humanized antibody that targets cells that overexpress the HER2/*neu* and has been successfully used in combination with chemotherapy to increase the efficacy of the antibody-based treatment. An anti-EGFR antibody known as IMC-225 is directed against cells that overexpress the EGFR oncoprotein.

Molecular Diagnosis of Breast Cancer

The assessment of DNA content (aneuploid, diploid) and cell cycle analysis (G0G1, S, G2, M) can be of prognostic use in certain solid tumors (e.g., breast cancer). Cell cycle analysis can be performed on fresh or frozen tissue. In breast cancer, research has indicated that low S phase and diploid DNA content are associated with a relatively good prognosis; a high S phase number of cells and aneuploid DNA content have a tendency to indicate a worse prognosis. The DNA content of a tumor is classified in order of worsening prognosis from diploid, near-diploid, tetraploid, aneuploid, hypertetraploid, and hypoploid. The ratio of tumor G0G1 DNA content to normal G0G1 DNA content is called the DNA index. Ploidy status and the S phase fraction should be combined with other indicators (e.g., hormone receptor status) to evaluate treatment options and prognosis.

In June 2011, the FDA approved the Inform Dual ISH, a genetic test developed by a Roche affiliate (Ventana Medical Systems, Tucson, Ariz). This test helps determine whether breast cancer patients are HER2-positive, which makes them candidates for trastuzumab therapy. The Dual ISH test was designed to detect amplification quantitatively by light microscopy of the *HER2* gene using two-color chromogenic in situ hybridization (ISH) in formal-fixed, paraffin-embedded human breast and gastric cancer. An advantage of this procedure is that it is possible to view *HER2* and chromosome 17 signals directly under a microscope and for a longer period.

Bladder Cancer

Bladder cancer tumor markers for the management of patients with bladder cancer have been actively investigated. Assays approved for clinical use include the following:
- Matritech nuclear matrix protein (NMP-22)
- Bard's BTA test

Almost all human tumors contain telomerase, a growth enzyme that promotes the malignant proliferation of cancer. Normal cells usually do not have this enzyme, but telomerase renews the DNA of tumor cells and permits indefinite replication.

Telomerase was first observed in ovarian cancer cells and its presence was later established in almost all cancers. It is not clear whether other vital cells need telomerase to function. For example, telomerase inhibition could adversely affect stem cells, which help produce blood cells and lymphocytes and may need the enzyme to function. Second, telomerase inhibition has not been proved or tested physiologically in human beings. Finally, a drug based on telomerase would have to reduce the ability of the cancer to spread. Screening for telomerase inhibitors and plans for future studies to discover and develop chemicals that block the action of telomerase may suggest a design of more effective anticancer drugs.

Monocyte Chemotactic Protein

Serum levels of a newer marker, monocyte chemotactic protein-1 (MCP-1) have been found to be helpful before and after vaccination with a HER2/*neu* E75 peptide plus granulocyte-macrophage colony-stimulating factor vaccine. Levels of serum MCP-1 higher than 250 pg/mL have correlated with favorable prognostic variables in breast cancer.

DNA MICROARRAY TECHNOLOGY

New developments in molecular genetics involve **DNA microarray technology** (see Chapter 14). Cancer can arise not only from mutations in oncogenes and tumor suppressor genes, but also from genes involved in cell cycle control, DNA repair, and apoptosis. Microarrays have the potential to uncover signature gene expression patterns for specific cancers and ultimately assist in the staging of tumors, prognosis, and treatment. Microarrays may help disclose global gene expression pattern differences between healthy and diseased cells as more sensitive and specific diagnostic markers are developed, such as CD44+/CD24- gene expression profile in breast cancer versus normal breast tissue. When differentially expressed genes were used to generate a 186-gene invasiveness gene signature (IGS), the IGS was strongly associated with metastasis-free survival and overall survival for four different types of tumors.

Proteomic technology uses two-dimensional polyacrylamide gel electrophoresis (2D-PAGE) and mass spectrometry. Although these techniques are not revolutionary, advances have improved their sensitivity. Expansion of computer-assisted bioinformatics has simplified the process of protein identification from mass spectra. Mass spectra are proving to be comparable to CA 125 for the detection of early-stage ovarian cancer.

In colorectal cancer, fecal DNA screening has been demonstrated to be useful. Oncogene mutations that characterize colorectal neoplasia are detectable in exfoliated epithelial cells in the stool. Neoplastic bleeding is intermittent but epithelial shedding is continual, potentially making fecal DNA testing more sensitive.

WHAT'S NEW IN CANCER DIAGNOSTIC TESTING?

Next Generation Sequencing (NGS)

Next Generation Sequencing (NGS) as described in Chapter 14, Molecular Techniques, is another step toward personalized cancer treatment. Three aspects of importance in NGS are:
1. Identification of somatic mutations
2. Detection of low levels of genomic alterations
3. Improved management of cancer treatment

Identification of Somatic Mutations

The genetic fingerprint reveals the somatic alteration of cancer genomes. Genetic changes that are associated with cancer include a single nucleotide change or structural chromosomal changes. Only some acquired genetic alterations are clinically significant.

Detection of Low Levels of Genomic Alterations

NCs has higher sensitivity of mutations in cells than traditional Sanger genome sequencing. This allows for better detection of changes occurring in only a small number of cells.

Improved Management of Cancer Treatment

Accurate diagnosis of cancer, including leukemias, is dependent on accurate molecular profiling. This contributes to improved treatment and the ability to predict prognosis.

The goal of NGS technology is to be able to quickly generate data from a small sample of tissue from a tumor.

Continuous Field-Flow Assisted Dielectropheresis (DEP)

The ability to isolate and characterize rare circulating tumor cells (CTCs) may provide critical insights into primary tumors, the process of metastasis, and monitor disease progression. Performing molecular analysis of CTCs offers a unique approach for genotyping patient-specific tumors and mutations as well as guiding treatment options.

To date, only one technology is FDA approved for use with only three tumor types: prostate, breast, and colorectal cancers. The new technology is antibody-dependent, that means the detection and capture of CTCs depends on antigen expression of the surface of cancer cells of epithelial origin, e.g., EpCAM. A new, next-generation antibody-independent technology has recently been developed. It relies on continuous field-flow assisted dielectropheresis (DEP) to isolate and recover CTCs from the blood of cancer patients. This technology has already proven to be successful in detecting and isolating a wider range of cancers in greater cells quantities, and research protypes are now being used in phase I, phase II, and phase III clinical studies. The isolation of rare cells from blood using DEP field-flow assist is based on the differences in dielectric properties between bloods, e.g., lymphocytes, monocytes, and granulocytes, and solid tissue-deprived cancer cells. This technology is revolutionary because:
1. It permits the isolation of cancer cells from all types of cancer, e.g., lung, prostate, melanoma, breast, pancreatic, and liver.
2. The higher CTC isolation and capture capability provides greater opportunities for downstream analysis of cancer cells for treatment options and monitoring of effectiveness.
3. DEP technology captures the cancer cells in a viable state that allows for additional biological testing.

Future applications of this technology are being explored to facilitate implementation of personalized medicine with improved clinical outcomes.

MODALITIES FOR TREATING CANCER

Many different modes of therapy, including angiogenesis inhibitors, which keep tumors from building new blood vessels to supply themselves with food and oxygen, have demonstrated effectiveness in the treatment of cancer (Table 33-10).

Chemotherapeutic Agents

Drugs are used in cancer therapy for cure, palliation, and research to develop more effective therapy. The mechanisms of drug action are linked to the mitotic cell cycle; thus, antitumor drugs may be placed in the following three classes:
- Cell cycle active, phase-specific
- Cell cycle active, phase-nonspecific
- Non–cell cycle active

Cell Cycle Active, Phase Specific

Drugs in the cell cycle active, phase-specific category act on the S, G2, or M phase of mitosis. S phase–active drugs are divided into antimetabolites, antifolates, and synthetic enzyme inhibitors. Antimetabolites act through the incorporation of a nucleotide analogue into DNA, resulting in an abnormal nucleic acid (e.g., 5-fluorouracil, 6-mercaptopurine, 6-thioguanine, fludarabine). The antifols act as competitive inhibitors of the enzyme dihydrofolate reductase, which is necessary for the generation of CH_3 groups required for thymidine synthesis (e.g., methotrexate). Synthetic enzyme inhibitors include DNA polymerase inhibitor (cytosine arabinoside) and nucleotide reductase inhibitor (hydroxyurea).

Table 33-10	**Immunotherapy in Malignant Disease**	
Approach	**Agent**	**Proposed Mechanism**
Active		
Specific	Modified or unmodified tumor cells, cell extract	Cellular and/or humoral response
Nonspecific systemic	Bacille Calmette-Guérin (BCG); methanol-extracted residue of mycobacterial skeletal wall, *Corynebacterium parvum, Pseudomonas* vaccine; levamisole, interferon	General immunocompetence; increased mononuclear phagocyte system activity; restores immunocompetence
Local	BCG; virus, hapten, dinitrochlorobenzene	Macrophage activation; killing of tumor with bystander effect
Passive		
Adoptive specific	Allogeneic organogenesis antibody; targeted monoclonal antibody; lymphocytes, lymphocyte extract (immune RNA transfer factor); lymphokine-activated killer cells	Removes soluble antigen or directly kills target cell; conjugated with antitumor drug or radioisotope; transfer of immunity; cytolysis of tumor cells

G2 phase active drugs include bleomycin, which is thought to cause fragmentation of DNA, and etoposide (Eposin, Etopophos, VePesid, VP-16), which is thought to cause double-stranded breaks in DNA by complexing with topoisomerase.

M phase active drugs include vinca alkaloids (e.g., vincristine, vinblastine), which are thought to inhibit the mitotic spindle apparatus, and paclitaxel (Taxol), which stabilizes microtubules.

Cell Cycle Active, Phase-Nonspecific

Drugs in the cell cycle active, phase-nonspecific category are intercalating agents, alkylating agents, and 5-fluorouracil. Examples of intercalating agents are anthracyclines (Adriamycin, Daunomycin, Idarubicin, Mitoxantrone) and actinomycin D (dactinomycin; Cosmegen, Lyovac). The alkylating agents in this category include cyclophosphamide and ifosfamide. These drugs act by distorting normal DNA through the insertion of flat, aromatic ring systems between the levels of base pairs into the DNA double helix.

Non–Cell Cycle Active

Drugs in the non–cell cycle active category can be divided into five types—alkylating agents, L-asparaginase, corticosteroids, hormone antagonists, and miscellaneous. Alkylating agents (e.g., nitrogen mustard and mustard derivatives—mechlorethamine [Mustargen], cyclophosphamide [Cytoxan], chlorambucil [Leukeran], and melphalan [Alkeran]) act by interstrand cross-linking of DNA, thereby preventing normal DNA replication. This interference is not only cytotoxic, but also potentially mutagenic and carcinogenic. L-Asparaginase inhibits protein synthesis.

Glucocorticosteroids are the most frequently used steroids. Steroids control the damaging inflammatory immune response. The target cells are monocytes and T lymphocytes. Monocytes block IL-1 production, block TNF-γ, and reduce chemotaxis. The consequences are inhibition of T cell activation, activation and recruitment of monocytes and neutrophils, and inhibition of the migration of cells to the site of inflammation. The steroids used in cancer oncology include glucocorticoids (prednisone), estrogens (diethylstilbestrol), androgens (testosterone propionate), and progestational agents (medroxyprogesterone, megestrol acetate).

Hormone estrogen antagonists (e.g., tamoxifen) competitively bind to specific cytoplasmic receptors.

Cytokines

Cytokines constitute another group of cancer chemotherapy drugs (see Chapter 5). IFN, IL-2, and colony-stimulating factors (CSFs) have been used to treat certain types of cancer in patients. Currently, IFNs are used to treat patients with hairy cell leukemia, chromic myelogenous leukemia, and multiple myeloma. IL-2 is used in the treatment of renal cell carcinoma and melanoma. CSFs decrease the duration of chemotherapy-induced neutropenia and may permit more dose-intensive therapy.

Interferon. The clinical development of recombinant IFN-α represents the most rapid development of any antineoplastic drug in the United States. IFN was first recognized as a naturally occurring antiviral substance in 1957 and identified for its antineoplastic properties. IFN-α appears to have activity in a wide range of malignancies.

Effects of Drug-Induced Immunosuppression

Drugs used to treat malignancies such as solid tumors or leukemia can have profoundly suppressive effects on the inflammatory response, delayed hypersensitivity, and specific antibody production (Table 33-11). Examples of the immune depression induced by drugs include depletion of T cells by corticosteroids, caused by the blocking of egress from the bone marrow into the circulation, and dysfunction of the antibody response, caused by folate antagonists and **purine analogues.** Thus, infection secondary to immune suppression is a major cause of death in cancer patients beginning therapy and those who are in clinical remission.

Recent Advances

Monoclonal antibody (MAb) technology began with the winning contribution of Köhler, Milstein, and Jerne, who won the Nobel Prize in Physiology or Medicine in 1984. This led to great expectation that MAbs would provide effective targeted therapy for cancer. After early enthusiasm for MAbs, clinical trials were disappointing in the 1980s and early 1990s with one exception, antiidiotype antibodies in follicular lymphoma. When success was finally observed in hematologic malignancies, the importance

Table 33-11	Effects of Chemotherapy on the Immune Response			
	Antibody		Delayed Hypersensitivity	
Chemotherapeutic Agent	Primary Response	Secondary Response	Primary Response (Initial)	Secondary Response (Recall)
Corticosteroid	0	0	+ +	+
Methotrexate	+ +	+	+	0
6-Mercaptopurine	0	+	+	0
Azathioprine	0	+	+	0
6-Thioguanine	0	+	+	0
Cytosine arabinoside	+	+ +	0	0
Cyclophosphamide	+ +	0	+	0
L-Asparaginase	+	0	0	0
Daunomycin	+	0	+	0

Table 33-12	Current FDA-Approved Antibodies for Cancer Treatment			
Generic Name	Trade Name	Composition	Antigen Target	Treatment Applications
Alemtuzumab	Campath	Humanized IgG1 monoclonal antibody with murine binding region for CD52	CD52	Chronic lymphocytic leukemia
Bevacizumab	Avastin	Humanized IgG1 monoclonal antibody with murine binding region for vascular endothelial growth factor	Vascular endothelial growth factor	Prevention of vascularity in tumor antiangiogenesis (e.g., colorectal and nonsmall cell lung cancers)
Cetuximab	Erbitux	Chimeric monoclonal-murine Fab variable portion and human IgG1 kappa Fc portion	Epidermal growth factor receptor	Colorectal, head and neck cancers
Rituximab	Rituxan	Chimeric monoclonal-murine Fab variable portion and human IgG1 kappa Fc portion	CD 20 on B-lymphocytes	Non-Hodgkin's lymphoma
Trastuzumab	Herceptin	Humanized IgG1 kappa monoclonal with murine binding region for HER2	HER2/*neu*	Breast cancer

of the antigen target specificity and developing humanized MAbs was recognized. The major success of mAB therapy has been seen with anti-CD20 MAbs. Anti-CD20 rituximab (Table 33-12) was the first MAb to be approved by FDA for use in relapsed indolent lymphoma. Today, rituximab is widely accepted to be the single most important factor leading to improved prognosis in a range of B cell lymphomas and, more recently, in B cell chronic lymphocytic leukemia (CLL). However, some patients develop resistance to rituximab, which provides a challenge for research.

Immunotherapy for tumors can take the form of active or passive therapy. Active host immune responses may be achieved by the following:

- Vaccination with killed tumor cells or with tumor antigens or peptides. New research studies have suggested that anti-CD20 MAb may induce an adaptive antitumor immune response or vaccination effect, which may underlie the durable remissions experienced by some patients after anti-CD20 MAb treatment.

- Enhancement of cell-mediated immunity to tumors by expressing costimulators and cytokines and treating with cytokines that stimulate the proliferation and differentiation of T lymphocytes and NK cells.
- Nonspecific stimulation of the immune system by the local administration of inflammatory substances or by systemic treatment with agents that function as polyclonal activators of lymphocytes.
- For the first time in the history of cancer treatment, gene therapy has apparently succeeded in shrinking and even eradicating large metastatic tumors. Inserting genes into a patient's cells enables the body to fight a disease on its own, without medication.

Passive immunotherapy consists of the following:
- Adoptive cellular therapy by transferring cultured immune cells with antitumor reactivity into a tumor-bearing host.
- Administration of tumor-specific MAbs for specific tumor immunotherapy.

Table 33-13	Targeted Therapeutic Agents in Cancer			
Classification	Gene	Genetic Alteration	Drug	Application
Nonreceptor tyrosine kinase	*ABL*	Translocation (*BCR-ABL*)	Imatinib	Chronic myelogenous leukemia
Receptor, tyrosine kinase	*ECFR*	Mutation, amplification	Gefitinib, erlotinib	Lung cancer, glioblastoma
Serine-threonine-lipid kinase	*PI3K*	*PIK3CA* mutations	BEZ235	Colorectal, breast, gastric cancer, glioblastoma
DNA damage or repair	*BRCA1* and *BRCA2*	Mutation (synthetic lethal effect)	Olaparib, MK-4827 (PARP inhibitor)	Breast, ovarian cancer

Adapted from McDermott U, Downing JR, Stratton MR: Genomics and the continuum of cancer care, N Engl J Med 364:340–350, 2011.

What's New in Drug Therapy?

The development of inhibitors to target proteins encoded by mutated cancer genes has now been achieved, with repeated success. The first victory was imatinib (Gleevec), approved by the FDA in 2001, a potent inhibitor of the Abelson (ABL) kinase in chronic myeloid leukemia (CML).

This is an important example of therapeutic targeting of the products of genomic alterations in a specific cancer. After the referencing of the genome sequence, cancer genomes have been identified for several new mutated cancer genes. Unfortunately, many mutated cancer genes do not make tractable targets for new drug development. The International Cancer Genome Consortium and the Cancer Genome Atlas are using next-generation sequencing technologies for tumors from 50 different cancer types to generate more than 25,000 genomes at genomic, epigenomic, and transcriptomic levels. This should generate a complete catalogue of oncogenic mutations, some of which may prove to be new therapeutic targets.

The list of drugs used for cancer therapy continues to grow. The new therapeutic agents target various modes of action and applications (Table 33-13).

CASE STUDY 1

LL, a 59-year-old white man, visited his primary care provider because of his need to urinate frequently and urgently. Over the last several years, his urine output had been in small volumes, with a decreasing flow rate.

On physical examination, the patient had an enlarged prostate with a smooth, uniform surface. A PSA assay was ordered. The results of the current and previous assays were as follows (reference range, 0-3.5 ng/mL):

* Current PSA level, 5.5 ng/mL
* PSA level 1 year ago, 2.3 ng/mL

Questions
1. Prostate specific antigen (PSA) is:
   a. A prostate cancer specific marker
   b. Prostate tissue specific marker

c. Indirectly proportional to tumor volume
d. Free PSA cannot distinguish cancer of the prostate from benign prostatic hypertrophy (BPH)
2. Tumor marker for prostate cancer can include:
   a. β-human chorionic gonadotropic hormone
   b. Ratio of free to total PSA
   c. Carcinoembryonic antigen (CEA)
   d. α-1 fetoprotein

See Appendix A for the answers to multiple choice questions.

Critical Thinking Group Discussion Questions
1. Is the change in the patient's PSA results in 1 year significant?
2. What is the clinical significance of the patient's results?
3. What is the expected follow-up regimen for a patient with this profile?
4. After a radical prostatectomy, what PSA values would be expected?

See instructor site ⊖volve for the discussion of the answers to these questions.

CASE STUDY 2

MS, a 65-year-old black woman, visited her primary care provider for an annual examination, including a routine pelvic examination. Although she had gained some weight since her last examination, she reported that her general health was good but that she had been experiencing some gastrointestinal problems over the last 6 weeks.

A palpable mass was discovered during her pelvic examination. A CA 125 assay and a transvaginal ultrasound examination were ordered.

The patient's CA 125 was 425 U/mL (reference range, <35 U/mL). The presence of a mass in the right side of the abdomen and abdominal ascites were confirmed.

The patient had a total abdominal hysterectomy with a bilateral salpingo-oophorectomy; 4 weeks after operation, she began a chemotherapy series. The patient was judged to be in remission for 6 months when recurrence of the tumor was noted with diagnostic imaging. Subsequent chemotherapy was ineffective, and the patient died 8 months later.

Question

1. The tumor marker of significance for ovarian cancer is:
   a. Carcinoembryonic antigen (CEA)
   b. α–1 fetoprotein (AFP)
   c. CA 125
   d. β-hCG human chorionic gonadotropic hormone

See Appendix A for the answers to multiple choice questions.

Critical Thinking Group Discussion Questions

1. Is CA 125 an effective diagnostic blood serum tumor marker?
2. Is CA 125 a specific tumor marker for ovarian cancer?
3. What is the major clinical use of CA 125?

See instructor site **volve** for the discussion of the answers to these questions.

✚ Prostate-Specific Antigen (PSA) Rapid Test of Seminal Fluid (SeraTEc, Goettingen, Germany)

Principle

The test is a chromatographic immunoassay (CIA) for the rapid semi-quantitative determination of PSA in body fluids. It contains two monoclonal murine anti-PSA antibodies as active compounds. One of these antibodies is immobilized at the test region on the membrane. A glass fiber pad downstream of the membrane is used for sample loading and transmission to a second fiber pad with the dried and gold labeled second monoclonal murine anti-PSA antibody. PSA at the sample will bind to the remobilized gold-labeled antibody and form a PSA-gold-labeled-anti-PSA-antibody-complex. The colored gold labeled anti-PSA-antibody will bind to the anti-mouse antibody at the control region and the region of the internal standard thus developing two red lines (one at the control region and one at the region of the internal standard). If the sample contains PSA, the PSA-gold-labeled anti-PSA-antibody complex will bind to the immobilized monoclonal antibody of the test result region that recognizes another epitope on the PSA molecule (sandwich complex). The binding is indicated by the formation of an additional line.

Clinical Applications

The current use of PSA is monitoring prostate cancer. This assay is also used as forensic crime scene testing for the presence of seminal fluid (semen).

CHAPTER HIGHLIGHTS

- Tumors are neoplasms described as benign or malignant. A benign neoplasm is a nonspreading tumor; a malignant neoplasm is a growth that infiltrates tissues, metastasizes, and often recurs after attempts to remove it surgically.
- A malignant neoplasm can be referred to as carcinoma or cancer.
- The incidence of cancer has been correlated with certain environmental factors (e.g., occupational exposure to known carcinogenic agents) and host susceptibility.
- Cancer often begins when a carcinogenic agent damages the DNA of a critical gene in a cell. The mutant cell multiplies and the succeeding generations of cells aggregate to form a malignant tumor.
- Proto-oncogenes act as central regulators of the growth in normal cells and are antecedents of oncogenes.
- The genetic targets of carcinogens, oncogenes, have been associated with various tumor types, largely from preexisting genes present in the normal human genome. Oncogenes are considered altered versions of normal genes that promote excessive or inappropriate cell proliferation.
- Various RNA and DNA viruses have been associated with human malignancies (e.g., Epstein-Barr virus, certain papillomaviruses).
- Viruses carry viral oncogenes into target cells, where they become firmly established. Clonal descendants then carry the viral genes, which maintain the malignant phenotype of the cell clones.
- A very different class of cancer genes was discovered rather recently. Tumor-suppressing genes (antioncogenes) in normal cells appear to regulate the proliferation of cell growth. When this type of gene is inactivated, a block to proliferation is removed and cells begin a program of deregulated growth, or the genetically depleted cell itself may proliferate uncontrollably.
- No single satisfactory explanation exists for the success of tumors in escaping the immune rejection process. It is believed that early clones of neoplastic cells are eliminated by the immune response.
- Cells, rather than immunoglobulins, are believed to dominate tumor immunity.
- Four types of identified tumor antigens are tumor-specific antigens on chemically induced tumors, tumor-associated antigens on virally induced tumors, carcinofetal antigens, and spontaneous tumor antigens.
- A tumor marker is a characteristic of a neoplastic cell that can be detected in plasma or serum. Markers may be useful in the diagnosis and selection of different treatment approaches, monitoring therapies, and determining prognosis.

- Tumor markers include CEA, AFP, β-hCG, neuron-specific enolase, prostatic acid phosphatase, and placental alkaline phosphatase.
- Various modalities are used to treat cancer. In addition to the classic therapies, newer therapies (e.g., monoclonal antibodies) are being used.

REVIEW QUESTIONS

1. Benign tumors are characterized as:
   a. Growing slowly
   b. Resembling the parent tissue
   c. Usually invading tissues (metastasizing)
   d. Both a and b

2-5. Match the following.

2. _____ Benign tumor arising from glands

3. _____ Benign tumor arising from epithelial surfaces

4. _____ Malignant tumor of connective tissue

5. _____ Malignant tumor of glandular epithelium (e.g., colon)
   a. Sarcoma
   b. Adenoma
   c. Adenocarcinoma
   d. Papillomas

6. Which of the following factors is not a risk factor in the development of cancer?
   a. Smoking
   b. Low-fat diet
   c. Obesity
   d. Sedentary lifestyle

7. Risk factors associated with breast cancer include:
   a. First-degree family history of breast cancer
   b. Pregnancy after 30 years of age
   c. Use of estrogen (oral contraceptives or hormone replacement)
   d. All of the above

8-10. Indicate true statements with the letter A and false statements with the letter B.

8. _____ Antibodies dominate body defenses against cancer.

9. _____ Tumors express antigens that can be recognized as foreign by the immune system of the tumor-bearing host.

10. _____ The normal immune response frequently fails to prevent the growth of tumors.

11. The cells involved in the immune response to tumors are:
    a. T lymphocytes, B lymphocytes, and macrophages
    b. Cytotoxic T lymphocytes, NK cells, and macrophages
    c. Neutrophils, lymphocytes, and monocytes
    d. CD8+ lymphocytes, monocytes, and basophils

12. Which of the following is not an environmental factor associated with carcinogenesis?
    a. Ultraviolet light
    b. Organically grown herbs
    c. Benzene
    d. Asbestos

13. The risk factor associated with the development of basal cell carcinoma or malignant melanoma is:
    a. Infrared light
    b. Sunless tanning lotions
    c. Ultraviolet light
    d. Strobe lights

14. Patients with Down syndrome have a higher incidence of:
    a. Leukemia
    b. Breast cancer
    c. Prostate cancer
    d. Teratomas

15. Tumor cells typically carry _____ genetic change(s).
    a. One
    b. Two
    c. Three to six
    d. Multiple

16. Cancer-predisposing genes may:
    a. Affect a host's ability to repair damage to DNA
    b. Increase cell cohesiveness
    c. Decrease cell motility
    d. Enhance the host's immune ability to recognize and eradicate incipient tumors

17. Oncogenes are:
    a. Genetic targets of carcinogens
    b. Altered versions of normal genes
    c. Detectable in 15% to 20% of a variety of human tumors
    d. All of the above

18 and 19. Match the following definitions.

18. _____ Mutation or overexpression of oncogenes

19. _____ Mutation or overexpression of tumor suppressor genes
    a. Results in the production of nonfunctional proteins that can no longer control cell proliferation
    b. Produces proteins that can stimulate uncontrolled cell growth

20. Which of the following is used to determine the risk of developing cancer?
    a. *p53* gene
    b. *c-erbB-2* gene
    c. Squamous cell carcinoma antigen
    d. Epidermal growth factor receptor (EGFR)

21. A tumor marker assay is most useful:
    a. To screen patients for malignancies
    b. To monitor a cancer patient for disease recurrence
    c. To determine the degree of tumor burden
    d. All of the above

22-24. Match the following.

22. _____ Tumor-specific antigens

23. _____ Tumor-associated antigens

24. _____ Carcinofetal antigens
   a. Cell surface molecules coded for by tumorigenic viruses
   b. Gene products resulting from gene derepression
   c. Antigens uniquely related to each tumor
   d. Probably do not produce unique antigens

25. Carcinoembryonic antigen is:
   a. An oncofetal protein, elevated in some types of cancer, that is found on normal fetal endocrine tissue in the second trimester of gestation
   b. An elevated oncofetal protein, strongly correlated with various malignancies, that is found on normal fetal endocrine tissue in the second trimester of gestation
   c. Used clinically to monitor tumor progress in some types of patients, persistently elevated even in residual disease or poor therapeutic response
   d. Both b & c

26. Alpha-fetoprotein (AFP):
   a. Is synthesized by the fetal liver and yolk sac
   b. Can be elevated in some nonneoplastic conditions
   c. Is a very reliable marker for monitoring a patient's response to chemotherapy and radiation therapy
   d. All of the above

27. β-hCG is not:
   a. Elevated in normal pregnancy
   b. A sensitive tumor marker
   c. Elevated in squamous cell carcinoma of the lung
   d. Elevated in teratocarcinoma and choriocarcinoma

28. Prostate-specific antigen is:
   a. Prostate tissue–specific
   b. Prostate cancer–specific
   c. Not useful for monitoring response to therapy in patients with prostate cancer
   d. Not directly proportional to tumor volume in prostate malignancies

29-33. Match the following tumor markers and applications.

29. _____ CEA

30. _____ AFP

31. _____ CA 125

32. _____ CA 19-9

33. _____ CA 27-29
   a. Frequently elevated in endometrially derived gastrointestinal neoplasms
   b. Most useful in ovarian and endometrial carcinomas
   c. Increased levels may indicate recurrent breast carcinoma.

   d. May be elevated in patients with gastrointestinal malignancies
   e. Should be quantitated with β-hCG initially in all patients with teratocarcinoma

34. Which tumor marker is used to monitor patients with breast cancer for recurrence of disease?
   a. CA 15-3
   b. Estrogen receptor (ER)
   c. Cathepsin-D
   d. CA 50

35-38. Match an example of a therapeutic intervention with the appropriate mode of action (an answer may be used more than once).

35. _____ 6-Mercaptopurine

36. _____ Corticosteroids

37. _____ Alkylating agents

38. _____ Vinca alkaloids
   a. Cell cycle active, phase-specific
   b. Cell cycle active, phase-nonspecific
   c. Non–cell cycle active
   d. b or c

39. Tamoxifen acts as a(an) _____ pharmaceutical agent.
   a. Cell cycle active, phase-specific
   b. Non–cell cycle active
   c. Estrogen receptor–blocking
   d. Both b and c

40. Active host immunotherapy responses may be achieved by:
   a. Transferring immune cells into host.
   b. Vaccination with killed tumor cells.
   c. Administration of tumor-specific MAbs.
   d. Administration of IFN-α.

41-45. Match the environmental factors and associated cancers.

41. _____ Benzene
42. _____ Estrogen
43. _____ Epstein-Barr virus
44. _____ Hepatitis B
45. _____ Asbestos

   a. Endometrial cancer
   b. Hepatocellular carcinoma
   c. Burkitt's lymphoma virus
   d. Leukemia
   e. Mesothelioma

BIBLIOGRAPHY

Alduaij W, Illidge TM: The future of anti-CD20 monoclonal antibodies: are we making progress? Blood 117:2993–3001, 2011.

Brugarolas J: Renal-cell carcinoma: molecular pathways and therapies, N Engl J Med 356:185–187, 2007.

Calle EE, et al: Organochlorines and breast cancer risk, CA Cancer J Clin 52:301–307, 2002.

Centers for Disease Control and Prevention: Division of Public Health Surveillance and Informatics, Epidemiology Program Office: sensitivity and predictive value of positive measurements for public health surveillance systems, 2012 (http://www.cdc.gov).

Check W: BRCA: what we now know, CAP Today 20(1):80–85, 78: 2006.

Christiani DC: Combating environmental causes of cancer, N Eng J Med 364, 791–791:2011.

Cohen HT, McGovern FJ: Renal cell carcinoma, N Engl J Med 353: 2477–2490, 2005.

Diamandis EP: Oncopeptidomics: a useful approach for cancer diagnosis? Clin Chem 531004–531006, 2007.

Eltzschig HK, Carmeliet P: Hypoxia and inflammation, N Eng J Med 364:656–665, 2011.

Friend SH, Dryja TP, Weinberg RA: Oncogenes and tumor-suppressing genes, N Engl J Med 318:618–623, 1988.

Herbst RS, Lippman SM: Molecular signatures of lung cancer, N Engl J Med 356:76–78, 2007.

Jelovac D, Armstrong DK: Recent progress in the diagnosis and treatment of ovarian cancer, CA Cancer J Clin 61:83–206, 2011.

Jordan CT, Guzman ML, Noble M: Cancer stem cells, N Engl J Med 356:1253–1260, 2006.

Karp JE, Broder S: Oncology, JAMA 270:237–240, 1993.

Kerbel RS: Tumor angiogenesis, N Engl J Med 358:2039–2049, 2008.

Kiluk J, Carter WB: Markers of angiogenesis in breast cancer, MLO Med Lab Obs 38(10):12–16, 2006.

Krontiris TG: Molecular medicine: oncogenes, N Engl J Med 333303–333306, 1995.

Liu R, et al: The prognostic role of a gene signature from tumorigenic breast-cancer cells, N Engl J Med 356217–356226, 2007.

Loeb S, Catalona WJ: PSA isoforms: the next generation of prostate cancer detection, Clin Lab News 33:12–13, 2007.

McDermott U, Downing JR, Stratton MR: Genomics and the continuum of cancer care, N Engl J Med 364:340–350, 2011.

Mehltretter S: Clinical cytogenetics, Adv Med Lab Prof 7:6–9, 20: 1995.

Oeffinger KC, Hudson MM: Long-term complications following childhood and adolescent cancer: foundations for providing risk-based health care for survivors, CA Cancer J Clin 54:237, 2004.

Pennisi E: Tumor suppressor's structure revealed, Sci News 146:36, 1994.

Plaut D: Unraveling the complexities of cancer, Adv Med Lab Prof 18:36–44, 2006.

Rhea JM, Singh HV, Molinaro RJ: Next generation sequencing in the clinical molecular diagnosis of cancer: Advantages and challenges to clinical laboratory implementation, Med Lab Obs 43:8–10, 2011.

Rhea JM, Molinaro RJ: Cancer biomarkers, MLO Med Lab Obs 43:10–18, 2011.

Roche: MabThera (Rituximab) product monograph, Hertfordshire, England, 2004, Roche.

Siegel R, Ward E, Brawley O, Jemal A: Cancer statistics, 2011, CA Cancer J Clin 61:212–236, 2011.

Thorn SH, Negrin RS, Contqg CH: Synergistic antitumor effects of immune cell–viral biotherapy, Science 311:1780–1784, 2006.

Van Dyke T: p53 and tumor suppression, N Engl J Med 356:79–81, 2007.

Woeste S: Diagnosing prostate cancer, Lab Med 36:399, 2005.

Woolf SH: A smarter strategy? Reflections on fecal DNA screening for colorectal cancer, N Engl J Med 351:2755–2758, 2005.

Wu JT: Circulating tumor markers of the new millennium, Washington, DC, 2002, American Association for Clinical Chemistry Press.

APPENDIX A

Answers to Case Study Multiple Choice Questions

CHAPTER 1: AN OVERVIEW OF IMMUNOLOGY

1. C
2. B

CHAPTER 2: ANTIGENS AND ANTIBODIES

1. B
2. D

CHAPTER 3: CELLS AND CELLULAR ACTIVITIES OF THE IMMUNE SYSTEM: GRANULOCYTES AND MONONUCLEAR CELLS

Case Study 1

1. D
2. C

Case Study 2

1. A
2. C

CHAPTER 4: CELLS AND CELLULAR ACTIVITIES OF THE IMMUNE SYSTEM: LYMPHOCYTES AND PLASMA CELLS

1. D
2. D

CHAPTER 5: SOLUBLE MEDIATORS OF THE IMMUNE SYSTEM

1. B
2. A

CHAPTER 6: SAFETY IN THE IMMUNOLOGY-SEROLOGY LABORATORY

1. D
2. C

CHAPTER 7: QUALITY ASSURANCE AND QUALITY CONTROL

1. B
2. B

CHAPTER 8: BASIC SEROLOGIC LABORATORY TECHNIQUES

1. C
2. C

CHAPTER 9: POINT-OF-CARE TESTING

1. D
2. A

CHAPTER 10: AGGLUTINATION METHODS

1. D
2. D

CHAPTER 11: ELECTROPHORESIS TECHNIQUES

1. B
2. B

CHAPTER 12: LABELING TECHNIQUES IN IMMUNOASSAY

1. C
2. C

CHAPTER 13: AUTOMATED PROCEDURES

1. A
2. D

CHAPTER 14: MOLECULAR TECHNIQUES

1. A
2. D

CHAPTER 15: THE IMMUNE RESPONSE IN INFECTIOUS DISEASES

1. C
2. A

CHAPTER 16: A PRIMER ON VACCINES

1. C
2. D

CHAPTER 17: STREPTOCOCCAL INFECTIONS

1. B
2. D

CHAPTER 18: SYPHILIS

1. D
2. B

CHAPTER 19: VECTOR-BORNE DISEASES

Case Study 1

1. A

Case Study 2

1. D

Case Study 3

1. A

Case Study 4

1. D

Case Study 5

1. C

CHAPTER 20: TOXOPLASMOSIS

1. D
2. C

CHAPTER 21: CYTOMEGALOVIRUS

1. D
2. B

CHAPTER 22: INFECTIOUS MONONUCLEOSIS

1. D
2. D

CHAPTER 23: VIRAL HEPATITIS

Case Study 1

1. A
2. D

Case Study 2

1. C
2. A

Case Study 3

1. D
2. C

Case Study 4

1. C
2. C

CHAPTER 24: RUBELLA INFECTION

1. B
2. A

CHAPTER 25: ACQUIRED IMMUNODEFICIENCY SYNDROME

1. B
2. D

CHAPTER 26: HYPERSENSITIVITY REACTIONS

Case Study 1

1. D

Case Study 2

1. B

Case Study 3

1. D

Case Study 4

1. A

Case Study 5

1. B

CHAPTER 27: IMMUNOPROLIFERATIVE DISORDERS

1. D
2. B

CHAPTER 28: AUTOIMMUNE DISORDERS

Case Study 1

1. D

Case Study 2

1. B

CHAPTER 29: SYSTEMIC LUPUS ERYTHEMATOSUS

Case Study 1

1. A
2. A

Case Study 2

1. D
2. D

CHAPTER 30: RHEUMATOID ARTHRITIS

Case Study 1

1. D
2. C

Case Study 2

1. C
2. D

CHAPTER 31: SOLID ORGAN TRANSPLANTATION

1. D
2. A

CHAPTER 32: BONE MARROW TRANSPLANTATION

1. D
2. C

CHAPTER 33: TUMOR IMMUNOLOGY

Case Study 1

1. B
2. B

Case Study 2

1. C

CHAPTER 1: AN OVERVIEW OF IMMUNOLOGY

1. e	8. b	15. a	22. a
2. a	9. d	16. a	23. a
3. b	10. b	17. a	
4. c	11. c	18. b	
5. d	12. d	19. b	
6. c	13. c	20. b	
7. a	14. b	21. b	

CHAPTER 2: ANTIGENS AND ANTIBODIES

1. b	14. d	27. d	40. b
2. a	15. c	28. b	41. a
3. d	16. b	29. d	42. d
4. d	17. a	30. b	43. c
5. a	18. c	31. d	44. a
6. c	19. b	32. b	45. b
7. a	20. c	33. c	46. d
8. d	21. a	34. a	47. c
9. b	22. d	35. a	48. d
10. e	23. d	36. e	49. b
11. b	24. b	37. c	50. d
12. e	25. c	38. b	
13. a	26. a	39. d	

CHAPTER 3: CELLS AND CELLULAR ACTIVITIES OF THE IMMUNE SYSTEM: GRANULOCYTES AND MONONUCLEAR CELLS

1. a	11. b	21. b	31. d
2. d	12. c	22. a	32. c
3. a	13. b	23. c	33. b
4. b	14. d	24. d	34. b
5. d	15. c	25. b	35. d
6. d	16. a	26. d	36. a
7. a	17. a	27. a	37. b
8. d	18. c	28. c	38. d
9. a	19. a	29. c	39. a
10. e	20. b	30. c	40. c

CHAPTER 4: CELLS AND CELLULAR ACTIVITIES OF THE IMMUNE SYSTEM: LYMPHOCYTES AND PLASMA CELLS

1. b	13. c	25. d	37. c
2. c	14. c	26. b	38. b
3. d	15. c	27. d	39. a
4. b	16. d	28. d	40. d
5. d	17. b	29. b	41. c
6. a	18. b	30. d	42. b
7. c	19. c	31. a	43. b
8. b	20. a	32. b	44. c
9. c	21. c	33. b	45. b
10. a	22. c	34. a	46. c
11. d	23. d	35. c	47. a
12. a	24. d	36. d	48. d

CHAPTER 5: SOLUBLE MEDIATORS OF THE IMMUNE SYSTEM

1. d	20. c	39. d	58. d
2. d	21. d	40. d	59. c
3. a	22. a	41. a	60. a
4. a	23. d	42. c	61. a
5. b	24. b	43. b	62. b
6. a	25. c	44. c	63. a
7. c	26. a	45. a	64. b
8. d	27. d	46. b	65. c
9. b	28. b	47. d	66. a
10. c	29. a	48. a	67. d
11. a	30. d	49. d	68. d
12. b	31. c	50. b	69. d
13. a	32. c	51. c	70. d
14. c	33. d	52. d	71. b
15. a	34. b	53. a	72. a
16. a	35. a	54. b	73. c
17. a	36. b	55. c	
18. b	37. a	56. a	
19. b	38. c	57. b	

CHAPTER 6: SAFETY IN THE IMMUNOLOGY-SEROLOGY LABORATORY

The Test Your Safety Knowledge

The crossword puzzle answers:

1. SAFETYHOOD (across)
2. ALCOHOLFOAMHANDANTISEPTIC (down)
3. 10%BLEACH
4. COLDWATER
5. TRIANGULAR, REDTAP
6. REDRIGIDCONTAINER
7. EYEWASH
8. FIREEXTINGUISHER
9. SHOWER
10. HEPAFILTERHOOD

1. a	5. b	9. d	13. d
2. d	6. a	10. b	
3. a	7. a	11. b	
4. c	8. a	12. d	

CHAPTER 7: QUALITY ASSURANCE AND QUALITY CONTROL

1. b	6. b	11. b	16. a
2. a	7. b	12. b	17. c
3. c	8. c	13. a	18. a
4. a	9. a	14. c	19. d
5. a	10. a	15. c	20. b

CHAPTER 8: BASIC SEROLOGIC LABORATORY TECHNIQUES

1. c	5. c	9. d	13. b
2. d	6. a	10. c	14. d
3. c	7. a	11. a	
4. d	8. d	12. b	

CHAPTER 9: POINT-OF-CARE TESTING

1. a	3. a	5. a	7. a
2. a	4. a	6. a	

CHAPTER 10: AGGLUTINATION METHODS

1. d	9. c	17. d	25. d
2. c	10. a	18. b	26. c
3. b	11. b	19. a	27. a
4. b	12. b	20. d	28. b
5. c	13. a	21. c	29. a
6. c	14. c	22. d	30. c
7. b	15. e	23. a	
8. d	16. d	24. b	

CHAPTER 11: ELECTROPHORESIS TECHNIQUES

1. c	5. a	9. b	13. d
2. d	6. b	10. d	14. a
3. c	7. a	11. d	15. d
4. b	8. a	12. c	16. a

CHAPTER 12: LABELING TECHNIQUES IN IMMUNOASSAY

1. d	5. a	9. a	13. a
2. a	6. b	10. c	14. b
3. b	7. b	11. b	15. c
4. d	8. c	12. a	16. d

CHAPTER 13: AUTOMATED PROCEDURES

1. b	4. c	7. b	10. b
2. c	5. a	8. a	11. d
3. b	6. b	9. c	12. d

CHAPTER 14: MOLECULAR TECHNIQUES

1. a	4. d	7. a	10. b
2. d	5. a	8. c	11. a
3. c	6. b	9. a	12. b

CHAPTER 15: THE IMMUNE RESPONSE IN INFECTIOUS DISEASES

1. d	7. c	13. a	19. c
2. b	8. d	14. d	20. a
3. d	9. c	15. c	21. b
4. a	10. b	16. d	22. c
5. c	11. c	17. d	23. a
6. a	12. a	18. a	24. b

CHAPTER 16: A PRIMER ON VACCINES

1. b	5. a	9. c	13. b
2. b	6. a	10. d	14. a
3. d	7. b	11. b	15. c
4. d	8. a	12. e	

CHAPTER 17: STREPTOCOCCAL INFECTIONS

1. b	6. b	11. c	16. c
2. a	7. d	12. a	17. b
3. d	8. a	13. b	18. b
4. b	9. b	14. b	19. b
5. a	10. d	15. a	20. c

CHAPTER 18: SYPHILIS

1. b	7. a	13. d	19. c
2. d	8. b	14. b	20. d
3. a	9. b	15. b	21. d
4. c	10. a	16. b	
5. c	11. a	17. b	
6. e	12. b	18. c	

CHAPTER 19: VECTOR-BORNE DISEASES

1. d	9. b	17. c	25. b
2. d	10. b	18. d	26. c
3. b	11. c	19. a	27. c
4. c	12. d	20. c	28. a
5. b	13. d	21. c	29. d
6. b	14. a	22. a	30. a
7. a	15. b	23. c	31. a
8. b	16. c	24. b	32. d

CHAPTER 20: TOXOPLASMOSIS

1. c	4. b	7. b
2. d	5. b	8. c
3. d	6. a	9. a

CHAPTER 21: CYTOMEGALOVIRUS

1. d	7. a	13. c	19. a
2. d	8. c	14. a	20. a
3. b	9. b	15. c	21. b
4. d	10. a	16. b	22. a
5. b	11. d	17. b	
6. c	12. b	18. d	

CHAPTER 22: INFECTIOUS MONONUCLEOSIS

1. d	6. d	11. c	16. a
2. b	7. d	12. d	17. b
3. b	8. d	13. c	
4. c	9. a	14. c	
5. d	10. c	15. c	

CHAPTER 23: VIRAL HEPATITIS

1. b	14. b	27. a	40. a
2. a	15. a	28. b	41. b
3. c	16. e	29. b	42. b
4. d	17. c	30. a	43. d
5. d	18. b	31. b	44. d
6. a	19. d	32. d	45. a
7. c	20. b	33. c	46. b
8. b	21. d	34. b	47. c
9. a	22. c	35. a	48. a
10. d	23. a	36. c	
11. b	24. b	37. a	
12. c	25. d	38. a	
13. d	26. b	39. a	

CHAPTER 24: RUBELLA INFECTION

1. c	5. c	9. d
2. b	6. c	10. b
3. d	7. c	11. d
4. a	8. d	

CHAPTER 25: ACQUIRED IMMUNODEFICIENCY SYNDROME

1. b	8. d	15. e	22. b
2. b	9. c	16. b	23. c
3. d	10. c	17. c	24. b
4. d	11. a	18. d	25. a
5. c	12. b	19. b	
6. b	13. d	20. c	
7. c	14. a	21. d	

CHAPTER 26: HYPERSENSITIVITY REACTIONS

1. d	8. d	15. d	22. d
2. a	9. b	16. b	23. d
3. c	10. b	17. c	24. d
4. b	11. c	18. a	25. d
5. d	12. a	19. a	
6. d	13. b	20. d	
7. d	14. a	21. b	

CHAPTER 27: IMMUNOPROLIFERATIVE DISORDERS

1. c	6. d	11. a	16. d
2. d	7. d	12. d	17. b
3. d	8. c	13. a	18. b
4. d	9. d	14. b	
5. c	10. c	15. a	

CHAPTER 28: AUTOIMMUNE DISORDERS

1. c	12. d	23. b	34. c
2. d	13. b	24. c	35. c
3. a	14. c	25. d	36. b
4. b	15. e	26. a	37. b
5. b	16. d	27. a	38. b
6. e	17. b	28. d	39. b
7. c	18. a	29. b	40. b
8. d	19. a	30. c	41. b
9. e	20. b	31. c	
10. a	21. a	32. d	
11. c	22. d	33. c	

CHAPTER 29: SYSTEMIC LUPUS ERYTHEMATOSUS

1. c	6. d	11. d	16. c
2. b	7. d	12. b	17. a
3. d	8. d	13. d	18. c
4. a	9. a	14. b	
5. c	10. d	15. a	

CHAPTER 30: RHEUMATOID ARTHRITIS

1. c	5. b	9. c	13. a
2. a	6. a	10. b	14. b
3. c	7. b	11. d	15. d
4. b	8. a	12. b	16. d

CHAPTER 31: SOLID ORGAN TRANSPLANTATION

1. b	7. c	13. a	19. c
2. a	8. e	14. a	20. b
3. c	9. d	15. c	21. b
4. d	10. d	16. b	22. d
5. b	11. d	17. d	23. b
6. a	12. b	18. a	24. c

CHAPTER 32: BONE MARROW TRANSPLANTATION

1. d	5. a	9. d	13. c
2. a	6. b	10. a	14. a
3. b	7. d	11. d	15. a
4. c	8. c	12. a	

CHAPTER 33: TUMOR IMMUNOLOGY

1. d	13. c	25. d	37. d
2. b	14. a	26. d	38. a
3. d	15. d	27. c	39. d
4. a	16. a	28. a	40. b
5. c	17. d	29. a	41. d
6. b	18. a	30. e	42. a
7. d	19. b	31. b	43. c
8. b	20. a	32. d	44. b
9. a	21. d	33. c	45. e
10. a	22. c	34. a	
11. b	23. a	35. a	
12. b	24. b	36. c	

APPENDIX C

Representative Diagnostic Assays in Medical Laboratory Immunology

Acetylcholine receptor (AChR) antibody: Three types of AChR antibodies exist—binding, blocking, and modulating.

Components	Reference Interval
AChR-binding antibody	Negative: 0.0-0.4 nmol/L Positive: ≥0.5 nmol/L
AChR-blocking antibody	Negative: 0%-15% blocking Indeterminate: 16%-24% blocking Positive: ≥25% blocking
AChR-modulating antibody	Negative: 0%-20% modulation Indeterminate: 21%-25% modulation Positive: ≥26% modulation

Approximately 10% to 15% of individuals with confirmed myasthenia gravis have no measurable binding, blocking, or modulating antibody.

Acetylcholine receptor (AChR)–binding antibody: Binding antibody can activate complement and lead to loss of ACh receptors at neuromuscular junctions of skeletal muscle. Useful in the diagnosis of myasthenia gravis; 85% to 90% of patients with myasthenia gravis express AChR; negative in ocular myasthenia, Eaton-Lambert syndrome, and generalized myasthenia gravis if treated or inactive.

Acetylcholine receptor (AChR)–blocking antibody: Measures antibody to AChRs that block binding of ^{125}I-α-bungarotoxin. Blocking antibody may impair AChR binding to the receptor, leading to poor muscle contraction; found in about one third of patients with myasthenia gravis.

Acetylcholine receptor (AChR)–modulating antibody: Modulating antibody causes receptor endocytosis, resulting in loss of AChR expression, which correlates most closely with clinical severity of disease.

Adrenal antibody: Measures antibody to adrenal cortex cells. High antibody titers are characteristic of autoimmune hypoadrenalism in about 75% of cases but are not found in tuberculous Addison's disease.

Alpha-fetoprotein (AFP): AFP is normally produced during fetal development by the liver and yolk sac, as well as in small amounts by the gastrointestinal (GI) tract. After birth, serum AFP levels in neonates drop rapidly and, by 6 months, the blood levels are very low. In pregnant females, AFP levels begin to rise at 12 to 14 weeks and peak during the third trimester.

AFP is a valuable tumor marker. Principal tumors that secrete AFP are endodermal sinus tumor (yolk sac carcinoma), neuroblastoma, hepatoblastoma, and hepatocellular carcinoma. In patients with AFP-secreting tumors, serum levels of AFP often correlate with tumor size. Resection is usually associated with decreased AFP levels and serum levels are useful in assessing response to treatment.

Increased AFP levels have been observed in patients with primary hepatocellular carcinoma, ataxia-telangiectasia, nonseminomatous testicular carcinomas, and ovarian carcinomas, as well as in other epithelial tumors, especially those of the GI tract. AFP is useful in the management of nonseminomatous testicular cancer patients when used with information from the clinical evaluation and other diagnostic procedures.

AFP is also increased in some benign (nonmalignant) hepatic diseases, such as acute viral hepatitis and chronic active hepatitis and cirrhosis. This result cannot be interpreted as absolute evidence of the presence or absence of malignant disease.

AFP Reference Interval

0-14 days	5000-105,000 ng/mL
15-30 days	300-60,000 ng/mL
1 month	100-10,000 ng/mL
2 months	40-1000 ng/mL
3 months	11-300 ng/mL
4 months	5-200 ng/mL
5 months	0-90 ng/mL
6 months and older	0-15 ng/mL
Adult males and nonpregnant females	0-15 ng/mL

NOTE: Results obtained with different assay methods or kits cannot be used interchangeably.

Alpha-fetoprotein (cerebrospinal fluid): Using the Roche Modular E170 AFP method, increased cerebrospinal fluid (CSF) AFP concentrations have been observed in ataxia-telangiectasia, hereditary tyrosinemia, primary hepatocellular carcinoma, teratocarcinoma, GI tract cancers, with and without liver metastases, and benign hepatic conditions such as acute viral hepatitis, chronic active hepatitis, and cirrhosis. The result cannot be interpreted as absolute evidence of the presence or absence of malignant disease. The result is not interpretable as a tumor marker in pregnant females.

AFP is a valuable aid in the management of nonseminomatous testicular cancer patients when used with information from the clinical evaluation and other diagnostic procedures. This test is approved by the U.S. Food and Drug Administration (FDA) but is not labeled for use with CSF. Results obtained with different assay methods or kits cannot be used interchangeably.

ANA: See antinuclear antibody.

ANCA: See antineutrophil cytoplasmic antibody.

Anticardiolipin antibody: Measures antibody directed to cardiolipin. The presence of antibody in systemic lupus erythematosus (SLE) is associated with arterial and venous thromboses, and in patients with placental infarcts in early pregnancy with or without SLE. Elevation of anticardiolipin antibody may be predictive of the risk of thrombosis or recurrent spontaneous abortions of early pregnancy.

Anticentromere antibody: Measures anticentromere (anti-kinetocore) to chromosomal centromeres. Most patients with CREST syndrome (*c*alcinosis, *R*aynaud's phenomenon, *e*sophageal dysfunction, *s*clerodactyly, *t*elangiectasia) demonstrate these antibodies. These antibodies are seen in about one third of patients with Raynaud's disease and approximately 10% of patients with systemic sclerosis.

Anti–DNase B antibody: High levels of neutralizing antibody to deoxyribonuclease B (DNase B) are typically found in patients after group A streptococcal infection. Because it persists longer than other streptococcal antibodies (2 to 3 months), DNase B antibody is the preferred test in patients with chorea suspected to be caused by rheumatic fever. Because it is not influenced by the site of infection, DNase B antibody is more reliable than the streptolysin O antibody test in providing evidence for streptococcal infection in patients with postimpetigo glomerulonephritis. Elevated titers strongly suggest recent or current infection with group A streptococci. Fourfold increases in titer between acute and convalescent samples taken approximately 2 weeks apart are confirmatory.

Anti-dsDNA antibody: Measures antibody to double-stranded deoxyribonucleic acid (dsDNA). Increased amounts (>25% by membrane assay) and decreased quantities of the C4 complement component confirm the diagnosis of systemic lupus erythematosus (SLE). These tests are useful in monitoring the activity and exacerbations of SLE. The absence of anti-DNA is demonstrated in about 25% of SLE patients; therefore, a negative test does not rule out SLE.

Antigliadin antibodies (IgA and IgG): Gliadin antibodies are immunoglobulin G (IgG) and IgA antibodies against a group of proteins found in the gluten of wheat and rye grains. The enzyme-linked immunosorbent assay (ELISA) for gliadin antibodies is a reliable screening test for the evaluation of asymptomatic celiac disease in prepubertal children with short stature. Celiac disease results from an intolerance to dietary gluten, resulting in small intestine villous atrophy with subsequent malabsorption and malnutrition. In celiac disease, IgG antibodies are more sensitive than IgA antibodies, but IgA antibodies are more specific than IgG antibodies. The level of IgA antibodies decreases with a gluten-free diet. IgA and IgG antibodies rise significantly during gluten challenge, sometimes several months before clinical relapse.

Anti–glomerular basement membrane antibody: Measures the amount of antibody to glomerular basement membrane (anti-GBM). High titers are suggestive of Goodpasture's syndrome (anti-GBM antibody disease) or anti-GBM nephritis. The test is useful for monitoring anti-GBM nephritis. Negative results, however, do not rule out Goodpasture's syndrome.

Anti–intrinsic factor (intrinsic factor antibody): Measures antibodies to intrinsic factor (IF). The presence of IF-blocking antibodies is diagnostic of pernicious anemia and occurs in about 60% of patients.

Anti–islet cell antibody: Measures antibodies to the islet cells of the pancreas. This test is useful as an early marker of beta pancreatic cell destruction.

Anti–Jo-1 antibody: Anti–Jo-1 antibody is found in patients with pure polymyositis, pure dermatomyositis, or myositis associated with another rheumatic disease or with interstitial lung disease.

Anti–liver-kidney microsomal (LKM) antibody: Measures antibodies to components of renal and hepatic microsomes. The presence of a high titer is diagnostic of hepatic illness and suggests aggressive disease.

Antimitochondrial (M2) antibody: Measures antibodies to cellular ultrastructures, the mitochondria. A high titer strongly suggests primary biliary cirrhosis (PBC); the absence of mitochondrial antibodies is strong evidence against PBC. Other forms of liver disease frequently exhibit low mitochondrial antibody titers.

Antimyelin antibody: Measures antibody to components of the myelin sheath of nerves of myelin basic protein. Antibodies to myelin are associated with multiple sclerosis (MS) or other neurologic diseases. Myelin antibodies are not detectable in the cerebrospinal fluid of MS patients.

Antimyocardial antibody: Measures antibody to components of the myocardium. The presence of myocardial antibodies is diagnostic of Dressler's syndrome (cardiac injury) or rheumatic fever.

Anti–native DNA: See anti-dsDNA antibody.

Antineutrophil antibody: Circulating antibodies to neutrophils can mediate neutropenia in a number of different disorders (e.g., SLE, Felty's syndrome, drug-induced neutropenia). Isoimmune destruction of neutrophils also occurs in febrile transfusion reactions and in isoimmune neonatal neutropenia. Antineutrophil antibodies may include anti-HLA antibodies.

Antineutrophil cytoplasmic antibody: Antineutrophil cytoplasmic antibodies (ANCAs) are autoantibodies specific for neutrophil lysosomal enzymes, particularly for proteinase 3 and myeloperoxidase. ANCA antibodies have been subdivided into c-ANCA (cytoplasmic) and p-ANCA (perinuclear). The p-ANCA pattern mimics antinuclear antibodies (ANAs). This perinuclear pattern reverts to c-ANCA, however, on formalin-fixed neutrophils. In about 80% of cases, c-ANCA has specificity for proteinase 3 and p-ANCA has specificity for myeloperoxidase.

Antinuclear antibody: Measures antibody to nuclear antigens. Antinuclear antibodies (ANAs) are found in 99% of patients with untreated systemic lupus erythematosus (SLE).

Anti–nuclear ribonucleoprotein antibody: Measures an antinuclear antibody (ANA), nuclear ribonucleoprotein (anti-nRNP). A high titer of this antibody is characteristic of mixed connective tissue disease (MCTD) or undifferentiated connective tissue disease. In MCTD, anti-nRNP is found in the absence of various other ANAs. Low titers of anti-nRNP are seen in about one third of SLE patients and are typically found in association with other ANAs (e.g., anti-DNA, anti-Sm).

Anti–parietal cell antibody: Measures antibody to parietal cells (large cells on margin of peptic glands of stomach). Most patients (80%) with pernicious anemia have parietal cell antibodies. In the presence of these antibodies, gastric biopsy almost always demonstrates gastritis. Low antibody titers to parietal cells are often found with no clinical evidence of pernicious anemia or atrophic gastritis and are sometimes seen in older patients.

Antiphospholipid antibody: See anticardiolipin antibody.

Antiplatelet antibody: Measures immunologically attached IgG on platelets. The presence of platelet antibodies, measured indirectly, is associated with immune thrombocytopenia and systemic lupus erythematosus (SLE).

Antireticulin antibody: Measures antibody to reticulin, an albuminoid or scleroprotein substance present in the connective framework of reticular tissue. Most patients (80%) with childhood gluten-sensitive enteropathy demonstrate reticulin antibodies. These antibodies can also be found in dermatitis herpetiformis and adult gluten-sensitive enteropathy and in about 20% of patients with chronic heroin addiction.

Anti–rheumatoid arthritis nuclear antigen (anti-RANA) antibody: Measures antibody to a component of the Epstein-Barr virus. Antibody is found in most patients with rheumatoid arthritis and in about 15% of SLE patients. Anti-RANA is not useful for the diagnosis or differential diagnosis of arthritis. Also called rheumatoid arthritis precipitin (RAP).

Antiribosome antibody: Measures the presence of antibodies to cellular organelles, the ribosomes. Ribosomal antibodies are found in about 10% of SLE patients.

Antiscleroderma (anti–Scl-70) antibody: Measures an antibody to a basic nonhistone nuclear protein. The presence of anti-Scl is diagnostic of systemic sclerosis; however, it is demonstrable in only about 20% of patients with systemic sclerosis.

Antiskin (dermal-epidermal) antibody: Measures antibody to the basement membrane area of the skin. Antibodies are present in more than 80% of patients with bullous pemphigoid, but the absence of antibodies does not rule out the disorder.

Anti-Smith (anti-Sm) antibody: Measures Sm (Smith) antibody to acidic nuclear protein. Sm antibody is demonstrated by about one third of patients with systemic lupus erythematosus (SLE). Presence of the antibody confirms the diagnosis of SLE, but the absence of antibody does not exclude the diagnosis.

Anti–smooth muscle antibody: Measures antibody to components of smooth muscle. A high and persistent titer suggests the autoimmune form of chronic active hepatitis. Anti–smooth muscle antibodies are also seen in viral disorders such as infectious mononucleosis.

Antisperm antibody: Evaluates the presence of reproductive cell, or sperm, antibodies. Half of vasectomized men and 40% of men and women with fertility problems demonstrate the antibody.

Anti–SS-A (SS-A precipitin, anti-Ro) antibody: Detects the presence of antibody to acidic nucleoprotein of human spleen extract. SS-A precipitins are demonstrable in more than 70% of patients with Sjögren's syndrome–sicca complex and are often found in a subset of these patients at risk for vasculitis. The antibody is also found in one third of patients with SLE or Sjögren's syndrome–rheumatoid arthritis, or the annular variety of subacute cutaneous lupus erythematosus (LE). In neonatal LE, autoantibodies to SS-A, discoid skin lesions, and congenital heart blocks are common.

Anti–SS-B (SS-B precipitin, anti-La) antibody: Detects antibody to acidic nucleoprotein thymus. Anti–SS-B is demonstrated by most patients with Sjögren's syndrome–SLE. Of patients with Sjögren's syndrome–sicca complex, 50% to 75% have the antibody; it is frequently found in a subset of these patients at risk for vasculitis.

Antistriational antibody: Measures antibody to components of striated muscle. Antibodies to striated muscle may be detected in patients with myasthenia gravis or thymoma or those receiving penicillamine treatment. Absence of the antibody in patients with myasthenia gravis generally rules out the presence of thymoma.

Antithyroglobulin and anti–thyroid microsome antibody: Evaluates the presence of antibody to the thyroid components: thyroglobulin, an iodine-containing protein secreted by the thyroid gland and stored within its colloid substance; and thyroid microsomes, particles derived from the endoplasmic reticulum. The presence of microsome antibodies is considered predictive of an elevated thyroid-stimulating hormone (TSH) level. A positive thyroid antibody test and an elevated TSH titer are associated with a risk of hypothyroidism. Absence of both antibodies is strong evidence against autoimmune thyroiditis.

α_1-Antitrypsin: Measures the quantity of α_1-antitrypsin, an acute-phase inflammatory reactant, in the blood. A deficiency of this protein is found if the alleles Z and S are present, moderate reduction is exhibited by the MS, and MZ phenotypes are increased in chronic or recurrent anterior uveitis and rheumatoid arthritis. The MZ phenotype is also associated with hepatoma and chronic hepatitis in adults. The ZZ phenotype predisposes an individual to the development of severe, early-onset pulmonary emphysema and liver disease in infancy and childhood.

Beta-glucuronidase: Measures the enzyme activity of the enzyme beta-glucuronidase in cerebrospinal fluid. Increased levels of enzyme activity are associated with bacterial or fungal meningitis; extremely elevated enzyme levels are encountered in untreated leptomeningeal (pia or arachnoid) metastases. Treated cases of leptomeningeal carcinoma may demonstrate decreased enzyme levels. Normal enzyme levels are usually seen in primary brain tumors and parenchymal metastases.

C1 esterase inhibitor (C1 inhibitor): Measures the activity and/or concentration of C1 inhibitor in serum. A deficiency of this protein is characteristic of hereditary angioedema. Some patients demonstrate catalytically inactive protein.

C1q: Evaluates the complement component C1q in serum. Decreased levels can be demonstrated in patients with hypocomplementemic urticarial vasculitis, severe combined immunodeficiency, or X-linked hypogammaglobulinemia.

C1q binding: Measures the binding of immune complexes containing IgG1, IgG2, IgG3, and/or IgM to the complement component C1q. High values of C1q binding are associated with circulating immune complexes that interact with the classic pathway of complement activation. This test can be useful as a prognostic tool at diagnosis and during remission of acute myelogenous leukemia.

C2: Measures the second component of complement. An extremely low level of C2 component is suggestive of a lupus-like disease that may be caused by a genetic deficiency associated with HLA-A25, B18, or DR2. Approximately 50% of those with decreased levels of C2 have autoimmune disease; the other 50% are apparently normal but have an increased susceptibility to bacterial infection.

C3: Measures the third component of complement. Extremely decreased levels are seen in patients with poststreptococcal glomerulonephritis or inherited (C3) complement deficiency. This component is also decreased in cases of severe liver disease and in patients with systemic lupus erythematosus who have renal disease.

C3b inhibitor (C3b inactivator): Measures the C3b component of complement. This component causes low complement C3 levels, the absence of C3PA in serum, and high C3b levels. A deficiency of C3b inhibitor is associated with an increased predisposition to infection.

C3PA (C3 proactivator, properdin factor B): Evaluates the level of the factor B component, which is consumed by activation of the alternate complement pathway. Assessment of C3PA indicates whether a decreased level of C3 is caused by the classic or alternate pathways of complement activation. A decreased level of complement components C3 and C4 demonstrates activation of the classic pathway. Decreased levels of C3 and C3PA with a normal level of C4 indicate complement activation via the alternate pathway.

Activation of the classic pathway (sometimes with accompanying alternate pathway activation) is associated with disorders such as immune complex diseases, various forms of vasculitis, and acute glomerulonephritis.

Activation of the alternate pathway is associated with many disorders, including chronic hypocomplementemic glomerulonephritis, diffuse intravascular coagulation, septicemia, subacute bacterial endocarditis, paroxysmal nocturnal hemoglobinuria, and sickle cell anemia.

In systemic lupus erythematosus, both the classic and the alternate pathway are activated.

C4a: Measures the level of component C4 of the classic complement activation pathway. A decreased C4 level with elevated anti-DNA and ANA titers confirms the diagnosis of systemic lupus erythematosus (SLE) in a patient. In SLE patients, the periodic assessment of C4 can be useful in monitoring the progress of the disorder. Patients with extremely low C4 and CH50 levels in the presence of normal levels of the C3 component may be demonstrating the effects of a genetic deficiency of C1 inhibitor or C4.

C4 allotypes: Evaluate the antigenically distinct forms of C4A and C4B, alleles located on the sixth chromosome in the major histocompatibility complex. Identification of C4 allotypes in conjunction with specific human leukocyte antigens (HLAs) is a marker for disease susceptibility.

C5b (C5b-9): Measures the concentration of the C5 complement component. A genetic deficiency of the C5 component is associated with increased susceptibility to bacterial infection and is expressed as an autoimmune disorder (e.g., SLE). In the case of dysfunction of C5 (Leiner's disease), the patient is predisposed to infections of the skin and bowel and the disease is characterized by eczema. In these patients, the level of C5 is normal, but the C5 component fails to promote phagocytosis.

C6: Measures the level of the C6 complement component. A decreased quantity of C6 predisposes an individual to significant *Neisseria* infections.

C7: Measures the quantity of the C7 complement component. A decreased level of this component is associated with severe bacterial infections caused by *Neisseria* spp., Raynaud's phenomenon, sclerodactyly, and telangiectasia.

C8: Measures the level of the C8 complement component. A decreased quantity of this component is associated with systemic lupus erythematosus. A deficiency of C8 makes patients highly susceptible to *Neisseria* infections.

CA 125: The CA 125 assay is useful for monitoring the response to therapy for patients with epithelial ovarian cancer. Serial testing for patient CA 125 values should be used in conjunction with other clinical methods for monitoring ovarian cancer. Elevations may be observed in patients with nonmalignant disease. A CA 125 assay result should not be interpreted as absolute evidence of the presence or absence of malignant disease.

CA 15-3: CA 15-3 is used to aid in the management of stages II and III breast cancer patients. Serial testing for patient CA 15-3 assay values should be used in conjunction with other clinical methods for monitoring breast cancer. Patients with confirmed breast carcinoma frequently have CA 15-3 assay values in the same range as healthy individuals and elevations may be observed in patients with nonmalignant disease. This assay should not be interpreted as absolute evidence of the presence or absence of malignant disease.

CA 19-9: CA 19-9 is useful in monitoring pancreatic, hepatobiliary, gastric, hepatocellular, and colorectal cancer. The CA 19-9 assay value should not be interpreted as absolute evidence of the presence or absence of malignant disease.

CA 27.29: The CA 27.29 assay is intended for use as an aid in monitoring patients previously treated for stage II or III breast cancer. Serial testing in patients who are clinically free of disease should be carried out in conjunction with other clinical methods used for the early detection of cancer recurrence. The test is also intended as an aid in the management of breast cancer patients with metastatic disease by monitoring the progression or regression of disease in response to treatment. Patients with confirmed breast carcinoma frequently have CA 27.29 levels within the reference interval. Elevated levels of CA 27.29 can be observed in patients with nonmalignant diseases. This assay cannot be interpreted as absolute evidence of the presence or absence of malignant disease and should always be used in conjunction with other diagnostic procedures, including information from the patient's clinical evaluation.

Carcinoembryonic antigen (CEA): Detects the presence of CEA in cerebrospinal fluid (CSF). An increased level of CEA in CSF is very suggestive of primary or secondary intradural malignancy. The level of CEA may decline with effective therapy.

Cardiolipin antibody: See anticardiolipin antibody.

Ceruloplasmin: Detects the level of the protein ceruloplasmin in blood. Although increased or decreased levels of this protein are associated with a variety of clinical conditions, a severely decreased or complete absence of ceruloplasmin can be demonstrated in most homozygous patients with Wilson's disease. The absence or gross deficiency of ceruloplasmin in heterozygous carriers of the gene responsible for Wilson's disease is rare.

Cold agglutinin: Evaluates the ability of antibodies to agglutinate group O erythrocytes at 4° C (39° F). The presence of an elevated titer of cold-reacting antibodies can cause acrocyanosis or hemolysis. These antibodies can be demonstrated in patients with primary (chronic) or secondary cold agglutinin syndromes caused by bacterial or viral disease (e.g., *Mycoplasma pneumoniae,* Epstein-Barr virus) or neoplasms (e.g., lymphoma, histiocytic lymphoma).

Complement activation product: Measures the protein fragments of C3 and C4 to reflect in vivo or in vitro activation. In vivo activation of complement (e.g., immune complex diseases) or in vitro activation (e.g., complement degradation) causes proteolytic digestion of these components and altered electrophoretic mobility. Assessment of these components is not considered to be of reliable diagnostic value.

Complement components (C1r, C1s, C2, C3, C4, C5, C6, C7, C8): Assess various components of complement. These components are often elevated in certain inflammatory conditions, acute illnesses such as myocardial infarction, trauma, and some infectious diseases, such as typhoid fever. Homozygous component deficiencies predispose an individual to autoimmune diseases such as systemic lupus erythematosus, chronic glomerulonephritis, infections, arthritis, and vasculitis. Determination of complement levels in synovial (joint) fluid is of value. Increased levels may be demonstrated in Reiter's syndrome; decreased levels (relative to plasma concentrations) may be observed in rheumatoid arthritis.

C-reactive protein: Assesses one of the acute-phase inflammatory proteins, C-reactive protein (CRP). CRP is increased in inflammatory conditions.

Cryofibrinogen: Evaluates cold-precipitable fibrinogen and similar plasma proteins. The presence of cryofibrinogen suggests primary or secondary disorders. Secondary disorders include acute and chronic inflammation, lymphoproliferative and connective tissue disorders, necrosis, and tumors.

Cryoglobulin: Detects the presence of cold-precipitable immunoglobulins in serum. The major types of cryoglobulins and associated conditions include the following:

- Monoclonal IgM, IgG, or IgA without known antibody specificity, or monoclonal Bence-Jones protein, associated with disorders such as Raynaud's phenomenon, myeloma, and macroglobulinemia.
- Monoclonal IgM, IgG, or IgA antibodies directed against polyclonal IgG associated with disorders such as Sjögren's syndrome, lymphoproliferative disorders, purpura, vasculitis, and macroglobulinemia.
- Mixed (usually IgM and IgG) polyclonal immunoglobulins associated with disorders such as Sjögren's syndrome, systemic lupus erythematosus, vasculitis, and purpura.

Diphtheria antibody: Measures the quantity of antibody present after the administration of diphtheria toxoid. The absence of antibody after immunization confirms a patient's inability to form new antibody (i.e., abnormal humoral immunity).

Ferritin: Evaluates the concentration of the storage form of iron, ferritin, in serum. In conjunction with abnormalities of erythrocyte tests (e.g., mean corpuscular volume, mean corpuscular hemoglobin), this assay is useful for establishing the diagnosis of iron deficiency anemia.

Histone antibody: Histone antibodies are the predominant autoantibody in patients with systemic or drug-induced lupus erythematosus (SLE). Histone autoantibodies have been detected in 20% to 55% of patients with systemic SLE and 80% to 95% of patients with drug-induced SLE. Patients with idiopathic SLE have various other autoantibodies in addition to histone autoantibodies. Histone antibodies of the IgG class have been shown to be SLE-specific, whereas IgM antibodies are found in normal healthy people and in some other non-SLE conditions. Histone antibodies occur in less than 20% of other types of connective tissue disorders.

HLA-B27: Assesses one of the human leukocyte antigens (HLAs) on the surface of lymphocytes. Detection of HLA-B27 is useful in establishing the diagnosis of ankylosing spondylitis (AS). Most white patients with AS are antigen-positive and about 50% of black patients with AS are antigen-positive.

HLA-DR: Assesses one of the human leukocyte antigens (HLAs) on the surface of lymphocytes. Detection of HLA-DR is useful in predicting a person's susceptibility to disease and in estimating adverse reactions to certain drugs (e.g., hydralazine).

Identification of combinations of HLA alleles at various loci, such as HLA-A, -B, -C, and -DR antigens, together with the inheritance of allotypes of C4 and allelic forms of C2 and properdin factor B (referred to as supratypes), has become a useful tool in diagnosing immunoregulatory abnormalities, as well as different types of clinical disease and susceptibility to infection.

HLA-DR3: Evaluates one of the human leukocyte antigens (HLAs) on the surface of lymphocytes. Detection of HLA-DR3 and an elevated titer of thyroid-stimulating hormone are prognostic for forms of Graves' disease that will not respond or relapse with antithyroid medication.

β–Human chorionic gonadotropin (β-hCG): β-Human chorionic gonadotropin (β-hCG) is found in normal concentrations during pregnancy. It can also be a valuable aid in the management of cancer patients with trophoblastic tumors, nonseminomatous testicular tumors, and seminomas when used with information from the clinical evaluation and other diagnostic procedures. Increased serum hCG concentrations have also been observed in melanoma, carcinomas of the breast, gastrointestinal tract, lung, and ovaries, and in benign conditions, including cirrhosis, duodenal ulcer, and inflammatory bowel disease.

Immunoglobulin: Measures the total immunoglobulin concentration in the serum. An increased concentration indicates hyperglobulinemia. A major decrease in concentration, immunodeficiency, causes recurrent infections, atypical arthritis, or persistent diarrhea.

Immunoglobulin A (IgA): Quantitates the concentration of IgA. Normal concentrations rule out agammaglobulinemias in childhood and selective IgA deficiency. Selective deficiencies of IgA are the most common type of immunodeficiency.

Immunoglobulin D (IgD): Quantitates the concentration of IgD). It is found in very low concentrations in serum but its functional role has not been well characterized.

Immunoglobulin E (IgE): Measures IgE. Greatly increased values can be found in patients with immunodeficient states, especially cell-mediated immunodeficiency and atopic eczema, systemic fungal infections such as allergic bronchopulmonary aspergillosis, and invasive parasitic infections.

Immunoglobulin G (IgG): Quantitates the concentration of IgG. It is the major antibacterial, antifungal, and antiviral antibody. A severe deficiency is manifested by repeated infections.

Immunoglobulin G (IgG) index: Compares the relative ratio of IgG to albumin in serum and cerebrospinal fluid. If the IgG index is increased (<0.7) and the IgG synthesis rate is increased in a specimen without oligoclonal immunoglobulins, plasma contamination may be present because of a leaky blood-brain barrier or a traumatic spinal tap.

Immunoglobulin G (IgG) rheumatoid factor: Measures the quantity of IgG antibodies reacting with human IgG. The role of IgG rheumatoid factor is considered of major pathogenic importance in rheumatoid arthritis.

Immunoglobulin G (IgG) subclass: Quantitates the subclasses IgG1, IgG2, IgG3, and IgG4 in serum. Increased levels of IgG4 can be demonstrated by patients with allergies who have normal IgE levels. A deficiency of IgG4 can be associated with severe recurrent sinopulmonary infections, symptomatic IgA deficiency, and common variable immunodeficiency (with pneumonia, bronchiectasis). In addition, elevated IgG4 is found in some highly allergic patients with normal IgE concentrations.

Immunoglobulin G (IgG) synthesis rate: Measures the rate of IgG synthesis in cerebrospinal fluid. Elevated rates are associated with demyelinating disease. Conditions associated with increased rates include multiple sclerosis, bacterial meningitis, subacute sclerosing panencephalitis, lupus-related central nervous system involvement, presenile dementia (Alzheimer's disease), IgG-synthesizing neoplasms, syphilis, cryptococcosis, chronic relapsing polyneuropathy, and acute cerebrovascular disease. If the immunoglobulin synthesis rate and IgG index are elevated, contamination of the specimen with plasma protein should be suspected.

IgM antibody (antigen-specific): Identifies antigen-specific IgM antibodies in the presence of antigen-specific IgG and rheumatoid factor. The separation of IgM and IgG antibodies is important in the serodiagnosis of congenital infections.

IgM rheumatoid factor: Measures IgM antibodies to human IgG fixed to latex particles. Elevated levels of rheumatoid factor (RF) are associated with rheumatoid arthritis, but these elevations may also be seen in other disorders. Increased RF levels in combination with high levels of C-reactive protein are predictive of aggressive rheumatoid disease. In the case of a negative RF assay, a patient may be diagnosed through clinical signs and symptoms as having seronegative rheumatoid disease. See also rheumatoid factor.

Intrinsic factor blocking antibody: See anti–intrinsic factor.

Islet cell antibody: See anti–islet cell antibody.

Jo-1 antibody: Detects precipitins to an acidic nuclear protein from calf thymus. Approximately one third of patients with uncomplicated polymyositis and some patients with dermatomyositis demonstrate Jo-1 antibody.

Ku antibody: Detects precipitins to an acidic nuclear protein from calf thymus. About 50% of patients with overlapping signs and symptoms of scleroderma and polymyositis demonstrate Ku precipitins.

Lyme disease testing: Centers for Disease Control and Prevention (CDC) recommendations for the serologic diagnosis of Lyme disease are to screen with the polyvalent enzyme-linked immunosorbent assay (ELISA) and confirm equivocal and positive results with Western blot (WB) testing. Both IgM and IgG WB tests should be performed on samples less than 4 weeks after the appearance of erythema migrans. Only the IgG WB test should be performed on samples more than 4 weeks after the disease onset. The IgM WB test in the chronic stage is not recommended and does not aid in the diagnosis of neuroborreliosis or chronic Lyme disease. Submit requests for appropriate WB testing within 10 days.

Lymphocyte mitogen stimulation: Measures the rate of DNA synthesis by isolated lymphocytes. Decreased proliferation and DNA synthesis are diagnostic of a defect in cellular immunity. Cellular immunity is frequently defective in immunodeficiency disorders, infectious diseases, carcinoma, and occasionally in autoimmune disorders.

Lymphocyte subset panel: Differentiates and measures (using monoclonal antibodies to identify cell surface markers) the quantities of T cells and B cells in the circulating blood; useful in distinguishing T and B cell leukemias and lymphomas. Determination of T cell subsets (helper-inducer, suppressor-cytotoxic) is helpful in monitoring treatment in patients with immunodeficiencies (e.g., HIV infection) or transplant recipients.

β_2-Microglobulin: Measures the quantity of β_2-microglobulin in serum or cerebrospinal fluid (CSF). Elevated levels of this protein are associated with central nervous system (CNS) involvement in patients with leukemia or lymphoma. Determination of β_2-microglobulin levels in serum and CSF are of value in the early diagnosis of CNS involvement and in monitoring intrathecal (within the spinal canal) therapy.

Myelin basic protein: Measures the concentration of myelin basic protein in cerebrospinal fluid. Elevated values indicate extensive and active demyelination of the central nervous system (CNS). Disorders in which the level of myelin basic protein can be increased include multiple sclerosis, subacute sclerosing panencephalitis, transverse myelitis, and optic neuritis. Increased values can also be observed in conditions that cause damage to nervous tissue but in which demyelination is not the primary process (e.g., radiation or chemotherapy of neoplasms in or near CNS).

Neutrophil oxidative burst assay (DHR): This is a semiquantitative flow cytometry method. Live leukocytes are incubated with dihydrorhodamine 123 (DHR) and catalas and then stimulated with phorbol 12-myristate 13-acetate (PMA). Dihydrorhodamine oxidation to thodamine by the respiratory burst of the leukocyte is measure by flow cytometry. The result is a stimulation index that is the ratio of stimulated cells versus unstimulated cells. The patient index is compared with a normal control specimen.

Oligoclonal banding—multiple sclerosis: Evaluates the presence of abnormal bands of immunoglobulins in cerebrospinal fluid (CSF). Abnormal bands of monoclonal immunoglobulins are associated with disorders such as multiple sclerosis (MS), subacute sclerosing panencephalitis, paraprotein disorders, and infections.

Oligoclonal bands are present in the CSF of approximately 90% of MS patients. A patient is considered positive for CSF oligoclonal bands if there are two or more bands in the CSF Ig region that are not present in the serum. To confirm local production of oligoclonal IgG in CSF, a matched serum sample is required. Oligoclonal bands present in CSF, but not in serum, indicate CNS production.

Oligoclonal bands and elevated levels of CSF IgG may be present in other disease states, including meningoencephalitis, neurosyphilis, Guillain-Barré syndrome, and meningeal carcinomatosis. Up to 10% of patients with clinically supported MS are negative for oligoclonal bands.

Platelet-associated IgG (PAIgG): Detects IgG found on the surface of platelets after thorough washing. Elevated levels of PAIgG with inversely proportional platelet counts are found in patients with immune thrombocytopenic purpura. Increased values can also be found in patients with systemic lupus erythematosus (SLE).

Platelet antibody: Evaluates the quantity of platelets with immunologically attached IgG by the use of fluorescein-tagged antihuman immunoglobulin specific for the Fc portion of IgG. Antibodies can be demonstrated by this indirect test in less than 50% of patients with immune thrombocytopenia and most SLE patients (82%).

PM-1 antibody: Detects antibodies to an acidic nuclear protein from calf thymus. These precipitins are found in most patients (87%) with polymyositis scleroderma. More than 50% of patients with polymyositis demonstrate the antibody, but it is detected in less than 20% of patients with dermatomyositis.

Prostate-specific antigen (PSA): Laboratory method approved as an aid in the detection of prostate cancer when used in conjunction with a digital rectal examination in men age 50 years and older. Serial measurement of PSA levels can be of value in the prognosis and management of patients with prostate cancer. Elevated PSA concentrations can only suggest the presence of prostate cancer until a biopsy is performed. PSA concentrations can also be elevated in benign prostatic hyperplasia or inflammatory conditions of the prostate. The PSA level is generally not elevated in healthy men or men with nonprostatic carcinoma.

Raji cell assay: Measures the binding of immune complexes to complement receptors on a lymphoblastoid cell line, Raji cells.

Rheumatoid factor (RF): RF may be found in patients with a variety of autoimmune diseases, as well as in up to 10% of apparently healthy individuals. RF assays may be positive in some patients with syphilis, viral infections, chronic liver diseases, sarcoidosis, leprosy, neoplasms, and other chronic inflammatory conditions. High concentrations of RF are found in patients with rheumatoid arthritis (RA) and Sjögren's syndrome. Juvenile-onset RA is seldom associated with a positive test for RF. The RF test should be used with caution in the diagnosis of RA because of its low predictive value for this disease. The percentage of positive RF assays in the normal population increases with age.

Streptolysin O antibody (ASO): In the past, the antistreptolysin O antibody (ASO) test was routinely used to provide serologic evidence of previous group A streptococcal infection in patients suspected of having complications (e.g., acute glomerulonephritis, acute rheumatic fever). Use of the ASO for diagnosis of an acute group A streptococcal infection is now rarely indicated unless the patient has received antibiotics that would render a culture negative.

An ASO performed on serum obtained during the presentation of a nonsuppurative complication that shows a titer two dilutions above the upper limit of normal indicates an antecedent streptococcal infection. It is recommended, however, to use a second test (e.g., anti–DNase B) to confirm antecedent infections. Elevated serum ASO titers are found in about 85% of individuals with rheumatic fever. When both ASO and anti–DNase B are used, the result is more than 95%.

Tetanus antibody: Measures antibody to tetanus toxoid. If a patient has a history of immunization and antibodies are not demonstrable, abnormal humoral immunity is suspected.

Thyroglobulin antibody: Aids in diagnosing Hashimoto's thyroiditis or substantiating thyroid disease in patients with nonthyroid illness using a quantitative chemiluminescent immunoassay. The assay may predict postpartum thyroditis.

Thyroid peroxidase (TPO) antibody: The thyroid microsomal antigen has been shown to be the enzyme thyroid peroxidase (TPO). The measurement of low levels of TPO antibodies in serum can be useful in the assessment of a number of thyroid disorders. More than 90% of patients with autoimmune thyroiditis (Hashimoto's thyroiditis) have thyroglobulin or TPO antibodies. Although not diagnostic, detection of TPO antibodies can aid in predicting the progression of chronic thyroiditis and in further substantiating thyroid disease in patients with nonthyroidal illness.

Antibodies to TPO have also been found in most patients with idiopathic hypothyroidism (85%) and Graves' disease (50%) and less frequently in patients with other thyroid disorders. Low titers may also be found in 5% to 10% of normal individuals.

Thyroid-stimulating hormone: Establishes the presence of hypothyroidism or hyperthyroidism, assesses and monitors thyroid status using a quantitative electrochemiluminescent immunoassay.

Thyroid-stimulating hormone receptor antibody (TRAb): A quantitative electrochemiluminescent immunoassay to discriminate between Graves' disease and toxic nodular goiter. The assay is diagnostic for Graves' disease with hyperthyroidism. In addition, it can be used to determine an appropriate course of therapy after diagnosis.

Thyroid-stimulating immunoglobulin: An assay used to detect thyroid antibodies for diagnosing Graves' disease, an autoimmune disorder.

Transplantation immune cell function assay: This assay (ImmuKnow, Cylex, Columbia, Md) quantifies the concentration of adenosine triphosphate (ATP) produced by circulating immune cells in response to phytohemagglutinin L (PHA-L) stimulation. However, this assay does not directly quantify the level of immunosuppression experienced by the patient.

BIBLIOGRAPHY

Ashwood ER, editor: Clinical testing: ARUP's guide to clinical laboratory testing. Salt Lake City: ARUP Laboratories, 2008.
Quest Diagnostics. Test menu: 2012 (http://www.specialtylabs.com).

A The nucleotide adenine.

abruptio placentae The premature separation of a normally situated placenta.

accelerated rejection Transplant rejection that occurs 1 to 5 days after a second exposure to tissue antigens because of reactivation of T or B lymphocytes.

accuracy Degree of conformity of a measurement to a true value.

acquired Incurred because of external factors; not inherited.

acquired immunity See adaptive immunity.

acquired immunodeficiency A defect in the normal immune response caused by external factors or an existing disease or condition; also called secondary immunodeficiency.

acquired immunodeficiency syndrome (AIDS) An immune disorder affecting T4 lymphocytes caused by the human immunodeficiency virus (HIV); previously called human T-lymphotropic retrovirus (HTLV) or lymphadenopathy-associated virus (LAV).

actinomycosis An infectious condition, usually of the mucosal surfaces (e.g., oral cavity) by *Actinomyces,* a bacterial genus.

activated partial thromboplastin time (aPTT) A coagulation procedure to detect factors active in the external mechanism (stage I) of blood coagulation.

activation unit The combination of complement components—C1, C4b and C2b—that forms the enzyme, C3 convertase, whose substrate is C3.

active immunity The form of immunity produced by the body in response to stimulation by a disease-causing organism (naturally acquired active immunity) or by a vaccine (artificially acquired active immunity).

acute Referring to a condition of sudden and short duration.

acute cellular rejection The type of transplantation rejection that takes place from days to weeks after the procedure due to cellular mechanisms and antibody formation.

acute glomerulonephritis A sudden inflammation of the small, convoluted mass of capillaries of the kidney, primarily the capsule.

acute graft-versus-host disease (GVHD) See graft-versus-host disease.

acute phase antibody Immune protein produced during the initial or early stage of infection.

acute-phase proteins Group of glycoproteins associated with nonspecific inflammation of body tissues (also called acute-phase reactants)

acute-phase response Form of natural immunity in which the levels of soluble proteins and other cells increase rapidly in response to the presence of an infectious agent.

acute rheumatic fever Condition in which there is cross-reactivity damage to cardiac tissue as the result of antibodies formed in response to group A streptococcal pharyngitis.

adaptive immunity The augmentation of body defense mechanisms in response to a specific stimulus, which can cause the elimination of microorganisms and recovery from disease. This response frequently leaves the host with a specific memory (acquired resistance), which enables the body to respond effectively if reinfection with the same microorganism occurs. Adaptive immunity is organized around T and B lymphocytes; also called adaptive immune response.

adaptive T regulatory 1 cells (TR1) CD4+ T lymphocytes induced from antigen-activated naïve T lymphocytes influenced by cellular regulators (e.g., interleukin-10 [IL-10]). These cells demonstrate suppressive actions.

adenocarcinoma A malignant new growth derived from glandular tissue or from recognizable glandular structures.

adenoma A tumor derived from glandular tissue.

adenopathy Swelling or enlargement of the lymph nodes.

adenosine A nucleoside found in ribonucleic acid (RNA).

adjuvant Pertaining to a substance that enhances the effect of an antigen when the substance is given along with the antigen.

adrenal medulla The inner core of the small endocrine gland that rests on top of each kidney.

afferent lymphatic duct The vessel that carries transparent liquids (unfiltered lymph) and antigens into the lymph node.

affinity Propensity; the bond between a single antigenic determinant and an individual combining site.

agammaglobulinemia The absence of plasma gamma globulin, caused by a congenital or acquired condition; also called common variable immunodeficiency.

agglutination Process whereby particulate antigens aggregate (clump) to form a larger complex in the presence of a specific antibody.

agglutination inhibition reaction A type of agglutination reaction based on competition between antigen-coated particles and soluble patient antigens. The competition is for a limited number of antibody-combining sites. Failure to exhibit agglutination (clumping) is interpreted as a positive result.

agglutinin Former term for antibody.

agglutinogen Former term for antigen.

aggregation See agglutination.

AIDS (acquired immunodeficiency syndrome) An immunologic disease caused by the human immunodeficiency virus (HIV); see earlier, acquired immunodeficiency syndrome.

albumin A water-soluble protein found in blood (serum), egg whites, and other substances.

aliquot A representative portion of a larger sample or specimen.

allele An alternate form of one or more genes that occur(s) at the same locus on homologous chromosomes.

allergen A substance that causes an allergic response when it enters the body.

allergic rhinitis Inflammation of the mucous membranes of the nose caused by a hypersensitivity reaction to environmental substances, such as pollen or mold.

allergy An abnormal or altered and often harmful response of the immune system to foreign substances, or antigens; also called atopy.

allergy march Progression of allergic disease.

alloantibody Immunoglobulin produced in response to exposure to foreign antigens of the same species.

alloantigen An antigen found in another member of the host's species. This type of antigen is capable of eliciting an immune response in the host.

allogenic (allogeneic) Genetically different individuals of the same species.

allograft A graft of tissue from a genetically different member of the same species (e.g., human kidney).

alloimmunization A recipient who is immunocompetent can mount an immune response to the donor antigens when exposed to foreign red blood cells, resulting in various clinical consequences depending on the type of blood cells and specific antigens involved. The antigens most commonly involved are classified in the following categories: (1) human leukocyte antigens [HLAs], class I, shared by platelets and leukocytes, and class II, present on some leukocytes; (2) granulocyte-specific antigens; (3) platelet-specific antigens (human platelet antigen [HPA]); and (4) red blood cell [RBC]–specific antigens.

allotype The protein of an allele that may be detectable as an antigen by another member of the same species.

alopecia Loss of hair; baldness.

alpha-fetoprotein A major plasma protein produced by the yolk sac and the liver during fetal development. It is thought to be the fetal form of serum albumin.

alternate pathway The pathway of complement activation triggered by constituents (e.g., toxins) of microorganisms. This pathway does not involve an antigen-antibody reaction to become activated.

alveolar Pertaining to an alveolus or alveoli; the thin-walled chambers of the lungs are referred to as pulmonary alveoli.

amniocentesis The process of removing fluid from the amniotic sac for study (e.g., for biochemical analysis).

amplicon A DNA fragment produced by amplification of a specific DNA sequence.

amplification A process to produce multiple copies of a specific DNA sequence.

amyloidosis A condition of intercellular deposition of an abnormal protein with a waxy translucent appearance in various tissues.

anaerobic metabolism The major non–oxygen-associated, energy-yielding pathway connected with the breakdown of glucose (glycolysis) in body cells; also referred to as the Embden-Meyerhof glycolytic pathway or TCA (tricarboxylic acid) cycle.

analyte The substance being assayed in an immunoassay.

anamnestic Pertaining to a memory response.

anamnestic antibody response An antibody memory response. This secondary type of response occurs on subsequent exposure to a previously encountered, recognized foreign antigen. It is characterized by the rapid production of IgG antibodies.

anaphylactic reaction A severe allergic reaction that can develop in IgA-deficient patients who have developed anti-IgA antibodies.

anaphylactic shock A severe allergic reaction.

anaphylactoid reaction A severe reaction to soluble constituents in donor plasma that produces edema.

anaphylatoxins Complement components C3a and C5a, which stimulate the release of their vasoactive amines by mast cells.

anaphylaxis An immediate (type I) hypersensitivity reaction characterized by local reactions such as urticaria (hives) and angioedema (redness and swelling), or by systemic reactions in the respiratory tract, cardiovascular system, gastrointestinal tract, and skin.

anaplastic tumor Tumor that is poorly differentiated by cell type but similar to embryonic or fetal tissue.

anergy A state of no immunologic response; absence of sensitivity to substances that would normally elicit an antigenic response

aneuploidy A deviation from the normal number of chromosomes.

angioedema Redness and swelling.

angiogenesis Formation and differentiation of blood vessels.

anicteric Without icterus, or lacking a yellow discoloration of the skin and sclera.

anion A negatively charged particle in solution.

anneal The bonding or hybridization of two complementary nucleic acid strands to one another.

anomaly Marked deviation from normal.

anorexia nervosa An eating disorder that occurs primarily in adolescent females.

antenatal Before birth.

antibody (*pl.,* antibodies) Specific glycoproteins (immunoglobulins) produced in response to an antigenic challenge. Antibodies can be found in blood plasma and body fluids (e.g., tears, saliva, milk). These serum globulins have a wide range of specificities for different antigens and can bind to and neutralize bacterial toxins or bind to the surfaces of bacteria, viruses, or parasites.

antibody affinity See affinity.

antibody-dependent cell-mediated cytotoxicity reaction (ADCC) A cellular activity exhibited by K cells and phagocytic and non-phagocytic myelogenous-type leukocytes. The target cell in ADCC is coated with a low concentration of IgG antibody.

antibody-mediated immunity See humoral immunity.

antibody-producing B cells See B lymphocytes.

antibody screen A laboratory procedure for testing recipient serum for the presence of antibodies to human leukocyte antigen (HLA) on potential donor transplant cells.

antibody titer See titer.

anticore window The period of time during which antigen cannot be detected in the circulating blood, such as in hepatitis B testing.

anti-DNase B (ADN-B) An antibody directed against anti-DNase B, a product secreted by group A streptococci.

antigen A foreign substance (immunogen) that can stimulate the production of antibodies (immune response).

antigen-antibody precipitin arcs A precipitin arc will form on a gel plate when a favorable antigen-to-antibody ratio exists (immunodiffusion).

antigenemia A foreign substance in the blood that can evoke an antibody response

antigenic determinant See epitope.

antigenic drift Movement of a foreign substance, an antigen, in populations of people.

antigenicity Ability of an antigen to stimulate an immune response.

antigen presentation The activity associated with conveying an altered antigenic molecule to T and B cells by macrophages. This process is necessary for most adaptive responses.

antigen-presenting cell (APC) Functionally defined cell capable of taking up antigens and presenting them to lymphocytes in a recognizable form.

antigen switching A protective mechanism invoked by parasites that involves variable synthesis of surface antigens to evade an immune response by the host.

anti-HBc Antibody to hepatitis B core antigen.

anti-HBe Antibody to hepatitis B capsid antigen.

anti-HBs Antibody to hepatitis B surface antigen.

anti–human globulin (AHG) reagent An enhancement medium to promote agglutination.

antimitochondrial antibody Antibody produced against the mitochondria of a cell.

antimyelin antibody Antibody produced against the sheath (covering) of axons and other nervous tissues.

antineoplastic agent Substance with reactive properties against new cellular or tissue growth.

antinuclear antibody Antibody produced in response to different components of the cellular nucleus in a variety of autoimmune disorders.

antinuclear factor A factor in serum that acts against the cellular nucleus.

antineutrophil cytoplasmic antibody An autoantibody divided into antineutrophil cytoplasmic antibody (c-ANCA) or antibody producing a perinuclear staining of ethanol-fixed neutrophils (p-ANCA).

antioncogene Tumor-suppressing gene that guards against unregulated cell growth.

antiparietal antibody Antibody against cells of the stomach. Parietal cells make and release a substance that the body needs to absorb vitamin B_{12}.

antiphospholipid syndrome A disorder in which the immune system mistakenly produces antibodies against certain normal proteins in the blood.

antiserum (*pl.***, antisera)** A serum containing antibodies or immune serum.

antistreptolysin O antibody (ASO) An antibody produced against streptolysin O, a hemolysin produced by streptococci, particularly group A.

antitoxin Antibody that interlocks with and inactivates toxins produced by certain bacteria.

α_1-antitrypsin An acute-phase protein.

apheresis The process of removing a specific component of the blood, such as platelets or plasma, and returning the remaining components (red blood cells) to the donor.

aplastic anemia A deficiency of blood cells (e.g., erythrocytes) caused by the lack of cell production (hematopoiesis) in the bone marrow. This form of anemia may result from exposure to toxic chemicals or drugs such as chloramphenicol.

apoptosis Programmed or normal cell death.

arteriole Small blood vessel

arteriosclerosis Loss of elasticity (hardening) in the walls of blood vessels (e.g., arteries).

arthralgia Pain in a joint.

arthritis Inflammation of a joint.

arthrocentesis Removal of fluid from a joint.

arthropathy Joint disease.

Arthus reaction A type III hypersensitivity reaction.

articular Related to a joint of the skeletal system.

arthrospore An asexual body capable of developing into another organism found in the conidia of various fungi.

ascites Abnormal accumulation of fluid in the spaces between tissues and organs of the abdominal cavity.

aseptic technique Handling of materials or specimens without the introduction of extraneous microorganisms.

aspergilloma A tumor-like growth caused by mold, *Aspergillus.*

asthma Respiratory condition characterized by recurrent attacks of dyspnea (difficult or painful breathing) and wheezing; caused by spasmodic constriction of the bronchi (larger air passages to or within the lungs).

astrocyte A nerve cell characterized by fibrous or protoplasmic processes. Collectively, these cells are called macroglia or astroglia.

asymptomatic Exhibiting no symptoms of a disease or disorder.

ataxia Irregularity of muscular action or faulty muscular coordination.

ataxia-telangiectasia Abnormal dilution of blood vessels near the surface of the skin.

atherosclerotic Pertaining to arteriosclerosis.

atopic eczema Inflammation of the epidermis (skin) characterized by redness, itching, and weeping; caused by a hypersensitivity reaction.

atopy Immediate hypersensitivity reaction caused by IgE antibody.

atrioventricular atrophy Wasting or lack of growth of tissues or organs.

autoantibody (autoagglutinin) An immunoglobulin produced against a self antigen.

autoantigen An antigen belonging to the host that normally does not elicit an immune response.

autoclaving A method of destroying microorganisms by the use of heat and pressure.

autodiluter An instrument used to make various concentrations of liquids.

autograph Tissue that is moved from one part of a person's body to another part of the same person's body.

autoimmune Against one's immune system.

autoimmune disorder A disorder that results from the immune system attacking the body's own tissue because of failure to recognize self.

autoimmune hemolytic anemia Destruction of erythrocytes by antibodies to self antigens.

autoimmunity Condition in which the body's own antigenic structures stimulate an immune response and react with self antigens in a manner similar to the destruction of foreign antigens. This process may cause autoimmune disease.

autologous A synonym for self or part of the same individual.

autonomic nervous system The branch of the nervous system that functions without conscious control.

autosomal dominant gene A genetic trait that expresses itself, if present; carried on one of the 22 pairs of (autosomal) chromosomes.

autosomal recessive gene A genetic trait carried on one of 22 pairs of chromosomes; expressed only if present in a homozygous state.

avascular necrosis Death of nonvascular cells or tissues.

avidity Strength with which a multivalent antibody binds to a multivalent antigen.

B cell See B lymphocyte.

B cell growth factor 2 See interleukin-5.

B cell–stimulating factor 1 See interleukin-4.

B cell–stimulating factor 2 See interleukin-6.

B lymphocyte Lymphocyte subset type that secretes antibody, the humoral element of adaptive immunity; also called B cell.

bacteremia Infection of the blood caused by bacterial microorganisms.

bare lymphocyte syndrome Infrequent cause of severe combined immunodeficiency (SCID).

base pair A nucleotide (adenine, guanine, cytosine, thymidine, or uracil) and its complementary base on the opposite strand.

BCG (bacille Calmette-Guérin) Tuberculosis vaccine also used to stimulate the immune system in patients with certain types of cancer.

Bence-Jones (BJ) protein The abnormal protein frequently found in the urine of patients with multiple myeloma. It precipitates at 50° C (122° F), disappears at 100° C, and reappears on cooling to room temperature.

benign Nonmalignant or noncancerous.

beta hemolysis A clearing or disruption of red blood cells in agar because of the exotoxins produced by certain bacteria (e.g., group A beta streptococci).

beta pancreatic cells Insulin-producing cells of the pancreas.

bilirubin A breakdown product of erythrocyte catabolism. If increased levels of this substance accumulate in the circulation, it will be deposited in lipid-rich tissues such as the brain and manifested by the skin and sclera as jaundice (icterus).

biohazard A dangerous condition caused by an infectious microorganism.

biologic response modifiers Substances that boost, direct, or restore normal immune defenses.

biometrics Refers in biologic studies to the collection, synthesis, analysis, and management of quantitative data on biological communities; also known as biologic statistics.

biosafety policies Rules to ensure safety when exposed to or working with disease-causing organisms.

blast transformation The conversion of a B lymphocyte into a plasma cell.

blotting Transfer or fixation of nucleic acids onto a solid matrix (e.g., nitrocellulose) so that the nucleic acids may be hybridized with a probe.

bond Physiochemical forces that hold atoms together to form molecules.

bone marrow The spongy material inside bones that contains hematopoietic (blood-forming) tissues.

bronchiectasis A chronic inflammatory condition of the airways (bronchi) caused by dilation and loss of elasticity of the vessel walls.

Bruton's disorder See X-linked agammaglobulinemia.

Burkitt's lymphoma An undifferentiated malignant neoplastic disorder of the lymphoid tissues.

bursa of Fabricius An outgrowth of the cloaca in birds that becomes the site of formation of lymphocytes with B cell characteristics.

C The nucleotide cytosine.

C1 complex Interlocking enzyme system consisting of C1q, C1r, and C1s.

C3 The most abundant and important component of complement; produces a small (C3a) and large peptide (C3b) when activated.

C5 The complement component split by C3b into C5a and C5b.

C6789 The lytic complement sequence that is activated by C5b and terminates in lysing the cell membrane; called the membrane attack complex (MAC).

cachexia Physical wasting away of the body (e.g., as in AIDS patients).

capture assay A type of immunoassay that uses two antibodies. The first antibody binds the antigen to solid phase; the second antibody has an enzyme label and acts as an indicator.

carboxy-terminal region A section of an antibody molecule.

carcinoma Another term for a malignant neoplasm of epithelial origin (cancer).

carcinoma in situ Cancer that has not spread beyond the origin tissue mass (organ) in which it is detected.

cardiolipid Antibody that is a subset of antiphospholipid antibodies; also referred to as lupus anticoagulant antibody.

carditis Inflammation of heart muscle.

carcinoembryonic antigen (CEA) A detectable tumor marker.

carrier molecule A molecule that when coupled to a hapten, makes the hapten capable of stimulating an immune response.

carrier state Asymptomatic condition of harboring an infectious organism. The term may also refer to a heterozygous individual or the carrier of a recessive gene, who does not have symptoms of a disease.

caseous necrosis Soft cheeselike tissue that forms as the result of tissue death.

catarrhal symptoms Term previously used to describe the manifestations of inflammation of the mucous membranes, particularly of the head or throat, with an accompanying discharge.

catecholamine Biologically active amine, such as epinephrine and norepinephrine, that has a marked effect on the nervous and cardiovascular systems, metabolic rate and temperature, and smooth muscle.

cation A positively charged particle in solution.

CD4 The protein receptor on the surface of a target cell to which the gp120 protein of the HIV viral envelope binds.

CD markers Molecules on the surface of lymphocytes that identify them to other immune system cells; also called cell surface markers.

cDNA Complementary DNA, produced from mRNA using reverse transcriptase.

cell adhesion molecule (CAM) Protein located on the cell surface involved with binding with other cells or with the extracellular matrix in a process called cell adhesion.

cell-mediated immunity The type of immunity dependent on the link between T cells and macrophages.

cell flow cytometry Procedure using computerized equipment for the separation, classification, and quantitation of particles (e.g., blood cells or antibodies). The technique is based on passing a monocellular stream of particles through a beam of laser light. The particles are categorized by size and then analyzed. Monoclonal antibodies can be used for the determination of specific subsets of cells. Subsets of cells can be identified by clusters of differentiation (CD) surface membrane markers; also called flow cell cytometry.

cell surface marker The expression of antigens on the membrane of a cell; detectable by flow cell cytometry.

cellulitis Inflammation within solid tissues, usually loose tissues beneath the skin; manifested by redness, pain, swelling (edema), and interference with function.

central tolerance Condition that develops in the thymus during fetal development and eliminates cells that react with self antigens.

centromere The constricted portion of a chromosome.

cerebrospinal fluid (CSF) The fluid formed by the choroid plexus in the ventricles of the brain; found within the subarachnoid space, central canal of the spinal cord, and four ventricles of the brain.

cerebrovascular accident (CVA) Stroke.

ceruloplasmin Substance often measured as copper in the blood.

cestode Tapeworm.

CH Constant region of the immunoglobulin heavy-chain gene locus.

chancre A lesion that begins as a papule and erodes into a red ulcer. It is the primary wound of syphilis; occurs at the site of entry of the spirochete.

Chédiak-Higashi syndrome A rare inherited autosomal recessive trait characterized by the presence of large granules and inclusion bodies in the cytoplasm of leukocytes.

chemiluminescence Luminescence in which the light emission is caused by the products of a specific chemical reaction.

chemokines A large family of homologous cytokines.

chemotactic factor See interleukin-8.

chemotaxis Release of substances that attract phagocytic cells as the result of traumatic or microbial damage.

chimera Organism whose bodies contain different cell populations of the same or different species, such as in the exchange of tissue between fraternal twins before birth so that each recognizes tissue antigens of the other and accepts them, or as the result of transplantation of donor cells such as bone marrow.

chimerism Different cell populations of the same or different species.

cholestasis Blockage or suppression of the flow of bile.

choreoathetosis A condition characterized by rapid, jerky, involuntary movements or slow, irregular, twisting, snakelike movements seen mostly in the upper extremities (e.g., hands, fingers).

chorioepithelioma A tumor arising from chorionic epithelium.

chorioretinitis Inflammation of the choroid (middle layer) and retina (innermost layer) of the eye.

chromaffin cell A deep-staining type of cell in adrenal tissue.

chromophore A chemical group that absorbs light at a specific frequency and consequently gives color to a molecule.

chromosomes Strands of DNA that carry all the genes, with 23 pairs of chromosomes in each human cell.

chronic Referring to a condition that persists for a long time.

chronic glomerulonephritis An inflammation of long duration of the small convoluted mass of capillaries of the kidney, primarily the capsule.

chronic GVHD See graft-versus-host disease (GVHD); chronic rejection of a transplanted graft over a longer period of time.

chyle A milky bodily fluid consisting of lymph and emulsified fats, or free fatty acids (FFAs); from the Greek *chylos,* meaning juice.

circulating immune complex Antigen-antibody in the blood flow.

class I MHC (HLA) molecules Proteins coded for by genes at three loci (A, B, C) in the major histocompatibility complex (MHC). These molecules are expressed on all nucleated cells and are important to consider in tissue typing for transplantation.

class II MHC (HLA) molecules Proteins coded for by the DR, DP, and DQ loci of the major histocompatibility complex (MHC). These molecules are found on B lymphocytes, activated T lymphocytes, monocytes, macrophages, dendritic cells, and endothelium.

class switching Change in isotype of antibody produced after a B lymphocyte has encountered an antigen.

classical pathway A pathway of complement activation that is launched with an antigen-antibody interaction.

clinical manifestations Observable abnormalities.

clonal expansion Multiplication of a clone of identical cells.

clonal selection Activation and proliferation of a lymphocyte when an individual lymphocyte encounters an antigen that binds to its unique antigen receptor site.

clone Group of cells descended from the same single cell (daughter cells), all having identical phenotypes and growth characteristics as the original precursor cell.

cluster of differentiation (CD) A surface marker that identifies a particular cell line or stage of cellular differentiation with a defined structure; can be identified with a group or cluster of monoclonal antibodies (MAbs).

coagglutination (CoA) A variation of latex agglutination. Visible agglutination of the coated particles indicate an antigen-antibody reaction.

coalesce A fusion of components.

coefficient of variation A statistical quality control calculation of variation from the average (mean).

collagen A protein found in skin, tendons, bone, and cartilage.

collagen disease Disease of the skin, tendons, bone, or cartilage, such as systemic lupus erythematosus and rheumatoid arthritis.

collecting tubule A small duct that receives urine from several renal tubules.

colloid A gelatinous or mucoid-like substance.

colloidal charcoal An insoluble indicator used in testing for syphilis.

colony-stimulating factors (CSFs) Molecular substances that stimulate hematopoietic progenitor cells to form colonies.

colorimetric reaction Chemical reaction that results in a change in color.

combining site The portion of the Fab molecule that possesses specificity.

common immunocyte Any cell of the lymphoid series that can react with an antigen to produce an antibody or participate in cell-mediated reactions.

common thymocyte Lymphocytes arising in the thymus that precede mature thymocytes (e.g., OKT 10, OKT 6 surface antigen) in development.

competitive immunoassay A form of immunoassay in which unlabeled and labeled antigens compete for a limited number of binding sites on a reagent antibody.

complement A group of soluble blood proteins (enzymes) consisting of C1 to C9. It is present in the blood and can produce inflammatory effects and lysis of cells when activated.

complement cascade The sequential activation of plasma proteins that cause lysis of a cell.

complement-dependent cytotoxicity (CDC) Killing of cells as the result of attachment of antibody with activation of complement.

complement fixation This traditional procedure detects the presence of a specific antigen-antibody reaction by causing the in vitro activation of complement. If complement is not fixed, lysis of the preantibody-coated reagent erythrocytes occurs.

complement receptor A part of the mediated innate immune system. Complement receptors are responsible for detecting pathogens by mechanisms not mediated by antibodies. Their activity can be triggered by specific antigens. Therefore, complement (a group of proteins in the serum that help achieve phagocytosis and lysis of antigens) is also part of the humoral immune system.

complete antibody Former term used for an IgM antibody.

concomitant Existing at the same time (a condition).

confidence limits Statistical standard deviations from a mean. Interval estimates are often desirable because the estimate of the mean varies from sample to sample.

congenital Pertaining to a condition present at birth.

congenital rubella syndrome See rubella syndrome.

conjugate Paired or joined; a laboratory substrate prepared by joining two substances, such as fluorescein to an immunoglobulin molecule.

conjugate vaccine A vaccine in which easily recognizable proteins are linked to the outer coat of the disease-causing organism to stimulate an immune response.

constant region The part of an antibody's structure that is the same in all antibodies of the same class.

control specimen A specimen such as serum with known assay values that is tested concurrently with patient specimens of unknown values.

convalescence The time of recovery from conditions such as illness, injury, or surgery; convalescent period.

convalescent phase antibodies A protein (antibody) response to an infectious agent after the acute phase has receded.

convalescent sera See convalescent phase antibodies.

convertase An enzyme associated with the complement system.

Coombs' test Traditional term for the anti–human globulin (AHG) test that can be performed as direct and indirect AHG procedures.

cooperativity Interaction of specific cellular elements (lymphocytes), cell products (immunoglobulins and cytokines), and nonlymphoid elements.

corpus luteum A yellow-colored mass of progesterone secreting endocrine tissue.

cortical-hypothalamic-pituitary axis Interrelated association among the outer layer of the brain, the structure located at the base of the cerebrum, small endocrine gland, and the pituitary gland.

corticosteroid Any hormone produced by the outer layer of the gland located on top of each kidney.

cosmopolitan Referring to a wide distribution.

counterimmunoelectrophoresis (CIE) A procedure in which oppositely charged antigen and antibody are propelled toward each other by an electrical field. This allows detection of concentrations of antigens and antibodies 10 times smaller than the lowest concentrations measurable by immunodiffusion or double diffusion.

covalent Pertaining to a type of chemical bond (*adv.*, covalently).

cranial nerve neuritis Inflammation of any of the nerves attached to the brain that pass through the openings of the skull.

C-reactive protein (CRP) A nonspecific, acute-phase, reactant glycoprotein.

cross-immunity A phenomenon that occurs when an antibody reacts with an antigen structurally similar to the original antigen that induced antibody production.

cross-reactivity A condition in which some of the determinants of an antigen are shared by similar antigenic determinants on the surface of apparently unrelated molecules, and a proportion of these antigens interact with the other kind of antigen.

cryoglobulin An abnormal protein that precipitates or forms a gel at 0° C (32° F) and redissolves at warm temperatures.

cryoglobulinemia Pertaining to a condition in which cold-reacting proteins (globulins) are found in the circulating blood.

cryptic plasmid A concealed or unrecognized extrachromosomal ring of DNA that replicates autonomously, especially in bacteria.

cryptogenic cirrhosis A condition of the liver with an obscure or doubtful cause.

cutaneous Referring to the skin (epidermis).

cutaneous systemic infection An infection involving all of the skin.

cutaneous T cell lymphoma Malignant neoplasm with epidermal manifestations that involves the T subset of lymphocytes.

cuvette A calibrated type of glass tube used for reading the color of a solution with a spectrophotometer.

cytogenetics The branch of genetics focusing on the study of chromosomes.

cytokine Polypeptide product of activated cells (lymphocytes or macrophages) that controls a variety of cellular responses and thereby regulates the immune system.

cytolysis Rupture of a cell membrane with release of the cellular cytoplasm.

cytomegalovirus A herpes family virus that can cause congenital infections in the newborn and a clinical syndrome resembling infectious mononucleosis.

cytopathology The study of abnormal cells.

cytopenia Severe decrease in the number of hematologic cells.

cytotoxic Able to kill cells.

cytotoxic T cell Subset type of lymphocyte that can kill other cells infected by viruses, fungi, and some types of bacteria or cells transformed by malignancy.

cytotoxicity A condition in which macrophages can kill some targets (possibly tumor cells) without phagocytizing them.

Dane particle The intact, double-shelled, hepatitis B virus.

darkfield microscopy A specialized type of microscopic examination.

Davidsohn differential test The classic laboratory reference test for the diagnosis of infectious mononucleosis.

definitive host A host in which the parasite reaches maturity and, if possible, reproduces sexually.

delta agent An RNA virus that causes hepatitis but requires the coexistence of hepatitis B infection.

delayed hypersensitivity An exaggerated immune response caused by chemicals released by sensitized T cells; usually peaks at 24 to 48 hours after reexposure to the antigen; also called a type IV hypersensitivity reaction.

dementia An irreversible condition of organic loss of mental function.

denaturation The process of heating and separating two DNA strands.

denatured DNA Double-stranded helix that separates into two single strands. Hydrogen bonds can break from heat, pH, nonphysiologic concentration of salts, organic solvents (e.g., alcohol), or detergents.

dendritic cells The weakly phagocytic Langerhans cell of the epidermis and similar nonphagocytic cells in the lymphoid follicles of the spleen and lymph nodes. These cells may be the main agent of T cell stimulation, but their precise region has not yet been determined.

deoxyribonucleic acid See DNA.

dermatitis An inflammation of the skin.

dermatome A section that produces skin.

dermatomyositis An inflammatory condition included in the collage disorders in which the skin, subcutaneous tissues, and muscles are involved. Necrosis of the muscles is characteristic.

desensitization A treatment for allergies such as hay fever that involves stimulating the buildup of IgG antibodies to block the effects of IgE; also called hyposensitization.

dextran A product produced by fermenting sucrose (sugar); used as a blood volume substitute.

DH Diversity region of the immunoglobulin heavy-chain gene locus.

diagnosis Determination of the nature of a disorder or disease.

diapedesis Ameboid movement of cells such as monocytes and polymorphonuclear neutrophils to a site of inflammation in phagocytosis.

DiGeorge syndrome An immunodeficiency disease resulting from failure of the parathyroid and thymus glands to develop before birth.

diluent One of two parts of a solution; also called the solvent. The solute is added as the second part of a solution.

dilution Reducing the concentration of a chemical constituent in a solution.

dimer A chemical structure formed from two subunits.

direct agglutination Macroscopic clumping that can be observed because particulate reagents are used to indicate the presence of an antigen-antibody reaction; a general term.

direct antiglobulin test (DAT) A test performed to detect the coating of erythrocytes with antibodies.

direct fluorescent antibody (DFA) test A microscopic technique that conjugates antibody to detect an antigen-antibody reaction.

discoid lupus Term used to differentiate the benign dermatitis of cutaneous lupus from the cutaneous involvement of systemic lupus erythematosus (SLE).

disease A pathologic condition characterized by a specific and unique set of signs and symptoms.

disorder An abnormality of body function.

distal tubules Ducts in the kidney located farthest from the center of the structure.

DNA A molecule found in a cell's nucleus that carries the cell's genetic information (genome); the nucleic acid that forms the main structure of genes. The sugar of this nucleic acid is deoxyribose. DNA (deoxyribonucleic acid) is the primary genetic material of all cellular organisms and DNA viruses.

DNA amplification Ultrasensitive polymerase chain reaction (PCR) technique for the detection of HIV that amplifies minute amounts of viral nucleic acid in the DNA of lymphocytes.

DNA dot blot hybridization A rapid molecular biology technique used to detect the presence of a specific DNA in a specimen.

DNA sequencing Determining the order of nucleotides in a segment of DNA.

domain Basic unit of an antibody structure. Variations among the domains of different antibody molecules are responsible for differences in antigen binding and in biologic function.

dot blot Technique used to determine whether a particular nucleotide sequence is present in a patient's specimen.

double immunodiffusion method Ouchterlony double immunodiffusion is a simple, rather dated method used to detect extractable nuclear antigens (also known as agar gel immunodiffusion or passive double immunodiffusion)

downregulation Reduction in the number of receptors on the surface of target cells, making the cells less sensitive to a hormone or another agent.

downstream Toward the 3′ end of a nucleic acid molecule.

dsDNA Double-stranded DNA.

Dᵘ An outdated term now referred to as weak D, a phenotype of the Rh blood group system.

Dᵘ rosette test An older procedure that uses D-positive indicator erythrocytes to form identifiable rosettes around individual D-positive fetal cells that may be in the maternal circulation.

dyscrasia A term formerly used to indicate an abnormal mixture of the "four humors"; now it is somewhat synonymous with a disease or pathologic condition.

dysgammaglobulinemia A disorder involving an abnormality in the structure, distribution, or frequency of serum gamma globulins.

dysplastic Pertaining to faulty or abnormal development of body tissue (dysplasia).

dyspnea Difficulty in breathing.

dysproteinemia An abnormality of the protein content of the blood.

early antigen (EA) An expressed by B lymphocytes infected with Epstein-Barr virus in infectious mononucleosis. EA consists of early antigen-diffuse (EA-D), which is found in the nucleus and cytoplasm of B cells, and early antigen-restricted (EA-R), which is usually found as a mass only in the cytoplasm.

early thymocyte Immature T cell in the thymus that precedes the common thymocyte in maturational development.

echinococcal Pertaining to a genus of tapeworm *(Echinococcus)*.

ectopic pregnancy The gestation of a fertilized egg outside the uterus, most often in the fallopian tube.

eczema An inflammatory condition of the skin (epidermis) characterized by redness, weeping, and itching.

edema (edematous) Accumulation of fluid in the tissues that produces swelling.

EDTA Ethylenediaminetetraacetic acid, disodium salt; a common in vitro anticoagulant.

effector cells Active cells of the immune system responsible for destroying or controlling foreign antigens.

effector T cells See effector cells.

efferent lymphatic duct The tubule through which semitransparent fluid (lymph) and possibly antigens exit the lymph node.

efficacy Ability of a vaccine to produce the desired clinical effect at the optimal dosage and schedule.

EIA See enzyme immunoassay.

electromagnetic spectrum Form of radiation, including visible light ranging from long to short wavelengths.

electrophoresis A method of separating macromolecules such as proteins on the basis of their net electrical charge and size (molecular weight). See also serum electrophoresis.

ELISA See enzyme-linked immunosorbent assay.

eluate The product obtained by purposely manipulating a red cell suspension to break an antigen-antibody complex, with the subsequent release of the antibody into the surrounding medium.

elution Removal of antibodies attached to antigen receptors on the red blood cell membrane.

embryogenesis The growth and development of a living organism. In human beings, this period is from the second to approximately the eighth week of gestation.

encephalopathy Any degenerative disease of the brain.

endemic Present at all times, such as the continual existence of a specific microorganism in a population of individuals or in a geographic location.

endocarditis An inflammation of the inner lining of the heart (endocardium).

endogenous Originating or produced within an organism, tissue, or cell.

endonuclease An enzyme that breaks down a nucleotide chain.

endoplasmic reticulum A component of a cell associated with protein production.

endosome A vesicle that has lost its coat.

endothelial cell The type of epithelial cell that lines body cavities such as the serous cavities, heart, and blood and lymphatic vessels.

endotoxemia A condition of having bacterial cell wall heat-stable toxins in the circulation. These toxins are pyrogenic and increase capillary permeability.

endotoxin A heat-stable toxin present in intact lipopolysaccharide complexes in the bacterial cell wall.

end-stage renal disease An irreversible pathologic condition of the kidneys.

enterocolitis An inflammation of the small intestine and colon.

env gene A structural gene of a retrovirus such as HIV that encodes for a polyprotein that contains numerous glycosylation sites. In HIV, the envelope proteins gp160, gp120 and gp41 are encoded.

enzyme immunoassay (EIA) A general term for quantitative testing of antigens and antibodies. The method uses color-changed products of an enzyme-substrate interaction or inhibition to measure the antigen-antibody reactions; also called ELISA.

enzyme-linked immunosorbent assay (ELISA) A quantitative method of laboratory analysis. Antigen or antibody can be measured using enzyme-labeled antibody or antigen bound to a solid support. A direct ELISA measures antigen using competition for antibody-binding sites between enzyme-labeled antigen and patient antigen. An indirect ELISA measures antibody concentrations using bound antigen to interact with specimen antibodies.

eosinophilia An increase in the numbers of certain blood cells, the eosinophils.

epidemic A situation where a condition extremely exceeds the usual number of cases (e.g., infectious diseases).

epidemiologic Pertaining to epidemiology.

epidemiology The study of an infectious disease or conditions in many individuals in the same geographic location at the same time.

epilepsy A transient disturbance of nervous system function caused by abnormal electrical activity in the brain.

episomal Pertaining to a replicating form; see episomal DNA.

episomal DNA An accessory, extrachromosome-replicating genetic element.

epithelial cell Cell of a type of body tissue that forms the covering of external and internal surfaces or composes a body structure, such as glandular epithelium.

epitope A single antigenic determinant. It is functionally the portion of an antigen that combines with an antibody paratope, the part of the antibody molecule that makes contact with the antigenic determinant.

Epstein-Barr virus (EBV) A human DNA herpesvirus found in association with leukocytes and B lymphocytes. It is the causative agent of infectious mononucleosis in the West countries and Burkitt's lymphoma in Africa.

equivalence The relative concentration of antibody and antigen that produces the maximal binding of antibody to antigen.

erysipelas A febrile disease caused by group A streptococci. The disease is manifested by inflammation and redness of the skin and subcutaneous tissues, fever, vomiting, and/or headache.

erythema Redness of the skin caused by inflammation, infection, or injury.

erythema migrans (EM) Characteristic red inflammation of *Borrelia* infection.

erythematous Characterized by erythema (redness).

erythrocyte The scientific term for a red blood cell (RBC).

erythrocyte sedimentation rate (ESR) A nonspecific measurement reflecting inflammation; rate at which red blood cells form a sediment in 1 hour.

erythrogenic toxin A substance producing redness.

erythropoiesis The process of producing red blood cells (RBCs).

estrogen A female sex hormone, such as estradiol, estriol, and estrone.

etiologic agent The substance, agent, or condition responsible for causing an abnormal condition.

etiology The study of the cause(s) of disease; also, the cause or origin of a disease.

exchange transfusion The replacement of an infant's coated erythrocytes with donor blood until the total blood volume is transferred.

excoriation Severe scratching leading to disruption of the integrity of the skin.

exocytosis Release of cellular substances contained in vesicles.

exogenous Pertaining to a source outside of a cell or system.

exogenous factors See exogenous.

exogenous insulin Insulin not produced by a person's own pancreas.

exogenous reservoir A storage place outside of a system.

exon polynucleotide Sequence coding for protein synthesis.

exotoxin A soluble poisonous substance produced by growth of microorganisms.

extra-articular Outside of a joint.

extracutaneous Outside of the skin.

extramedullary hematopoiesis Production of erythrocytes outside the bone marrow, which can result in enlargement of the liver and spleen.

extrathecal synthesis Produced outside an enveloping sheath.

extravasation Forcing out of a vessel or channel (extravasating).

extravascular destruction The destruction of an erythrocyte through phagocytosis and digestion by macrophages of the mononuclear phagocyte system.

extravascular hemolysis The phagocytizing and catabolizing of erythrocytes by the mononuclear phagocyte system.

F(ab)2 Portion of an IgG molecule produced by pepsin digestion that contains two Fab fragments; two light chains and portions of two heavy chains are joined by disulfide bonds in the hinge region; has two antigen-combining sites.

Fab fragments Two of the three fragments formed if a typical monomeric IgG is digested with a proteolytic enzyme (e.g., papain). These fragments retain the ability to bind antigens (specific receptors on cells) and are called antigen-binding fragments.

factor H Major controlling factor of the alternate complement pathway. Factor H acts as a cofactor with factor I to break down complement component, C3b, which is formed during complement activation.

factor I A serine protease that cleaves the complement components, C3b and C4b, that are formed during complement activation. Separate cofactors are required for each of these reactions.

Fc portion (Fc fragment) The third fragment formed in addition to the two Fab fragments if a typical monomeric IgG is digested with a proteolytic enzyme (e.g., papain). This fragment is relatively homogeneous and sometimes crystallizable.

Fc receptor The portion of an antibody responsible for binding to antibody receptors on cells and the C1q component of complement.

Fd fragment The fragment consisting of a light chain and half of a heavy chain if the interchain disulfide bonds in the Fab fragment are disrupted.

febrile Hot or heat-producing.

febrile agglutinin Antibody demonstrated in microbial diseases that produce a high fever.

febrile disease A pathologic process in which an extremely high fever is a characteristic manifestation.

febrile purpura Discoloration of the skin associated with a high temperature or fever.

femur Bone of the leg that extends from the pelvic girdle to the knee (the thigh bone).

fibrin A mesh protein clot formed by the action of thrombin on fibrinogen.

fibroblast An immature fiber-producing cell of connective tissue capable of differentiating into a cartilage-forming cell (chondroblast), collagen-forming cell (collagenoblast), or bone-forming cell (osteoblast).

fimbriae Fringed or finger-like structures.

FISH See fluorescent in situ hybridization.

flocculation Clumping together of particles to form visible masses over a narrow range of antigen concentration (*v.,* flocculate).

flow cytometry See cell flow cytometry.

fluorescence Property of some compounds that can absorb energy from an incident light source and convert that energy into light of a longer wavelength.

fluorescence polarization immunoassay (FPIA) A type of immunoassay based on the change in polarization of fluorescent light emitted from a labeled molecule when it is bound by antibody.

fluorescent antibody A dye-antibody combination that emits light of another, longer wavelength.

fluorescent antibody (FA) assay General term describing a procedure using fluorescent microscopy that uses the visual detection of fluorescent dyes coupled (conjugated) to antibodies that react with the antigen, when present.

fluorescent antinuclear antibody (FANA) test An assay that detects antibody to nuclear antigens using nucleated cells and a fluorescence-labeled antihuman immunoglobulin.

fluorescent in situ hybridization (FISH) A laboratory technique for demonstrating the presence of HIV-1 in lymphocytes in primary lymph nodes and in peripheral blood from HIV-infected patients.

fluorochrome dye A stain for specific component or other markers.

follicle-stimulating hormone (FSH) A protein that stimulates follicles in the ovary.

follicular Referring to follicles.

Forssman antibody A heterophil type of immunoglobulin that is stimulated by one antigen and reacts with an entirely unrelated surface antigen present on cells from a different mammalian species. It can be absorbed from human serum by guinea pig kidney cells.

forward angle light scatter The type of light scattered at an angle of less than 90 degrees that indicates overall cell size.

Franklin's disease A dysproteinemia synonymous with gamma heavy-chain disease. This abnormality is characterized by the presence of monoclonal protein composed of the heavy-chain portion of the immunoglobulin molecule.

FTA-ABS test Fluorescent treponemal antibody absorption test, a confirmatory test for syphilis. This test detects antibodies to the bacterial spirochete, *Treponema pallidum*, using antihuman immunoglobulin and a fluorescent label (tag).

fulminant To occur suddenly with great intensity, such as lightning-like flashes of pain.

fulminant disease Sudden and severe onset of an abnormal condition.

G The nucleotide guanine.

gag gene A gene of a retrovirus such as HIV that encodes for the major core structural protein.

gait disturbance Walking in an unusual or abnormal manner.

gamma heavy-chain disease See Franklin's disease.

GALT See gut-associated lymphoid tissue.

gammopathy A disorder manifested by abnormality of gamma globulins.

gastroenteritis An inflammation of the lining of the stomach and intestine.

Gaussian curve A frequency distribution curve represented by a deviation from the mean (average) of a test sample.

gel electrophoresis A method for separating proteins or DNA based on size and electrical charge. Specimens are placed into wells made in a gel and subjected to an electrical current.

gene A unit of genetic material that codes for hereditary traits.

gene cloning A method for producing quantities of a specific DNA sequence.

gene expression profiling A method that can, for example, distinguish between cells that are actively dividing or show how the cells react to a particular treatment. Microarray technology measures the relative activity of previously identified target genes.

genitalia The female and male reproductive organs and associated external structures such as the penis.

genome The complete DNA composition (hereditary factors).

genomics Study of an organism's entire genome.

genotype Actual alleles, coding for a specific trait, that are inherited.

germinal center The interior location of secondary follicles where B lymphocytes undergo blast transformation.

gestation The period of development and growth of the unborn in viviparous animals (e.g., human beings), from fertilization of the ovum to birth.

giant cell Macrophage-derived cell typically found at sites of chronic inflammation. A giant multinucleated cell is formed by the coalescing of cells into a solid mass, or granuloma; also called an epithelioid cell.

giardiasis A parasitic infection associated with the unicellular *Giardia* species.

glial cell The non-nervous or supportive tissue of the brain and spinal cord known to produce minute amounts of CD4 or an alternate receptor molecule, which allows it to be infected with HIV virus; also known as a neuroglial cell.

glomerulonephritis See acute glomerulonephritis or chronic glomerulonephritis.

glomerulus (*pl.*, glomeruli) The small structure(s) in the malpighian body of the kidney composed of a cluster of capillary blood vessels enveloped in a thin wall.

glycolipids A molecule consisting of a carbohydrate plus a lipid.

glycoprotein A molecule consisting of a carbohydrate plus a protein.

goodness of fit The complementary matching of antigenic determinants and antigen-binding sites of corresponding antibodies that influences the strength of bonding between antigens and antibodies.

grading Strength of agglutination rated from negative (0) to 4+.

grafting The transfer of cells or organs from one individual to another or from one site to another in the same individual.

graft-versus-host disease (GVHD) An intense and frequently fatal immunologic reaction of engrafted cells against the host caused by the infusion of immunocompetent lymphocytes into individuals with impaired immunity; can be acute or chronic.

grand mal seizure A major epileptic attack, with or without loss of consciousness.

granzyme A/B Enzyme in granules.

gram-negative organism Bacteria that appear red when stained with Gram stain and examined under the microscope.

granulocyte A type of leukocytic white blood cell.

granuloma A macrophage-derived lesion containing sequestered noxious agents such as foreign bodies, some types of bacteria, and others that cannot be eliminated.

granulomatous lesion A wound composed of a granuloma.

Graves' disease An autoimmune disorder of the thyroid gland.

Guillain-Barré syndrome A relatively rare disease of the nerves; also called acute idiopathic polyneuritis.

gumma A granuloma that may result from delayed hypersensitivity. It is the soft tumor of tissues characteristic of the tertiary stage of syphilis.

gut-associated lymphoid tissue (GALT) GALT and bone marrow may play a role in the differentiation of stem cells into B lymphocytes; functions as the bursal equivalent in humans.

HAART Highly active antiretroviral therapy. This regimen consists of multiple drugs; it is conventional therapy for HIV infection and AIDS.

haptoglobin A protein produced by the liver.

haplotype A single chromosome's set of genetic determinants.

hapten(s) Very small molecule(s) that can bind to a larger carrier molecule and behave as an antigen.

harmonization To be in agreement; compatible interfacing.

HBeAg Antigen associated with capsid of hepatitis B virus (HBV).

HbsAg Surface antigen of hepatitis B virus (HBV), the initially detectable evidence of hepatitis B infection.

heavy (H) chain One of the polypeptide units of an immunoglobulin molecule. Each monomer of an immunoglobulin consists of two heavy chains paired with two light chains.

helper-inducer T cell subset A major phenotypic lymphocyte subset of T lymphocytes; also referred to as T4 subset, helper T cells.

hemagglutination A laboratory technique for the detection of antibodies that involves the agglutination of red blood cells.

hemagglutination assay A testing method that uses red blood cells to indicate clumping in an antigen-antibody reaction.

hemagglutination inhibition technique (HAI) A laboratory technique for detecting antibodies that involves the blocking of agglutination of red blood cells.

hematology The study of blood.

hematopoiesis (hematopoietic tissues) Blood-producing structures of the body, such as the liver, spleen, and bone marrow.

hematopoietic cells Blood-producing cells.

helminth A parasitic worm.

hemodynamic shock A physiologic condition (e.g., decreased blood pressure) resulting from the rapid loss of 15% to 20% or more of the blood volume.

hemoflagellate A protozoan parasite found in the blood and body tissues.

hemolysin A substance such as streptolysin O and streptolysin S produced by most group A strains of streptococci that disrupts the membrane integrity of red blood cells, causing the release of hemoglobin.

hemolysis Rupturing of the cell membrane (e.g., erythrocyte), with subsequent release of cytoplasmic contents (hemoglobin).

hemolytic Pertaining to rupturing of circulating erythrocytes.

hemolytic anemia A condition manifested by a severe decrease in circulating erythrocytes, with associated findings caused by the rupturing of circulating erythrocytes.

hemolytic disease of the newborn (HDN) An immunologic incompatibility between mother and fetus that can produce severe or fatal consequences in the unborn or newborn; caused by destruction of erythrocytes and the accumulation of breakdown products; previously referred to as erythroblastosis fetalis.

hemolytic titration (CH50) assay A now obsolete assay used to measure complement-activating ability.

hemolyzed Pertaining to ruptured erythrocytes.

hemoptysis Coughing and spitting up of blood as the result of bleeding from any part of the respiratory system.

hemostatic Pertaining to cessation of bleeding.

hemostasis Process that causes bleeding to stop.

hepatitis Inflammation of the liver caused by a virus, other agents (e.g., drugs), or sexual contact.

hepatitis B virus (HBV) A DNA virus transmitted by the parenteral route or sexual contact.

hepatitis C virus (HCV) Virus transmitted by blood or sexual contact; can be an acute or chronic form.

hepatomegaly Excessive enlargement of the liver.

hepatosplenomegaly An enlarged liver and spleen.

herpesvirus Any of a large group of DNA viruses such as herpes simplex and varicella.

heterodimer A protein composed of two polypeptide chains differing in composition and in the order, number, and/or type of their amino acid residues.

heterogeneous Different; a mixed or dissimilar population such as different types of cells or different ethnic groups mixed together.

heterosexual disease A pathologic condition transmitted between individuals of the opposite gender.

heterozygous Genetic state of having two dissimilar genes for the same trait.

heterophile antigen An identical or closely related antigen in unrelated plants or animals. Antibodies produced to one heterophile antigen will cross-react with antibodies to the other.

hinge region The area of an antibody molecule between the Fc and Fab regions that allows the two regions to operate independently.

histamine An amine produced by the catabolism of histidine, which causes dilation of blood vessels.

histoplasmosis A severe respiratory infection caused by a fungus, *Histoplasma capsulatum.*

histiocyte A large phagocytic interstitial cell of the mononuclear phagocyte system; a macrophage.

histocompatibility (HLA) antigen Cell surface protein antigen found on blood and body cells (e.g., leukocytes, platelets); readily provokes an immune response if transferred into a genetically different (allogenic) individual of the same species.

histone A simple protein found in combination with acidic substances such as nucleic acids.

histoplasmosis Disease caused by the inhalation of spores of the fungus *Histoplasma capsulatum.*

HIV Causative agent of acquired immunodeficiency syndrome (AIDS), also called human immunodeficiency virus type 1 (HIV-1); formerly referred to as human T-lymphotropic virus (retrovirus) type III (HTLV-III) and lymphadenopathy-associated virus (LAV).

HLA genotype Actual inherited alleles for HLA antigens.

HLA match The pairing or matching of a transplant donor and recipient based on HLA antigens.

HLA phenotype HLA genes expressed as proteins on cells.

Hodgkin's lymphoma A major form of malignant lymphoma; also called Hodgkin's disease.

homogeneous Uniform; the same. All of the individual cells or organisms are the same.

homogeneous enzyme immunoassay An assay requiring no separation steps based on the principle of a decrease in enzyme activity when specific antigen-antibody combinations occur.

homologous The same.

homozygous In genetics, when the genes for a trait on homologous (paired) chromosomes are the same.

human B cell lymphotropic virus (HBLV) A herpesvirus that can interact with HIV in a way that might increase the severity of HIV infection.

human gonadotropic hormone (hCG) A glucoprotein hormone secreted by the trophoblast of a developing embryo in early pregnancy.

human herpesvirus 6 (HHV-6) A herpesvirus that can interact with HIV in a way that might increase the severity of HIV infection.

human immunodeficiency virus (HIV) See HIV.

human leukocyte antigen (HLA) Antigen on the cell surface that identifies the cells as belonging to a specific body, rather than being foreign substances.

human T-lymphotropic virus type III (HTLV-III) See human immunodeficiency virus.

humoral Pertaining to any fluid or semifluid in the body.

humoral immunity A form of body defense against foreign substances represented by antibodies and other soluble extracellular factors in the blood and lymphatic fluid.

hutchinsonian triad The characteristic manifestation of congenital syphilis. The three major features are notched teeth, interstitial keratitis, and nerve deafness.

hyaluronidase An enzyme that breaks down hyaluronic acid found in connective tissue; also called spreading factor.

hybridization Interaction between two single-stranded nucleic acid molecules to form a double-stranded molecule.

hybridoma A cell line created in vitro by fusion of two different cell types. A hybridoma is usually formed from lymphocyte or plasma cells, one of which is a tumor cell.

hydatid cyst A parasitic infestation by a tapeworm of the genus *Echinococcus.*

hydatidiform mole An abnormal condition of degenerated chorionic villi in the uterus.

hydrophilic Water-loving.

hydrophobic Water-hating.

hyperacute rejection A type of transplant rejection that occurs rapidly (minutes to hours) after transplantation because of the presence of antibodies to blood group ABO or HLA antigens.

hypercalcemia A marked increase in ionized calcium in the circulating blood.

hypergammaglobulinemia An increased gamma globulin fraction of plasma protein.

hyperkeratosis A condition of increased growth of the upper layer of the skin (epidermis) or overgrowth of the cornea.

hyperplastic Abnormally increased cell growth.

hypersensitivity An unpleasant or damaging condition of the body tissues caused by antigenic stimulation. Hypersensitivity reactions include allergies such as hay fever.

hypervariable region A part of an antibody molecule that enables the antibody to single out one antigen to attack.

hyperviscosity An increase in the thickness (viscosity) of substances such as blood plasma.

hyperviscosity syndrome A collection of symptoms resulting from increased resistance (viscosity) of the flow of blood in the circulation.

hypervolemia An increase of total blood volume.

hypocomplementemia A decrease or deficiency of complement in the blood circulation.

hypogammaglobulinemia A decrease in the gamma globulin fraction of plasma protein.

hypoplastic Defective or incomplete development of a tissue or organ.

hypothalamus The portion of the brain beneath the thalamus at the base of the cerebrum that forms the floor and part of the walls of the third ventricle.

icteric Pertaining to icterus.

icterus Synonym for jaundice, the yellow appearance of the skin and mucous membranes caused by accumulation of bilirubin (a product of red cell breakdown).

idiopathic Pertaining to a disorder or disease without an identifiable external cause, or self-originated.

idiotope An epitope in the variable region of an antibody.

idiotype The antigenic characteristic of the antibody-variable region.

IgA The second most abundant immunoglobulin in serum; the predominant form in tears, saliva, and colostrum.

IgD An immunoglobulin found in B cell membranes; thought to play a role in B cell response to antigens.

IgE The immunoglobulin responsible for allergic reactions.

IgG The most abundant immunoglobulin in serum; responsible for protection against viruses and bacteria.

IgM The largest immunoglobulin molecule and the first antibody produced in response to an antigen.

iliac node Small rounded structure located in the lower 60% of the small intestines, from the jejunum to the ileocecal valve or in the inguinal region.

immature B cell The receptor cell that is finally programmed for insertion of specific IgM molecules into the plasma membrane.

immediate early antigen A marker for Epstein-Barr virus infection in infectious mononucleosis.

immediate hypersensitivity A subset of the body's antibody-mediated mechanisms.

immune adherence The ability of phagocytic cells to bind complement-coated particles, such as bacteria.

immune complex The noncovalent combination of an antigen with its specific antibody. An immune complex can be small and soluble or large and precipitating, depending on the nature and proportion of the antigen and antibody.

immune response The reaction of the immune system to foreign antigens in the body.

immune senescence Aging of the immune system, particularly its effect on changes in lymphocyte development and function, particularly in older adults.

immune status The ability of a host (an individual) to recognize and respond to foreign (nonself) substances (e.g., antigens).

immune system The structures (e.g., bone marrow, thymus, lymph nodes), cells (e.g., macrophages, lymphocytes), and soluble constituents of the circulating blood (e.g., complement) that allow the host to recognize and respond to foreign (nonself) substances, such as antigens.

immunity The process of being protected against foreign antigens.

immunization A process of exposing the body to specific antigens to stimulate immunity.

immunoassay A laboratory procedure for analyzing immunoglobulins.

immunoblot See Western blot.

immunochromatographic Pertaining to an analytic method used in immunology.

immunocompetent The ability to mount an immune response. A host is able to recognize a foreign antigen and produce specific antigen-directed antibodies. The term refers to lymphocytes that acquire thymus-dependent characteristics, which allow them to function in an immune response.

immunocompromised Pertaining to the condition that occurs when the immune system is unable defend itself because of existing conditions.

immunodeficiency A dysfunction in body defense mechanisms that cause a failure to detect foreign antigens and produce antibodies against these foreign (nonself) substances.

immunodeficiency disease A condition in which a defect exists in the ability to detect antigens and/or produce antibodies against foreign antigens.

immunodeficiency syndrome A condition in which the immune system is not responding in an expected fashion.

immunodiffusion A laboratory method for the quantitative study of antibodies (e.g., radial immunodiffusion [RID]) or qualitative identification of antigens (e.g., Ouchterlony technique); also called double diffusion. This classic technique is used to detect the presence of antibodies and determine their specificity by visualizing lines of identity (precipitin lines).

immunoelectrophoresis (IEP) Two-step procedure involving the electrical separation of proteins, followed by the linear diffusion (immunofixation) of antibodies into the electrophoretic gel from a trough that extends through the length of the gel adjacent to the electrophoretic path. The reactions produce precipitin arcs at positions of equivalence.

immunofixation electrophoresis A procedure in which specific antibodies help produce sensitive and specific qualitative visual identification of paraproteins by electrophoretic position.

immunofluorescent assay (IFA) A laboratory method that uses a fluorescent substance in immunologic studies. For example, particular antigens can be identified microscopically in tissues or cells by the binding of a fluorescent (light-emitting) antibody conjugate.

immunogen A large organic molecule that is a protein or large polysaccharide and rarely, if ever, a lipid.

immunogenic Pertaining to antigen.

immunoglobulin (immune globulin; Ig) Protein produced by the immune system (i.e., antibodies); a synonym for antibody. The term has replaced the term *gamma globulin* because not all antibodies have gamma electrophoretic mobility. Immunoglobulins are divided into five classes: IgM, IgG, IgD, IgA, and IgE. IgG is the most abundant.

immunohematology The study of antigen and antibody as related to blood transfusions and associated blood conditions.

immunohistochemistry The use of labeled antibodies to detect tumor markers in stained tissue specimens directly.

immunologic Related to antigens and antibodies.

immunologic dysfunction See immunodeficiency disease.

immunology The study of molecules, cells, organs, and systems responsible for the recognition and disposal of nonself materials and how they work, or can be manipulated. All aspects of body defense, such as antigens and antibodies, allergy, and hypersensitivity, are included.

immunomodulators Substances that influence regulation of the immune system.

immunophenotyping Procedure for identifying cells according to the presence of surface antigen expression.

immunoproliferation Overexpansion of cells or their products related to the immune system.

immunoprophylaxis Prevention of an immune response.

immunoregulation Control of the immune system.

immunoregulatory cells Specific cells that influence the operation of the immune system.

immunosorbent agglutination assay (ISAGA) An assay for the detection of IgM antibodies against *Toxoplasma gondii*.

immunosuppression Prevention of the recognition of antigen and/or production of antibody by repressing the normal adaptive immune response with drugs, chemicals, or other means. This process is frequently necessary before and after bone marrow or solid organ transplantation, or to alter a severe hypersensitivity reaction.

immunosuppressive agent Drug, chemical, or other mechanism that prevents the immune system from recognizing and responding to nonself.

immunosurveillance A mechanism whereby the body rids itself of abnormal or transformed cells.

immunotherapy Desensitization or stimulation of a patient's own immune system to fight a tumor.

immunotoxin Antibodies conjugated to toxins to help destroy cancer cells.

impetigo A skin infection caused by streptococci that begins as a papule.

innate immune system Nonspecific immune system.

in situ In place, or existing within the tissue itself.

in situ hybridization The binding of a nucleic acid probe to target DNA located within intact cells.

in vitro A term indicating outside the body (i.e., in a test tube).

in vivo A term indicating occurring in the living organism.

inactivated toxins Toxins produced by bacteria and viruses that have been killed and are no longer capable of causing disease.

inactivated vaccine (killed vaccine) A vaccine made from a whole microorganism (bacteria or virus) whose biologic ability to grow or reproduce is ended.

inactivation Blocking the activity of a substance (e.g., complement).

incomplete antibody Formerly used term that refers to IgG-type antibodies.

indirect allorecognition pathways Presentation of processed donor HLA peptides bound to HLA class II molecules to CD4+ lymphocytes. The result is antibody formation directed against the donor graft.

indirect fluorescent assay (IFA) Procedure used to detect homogeneous antigen plus antigen with antiimmunoglobulins using fluorescent microscopy.

indirect hemagglutination technique Laboratory method that uses erythrocytes passively coated with substances such as extracts of bacterial cells, rickettsiae, pathogenic fungi, protozoa, purified polysaccharides, or proteins to detect antibody; also called passive hemagglutination technique.

indirect immunofluorescent assay A method to identify antigen by using two antibodies—one specific to the antigen and one that is an antihuman immunoglobulin with a fluorescent tag.

indolent Slow-growing; causing little pain.

induction A therapeutic phase during which cells are exposed to a variety of drugs or radiation so that they can be destroyed.

infarction Tissue death. An area of tissue, such as heart muscle, that undergoes necrosis (tissue breakdown) because of the lack of oxygen from the circulating blood. A condition of oxygen deprivation may be caused by narrowing of blood vessels (stenosis) or blockage of the blood circulation in the vessel (occlusion).

infection A pathogenic condition caused by microorganisms (e.g., viruses, bacteria, fungi) that produce injurious effects.

infectious material Body fluids or excretory products, or nonhuman substances contaminated with body fluids, that contain disease-causing microorganisms.

infectious waste Contaminated discarded products that can cause infectious disease.

infectious mononucleosis A benign lymphoproliferative disorder.

inflammation Tissue reaction to injury caused by physical or chemical agents, including microorganisms. Symptoms include redness, tenderness, pain, and swelling.

inflammatory response See inflammation.

inguinal adenopathy Enlarged lymph nodes in the region of the groin.

innate immunity Natural or inborn resistance to infection after microorganisms have penetrated the first line of resistance; innate immune system.

innate resistance Natural or inborn ability to resist infection.

interferons Cytokines produced by T lymphocytes and other cells lines that inhibit viral synthesis or act as immune regulators.

interferon-α (IFN-α) A protein that may be an immunosuppressive agent important in controlling the immune response in a negative manner; originally called leukocyte interferon.

interferon-β (IFN-β) Originally called fibroblast interferon or B cell stimulatory factor-2; now reclassified as interleukin-6 (IL-6).

integrin Transmembrane glycoproteins receptor that mediates attachment between a cell and the tissues surrounding it.

interleukin (IL) Cytokine or chemical messenger produced by leukocytes that affect the inflammatory process through an increase in soluble factors or cells.

interleukin-1 (IL-1) A cytokine whose most prominent biologic activity is activation of resting T cells; originally called lymphocyte-activating factor.

interleukin-2 (IL-2) A cytokine best known for its ability to initiate proliferation or clonal expansion of activated T cells. IL-2 also dramatically enhances the cytolytic activity of a population of natural (lymphokine-activated) killer cells against certain tumor cells; originally called T cell growth factor.

interleukin-3 (IL-3) A cytokine that principally promotes the growth of early hematopoietic cell lines; originally called multicolony-stimulating factor (mCSF).

interleukin-4 (IL-4) A growth factor for the early activation of resting B cells that influences the synthesis of some immunoglobulins; originally called B cell–stimulating factor-1.

interleukin-5 (IL-5) IL-5 shares many activities with IL-4, but it is not active on early lymphoid cells; originally called T cell–replacing factor or B cell growth factor-2.

interleukin-6 (IL-6) A cytokine that induces secretion of immunoglobulin and is a major factor in induction of the acute-phase reaction; originally called interferon-β2 or B cell–stimulating factor-2.

interleukin-7 (IL-7) A cytokine that stimulates early B cell progenitor cells; originally called lymphopoietin-1.

interleukin-8 (IL-8) An inflammatory cytokine that is chemotactic for neutrophils and T cells; originally called monocyte-derived neutrophil chemotactic factor.

interleukin-9 (IL-9) A cytokine that is a potent lymphocyte growth factor.

interleukin-10 (IL-10) A cytokine that inhibits cytokine synthesis in various cells.

interleukin-11 (IL-11) A regulator of hematopoietic stroma that stimulates the production of megakaryocyte and myeloid progenitors; increases the number of immunoglobulin-secreting B lymphocytes.

interleukin-12 (IL-12) Enhances the activity of cytotoxic effector T cells; acts as a growth factor for natural (lymphokine-activated) killer cells and for activated T cells of the CD4+ and CD8+ subsets.

interleukin-13 (IL-13) IL-13 possesses many biologic effects similar to those of IL-4. The major action of IL-13 on macrophages is to inhibit their activation and antagonize interferon-γ (IFN-γ).

interleukin-14 (IL-14) IL-14 acts as a B cell growth factor (BCGF).

interleukin-15 (IL-15) IL-15 is biologically similar to IL-2. Endogenous IL-15 is a key condition for IFN-γ synthesis.

interleukin-16 (IL-16) IL-16 acts as a T cell chemoattractant and participates in the regulation of many cytokines (e.g., IL-1, IL-4, IL-6, IL-10, IL-12, IFN-γ). Histamine and serotonin increase the production of IL-17. It mimics many of the proinflammatory actions of tumor necrosis factor-α (TNF-α) and TNF-β.

interleukin-18 (IL-18) IL-18 acts as a synergist with IL-12 in some of their effects, especially in the induction of IFN-γ production and inhibition of angiogenesis. It stimulates the production of IFN-γ by natural killer cells and T cells and synergizes with IL-12 in this response.

interleukin-19 (IL-19) The biologic function of IL-19 is similar to that of IL-10. It regulates the functions of macrophages and suppresses the activities of T helper cells (Th1 and Th2).

interleukin-20 (IL-20) IL-20 plays an important role in skin inflammations.

interleukin-21 (IL-21) IL-21 regulates hematopoiesis and immune response and influences the development of lymphocytes; similar to the actions of IL-2 and IL-15 in regard to the antitumor defense system.

interleukin-22 (IL-22) IL-22 is similar to IL-10 but does not prevent the production of proinflammatory cytokines through monocytes.

interleukin-23 (IL-23) Cytokine that shares some in vivo functions with IL-12, including the activation of STAT-4 (signal transducer and activator of transcription factor 4).

interleukin-25 (IL-25) A secreted bone marrow stroma–derived growth factor; also called SF-20.

internal defense system Defense mechanism in the body in which cells and soluble factors play essential roles.

interstitial pneumonitis An inflammation situated between or in the interspaces of the lung tissue.

intradermal Pertaining to forcing a liquid into a part of the body, as into the subcutaneous tissues, vascular tree, or organ.

intrahepatic cholestasis Failure of bile to flow in the liver.

intraperitoneal fetal transfusion (IPT) Administration of blood to a fetus (unborn infant) via the abdominal cavity.

intrarenal obstruction Blockage within the kidney.

intrathecal Pertaining to something introduced into or occurring in the space under the arachnoid membrane of the brain or spinal cord.

intrathecal synthesis A process whereby something is introduced into or produced in the space under the arachnoid membrane of the brain or spinal cord.

intratubular precipitation Formation of a solid mass from soluble substances in the tubules of the kidney.

intrauterine Within the uterus.

intravascular coagulation Formation of a clot within a vessel (i.e., blood vessels of the circulatory system).

intravascular destruction An alternate pathway for erythrocyte breakdown, which normally accounts for less than 10% of red cell destruction.

intravascular hemolysis An alternate pathway of red cell destruction in which the cells are lysed in the vessels of the circulatory system.

intravascular thrombosis The formation of a clot in a blood vessel.

intravenous Pertaining to the administration of drugs or fluids directly into the veins.

intravenous urography Radiologic study of any part of the urinary tract by the administration of an opaque medium through a vein, which is rapidly excreted in the urine.

intrinsic coagulation mechanism Initial stage of blood coagulation that can be activated by antigen-antibody complexes.

intrinsic factor (IF) A substance secreted by the parietal cells of the mucosa in the fundus region of the stomach.

intron A polynucleotide sequence that does not code for protein synthesis.

ischemic Pertaining to a decrease in the blood supply to a bodily organ, tissue, or part caused by constriction or obstruction of the blood vessels; causes death of cells not receiving oxygen.

islet cell Insulin-producing cell in the pancreas.

isoagglutinin An antibody type that reacts (agglutinates) erythrocytes of other persons of the same species; also called isohemagglutinin.

isoelectric focusing Separation of molecules on the basis of their charge. Each molecule migrates to the point in the pH gradient at which it has no net charge.

isoimmune Possessing antibodies to antigens of the same system.

isotype A term that refers to genetic variation in a family of proteins or peptides so that every member of the species will have each isotype of the family represented in its genome (e.g., immunoglobulin classes).

isotypic variant The heavy-chain constant region structure associated with the different classes and subclasses. Isotopic variants are present in all healthy members of a species.

jaundice A yellowish appearance of the skin, sclerae, and body excretions; see also icterus.

Kahler's disease An alternate term for multiple myeloma.

Kaposi's sarcoma A rare, malignant, metastasizing disorder chiefly involving the skin. An increased incidence of this malignancy has been observed in patients with AIDS.

kappa (κ) chain One of two types of immunoglobulin light chains present in two thirds of all immunoglobulin molecules.

keratinization Development of or conversion into keratin, an extremely tough scleroprotein found in structures such as hair and nails.

kernicterus Deposition of increased bilirubin, a red cell breakdown product, in lipid-rich nervous tissue such as the brain, which can produce mental retardation or death in the newborn. This condition can occur when circulating plasma bilirubin levels reach 20 mg/dL in a full-term infant and a lower level in a premature infant.

killer T cells Subset of lymphocytes that can kill cancer cells and cells infected with viruses, fungi, or certain bacteria; also referred to as cytotoxic T cells and cytotoxic lymphocytes (CTLs).

kinetochore A term for the centromere, the constricted area of the chromosome that demarcates the upper and lower arms of the structure.

kinetoplast An accessory structure/body found in many protozoa; also called micronucleus.

kinin A small, biologically active peptide.

kinin system A series of serum peptides sequentially activated to cause vasodilation and increased vascular permeability.

Kleihauer-Betke test A testing method based on the differences in solubility between adult and fetal hemoglobin. The test is performed on a maternal blood specimen for the detection of fetal-maternal hemorrhage.

Kupffer cell A phagocytic type of cell that lines the minute blood vessel (sinusoids) of the liver.

lag period The period of time between a stimulus (e.g., antigenic stimulation) and a reaction (e.g., immunoglobulin response).

lambda (λ) light chain One of two types of immunoglobulin light chains that are present in about one third of all immunoglobulin molecules.

Langerhans cell A macrophage found in the skin.

large granular lymphocyte (LGL) Synonym for natural killer (NK) cell. About 75% of LGLs function as NK cells and appear to account fully for the NK activity in mixed-cell populations.

laser *L*ight *a*mplification by *s*timulated *e*mission of *r*adiation; used in flow cell cytometry to identify cells.

latent Hidden or inactive.

latent infection Persistent infections characterized by periods of reactivation of the signs and symptoms of the disease.

latex agglutination A technique similar to hemagglutination except that smaller, antigen-coated latex particles are substituted for erythrocytes for the detection of antibodies. Antibodies can be absorbed into the latex particles by binding to the Fc region of antibodies, leaving the Fab region free to interact with antigens present in the patient specimen.

lattice formation The establishment of cross-links between sensitized particles such as erythrocytes.

lattice hypothesis A theoretical step in the production of agglutination.

lecithin A waxy phospholipid.

lecithin pathway A pathway for activation of complement based on the attachment of mannose-binding protein to components of bacterial cell walls.

lesion A localized pathologic change in a bodily organ or tissue, such as a cut, abrasion, or sore.

leukocyte A white blood cell (WBC) that functions in antigen recognition and antibody formation.

leukocyte integrin Glycoprotein on the cell surface of white blood cells.

leukocytosis A marked increase in the total circulating white blood cell concentration.

leukopenia A marked decrease in the total circulating white blood cell concentration.

leukotriene Class of compounds that mediate the inflammatory functions of leukocytes. These substances are a collection of metabolites of arachidonic acid, with powerful pharmacologic effects.

ligand A linking or binding molecule.

ligase chain reaction (LCR) A means of increasing signal probes through the use of an enzyme called ligase, which joins two pairs of probes only after they have bound to a complementary target sequence.

light (L) chain Small chain in an immunoglobulin molecule that is bound to the larger chain by disulfide bonds. There are two types of light chains, kappa and lambda.

light-chain disease (LCD) A dysproteinemia of the monoclonal gammopathy type. In LCD, only kappa or lambda monoclonal light chains, or Bence-Jones proteins, are produced.

linear epitope Amino acids that follow one another on a single chain that act as a key antigenic site; linear antigenic determinant.

lipemia Visibly cloudy blood serum.

lipemic Pertaining to lipemia.

lipopolysaccharide (LPS) The major component of some gram-negative bacterial cell walls, which protects them from phagocytosis but activates C3 directly. LPS can also act as a B cell mitogen.

liposome A particle of fatlike substance held in suspension in tissues.

liposome-enhanced testing A variation of latex testing.

live attenuated vaccine A vaccine whose biologic activity has not been inactivated, but whose ability to cause disease has been weakened.

localized Confined to a specific area.

localized inflammatory response A tissue reaction confined to a specific area. This response is caused by physical or chemical agents, including microorganisms. The manifestations of the response include redness, tenderness, pain, and swelling.

LOCI Luminescent oxygen–channeling immunoassay.

long terminal redundancy (LTR) A structure that exists at each end of the proviral genome and plays an important role in the control of viral gene expression and the integration of the provirus into the DNA of the host.

lupus erythematosus An autoimmune disorder.

luteal phase A period of the menstrual cycle.

luteinizing hormone A hormone associated with ovulation.

lymphadenopathy Disease of the lymph nodes.

lymphoblast The most immature stage of the lymphocyte type of leukocyte.

lymphocyte A small white blood cell found in lymph nodes and circulating blood. Two major populations of lymphocytes are recognized, T and B cells.

lymphocyte-activating factor See interleukin-1.

lymphocyte recirculation Process that enables lymphocytes to come into contact with processed foreign antigens and disseminate antigen-sensitized memory cells throughout the lymphoid system.

lymphocytopenia A severe decrease in the total number of lymphocytes in the peripheral blood.

lymphocytosis A significant increase in the total number of lymphocytes in the peripheral blood.

lymphokine A soluble protein mediator released by sensitized lymphocytes on contact with an antigen. See soluble mediator.

lymphokine-activated killer (LAK) cells A population of natural killer (NK) cells with enhanced cytolytic activity resulting from the addition of IL-2.

lymphoma Solid malignant tumor of the lymph nodes and associated tissues or bone marrow.

lymphopoietin-1 See interleukin-7.

lymphoproliferative disorder A group of diseases characterized by the proliferation of lymphoid tissues and/or lymphocytes.

lymphosarcoma Malignant neoplastic disorders of the lymphoid tissues, excluding Hodgkin's disease.

lyse To break apart or dissolve.

lysis Irreversible leakage of cell contents that occurs after membrane damage.

lytic Refers to lysis.

lysozyme (muramidase) An enzyme secreted by macrophages that attacks the cell walls of some bacteria.

M protein See monoclonal protein.

macroglobulin A high-molecular-weight protein of the globulin type.

macroglobulinemia See Waldenström's primary macroglobulinemia.

macrophage A large mononuclear phagocytic cell of the tissues that exists as a wandering or fixed type; lines the capillaries and sinuses of organs such as the bone marrow, spleen, and lymph nodes. This cell phagocytizes, processes, and presents antigens to T cells and is also responsible for removing damaged tissue, cells, bacteria, and other substances from the host.

macrophage migration inhibitory factor (MIF) A lymphocyte product that is chemotactic for monocytes. Other similar factors stimulate monocyte and macrophage functions.

macular lesion A discolored unraised (flat) spot on the skin.

maculopapular A lesion with macular and papular characteristics.

major histocompatibility complex (MHC) A genetic region in human beings and other mammals responsible for signaling between lymphocytes and antigen-bearing cells. It is also the major determinant of transplant compatibility (or rejection).

malaise A general feeling of tiredness or discomfort.

malignant (malignancy) Cancerous.

malignant neoplasm A cancerous new growth.

manifestation The development of the signs and symptoms of a disease or disorder.

mannose-binding lectin A pattern recognition molecule of the innate immune system.

mannose-binding lectin pathway A complement activation pathway.

margination The process of white blood cells clinging to the lining of blood vessels.

mass spectrometry An analytic technique that identifies the chemical composition of a specimen on the basis of the mass-to-charge ratio of charged particles.

mast cell A large tissue cell with basophilic granules containing vasoactive amines and heparin. When the cell is damaged, the granules release these inflammatory mediators, which increase vascular permeability and allow complement and phagocytic cells to enter damaged tissues from the circulating blood.

material safety data sheet (MSDS) A required informational sheet that describes various characteristics and cautions related to the product.

mature B cell A cell concerned with synthesis of circulating antibodies.

mean Statistical (arithmetic) average.

median A numerical value separating the halves of a sample; half the numbers in a series are above the mean and half the numbers in the series are below the mean.

mediastinum The tissues and organs such as the heart, trachea, esophagus, and lymph nodes that separate the sternum in the front (ventral side) from the vertebral column in the back (dorsal side) of the body.

medullary Refers to the middle of something; pertaining to a medulla, bone marrow, or spinal cord.

megakaryocyte A platelet cell.

megakaryocytic thrombocytopenic purpura A severe deficiency of cells (e.g., thrombocytes, platelets) related to blood clotting that causes large purple discolorations of the skin.

melanocyte A cell that produces melanin, the dark pigment normally found in structures such as the hair, eyes, and skin. It can also occur abnormally in certain tumors, called melanomas.

membrane attack complex (MAC) A unit created by action of the complement components (C7-C9) that punctures the wall of a cell and allows cytoplasm and organelles to flow out.

memory The immunologic response to an antigenic stimulus that usually leaves the immune system changed.

memory cells Long-lived T or B lymphocytes that have been stimulated by a specific antigen and recall prior antigen exposure.

meningoencephalitis An inflammation of the brain and its membranous covering (the meninges).

meningovascular A term that refers to the blood vessels of the covering of the brain and spinal cord (meninges).

mesothelium A type of epithelium, originally derived from the mesoderm lining the primitive embryonic body cavity, that becomes the serous membrane of body surfaces, such as the peritoneum (membrane viscera and lining of the abdominal cavity, except the kidneys), pleura (membrane covering the lungs), walls of the thoracic cavity (chest and diaphragm), and pericardium (sac enclosing the heart).

metastasis Spreading of malignant cells from the primary site of malignancy.

meniscus The upside-down, half-moon shape of aqueous liquids in a glass vessel such as a pipette or flask.

mentation Mental activity.

MHC See major histocompatibility complex.

microbial antigen A carbohydrate structure on a cell wall of a microorganism.

microbiology The study of microorganisms.

microencephaly Abnormally small brain.

microglia The phagocytic cells of the brain, thought to be derived from incoming blood monocytes.

microplate A compact plate of rigid or flexible plastic with multiple wells.

microspheres Tiny (microscopic) spheres that can carry vaccines or drugs and can pass easily through the body's tissues.

mitogen A substance that stimulates cell division (mitosis).

mixed-field agglutination An observation of some cells or particles clumping together whereas others do not clump.

mobility The ability of specific and nonspecific cells of the immune system to circulate.

mode The most frequent number in a group of numbers.

molecular mimicry Similarity between an infectious agent and a self antigen that causes antibody formation in response to the infectious agent to cross-react with self.

molecule The smallest unit of a specific chemical substance that can exist alone.

monoclonal antibody (MAb) Purified immunoglobulin produced by cells cloned from a single fusion-type hybridoma cell. Monoclonal antibodies are directed against antigens derived from a single cell line.

monoclonal gammopathy A dysproteinemia in which the level of a single type of immunoglobulin is increased. This immunoglobulin is secreted by a single clone of plasma cells.

monoclonal protein A protein characterized by a narrow peak or a localized band on electrophoresis, by a thickened bowed arc on immunoelectrophoresis, and by a localized band on immunofixation; also called M protein, paraprotein.

monoclonal antiserum (*pl.*, antisera) Specific antibodies directed against antigens.

monocyte A type of leukocyte found in the peripheral blood.

monocyte-macrophage Related cell types.

monocytic Referring to monocyte(s).

monokine A soluble protein mediator.

monogenetic Refers to the theory that all living organisms are descended from a single cell or organism.

mononuclear cell Cell type that includes monocytes, promyelocytes, myelocytes, and blasts.

mononuclear phagocyte system (MPS) The body defense system composed of macrophages and a network of specialized cells of the spleen, thymus, and other lymphoid tissues; formerly called the reticuloendothelial system (RES).

monospecific Directed against one antigen site.

monovalent An antigen with only one antigenic determinant.

morbidity A condition of being diseased; the ratio of sick to healthy persons or the number of cases of a specific illness in a designated population.

morphologic Refers to the appearance of a structure.

mortality The rate of death or ratio of the number of deaths to living individuals in a designated population.

mucopurulent Refers to an exudate containing mucus and pus.

mucosal-associated lymphoid tissue (MALT) Lymphoid tissue found in the lining of the respiratory, gastrointestinal, and genitourinary tracts.

multimolecular lattice Cross linkages of molecules.

multiple myeloma A malignant disorder of plasma cells, also known as plasma cell myeloma or Kahler's disease.

multiple sclerosis (MS) An autoimmune disorder of the myelin sheath of nerve cell axons.

multipotential stem cell (MSC) Precursor cells in the bone marrow capable of differentiating into various blood cell (hematopoietic) types.

multivalent Having many charges.

murine hybridoma The fusion product of a malignant and normal cell that produces large quantities of monoclonal antibodies.

myalgia Pain or tenderness in the muscles.

myelin Covering of axons and other areas of the nervous system, such as the sheath of the spinal cord.

myelitis An inflammation of the spinal cord or bone marrow.

myeloablation Total destruction of bone marrow.

myeloma cell Plasma cells derived from malignant tumor strains.

myeloma clone A group of neoplastic cells that are descendants of a single neoplastic cell.

myeloma kidney disorders Abnormalities of the kidney associated with the neoplastic disorder multiple myeloma.

myelomatosis A term for multiple myeloma.

myeloperoxidase An important enzyme in the process of phagocytosis.

myelosuppressive An action to depress the growth of bone marrow cells.

myocarditis An inflammation of the cardiac muscle tissue.

myopericarditis Inflammation around the heart muscle.

myosin One of the two main contractile proteins found in muscles.

naked DNA vaccine Vaccine made up of deoxyribonucleic acid that is not encased or encapsulated.

nasopharyngeal carcinoma A malignancy involving the nose and throat.

natural immune system See innate immune system.

natural killer (NK) cells A population of effector lymphocytes that produce mediators as such interferon and IL-2; previously called null cells.

natural resistance Body resistance that is innate or inborn.

natural T regulatory (Treg) cells A subclass of CD4+ T lymphocytes that plays a key role in establishing tolerance to self antigens, tumor cells, transplant antigens, and allergens.

necrosis The death of cells or a localized group of cells.

necrotic Dead.

necrotizing fasciitis Dying covering of muscles.

necrotizing vasculitis Inflammation of a vessel (e.g., blood vessel) that results in tissue destruction.

negative selection The process whereby T lymphocytes that are capable of responding to self antigen are destroyed in the thymus gland.

neoantigens New antigens.

neonatal lupus An autoimmune disorder in a newborn.

neonatal septicemia Systemic disease caused by pathogenic microorganisms or their toxins in the blood of an infant up to 4 weeks old.

neonate An infant up to 4 weeks old.

neoplasm Any new and abnormal tissue, such as a tumor.

neoplasia (neoplastic) Referring to new abnormal tissue growth.

nephelometry A laboratory assay method based on the measurement of the turbidity of particles in suspension. A nephelometer can be used for assays such as quantitating immunoglobulin concentrations in serum.

nephritis An inflammation of the kidney.

nephritogenic An agent or microorganism capable of causing an inflammation of the kidney.

nephrolithiasis Disorder characterized by the formation of a kidney stone.

nephropathy Any inflammatory, degenerative, or sclerotic disease of the kidneys.

nephrosis A condition of the kidneys, particularly tubular degeneration, without the signs and symptoms of inflammation.

nephrotic syndrome A disorder of the kidneys characterized by a decreased concentration of albumin in the circulating blood, marked edema (swelling), increased protein levels in the urine (proteinuria), and increased susceptibility to infection.

nephrotoxic Refers to an agent, such as a specific toxin, that is destructive to kidney cells.

NETS Neutrophil extracellular traps.

neuralgia Acute pain radiating along the course of a nerve.

neurologic sequelae Morbid nervous system signs and symptoms that follow or are caused by a disease.

neurotoxic cytokine A substance able to destroy nervous tissue.

neutralization Procedure similar to complement fixation, but can be used only when the antibody being measured is directed against a hemolysin (bacterial toxin capable of directly lysing red blood cells).

neutropenia A marked decrease in the neutrophil type of leukocytes.

neutrophil A granulocyte-containing type of leukocyte.

neutrophil chemotactic factor A preformed mediator whose function is to attract neutrophils to an inflammatory area.

noncompetitive assay An assay in which an excess of binding sites is present in order for all the specified analytes in the specimen to be bound and measured.

non-Hodgkin's lymphoma (NHL) A condition of solid malignant tumors of the lymph nodes and associated tissues or bone marrow that is not of the Hodgkin's type.

nonhistone In chromatin, refers to those proteins that remain after the histones have been removed.

nonintact Broken or disrupted, such as a cut in the skin.

nonmicrobial antigen A structure not related to microorganisms.

nonself Recognition of foreign material in body defenses; antigenically dissimilar from self.

nonsymptomatic An abnormal condition, such as an infectious disease, that does not manifest the signs and symptoms of the disorder.

nontreponemal antibody assays Serologic assays for syphilis that detect antibody to cardiolipin and not specific antitreponemal antibody.

normal flora Microorganisms that normally inhabit areas of the body such as the skin, mucous membranes, and intestinal tract; also called normal biota.

normocytic normochromic anemia A deficiency of erythrocytes. However, the erythrocytes present in the circulation are of normal size and color.

Northern blot A molecular biology technique similar to the Southern blot, except that messenger RNA (mRNA) from the specimen is separated and blotted. If specific RNA is present, the radiolabel can be detected.

nosocomial Pertaining to a hospital; a nosocomial infection is a hospital-acquired infection.

NSAID Nonsteroidal antiinflammatory drug.

nucleic acid probe Short strand of DNA or RNA of a known sequence used to identify a complementary nucleic acid strand in a patient sample.

nucleic acid sequence–based amplification (NASBA) A technique for amplifying RNA by first making a DNA copy and then making RNA transcripts from this template.

nucleocapsid Nucleic acid and surrounding protein coat of a virus.

null cell See natural killer cell.

occlusive Blocking.

Occupational Safety and Health Administration (OSHA) A government regulatory agency that helps ensure safe and healthful working conditions.

oligonucleotide probe A small portion of a single string of nucleotides used to detect the presence of a complementary nucleic acid sequence.

oncofetal protein Gene product whose level is increased in malignant transformation.

oncogene A transforming gene of cellular origin found in retroviruses and associated with acute leukemias.

oncogenic Associated with tumor formation.

oncology The study of malignancy (diagnosis and treatment).

oncopeptidomics Protein profiling in cancer patients to determine the presence of new tumor markers or proteins that are consistent with cancer.

oocyst The encysted form of a fertilized gamete occurring in certain sporozoa; an immature ovum.

opportunistic infection A microbial disease that infects a debilitated host.

opsonin A chemical substance that binds to antigens and increases the rate and quality of action by phagocytes to destroy invading organisms.

opsonization A process in which the complement component C3b is attached to a particle, which promotes the adherence of phagocytic cells because of the C3 receptors. Antibody, if present, augments this by binding to Fc receptors.

oropharynx The part of the throat between the soft palate and upper edge of the epiglottis.

osmosis The movement of water through a semipermeable membrane.

osmotic-cytolytic reaction Rupture of a cell due to water intrusion that creates pressure on the cellular membrane.

osteoclast A giant multinucleated cell formed in the bone marrow of growing bones. This cell is associated with reabsorption and removal of unwanted tissue.

osteomyelitis An inflammation of bone or bone marrow.

osteonecrosis Accelerated destruction of bone tissue.

osteoporosis Increased porosity of bone that causes softening and thinning of the bone.

otitis media Inflammation of the middle ear.

Ouchterlony double diffusion A classic gel precipitation method in which antigen and antibody diffuse out from wells cut into the gel. The pattern indicates whether or not antigens are identical.

oxidative burst A state of increased oxygen consumption in phagocytic cells in which generated oxygen radicals kill engulfed (phagocytized) bacteria or parasites.

p24 A structural core antigen that is part of the human immunodeficiency virus (HIV).

PAMPs (pathogen-associated molecular patterns) Antigens on a few large groups of microorganisms.

pancreatitis An inflammation of the pancreas, with endocrine and exocrine functions located behind the stomach, between the spleen and duodenum.

papilloma Polyp of epithelial surfaces.

papule A small, solid, elevated lesion of the skin.

paracortical Around the cortex (outer portion) of an organ or gland.

paraprotein See monoclonal protein.

parenchymal Referring to the functional constituents of an organ as opposed to the framework (stroma).

parenteral Administered subcutaneously (beneath the skin), intramuscularly, or intravenously.

parotid gland The largest of the three salivary glands, located near the ear.

paroxysmal cold hemoglobinuria (PCH) A form of destruction of erythrocytes (red blood cells) caused by an IgG protein that reacts with the erythrocytes in colder parts of the body and subsequently causes complement components to bind to erythrocytes irreversibly. It is typically seen as an acute transient condition secondary to viral infection.

paroxysmal nocturnal hemoglobinuria (PNH) A disorder in which the patient's erythrocytes act as a complement activator. The activation of complement results in excessive lysis of the patient's erythrocytes.

passive hemagglutination technique See indirect hemagglutination technique.

passive immunity Temporary immune protection resulting from the transfer of antibodies from another individual who has actively formed antibodies; for example, transfer from a mother to her unborn child. Also, it can be a transfer of lymphocytes from another individual known to be immune to a specific antigen.

passive immunodiffusion A precipitation reaction in a gel medium in which an antigen-antibody combination can result because of diffusion.

pathogen A disease-causing microorganism or agent.

pathogenesis The origin of disease.

pathogenic Refers to the disease-producing potential of a microorganism (pathogenicity).

pathologic Disease-causing.

pattern recognition receptors Receptors of the innate immune system that recognize PAMPs.

PCR Polymerase chain reaction.

peptide Short polymer of amino acid monomers linked by peptide bonds.

percutaneous (parenteral) Infused into a blood vessel.

perforation A hole or break in the wall or membrane of an organ or body structure.

periarteritis nodosa An inflammation of the layers of small and medium-sized arteries. This condition is manifested by a variety of systemic signs and symptoms, including febrile manifestations.

pericarditis An inflammation of the serous membrane lining of the sac surrounding the heart and origins of the great blood vessels.

perifollicular Around a follicle.

perinatal Refers to the period preceding, during, or after birth.

perineal region External region between the vulva and anus in the female or between the scrotum and anus in the male.

peripheral blood stem cell (PBSC) Progenitor cell or the earliest form of an undifferentiated blood cell.

peripheral tolerance Process involving mature lymphocytes that occurs in the blood circulation.

peritonitis An inflammation of the serous membrane covering the intestines and abdominal organs (viscera) and abdominal cavity.

pernicious anemia An erythrocytic disorder associated with defective vitamin B_{12} uptake.

personal protective equipment (PPE) Clothing or accessories worn to protect or reduce the risk of transmission of infectious agents.

petechiae Small, purple hemorrhagic spots on the skin or mucous membranes.

phagocyte Any cell capable of engulfing and destroying foreign particles, such as bacteria.

phagocytic Capable of engulfment.

phagocytosis A form of endocytosis. This important body defense mechanism is the process whereby specialized cells engulf and destroy foreign particles, such as microorganisms or damaged cells. Macrophages and segmented neutrophils (PMNs) are the most important phagocytic cells.

phagolysosome A vacuole (secondary lysosome) formed by the fusion of a phagosome and primary lysosome(s) in which microorganisms are killed and digested.

phagosome A membrane-bound vesicle in a phagocyte containing the engulfed material.

pharyngeal pouch An embryonic structure.

pharyngitis An inflammation of the throat.

pharynx The throat.

phlebotomy A procedure in which blood is drawn from a blood vessel.

phenotype Visual expression of genetic makeup.

photon A basic unit of radiation.

phototherapy Process that uses ultraviolet light to accelerate the breakdown of bilirubin that has abnormally accumulated in the skin.

phytohemagglutinin A specific substance, a lectin, that is derived from plants and has the ability to agglutinate erythrocytes.

picornavirus A single-stranded RNA virus.

pipetting A method of measuring and transferring liquids via a calibrated tube.

plasma The straw-colored fluid component of blood in circulating or anticoagulated blood.

plasma cell A few mature blood plasma cells can be found in the bone marrow, but they are not normally seen in the circulating blood.

plasma cell myeloma See multiple myeloma.

plasmacytoid Resembling or similar to a plasma cell.

plasmacytoid lymphocyte A cell that resembles a plasma cell.

plasmin A proteolytic enzyme with the ability to dissolve formed fibrin clots.

plasminogen The inactive precursor to plasmin, which is converted to plasmin by the action of substances such as urokinase.

platelet factor 3 An important blood coagulation factor associated with thrombocytes (platelets).

pleiotropy Many different actions of a single cytokine. It may affect the activities of more than one type of cell and have more than one type of effect on the same cell.

pleura The membrane covering the lungs, walls of the thoracic cavity (chest), and diaphragm.

pleuritis An inflammation of the serous membrane lining, the pleura.

pluripotent See multipotential stem cells.

Pneumocystis jiroveci A protozoan that causes interstitial plasma cell pneumonia. This microorganism is frequently observed as an opportunistic pathogen in patients with AIDS; formerly called *Pneumocystis* carinii.

PMN See polymorphonuclear leukocyte.

point-of-care testing (POCT) A term used to designate laboratory testing at or near the patient.

pol gene A gene of a retrovirus (e.g., HIV) that encodes for reverse transcriptase, endonuclease, and proteases activities.

polyagglutinable RBCs Capable of reacting with many red blood cells.

polyarthritis Inflammation of several joints.

polyclonal antiserum (*pl.,* antisera) Antibody directed against more than one antigen.

polyclonal gammopathy A dysproteinemia in which the products of a number of different cell types are demonstrated.

polyendocrinopathy A disease condition that involves several endocrine glands.

polymerase chain reaction (PCR) A molecular biology technique that uses amplification of low levels of specific DNA sequences in a sample to reach the threshold of detection. The reaction products are hybridized to a radiolabeled DNA segment complementary to a short sequence of the amplified DNA. After electrophoresis, the radiolabeled product of specific size is detected by autoradiography.

polymerization Coming together of many molecules.

polymorphonuclear leukocyte (PMN) A short-lived scavenger blood cell whose granules contain powerful bactericidal enzymes; also called polymorphonuclear neutrophil leukocyte.

polymyositis Inflammation of several muscles at the same time. This condition is manifested by a number of signs and symptoms, including pain, edema, deformity, and sleep disturbance.

polyneuropathy A disease involving several nerves.

polyserositis A condition of general inflammation of the serous membranes with effusion (escape of fluid). The inflammation is progressive and especially prevalent in the upper abdominal cavity.

polyspecific Refers to many antigen or antibody reactions.

posterior cervical In the back (dorsal surface); associated with the vertebral bone of the neck.

posterior pharynx Back of the throat.

positive selection The process of selecting immature T lymphocytes for survival on the basis of expression of high levels of CD3 cell surface markers and the ability to respond to self MHC antigens.

postexposure prophylaxis A treatment protocol used after exposure to a potentially infectious microorganism.

postnatal After birth.

postoccipital lobe The back portion (lobe) of the cerebral hemisphere that is shaped like a three-sided pyramid.

postpartum After birth.

poststreptococcal glomerulonephritis An inflammation of a renal structure after an infection with streptococci.

postzone Excess of antigen resulting in no lattice formation in an agglutination reaction.

potency The strength of a substance.

preanalytic Before testing (preevaluation).

pre–B cell An early, rapidly dividing, mature B cell precursor.

precipitation Formation of a solid mass (precipitate) from previously soluble components. An alternate definition is a process that occurs suddenly or unexpectedly.

precipitin lines Observable lines of insoluble particulate matter.

precipitin Soluble particle that becomes insoluble particulate matter.

precision The degree to which further measurements or analysis produce the same or very similar results; also called reproducibility or repeatability.

predictive value An expression of the probability that a given test result correlates with the presence or absence of disease. A positive predictive value is the ratio of patients with the disease who test positive to the entire population of individuals with a positive test result; a negative predictive value is the ratio of patients without the disease who test negative to the entire population of individuals with a negative test.

prenatal Before birth.

primary antibody response An immunologic (IgM antibody) response that occurs after a foreign antigen challenge.

primary biliary cirrhosis Cirrhosis (interstitial inflammation of an organ) of the liver caused by chronic retention of bile. The causative agent is unknown in the primary form of the disorder.

primary disorder An initial or first condition.

primary follicle A cluster of B lymphocytes that have not yet been stimulated by antigen.

primary immunodeficiency Dysfunction in an immune organ such as the thymus.

primary immunoglobulin deficiency A genetically determined disorder associated with certain diseases.

primary infection The first or original infection.

primary lymphoid tissue or organ The bone marrow and thymus gland are classified as primary or central lymphoid tissues.

primary response An initial antibody reaction to a foreign antigen.

prime To give an initial sensitization to antigen.

primer Short sequences of DNA, usually 20 to 30 nucleotides in length, used to hybridize specifically to a particular target DNA to help initiate replication of the DNA.

primitive stem cell The early form of uncommitted, multipotential blood cells that replicate themselves and generate more differentiated daughter cells.

procainamide A drug that functions as a cardiac depressant; used in the treatment of cardiac arrhythmias.

prodromal period Earliest or initial sign or symptom of a developing disease or disorder. For example, the prodromal period (prodrome) of an infectious disease manifested by rash would be the time between the earliest symptoms and the appearance of the rash or fever.

proficiency testing A comparison of in-house laboratory assay results with results from external laboratories; a valuable continuous improvement (quality assurance) tool.

progenitor cell Precursor (immature) blood cell.

prognosis A forecast of the probable outcome of a condition, disorder, or disease.

prognostic To predict an outcome.

progressive systemic sclerosis (PSS) A disorder of loss of tissue elasticity throughout the body that advances in severity over time.

properdin A normal protein of human plasma or serum.

prophylaxis A synonym for prevention.

prostaglandin Naturally occurring, unsaturated fatty acid that stimulates and suppresses the effects of many inflammatory processes and stimulates the contraction of uterine and other smooth muscle tissues; pharmacologically active derivative of arachidonic acid. Different prostaglandins are capable of modulating cell mobility and immune responses.

prostate-specific antigen (PSA) A cancer tumor marker for prostate cancer.

prostration A condition of extreme exhaustion (lack of strength or energy).

proteinase Enzyme that can act on proteins.

protein Large molecule, composed of amino acids, that is a major constituent of cells.

proteinuria Protein (albumin) in the urine.

proteolysis The breaking apart of a protein molecule.

proteolytic enzyme A substance able to break apart a protein molecule.

proteomics Large-scale study of proteins, particularly their structures and functions.

prothrombin time (PT) A blood coagulation test that assesses the process of clotting, beginning with the formation of factor X.

protocol The steps usually followed in a situation such as laboratory testing or patient treatment.

proto-oncogene Regulatory gene that promotes cell division.

proximal humerus The end portion of the upper bone of the arm nearest the center of the body (shoulder).

prozone phenomenon A possible cause of false-negative antigen-antibody reactions caused by an excessive amount of antibody.

pruritus Itching.

pseudoagglutination False clumping of cells or particles.

psychoneuroimmunology The relationship between the mind and body that combines research in basic science with psychological and psychosocial factors.

psychosocial factors Related to both psychological and social factors.

PT See prothrombin time.

purine Nitrogenous bases, adenine and guanine, incorporated into DNA or RNA, which represent a portion of the genetic code (genome).

purulent Containing, discharging, or causing the production of pus.

purpura An extensive area of red or dark purple discoloration of the skin.

pyelonephritis An inflammation of the kidney and pelvis region of the kidney, funnel-shaped expansion of the upper end of the ureter into which the renal calices open.

pyoderma Any purulent (pus-producing) skin disease.

pyogen Microorganism causing fever.

pyogenic Producing pus.

pyrimidine Nitrogenous bases, cytosine and thymidine, in DNA, and cytosine and uracil in RNA, which form a portion of the genetic code (genome).

pyrogenic Inducing fever.

pyroglobulin An abnormal (IgM) globulin that precipitates on heating to 50° to 60° C (122° to 140° F) but does not redissolve on cooling or intensified heating, as do typical Bence-Jones pyroglobulins.

pyroglobulinemia Presence in the blood of pyroglobulins.

quality assurance (QA) Planned or systematic action necessary to provide confidence that a laboratory assay result will satisfy the given requirements for quality.

quality control A process used to ensure a certain level of quality in laboratory testing, including control of preanalytic, analytic, and postanalytic factors. The basic goal of quality control is to ensure that the results meet specific requirements and are dependable and satisfactory.

quantitation Process that measures the concentration of a substance.

radial immunodiffusion (RID) A quantitative variation of immunodiffusion. The diameter of the precipitin ring formed from evenly distributed antigen (or antibody) and its counterpart from the test sample diffuses into agar gel from a single well, resulting in a circular ring of precipitin around the sample well. The diameter of the precipitin ring is proportional to the concentration of specific antibody (or antigen) present in the test specimen. A comparison to a known standard allows for quantitation of the test specimen.

radioallergosorbent test (RAST) This procedure detects the presence of IgE (and IgG) antibodies to allergens; a method used to measure antigen-specific IgE by means of a noncompetitive solid-phase immunoassay.

radioimmunoassay (RIA) An older and less frequently used laboratory technique using radioactive substances to evaluate immunoglobulins. Traditional RIA is done with specific antibodies in liquid solution. Solid-phase RIA uses antibody bound to a solid support (e.g., tube, glass beads).

RAST See radioallergosorbent test.

Raynaud's phenomenon (Raynaud's disease) A condition of episodic constriction of small arteries of the extremities (usually fingers or toes) induced by cold temperatures or emotional stress that would not affect a nonafflicted person. The signs and symptoms of the condition include two forms, a pale appearance and numb feeling followed by redness and tingling or a swollen, red, and painful condition. Heat relieves the condition if the stimulus was cold-induced.

reactivated infection Another appearance of an infection.

reagent A chemical solution used in laboratory testing.

reactive oxygen species (ROS) Chemically reactive molecules containing oxygen, such as H_2O_2.

reagin An antibody-like protein that binds to a test antigen such as cardiolipin lecithin–coated cholesterol particles in the Venereal Disease Research Laboratory (VDRL) serologic method of testing for syphilis, a rapid plasma reagin (RPR) test; also, a former term for IgE with a specificity for allergens.

reagin antibody Nontreponemal antibody produced by a patient infected with *Treponema pallidum* against components of their own or other mammalian cells.

real-time PCR A sensitive technique for measuring amplification of DNA by using fluorescent dyes or probes to take readings after each cycle instead of waiting until all the cycles have been completed.

re-anneal To reassemble or recombine two nucleic acid strands.

receptor A cell surface molecule that binds specifically to particular proteins or peptides in the fluid phase.

recessive The term used to describe a gene that is not expressed unless it is in the homozygous form.

recirculation Lymphocytes, mostly T cells, which pass from the circulating blood through the lymphatic system back to the circulating blood.

recognition unit The complement component that consists of the C1qrs complex. This unit must bind to at least two Fc regions to initiate the classic complement cascade.

recombinant DNA technology The technique whereby genetic material from one organism is inserted into a foreign cell or another organism to mass produce the protein encoded by the inserted genes; also called recombinant genetic engineering.

recombinant vector vaccine A vaccine that combines a vector, a harmless bacterium or virus, used to transport an antigen into the body to stimulate protective immunity and an antigen or immunogen from an organism other than the vector.

redundant Refers to different cytokines that have the same effect.

reference range Typical laboratory results for specific groups of patients, such as gender- or age-related average values. This term was previously referred to as normal values.

refractory anemia A form of anemia (decreased erythrocytes in the circulation) resistant to ordinary treatment.

regimen A schedule of treatment.

regional adenopathy Swelling or enlargement of the lymph nodes in a certain area or areas of the body.

reinfection A second or more incidence that manifests a prior infection.

relative lymphocytosis An increase of lymphocytes in the circulating blood in relationship to the total number of leukocytes in the circulation.

reliability Dependability of results.

remission Withdrawal of symptoms of a disease or disorder; a temporary cure.

renal impairment Dysfunction of the kidneys.

renal insufficiency Inadequate functioning of the kidneys.

replicability The ability of specific and nonspecific cells of the immune system to produce daughter cells.

reproducibility The ability to obtain similar results when the same specimen is repeatedly tested.

restriction endonuclease Bacterial enzyme that recognizes short sequences of DNA and cleaves the DNA near this restriction site. Each enzyme is named after the bacteria from which it has been isolated.

respiratory burst The increase in oxygen consumption that occurs in a phagocytic cell as it begins to engulf a particle.

restriction endonuclease Enzymes that cleave DNA at specific recognition sites that are typically four to six base pairs long.

restriction fragment length polymorphism (RFLP) Variation in nucleotides in DNA that change where restriction enzymes cleave the DNA. Where mutations occur, different-sized segments of DNA are obtained, producing an altered electrophoretic pattern.

reticuloendothelial system (RES) See mononuclear phagocyte system (MPS).

retinal hemorrhage Extreme bleeding from the inner layer of the eye (retina) into the fluid-filled interior of the eye.

retinitis An inflammation of the inner layer (retina) of the eye.

retroauricular Behind the protruding portion of the external ear that surrounds the opening (auricle).

retrovirus A type of virus that carries a single, positive-stranded RNA and uses a special enzyme, reverse transcriptase, to convert viral RNA into DNA.

reverse passive hemagglutination A laboratory method that uses erythrocytes as indicator cells to observe the absence of agglutination in the presence of antibodies. Carrier particles coated with antibody clump together because of a combination of antigen.

reverse transcriptase (RT) An enzyme found in the single, positive-stranded RNA core of a retrovirus. This enzyme converts (copies) RNA to DNA.

Reye's syndrome An acute and frequently fatal childhood disease that may follow a variety of common viral infections within several hours or days. The signs and symptoms of disease include persistent vomiting, followed by delirium caused by edema of the brain, hypoglycemia, dysfunction of the liver, convulsions, and coma.

RFLPs (restriction fragment length polymorphisms) A variation in the DNA sequence of a genome that can be detected by a laboratory technique known as gel electrophoresis. Analysis of RFLP variation is an important tool in genome mapping, localization of genetic disease genes, and determination of risk for a disease.

Rh factor This blood group antigen, named for the rhesus monkey, was originally identified because an antibody agglutinated the erythrocytes of all rhesus monkeys and 85% of human beings. The antibody was later discovered to be the Landsteiner-Wiener antibody, which is different than the Rh antibody.

rheumatic disease A collection of rheumatoid disorders.

rheumatic fever A disease caused by the toxins produced by group A beta streptococci.

rheumatoid factor An IgM class antibody directed against IgG; detectable in patients with rheumatoid arthritis.

rhinitis Inflammation of the nose.

rhinorrhea Watery discharge from the nose.

RIA See radioimmunoassay.

ribonucleic acid (RNA) The nucleic acid containing the carbohydrate, ribose.

RIST Radioimmunosorbent test used to measure total IgE using a solid phase immunoassay with anti-IgE.

rocket immunoelectrophoresis A classic method used to quantify antigens on the basis of the height of a rocket-shaped precipitin band obtained when radial immunodiffusion is combined with electrophoresis.

rouleaux, rouleaux formation Pseudoagglutination or the false clumping of erythrocytes when the cells are suspended in their own serum. This phenomenon is caused by an abnormal protein in the serum, plasma expanders (e.g., dextran), or Wharton's jelly from cord blood samples. Rouleaux formation appears as rolls resembling stacks of coins on microscopic examination.

RPR (rapid plasma reagin) test A serologic test for venereal disease (syphilis).

rubella The RNA viral cause of German or 3-day measles.

rubella syndrome A term for a number of congenital anomalies such as mental retardation and cardiovascular defects caused by the rubella virus.

rubeola The single-stranded RNA virus that cause measles.

sandwich format immunoassay An immunoassay method based on the ability of antibody to bind with more than one antigen.

sandwich hybridization A nucleic acid detection method using two probes, one of which is placed on a solid support (e.g., a membrane or microtiter plate) to capture the target DNA. A second labeled probe, which binds to a second site on the target DNA, is added to detect specific gene sequences.

sarcoma Malignant tumor of connective tissue origin.

scarlet fever An acute infectious disease caused by group A streptococcus. The rash and other signs and symptoms are caused by the erythema-producing toxin produced by the streptococci.

schistosomiasis An infectious disease caused by trematode worms.

sclerodactyly A chronic disorder characterized by progressive fibrosis of the fingers and toes.

scleroderma A progressive fibrosis beginning with the skin.

sebum The oily secretion of the sebaceous glands whose ducts open into the hair follicles.

second follicle A cluster of B lymphocytes that are proliferating in response to a specific antigen.

secondary immune response The second and subsequent response by the immune system to the same antigen encountered; the secondary response is shorter, faster, and wider than the primary response.

secondary immunoglobulin deficiency An acquired disorder associated with certain diseases.

secondary lymphoid tissue, secondary lymphoid organs These secondary tissues include the lymph nodes, spleen, and Peyer's patches in the intestine.

secretory component A protein in secretory IgA and IgM thought to protect against enzyme damage.

selectin A Sugar-binding lectin on the surface of cells.

self-limiting, self-limited Confined; able to resolve over time.

senescence The process of growing old.

sensitivity The frequency of positive results obtained in testing a population of individuals who are positive for antibody.

sensitization Physical attachment of antibody molecules to antigens on the erythrocyte membrane.

sepsis Microbial infection throughout the systemic circulation.

septic arthritis An inflammation of the joints caused by the presence of pathogenic microorganisms.

septicemia The presence of pathogenic microorganisms in the blood.

sequela (*pl.*, sequelae) A disease or condition occurring after or as a consequence of another condition or event.

serial dilution The stepwise decreasing strength (dilution) of a substance in solution.

seroconversion The development of a demonstrable antibody response to a disease or vaccine.

serodiagnostic test Assay of substances (Ag tab) in serum

seroepidemiologic Pertaining to the evidence of antibodies to a disease in a defined population.

serologic Pertaining to serology.

serologic testing Assay of constituents of serum.

serology The study of constituents of serum, the straw-colored fluid component of whole blood.

seronegative The lack of evidence of an antibody to a disease.

seronegative spondyloarthropathy Antibody negative in a condition affecting the joints of the spine.

seropositive The presence of antibodies in a specimen.

seroprevalence The frequency of occurrence of a specific antibody in a specified population.

serositis An inflammation of the membrane consisting of mesothelium, a thin layer of connective tissue, manifested by lines enclosing the body cavities.

serotype A group of closely related microorganisms distinguished by a characteristic set of antigens.

serum Straw-colored fluid present in whole blood; seen after blood clots.

serum electrophoresis A technique for separating ionic molecules, principally proteins, into five fractions on a medium such as paper or cellulose acetate. The separation is based on the rate of migration, depending on size and ionic charge of the individual components in an electrical field. The components can be visualized by staining and quantitated using a densitometer.

serum sickness A type III hypersensitivity reaction occurring after a single large injection of serum from an animal of another species (passive immunization).

severe combined immunodeficiency disease (SCID) A life-threatening condition that results when a child is born without any major immune defenses.

sex-linked trait A genetic trait associated with the X chromosome.

sharps Objects that can cut.

sialic acid Found on red blood cell membranes; produces a negative surrounding charge.

sialoglycoprotein A sialic acid containing carbohydrate and a protein molecule.

sickle cell anemia An inherited form of anemia caused by genetically defective hemoglobin.

silent carrier A carrier of a disease who manifests no clinically obvious symptoms or signs.

single diffusion A precipitation reaction in which one of the reactants is incorporated in the gel and the other reactant diffuses out from the point of application.

single-strand conformational polymorphism assay A technique used to detect subtle differences in nucleotide sequences; typically used to compare sequences from two or more individuals to determine whether they are identical or if a mutation has occurred.

sinusitis An inflammation of the cavity in a bone, such as in the paranasal sinuses.

sinusoid A specialized capillary found in locations such as the bone marrow, spleen, and liver through which blood passes to reach the veins, allowing the lining macrophages to remove damaged or antibody-coated cells.

Sjögren's syndrome An autoimmune disorder manifested by enlargement of the parotid glands, chronic polyarthritis, and dryness of the conjunctiva, throat, and mouth.

SLE See systemic lupus erythematosus.

solid-phase assay A laboratory method in which one of the reactants is bound to the surface.

soluble Able to be dissolved in a liquid, or as if in a liquid, especially water.

soluble mediator A substance secreted by monocytes, lymphocytes, and neutrophils that provides the mechanism of cell to cell communication.

somnolence A condition of prolonged drowsiness or a state resembling a trance.

sor gene A gene of a retrovirus such as HIV. The product of the small, open-reading frame is a protein that induces antibody production in the natural course of infection.

Southern blot A molecular biology laboratory technique used in DNA analysis. DNA from a patient specimen is denatured and treated with enzymes to produce DNA fragments. The single-stranded DNA fragments are then separated by electrophoresis. The fragments are further treated and radiolabelled. The resulting DNA with the radiolabel, if present, is then detected by autoradiography. Applications include studying the HIV sequence in peripheral blood cells and tissues such as lymph nodes, liver, and kidney.

specificity Ability of a particular antibody to combine with one antigen instead of another; also, the proportion of negative test results obtained in the population of individuals who actually lack the antibody in question.

spectrophotometry A method of measurement of the passage of colored light by reflection or transmission.

spirochete A type of bacteria with a twisted or spiral appearance when viewed microscopically.

spirochetemia The presence of spirochetes (e.g., in the disease, syphilis) in the circulating blood.

spleen A large glandlike organ located in the upper left quadrant of the abdomen, under the ribs. The spleen is the body's largest reservoir of mononuclear phagocytic cells.

splenomegaly A disorder characterized by a greatly enlarged spleen.

spontaneous tumor antigen A unique antigen expressed by a tumor.

sporotrichosis An infection with or disease caused by a fungus.

sporotrichotic Pertaining to sporotrichosis.

S protein A control protein in the complement cascade that interferes with binding of the C5b67 complex to a cell membrane, thereby preventing lysis.

SQUID See superconducting quantum interference device.

Standard Precautions Specific regulations and practices, such as wearing gloves, that conform to current state and federal requirements. These precautions assume that all specimens (e.g., blood) have the potential for transmitting disease; also called Universal Blood and Body Fluid Precautions (CDC), previously Uniform Precautions.

stasis Cessation of bleeding.

steric hindrance Mutual blocking of dissimilar antibodies with the same binding constant directed against antigenic determinants located in close proximity on a cell's surface.

stillborn Dead at birth.

strand displacement amplification A technique for amplifying DNA by using a DNA primer that is nicked by an endonuclease, allowing for displacement of the amplified strands.

streptococcal pharyngitis Sore throat caused by group A streptococcus.

Streptococcus pyogenes A species of streptococcus.

streptokinase An enzyme that dissolves clots by converting plasminogen to plasmin.

streptolysin O (SLO) A protein capable of lysing erythrocytes and leukocyte produced by some types of streptococci as they grow.

streptolysin S Associated with group A streptococcus.

stroma The connective, functionally supportive framework of a biologic cell, tissue, or organ.

subclinical infection An early or mild form of a disease without visible signs.

substrate A substance on which another substance acts, such as an enzyme.

superantigens A class of antigens that cause nonspecific activation of T cells resulting in oligoclonal T cell activation and massive cytokine production.

superconducting quantum interference device (SQUID) Very sensitive magnetometer used to measure extremely small magnetic fields, based on superconducting loops containing Josephson junctions.

superinfection An infection on top of another infection.

supernatant Fluid above the solid portion (e.g., cells in a centrifuged or sedimented specimen).

suppressor (cytotoxic) lymphocytes A major phenotypic lymphocyte subset of T lymphocytes; also referred to as T8 cells.

supraglottic larynx The area above the true vocal cords.

surface immunoglobulin (sIg) An immunoglobulin, at first cytoplasmic and later surface-bound, that is the key feature of B cells whereby they recognize specific antigens.

surgical pathology The study of tissue or organs removed from the body.

surrogate testing Procedures performed in place of specific tests for an infectious agent such as non-A, non-B hepatitis.

susceptibility Having little resistance, such as resistance to infectious disease.

symptom An indication of a disorder or disease or a variation in normal body function.

symptomatic A deviation from usual function or appearance.

syncope Loss of balance.

syncytia Giant multinucleated groups or masses of cells.

syndrome A collection of symptoms that occur together.

synergistic The action of two or more agents that frequently produces a much greater effect than the expected sum of the individual agents.

synovial fluid A viscous fluid in the joints.

synovitis Inflammation of the synovium.

synovium Synovial membrane (synovium) is the soft tissue found between the articular capsule (joint capsule) and joint cavity of synovial joints.

systematic errors Errors in testing that occur on a repeated and regular basis.

systemic Throughout the body.

systemic circulation Blood circulation throughout the body.

systemic inflammatory response syndrome (SIRS) An inflammation that overwhelms the whole body.

systemic lupus erythematosus (SLE) An autoimmune disorder expressed as a group of multisymptom disorders that can affect almost every organ of the body.

systemic sclerosis Loss of tissue elasticity of vessels, such as blood vessels, throughout the whole body.

T cell See T lymphocyte.

T cell receptor (TCR) A T lymphocyte surface membrane marker.

T-independent antigen Not dependent on T-cell recognition.

T lymphocyte The cell responsible for the cellular immune response and involved in the regulation of antibody reactions; also called a T cell.

tabes dorsalis A slowly progressive degeneration of the nervous system caused by syphilis. In untreated patients, this condition may appear from 5 to 20 years after the initial infection with *Treponema pallidum*.

tachycardia An abnormally fast heart rate.

tachyarrhythmia Accelerated rhythm of the heartbeat.

tachypnea Accelerated breathing.

tart cell Cells that usually represent monocytes that have phagocytized another whole cell or nucleus, often a lymphocyte. When a blood preparation is microscopically examined for the presence of cells associated with systemic lupus erythematosus (SLE), tart cells may be seen. These cell formations can be mistaken for the classic LE cell connected with SLE.

TdT See terminal deoxynucleotidyl transferase.

telangiectasia A vascular lesion formed by the dilation of a group of capillaries and occasionally of terminal arteries.

teratocarcinoma A malignancy (see teratoma).

teratoma Malignant tumor derived from three germ layers.

terminal deoxynucleotidyl transferase (TdT) An intracellular DNA polymerase found mainly in cortical, and therefore young, thymocytes. These cells are lost from the thymus after corticosteroid treatment.

T helper (Th) cells CD4+ lymphocytes. Their function is assist B lymphocytes in the recognition of foreign antigens.

thrombocytopenia A severe deficiency of circulating blood platelets (thrombocytes).

thrombocytopenia purpura Red discoloration of the skin due to patient deficiency.

thrombophlebitis An inflammation of a vein that develops before the formation of a thrombus (clot).

thrombosis Formation of a blood clot or thrombus.

thrombus A clot.

thymocyte Immature lymphocyte, found in the thymus gland, that undergoes differentiation to become a mature T cell.

thymoma A tumor derived from the epithelial or lymphoid elements of the thymus.

thymosin A humoral factor secreted by the thymus that promotes the growth of peripheral lymphoid tissue; also called thymic hormone.

thymus A primary or central lymphoid tissue responsible for processes of lymphocytes into the T type of cell. This ductless glandlike structure is located beneath the sternum (breastbone).

titer The concentration or strength of an antibody expressed as the highest dilution of the serum that produces agglutination (e.g., 1:4, 1:8).

Todd unit A unit that expresses antibody concentration when testing for antistreptolysin antibodies.

tolerance Lack of immune response to self antigens initiated during fetal development.

TORCH A group of tests for infectious microorganisms. TORCH stands for *Toxoplasma*, *o*ther (viruses), *r*ubella, *C*MV (cytomegalovirus), and *h*erpes.

toxic shock syndrome A serious and potentially fatal disorder caused by toxins produced by *Staphylococcus aureus.*

toxicology The study of drugs and related substances.

Toxoplasma gondii A protozoal microorganism that can be transmitted from an infected mother to an unborn infant. The disease can result in encephalomyelitis.

trans- A prefix meaning across, over, or through.

transaminase An enzyme (alanine transaminase [ALT], serum glutamic pyruvic transaminase [SGPT]) used in a surrogate test for non-A, non-B hepatitis.

transcription The process of generating a messenger RNA strand from DNA, used to code for proteins.

transcription-mediated amplification (TMA) A method of increasing target DNA through the use of two enzymes, an RNA polymerase and a reverse transcriptase, to synthesize new strands of DNA.

transferrin A plasma protein that transports iron through the blood to the liver.

transforming growth factor (TGF) Cytokine identified as product of virally transformed cells (e.g., TGF-β). These molecules can induce phenotypic transformation in non-neoplastic cells.

translation The process whereby messenger RNA is used to make functional proteins.

transplacental hemorrhage The entrance of fetal blood cells into the maternal circulation across the placenta.

transporter associated with antigen processing (TAP) A term used for proteins responsible for the ATP-dependent transport of newly synthesized short peptides from the cytoplasm to the lumen of the endoplasmic reticulum for binding to class I HLA antigens.

treponeme Spirochete of the genus *Treponema.*

trophoblast The outer layer of the blastocyst.

trophoblastic neoplasm A new growth involving trophoblastic tissue.

tubular cell injury Damage to cells of the renal tubules.

tumor Proliferation of cells that produce a mass rather than a reaction or inflammatory condition.

tumor-associated antigen Antigen found on tumor cells that is not unique to those cells but that can be used to distinguish them from normal cells.

tumor necrosis factor (TNF) A cytokine that can destroy tumor cells.

tumor-specific antigen (TSA) A tumor marker, an antigen that is only associated with a specific type of tissue.

tumor suppressor gene Gene that inhibits the growth of tumors.

tumorigenesis Formation of tumors.

turbid Cloudy.

turbidimetry See nephelometry.

ubiquitous Existing everywhere.

ulcerative lesion An open sore.

unilateral blindness The lack of vision in one eye.

Universal Blood and Body Fluid Precautions See Standard Precautions.

upregulation An increase in the number of receptors on the surface of target cells, making the cells more sensitive to a hormone or other agent.

urticaria Hives.

vaccination A method of stimulating the adaptive immune response and generating memory and acquired resistance without contracting disease; a form of artificial, active-acquired immunity.

vaccine A suspension of killed or attenuated (inactivated) infectious agents administered to establish resistance to the disease.

variable region The antigen-binding portion of an immunoglobulin molecule.

variable lymphocyte A type of white blood cell that lacks the characteristics of a normal lymphocyte.

varicella A virus that causes chickenpox.

varicosity A condition of having distended veins.

vasculitis An inflammation of a vessel such as a blood vessel.

vasoamine Produced by mast cells, basophils, and platelets, vasoactive amines (e.g., histamine, 5-hydroxytryptamine) cause increased capillary permeability.

vasodilation Expansion of blood vessels.

vector A bacterium or virus that does not cause disease in humans and is used in genetically engineered vaccines, or an organism, such as a mosquito or tick, that carries disease-causing microorganisms from one host to another.

venereal route A sexually transmitted mode of infection.

viral capsid antigen (VCA) An antigen expressed by B lymphocytes infected with Epstein-Barr virus in infectious mononucleosis.

viral load testing A quantitative measurement for HIV nucleic acid that is used principally to monitor the effects of antiretroviral therapy.

viremia A systemic (blood) infection caused by a virus.

virion A complete virus particle.

virulence The degree of pathogenicity or ability to cause disease of a microorganism.

Waldenström's primary macroglobulinemia A neoplastic proliferation of the lymphocyte–plasma cell system; also called Waldenström's macroglobulinemia.

Wasserman test The first diagnostic serologic test for syphilis; no longer in use.

Western blot (WB) A molecular biology diagnostic technique similar to the Northern blot and Southern blot procedures. WB is used to detect antibodies to specific epitopes of electrophoretically separated subspecies of antigens. WB is often used to confirm the specificity of antibodies detected by an ELISA screening procedure.

window period A period of undetectable evidence of infectious disease.

Westcott-Aldrich syndrome A genetic disorder passed to males through the X chromosome; results in decreased production of specific antibodies and abnormal cellular immunity.

X-linked agammaglobulinemia An inherited form of agammaglobulinemia, transmitted to males through the X chromosome, in which B cells fail to mature and to secrete immunoglobulins.

xenograft A transplant (graft) between different species, such as pigs to humans.

zeta potential An electron cloud surrounding a red blood cell in a solution (e.g., plasma zone electrophoresis).

zone of equivalence Area in which optimum precipitation occurs because the number of multivalent sites of antigen and antibody are approximately equal.

zoonosis Any infectious disease that can be transmitted (by a vector) from other animals, wild and domestic, to or from human beings to animals (the latter is sometimes called reverse zoonosis).

zymosan A glucan with repeating glucose units connected by β-1,3-glycosidic linkages.

Index

Note: Page numbers followed by "f" refer to illustrations; page numbers followed by "t" refer to tables; page numbers followed by "b" refer to boxes.